Medical Radiology

Diagnostic Imaging

Series Editors

Hans-Ulrich Kauczor
Paul M. Parizel
Wilfred C. G. Peh

The book series *Medical Radiology – Diagnostic Imaging* provides accurate and up-to-date overviews about the latest advances in the rapidly evolving field of diagnostic imaging and interventional radiology. Each volume is conceived as a practical and clinically useful reference book and is developed under the direction of an experienced editor, who is a world-renowned specialist in the field. Book chapters are written by expert authors in the field and are richly illustrated with high quality figures, tables and graphs. Editors and authors are committed to provide detailed and coherent information in a readily accessible and easy-to-understand format, directly applicable to daily practice.

Medical Radiology – Diagnostic Imaging covers all organ systems and addresses all modern imaging techniques and image-guided treatment modalities, as well as hot topics in management, workflow, and quality and safety issues in radiology and imaging. The judicious choice of relevant topics, the careful selection of expert editors and authors, and the emphasis on providing practically useful information, contribute to the wide appeal and ongoing success of the series. The series is indexed in Scopus.

Mark Davies • Rajesh Botchu
Karthikeyan. P. Iyengar
Editors

Imaging of the Hand and Wrist

Techniques and Applications

Second Edition

Springer

Editors
Mark Davies
Department of Musculoskeletal
Radiology
Royal Orthopaedic Hospital
Birmingham, UK

Rajesh Botchu
Department of Musculoskeletal
Radiology
Royal Orthopaedic Hospital
Birmingham, UK

Karthikeyan. P. Iyengar
Department of Orthopaedics,
Southport and Ormskirk Hospital
Mersey and West Lancashire
Teaching, NHS Trust
Southport, Merseyside, UK

ISSN 0942-5373 ISSN 2197-4187 (electronic)
Medical Radiology
ISSN 2731-4677 ISSN 2731-4685 (electronic)
Diagnostic Imaging
ISBN 978-3-032-05338-1 ISBN 978-3-032-05339-8 (eBook)
https://doi.org/10.1007/978-3-032-05339-8

This Springer imprint is published by the registered company Springer Nature Switzerland AG
The registered company address is: Gewerbestrasse 11, 6330 Cham, Switzerland

Preface

Imaging studies of the hand and wrist represents a keep step in the diagnostic algorithm of management of patients with symptomatic hand and wrist joint. Musculoskeletal imaging continues to evolve since the first edition of this book published 20 years ago.

The hand and wrist is a common anatomical site imaged by orthopedic surgeons, rheumatologist, and other musculoskeletal clinicians.

This edition of the *Imaging of the Hand and Wrist* simplifies the complex field of musculoskeletal imaging. Since knowledge and skills update is integral for clinical practice, the book provides up-to-date developments and directions to select the most appropriate imaging modality in the diagnostic investigation of musculoskeletal conditions of hand and wrist

As before, the book takes a dual approach with the *First* section dealing with full range of techniques available for imaging hand and wrist pathologies including contributions on radiographs, ultrasound, computed tomography, and MR imaging. The *Second section* comprising 13 chapters discusses the optimal application of these techniques to specific pathologies highlighting practical solutions to every day clinical problems noticed in day-to-day radiology practice.

The editors are grateful to the international panel of authors for their contribution to this ***Second Edition*** of the ***Imaging of the Hand and Wrist*** that aims to provide a comprehensive overview of current imaging of the hand and wrist.

Birmingham, UK	Mark Davies
Birmingham, UK	Rajesh Botchu
Southport, Merseyside, UK	Karthikeyan. P. Iyengar

Contents

Radiography and Arthrography

Drushi Patel, Ankur Shah, Ojasvi Vemuri,
S. G. Davies, and Rajesh Botchu

Contents

D. Patel
Gujarat Imaging Centre, Ahmedabad, India

A. Shah (✉)
Gujarat Imaging Centre, Ahmedabad, India

Sadbhav Imaging Centre, Ahmedabad, India

GIC Prime, Ahmedabad, India

O. Vemuri
Siddhartha Medical College, Viajyawada, India

S. G. Davies
Radiology Department, Royal Glamorgan Hospital, Rhondda Cynon Taf, Llantrisant, UK
e-mail: Stephen.Davies1@wales.nhs.uk

R. Botchu
Royal Orthopedic Hospital, Birmingham, UK

Abstract

The main emphasis of this chapter is a description of basic radiography of the wrist and hand with detailed description of radiographic technique and evaluation of the different projections. Static and dynamic carpal instability evaluation is vital for the assessment of ligamentous disruption. Various measurement techniques which can be used in the assessment of wrist pathology, following distal radial fracture, radial inclination, radial length, and palmar tilt have also been described. Ulnar variance is also assessed following distal radial fracture and in the context of ulnar-sided wrist pain. The scapholunate angle and capitate–lunate angle are assessed when intercalated instability is suspected. Finally, the carpal height is a measurement which is applied when there is evidence of carpal collapse or loss of joint space. Arthrography still has a place in the modern assessment of the wrist. Radiocarpal and to a lesser extent midcarpal injection techniques may be employed.

Med Radiol Diagn Imaging (2025)
https://doi.org/10.1007/174_2025_600,
Published Online: 02 August 2025

1 Introduction

Plain film radiography has a fundamental role in the evaluation of the hand and wrist following trauma, in cases of suspected arthropathy, as well as for evaluation of systemic disorders with hand manifestations and in other miscellaneous situations such as tumor masses and pain. Optimal radiographic technique is essential because decisions about injuries, especially around the elbow and wrist affect future dexterity, employment, and earnings of the patient.

To ensure maximum of radiation protection, the patient should be seated at the side or end of the table with the lower limbs and gonads away from the primary beam, obtained by placing the legs to the side of the table rather than under it. The beam should be collimated within the margins of the cassette. It is possible to obtain more than one projection in the same cassette by masking the half of the unused cassette by a lead rubber mask. The importance of relaxed and comfortable position of the limb to obtain a still image cannot be over emphasized and hence non-opaque pads can be used for immobilization within the radiation field and sand bags outside the field. When the hand or wrist is being examined, the patient's forearm and hand should be resting on the table. It is of utmost importance to ensure correct registration of right or left markers.

2 Radiographic Projections

2.1 Radiographic Projections of the Wrist

The standard wrist projections are posteroanterior (PA), lateral, and anterior oblique projections (Whitley et al. 2005). All the three projections may be taken on the same cassette using lead rubber mask.

2.1.1 PA Projections of the Wrist

Position of the patient and cassette

The PA projection is performed with the patient seated. The shoulder is 90° abducted and the elbow is 90° flexed. The forearm is held in a neutral position with the palm of the hand resting on the tabletop. The tabletop should be at the same height as the forearm. The field of projection should include the distal half of the radius and ulna extending distantly to include the proximal two-thirds of the metacarpals (Fig. 1).

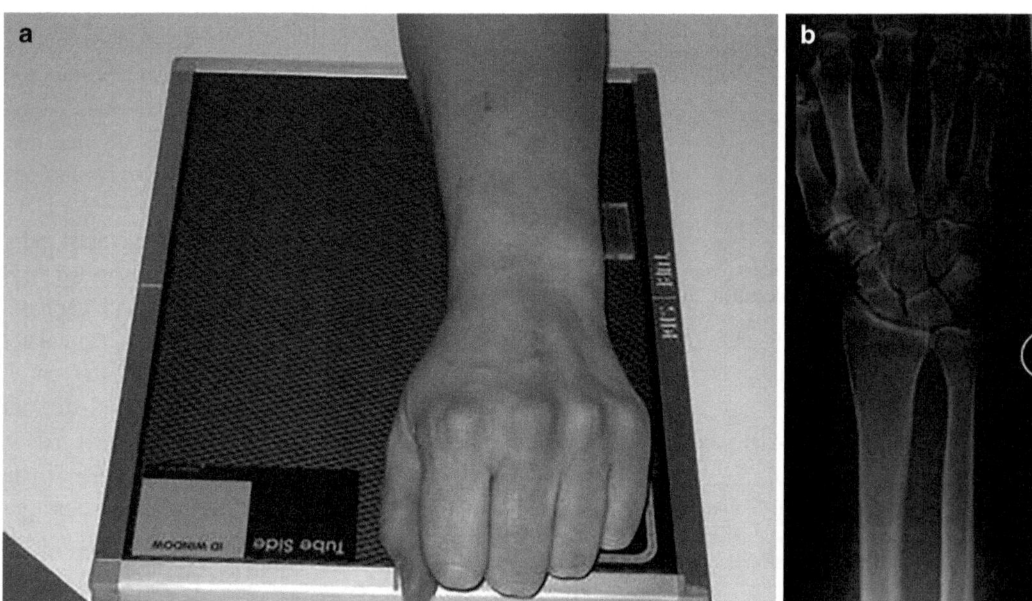

Fig. 1 (**a**) Patient positioning for posteroanterior (PA) wrist radiograph. (**b**) PA radiograph of wrist

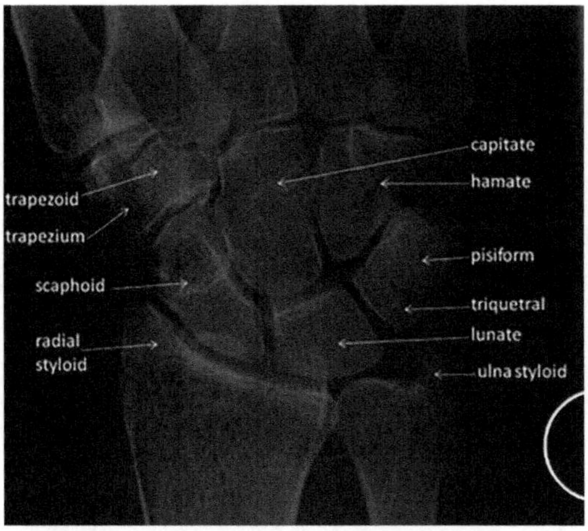

Fig. 2 Carpal anatomy

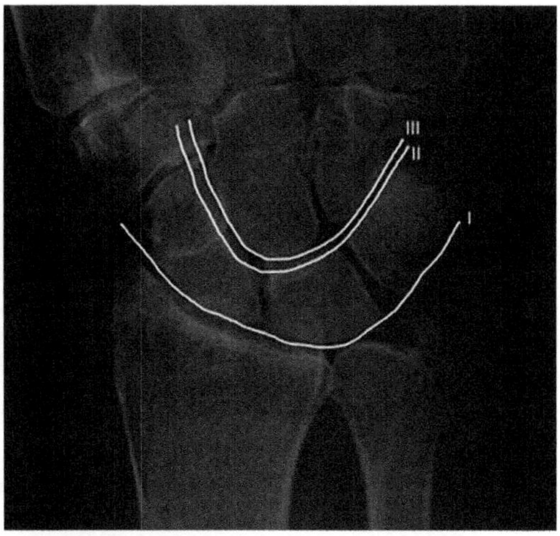

Fig. 3 Carpal arcs

The fingers are flexed slightly to bring the anterior aspect of the wrist in contact with cassette.

Wrist joint is adjusted to ensure that the radial and ulnar styloid processes are equidistant from the cassette

Forearm is immobilized using a sand bag.

Direction and centering of the X-ray beam
The centering point is midway between the radial and ulnar styloid.

Evaluation criteria
The PA projection of the wrist is useful in the evaluation of injuries to the distal radius and ulna, carpus, and proximal metacarpals. It is also helpful in the evaluation of pathology such as erosions to the distal radius and ulna and carpus.

The PA wrist should profile the extensor carpi ulnaris tendon groove which should be at the level of, or radial to the base of the ulnar styloid (Fig. 1) (Goldfarb and Yin 2001)

The PA view of the wrist displays the carpal anatomy (Fig. 2). The carpal bones are arranged in proximal (scaphoid, lunate, and triquetral) and distal (trapezium, trapezoid, capitate, and hamate) rows (Resnik 2000). The normal anatomic relationships of the wrist should demonstrate parallel opposing articular surfaces with symmetrical width of all intercarpal joints. The articular surfaces of the carpal bones should be normally aligned in three arcs (Gilula Arcs) (Fig. 3). Arc I describes the outer proximal convexities of scaphoid, lunate, and triquetrum. Arc II describes the distal concavities of the scaphoid, lunate, and triquetrum. Arc III describes the proximal convexities of the capitate and lunate. For optimal demonstration, the wrist must be imaged PA in the neutral position (Gilula et al. 1984).

Two normal anatomical variants of the arcs are recognized. The first variant is that the triquetrum may be shorter in its proximal–distal dimension than the adjacent lunate. This gives rise to discontinuity of arc I. The second variant is that the proximal hamate may be unusually prominent and rounded thereby creating discontinuity of arc III (Loredo and Sorge 2005).

Evaluation of the integrity of the arcs is important when assessing for fractures, dislocations, and instability. An arc is disrupted if it cannot be traced smoothly. A break in one of the arcs indicates a fracture or the disruption of a ligament leading to a subluxation or dislocation (Gilula et al. 1984).

2.1.2 Lateral Projections of the Wrist

Position of the patient and cassette
There are two different methods for obtaining the lateral projection of the wrist. The simplest method is to rotate the hand 90° maintaining the elbow in a flexed position. With this method, the ulna stays in a fixed position and the radius rotates through 90° along with the carpus.

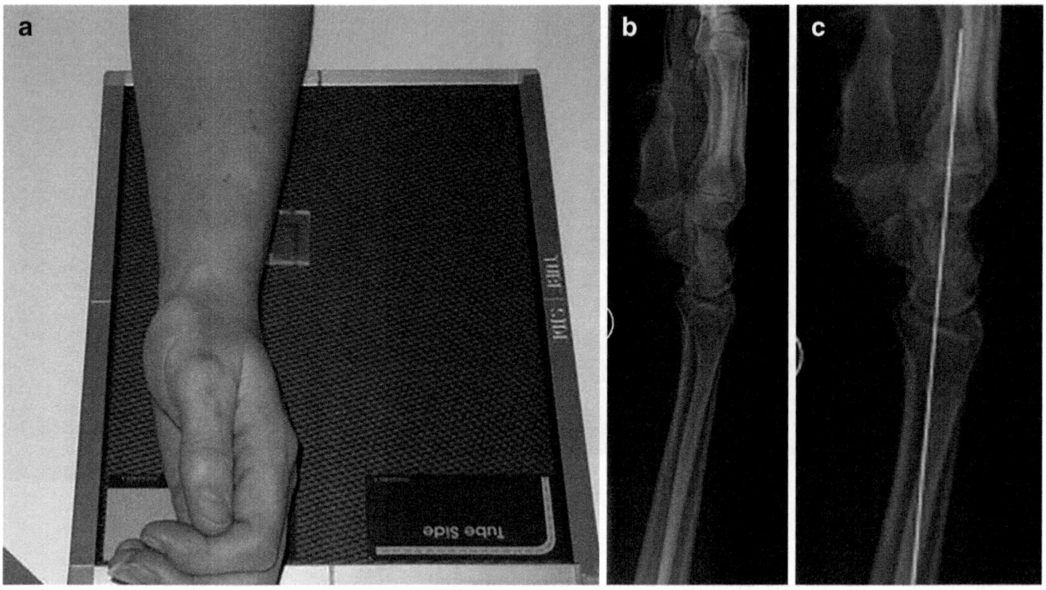

Fig. 4 (**a**) Patient positioning for lateral wrist radiograph. (**b**) Lateral radiograph of wrist. (**c**) Lateral wrist demonstrating axis for lateral alignment (not co-axial in this case)

The second method involves rotation of both ulna and radius through 90°. This is achieved by extending the elbow and externally rotating the humerus through 90°. This latter method has the benefit of enabling a second projection at 90° to the first of the ulna.

Direction and centering of the X-ray beam
The centering point for both methods is the radial styloid (Fig. 4).

Evaluation criteria
The positioning of the lateral projection of the wrist is evaluated with reference to the palmar cortex of the pisiform. A well-positioned and centered lateral projection results in the palmar cortex of the pisiform lying between the palmar cortices of the distal scaphoid and capitate (Fig. 4).

An important feature of the lateral wrist is the alignment of the radius, lunate, and capitate (Fig. 4). These structures should be within 10° of co-axial alignment. It is noted that they are truly co-axial in only 11% of cases (Mann and Wilson 1992).

2.1.3 Anterior Oblique Projection of the Wrist

Position of the patient and cassette
With the elbow in 90° flexion and arm abducted such that the anterior aspect of forearm and palm of the hand rest on the table. If possible, shoulder joint should be at the same height as the forearm (Ballinger and Frank 1999).

The hand is externally rotated through 45° (Fig. 5) and supported in a position using non-opaque foam pad and the forearm is immobilized with sand bags.

Direction and centering of the X-ray beam
The central ray is directed midway between radial and ulnar styloid processes.

Evaluation criteria
The image shows proximal 2/3rd of metacarpal, carpal bones and distal third of radius and ulna

2.1.4 Carpal Tunnel View of the Wrist

Carpal tunnel
The carpal bones form a shallow concavity, which, with the bridging flexor retinaculum,

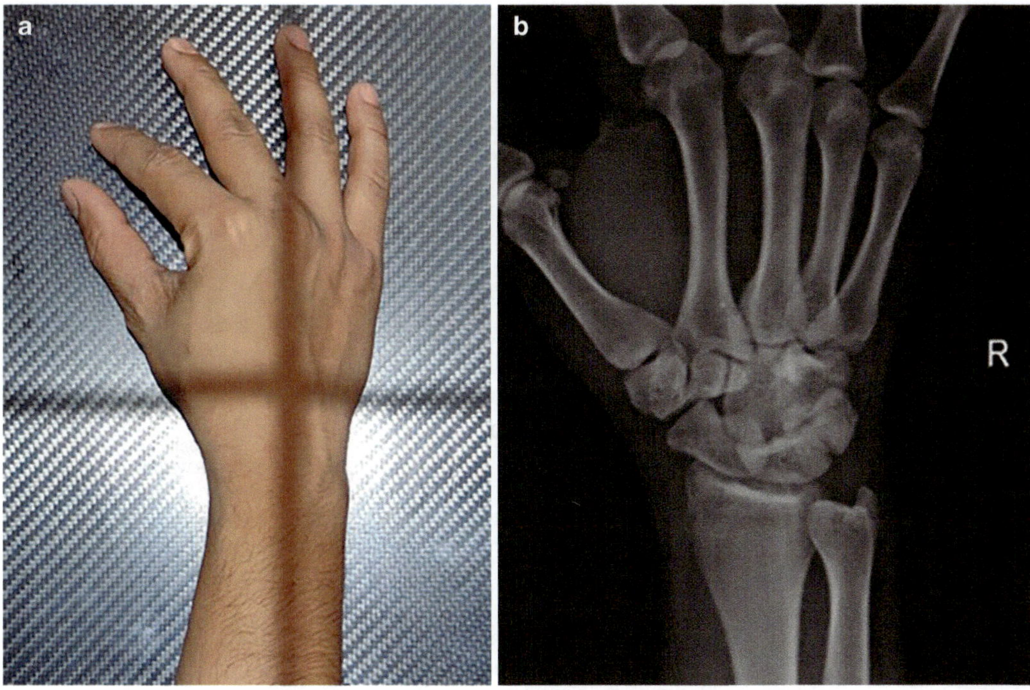

Fig. 5 Panel (**a**, **b**) displays a photo and radiograph of a hand with fingers slightly spread

forms the carpal tunnel. The flexor retinaculum is attached to the two medial prominences (the pisiform and the hook of the hamate) and to the two lateral prominences (the tubercle of the scaphoid and the tubercle of the trapezium). The median nerve along with the flexor tendons passes through the tunnel, and any swelling here can cause compression of the median nerve, giving rise to the carpal tunnel syndrome.

Radiographic examination of the bony part of the tunnel is performed by an axial projection to demonstrate the medial and lateral prominences and the concavity. This examination is requested less often nowadays due to improved electrophysiological technique.

Two alternative positions are described depending upon the condition of the patient (Whitley et al. 2005).

Axial method 1 (Fig. 6a)

Position of patient and cassette

Patient is in the standing position with back toward the table and the cassette is placed level with the edge of the tabletop. The palm of the hand is rest onto the cassette with the wrist joint dorsiflexed to approximately 135°. The fingers can be curled around under the table to assist in immobilization.

Direction and centering of the X-ray beam

Vertical central ray is centered between the pisiform and the hook of hamate medially and the tubercle of scaphoid and ridge of trapezium laterally.

Axial method 2 (Fig. 6b)

Position of patient and cassette

The patient is seated alongside the table and the cassette is placed on top of a plastic block approximately 8 cm high. The lower end of the forearm rests against the edge of the block, with the wrist adducted and dorsiflexed to 135°.This position is assisted using a traction bandage held by the patient's other hand.

Direction and centering of the X-ray beam

The vertical central ray is centered between the pisiform and hook of the hamate medially and the tubercle of the scaphoid and the ridge of the trapezium laterally.

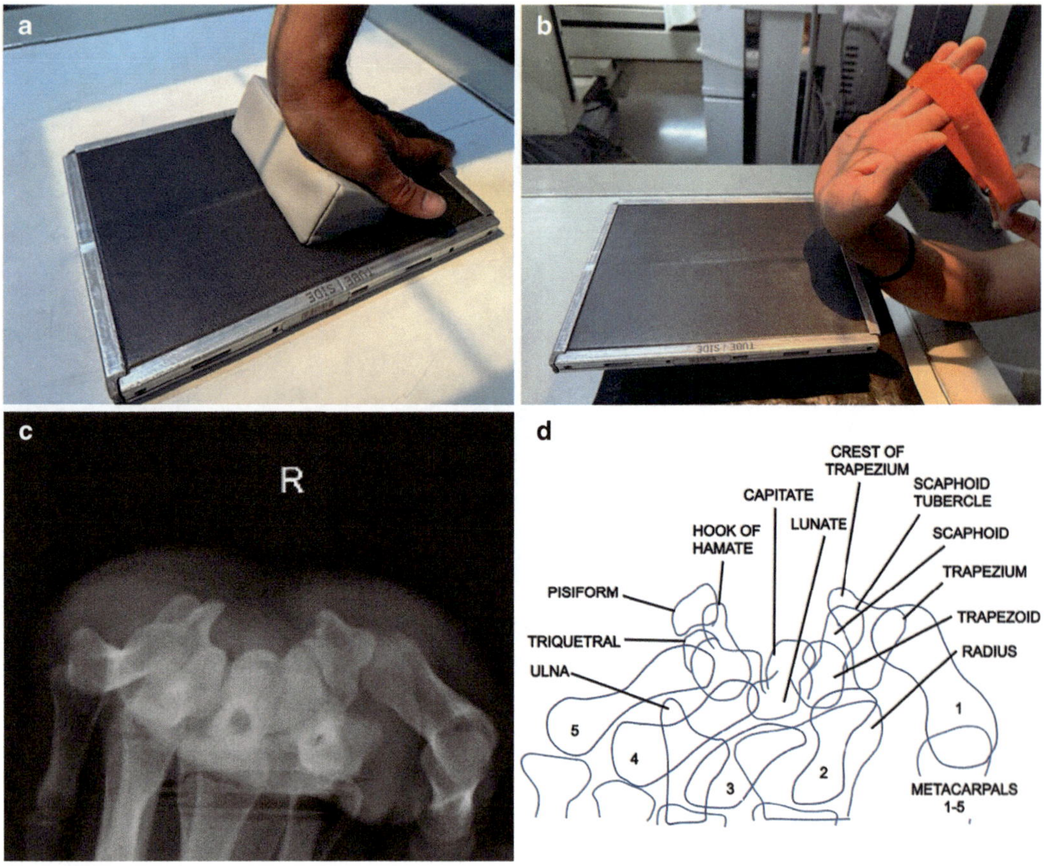

Fig. 6 Patient positioning for carpal tunnel view of wrist joint. (**a**) Method 1. (**b**) Method 2. (**c**) Radiograph of carpal tunnel. (**d**) Line diagram of carpal tunnel

Evaluation criteria

The image should clearly demonstrate the pisiform and the hook of hamate medially and scaphoid and the prevertebral of adhesion laterally (Fig. 6c, d).

2.2 Radiographic Projections of the Scaphoid Carpus

There are four standard projections for radiography of the scaphoid: AP with ulnar deviation (plus or minus tube angulation), anterior oblique (pronated oblique), posterior oblique (supinated oblique), and lateral.

This series is designed to provide tangential projections of the carpal bones with particular emphasis on evaluation of the scaphoid. The prime indication for these projections is the presence of trauma to the carpus particularly if there is associated tenderness in the region of the scaphoid.

2.2.1 PA with Ulnar Deviation

Position of the patient and cassette

The patient is seated alongside the table with the affected side nearest the table. The arm is extended across the table with the elbow flexed and the forearm pronated. If possible, the shoulder, elbow, and wrist should be at the level of the tabletop. The hand is adducted and deviated in the ulnar direction to reduce the foreshortening of the scaphoid seen on the standard PA projection (Fig. 7). Radial and ulnar styloid processes should be equidistant from cassette and immobilized with sandbags.

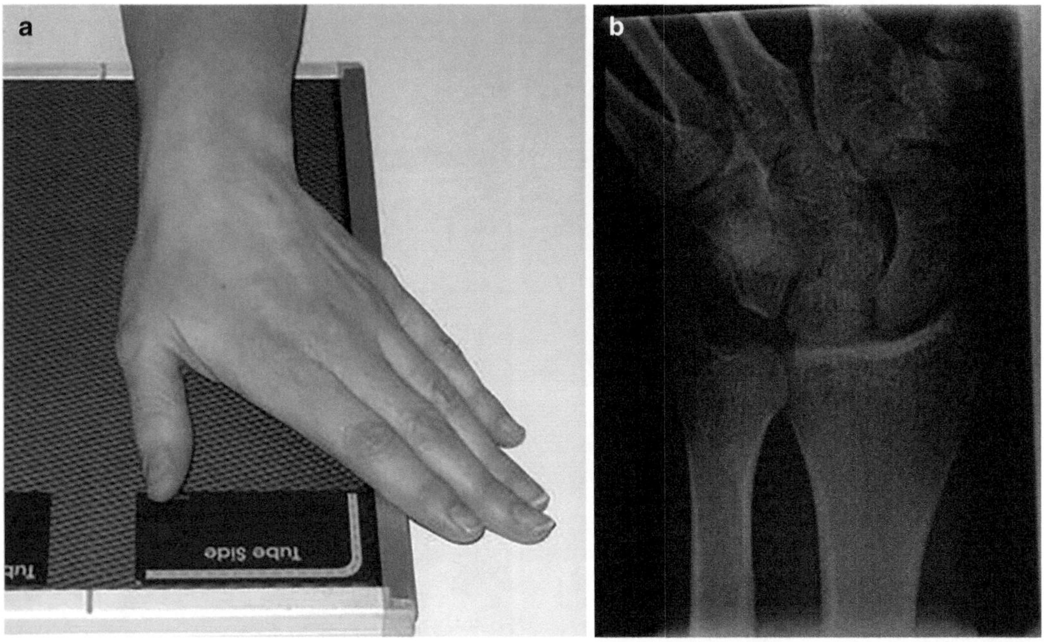

Fig. 7 (**a**) Patient positioning for PA carpus with ulna deviation. (**b**) PA radiograph with ulna deviation of carpus

When the wrist is in the normal neutral position, the scaphoid is tilted. Additionally, the X-ray tube may be angled toward the elbow by 20° (Fig. 8) which further compensates for the normal scaphoid tilt (Lampignano and Kendrick 2017).

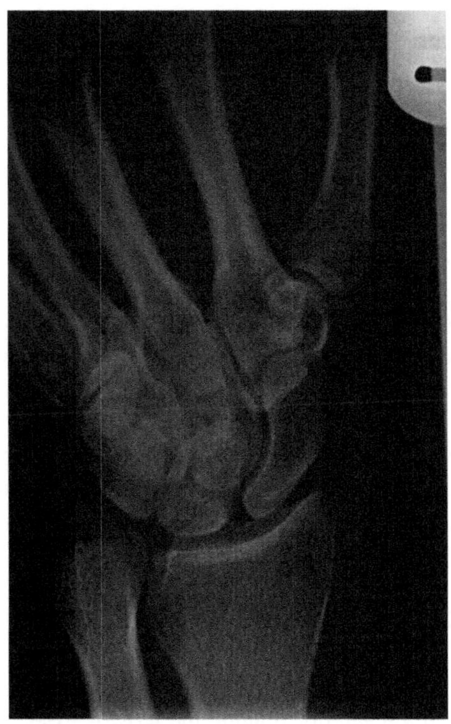

Fig. 8 PA radiograph with ulna deviation and 20° of tube angulation

Direction and centering of the X-ray beam
The centering point is midway between the ulna and radial styloid processes.

Evaluation criteria
The image should include the distal radius and ulna and proximal metacarpals. The PA projection should produce a good projection of the length of the scaphoid aiming at visualization of clear joint space around the whole of the scaphoid (Fig. 7). Occasionally, there is some distal overlap (Whitley et al. 2005).

2.2.2 Anterior Oblique (Pronated Oblique)

Position of the patient and cassette
The wrist is externally rotated from the PA neutral position by 45° (Fig. 9). The hand showed

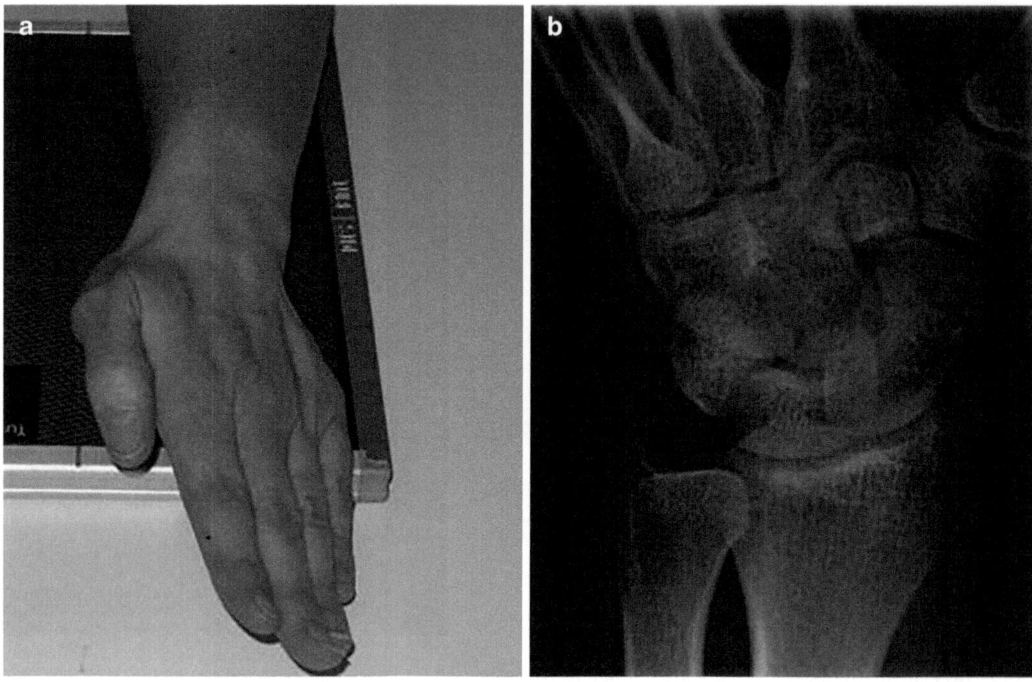

Fig. 9 (**a**) Patient positioning for anterior oblique of the carpus. (**b**) Anterior oblique radiograph of the carpus

remain adducted in ulnar deviation. The radial styloid is, therefore, elevated from the tabletop (Ballinger and Frank 1999).

Direction and centering of the X-ray beam
The centering point is midway between the ulnar and radial styloid.

Evaluation criteria
This projection (Fig. 9) gives a good demonstration of the distal scaphoid and trapezium. It is also a useful projection for evaluating the trapezoid and bases of the first and second metacarpals. The radial styloid and dorsal surface of the triquetrum is visible (Ballinger and Frank 1999).

2.2.3 Posterior Oblique (Supinated Oblique)

Position of the patient and cassette
From the anterior oblique the wrist is externally rotated a further 90° (Fig. 10) such that posterior aspect of hand and wrist are at 45° to the cassette. The fingers are held together. The wrist may be supported on 45° non-opaque foam pad.

Direction and centering of the X-ray beam
The centering point is the ulnar styloid.

Evaluation criteria
This projection demonstrates the pisiform in-profile, situated anterior to triquetral bone and the piso-triquetral joint (Fig. 10). It is also useful for evaluating the hook of the hamate and bases of the fourth and fifth metacarpals. The long axis of the scaphoid lies perpendicular to the cassette.

2.2.4 Lateral

Position of the patient and cassette
From the PA position, the hand and wrist are rotated internally to 45° such that the medial aspect of wrist is in contact with the cassette. The hand is adjusted to ensure superimposition of radial and ulnar styloid processes and immobilized with sand bands.

The above-mentioned technique is as described for the standard lateral view of the wrist (Sect. 2.1). However, a narrower field of view is generally used including only the distal aspect of the radius and ulna and proximal metacarpal bases (Fig. 11) (Ballinger and Frank 1999).

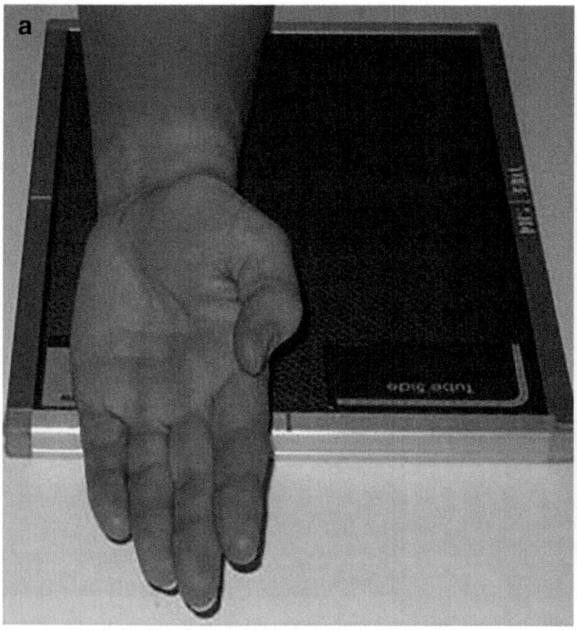

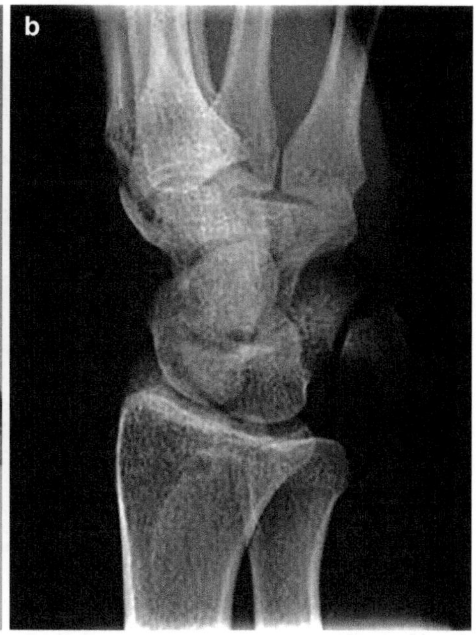

Fig. 10 (**a**) Patient positioning for posterior oblique of carpus. (**b**) Posterior oblique radiograph of carpus

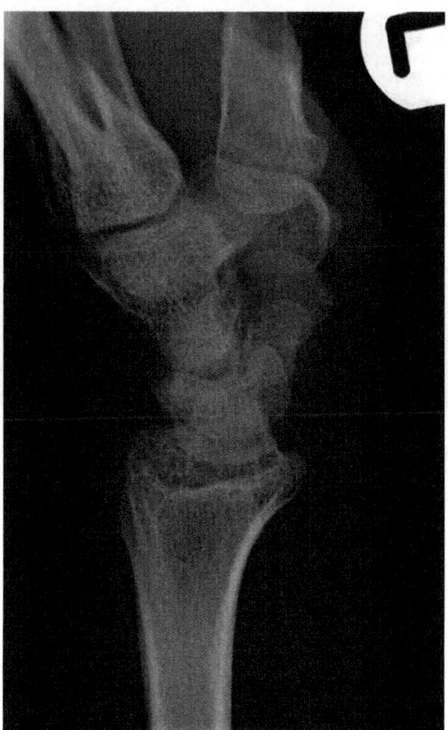

Fig. 11 Lateral radiograph of carpus

Direction and centering of the X-ray beam
The centering point is the radial styloid.

Evaluation criteria
The lateral projection is particularly valuable in assessing the dorsal surface of distal radius for fracture. This projection enables an evaluation of the alignment of the distal radius, lunate and capitate (Fig. 11). This projection is useful when assessing for dislocation and carpal instability.

2.3 Radiographic Projections of the Hand

There are two standard projections for the hand which are the PA and anterior oblique projections. Supplementary projections include the lateral projection and the posterior oblique projection.

2.3.1 PA Hand

Position of the patient and cassette
Elbow joint is flexed to 90° and, forearm is pronated and the palm of the hand rest on the cas-

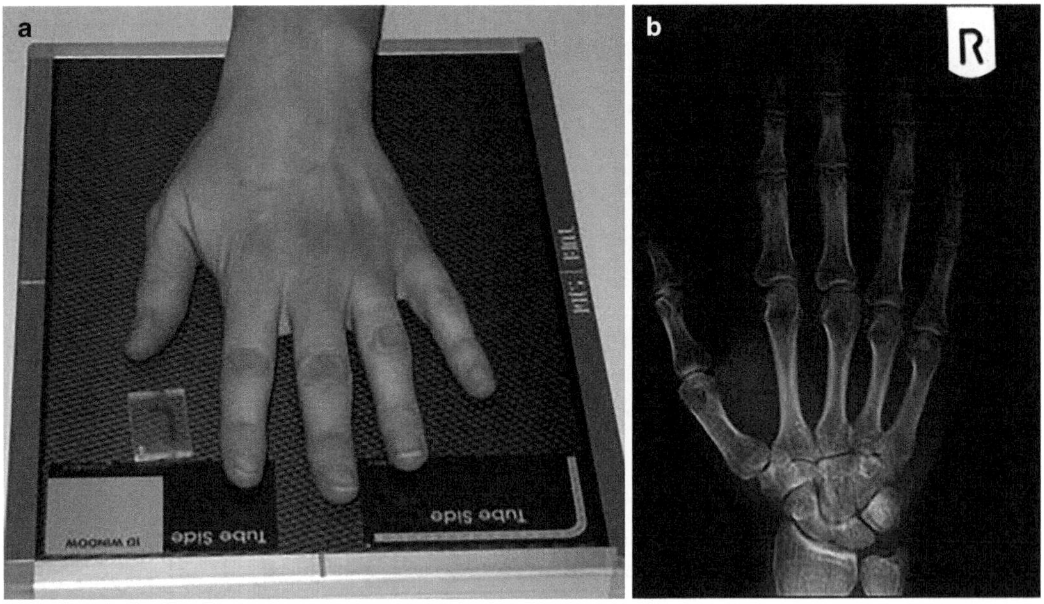

Fig. 12 (**a**) Patient positioning for PA hand. (**b**) Radiograph of PA hand

sette (Fig. 12). If mobility of the patient permits, the shoulder joint should be at the same height as the forearm. The ulnar styloid and radial styloid should lie equidistant from the tabletop. Fingers are separated and extended but relaxed to ensure that they remain in contact with cassette.

Direction and centering of the X-ray beam
The centering point is the third metacarpal head.

This projection should include the whole of the fingers (phalanges), metacarpals, carpus together with distal ends of the radius and ulna.

Evaluation criteria
The PA hand projection should demonstrate all of the joints of the hand, carpus, and wrist (Fig. 12). The joint spaces should be symmetrical and parallel without any rotation. This projection is used in the evaluation of trauma, arthropathy, and a range of miscellaneous conditions. The carpometacarpal joint may be evaluated with a line drawn between the distal articular surfaces of the trapezoid, capitate, and hamate and the parallel articular surfaces of the second-fifth metacarpals (Fig. 13). Discontinuity of this line should raise a suspicion of fracture and or dislocation.

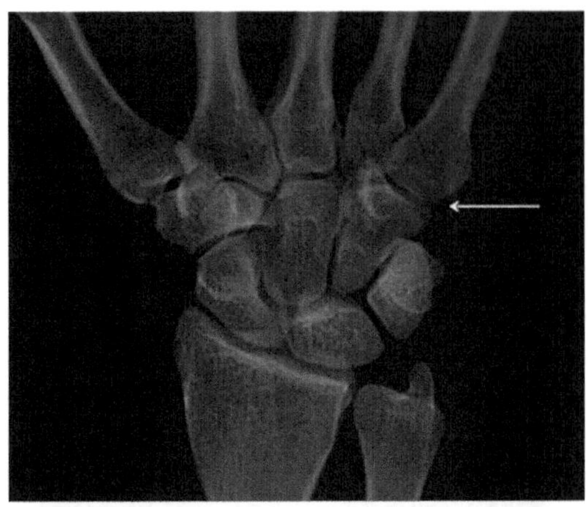

Fig. 13 PA hand radiograph showing level for assessment of parallelism across carpometacarpal joint (*white arrow*)

2.3.2 PA Anterior Oblique Hand

Position of the patient and cassette
The hand is externally rotated by 45° from the PA projection (Fig. 14). The fingers should be

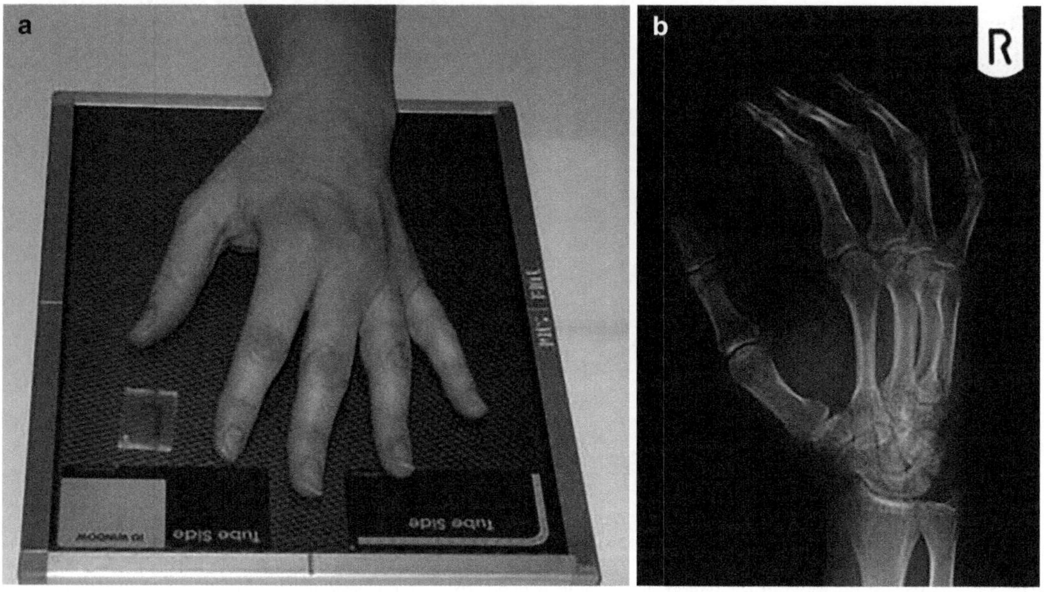

Fig. 14 (**a**) Patient positioning for PA anterior oblique of hand. (**b**) Radiograph of PA anterior oblique of hand

extended and separated and the hand supported on of 45° foam pad.

Direction and centering of the X-ray beam
The film is centered over the third metacarpal head.

Evaluation criteria
This projection is very useful for evaluating the shafts and necks of the metacarpals (Fig. 14). The phalanges are seen in an oblique plane. The first and second metacarpals are usually separated while there is an overlap of the fourth and fifth metacarpals (Yochum and Rowe 2005).

2.3.3 Lateral Hand

This projection (Fig. 15) is useful for evaluating the carpal–metacarpal region. It is helpful in evaluating the fifth metacarpal shaft fractures. This projection is also used for foreign body assessment and to demonstrate fracture or dislocation of carpal bones. If the projection has been undertaken to identify position of the foreign body, the kVp should be lowered to demonstrate or exclude its presence in the soft tissues. A metal marker placed adjacent to the puncture site is commonly used to aid localization of the foreign body.

Position of the patient and cassette
The hand is placed in the lateral position on the cassette with the medial border of the wrist and hand resting on the cassette. The fingers are extended. The thumb is abducted and placed clear of the rest of the hand (Fig. 15). The radial and the ulnar styloid processes are superimposed.

Direction and centering of the X-ray beam
The centering point is the head of the second metacarpal.

Evaluation criteria
The image should include fingertips including soft tissue and radial and ulnar styloid processes. The heads of the metacarpals should be superimposed. The thumb should be demonstrated clearly without superimposition of other structures.

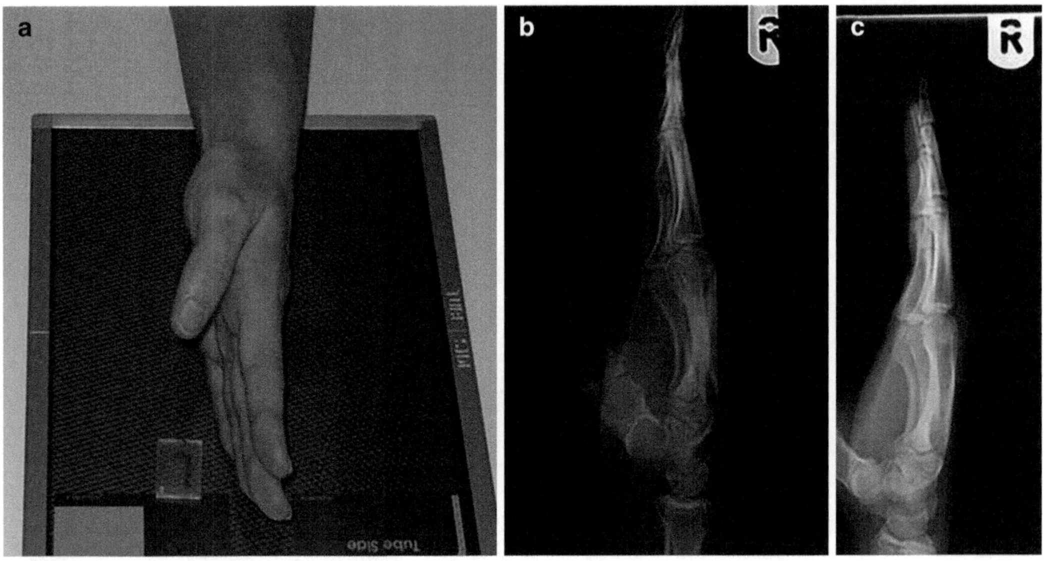

Fig. 15 (**a**) Patient positioning for lateral radiograph of hand. (**b**) Lateral radiograph of hand. (**c**) Soft tissue lateral radiograph of hand

2.3.4 Posterior Oblique of Both Hands or Norgaard View or "Ball Catcher's" View

Position of the patient and cassette

Both hands are placed symmetrically on the cassette with the forearm in supination and dorsal surface of the hands in contact with cassette. From this position, both hands are rotated internally (medially) 45° in "ball catching" position. Fingers and thumb are separated and extended but relaxed to ensure that they remain in contact with the cassette. The radial styloid is elevated from the cassette on both sides (Goldfarb and Yin 2001).

If it has been necessary to position the patient facing the table, it is essential to provide radiation protection for the lower limbs and gonads. A lead rubber sheet must be placed underneath the cassette to attenuate the primary beam.

Direction and centering of the X-ray beam

The centering point is midway between the hands at the level of the fifth metacarpal head.

Evaluation criteria

The metacarpal heads should all be clearly seen and separated without superimposition (Fig. 16). The purpose of this projection is to evaluate the metacarpal heads for bone erosion. This projection has also been termed the Norgaard view or "ball catcher's" view. The obliquity of the projection enables a different part of the metacarpal head to be shown in profile. It is considered that this improves the visualization of bone erosions from rheumatoid disease as more of the beam is tangential to the bare area of the metacarpal head, the area susceptible to erosions. This is when compared with the conventional PA projection. However, two studies have demonstrated that there is limited additional information with this projection. This projection is also used to demonstrate the fracture of the base of fifth metacarpal.

2.4 Radiographic Projections of the Phalanges

The standard projections are PA and lateral. Supplementary oblique views either of individual phalanges or as part of a PA oblique hand examination may also be undertaken. The oblique projection does not substitute for the lateral view which is an essential projection when evaluating trauma.

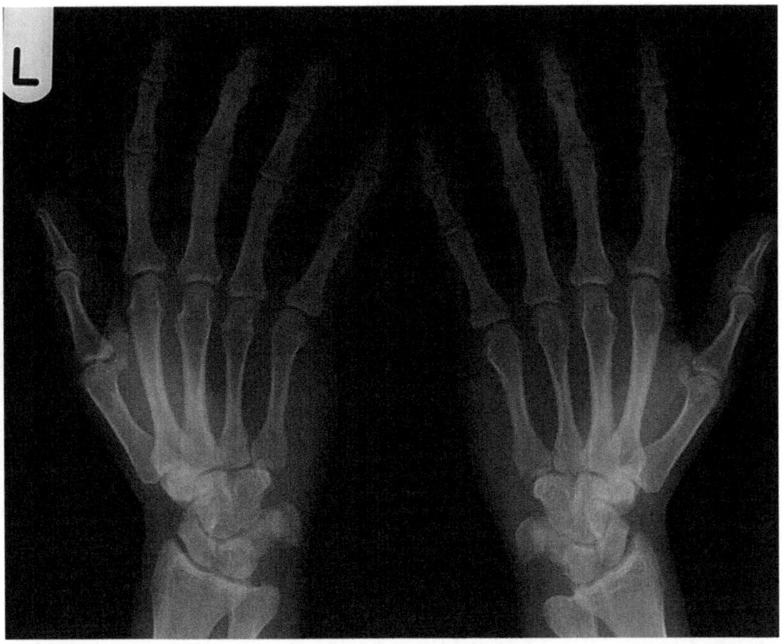

Fig. 16 Posterior oblique (ball catcher's) radiograph of the hands

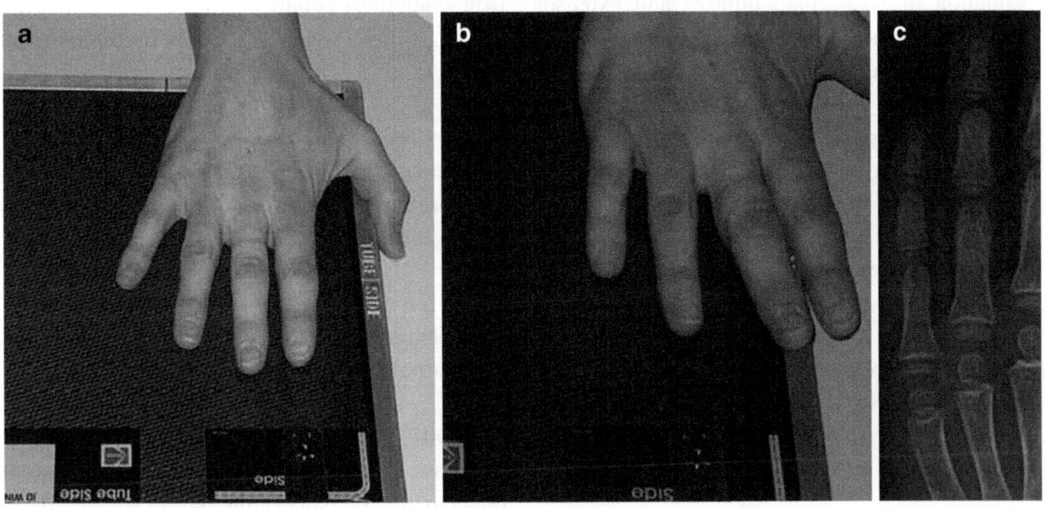

Fig. 17 (**a**) Patient positioning for PA second and third fingers. (**b**) Patient positioning for PA fourth and fifth fingers. (**c**) Radiograph of PA fingers

2.4.1 PA Phalanges

Position of the patient and cassette

The phalanges may be X-rayed individually or in pairs. For example, the second and third phalanges are imaged together or the fourth and fifth are imaged together. The fingers are extended and separated and placed on the cassette with a hand in the neutral PA position (Fig. 17).

Direction and centering of the X-ray beam

The centering is directed over the PIP joint of the relevant finger.

Evaluation criteria

The X-ray should include the distal third of the metacarpal as far as the soft tissue of the fingertip. The joint spaces should be uniform and parallel (Fig. 17).

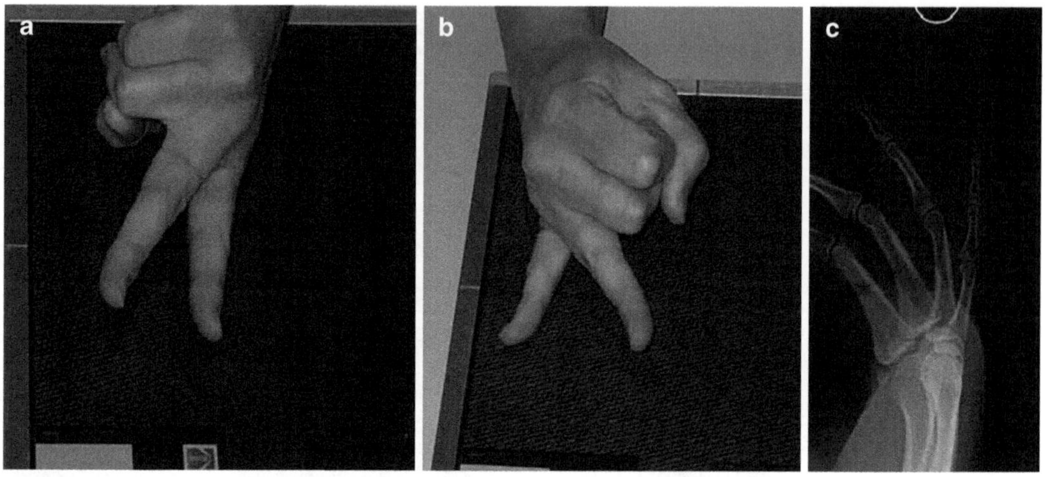

Fig. 18 (**a**) Patient positioning for lateral of second and third fingers. (**b**) Patient positioning for lateral of fourth and fifth fingers. (**c**) Lateral radiograph of fingers

2.4.2 Lateral Phalanges

The lateral view is especially important in the evaluation of volar plate injuries and extensor avulsion injuries. The phalanx must be X-rayed in the true lateral position (Fig. 18).

Position of the patient and cassette

The phalanges may be X-rayed individually or in pairs. Typically, the second and third are imaged together or the fourth and fifth phalanges. The phalanges are extended and separated so that both are visible on the film.

Direction and centering of the X-ray beam

The centering point is directed tangential to the proximal interphalangeal joint of the affected finger (Fig. 18).

Evaluation criteria

The image should include fingertip and distal third of the metacarpal bone. The condyles should be superimposed to avoid obscuring volar plate fractures.

2.5 Radiographic Evaluation of the Thumb

The conventional projections of the thumb are AP and lateral. They are performed separately from the examination of the hand. The PA projection may be substituted for the AP projection when there is pain or difficulty in achieving the appropriate position (Keats and Sistrom 2001).

2.5.1 AP Thumb

Position of the patient and cassette

The forearm is over-pronated such that the thumb lies on the cassette (Fig. 19).

Direction and centering of the X-ray beam

The centering point is the base of the first metacarpal.

Evaluation criteria

The base of the first metacarpal and the base of the proximal phalanx of the thumb are well demonstrated and can be assessed for fracture (Fig. 19).

2.5.2 Lateral Thumb

Position of the patient and cassette

The thumb is rested on the cassette in the lateral position. The palm of the hand is slightly rotated to bring thumb into it through lateral profile.

Direction and centering of the X-ray beam

The centering point is the metacarpophalangeal joint (Fig. 20).

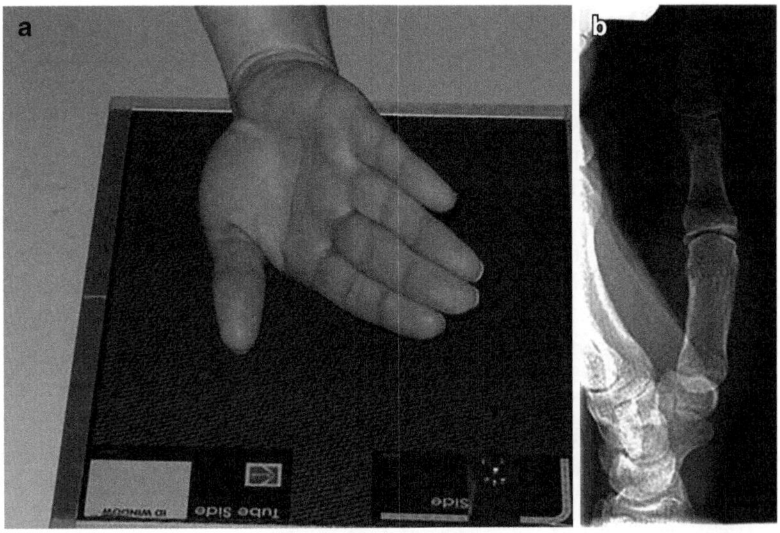

Fig. 19 (a) Patient positioning for AP thumb. (b) AP radiograph of thumb

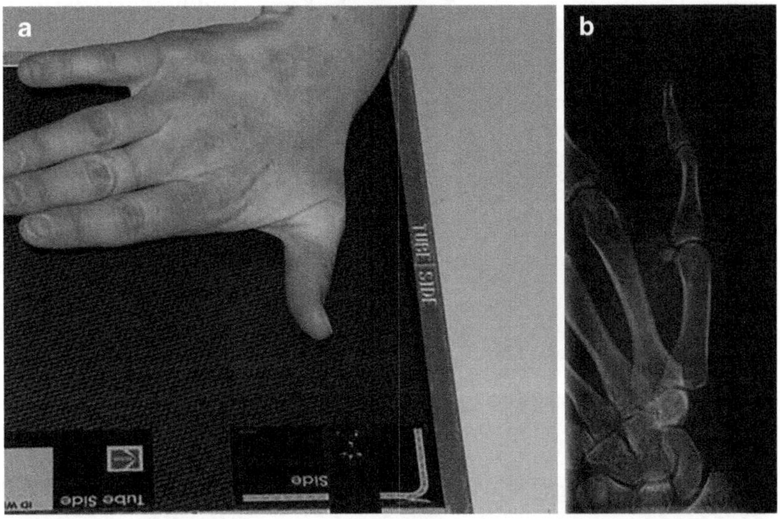

Fig. 20 (a) Patient positioning for lateral thumb. (b) Lateral radiograph of thumb

Evaluation criteria

This projection is important for evaluation of the base of the first metacarpal for fracture (Fig. 20).

2.5.3 PA Thumb

Position of the patient and cassette

The medial border of the hand is rested on the cassette. The hand is rotated forward with the thumb extended until a PA view of the thumb is obtained (Fig. 21). It is important that the thumb is extended; otherwise, there is overlap at the metacarpal phalangeal joint. This projection is used when it is not possible for the patient to achieve the over-pronation of the forearm required for the AP projection.

Direction and centering of the X-ray beam

The centering point is the base of thumb.

Evaluation criteria

Care must be taken to obtain a good PA view and to assess for parallelism at the metacarpal–phalangeal joint.

2.5.4 Bilateral PA Stress Radiograph of MCP Joint of Thumb

Hypermobility at the thumb carpometacarpal (CMC) joint has been proposed as an explanation for abnormal loading and subsequent development of osteoarthritis. Radiographic evaluation of CMC joint of thumb is difficult owing to the obliquity of the articulation. This is a modified bilateral stress PA radiograph of the thumbs to measure CMC joint laxity (Wolf et al. 2009).

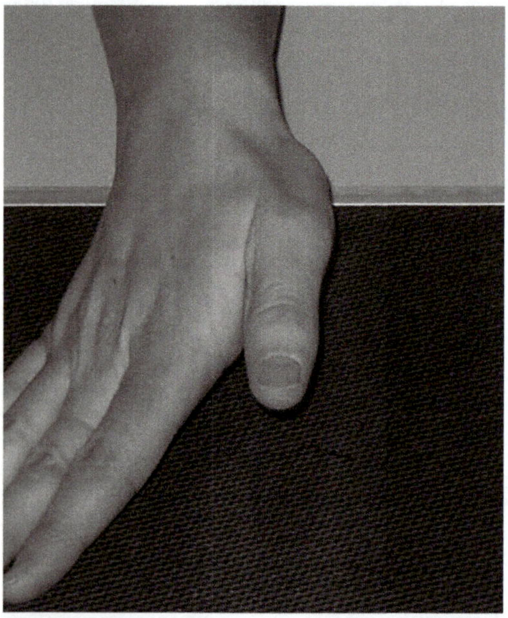

Fig. 21 Patient positioning for PA thumb

Position of the patient and cassette
Patient is seated at the end of the table with arm on the table and elbows flexed. Ideally, upper arm, elbow, and forearm are all resting on the table. Both hands are placed such that the medial aspects of both hands abut each other and both thumbs are in a PA plane with thumbnails parallel to the cassette. The patient is asked to press their thumbs together using a foam hand support (Fig. 22a).

Direction and centering of the X-ray beam
Perpendicular to the image receptor between both hands.

Evaluation criteria (Fig. 22b)
This view adequately demonstrates the first CMC joint spaces. It shows also the first metacarpals and the first MCP joint. This view is useful for the diagnosis of ulnar collateral ligament rupture.

3 Additional Projections and Fluoroscopy

The radiographic evaluation of carpal instability includes a static series and dynamic fluoroscopy. The objective of these examinations is to demon-

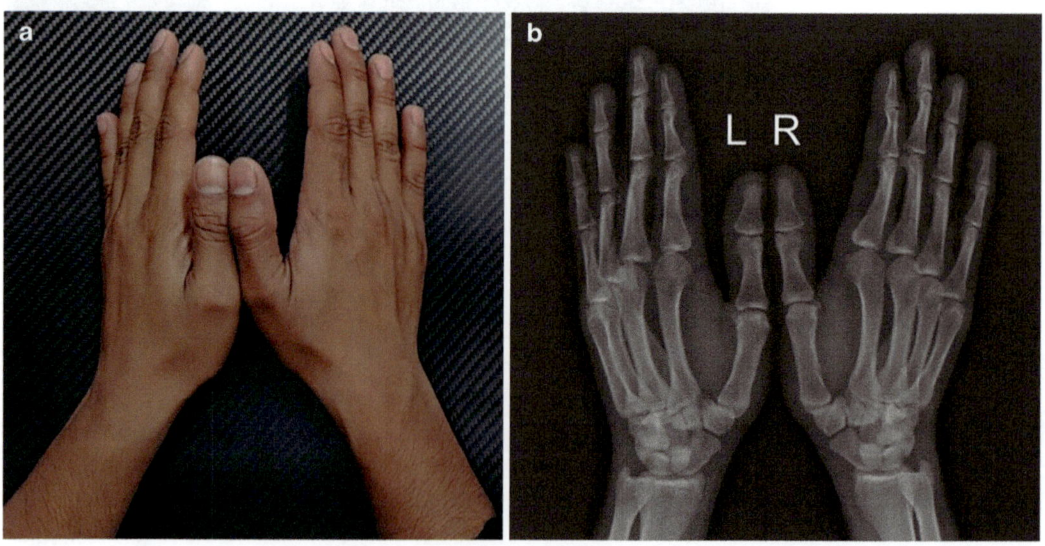

Fig. 22 (**a**) Positioning of patient for PA stress radiograph of MCP joint of thumb. (**b**) Bilateral PA stress radiograph of MCP joint of thumb

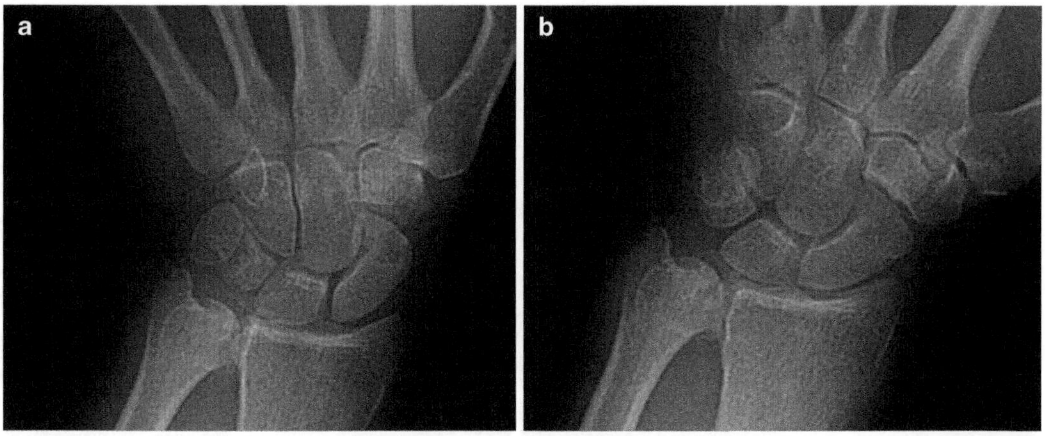

Fig. 23 Fluoroscopy images of PA wrist: (**a**) ulna deviation and (**b**) radial deviation

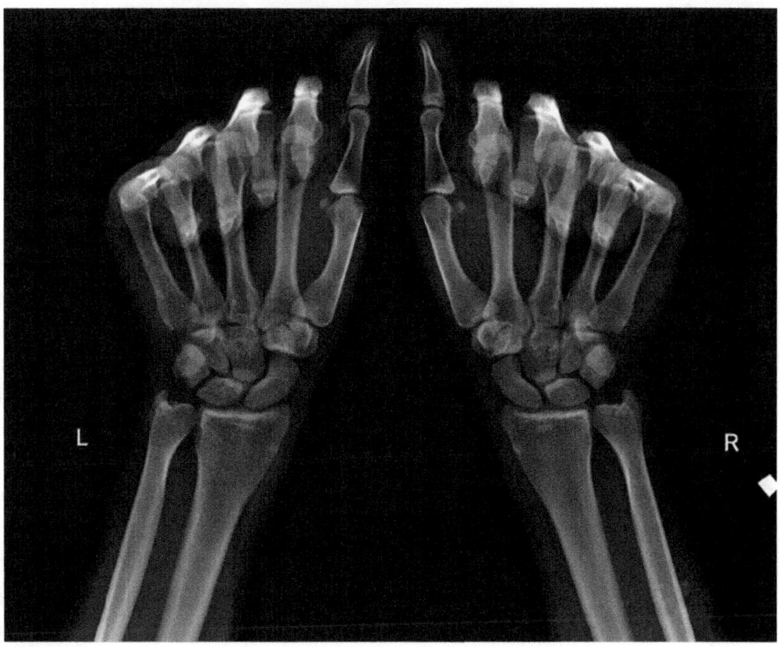

Fig. 24 Clenched fist radiograph of both wrists

strate malalignment of the carpal bones either in a static position or alternatively as part of a dynamic examination. The dynamic examination also provides the opportunity to assess for dysynchronous movement between the carpal bones. Malalignment or dysynchronous movement is likely to be a consequence of ligament disruption. Of particular importance in this regard are the scapholunate and lunotriquetral ligaments. Both have strong anterior and posterior components with a thin "membranous" central portion.

3.1 Carpal Instability Series—Static Evaluation

3.1.1 Technique

The standard series would include the following projections. Initially, the wrist is placed in the neutral PA position. From this, the wrist is deviated in the ulnar and then radial directions (Fig. 23). Images are taken in all three positions. Following this, this series is repeated with the fist clenched (Fig. 24). In some cases, the technique

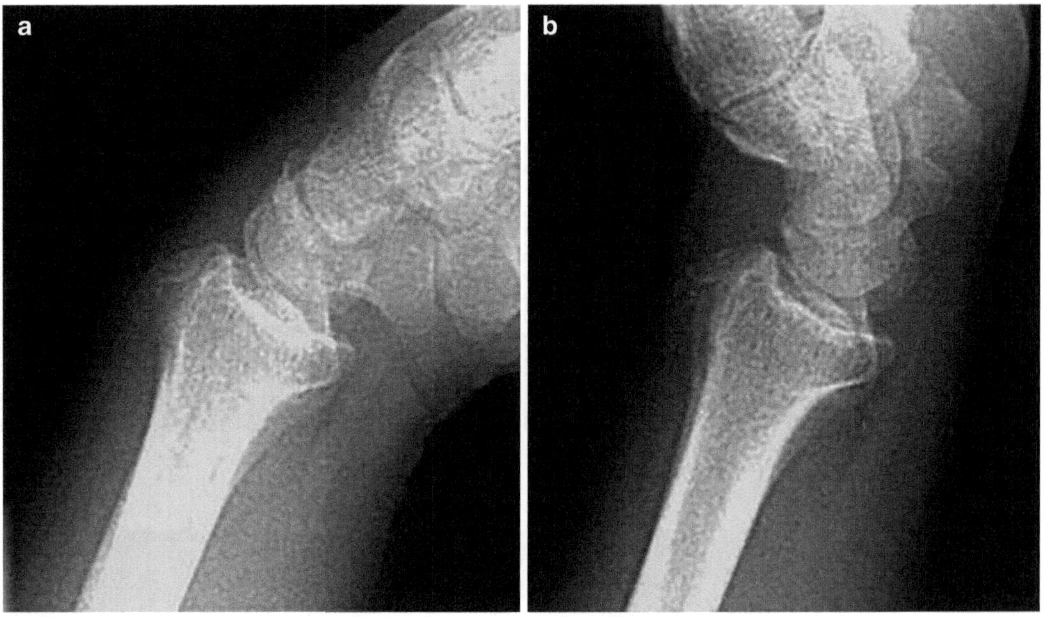

Fig. 25 Fluoroscopy images of lateral wrist in (**a**) flexion and (**b**) extension

may be conducted with the fist clenched around a pencil or a tennis ball. Then three further views are performed with the wrist in the lateral position: neutral, full extension, and full flexion (Fig. 25). An additional view which is performed for evaluation of the piso-triquetral joint is the 30° supinated view of the wrist.

3.1.2 Evaluation

The integrity of the carpal arcs is assessed. Congruency of the intercarpal joints and the width of these joints are also assessed. Of particular importance with regard to the proximal carpal row is the relationship of the lunate relative to the radius. The proximal surface of the lunate should not move more than half of its width on the distal surface of the radius (Fig. 25).

3.2 Dynamic Evaluation—Fluoroscopy or Image Intensifier Television (IITV)

3.2.1 Technique

A dynamic study provides a further opportunity to assess for carpal instability in the situation where the static views are negative. Essentially, the static series are repeated with movement. Therefore, from the PA neutral position the wrist is deviated in the ulnar direction and then back through the neutral position to the radial position. This movement is repeated. From the lateral position, the wrist is fully flexed and then fully extended. This is also repeated as required. A further, non-standard part of the study follows enquiry of the patient with regard to the movement causing symptoms. The patient undertakes this movement which is recorded with fluoroscopy. This study may be recorded and therefore replayed at normal and reduced speeds.

3.2.2 Evaluation

The alignment of the carpal bones in all the positions is evaluated. In addition, careful viewing of the relative movements within each carpal row and then between carpal rows is important. For the proximal carpal joint, the movement of the lunate relative to the distal radius is important. For the metacarpal joint, the movement of the hamate relative to the lunate is important.

4 Measurements

There are a number of measurements that are useful in the assessment of the wrist, which can be performed on plain radiographs (Rosner and Zlatkin 2004). Ulna variance is useful in a range of conditions including assessment following fracture and ulna-sided wrist pain. Distal radial measurements useful in the assessment of distal radial fractures include radial inclination, radial length, and palmar tilt (Schmitt and Froehner 2006). The scapholunate and capitate–lunate angles are calculated when carpal instability is suspected. Finally, carpal height is measured when collapse of the carpus is suspected, for example, as a consequence of carpal instability or previous fracture.

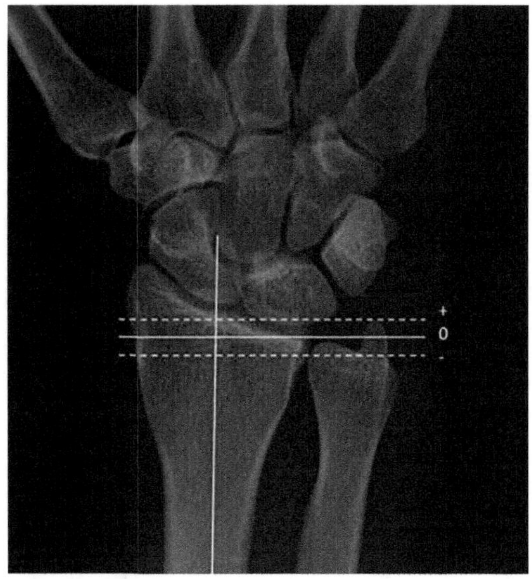

Fig. 26 Measurement of ulna variance. Solid line is ulna neutral (normal). + is positive ulna variance and – represents negative ulna variance

4.1 Ulna Variance

Ulna variance is the difference in length between the distal radius and the distal ulna. This measurement is relevant in a number of carpal disorders including fracture assessment and abnormalities of the proximal carpal row such as chondromalacia of the lunate. The wrist is assessed in a neutral PA position. A technique for the assessment of ulna variance involves first identifying the long axis of the radius at 2.0 and 5.0 cm from the distal radial cortex. A perpendicular running tangential to the most ulna portion of the distal radial articular cortex is then drawn to this line. Second, the line is drawn tangential to the distal ulna and parallel to the line described above (Fig. 26). In negative ulna variance (ulna minus), the ulna is shorter than the radius. In positive ulna variance (ulna plus), the ulna is longer than the radius. Normally, the radius and ulna are of the same length or there is mild negative ulna variance.

4.2 Radial Inclination

Radial inclination describes the slope of the radius between the tip of the radial styloid and the ulnar border of the radius in the frontal or PA plane. Its assessment is important following distal radial fractures. The technique for obtaining the measurement is first to identify the long axis of the radius as described above (Sect 4.1) (Goldfarb and Yin 2001; Mann and Wilson 1992). Second, a line is drawn from the tip of the radial styloid to the ulnar border of the distal radius. The third line is drawn through the intersection of these lines, perpendicular to the long axis of the radius. The radial inclination is the angle between the perpendicular and the line running tangential to the radial styloid and ulnar border of radius (Fig. 27). The normal inclination is 23° (21–25°).

4.3 Radial Length (Radial Height)

Radial length (radial height) is a method for assessing shortening of the radius, for example, following a fracture. The measurement involves identification of the long axis of the radius. Two lines perpendicular to this are then constructed: first, tangential to the tip of the radial styloid and second tangential to the ulnar border of the distal radius (Fig. 28). The distance between these two lines is the radial length. A normal value of 10–13 mm is expected.

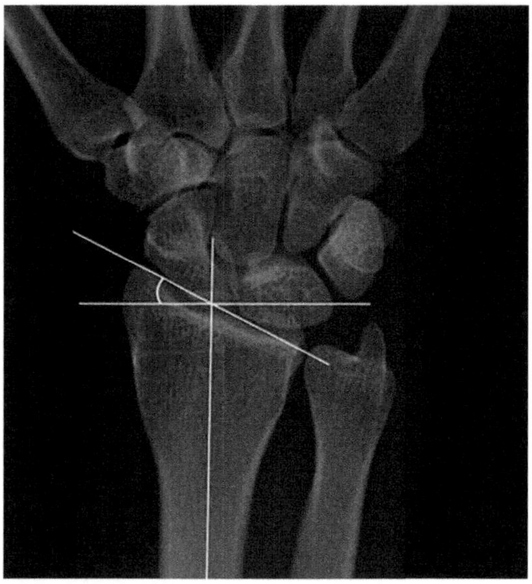

Fig. 27 Measurement of radial inclination. Normal inclination is 21–25°

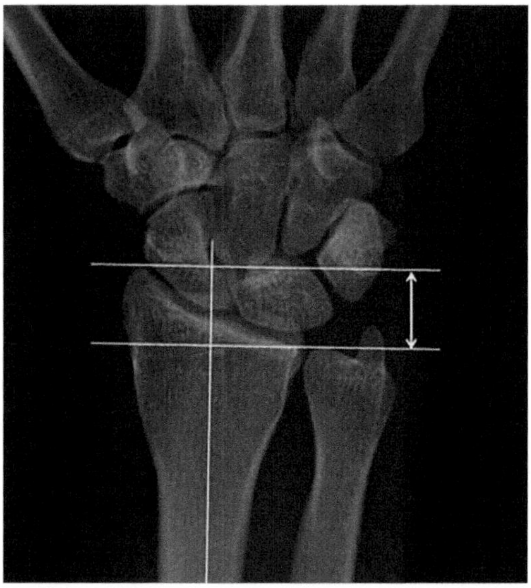

Fig. 28 Measurement of radial length. Normal measurement is 10–13 mm

4.4 Palmar Tilt (Volar Tilt or Volar Inclination)

This measurement assesses the tilt of the distal radius at the radiocarpal joint. The central axis of the radius is identified in the lateral plane using points at 2 and 5 cm from the midpoint of the distal articular surface. A perpendicular is drawn to this line at the articular surface. A third line is drawn from the dorsal lip of the distal radius to the volar lip of the distal radius. The palmar tilt is the angle between the third line and the perpendicular (Fig. 29). It is normally between 0° and 22°. This is an important measurement in the assessment of distal radial fractures.

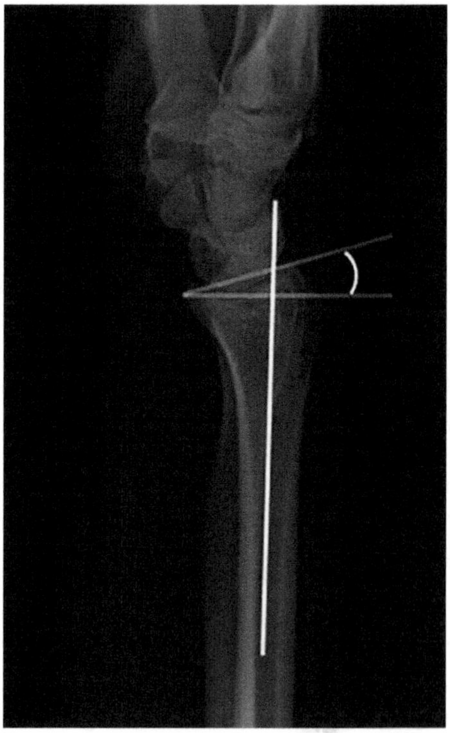

Fig. 29 Measurement of palmar tilt (volar inclination). Normal value 0–22°

4.5 Scapholunate Angle

This angle is calculated when carpal instability is suspected. It is particularly pertinent in the assessment of dorsal intercalated instability (DISI). The angle is measured from the lateral view of the wrist. The angle is calculated by drawing two lines. A line is drawn through the proximal and distal volar convexities of the scaphoid. This defines the scaphoid axis (Fig. 30a). The lunate axis is perpendicular to a line drawn between the distal poles of the lunate

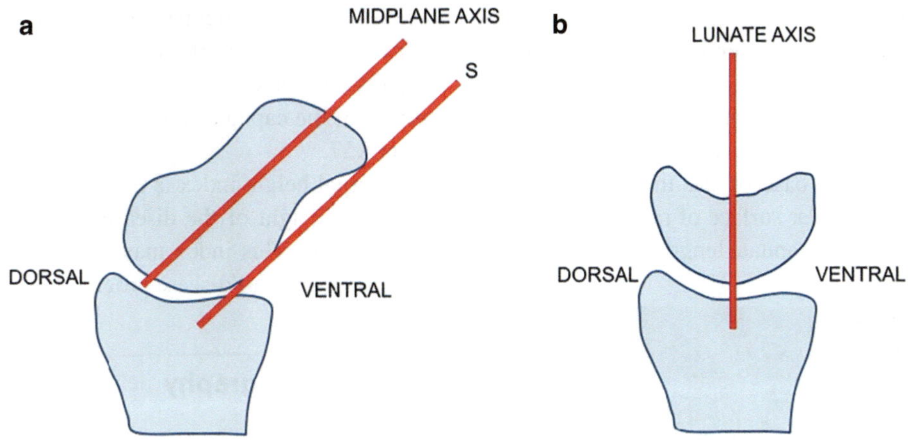

Fig. 30 (**a**) Scaphoid axis. (**b**) Lunate axis

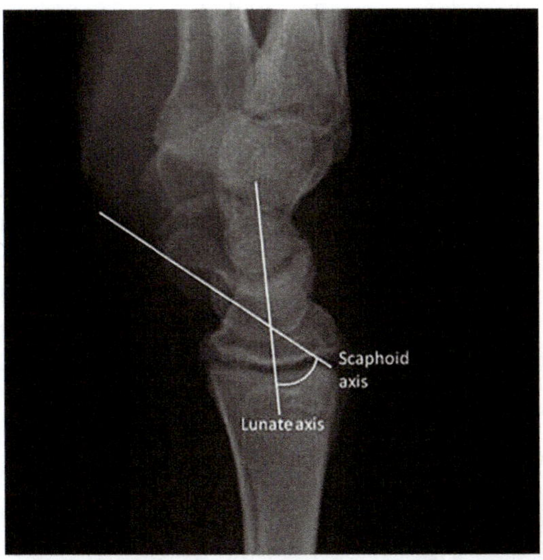

Fig. 31 Scapholunate angle. White lines represent long axis of scaphoid and lunate. Normal range is 30–60°

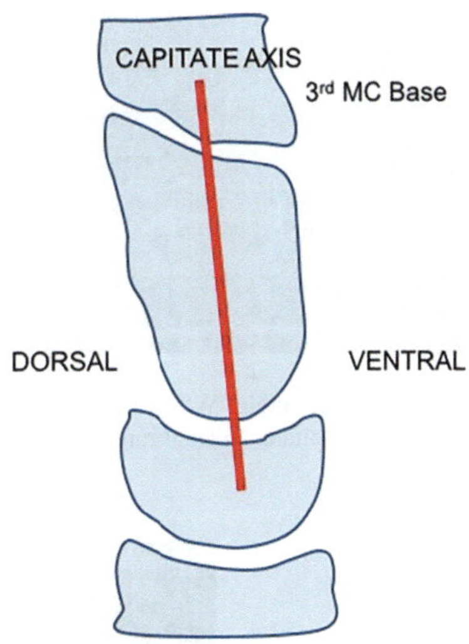

Fig. 32 Capitate axis

(Fig. 30b). The normal scapholunate angle lies between 30° and 60° (Fig. 31) (Linkous and Pierce 2000).

4.6 Capitate–Lunate Angle

This angle is calculated when the volar instability pattern (VISI) of carpal instability is suspected. The angle is measured from the lateral view of the wrist. The long axis of the lunate is drawn as described above (Sect 4.5). The long axis of the capitate is drawn from the center of its distal articular surface to the center of the proximal articular surface (Fig. 32). The normal capitate–lunate angle lies between 0° and 30° (Fig. 33).

4.7 Carpal Height

Carpal height provides quantification of the degree of carpal collapse, for example, in scapholunate advanced collapse (SLAC). Two methods have been described. The first method describes a ratio between the distance from the base of the third metacarpal to the proximal articular surface of the radius and the length of the third metacarpal. The line drawn extends from the long axis of the third metacarpal (Fig. 34a). With this method, the normal carpal height ratio is 0.54.

The second method divides the carpal height (distance from base of the third metacarpal to proximal articular surface of radius) by the capitate length. The capitate length is calculated from the distal angular articular surface of the capitate (between the bases of the second and third metacarpals) and the center of the proximal articular surface of the capitate (Fig. 34). The normal figure is 1.57.

A carpal height index is obtained by dividing the carpal height of the diseased wrist with the normal wrist. This index may be followed with time as a marker of disease progression.

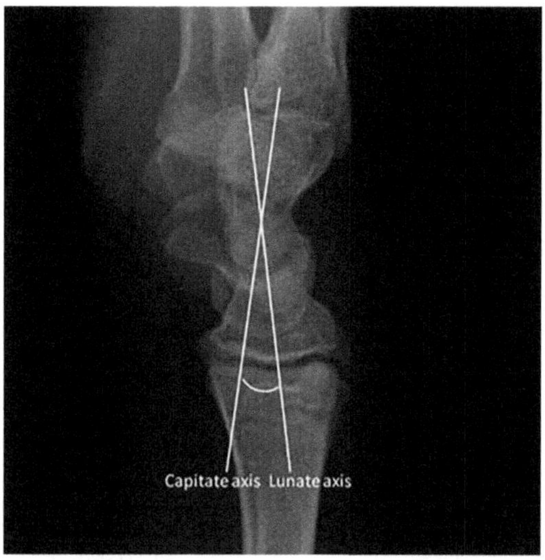

Fig. 33 Capitolunate angle. White lines represent long axis of lunate and capitate. Normal range is 0–30°

5 Arthrography

Arthrography of the wrist is performed in the assessment of interosseous (scapholunate and lunotriquetral) wrist ligaments and the triangular fibrocartilage complex. With the advent of cross-sectional imaging techniques, it is more frequently undertaken now as part of an MRI or CT arthrographic study. The basic technique is that of a proximal row or radiocarpal injection. A more complex study will involve injection of two or three wrist compartments (Braunstein and Louis 1985).

Unicompartmental injection to the radiocarpal may be undertaken by injection at two different points. The first is a dorsal approach to the junc-

Fig. 34 Measurement of carpal height: (**a**) method 1 and (**b**) method 2

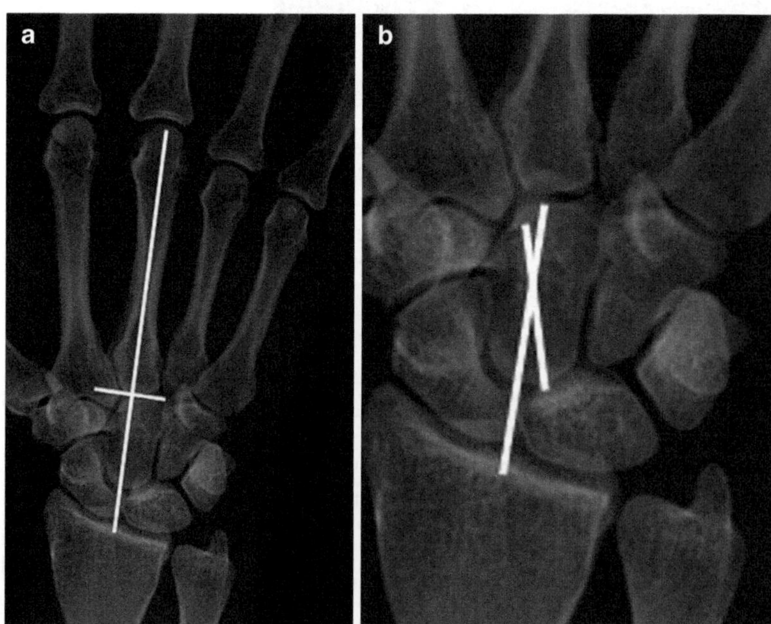

tion between the scaphoid and lunate just proximal to the scapholunate ligament. The second is between the scaphoid and distal radius. The wrist is gently flexed and a 22G needle introduced under fluoroscopic guidance (Wilson and Gilula 1991). Care must be taken not to damage the scapholunate ligament. Note should be taken of the normal radial inclination and allowance made for the dorsal lip of the radius when introducing the needle. Contrast is injected into the radiocarpal space. The usual filling volume is between 2 and 4 ml. The end of the injection is signified by gentle resistance to further filling and distribution of contrast across the radiocarpal joint. Generally, contrast of 240 IU/l is sufficient for good radiographic imaging. The mixture injected will alter for CT arthrography and MRI arthrography.

Contrast should be injected slowly, carefully observing the filling of the radiocarpal space and looking for contrast tracking into the scapholunate space, lunotriquetral space, or distal radioulnar joint. Spot films are taken during injection (Fig. 35). At the end of the injection when there is good filling of the radiocarpal space, a further series of films is taken following gentle exercise of the wrist. A typical series of films would include PA in the neutral, ulnar deviation, and radial deviation positions followed by a lateral view. It is commonplace to have performed a static and dynamic instability series (as outlined earlier in this chapter) prior to injection of contrast. Fluoroscopy and videotaping the procedure enabled further retrospective analysis.

The normal pattern of filling (Fig. 30) outlines the radiocarpal joint. Age-related degenerate perforations of the central portion of the scapholunate and lunotriquetral ligaments are well recognized (Linkous and Pierce 2000). Similarly, age-related degenerate perforations of the radial side of the triangular fibrocartilage complex with filling of the distal radioulnar joint may also be observed. Small volar outpouchings (radial recesses) of the capsule are well recognized (Fig. 35). On the ulnar side, there is a small prestyloid recess above which the meniscus homologue and a further collection of contrast may be identified. Filling of the piso-triquetral space is a normal variant.

Midcarpal injection involves injection between the distal scaphoid and capitate with the wrist in gentle flexion (Fig. 36). Careful injection with fluoroscopic guidance is undertaken until good filling of the space has been obtained. Careful observation of the scapholunate and lunotriquetral spaces is undertaken, looking for evidence of filling of these spaces. This is considered an easier method for establishing the integrity of the scapholunate and lunotriquetral ligaments. A static and dynamic instability series would be obtained (Tirman and Weber 1985).

Triple compartment arthrography is regarded as being of superior diagnostic quality (Levinsohn and Rosen 1991). However, single radiocarpal joint injection has an advantage of evaluation of scapholunate ligament, lunotriquetral ligament, and triangular fibrocartilage complex in a single injection. It also avoids the time-consuming wait between each of the three compartment injections while awaiting absorption of contrast. However, the diagnostic yield is greater with a midcarpal injection based on an analysis of unidirectional joint communications. It was proposed that if a scapholunate or lunotriquetral ligament disruption was suspected, then a midcarpal injection should be performed first. If a triangular fibrocartilage complex disruption was suspected, then a radiocarpal injection should be performed first.

Full triple compartment arthrography also involves injecting the distal radioulnar joint looking for communication with the proximal carpal joint.

3.0 T MR without arthrography allows adequate evaluation of ligaments and has limited the use of arthrography in current practice (Saupe 2009; Magee 2009).

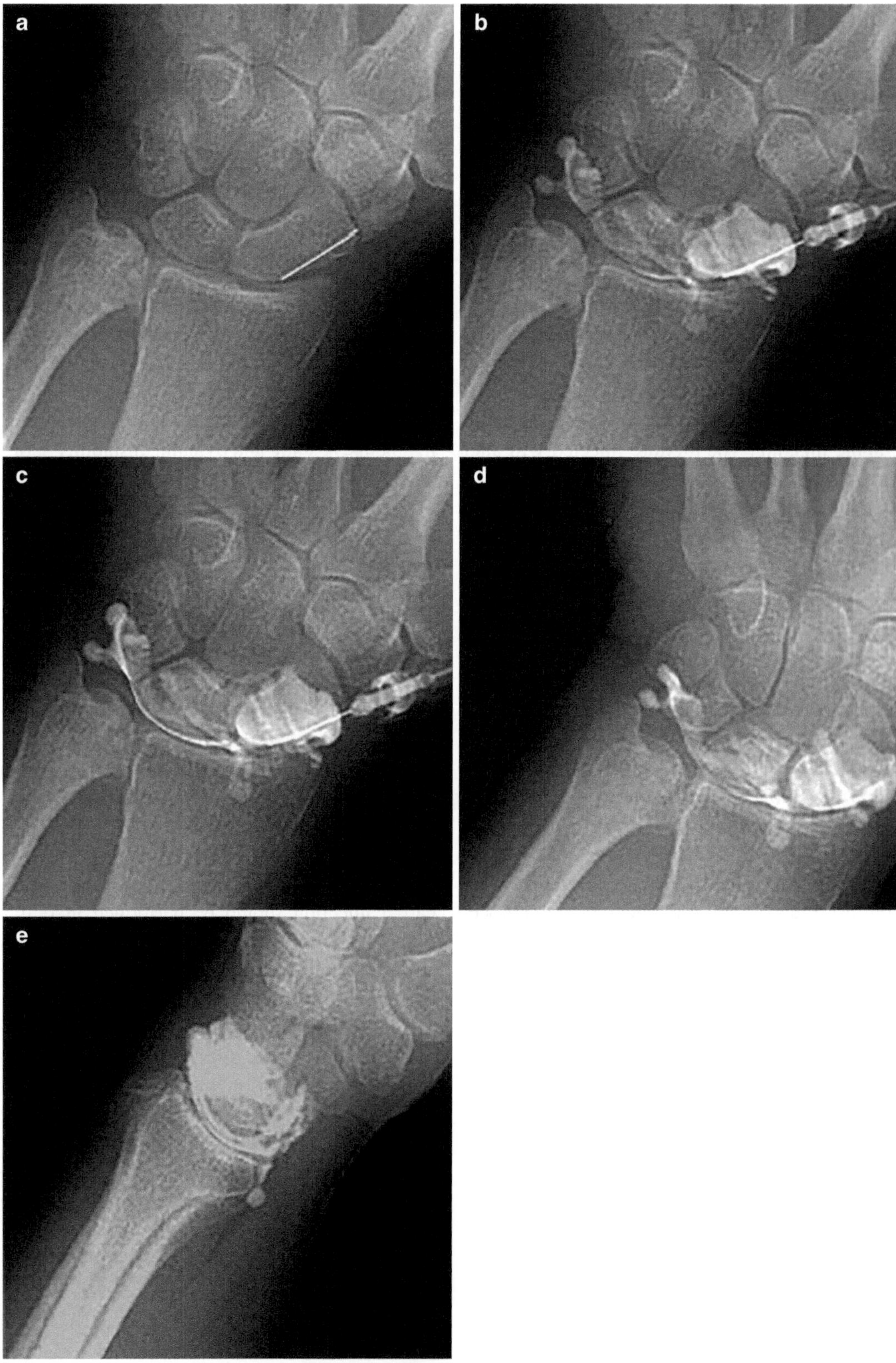

Fig. 35 Fluoroscopy images from radiocarpal arthrogram: (**a**) needle position, (**b**) early filling with contrast, (**c**) mid-filling phase, (**d**) late-filling phase (complete), and (**e**) lateral view post exercise

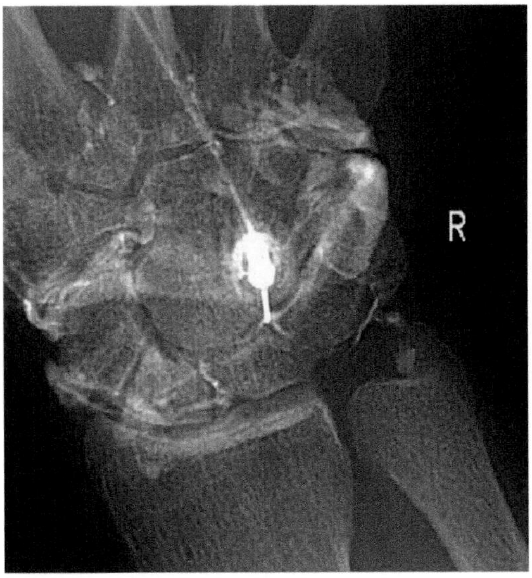

Fig. 36 Fluoroscopy image from midcarpal arthrogram demonstrating needle position and filling of radiocarpal space

Acknowledgments We thank authors of previous edition of this chapter for their valuable contribution.

We thank Mr. Mahammad Yunus Shaikh, Radiography Technician, and Dr. Sushant Bhat, DNB Radiology Resident, for assistance in obtaining the radiographic projections.

References

Ballinger WP, Frank ED (1999) Merrill's atlas of radiographic positions and radiologic procedures, 9th edn. Mosby, St Louis

Braunstein EM, Louis DS (1985) Fluoroscopic and arthrographic evaluation of carpal instability. AJR Am J Roentgenol 144(6):1259–1262

Gilula LA, Destouet JM et al (1984) Roentgenographic diagnosis of the painful wrist. Clin Orthop Relat Res 187:52–64

Goldfarb CA, Yin Y (2001) Wrist fractures: what the clinician wants to know. Radiology 219(1):11–28

Keats TE, Sistrom C (2001) Atlas of radiologic measurement. ISBN: 0323001610 – Google Books

Lampignano J, Kendrick LE (2017) Bontrager's textbook of radiographic positioning and related anatomy. ISBN: 9780323399661

Levinsohn EM, Rosen ID (1991) Wrist arthrography: value of the three-compartment injection method. Radiology 179(1):231–239

Linkous MD, Pierce SD (2000) Scapholunate ligamentous communicating defects in symptomatic and asymptomatic wrists: characteristics 1. Radiology 216(3):846–850

Loredo RA, Sorge DG (2005) Radiographic evaluation of the wrist: a vanishing art. Semin Roentgenol 40(3):248–289

Magee T (2009) Comparison of 3-T MRI and arthroscopy of intrinsic wrist ligament and TFCC tears. AJR Am J Roentgenol 192(1):80–85

Mann FA, Wilson AJ (1992) Radiographic evaluation of the wrist: what does the hand surgeon want to know? Radiology 184(1):15–24

Resnik CS (2000) Wrist and hand injuries. Semin Musculoskelet Radiol 4(2):193–204

Rosner JL, Zlatkin MB (2004) Imaging of athletic wrist and hand injuries. Semin Musculoskelet Radiol 8(1):57–79

Saupe N (2009) 3-Tesla high-resolution MR imaging of the wrist. Semin Musculoskelet Radiol 13(1):29–38

Schmitt R, Froehner S (2006) Carpal instability. Eur Radiol 16(10):2161–2178

Tirman RM, Weber ER (1985) Midcarpal wrist arthrography for detection of tears of the scapholunate and lunotriquetral ligaments. AJR Am J Roentgenol 144(1):107–108

Whitley AS, Sloane C, Hoadley G, Moore AD, Alsop CW (2005) Clark's positioning in radiography, 12th edn. Hodder Arnold, London

Wilson AJ, Gilula LA (1991) Unidirectional joint communications in wrist arthrography: an evaluation of 250 cases. AJR Am J Roentgenol 157(1):105–109

Wolf J, Oren T, Ferguson B, Williams A, Peterson B (2009) The carpometacarpal stress view radiograph in the evaluation of trapeziometacarpal joint laxity. J Hand Surg 34(8):1402–1406

Yochum TR, Rowe LJ (2005) Essentials of skeletal radiology. ISBN: 9780781739467 – Google Books

Computed Tomography of Hand and Wrist

Sri Priya Suresh and Tishi Ninan

Contents

S. P. Suresh
Department of Radiology, Plymouth Hospitals NHS Trust, Crownhill, Devon, UK

T. Ninan (✉)
Department of Radiology, Swansea Bay University Health Board,
Heol Maes Eglwys, Morriston, Swansea, UK
e-mail: Tishi.ninan@wales.nhs.uk

Abstract

Computed tomography (CT) scanning has transformed medical imaging over the past five decades, evolving from a pioneering technology to a cornerstone of modern diagnostics. The first CT scan on a human patient was conducted on 1 October 1971 at Atkinson Morley Hospital in Wimbledon, England, marking the beginning of a new era in noninvasive imaging. Innovations such as multidetector systems, faster gantry rotation speeds, spectral imaging, dose-reduction algorithms, and the integration of artificial intelligence have significantly expanded CT capabilities. These developments, bolstered by advances in computer technology and engineering, have enhanced image quality and broadened clinical applications.

Today, CT is widely used for evaluating bony abnormalities in the hand and wrist, benefiting from its high resolution and increasing accessibility. Recent technological breakthroughs have further expanded its utility to soft tissue assessment and dynamic imaging. With optimised workflows, a wrist CT scan can now be performed in the time it takes to obtain plain radiographs in multiple views, often with a comparable radiation dose.

Med Radiol Diagn Imaging (2025)
https://doi.org/10.1007/174_2025_612,
Published Online: 25 September 2025

1 Introduction

Over the past half-century, computed tomography (CT) has evolved dramatically, alongside other imaging techniques. Most radiology departments now have access to a wide range of imaging modalities. However, this abundance sometimes leads to over-utilisation, where multiple imaging tests are performed unnecessarily, or advanced modalities are employed without clear clinical justification.

The guiding principle should always be to select the imaging modality that most effectively addresses the clinical question with the fewest steps, lowest radiation exposure (in line with ALARA), and minimal cost. CT is invaluable in many situations, sometimes serving as a first-line modality, at other times as complementary to other studies, and often as a second-line tool when other options are contraindicated or inconclusive.

In this chapter, we will highlight scenarios in which CT is the preferred first-line investigation. We will explore its advantages over other imaging modalities in specific clinical contexts while briefly touching upon conditions where alternative techniques may be more appropriate as the initial imaging choice.

2 Computed Tomography Techniques

2.1 Patient Positioning

For wrist and hand CT scans, patients typically lie in a prone position with the affected arm extended above their head in the so-called "Superman" position, with the palm facing downwards. This positioning minimises radiation exposure to radiosensitive organs such as the eyes, breasts, chest, and abdomen. It also helps to reduce beam-hardening artefacts that can occur if the hand is scanned close to the torso.

2.2 Scan Technique

Modern multi-detector CT (MDCT) scanners enhance both spatial resolution and scan speed, particularly valuable in evaluating wrist trauma. Scan parameters—including voltage (kV), tube current (mA), pitch, and field of view—are tailored to individual patient factors such as body habitus, the presence of a cast, and the clinical indication.

Radiation doses are generally lower for wrists without casts, although imaging may still be performed with casts or dressings in place for unstable, complex fractures or open injuries. During scanning, the wrist should be centred in the gantry with the upper arm fully extended to avoid wrist deviation. Excessive wrist dorsiflexion should be avoided to maintain accurate anatomical alignment.

Technical optimisation includes the use of:

- Dose and noise reduction algorithms
- Deep learning-based image reconstruction (as per departmental protocol)
- Isotropic data acquisition, enabling high-quality multiplanar reconstructions (MPR) in axial, sagittal, and coronal planes

Reconstructions are typically aligned along the axis of the capitate bone, and high-resolution bone algorithms with edge enhancement are used to maximise osseous detail.

2.3 CT Arthrogram

In selected cases, a CT arthrogram may be performed to enhance visualisation of intra-articular structures, particularly ligaments and cartilage. This involves the intra-articular injection of contrast before scanning. Specific techniques and indications for CT arthrography are discussed in a later section of this chapter.

3 Clinical Applications

3.1 Fractures

While some institutions utilise MRI, CT has become the primary cross-sectional imaging modality for wrist trauma in many centres. This section reviews the role of CT in evaluating and managing various hand and wrist fractures.

3.1.1 Fractures of the Distal Radius and Ulna

Distal radius fractures are common presentations in emergency settings. As surgical management options expand, detailed imaging of fracture configuration, angulation, and comminution is increasingly essential for treatment planning (Fig. 1). CT provides superior assessment of:

- Radial inclination
- Radial shortening
- Radial tilt
- Articular incongruity
- Degree of comminution

For distal ulnar fractures, CT may be indicated in cases involving severe comminution or shortening, which are challenging to assess on plain radiographs.

3.1.2 Fractures of Carpal Bones

Evaluating carpal bone fractures is crucial due to the complex anatomy and risk of missed injuries, which may result in complications such as nonunion and chronic pain.

Plain radiography is typically the first-line modality due to its accessibility and cost-effectiveness.

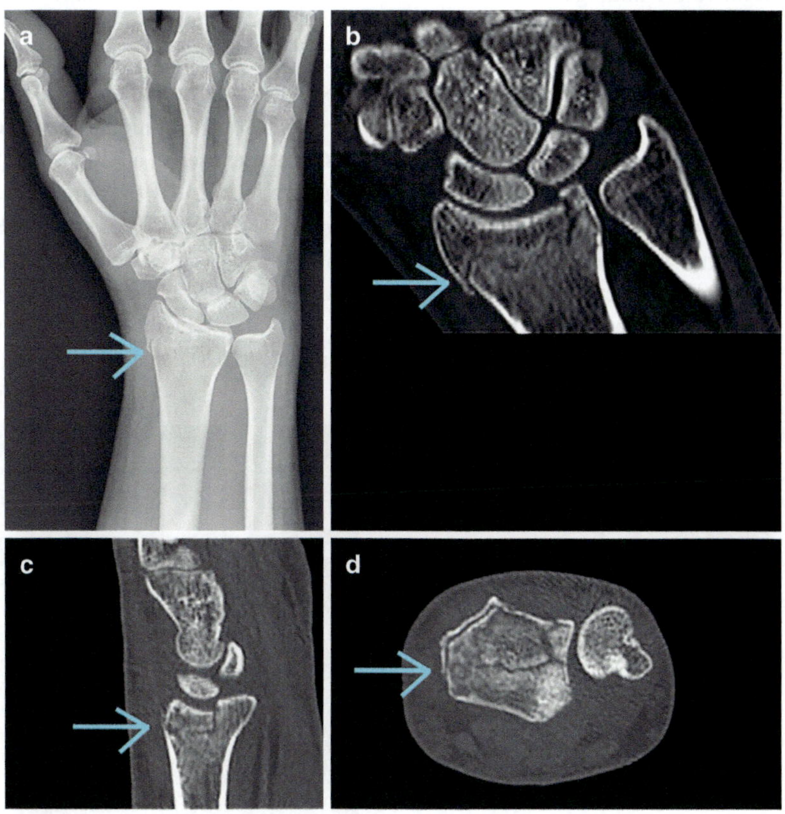

Fig. 1 Radiograph of wrist (**a**) demonstrating an intra-articular fracture of the distal radius (Blue arrow). Starting at the top right-hand corner and clockwise, images show coronal (**b**), transverse (**d**) and sagittal (**c**) CT reconstructions in the same patient. The degree of comminution and extent of articular depression are difficult to appreciate on the plain radiograph

However, multiple studies have demonstrated its limitations, particularly in detecting occult scaphoid fractures (Slaar et al. 2012).

CT scanning significantly enhances the detection of subtle or occult fractures following inconclusive radiographs. It provides excellent spatial resolution and facilitates multi-planar reconstruction (MPR) using MDCT, allowing for detailed assessment of complex fracture patterns (Balcı et al. 2014; Refaat et al. 2020; Amin et al. 2022).

CT signs of fracture include:

- Sharp, lucent lines within trabecular bone
- Cortical disruption or misalignment
- Fragment displacement or dislocation

Noncontrast CT is less effective than MRI in assessing soft tissue or ligamentous injuries, which may account for persistent pain despite negative CT findings.

3.1.2.1 Scaphoid Fractures

The scaphoid is the largest bone in the proximal carpal row and serves as a key stabiliser between the proximal and distal carpal rows. It is also the most fractured carpal bone, accounting for approximately 70% of all carpal fractures (Fig. 2), with the waist being the most frequent site of injury (Welling et al. 2008). The proximal pole of the scaphoid receives blood supply from the distal pole, making it vulnerable to avascular necrosis. Early and accurate detection is essential to reduce the risk of non-union and avascular necrosis.

Scaphoid fractures that are not visible on initial radiographs, known as radiographically occult fractures, present a diagnostic challenge due to the limited sensitivity of conventional X-rays, which is approximately 70% (Gäbler et al. 2001). MRI is the most accurate modality for detecting these fractures, with a reported sensitivity of 94.2% and specificity of 97.9% (Bäcker et al. 2020). CT offers high spatial resolution and is effective in identifying cortical breaks and trabecular injuries. It is also more readily available and faster to perform than MRI. However, CT is less sensitive (81.5%) and slightly less specific (96%) than MRI. Moreover, CT has limited capability in detecting soft tissue injuries and bone marrow abnormalities. In contrast, MRI is superior in identifying occult fractures, bone marrow oedema, and associated ligamentous or cartilaginous injuries (Sahu et al. 2021; Dreckmann et al. 2019).

The choice between CT and MRI often depends on institutional resources and workflow logistics (Smith et al. 2016; Wijetunga et al. 2018; Chunara et al. 2019). A practical approach is to use CT as a triage tool, reserving MRI for cases with persistent clinical suspicion despite negative CT findings. This helps to prevent unnecessary immobilisation and facilitates early intervention (Daniels et al. 2020; Dean 2021).

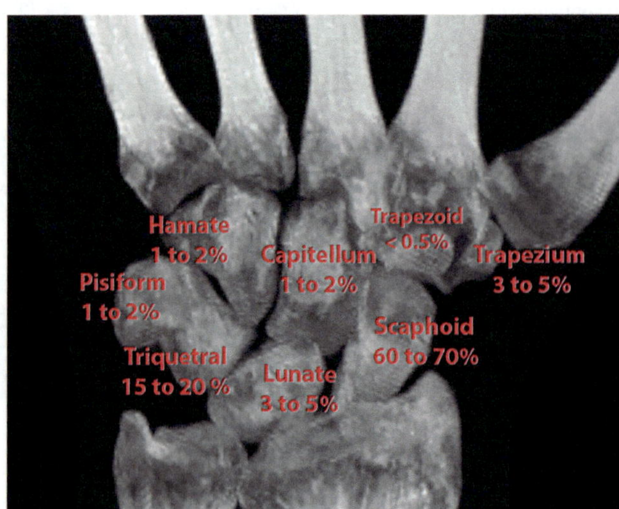

Fig. 2 Illustrates the relative frequency of fractures in the different carpal bones quoted by various sources

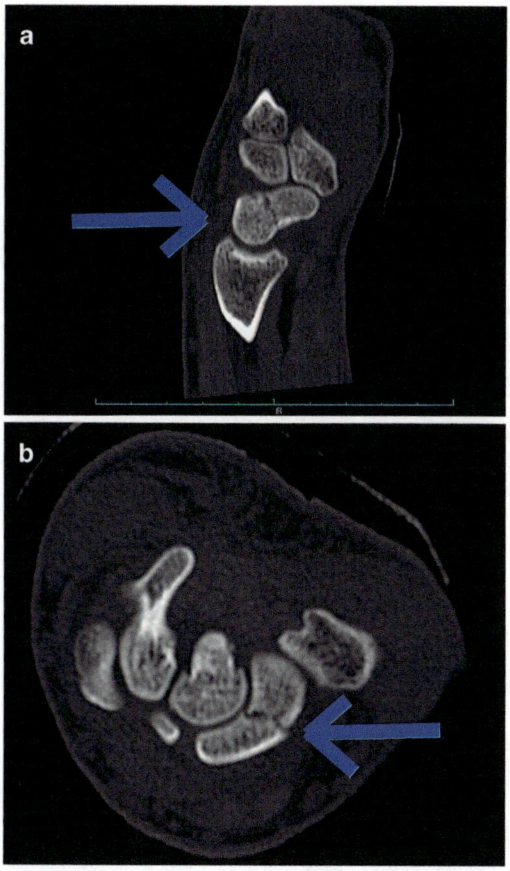

Fig. 3 (**a**) Sagittal CT section through scaphoid demonstrating fracture of the scaphoid waist. (**b**) Axial CT section through scaphoid demonstrating fracture of the scaphoid waist

Emerging technologies such as low-dose CT, dual-energy CT, and spectral imaging demonstrate promise in improving diagnostic accuracy while reducing radiation exposure. Nonetheless, these methods are not yet widely validated or accessible.

Scaphoid fractures typically result from a fall onto an outstretched hand, causing dorsiflexion of the wrist. The waist of the scaphoid is the most common site of injury (Fig. 3). Less commonly, injuries such as tuberosity avulsions or proximal pole avulsions may occur from traction on the scapholunate ligament.

3.1.2.2 Lunate Fractures

Lunate fractures account for approximately 4% of carpal fractures (Fig. 2). Centrally located in the proximal carpal row, a missed or delayed diagnosis of lunate fractures can lead to carpal instability, nonunion, and avascular necrosis.

Due to overlapping structures, lunate fractures are often challenging to detect on plain radiographs. CT effectively reveals various fracture patterns, which are typically classified by location (body, dorsal pole, volar pole) and fracture orientation (transverse or sagittal) (Fig. 4a). Coronal plane fractures are uncommon, with volar pole fractures being the most frequently encountered. These typically result from axial compression by the capitate when the wrist is positioned in dorsiflexion and ulnar deviation. Additionally, these injuries may also be associated with volar intercalated segment instability (VISI).

Similar to the scaphoid and capitate, the proximal portion of the lunate is particularly susceptible to vascular compromise following trauma. In approximately 20% of individuals, the lunate receives its entire blood supply from a single palmar nutrient artery, rendering it vulnerable to osteonecrosis in the event of injury.

3.1.2.3 Triquetral Fractures

Triquetral fractures are the second most common type of carpal fracture, accounting for about 20% of cases. The most frequent variant is the dorsal ridge fracture, typically caused by ulnar styloid impaction or ligamentous avulsion during wrist hyperextension and ulnar deviation (Fig. 4c, d). These fractures are usually visible on plain radiographs. However, body fractures or those associated with perilunate dislocations may necessitate a CT scan for thorough assessment.

3.1.2.4 Pisiform Fractures

Pisiform fractures are rare, accounting for approximately 2% of carpal fractures. They typically result from a direct blow and are challenging to identify on plain radiographs due to overlapping ossification centres and bony structures.

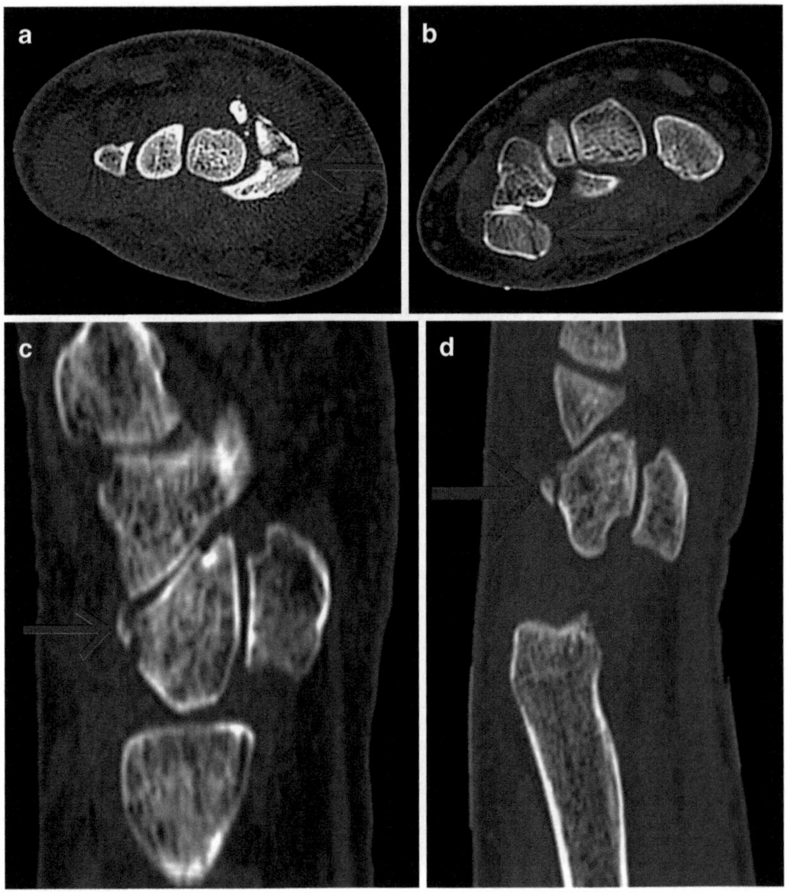

Fig. 4 (**a**) CT transverse section through the lunate demonstrating comminution that is difficult to appreciate on the plain radiograph. (**b**) CT transverse section demonstrating a minimally displaced fracture of the pisiform. (**c, d**) CT sagittal sections through the triquetral demonstrating dorsal ridge fractures (*arrows*) that were occult on the initial plain radiograph

CT is particularly useful in confirming the diagnosis and assessing associated injuries (Fig. 4b).

3.1.2.5 Trapezium and Trapezoid Fractures

The trapezium, the most mobile bone in the distal row, is most often fractured at the trapezial ridge, where the flexor retinaculum attaches. Fractures usually occur due to direct trauma or avulsion.

The trapezoid is the least commonly fractured carpal bone (Fig. 2, approximately 0.5% of cases), typically resulting from high-energy trauma and usually associated with other injuries. CT is highly effective in identifying these fractures, especially when they are occult on radiographs.

3.1.2.6 Capitate Fractures

The capitate, the largest of the carpal bones, is often involved in high-energy trauma. Its proximal third is nearly entirely covered in articular cartilage, which can obscure fracture lines on plain radiographs, making CT imaging essential for precise assessment, particularly in cases of suspected articular involvement. Although isolated capitate fractures are uncommon, they can occur. Similar to the scaphoid, the capitate receives retrograde blood supply from its distal pole, putting its proximal portion at risk of avascular necrosis following fracture.

Capitate fractures are classified based on fracture orientation and location. These include:

- Transverse fractures of the pole, body, or neck
- Vertico-frontal and parasagittal fracture patterns

Among these, transverse fractures of the capitate body are the most common.

A particularly rare and complex injury involving the capitate is *Fenton's syndrome*, also known as scaphocapitate fracture syndrome. This condition features simultaneous transverse fractures of the scaphoid and capitate, typically occurring as part of a trans-scaphoid, trans-capitate, perilunate fracture-dislocation. The proximal capitate fragment may rotate by 90° or 180°, leading to malalignment even after spontaneous reduction of the dislocation. These injuries are often associated with additional carpal trauma. CT is recommended to evaluate alignment, fracture union, and to assess for complications such as non-union or avascular necrosis.

3.1.2.7 Hamate Fractures

Hamate fractures are commonly observed in athletes engaged in sports that involve clubs or racquets (e.g., golf, tennis). Fractures of the hook of the hamate are especially subtle and can be overlooked on radiographs.

A delayed diagnosis or malunion may lead to ulnar nerve palsy. CT offers excellent visualisation and is crucial for confirming the diagnosis.

3.1.3 Fractures of the Metacarpals

While metacarpal shaft fractures are usually apparent on radiographs, fractures at the base, particularly fracture-dislocations, may be overlooked. This is especially pertinent in young, active patients, where a missed injury can result in significant morbidity.

Plain films may underestimate comminution and angulation. CT is frequently used for both diagnosis and surgical planning, especially in intra-articular fractures. Even when fractures of the base of the first metacarpal are visible on plain films, CT can be useful for assessing fragmentation and joint involvement. If not managed appropriately, these injuries can result in early osteoarthritis and long-term functional impairment.

3.2 Dislocations

3.2.1 Distal Radioulnar Joint

The distal radioulnar joint (DRUJ) is essential for facilitating forearm rotation, particularly pronation and supination. DRUJ instability may arise from trauma, distal radius fractures, ulnar styloid injuries, or degenerative changes. CT imaging proves invaluable for evaluating DRUJ alignment and congruity, especially when conventional radiographs prove inconclusive.

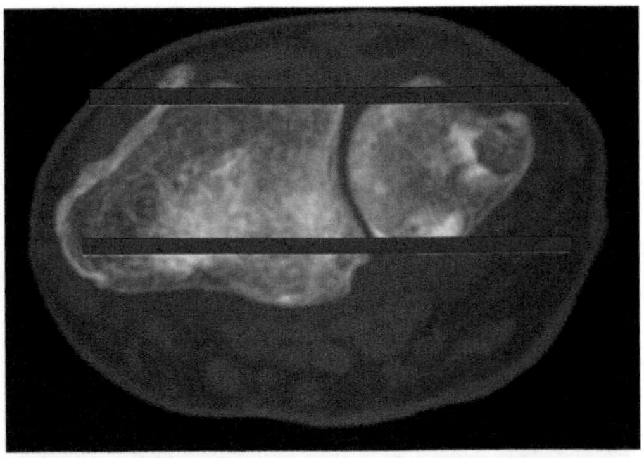

Fig. 5 Illustration of the Mino method for assessing DRUJ subluxation. If more than 50% of the ulnar head is within the sigmoid notch, it indicates a stable joint. Less than 50% signifies subluxation or instability

To evaluate DRUJ stability, both symptomatic and contralateral (asymptomatic) wrists are typically imaged in neutral, pronation, and supination positions. This facilitates a comparison between sides and helps identify abnormal joint relationships in various functional positions.

When plain radiographs yield subtle or indeterminate findings, CT provides enhanced detail for evaluating alignment. Several well-established methods are employed to assess the DRUJ:

3.2.1.1 Mino Method

This method is best used when the wrist is imaged in a neutral position. The position of the ulnar head is assessed on an axial slice by determining whether it lies between two parallel lines drawn along the volar and dorsal rims of the sigmoid notch. If the ulnar head is situated between these lines, the joint is regarded as stable (Fig. 5).

3.2.1.2 Congruency Method

This method is best employed when the wrist is in pronation. The congruence of the joint is evaluated by assessing how well the ulnar head aligns with the sigmoid notch. Normal congruence suggests stable articulation (Fig. 6).

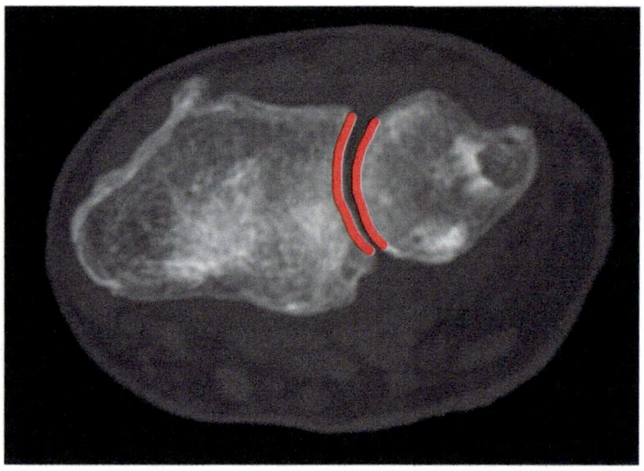

Fig. 6 Illustration of the congruency method for the assessment of DRUJ subluxation. Greater articular overlap suggests a congruent, stable joint. Reduced overlap or articular mismatch implies incongruency and potential instability. This method is particularly useful when assessing chronic degenerative changes or congenital variations of the DRUJ

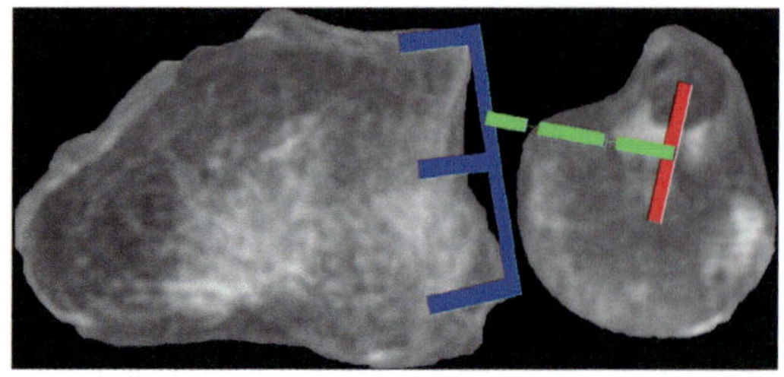

Fig. 7 Illustration of the epicentre method for evaluating distal radioulnar joint (DRUJ) alignment. A reference line (red) is drawn connecting the centre of the ulnar styloid and the centre of the ulnar head. From this, a perpendicular line (dashed green) is extended towards a chord drawn across the sigmoid notch. The DRUJ is considered normally aligned when this perpendicular line passes close to the central portion of the sigmoid notch. In a stable joint, the centre of rotation lies close to or within the confines of the sigmoid notch chord. If the centre of rotation lies significantly outside this region, it indicates a malalignment or subluxation of the ulnar head relative to the sigmoid notch. The method allows for an anatomical and reproducible assessment that is less affected by patient positioning than some other techniques

3.2.1.3 Epicentre Method

This method is best used when the wrist is in supination. In this technique, a line is drawn between the centre of the ulnar styloid and the centre of the ulnar head. A perpendicular line is then dropped from this axis to intersect the sigmoid notch. If this line passes centrally through the sigmoid notch, it indicates a normal joint relationship (Fig. 7).

Each method has its strengths and limitations. Reported sensitivities range from 55% to 100%. However, care must be taken when interpreting these signs, as the presence of distal radius malunion can result in false positives—particularly with the Mino and Congruency methods. Among the available techniques, the Epicentre method is often regarded as the most specific for identifying true DRUJ dislocation or subluxation.

3.2.2 Carpal Bone Dislocations

Carpal bone dislocations are broadly categorised based on the alignment between the distal radius articular surface and the carpal bones. According to Gilula and Minnie (1979), these can be classified as lunate dislocations, perilunate dislocations, or mid-carpal dislocations. In a lunate dislocation, the lunate is displaced relative to the distal radius, while the remaining carpal bones—centred around the capitate—maintain alignment with the radius. In contrast, during a perilunate dislocation, the lunate remains aligned with the distal radius, but the other carpal bones are displaced. When both the lunate and the capitate are displaced relative to the distal radius, the injury is referred to as a mid-carpal dislocation.

CT scanning is often used to assess any damage associated with lunate or pericarpal dislocations. CT can reveal small flake fragments indicative of avulsion injuries and aid in evaluating comminution of the articular surfaces, although MRI is superior for detecting ligamentous injuries. In cases of significant trauma, it is common practice to utilise both CT and MRI together.

Perilunate dislocations are the most common type, usually resulting from high-energy trauma that causes the wrist to hyperextend and deviate towards the ulna. These injuries form a continuum ranging from minor ligament strains to complete carpal dislocations and are often accompanied by carpal instability.

The Mayfield classification (Table 1) outlines a progressive sequence of perilunate instability, which typically results from high-energy trauma. The injury progresses from the radial side to the

Table 1 Mayfield classification of wrist injury

Stage	Description	Structures involved	CT imaging findings	Clinical relevance
I	Scapholunate dissociation	Scapholunate ligament	CT may show *widened scapholunate gap* and early *rotary subluxation* of the scaphoid	Missed injuries can lead to *scapholunate advanced collapse (SLAC wrist)* if untreated
II	Perilunate dislocation	Capitohamate and radiocapitate ligaments	Capitate is dislocated *dorsally* while the lunate remains in place. CT shows malalignment of the capitate-lunate axis	May be misdiagnosed on plain films; *CT confirms displacement*, essential before surgery
III	Triquetrum dislocation	Lunotriquetral ligament	Disruption between lunate and triquetrum; CT may show *volar shift of triquetrum* and carpal collapse	Risk of progressive carpal instability; surgical repair of the lunotriquetral ligament may be required
IV	Lunate dislocation	Lunate dislocates volarly from the lunate fossa	CT shows *lunate completely dislocated volarly*, no longer articulating with radius. May have "*spilled teacup*" appearance on sagittal reconstructions	Urgent surgical reduction needed to avoid *median nerve compression* and *avascular necrosis of the lunate*

ulnar side through predictable stages of ligament disruption, making it crucial for guiding both diagnosis and management.

CT is used for the following reasons:

- Detects occult fractures (e.g., radial styloid, scaphoid, capitate) not seen on X-rays.
- Precisely maps carpal alignment in three planes.
- Aids pre-operative planning by clearly defining the extent and complexity of dislocation or instability.
- Identifies subtle intra-articular fragments that might affect outcomes if left untreated.

3.3 Fracture Union

As early as 1987, Bush et al. demonstrated that CT imaging is far superior to plain radiographs in assessing fracture union. CT allows for precise visualisation of:

- Fracture gaps
- Bony bridging
- Callus formation

While MRI and ultrasound have been explored as alternatives, *CT remains the modality of choice* for evaluating union, malunion, and nonunion. This is particularly true in complex fractures and postoperative settings (Figs. 8 and 9).

Recent technological advances have further enhanced CT's ability to visualise both *cortical and cancellous bone*, even in the presence of *metal implants*, making it a reliable tool throughout the fracture healing process (Fig. 9).

3.4 Assessment of Metalwork

In the context of evaluating orthopaedic implants, CT is the preferred imaging modality over MRI, particularly for assessing hardware integrity and complications. This is due to the superior performance of metal artefact reduction techniques in CT, which generally provide clearer and more reliable visualisation of metal components compared to MRI.

From a radiological perspective, CT allows high-resolution assessment of both the implant and adjacent osseous structures (Fig. 10). It is particularly effective in detecting:

- Fractures or mechanical failure of the implant
- Malpositioned screws, especially those breaching the articular surface
- Impingement of hardware on adjacent bones or joint spaces

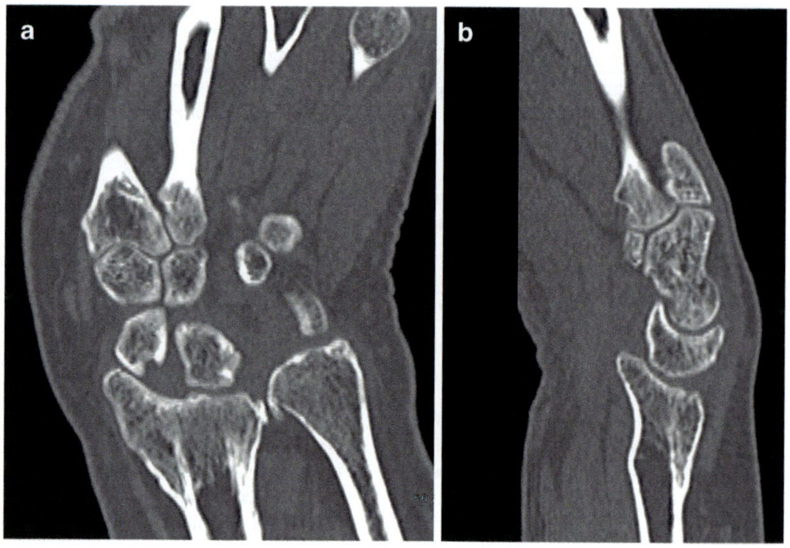

Fig. 8 (**a**) Coronal reconstruction showing healed distal radius fracture with irregularity of the distal radial articular surface. (**b**) Malunion—sagittal reconstruction showing a healed distal radius fracture that demonstrates dorsal angulation of the radial articular surface

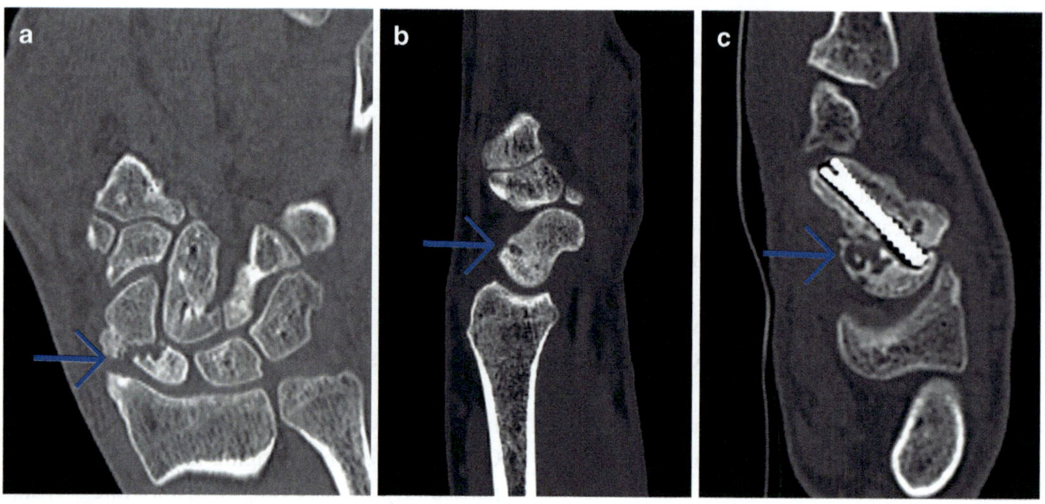

Fig. 9 (**a**) Nonunion of scaphoid with increased density of the proximal pole suggestive of avascular necrosis. (**b**) Partially united scaphoid; a gap is visible in the dorsal cortex. (**c**) Scaphoid fracture fixed with interfragmentary screw. The fracture is still nonunited, and there is cystic degeneration in the proximal fragment

- Loosening or osteolysis around the implant interface
- Early signs of peri-implant infection such as cortical erosion or soft tissue changes

While MRI can provide valuable information regarding soft tissue complications, such as fluid collections, synovitis, or bone marrow oedema, its utility near metallic implants is often limited by artefact. Techniques like MAVRIC (Multi-Acquisition Variable-Resonance Image Combination) and SEMAC (Slice Encoding for Metal Artefact Correction) have improved MRI evaluation in these settings, but they still do not match the artefact suppression and spatial resolution offered by CT (Fig. 10).

CT with metal artefact reduction algorithms (e.g., iterative reconstruction or dual-energy techniques) should be the first-line modality when evaluating the structural integrity and positioning

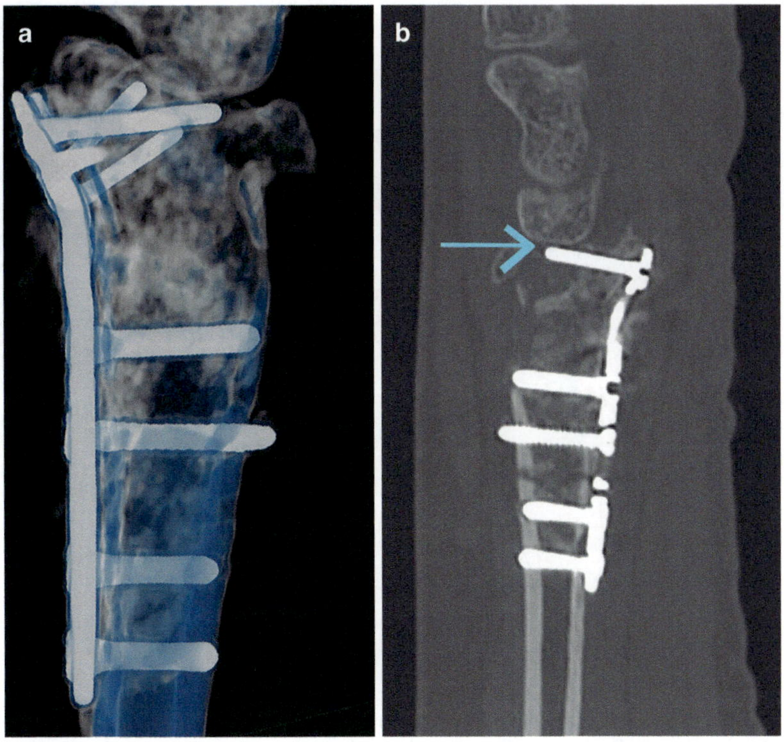

Fig. 10 (**a**) Three-dimensional volume-rendered and sagittal CT reconstructions acquired using *metal artefact reduction techniques*. Note the *minimal artefact from orthopaedic hardware*, allowing clear visualisation of surrounding structures. In image **b**, *breach of the articular surface* is evident, with the tip of the screw *abutting the lunate*

of orthopaedic hardware. MRI should be reserved for specific indications where soft tissue or marrow pathology is suspected and when advanced metal artefact reduction sequences are available.

3.5 Carpal Instability

While ligament injuries are best visualised on MRI, CT of the wrist can demonstrate bony signs of ligament injuries, and it is useful to understand them.

3.5.1 Normal Alignment

The scapholunate angle is created by a line along the volar surface of the scaphoid and the lunate axis. Typically, this angle measures between 30° and 60°. The capitolunate angle is determined between the lunate axis and the capitate axis. In a healthy wrist, these structures align closely, yielding a capitolunate angle of under 30°, ideally close to 0°, indicating neutral alignment (Fig. 11).

3.5.2 Carpal Instability Patterns

Carpal instability (CI) is a broad term that encompasses various abnormal kinematic patterns of the wrist and can be classified into four main categories: dissociative (CID), non-dissociative (CIND), combined/complex (CIC), and adaptive (CIA). These classifications are useful in understanding the mechanisms behind specific instability presentations such as DISI and VISI (Okoro et al. 2023).

3.5.2.1 Dissociative Carpal Instability (CID)

This involves a disruption among the carpal bones within the same row, typically due to intrinsic ligament injuries. It is most often seen in the proximal carpal row, with examples including scapholunate dissociation (SLD) associated with DISI and lunotriquetral dissociation (LTD) associated with VISI. Other causes include unstable scaphoid fractures and Kienböck disease. Dissociative instability in the distal carpal row is rare.

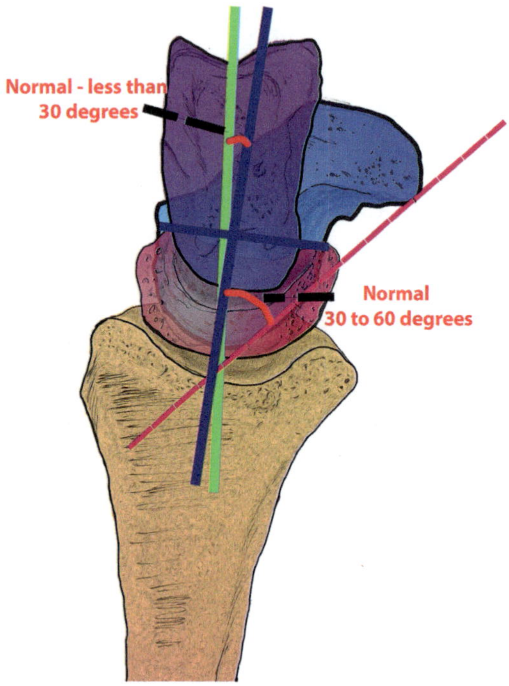

Fig. 11 Colour-coded anatomical illustration of the wrist showing the scaphoid (blue), lunate (pink), and capitate (purple). The scapholunate angle is formed between a line drawn along the volar surface of the scaphoid (pink dashed) and the axis of the lunate (vertical blue line). This angle normally ranges between 30° and 60°. The capitolunate angle is measured between the lunate axis (vertical blue line) and the capitate axis (green line). In a healthy wrist, these structures are nearly aligned, resulting in a capitolunate angle of less than 30°, typically approaching 0°, indicating neutral alignment

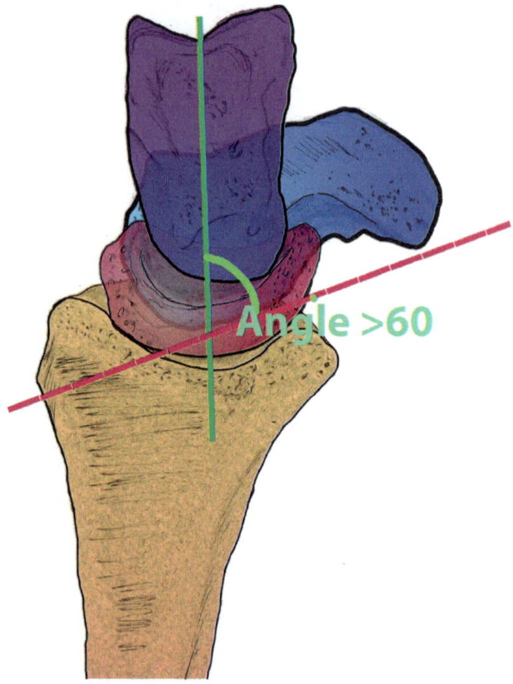

Fig. 12 Illustration demonstrating excessive volar flexion of the scaphoid relative to the lunate, resulting in an increased scapholunate angle. The red line outlines the volar border of the scaphoid, while the green line traces the longitudinal axis of the lunate

Dorsal Intercalated Segment Instability (DISI)

DISI occurs following disruption of the scapholunate ligament (SLL), resulting in abnormal alignment of the proximal carpal row. These bones, particularly the scaphoid, lunate, and triquetrum, act as a passively moved intercalated segment due to the absence of direct muscular attachments (Fig. 12).

CT Imaging Findings

- Scapholunate gap >3 mm ("Terry Thomas sign") on coronal CT
- Volar tilt of scaphoid on sagittal CT; scapholunate angle >60° (Fig. 12)
- Secondary changes: Joint space narrowing, osteophytes, and early degenerative signs in chronic DISI
- CT arthrography: Contrast leakage through the scapholunate interval confirms ligament disruption
- 3D CT: Assesses scaphoid rotation and malalignment
- Dynamic CT: Demonstrates abnormal scaphoid-lunate motion during movement. The scaphoid and lunate fail to move synchronously. The scaphoid flexes excessively during wrist flexion-extension or radial-ulnar deviation. The lunate remains in extension or moves out of phase with the scaphoid.

Scapholunate Advanced Collapse (SLAC) Wrist

This outlines the distinct pattern of degenerative arthritis seen in chronic dissociation between the scaphoid and lunate. Consequently, the capitate dorsiflexes and moves proximally, resulting in DISI alignment and ultimately causing progressive arthritis. The Watson clas-

Table 2 Watson classification of wrist arthropathy

Stage	Description	Arthritic involvement
Stage I	Isolated arthritis between the radial styloid and scaphoid	Radioscaphoid joint (radial styloid only)
Stage II	Arthritis extends across the entire radioscaphoid joint	Full radioscaphoid joint
Stage III	Involvement of the midcarpal joint	Radioscaphoid + capitolunate joint
Stage IV	Pan-carpal arthritis, including the radiolunate joint	Entire carpus, including radiolunate articulation

sification (Table 2) is utilised to stage the advancement of wrist arthritis resulting from chronic scapholunate instability.

Scaphoid Nonunion Advanced Collapse (SNAC) Wrist

Follows scaphoid non-union, leading to similar mechanics and degeneration as SLAC wrist. Stages of disease in SNAC wrist are as follows:

- Stage I: Degeneration between scaphoid and radial styloid
- Stage II: Widespread radiocarpal joint involvement
- Stage III: Scaphocapitate and/or capitolunate arthritis

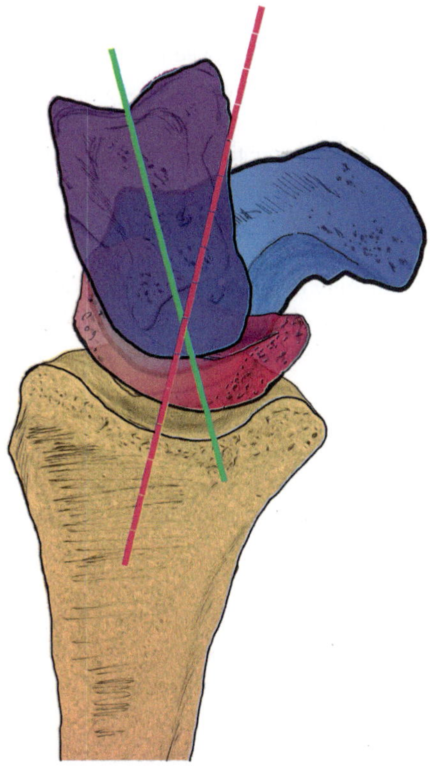

Fig. 13 Illustration showing excessive volar flexion of the lunate (pink) relative to the capitate (purple), resulting in an increased capitolunate angle exceeding 30°. A green line marks the axis of the capitate, while a red line highlights the longitudinal axis of the lunate. Other carpal bones shown include the scaphoid (blue)

Volar Intercalated Segment Instability (VISI)

VISI is associated with lunotriquetral ligament disruption, leading to a volar tilt of the lunate and an increased capitolunate angle exceeding 30° (Fig. 13). Often related to ulnar-sided trauma or ligamentous laxity, patients may experience pain, instability, and weakness.

CT Imaging Findings

- Volar lunate angulation seen on sagittal images
- Increased capitolunate angle exceeding 30°
- Subtle lunotriquetral diastasis or overlap on coronal images
- Detection of associated injuries like from ears or ulnar-sided fractures
- CT arthrography shows contrast extravasation through lunotriquetral interval
- Dynamic CT captures abnormal motion of the lunate during ulnar deviation. The lunate does not function as a central stabiliser, as it should. The proximal carpal row loses its coordinated "row-like" movement. The lunate drops into flexion throughout the motion cycle, particularly during wrist extension. One may observe asynchronous or paradoxical motion between the lunate and triquetrum.

CT assists in evaluating instability severity, guiding treatment from splinting to surgical fusion. CT arthrography improves diagnostic accuracy when MRI is contraindicated.

Lunotriquetral Advanced Collapse (LTAC)

LTAC is a rare degenerative condition of the wrist caused by chronic instability or injury to the lunotriquetral (LT) ligament. This results in abnormal movement between the lunate and triquetrum, leading to progressive cartilage loss, joint space narrowing, and osteoarthritic changes in the LT joint. Over time, the degenerative process may extend to the midcarpal and radiocarpal joints, causing pain, stiffness, and reduced wrist function.

CT imaging is particularly useful for identifying LT joint space narrowing, subchondral sclerosis, and osteophytes, while also assessing carpal alignment and guiding surgical interventions such as LT fusion or proximal row carpectomy.

CT arthrography also assists in evaluating ligamentous integrity in patients unsuitable for MRI.

3.5.2.2 Non-dissociative Carpal Instability (CIND)

This refers to abnormal movement between the proximal and distal carpal rows, or between the radius and the proximal carpal row, and is usually a result of extrinsic ligament failure. These often present as midcarpal or radiocarpal instability patterns.

Midcarpal Instability (MCI)

MCI involves abnormal kinematics between the proximal and distal carpal rows. It may be intrinsic (ligamentous laxity) or extrinsic (e.g., secondary to distal radius malunion). Clinically, patients may experience a "catch-up clunk" with ulnar deviation.

CT Imaging Findings

- Abnormal alignment of the capitate or hamate with the proximal row
- Extrinsic causes: Distal radius malunion with altered radial inclination or dorsal angulation
- 3D CT reveals subtle bony abnormalities and malalignments
- Midcarpal subluxation is visible on dynamic or 4D CT
- CT arthrography may show capsular or ligamentous laxity

3.5.2.3 Combined or Complex Carpal Instability (CIC)

This includes elements of both CID and CIND. It reflects disruption within a carpal row as well as between rows. Examples include perilunate dislocations, fracture-dislocations, isolated carpal bone dislocations, and axial carpal dislocations.

3.5.2.4 Adaptive Carpal Instability (CIA)

This occurs secondary to conditions external to the carpus itself. These changes alter carpal mechanics without direct ligamentous or bony injury. Examples include Madelung deformity and malunited distal radius fractures, where the carpus adapts to altered loading or biomechanics.

While MRI offers superior soft tissue contrast for ligament evaluation, CT remains crucial for assessing associated osseous abnormalities, joint alignment, and carpal bone orientation. CT arthrography (described in Sect. 3.5.2) can be used for evaluating.

3.5.3 CT Arthrography

The wrist comprises three functional compartments: the DRUJ, radiocarpal joint, and midcarpal joint. The proximal carpal row, stabilised by the scapholunate (SL) and lunotriquetral (LT) ligaments, is critical for coordinated motion (Berger 1996). The SL and LT ligaments form a horseshoe configuration, with their palmar and dorsal portions being biomechanically significant (Boabighi et al. 1993). The Triangular Fibrocartilage Complex (TFCC) stabilises the DRUJ, separating it from the radiocarpal joint.

3.5.3.1 Technique

Under fluoroscopic guidance, a 24-gauge needle is inserted into the dorsal wrist, and 5 mL of iodinated contrast (<250 mg iodine/mL) is injected to minimise beam-hardening artefacts. CT images are acquired immediately to prevent contrast dilution (Fig. 14).

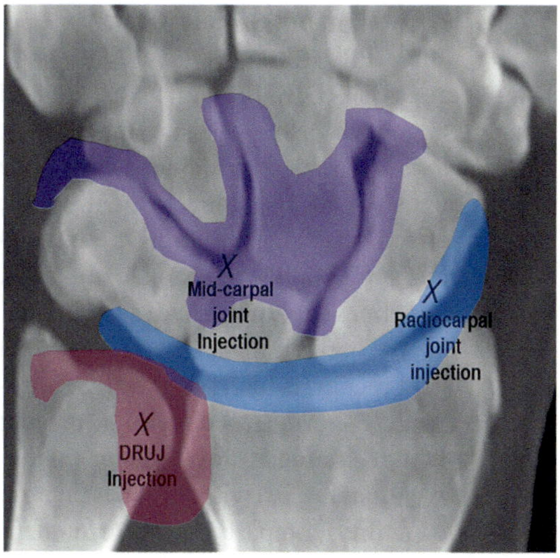

Fig. 14 Image representing the various joint capsules and sites for injection. *Purple*: mid carpal joint with injection site between the carpals *Blue*: Radiocarpal joint with preferred injection site being over the proximal articular surface of scaphoid. *Pink*: Distal radio-ulnar joint with preferred injection site over the distal ulna

3.5.3.2 Ligament Tears

CT arthrography identifies tears when contrast passes through the ligament, distinguishing full-thickness (communicating) from partial-thickness (non-communicating) tears. Studies report CT arthrography's sensitivity and specificity for SL ligament tears at up to 100%, and for LT tears, 85% sensitivity and 100% specificity (Theumann et al. 2001; Schmid et al. 2005). Its advantages include a small field of view, excellent spatial resolution, and rapid scan times that minimise motion artefacts.

3.6 Infection

Computed tomography (CT) plays a vital role in evaluating musculoskeletal infections, especially when radiographic findings are inconclusive or when MRI is contraindicated or unavailable. Although MRI remains the modality of choice for assessing most aspects of infection due to its superior soft tissue contrast and sensitivity to bone marrow changes, CT provides valuable complementary information, particularly regarding bony involvement.

Advantages of CT in infection include:

- High spatial resolution for detecting early cortical erosion, sequestrum, and cloaca formation
- Clear delineation of periosteal reaction and involucrum in chronic osteomyelitis
- Better evaluation of gas within soft tissues, which may indicate gas-forming organisms or necrotising fasciitis
- Assessment of bone destruction and deformity associated with chronic infection
- Detection of calcifications or foreign bodies that may serve as a nidus for infection

In acute settings, CT is advantageous when subtle cortical breaches are suspected but not visible on plain radiographs. However, MRI remains superior for detecting bone marrow oedema, subperiosteal abscesses, joint effusions, synovial thickening, and cartilage loss in septic arthritis. MRI also reveals soft tissue cellulitis, fasciitis, and myositis associated with the spread of infection. When septic arthritis is strongly suspected and clinical signs are evident, MRI would be the investigation of choice.

CT-guided aspiration or *biopsy* can provide a valuable interventional role, especially when sampling is needed from difficult-to-access areas such as the carpus.

In chronic osteomyelitis, CT can identify complex sequestra, fistulous tracts, and bone remodelling, aiding in preoperative planning and surgical debridement.

3.7 Arthropathies

3.7.1 Initial Diagnosis

Accurate early diagnosis is critical for initiating therapy to prevent joint damage. In practice, CT is not a first-line diagnostic tool for inflammatory arthritis, but it can provide complementary information in specific scenarios:

3.7.1.1 Rheumatoid Arthritis (RA)

The hallmark of RA is bone erosions in the wrists, MCP, and PIP joints. The high resolution of CT makes it extremely sensitive for detecting bone erosions, often identifying cortical breaks that are not yet visible on X-ray (Perry et al. 2005). Studies using CT as a reference standard have shown that MRI and US, while more sensitive than radiographs, still miss some small erosions that CT can detect. Multiplanar CT is considered *perhaps the most sensitive modality* for bone erosion detection due to its 3D visualisation of bone structure. However, guidelines do not generally recommend routine CT for initial RA diagnosis. Notably, CT may be considered if radiographs are normal but there is a high suspicion of erosive disease, *and* MRI/US cannot be performed. Otherwise, *CT is not routinely used* for diagnosing rheumatoid arthritis.

3.7.1.2 Psoriatic Arthritis (PsA)

PsA in the hands can lead to a combination of erosive damage and bone proliferation (e.g., periostitis, ankylosis) in the distal interphalangeal (DIP) joints, proximal interphalangeal (PIP) joints, and wrists. Conventional X-rays readily display classic PsA changes, such as "pencil-in-cup" erosions and joint fusion. CT can delineate these structural changes in fine detail, including the size of erosions and new bone formation. For instance, CT can better visualise periosteal new bone (which is more common in PsA) and complex erosions or ankyloses in the carpus. However, similar to RA, *CT is not generally indicated* as a first-line test for PsA. Ultrasound and MRI are more effective for detecting enthesitis and synovitis in early PsA, which supports an early diagnosis of a seronegative spondyloarthritis.

3.7.1.3 Juvenile Idiopathic Arthritis (JIA)

In paediatric patients, limiting radiation is paramount, so *CT is rarely used for JIA diagnosis*. The EULAR–PReS consensus "points to consider" on imaging in JIA emphasises radiography, US, and MRI. Paediatric guidelines recommend avoiding CT in favour of MRI/US due to safety concerns, unless detailed bone anatomy from CT is absolutely required for management.

3.7.1.4 Crystal Arthropathies (Gout and CPPD)

Dual-energy CT (DECT) has revolutionised imaging in gout and other crystal arthropathies. DECT can directly identify monosodium urate crystal deposits and colour-code them on the post-processed images, facilitating a noninvasive diagnosis of gout (Glazebrook et al. 2011). Current guidelines incorporate advanced imaging for diagnosing crystal arthritis. The 2018 EULAR gout recommendations state that ultrasound or DECT can be used to confirm gout when crystal aspiration is not feasible. In contrast, conventional CT (without dual-energy) has limited utility compared to these modalities. DECT possesses high specificity (~90–93%) for urate crystals and good sensitivity (~81–88%) in established gout. It may miss some cases in very early disease (sensitivity drops to ~36–80% in acute gout of <6 weeks), but a positive DECT (urate signal in tophi or cartilage) is virtually diagnostic of gout. In the hands and wrists, DECT can reveal urate deposits at atypical sites (e.g., RC joint, TFCC cartilage) that might be overlooked on radiographs. For CPPD (pseudogout), CT can show calcifications in cartilage and tendons. DECT is useful for distinguishing between urate and calcium. It will not label CPPD calcifications as urate (no coloured images), helping to differentiate gout from CPPD in uncertain situations.

3.7.1.5 Osteoarthritis (OA)

OA most commonly affects the first carpometacarpal (CMC) joint in the hand, followed by the distal interphalangeal joints. CMC joint OA can be particularly debilitating, especially among postmenopausal women, and is the most frequent site for hand surgery due to arthritis. While CT is rarely used as a first-line investigation, akin to RA and PsA, it can assist in detecting early changes such as loss of joint space, subchondral sclerosis, small osteophytes, and small subchondral cysts. Additionally, CT can help distinguish CMC joint OA from RA and PsA because of the absence of erosions and periostitis.

3.7.2 Monitoring Disease Progression

Inflammatory arthropathies require continuous monitoring of joint damage and disease activity to guide therapeutic decisions. Radiographs have traditionally been employed to assess structural progression, such as erosion scores and joint space narrowing in RA and PsA, due to their affordability and standardisation (e.g., Genant or Van der Heijde modified Sharp scoring in RA). MRI and US are effective in detecting active inflammation and are routinely employed to monitor subclinical disease activity or remission. CT may be considered in certain scenarios, as mentioned below.

3.7.2.1 Bone Erosion Progression

CT can detect structural progression such as new erosions, osteophytes, or ankylosis in PsA more accurately and earlier than X-ray; however, its use is typically reserved for research settings or specific clinical queries due to practical considerations. Recent studies have employed *ultra-low-dose* CT scans of the hand to track erosion changes over time, which correlate well with MRI scores. Nevertheless, the *routine use of CT for serial monitoring is not yet standard practice*.

3.7.2.2 Disease Activity and Inflammation

Traditional CT has a limited ability to monitor active inflammation. Contrast-enhanced CT with subtraction and DECT iodine mapping can visualise inflamed synovium and tendon sheaths by highlighting areas of hyperaemia. A recent prospective study comparing DECT with iodine contrast maps to MRI in patients with hand arthritis found that enhanced CT techniques could detect synovitis nearly as well as MRI. At the patient level, DECT iodine maps achieved approximately 93–100% sensitivity for synovitis in comparison to MRI. Although promising, these advanced CT methods for inflammation are still undergoing validation.

3.7.2.3 Paediatric Monitoring

In JIA, the avoidance of radiation generally means that *CT is not used for serial monitoring*.

3.7.3 Treatment Planning and Management

Though not routinely used for day-to-day disease activity assessment, CT can be valuable in *planning interventions* and tailoring management in several ways:

3.7.3.1 Surgical Planning

CT provides exquisite 3D detail of bone anatomy, which is helpful for orthopaedic planning. In RA patients with severe wrist destruction, for instance, CT can delineate the extent of carpal collapse, erosions, and subluxations to guide surgeons considering a wrist fusion or arthroplasty. In the small finger joints, CT can help assess fragment positions for possible arthrodesis or implant arthroplasty. In JIA, if surgery is needed (which is less common in the biologic era but still done for severe contractures or limb length discrepancies), CT may be employed to map bony deformities or to create custom prostheses. Similarly, in PsA, tendon ruptures or fixed deformities in the hand might be better evaluated in 3D by CT before reconstructive surgery. Overall, whenever high-precision knowledge of bone geometry is needed to guide an orthopaedic procedure, CT is often the imaging of choice. *In osteoarthritis* CT imaging provides valuable detail for both surgical planning and postoperative follow-up.

3.7.3.2 Guiding Injections or Aspirations

Generally, ultrasound is used to guide injections in the wrist and hand joints due to its convenience. CT guidance is rarely necessary for superficial joints. For wrists, CT guidance is infrequently used, except perhaps in unusual scenarios, such as guiding a needle into a small erosional cavity or to aspirate a tophus. Thus, this represents a minor role in peripheral arthritis.

3.7.3.3 Assessing Treatment Efficacy

In gout management, DECT is increasingly utilised to *quantify tophus burden* and monitor response to urate-lowering therapy. For example, serial DECT scans can measure the volume of urate deposits and confirm that tophi are dissolving with treatment. This can guide the duration of therapy or identify patients who are not responding.

3.7.3.4 Patient Education

Finally, *patient education* can sometimes be enhanced with the use of CT images. Seeing a 3D rendering of eroded joints (or gout crystals in vivid colour on DECT) can help patients understand the damage caused by their disease and the importance of adhering to therapy. While not a formal aspect of treatment planning, this use of imaging can support shared decision-making.

3.8 Osteonecrosis

Osteonecrosis of the carpal bones is a condition in which bone tissue dies due to impaired blood supply, leading to structural collapse and potential long-term dysfunction of the wrist. The carpal bones are particularly vulnerable because of their limited vascular supply and the mechanical stresses they endure. The lunate is most commonly affected osteonecrosis can also involve the scaphoid and capitate, among others. These cases often arise following trauma, vascular compromise, or underlying systemic conditions, and may result in progressive degeneration if not promptly addressed.

3.8.1 Kienböck's Disease (Lunate Osteonecrosis)

Kienböck's disease involves avascular necrosis of the lunate, typically affecting young adults aged 20–40 years, with a male predominance. The exact aetiology remains multifactorial, primarily linked to compromised vascular supply and mechanical factors. The blood supply to the lunate often depends on a single nutrient artery in 20% of individuals, rendering it vulnerable to ischaemia. Mechanical contributors include negative ulnar variance, which increases shear stress on the lunate, and repetitive microtrauma from activities such as manual labour or sports. Additional risk factors encompass anatomical variations (e.g., a single vascular pedicle), systemic conditions (e.g., sickle cell disease, corticosteroid use), and trauma that disrupts blood flow.

Patients typically present with progressive wrist pain, stiffness, and swelling, which worsen with activity. Grip strength decreases, and tenderness over the lunate (dorsal midline) is common. In advanced stages, patients may experience limited wrist motion, a palpable clunk, and associated signs. In advanced cases, carpal collapse and secondary osteoarthritis may develop, leading to significant functional impairment.

3.8.1.1 Lichtman Classification

The Lichtman classification stages Kienböck's disease according to imaging findings, which guide treatment:

- *Stage I*: Normal radiographs but MRI shows lunate oedema; no sclerosis or collapse.
- *Stage II*: Lunate sclerosis on radiographs/CT; no collapse; early bone changes.
- *Stage IIIA*: Lunate collapse without carpal collapse; sclerosis and fragmentation.
- *Stage IIIB*: Lunate collapse with carpal collapse (e.g., fixed scaphoid rotation, proximal capitate migration).
- *Stage IV*: Advanced lunate collapse with secondary radiocarpal or midcarpal osteoarthritis.

CT Imaging Findings

CT plays a critical role in assessing Kienböck's disease, particularly for evaluating bony architecture and staging disease progression:

- *Early Stages (I–II)*: CT may appear normal or show subtle lunate sclerosis (increased density compared to adjacent bones). Coronal reconstructions can quantify negative ulnar variance, a key risk factor.
- *Intermediate Stages (IIIA–IIIB)*: CT reveals lunate collapse, characterised by fragmentation, irregular contours, and decreased lunate height. Sagittal views assess carpal alignment, detecting scaphoid rotation or capitate migration.
- *Advanced Stages (IV)*: CT demonstrates severe lunate collapse, carpal height loss, and secondary degenerative changes (e.g., joint space narrowing, osteophytes) in the radiocarpal or midcarpal joints.
- *Dynamic CT*: In select cases, dynamic or 4D CT can evaluate carpal kinematics, identifying instability patterns like VISI or DISI associated with lunate collapse.

CT's high resolution complements MRI, which is superior for the early detection of marrow oedema. However, CT excels in assessing bony collapse and carpal alignment, both of which are critical for surgical planning.

3.8.2 Scaphoid (Preiser's Disease)

Preiser's disease is characterised by idiopathic avascular necrosis of the scaphoid, frequently affecting the proximal pole due to its retrograde blood supply, with dorsal vessels supplying 70–80% of the bone from distal to proximal. This condition may develop after trauma, such as a non-union of a scaphoid fracture, or arise idiopathically. Contributing risk factors include the use of corticosteroids, systemic lupus erythematosus, and chemotherapy, all of which can impact blood flow.

Patients present with radial-sided wrist pain, swelling, and diminished grip strength. Symptoms aggravate with wrist extension or radial deviation. In chronic cases, scaphoid collapse may result in radiocarpal arthritis, which resembles scapholunate advanced collapse (SLAC).

CT Imaging Findings

- *Early Stage*: CT may show proximal pole sclerosis or subtle density changes compared to the distal pole.
- *Progressive Stage*: Fragmentation and collapse of the proximal pole, exhibiting irregular contours and reduced bone height.
- *Late Stage*: Secondary degenerative changes in the radiocarpal joint, including joint space narrowing and osteophytes. Coronal CT may reveal associated scapholunate dissociation.

3.8.3 Capitate Osteonecrosis

Capitate osteonecrosis is rare, often linked to high-energy trauma disrupting its intraosseous blood supply, which enters primarily through the distal aspect and may be limited in 30% of individuals. Repetitive microtrauma (e.g., in golfers or gymnasts) or systemic conditions like vasculitis can also contribute.

Patients report central wrist pain, exacerbated by gripping or loading activities, with reduced range of motion. Late stages may involve midcarpal instability or collapse, leading to degenerative changes.

CT Imaging Findings

- *Early Stage*: Increased capitate density.
- *Progressive Stage*: Capitate collapse with fragmentation, often involving the proximal articular surface.
- *Late Stage*: Midcarpal joint degeneration, with subchondral cysts and osteophytes. Dynamic CT may reveal abnormal capitate motion, which contributes to instability.

3.8.4 Other Carpal Bones

Osteonecrosis of the triquetrum, pisiform, trapezium, trapezoid, or hamate is exceedingly rare, typically following direct trauma or systemic conditions affecting vascularity (e.g., sickle cell disease). CT findings mirror those of other carpal bones, with sclerosis, fragmentation, and eventual collapse, often accompanied by secondary arthritis in adjacent joints. Management depends on the extent of necrosis and collapse, ranging from conservative measures to surgical intervention, with CT providing critical anatomical detail for planning.

3.9 Tumour Imaging

CT plays a complementary role to MRI—the primary imaging modality for staging bone tumours—in the evaluation of osseous lesions. When a bone tumour is suspected, imaging usually begins with plain radiographs, followed by MRI to evaluate intraosseous and soft tissue involvement. However, CT is particularly valuable for:

- Clarifying patterns of bone destruction
- Identifying periosteal reactions
- Visualising matrix mineralisation

Osteoid osteoma is a benign but painful bone tumour that represents around 10% of benign osseous lesions and most frequently occurs in the lower limbs. In the hand, it accounts for approxi-

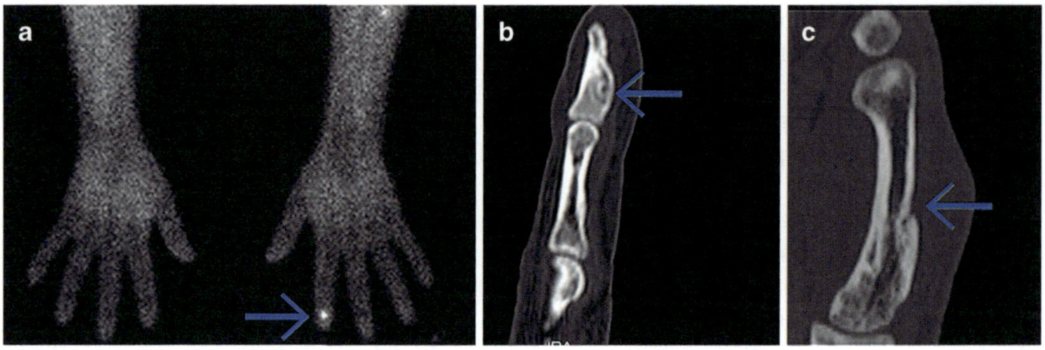

Fig. 15 (**a**) Bone scintigraphy demonstrates a "hot spot" which, upon subsequent CT (**b**), was identified as an osteoid osteoma with smooth, round margins and a central nidus. In contrast, (**c**) shows a cortical breach and margin irregularity, consistent with a more aggressive lesion; in this case, osteomyelitis

mately 8% of cases, primarily affecting the phalanges and carpal bones (Ambrosia et al. 1987).

CT is highly effective in diagnosing osteoid osteoma (Allieu and Lussiez 1988; Chai et al. 2010) due to its ability to clearly depict the nidus, which typically appears as:

- A well-circumscribed, round or oval lucent lesion
- Often containing a central calcified focus representing mineralised osteoid

This appearance allows CT to differentiate osteoid osteoma from other lesions such as intracortical abscess or inflammatory arthritis (Fig. 15).

4 Modern Advances

Traditionally, CT scanning was limited by high radiation doses, low temporal resolution, and metal artefacts. Furthermore, CT's static nature meant it could not capture dynamic joint movements—a disadvantage when evaluating complex structures like the wrist. Modern CT technologies are addressing past limitations and opening new frontiers in imaging:

4.1 Dual-Energy CT (DECT)

DECT is now routinely employed for gout, as it can accurately identify urate crystals by colouring them on CT images. Additionally, it assists in quantifying crystal burden through software that calculates the volume of urate in a tophus, facilitating longitudinal monitoring. Its use has been detailed in Sect. 3.7.1.4.

Beyond gout, DECT is being explored in rheumatoid arthritis and psoriatic arthritis. Studies have demonstrated that iodine maps on DECT can detect synovitis with comparable sensitivity to MRI (Ulas et al. 2022).

DECT can also differentiate urate from calcium in the same scan, which is beneficial for patients who may have both gout and CPPD or have osteophytes rather than tophi. Overall, DECT exemplifies CT's "theranostic" evolution in arthritis—from pure morphology to identifying the chemical composition of deposits and inflammation.

Another application involves generating virtual non-calcium images. Preliminary research indicates that DECT can detect bone marrow oedema by differentiating the calcium signal from water, potentially revealing bone changes similar to those seen on MRI. This capability can enhance the sensitivity in diagnosing fractures (Müller et al. 2020; Xie et al. 2020).

4.2 Low-Dose and Ultra-Low-Dose CT

Reducing radiation dose has been a primary technical focus of numerous research studies involving CT scans. Modern scanners with enhanced detectors and iterative reconstruction algorithms can obtain diagnostic hand and wrist CT images at a fraction of the previous doses (Alagic et al. 2019).

Researchers have reported a contrast-enhanced ultra-low-dose CT (ULD-CT) protocol for RA hands with a dose of less than 0.01 mSv, which is ten times less than a chest radiograph and comparable to an X-ray of the hands and feet. Despite the minuscule dose, this ULD-CT successfully depicted synovitis after contrast and correlated strongly with MRI scores ($r = 0.94$). The ULD-CT reliably detected severe synovitis and tenosynovitis, even though it exhibited limited sensitivity for mild inflammation (Diekhoff et al. 2019).

Additionally, specialised extremity cone-beam CT scanners are emerging, which can perform high-resolution scans of hands with a much lower dose than conventional CT. Low-dose protocols make CT far more feasible for routine monitoring of structural damage, potentially replacing serial radiographs in the future for more precise tracking. Guidelines have begun to acknowledge that low-dose CT could replace radiography in many circumstances and might supplement MRI for arthritis imaging. While that is forward-looking, it underlines the progress in dose reduction.

4.3 High-Resolution Peripheral Quantitative Computed Tomography (HR-pQCT)

Although this technique has been in existence for over two decades, it remains primarily a research method due to challenges such as availability, regulatory approvals, and the need for demonstrated cost-effectiveness (Boyd 2024). Essentially, it serves as a micro-CT for patients, utilised in certain centres to examine bone microarchitecture. It can visualise changes in trabecular and cortical bone at the micro level (voxel size ~100 microns) in the metacarpals and wrists. Studies have employed HR-pQCT to detect very early, minute erosions and to quantify changes in bone density around joints in RA. Additionally, it can assess bone strength through finite element analysis, potentially predicting fracture risk. While not routinely used in clinical practice, findings from HR-pQCT are enhancing our understanding of arthritis bone pathology and may ultimately translate into improved care, possibly through the implementation of smaller dedicated scanners in clinics.

4.4 4D CT and Motion Analysis

The advent of fast multislice CT scanners enables imaging of the entire wrist joint throughout its full range of motion (Leng et al. 2011). 4D CT can capture the dynamic movement of the carpal bones, which is beneficial for detecting ligament injuries or instability that static images may overlook. This is particularly useful in cases of carpal instability syndromes, as detailed in Sect. 3.5.2. In cases of inflammatory arthritis, chronic damage can lead to altered biomechanics (e.g., caput ulnae syndrome in RA with distal ulna subluxation). 4D CT may assist in assessing these abnormal kinematics and guiding surgical repairs. Although this represents a niche application, it demonstrates how CT can provide unique information.

4.5 Photon-Counting CT

A cutting-edge CT technology that employs photon-counting detectors can enhance image resolution and contrast at lower doses. Photon-counting CT can also inherently perform spectral imaging, such as dual-energy, in a single scan. For arthritis, this could result in ultra-clear images of both bone and soft tissue at a low dose, potentially enabling better visualisation of cartilage or inflammation. Although it remains in the early stages clinically, experts are optimistic that photon-counting CT will further enhance CT's role in musculoskeletal imaging.

These capabilities make modern CT a powerful, versatile tool in wrist imaging, offering detail comparable to MRI in some cases, with faster acquisition and broader availability.

5 Conclusion

Over the past five decades, CT has transformed from a groundbreaking tool into a fundamental element of musculoskeletal imaging. With ongoing advancements in detector design, dose reduction, and image reconstruction, CT now provides high-resolution, low-dose imaging with an expanding range of clinical applications.

In the wrist, CT is essential not only for detailed assessment of fractures and bony alignment but also for evaluating arthropathies, ligament injuries, and complex carpal instabilities. Innovations such as spectral imaging, dynamic 4D acquisitions, and dual-energy analysis are pushing the boundaries of diagnostic accuracy.

As technology evolves, CT is poised to further expand its role across musculoskeletal imaging, supplementing and, in some scenarios, rivalling the diagnostic utility of both MRI and conventional radiography.

Acknowledgements Thanks to Mrs. Teena Ninan for the illustrations.

References

Alagic Z et al (2019) Ultra-low-dose CT for extremities in an acute setting: initial experience with 203 subjects. Skeletal Radiol 49(4):531–539

Allieu Y, Lussiez B (1988) Osteoid osteoma of the hand: apropos of 46 cases. Ann Hand Surg 7:298–304

Ambrosia JM et al (1987) Osteoid osteoma of the hand and wrist. J Hand Surg [Am] 12:794–800

Amin M et al (2022) Role of multidetector computed tomography (MDCT) with MPR in assessment of fracture patterns around the wrist joint. Minia J Med Res 31(4):101–109

Bäcker H et al (2020) Systematic review of diagnosis of clinically suspected scaphoid fractures. J Wrist Surg 9(1):81–89

Balcı A et al (2014) Wrist fractures: sensitivity of radiography, prevalence, and patterns in MDCT. Emerg Radiol 22(3):251–256

Berger RA (1996) The gross and histologic anatomy of the scapholunate interosseous ligament. J Hand Surg 21(2):170–178

Boabighi A et al (1993) The distal ligamentous complex of the scaphoid and the scapho-lunate ligament: an anatomic, histological and biomechanical study. J Hand Surg 18(1):65–69

Boyd SK (2024) Two decades of high-resolution peripheral quantitative computed tomography: present and future clinical perspectives. Semin Musculoskelet Radiol 28(5):560–575. Thieme Medical Publishers, Inc

Bush CH et al (1987) High-resolution CT of the wrist: initial experience with scaphoid disorders and surgical fusions. Am J Roentgenol 149(4):757–760

Chai JW et al (2010) Radiologic diagnosis of osteoid osteoma: from simple to challenging findings. Radiographics 30:737

Chunara MH et al (2019) Current imaging practice for suspected scaphoid fracture in patients with normal initial radiographs: UK-wide national audit. Clin Radiol 74:450–455

Daniels AM et al (2020) The interobserver reliability of the diagnosis and classification of scaphoid fractures using high-resolution peripheral quantitative CT. Bone Joint J 102-B:478–484

Dean B (2021) The management of suspected scaphoid fractures in the UK: a national cross-sectional study. Bone Joint Open 2(11):997–1003

Diekhoff T et al (2019) Ultra-low-dose CT detects synovitis in patients with suspected rheumatoid arthritis. Ann Rheum Dis 78(1):31–35

Dreckmann S et al (2019) Utility of specialized imaging for diagnosis of chronic wrist pain. J Wrist Surg 8(6):497–502

Gäbler C et al (2001) Diagnosis of occult scaphoid fractures and other wrist injuries: are repeated clinical examinations and plain radiographs still state of the art? Langenbeck's Arch Surg 386:150–154

Gilula LA, Minnie A (1979) Review carpal injuries: analytic approach and case exercises. Am J Roentgenol 133:503–517

Glazebrook KN et al (2011) Identification of intraarticular and periarticular uric acid crystals with dual-energy CT: initial evaluation. Radiology 261(2):516–524

Leng S et al (2011) Dynamic CT technique for assessment of wrist joint instabilities. Med Phys 38(S1):S50

Müller FC et al (2020) Dual-energy CT for suspected radiographically negative wrist fractures: a prospective diagnostic test accuracy study. Radiology 296:596–602

Okoro CK et al (2023) Imaging diagnosis and management of carpal trauma and instability—an illustrated guide. Life 13(7):1426

Perry D et al (2005) Detection of erosions in the rheumatoid hand: a comparative study of multidetector computerized tomography versus magnetic resonance scanning. J Rheumatol 32(2):256–267

Refaat M et al (2020) Role of multi-detector CT in evaluation of carpal bone fracture in wrist injuries. Benha Med J 37 (special issue (Radiology)): 54–62

Sahu A et al (2021) Prospective comparison of magnetic resonance imaging and computed tomography in diagnosing occult scaphoid fractures. Acta Radiol 64(1):201–207

Schmid MR et al (2005) Interosseous ligament tears of the wrist: comparison of multi-detector row CT arthrography and MR imaging. Radiology 237(3):1008–1013

Slaar A et al (2012) The role of plain radiography in paediatric wrist trauma. Insights Imaging 3(5):513–517

Smith JE et al (2016) The management of suspected scaphoid fractures in English hospitals. Eur J Emerg Med 23:190–193

Theumann N et al (2001) Wrist ligament injuries: value of post-arthrography computed tomography. Skeletal Radiol 30(2):88–93

Ulas ST et al (2022) Contrast-enhanced CT techniques and MRI perform equally well in arthritis imaging of the hand: a prospective diagnostic accuracy study. Eur Radiol 32(9):6376–6383

Welling RD et al (2008) MDCT and radiography of wrist fractures: radiographic sensitivity and fracture patterns. Am J Roentgenol 190(1):10–16

Wijetunga A et al (2018) The utility of cross-sectional imaging in the management of suspected scaphoid fractures. J Med Radiat Sci 66(1):30–37

Xie C et al (2020) Dual-energy CT in the diagnosis of occult acute scaphoid injury: a direct comparison with MRI. Eur Radiol 31(6):3610–3615

MR Imaging of the Hand and Wrist: Techniques and Applications

Michail E. Klontzas, Evangelia E. Vassalou, Matthaios Triantafyllou, and Apostolos H. Karantanas

Contents

M. E. Klontzas · M. Triantafyllou · A. H. Karantanas (✉)
Department of Medical Imaging, Heraklion University Hospital, Heraklion, Greece

Department of Radiology, School of Medicine, University of Crete, Heraklion, Greece

E. E. Vassalou
Department of Medical Imaging, Heraklion University Hospital, Heraklion, Greece

Abstract

Magnetic resonance imaging (MRI) has been established as an important diagnostic tool for hand and wrist disorders. Its major advantages include high spatial and contrast resolution, multiplanar imaging, and lack of ionizing radiation. MRI combined with arthrography provides additional information on intra-articular disorders such as ligamentous tears, articular cartilage degradation, and triangular fibrocartilage complex tears. In acute trauma, MRI has a complementary role to plain radiographs and computed tomography, whereas regarding bone marrow disorders, it is the method of choice. A proper technique on the patient's positioning, coil selection, and sequence application is required to extract all the capabilities of MRI. Each MRI examination should be tailored to the specific clinical question. The increased prominence of artifacts in high-field scanner images necessitates their recognition and technical alleviation to avoid diagnostic errors.

1 Introduction

The wrist and hand are intricate structures with a high degree of mobility and function, yet they are prone to various injuries and degenerative disorders. For accurate assessment and diagnosis of pathologies in this region, MR imaging (MRI)

Med Radiol Diagn Imaging (2025)
https://doi.org/10.1007/174_2025_599,
Published Online: 03 September 2025

and MR arthrography (MRa) are invaluable imaging techniques. These techniques provide exceptional soft tissue contrast, allowing for detailed evaluation of the joints, ligaments, tendons, cartilage, and bones of the wrist and hand. Proper technique is crucial in obtaining high-quality images that reflect the true anatomy and pathology of these regions. A thorough understanding of the normal anatomy of the wrist and hand is essential for interpreting MRI findings accurately. Knowledge of normal variants that can mimic pathology will also be discussed.

Despite the technical advancements of the MR scanners, there are potential pitfalls that may complicate interpretation. By the end of this chapter, readers will gain a comprehensive understanding of the techniques, normal anatomy, variants, and potential pitfalls in MRI and MRa of the wrist and hand, ensuring a more effective and precise approach to diagnosing and managing disorders of this complex and essential part of the body.

2 MRI Technique

The patients should be placed in the prone position with the affected arm elevated ("superman position") and the wrist positioned at the center of the scanner. Adapted dedicated wrist or small surface wrist coils, designed for high-resolution wrist imaging, optimize spatial and contrast resolution for a small field of view (3–10 cm) and thin slice thickness (1–2 mm). Coronal images are oriented between radial and ulnar styloid processes, sagittals are oriented 90° to coronals, and axial images include a volume of 2–3 cm proximal to the radiocarpal and 1 cm distal to the carpometacarpal joints (ESSR 2016).

The *European Society of Musculoskeletal Radiology* has issued guidelines on the MRI of the hand and wrist. A complete protocol includes proton density—weighted (w) images with fat suppression (FS PD-w) at three orthogonal planes (coronal, sagittal, and transverse) and T1-w images in at least two planes (coronal and sagittal). All sequences should be acquired with a field of view of 10 cm, a minimum matrix of 240 × 320 px and a maximum slice thickness of 3 mm. If possible a slice thickness of 2 mm should be preferred. A 3D T2-w gradient echo sequence can also be added to the protocol, allowing multiplanar reconstructions, which is particularly assessment of articular surfaces and the evaluation of potential bony erosions. This sequence should be obtained with thinner slices of 1.5–2 mm and a minimum matrix of 320 × 450 px (ESSR 2016). A dedicated high-resolution wrist coil (e.g., 8 channel) should be used (Dallaudière et al. 2015).

3 MR Arthrography

MRa merges the benefits of standard MRI imaging with arthrography, allowing for improved detection of even minimal intra-articular abnormalities and their precise delineation (Elentuck and Palmer 2004). The interosseous scapholunate and lunotriquetral ligaments and the triangular fibrocartilage complex (TFCC) are the most important structures to consider.

3.1 Contrast Material

For wrist MRA, a concentration range of the diluted gadolinium-based contrast agent between 1.25 and 2.5 mmol/L is considered ideal for optimum signal-to-noise ratio (Ugas et al. 2014). As the most common commercially available concentration of the gadolinium agents is 0.5 mol/L, a dilution ratio of ~1:200 or ~1:250 would produce a final concentration of 2.5 mmol/L and 2 mmol/L, respectively. This mixture can be prepared using sterile saline, iodinated contrast medium, and/or a local anesthetic. Addition of anesthetics in the injectate has been linked to significantly reduced periprocedural and postprocedural pain (Andreisek et al. 2007). Low concentrations of bupivacaine (0.0625%), ropivacaine (0.1% and 0.2%), and mepivacaine (0.5%) have no established significant chondrotoxic effect and could be safely used (Kreuz et al. 2018). The addition of iodinated contrast to the mixture aids in confirmation of appropriate needle position, if fluoroscopic guidance is utilized, and allows for conversion to CT arthrography if necessary. When simultaneous CT and MRa is a consideration, a mixture of 1:25 mmol/L of gadolinium agent and 25% iodinated contrast is the suggested optimal mixture ratio (Choi et al. 2008). For this purpose, a solution of 0.1 mL gadolinium diluted in 20 mL of a solution composed of 10 mL of saline, 5 mL of iodinated contrast material, and 5 mL of local anesthetic is suggested (Cerezal et al. 2005). Scanning should be performed within 30 min after the intra-articular injection (Andreisek et al. 2007). Importantly, gadolinium-based contrast agents enter the environment through the disposal of unused substances and excretion following intravenous administration, mainly via liquid dispersion. Although the extent of gadolinium environmental excretion following intra-articular administration of gadolinium has not been studied, it is possible that it is exerted to some degree after it enters the bloodstream through capsular resorption. This human-induced release of gadolinium, known as *anthropogenic gadolinium*, has been linked to its presence in water sources, raising concerns about potential environmental effects and prompting efforts to reduce its impact (Lenkinski and Rofsky 2024). This is of particular relevance where the raw water for drinking water production has a higher proportion of recycled wastewater.

3.2 Volume of Contrast Material

For the radiocarpal joint, a total injected volume of 3–4 mL is usually adequate to achieve optimal distention (Chang et al. 2024). If communication with the midcarpal or distal radioulnar joints is detected, additional 3 mL or 1 mL, respectively, should be injected (Chang et al. 2024). For individual injection of the distal radioulnar and the midcarpal joints, a total volume of 1–2 mL and 2–3 mL, respectively, is suggested for optimal joint distension and opacification (Rastogi et al. 2016).

3.3 Injection Techniques

A single-compartment (radiocarpal joint), double-compartment (radiocarpal plus either a midcarpal or distal radioulnar joint), or triple-compartment injection technique may be used depending on the diagnostic indications and structures of interest. Image-guided injections have been proved significantly more accurate than landmark-based injections (Ali et al. 2022). The type of imaging guidance largely depends on operator experience and preference as well as equipment availability. Although ultrasound (US) and fluoroscopy have shown similar accuracy rates reaching 100%, US-guided interventions have been associated with significantly reduced pain and procedure duration compared to fluoroscopic-guided interventions (Ali et al. 2022). US-guidance may also be superior in patients with osteoarthritic changes of the radiocarpal joint space. Ordinary skin antisepsis should be applied over the dorsal aspect of the wrist before the procedure. The use of sterile gloves, fenestrated drape, and sterile probe cover with sterile gel, when US-guidance is used, is suggested. A high-frequency (15–18 MHz) linear or hockey-stick transducer and small-bore needles, usually 1.5-inch (3.8-cm) 23–25 gauge, are needed. We do not normally apply local anesthesia because of the small needle caliper.

For the US-guided radiocarpal joint injection, the hand is positioned prone resting on a roll of gauze to maintain a position of mild flexion and mild ulnar deviation. The transducer is placed along the short axis of the distal radius and moved distally until the Lister's tubercle is identified. The extensor pollicis longus (EPL) can be seen on the ulnar side of the tubercle followed by the extensor digitorum communis (EDC). The interval between EPL and EDC tendons is centered on the screen, and the transducer is moved distally until the cortex of the radius does not appear on the screen. Then, a transducer rotation by 90° enables visualization of the underlying radial-scaphoid joint in the long axis. The needle should be inserted in-plane from distal to proximal into the radiocarpal joint. Alternatively, the needle may be inserted out-of-plane, vertically into the joint space (Patel et al. 2023). For injecting the distal radioulnar joint under US guidance, the Lister's tubercle is identified through scanning along the distal forearm in the short axis. The extensor digiti minimi, running through the fifth extensor compartment at the ulnar side of the EDC, is detected and the needle is advanced along the ulnar aspect of this tendon. This reduces the risk of injury to neurovascular structures (e.g., the interosseous artery, the cutaneous branch of the ulnar nerve) and provides access to the largest recess of the distal radioulnar joint (Smith et al. 2011). A midcarpal injection is typically performed as part of a triple-compartment injection in patients with confounding symptoms and an indeterminate source of pain at clinical examination. For injection of the midcarpal joints, the transducer is placed in the long axis at the dorsal recess of the midcarpal joint. The needle is inserted in-plane from proximal to distal and is advanced toward the articular surfaces until bone contact, ensuring intra-articular placement. For fluoroscopically guided arthrography of the radiocarpal joint, the wrist is positioned prone with mild ulnar deviation allowing enhanced depiction of the scaphoid. The injection site should be opposite to the side of symptoms on the patient's wrist to avoid interpreting iatrogenic spill into the dorsal soft tissues as a true capsular disruption. For radial-side injections, the needle is advanced to the proximal cortex of the scaphoid, ulnar to the tubercle. Because of the natural volar tilt of the distal radius, a slight angulation of the fluoroscope in the cranial direction prevents the needle-tip from striking the dorsal lip of the radius, which frequently overlays the radioscaphoid space on a true posteroanterior projection. For ulnar side injections, the target is the space between the radial side of the pisiform and the proximal triquetrum. The needle is inserted in a slight caudocranial direction upon bone contact. Flow of contrast medium away from the needle tip and opacification of the periscaphoid recess confirm adequate position (Cerezal et al. 2005; Moser et al. 2008). For injecting the distal radioulnar joint, the target is the radial and distal aspect of the ulnar head just proximal to its physeal scar. The needle is inserted until bone contact. Flow of contrast media away from the needle tip and opacification of the compartment confirm adequate position (Cerezal et al. 2005). To inject into the midcarpal compartment under fluoroscopic guidance, the needle puncture site is through the dorsal aspect of the wrist into the midcarpal space at the junction between the scaphoid and capitate or between the triquetrum and hamate. Following needle advancement till bone contact, injection should continue until the contrast is readily visualized in the capitolunate joint space.

3.4 Scanning Technique

MRa of the wrist can be performed at 1.5T or 3T field strengths. FS T1-w fast or turbo spin echo (FSE/TSE) sequences in all three planes could be used. To enhance bone marrow and soft tissue fat plane evaluation, some protocols omit fat suppression in one plane or include an additional non-fat-suppressed T1-w sequence. At least one fluid-sensitive sequence such as a FS PD-w or FS Intermediate-weighted (IW) sequence should be also added to assess the presence of bone marrow edema and extra-articular tissue abnormalities (Elentuck and Palmer 2004; Omoumi et al. 2009). A 3D gradient echo sequence can be also added (Andreisek et al. 2007). Under specific clinical indications, MRa images may be combined with FS contrast enhanced T1-w images to assess the bone marrow. The latter is the sequence of choice in order to evaluate bone marrow viability following a previous scaphoid fracture (Fig. 1) (Karantanas et al. 2007; Taljanovic et al. 2012). Additionally, 3D gradient echo (spoiled or steady-state) or FSE/TSE sequences with thin slices are optimal as they enable multiplanar reformatting (Chang et al. 2024).

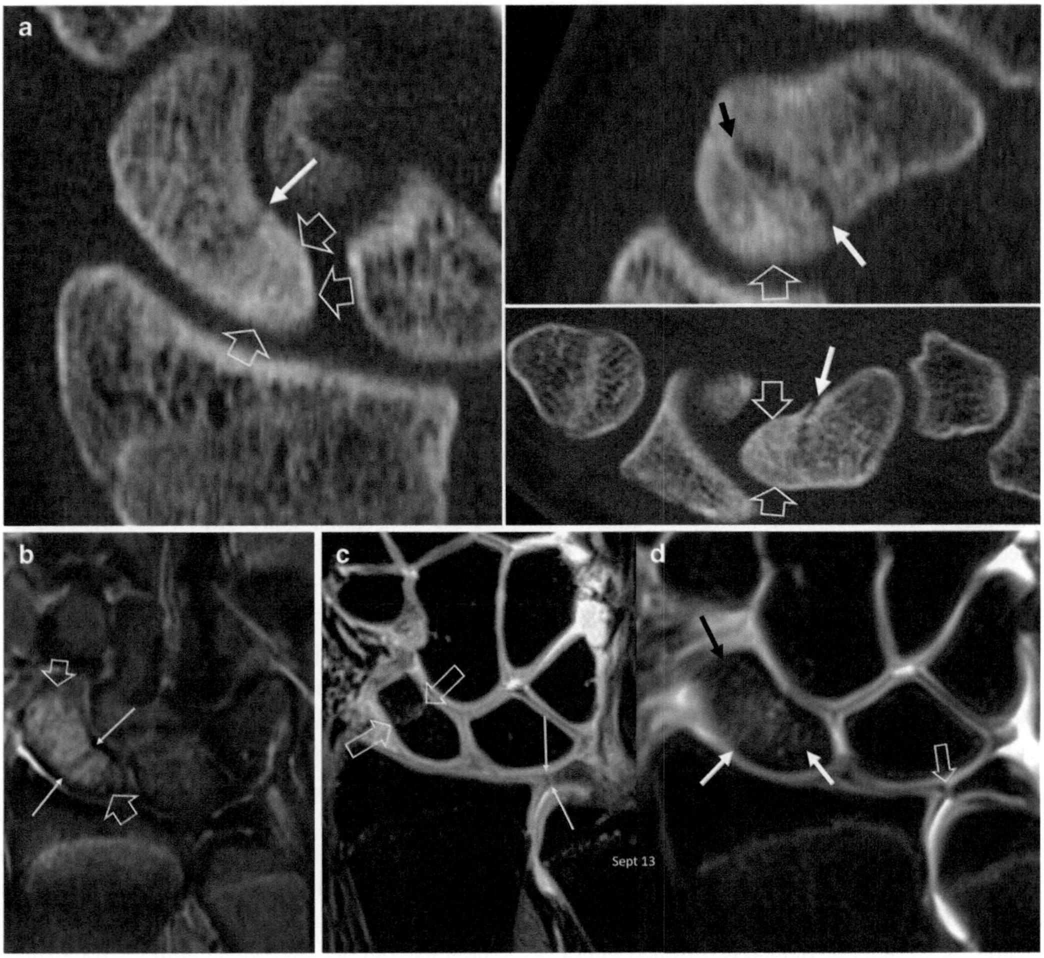

Fig. 1 A 15-year-old male patient underwent a wrist injury. Initial plain radiographs were unremarkable. (**a**) Two weeks following injury, CT in multiple reconstructions, shows a non-displaced scaphoid waist fracture (arrows) and proximal pole osteosclerosis (open arrows) in keeping with osteonecrosis. (**b**) Coronal fat-suppressed PD-w MR image 2 weeks after CT shows the fracture line (arrows) and the diffuse bone marrow edema within the scaphoid bone (open arrows). (**c**) Coronal 3D T1-w gradient echo (0.3 mm slice thickness) MR arthrographic image 4 weeks after CT, showing the fracture line (open arrows) and a tear in the radial aspect of the TFC (arrows), which allows contrast to fill the distal radioulnar joint. The bone marrow cannot be appreciated with this sequence. (**d**) Coronal fat-suppressed contrast-enhanced T1-w MR image, showing the enhancing bone marrow edema (arrows) in keeping with viability with no evidence of osteonecrosis. The TFC tear is not seen as clearly as in **c** (open arrow)

4 Normal Anatomy

MRI of the wrist and hand is an essential tool for evaluating musculoskeletal pathologies, offering superior soft tissue contrast and detailed anatomical visualization. The wrist and hand comprise a complex network of bones, ligaments, tendons, and neurovascular structures, all working in unison to provide mobility, dexterity, and stability. Given this intricate anatomy, precise imaging assessment is crucial for diagnosing conditions such as fractures, ligament injuries, arthritis, tendinopathies, and nerve compression syndromes. A systematic approach to wrist and hand MRI interpretation involves evaluating different anatomical planes. The axial (transverse) plane is best for assessing tendon compartments, neurovascular structures, and intrinsic wrist ligaments.

The coronal plane provides excellent visualization of carpal bone alignment, ligament integrity, and joint congruency. The sagittal plane is useful for evaluating joint spaces, flexor and extensor tendons, and carpal instability (Stein et al. 2011).

4.1 Osseous Structures

The radius and ulna form the primary osseous framework of the forearm, articulating distally with the carpal bones to contribute to wrist mobility and stability. These bones play crucial roles in load transmission, forearm rotation, and ligamentous attachment, influencing both function and pathology in the wrist and hand. The ulna is the medial bone of the forearm, primarily stabilizing the distal radioulnar joint. The fovea of the ulna is an important anatomical landmark, serving as the primary articulation point for the triangular fibrocartilage complex (TFCC), a crucial stabilizer of the wrist. The posterior groove of the ulna provides a passage for the extensor carpi ulnaris (ECU) tendon, which is essential for wrist stability, particularly during supination and ulnar deviation. The styloid process of the ulna changes its orientation based on wrist position: dorsally in supination, volarly in pronation, and laterally in a neutral position. The radius, positioned laterally in the forearm, is the primary load-bearing bone of the wrist. The Lister's tubercle, a prominent dorsal ridge of the distal radius, acts as a pulley for the extensor pollicis longus (EPL) tendon, influencing thumb extension mechanics and playing a key role in distinguishing the extensor compartments of the wrist. The proximal carpal bones form a critical articulating unit between the radius, ulna, and distal carpal row, allowing for wrist motion while maintaining stability (Fig. 2). The scaphoid is a vital bone for wrist stability, articulating with the radius, capitate, and trapezium. It is divided into three key regions: the proximal pole, waist, and distal pole. Due to its retrograde blood supply, the proximal pole is at high risk of osteonecrosis following fractures, making scaphoid injuries particularly concerning in clinical practice. The lunate is a crescent-shaped bone that articulates with the radius and triquetrum while cupping the capitate. Its central position within the proximal row makes it integral to wrist biomechanics. The triquetrum serves as an important stabilizer on the ulnar side, articulating with both the lunate and the pisiform. The pisiform, a sesamoid bone embedded within the flexor carpi ulnaris (FCU) tendon, functions primarily as a pulley, enhancing the mechanical efficiency of wrist flexion. The pisotriquetral joint is a small articulation between the pisiform and triquetrum, often overlooked in wrist assessments but significant in cases of ulnar-sided wrist pain. The pisotriquetral recess, located volarly, is frequently visible on MRI and contains synovial fluid. Mild fluid presence in this recess can be normal and should not be misinterpreted as pathology.

The distal carpal bones serve as a transition between the proximal carpal row and the metacarpals, providing stability and facilitating motion at the wrist and hand joints. These bones contribute to load transmission, mobility, and precise articulation for grip and dexterity. The trapezium is an essential bone for thumb function, forming the first carpometacarpal (CMC) joint with the first metacarpal. This highly mobile joint allows thumb opposition, a fundamental movement for grasping and precision handling. The trapezoid, located adjacent to the trapezium, articulates primarily with the second metacarpal and plays a less dynamic but structurally important role in wrist stability. The capitate is the largest of the carpal bones and serves as the central stabilizer of the wrist. It articulates proximally with the lunate and distally with the third metacarpal, forming a keystone structure that provides strength and support to wrist movements. The hamate is distinguished by its hook (hamulus), a palpable prominence on the volar aspect of the wrist. This hook serves as a crucial anatomical landmark, providing a protective passage for the ulnar nerve. Guyon's Canal, also known as the ulnar tunnel, is a fibro-osseous passage that allows the ulnar nerve and ulnar artery to transition from the forearm into the hand. It is clinically significant as a common site of ulnar nerve compression. The anatomical boundaries of Guyon's Canal include the pisiform bone medi-

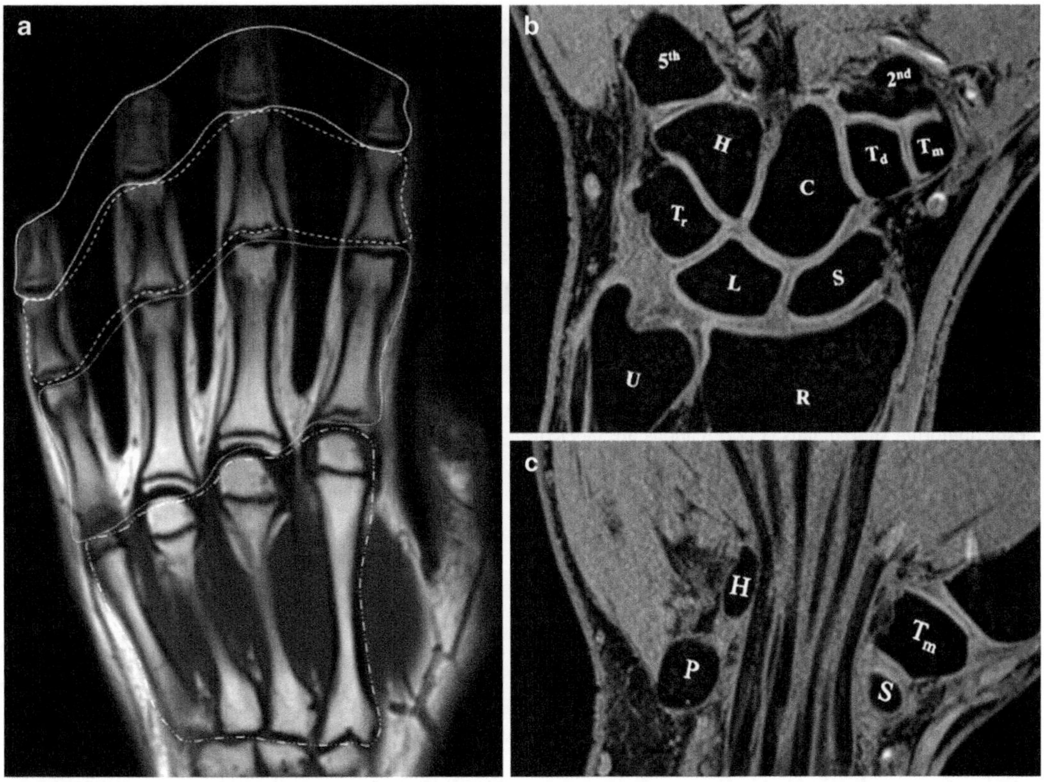

Fig. 2 (**a**) Coronal T1-w image of the hand demonstrating the second to fifth metacarpal bones along with their associated proximal, middle, and distal phalanges. (**b**, **c**) Coronal 3D FS T1-w Gradient Echo image depicting osseous structures including the ulna (U), radius (R) with its articular surfaces for the scaphoid (S), lunate (L), triquetrum (Tr), hamate (H), capitate (C), trapezoid (Td), trapezium (Tm), and the bases of the 2nd and 5th metacarpal bones. On the volar surface, the pisiform (P), hook of the hamate, trapezium, and scaphoid tubercle, which contribute to the structural framework guiding the passage of the flexor tendons, are shown

ally, the hook of the hamate laterally, the flexor retinaculum forming the floor, and the palmar carpal ligament along with the palmaris brevis muscle forming the roof. Its contents consist of the ulnar nerve, which provides motor innervation to the intrinsic hand muscles and sensory input to the medial hand and the ulnar artery, supplying blood to the ulnar aspect of the hand (Fig. 3) (Vassa et al. 2020).

The bones of the hand form a complex yet stable structure, with ligaments, tendons, and joint congruency maintaining proper alignment. The phalanges consist of 14 bones, with each finger containing a proximal, middle, and distal phalanx, except for the thumb, which lacks a middle phalanx. Their concave base and convex head at the joints allow for smooth articulation, facilitating precise finger movements. The sesamoid bones are located at the first metacarpophalangeal (MCP) joint, embedded within the flexor pollicis brevis and adductor pollicis tendons. They enhance leverage for thumb flexion but can be displaced in MCP dislocations, leading to functional impairment.

4.2 Ligaments

The ligaments of the wrist are classified into extrinsic ligaments, which connect the radius and ulna to the carpal bones, and intrinsic ligaments, which interconnect the carpal bones, contributing to the wrist's stability and function. The TFCC is a critical structure in wrist biomechanics, providing stability to the distal radioulnar joint (DRUJ) and contributing to load transmission across the wrist

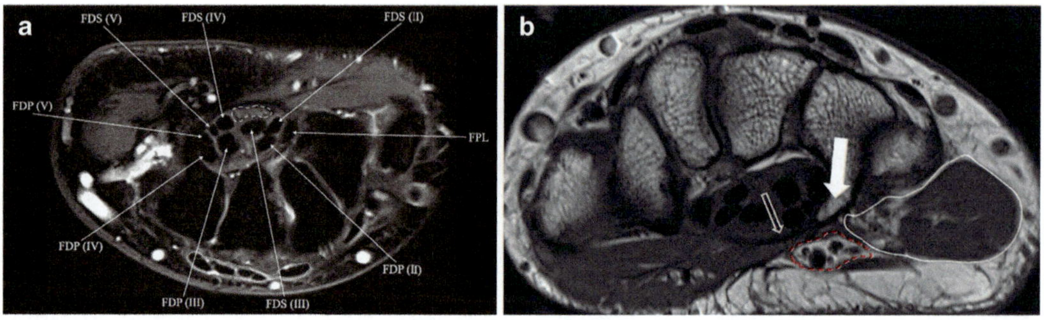

Fig. 3 (**a**) Axial FS PD-w MR image of the wrist at the level of the carpal tunnel, with long arrows indicating the flexor tendons. The flexor digitorum profundus (FDP) and flexor digitorum superficialis (FDS) tendons are labeled. The median nerve, enclosed by the dashed white line, exhibits its characteristic honeycomb fascicular pattern. The thin dotted white line delineates the extensor tendons for the second, third, and fourth fingers, showing that the extensor digitorum communis (EDC) may appear bifid (split) on MRI, a normal anatomical variant rather than a pathological finding. (**b**) Axial T1-w MR image of the wrist at the level of the hook of the hamate. The solid arrow identifies the hook of the hamate, while the thin arrow marks the flexor retinaculum. The red dashed line highlights the ulnar nerve and artery, demonstrating their close anatomical relationship with the hook of the hamate. The solid line delineates the hypothenar muscles, which are positioned along the ulnar aspect of the palm

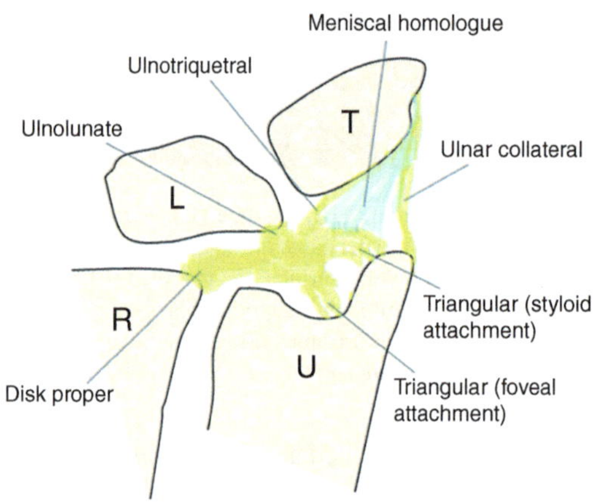

Fig. 4 Illustration of the central portion of the triangular fibrocartilage complex (TFCC), displayed in a slightly volar perspective to highlight the ulnolunate and ulnotriquetral ligaments. The dorsal and volar radioulnar ligaments, which are also key stabilizers of the TFCC, are not shown in this view

(Fig. 4). It consists of multiple interconnected structures (Bateni et al. 2013). The disc proper is a fibrocartilaginous, biconcave-shaped structure that attaches to the hyaline cartilage of the sigmoid notch of the distal radius. The dorsal and volar radioulnar ligaments form the borders of the TFCC, attaching from the dorsal and radial part of the sigmoid notch to the base of the ulnar styloid process. The ulnolunate and ulnotriquetral ligaments extend centrally and volarly, reinforcing the lunotriquetral ligament. The triangular ligament consists of two laminae, with the upper lamina attaching to the fovea of the ulna and the lower lamina attaching to the styloid process of the ulna, with connective tissue known as the ligamentum subcruentum interposed between them. A meniscus homologue, a fibrous structure, extends from the ulnar styloid to the ulnar surface of the triquetrum. Additionally, the ulnar collateral ligament, a thickened part of the joint capsule, is in continuity with the meniscus homologue and the ECU tendon sheath.

Apart from the TFCC-associated ligaments, other extrinsic ligaments of the wrist on the volar and dorsal side provide crucial stability and regulate motion. They can be depicted with thin slice 3D gradient echo MR images, but further analysis is beyond the scope of this chapter.

The intrinsic ligaments of the wrist primarily contribute to carpal stability by directly connecting adjacent carpal bones. The scapholunate ligament is the major stabilizer of the scapholunate joint and has a distinctive C-shaped structure composed of three parts: a dorsal portion made of thick collagen fibers, which is the strongest and most crucial for preventing scapholunate dissociation; a central fibrocartilaginous membranous segment that exhibits a variable trapezoidal shape depending on wrist positioning, best visualized in the coronal plane;

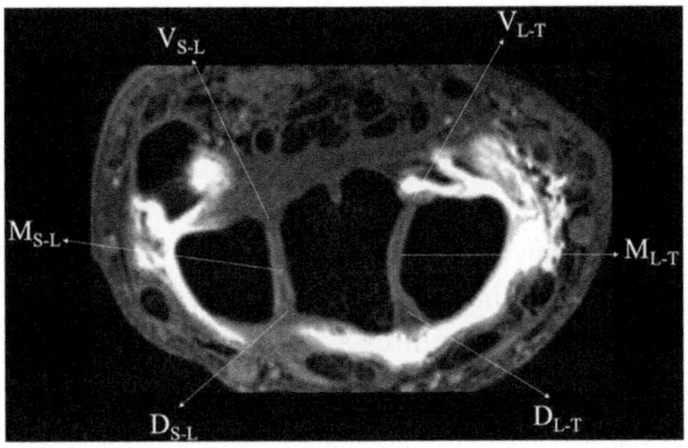

Fig. 5 Axial 3D T1-w gradient-echo MR arthrography image of the wrist at the level of the proximal carpal row, highlighting the scapholunate and lunotriquetral ligaments. The dorsal portion of the scapholunate ligament (DS-L) appears thicker than its volar portion (VS-L), while the lunotriquetral ligament demonstrates the reverse pattern, with a thicker volar portion (VL-T) compared to its dorsal portion (DL-T). The central C-shaped membranous fibrocartilaginous components of both ligaments are also visible, identified as the membranous portion of the scapholunate ligament (MS-L) and the membranous portion of the lunotriquetral ligament (ML-T)

and a thin volar portion that provides additional reinforcement (Stein et al. 2011). The lunotriquetral ligament plays a similar stabilizing role in the lunate-triquetrum articulation, attaching to the proximal surfaces of both bones. Like the scapholunate ligament, it consists of three parts: a dorsal and volar portion composed of collagen fibers and a wide central fibrocartilaginous membranous segment, which has a variable shape that is even smaller and more difficult to visualize (Bateni et al. 2013). Due to these structural characteristics, the lunotriquetral ligament is best assessed on coronal images. Axial images can provide additional insight into the integrity of both the scapholunate and lunotriquetral ligaments (Fig. 5). Other intrinsic ligaments serve to connect adjacent carpal bones and maintain structural integrity. They can be depicted with thin slice 3D gradient echo MR images, but further analysis is beyond the scope of this chapter.

4.3 Tendons

Four structures lie volarly and peripherally, creating a passage for the flexor tendons in the volar wrist, situated deep to the flexor retinaculum: the trapezoid, scaphoid, hook of the hamate, and pisiform (Fig. 3). These structures contribute to the formation of the carpal tunnel, guiding and protecting the flexor tendons as they pass into the hand. Additionally, the transverse carpal ligament (flexor retinaculum) spans these bony landmarks, securing the tendons and preventing bowstringing during flexion. The median nerve, which also courses through this tunnel, is particularly vulnerable to compression, leading to disorders such as carpal tunnel syndrome.

The flexor tendons of the wrist and hand primarily function to facilitate finger flexion and are mostly contained within the carpal tunnel, running deep to the flexor retinaculum, which is located between the tubercle of the trapezium and the hook of the hamate. The flexor digitorum superficialis (FDS) and flexor digitorum profundus (FDP) serve as the primary flexors of the fingers, while the flexor pollicis longus (FPL) is responsible for thumb flexion. These tendons are enveloped in synovial sheaths, reducing friction and allowing smooth gliding movements during hand function. The FDS tendon to the 5th finger exhibits anatomical variability and may be missing (Yilmaz et al. 2009). The median nerve courses through the carpal tunnel, dividing into motor and sensory branches. MRI can assess fibrillar patterns, internal signal changes, and flattening of the nerve, though ultrasound provides more precise cross-sectional area measurements, making it the superior imaging modality for carpal tunnel syndrome diagnosis (Hersh et al. 2019).

The extensor tendons of the wrist and hand are organized into six extensor compartments, each containing specific tendons responsible for wrist and finger extension (Fig. 6). These tendons are held in place by the extensor retinaculum, preventing bowstringing and ensuring smooth gliding over the dorsal aspect of the wrist (Plotkin et al. 2016). The first extensor compartment, located most laterally, contains the abductor pollicis longus (APL) and extensor pollicis brevis (EPB) tendons, which contribute to thumb abduction and extension. The second compartment houses the extensor carpi radialis longus (ECRL) and extensor carpi

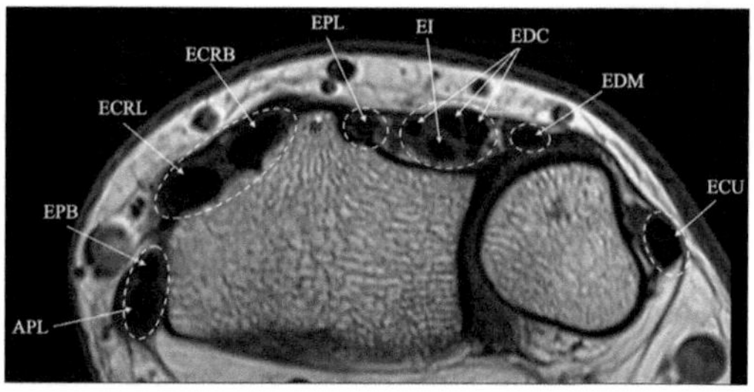

Fig. 6 Axial T1-w MR image of the wrist, illustrating the six extensor compartments. The first compartment contains the abductor pollicis longus (APL) and extensor pollicis brevis (EPB). The second compartment consists of the extensor carpi radialis longus (ECRL) and extensor carpi radialis brevis (ECRB). Lister's tubercle, marked by the red asterisk, serves as a bony landmark separating the second and third compartments. The third compartment houses the extensor pollicis longus (EPL). The fourth compartment contains the extensor indicis (EI) and extensor digitorum communis (EDC). The fifth compartment consists of the extensor digiti minimi (EDM), while the sixth compartment contains the extensor carpi ulnaris (ECU)

radialis brevis (ECRB), which are primary wrist extensors. Lister's tubercle, a bony prominence on the distal radius, lies between the second and third compartments, serving as a pulley for the extensor pollicis longus tendon. The third compartment contains the extensor pollicis longus (EPL), which courses medially over Lister's tubercle before angling toward the thumb, facilitating thumb extension. The fourth compartment consists of the extensor digitorum communis (EDC) and extensor indicis (EI) tendons, responsible for extending the fingers. The fifth compartment contains the extensor digiti minimi (EDM), which extends the little finger. The sixth compartment, positioned most medially, houses the extensor carpi ulnaris (ECU), which has a close anatomical relationship with the TFCC and the ulnar collateral ligament, playing a crucial role in wrist stabilization. The extensor hood mechanism, also known as the dorsal aponeurosis, provides structural support for digital extension. It ensures coordinated finger movement by distributing force from the extensor tendons to the proximal and distal interphalangeal joints (PIP and DIP), allowing for precise extension and stabilization of the fingers during functional activities.

4.4 Muscles of the Hand

The muscles of the hand play a critical role in fine motor control, grip strength, and dexterity. They can be categorized into thenar, hypothenar, intrinsic, and interossei muscles, each serving distinct functions in hand movement. MRI evaluation of these muscles requires assessing signal intensity on FS PD/T2-w images for pathology on T1-w images to detect chronic denervation and fatty atrophy (Fig. 7).

The thenar muscles, responsible for thumb mobility, are primarily innervated by the median nerve. The abductor pollicis brevis abducts the thumb, the flexor pollicis brevis contributes to thumb flexion, and the opponens pollicis enables opposition, a crucial movement for grasping and manipulating objects. The hypothenar muscles, controlled by the ulnar nerve, allow for independent movement of the fifth digit. The abductor digiti minimi abducts the pinky, the flexor digiti minimi brevis facilitates flexion, and the opponens digiti minimi enables opposition, aiding in grasping and cupping motions of the hand.

The lumbricals, originating from the FDP tendons and inserting into the extensor expansion, play a key role in MCP flexion and PIP/DIP extension, essential for fine motor coordination. The first and second lumbricals are innervated by the median nerve, while the third and fourth lumbricals are controlled by the ulnar nerve. On MRI, lumbricals appear as small, elongated, intermediate- to low-signal intensity structures adjacent to the flexor tendons, best visualized on axial and coronal T1-w and T2-w sequences.

The palmar interossei and dorsal interossei are named based on their function and numbering system. The palmar interossei, consisting of three muscles, are located on digits 2, 4, and 5 and function to adduct the fingers toward the midline (PAD: Palmar ADduct). The third digit (middle finger) does not require a palmar interosseous muscle as it is already in the midline, while the thumb has its own adductor pollicis, eliminating the need for a palmar interosseous muscle. The dorsal interossei, composed of four muscles, are found on digits 2, 3, and 4, with the third digit having two dorsal interossei (Andreisek et al.

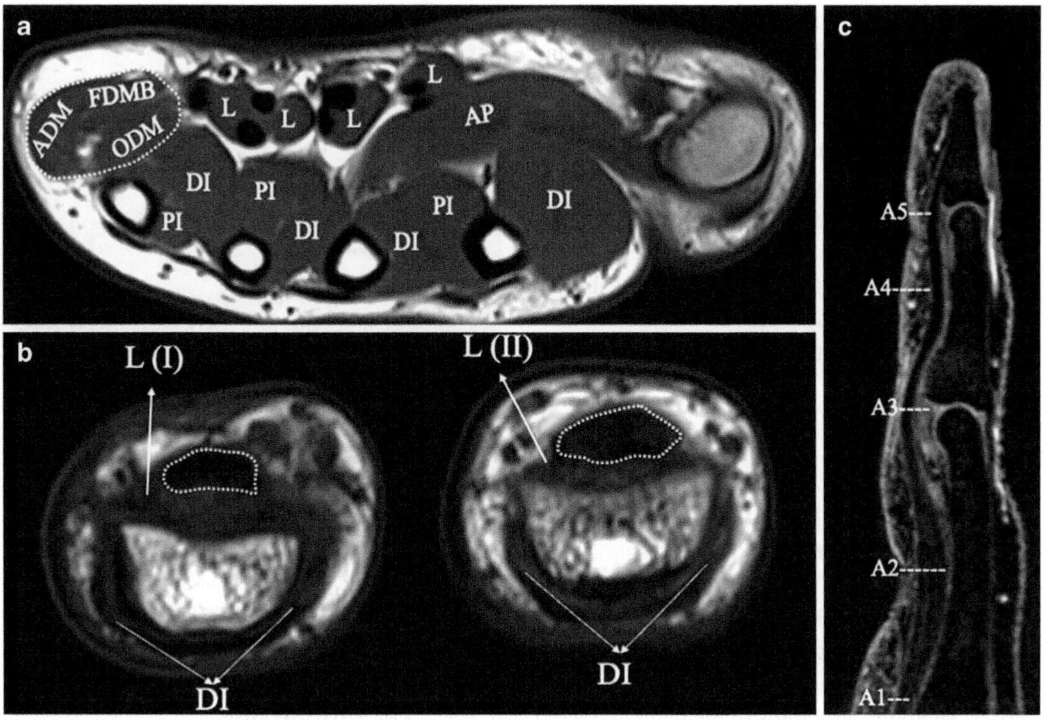

Fig. 7 (**a**) Axial T1-w MR image at the level of the metacarpal bones, depicting the dorsal interossei (DI), palmar interossei (PI), and lumbrical muscles (L). More distally, at the PIP joint level, the lumbricals can be seen merging with the dorsal interossei as they approach the extensor tendon. The dotted line delineates the hypothenar muscles, including the abductor digiti minimi (ADM), flexor digiti minimi brevis (FDMB), and opponens digiti minimi (ODM). The adductor pollicis (AP) muscle is also labeled. (**b**) Axial T1-w MR image at the level of the mid-metacarpal bone diaphysis, illustrating the dorsal interossei (DI) positioned dorsally to the digits. The dotted lines enclose the flexor digitorum superficialis and flexor digitorum profundus tendons, with the lumbrical muscles seen adjacent to these tendons. (**c**) Sagittal 3D FS gradient echo T1-w MR image displaying the annular pulley system (A1–A5) in relation to the flexor tendons. The A2 and A4 pulleys are critical for maintaining the proximal and middle phalanx diaphyses well-opposed to the bone and periosteum. The A1, A3, and A5 pulleys are located at the MCP, PIP, and DIP joints, respectively

2005). These muscles function to abduct the fingers away from the midline (DAB: Dorsal ABduct). The thumb and pinky have their own abductor muscles (abductor pollicis brevis and abductor digiti minimi, respectively), meaning they do not require dorsal interossei. The middle finger, which can move in both directions, has two dorsal interossei.

The flexor pulley system consists of annular (A1–A5) and cruciform (C1–C3) pulleys, which stabilize the flexor tendons and prevent bowstringing during flexion. The A2 and A4 pulleys are the most critical in preventing tendon displacement, whereas the A1 pulley is frequently involved in trigger finger, a condition where thickening of the pulley restricts smooth tendon gliding. Although pulleys are difficult to visualize on MRI, their integrity can be inferred from the flexor tendon trajectory (Hauger et al. 2000). Normally, the tendons should remain well-opposed to the bone and periosteum. Volar displacement of the FDP or FDS tendon at a specific level may indicate pulley rupture, particularly in cases of excessive bowstringing. The cruciform (C) pulleys, arranged in an X-pattern, provide flexibility while stabilizing movement. The C1 pulley is located between the A2 and A3 pulleys, the C2 pulley between A3 and A4, and the C3 pulley between A4 and A5. Unlike the A2 and A4 annular pulleys, which are thick and rigid, cruciform pulleys are thinner and more flexible, ensuring smooth tendon gliding during finger motion.

The volar plate, a thick fibrocartilaginous structure, prevents hyperextension at the MCP and PIP joints (Petchprapa and Vaswani 2019). The collateral ligaments at the MCP, PIP, and DIP joints provide lateral stability, resisting valgus, and varus forces. The deep transverse metacarpal ligament unites the metacarpal heads, limiting excessive finger spread while maintaining structural integrity. The thumb ulnar collateral ligament (UCL) plays a critical role in grip strength.

5 Artifacts, Pitfalls, and Variants

Although high spatial and contrast resolution are providing superb diagnostic information, numerous pitfalls may arise due to the small size of the various anatomic structures in the hand and wrist and the presence of air between these structures and the wrist coil. In addition, many anatomical variants exist. Both pitfalls and variants are more pronounced on MR imaging with 3T scanners.

5.1 MRI Artifacts

Various artifacts may occur during an MRI examination, in the hand and wrist (Morelli et al. 2011).

5.1.1 Chemical Shift

This artifact is related to the differences in the resonance frequencies of water and fat and results in their spatial misregistration. Concerning wrist and hand MRI, this artifact occurs at the interface between cartilage and bone marrow and may lead to over- or underestimation of the cartilage thickness. It occurs in the frequency-encoding direction, thus switching this direction when rescanning will shift the appearance of the artifact (Fig. 8). The artifact is more pronounced with high field scanners and is reduced or even eliminated by increasing the receiver bandwidth or by applying fat suppression (Fig. 9).

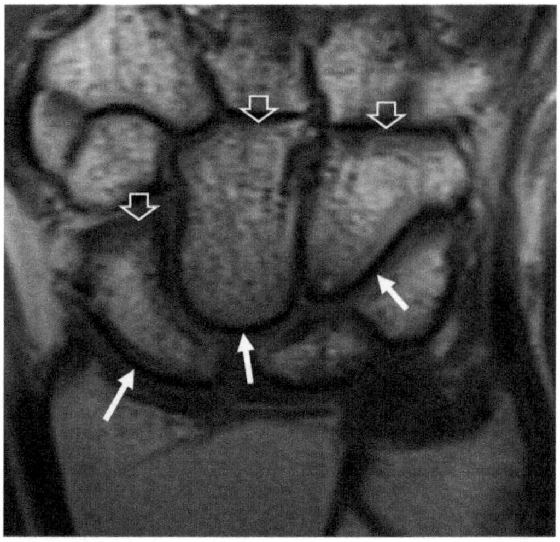

Fig. 8 Coronal T1-w MR image in a 35-year-old male patient, showing the "chemical shift" artifact in the frequency encoding direction, demonstrated as an artifactual thickening of the subcondral bone proximally (arrows) as opposed to almost vanished cortex distally (open arrows)

5.1.2 Fat Suppression

The most commonly used fat suppression (FS) techniques in musculoskeletal imaging include the chemical shift/spectral selective, the short tau inversion recovery (STIR), hybrid sequences such as the combined spectral and STIR, and finally DIXON and spatial-spectral sequences such as water excitation. FS utilizing a chemically/spectral selective radio frequency pulse with a narrow bandwidth adjusted on the fat resonance frequency works better with higher magnetic fields (Del Grande et al. 2014). Prerequisites for successful spectral FS include the homogeneity of both the main (Bo) and gradient (B1) fields. Spectral FS is used with PD/T2-w (w), T1-w SE/TSE combined with arthrography and contrast agent-enhanced, T1-w SE/TSE sequences. Spectral FS failure may result from field inhomogeneities but also from the use of large field of view, off-center imaging, and anatomic structures with abrupt tissue-air transition, as in the hand and wrist (Fig. 10). Spectral FS should not be applied in the presence of metals in the field of view. In cases where pathology cannot be discriminated from an artifact, repeated scanning with STIR sequences, which is not influenced by field inhomogeneities, will clarify the findings.

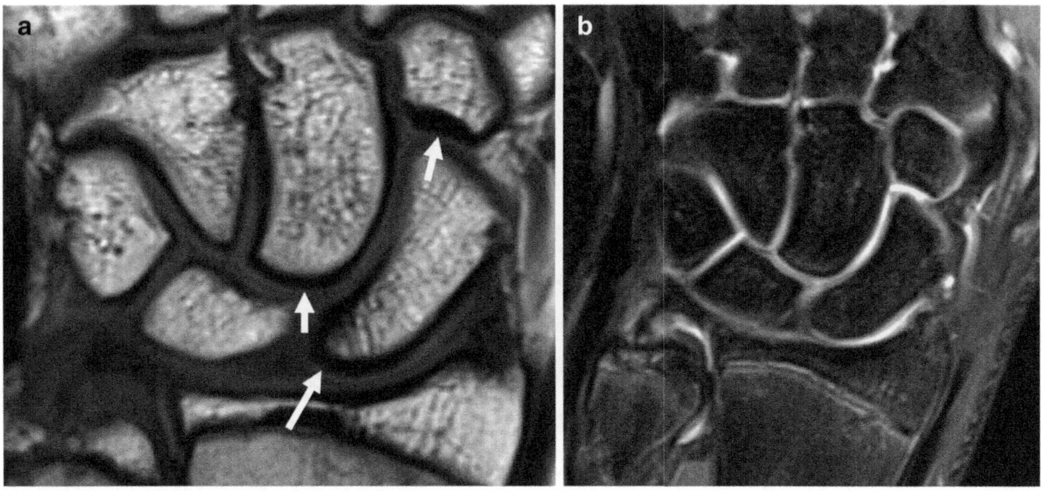

Fig. 9 (**a**) Coronal T1-w MR image in a 17-year-old male athlete. Chemical shift artifact artificially thickens the dark line of the subchondral bone (arrows). This is more pronounced with the high field scanners. (**b**) Coronal fat-suppressed PD-w MR image. The artifact is eliminated with the application of fat suppression

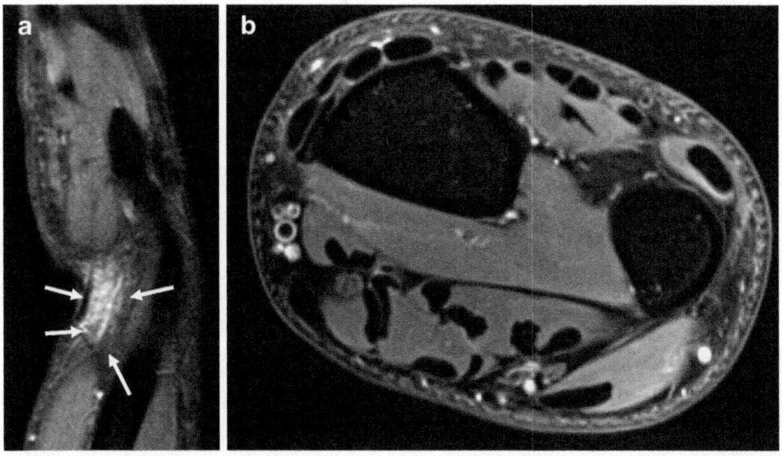

Fig. 10 (**a**) Sagittal fat-suppressed PD-w MR image (1.5 Tesla) in a 30-year-old male patient with dorsal pain, showing an artifactual abnormal area with increased signal palmarly, resulting from field inhomogeneity (arrows). (**b**) Axial fat-suppressed PD-w MR image (3 Tesla scanner with very good field homogeneity) in a 44-year-old female patient shows excellent fat suppression throughout the field of view

STIR sequences are however limited by the longer scanning time and the inherent low signal-to-noise ratio (Fig. 11). In addition, repositioning the patients will alter the artifact.

5.1.3 Magic Angle Effect

The magic angle effect is seen in sequences with short time echo (TE) (T1-w and PD-w) and is related to collagen fibers anisotropy in tissues such as tendons, menisci, and hyaline cartilage. The effect may also be seen on T1-w 3D gradient echo sequences. The magic angle effect may lead to abnormally high signals within cartilage or tendons in the wrist area and, thus, create the erroneous impression of cartilage degeneration or tendinopathy. The abnormal signal is maximized if the collagen fibers have an orientation of 55° with respect to

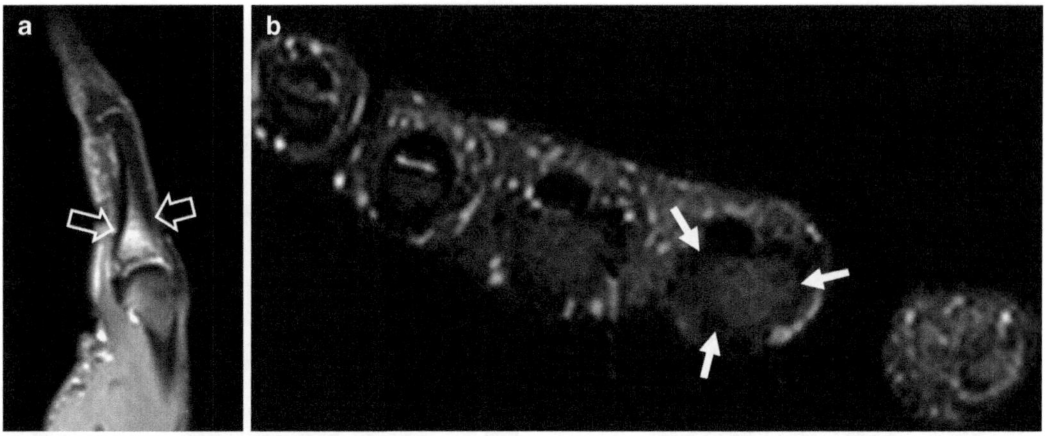

Fig. 11 (**a**) Sagittal fat-suppressed PD-w MR image (1.5 Tesla) in a 35-year-old male patient with carpometacarpal pain, showing failure of fat suppression in the proximal 2nd phalanx, resulting from field inhomogeneity (open arrows). (**b**) Corresponding axial fat-suppressed STIR MR image shows excellent fat suppression in the proximal phalanx (arrows)

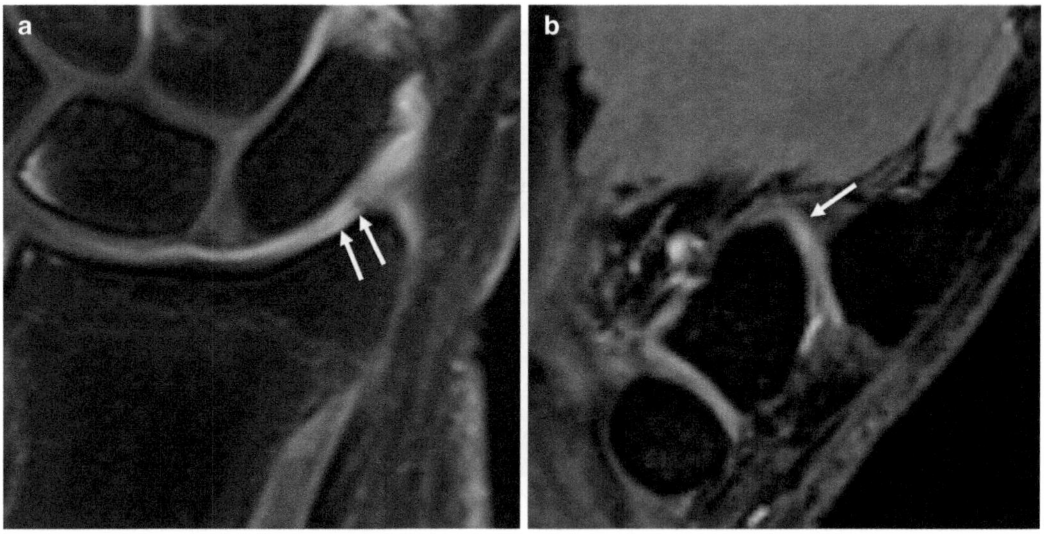

Fig. 12 Coronal contrast enhanced fat-suppressed T1-w (TR/TE: 800/11 ms) MR image (**a**) and 3D fat-suppressed T2* (TR/TE: 13/5 ms) MR image (**b**), showing high signal intensity of the hyaline cartilage due to the "magic angle" effect (arrows)

the main magnetic field axis (Fig. 12). In the wrist area, the flexor pollicis longus and the extensor pollicis longus tendons commonly demonstrate this artifact (Fig. 13). The magic angle effect can be corrected by using images with long TE, i.e., T2-w, by applying FS or by repositioning and repeating scanning.

5.1.4 Other Artifacts

Other artifacts, including the *flow or motion*, *wraparound or aliasing*, *partial volume*, *Gibbs*, and *shading*, are not difficult to depict and are rarely seen with modern scanners that provide the capability of short acquisition times and specifically designed coils and sequences. When images

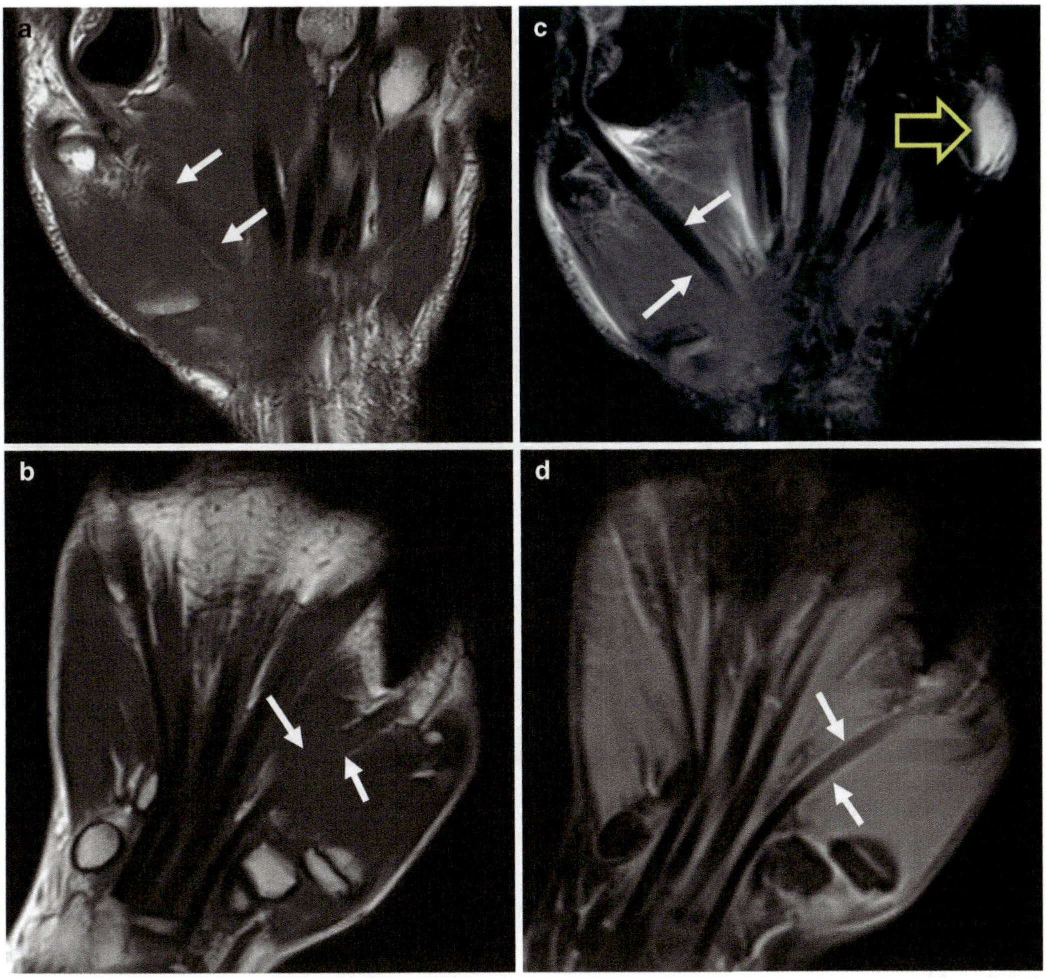

Fig. 13 "Magic angle" effect in two patients. (**a**, **b**) Coronal T1-w MR images (TR/TE: 640/8 ms in **a** and 500/10 ms in **b**) showing lack of visualization of the oblique part of the flexor pollicis longus tendon (arrows). By increasing the TR and the TE (TR/TE: 2850/33 ms in **c** and 2800/37 ms in **d**), the tendon reappears (arrows). A "pseudolesion" is shown in **c** (open arrow) due to failed fat suppression

show severe motion artifacts, rescanning is the only means of amendment, often with the use of immobilizing devices (Fig. 14). The use of a larger field of views, but primarily selection of the phase direction along the minor axis of the object to be imaged, can lead to correction of the wraparound artifact. The partial volume artifact can be reduced by rescanning with increased matrix size and slice thickness. The *Gibbs* artifact, also known as *truncation* artifact or *ringing* artifact, refers to the presence of lines in the MR image parallel to abrupt and intense changes. It can be reduced by increasing the matrix size (Block et al. 2008). The "*shading*" artifact is eliminated using larger coils instead of surface coils.

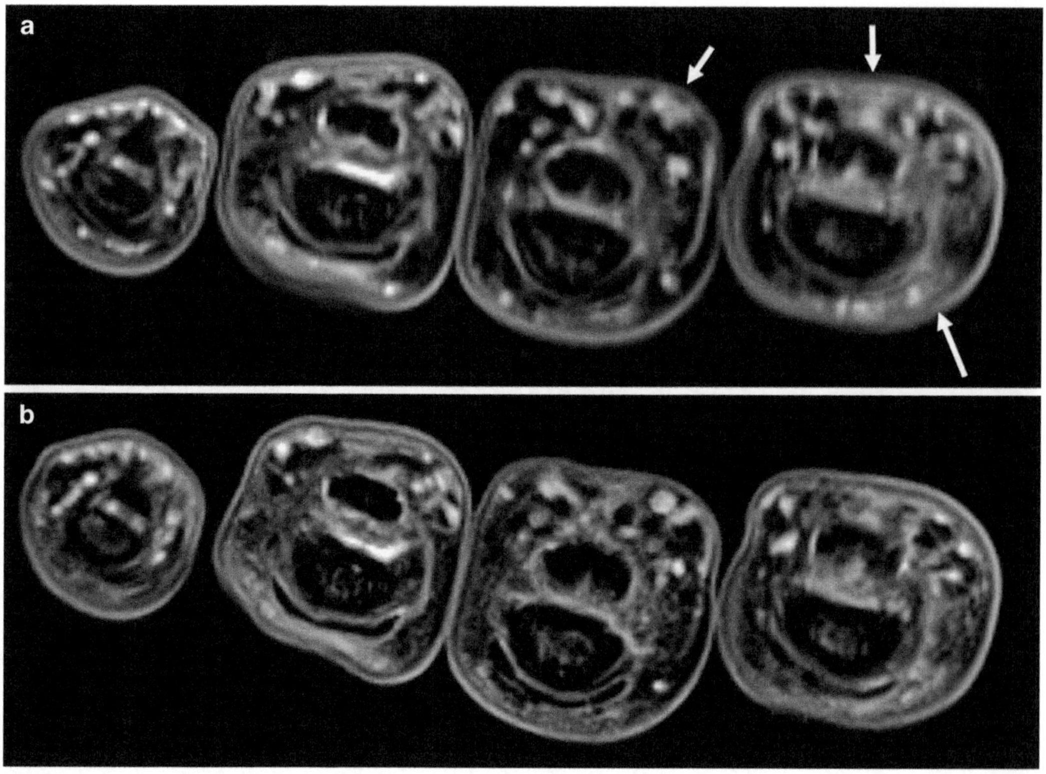

Fig. 14 Axial fat-suppressed PD-w MR images in the hand. (**a**) Motion artifact results in blurring of the anatomic structures (arrows). (**b**) Rescanning with use of immobilizing devices results in better quality images

5.2 Pitfalls

5.2.1 Alignment

The position of the wrist during an MRI examination may vary either being at the patient's side or in an overhead position ("Superman" position). The former is comfortable, but the wrist is out of the center of the bore, decreasing thus the signal-to-noise and often leading to failure of fat suppression. The latter position offers better visualization, by placing the wrist in the center of the magnet. However, elderly and high BMI patients as well as those suffering from respiratory problems cannot endure it. Apart from positioning, other parameters, such as the degree of pronation and supination and ulnar and radial deviation, differing among patients, may affect the final outcome and lead to misinterpretation of normal imaging findings. The diagnostic approach of carpal instability is based on the evaluation of anatomic correlations on plain radiographs (Zlatkin et al. 1989). The most significant types are volar intercalated segmental instability (VISI) and dorsal intercalated segmental instability (DISI) (Gilula and Weeks 1978; Zanetti et al. 1998). It is virtually impossible to achieve a perfectly neutral position of the wrist during MRI, particularly when scanning in the "Superman" position where ulnar tilting occurs secondarily to asymmetric mechanical load. On sagittal MR images, the lunate is then mostly more dorsally tilted than on standard lateral radiographs, and thus, a "pseudo DISI" appearance may be encountered (Fig. 15). Correlation with standard lateral radiographs is strongly advised before proposing diagnosis of DISI or VISI on MRI (Zanetti et al. 1998).

Another normal variation, which may be misinterpreted as abnormality, is seen on axial MR images of the DRUJ. Normally, the ulna projects dorsally in pronation, and volarly in supination, in relation to the radius (Fig. 16) (Timins 1999a).

Taking into consideration that pronation is the common position of the wrist for MRI, radiologists must be careful not to overestimate this normal alignment as dorsal subluxation when evaluating DRUJ integrity (Ehman et al. 2015). Repeated scanning with the wrist in supine position will support the correct interpretation.

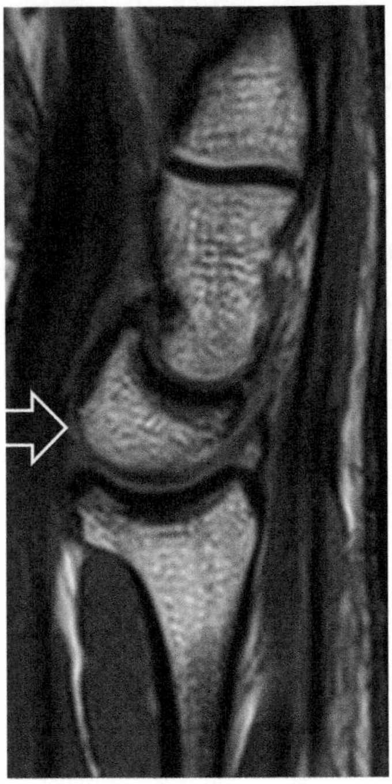

Fig. 15 Pseudo DISI in a 57-year-old male who had no clinical findings of instability. The sagittal T1-w, MR image shows dorsal tilting of the lunate (open arrow)

5.2.2 MR Arthrography Pitfalls

During the intra-articular injection of contrast medium for an MR arthrography, gas may be injected unintentionally. This leads to the presence of low signal intensity pseudolesions within the joint fluid, which may be misinterpreted as intra-articular loose bodies (Fig. 17). The gas bubbles are located at the dorsal aspect of the joint when the wrist is scanned in the prone position. A low signal intensity line between the car-

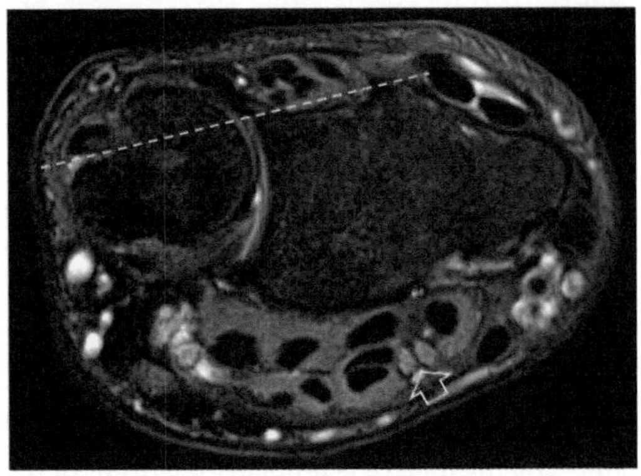

Fig. 16 Pseudosubluxation of the distal radioulnar joint in a 25-year-old male who had no clinical findings of instability. The axial PD-w, fat-suppressed MR image with the wrist in the prone position shows dorsal subluxation of the ulna (dashed line). Bifid median nerve is also shown (arrow)

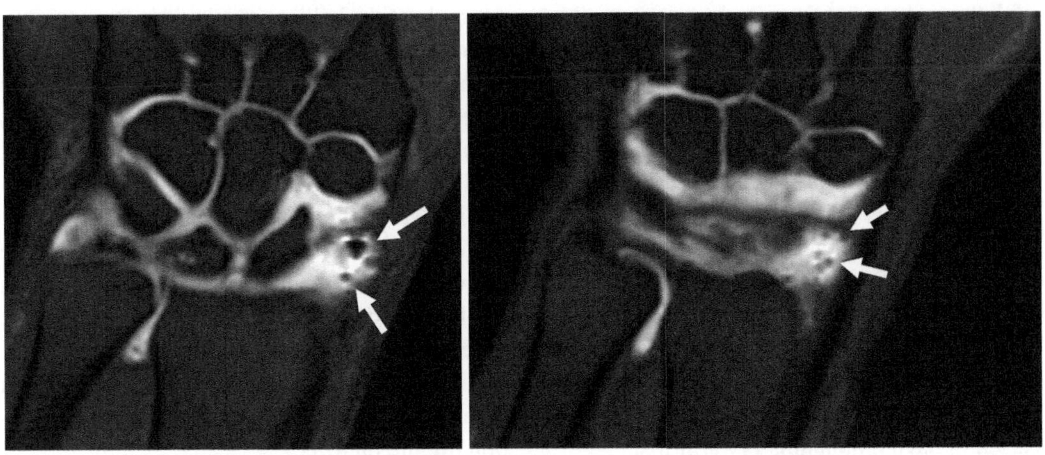

Fig. 17 Intra-articular air bubbles in MR arthrography. The bubbles are shown as low signal intensity structures on these consecutive coronal fat-suppressed T1-w MR images (arrows)

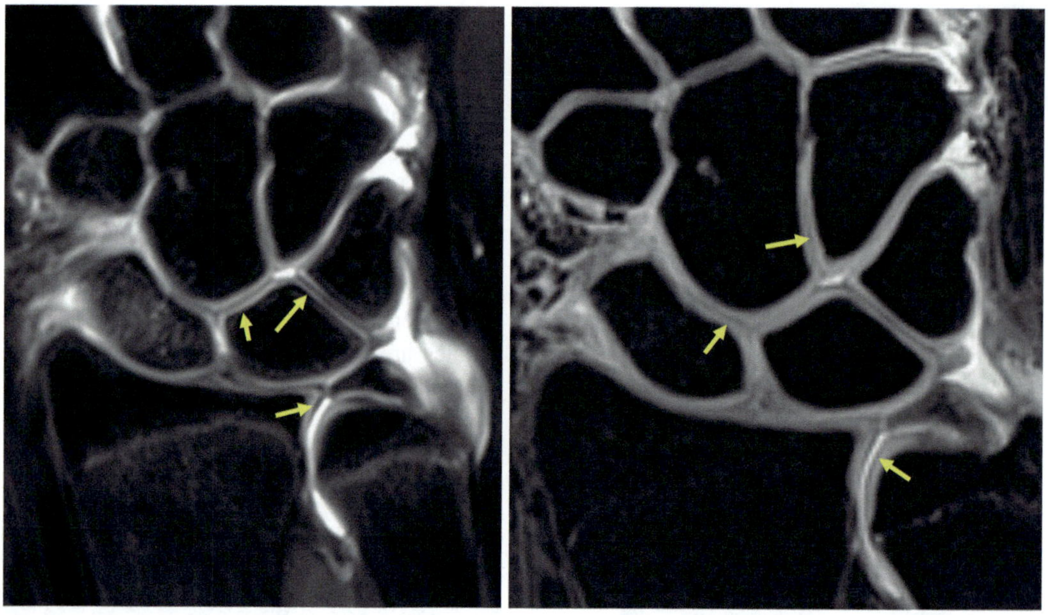

Fig. 18 Fat-suppressed coronal MR arthrographic images (T1-w TSE/FSE left and 3D T1-w gradient echo right) in different patients, showing a pitfall demonstrated as a low signal intensity line (arrows). The pitfall is attributed to the tightly packed collagen fibers of the superficial zone (primarily, type II and IX collagen) which are aligned parallel to the articular surface

pal bones on high-resolution fat-suppressed arthrographic images is probably the result of the tightly packed collagen fibers of the superficial zone of both opposing articular surfaces (Fig. 18). This pitfall is more often seen with 3-Tesla scanners.

5.2.3 Vascular Remnants

With the wide use of three Tesla scanners, which achieve thin slice images, "pseudo-erosion" or "pseudo-cyst" lesions are very common. This is a finding representing prominent vascular remnants, not reported yet, similar to the ones seen in the calcaneus (Fleming 2nd et al. 2005). Clue to correct diagnosis in order to avoid misinterpretation is the connection of the subcortical lesion with the joint (Fig. 19). The presence of contrast within the "pseudo-erosion" on arthrographic images confirms the presence of this variant (Fig. 20). Recognition of this variant is of substantial significance when scanning patients suspected of having inflammatory arthritis.

5.2.4 Tendons

A focus of abnormal signal within the extensor carpi ulnaris tendon along its course by the ulnar styloid is one of the most common pitfalls related to tendon imaging in the hand and wrist (Fig. 21). This finding can be attributed to the fact that the central part of the tendon histologically shows fibrovascular tissue surrounded by spiral fibers from the two bellies which form the muscle. Intratendinous signal alteration can also be seen in the abductor pollicis longus, resulting from the several bundles, which form the muscle (Fig. 21) (Malone et al. 2010; Pfirrmann and Zanetti 2005). The FDS tendon to the 5th finger exhibits anatomical variability and is frequently hypoplastic, partially absent, or completely missing in some individuals. In many cases, people rely solely on the FDP tendon for 5th finger flexion due to the absence of an independent FDS contribution (Yilmaz et al. 2009). This is a normal anatomical variant and should not be misinterpreted as a tendon rupture on MRI.

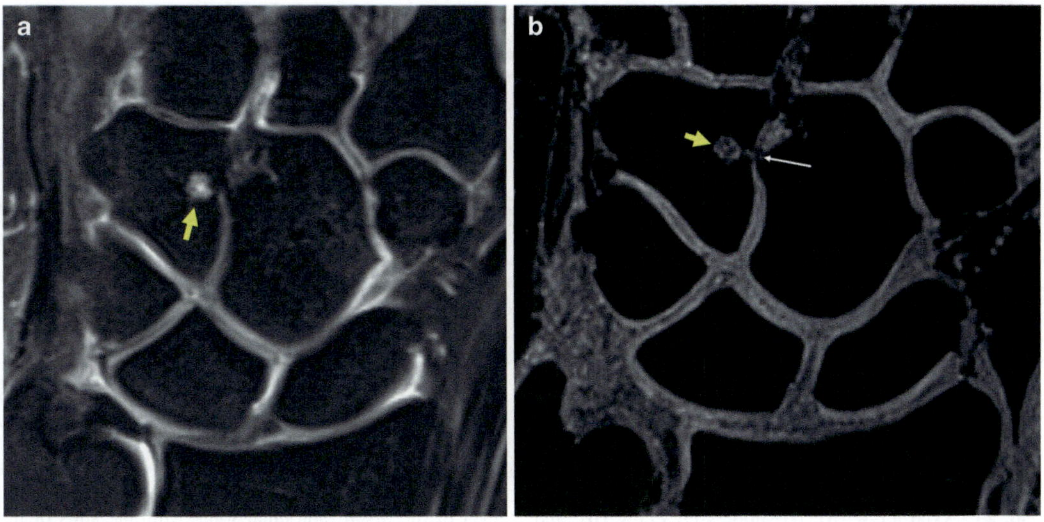

Fig. 19 (**a**) Coronal fat-suppressed PD-w MR image with a slice thickness of 2.5 mm shows a subcortical cyst in the hamate (arrow). (**b**) Coronal fat-suppressed 3D T1-w gradient echo image with a slice thickness of 0.3 mm shows that the cyst (short arrow) is connected to the joint with a thin channel (thin long arrow)

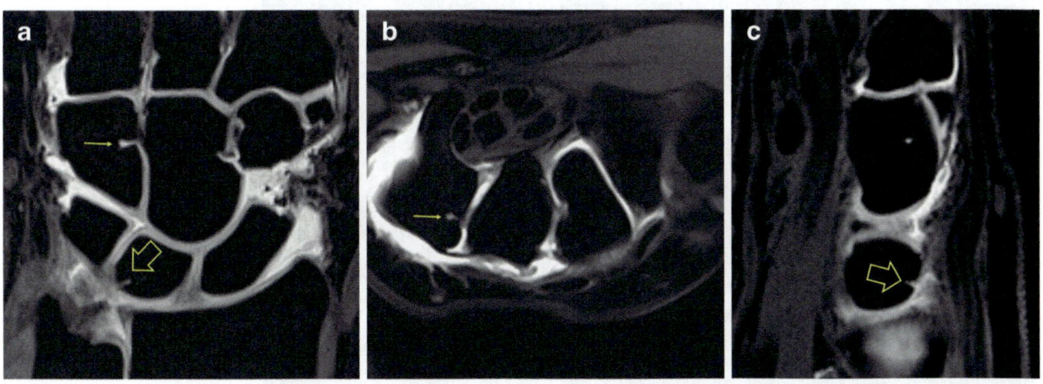

Fig. 20 Coronal fat-suppressed 3D T1-w gradient echo arthrographic MR image with a slice thickness of 0.3 mm in coronal (**a**), axial (**b**), and sagittal (**c**) planes shows the presence of contrast into the vascular defects in the hamate (arrows) and the lunate (open arrows)

5.2.5 Ligaments

The intrinsic carpal ligaments originate and insert onto the carpal bones. In asymptomatic wrists, defects may occur within the two most important interosseous ligaments, namely, the scapholunate (Fig. 22) and the lunotriquetral (Fig. 23). Degenerative perforations through the thinner central, membranous part of both ligaments should be considered a part of the normal ageing process.

5.2.6 Triangular Fibrocartilage Complex

The triangular fibrocartilage complex (TFCC) is an important stabilizer of the ulnar side of the wrist and particularly of the DRUJ. The triangular fibrocartilaginous disc (TFC proper) represents its most important structure, is triangular in shape with a rather broad ulnar side and a narrow radial side, and is thinner at its central part. TFC shape alters slightly

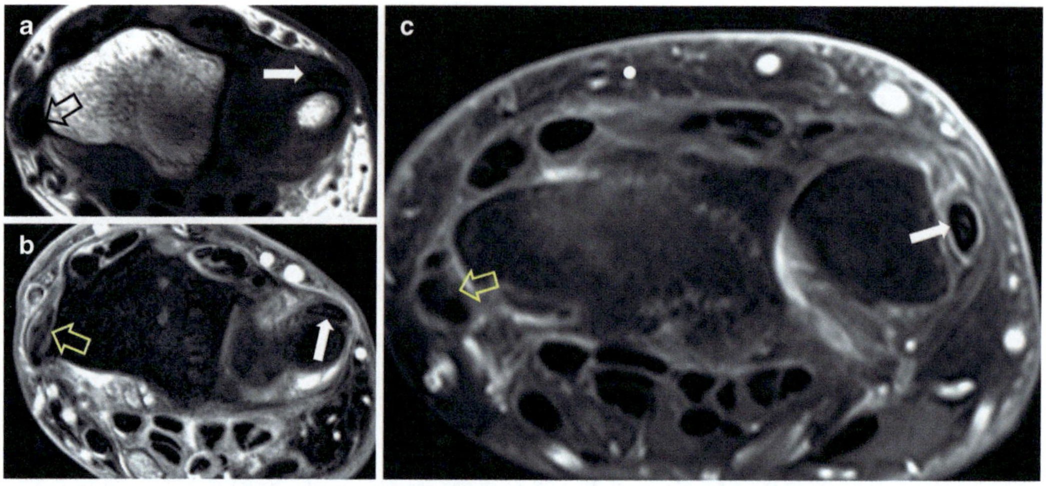

Fig. 21 Axial T1-w (**a**), fat-suppressed PD-w (**b**), and fat-suppressed contrast enhanced T1-w (**c**) MR images in a second patient, showing centrally increased signal (arrow) within the extensor carpi ulnaris tendon at the level of the distal radioulnar joint. Multiple slips of the abductor pollicis longus tendon (open arrow) are seen. They represent normal findings

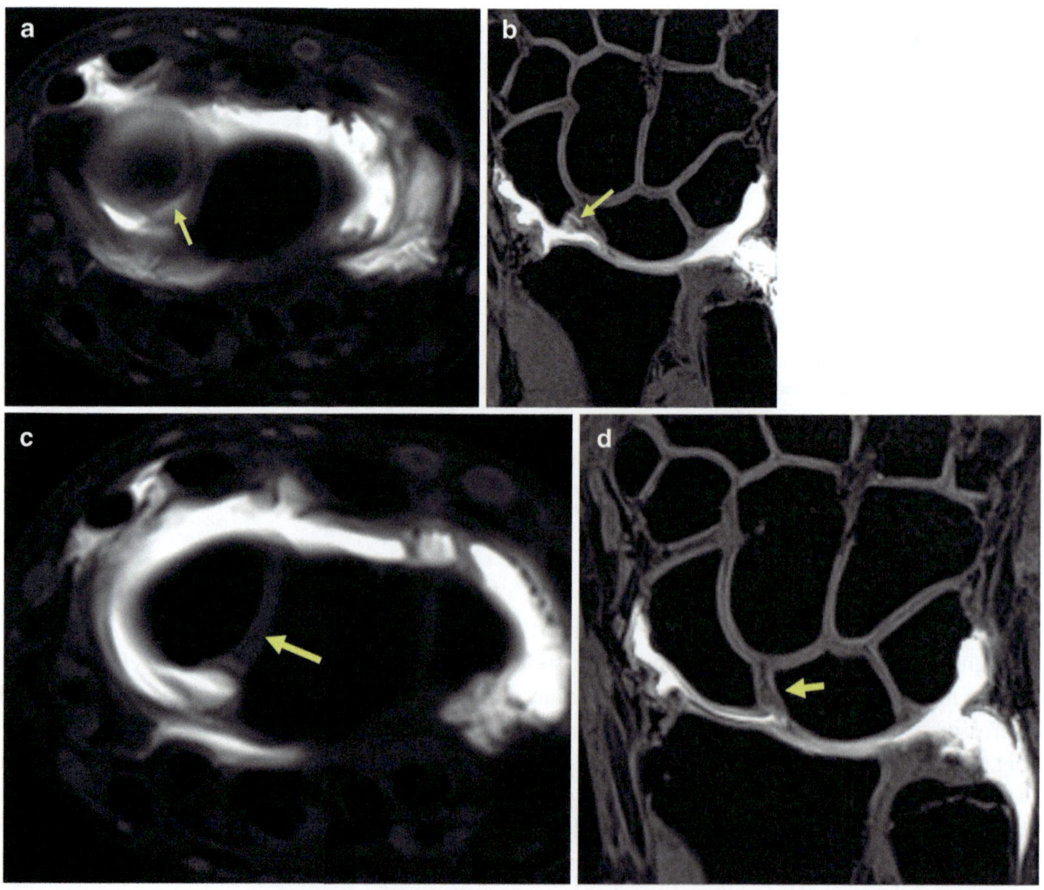

Fig. 22 Fat-suppressed axial T1-w (**a**) and coronal T1-w 3D Gradient echo (**b**) MR arthrographic images showing an asymptomatic defect of the palmar aspect of the scapholunate ligament (arrows). (**c, d**) corresponding images at the central part of the ligament show a normal appearance (arrows)

when the wrist is in different rotational positions (Pfirrmann and Zanetti 2005). Normally, the TFC proper returns low signal intensity on all pulse sequences (Pfirrmann and Zanetti 2005). However, the gradient echo sequences due to inherent lower S/N ratio and the thinner slices demonstrate the TFC proper with higher than the spin echo-based sequences signal, which is normal (Fig. 24). The thin central disc may not be seen in low-resolution images, producing the appearance of a perforation, and thus can be mistaken for a tear. Repeating the scan with higher-resolution images will reveal a thin but intact TFC. The TFC proper has one radial and two ulnar insertions. The radial attachment inserts to the styloid notch of the distal radius. The presence of hyaline cartilage on the tip of the radius may be misinterpreted as a tear (Fig. 24). The ulnar attachments of the TFC insert at the ulnar styloid and the ulnar fovea. The space between the ulnar insertions of the TFC is filled with vascularized connective tissue, shows normally intermediate to high signal intensity, which may be erroneously interpreted as an abnormality, and is referred to as ligamentum subcruentum (Fig. 24) (Burns et al. 2011; Zlatkin and Rosner 2004).

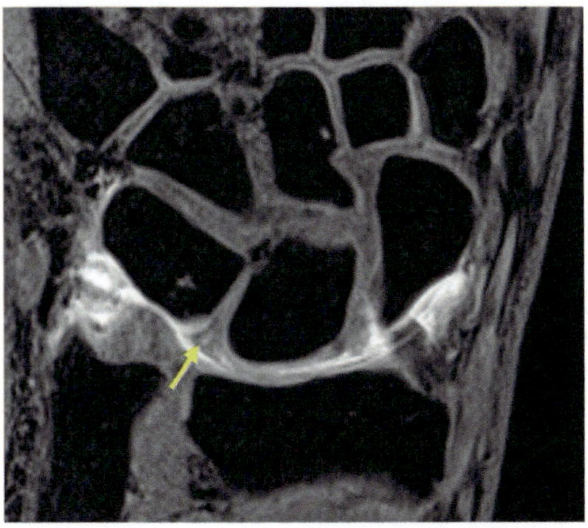

Fig. 23 Coronal T1-w 3D Gradient echo MR arthrographic images showing an asymptomatic defect of the lunotriquetral ligament (arrow)

5.3 Variants

5.3.1 Osseous Variants

5.3.1.1 Distal Radioulnar Joint

The distal radioulnar joint is a synovial pivot joint consisting of the sigmoid notch of the distal radius and the ulnar head. Coronal anatomy of

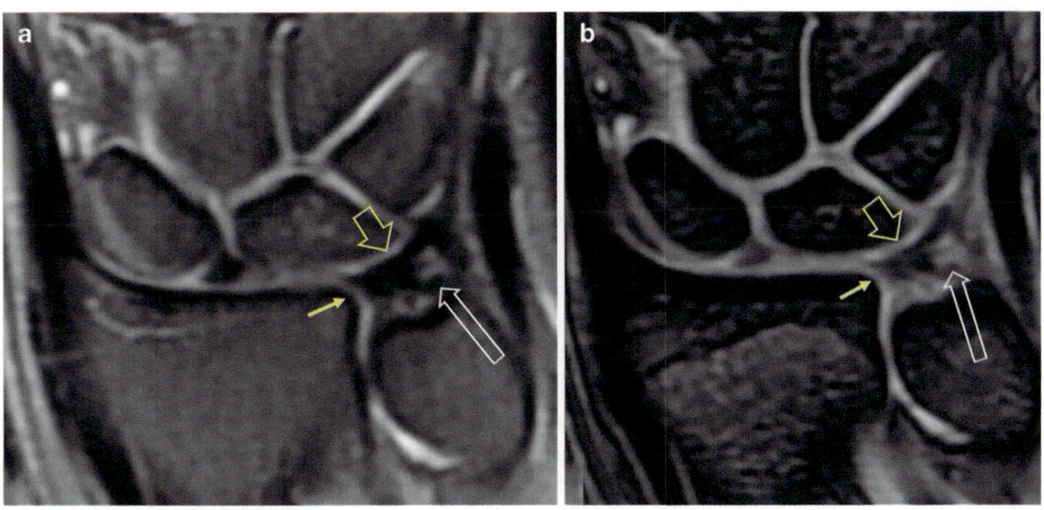

Fig. 24 Coronal fat-suppressed PD-w (**a**) and T2*-w (**b**) MR images. The radial attachment of the triangular fibrocartilaginous disc on the tip of the radius may be misinterpreted as a tear (small arrows). The signal of the disc is increased on the gradient echo sequence as compared to the PD-w (open arrows). The presence of vascularized connective tissue in the space between the ulnar insertions shows normally intermediate to high signal intensity, which may be erroneously interpreted as an abnormality (long open arrow)

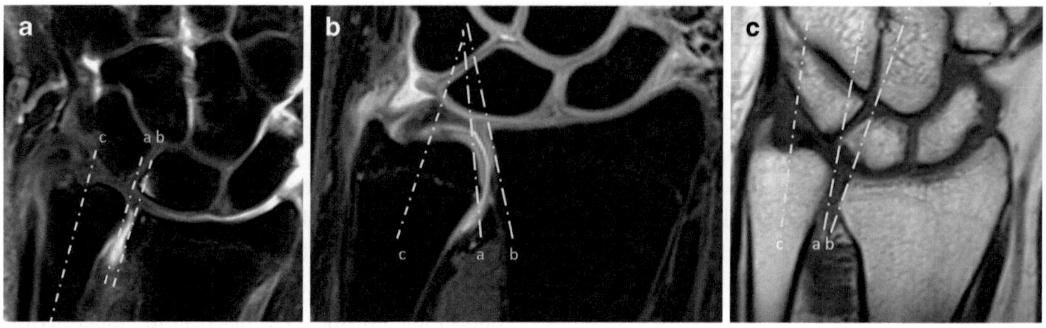

Fig. 25 Types of the distal radioulnar joint. (**a**) Type I: The opposing joint surfaces (a & b) are parallel to the long axis of the ulna (c). (**b**) Type II: The opposing joint surfaces (a & b) are oblique and have an ulnar deviation with respect to the long axis of the ulna (c). (**c**) Type III: The opposing joint surfaces (a & b) are oblique and have a radial deviation with respect to the long axis of the ulna (c)

the DRUJ varies significantly among individuals and is best assessed with plain radiographs. However, coronal MR images can classify the variants of the DRUJ anatomy, namely, type I or vertical seen in 38%, oblique or type II seen in 50%, and reverse or type III seen in 12% of cases (Fig. 25) (Tolat et al. 1992). In our practice (unpublished data), type I is seen in 4%, type II in 95%, and type III in 1%. Types II and III may result in impingement between the radial sigmoid notch and the ulnar articular surface followed by osteoarthritis, particularly in the setting of ulnar variance.

5.3.1.2 Ulnar Variance and Styloid

The ulnar variance denotes the relative length of the ulnar articular surface with respect to the articular margin of the radius, as measured on standard PA radiographs. MR imaging is not as accurate as plain radiographs in evaluating ulnar variance because of the variability of wrist positioning during scanning. Nevertheless, a rough estimation can be done on coronal T1-w images. A negative ulnar variance indicates that the ulna is >2 mm shorter than the radius, and a positive ulnar variance indicates >2 mm increase in length compared to the radius (Fig. 26). Neutral variance occurs when both bones are equal or differ in length by a maximum of 1 mm (Mellado et al. 2003). Thus, subtle alterations of ulnar variance should not be assessed without first evaluating the plain radiographs (Cerezal et al. 2002). The short ulna predisposes to Kienbock's disease and the long ulna to ulnar side impaction syndrome (Imaeda et al. 1996). The latter may result not only from a long ulna but can also be the result of an elongated styloid process if the latter has a length of ≥6 mm (Figs. 27 and 28). Absence of the ulnar styloid has been observed, but this is often attributed to previous trauma rather than developmental anomaly.

5.3.1.3 Lunate

Two distinct types of lunates have been described. Type I lunate bone articulates with the radius proximally, the scaphoid radially, the triquetrum ulnarly, and the capitate distally (Fig. 29a). Type II lunate has an additional facet as opposed to type I, articulating with the hamate (Fig. 29b) (Malik et al. 1999). The reported incidence for type I lunate ranges from 27% to 34.5% and for type II from 65.5% to 73%. The size of this extraarticular facet ranges in the majority of cases from 2 to 4.5 mm (Malik et al. 1999). Type II lunate predisposes to chondromalacia and osteoarthritis and can be a cause of ulnar-sided wrist pain (Sagerman et al. 1995). Arthroscopy and gross specimen analysis have shown that the prevalence of proximal hamate chondromalacia is higher than that reported solely on MRI, denoting that many cases remain occult on imaging (Malik et al. 1999). This may be attributable to the low hyaline articular cartilage thickness of the intercarpal joints, resulting in visualization difficulties (Zanetti et al. 2007). Chondromalacia should be strongly suspected when marrow

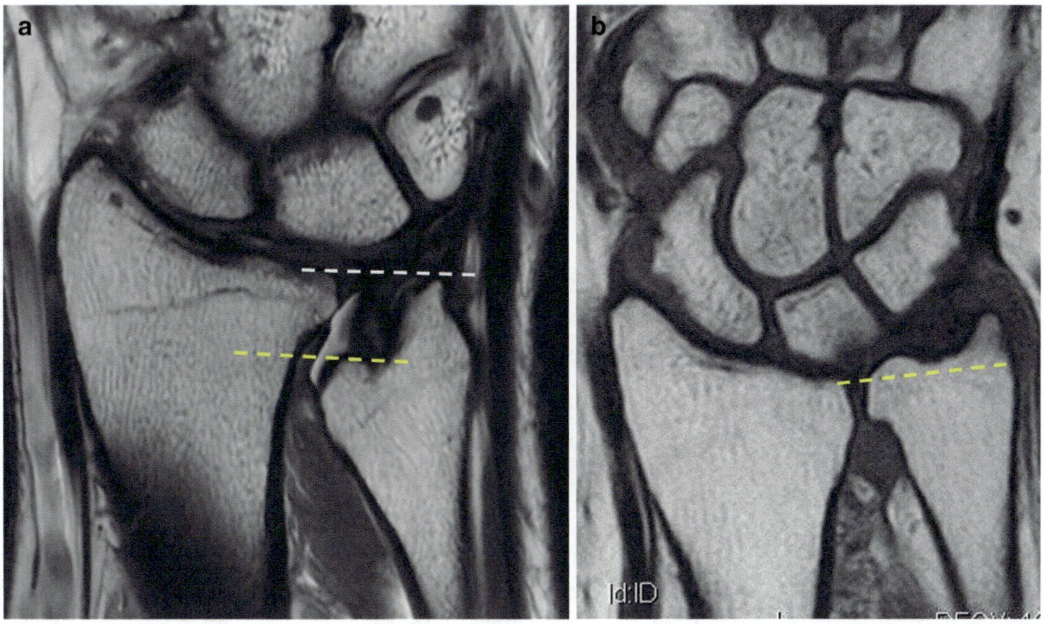

Fig. 26 Coronal T1-w MR images showing a negative ulnar variance (**a**) and a positive ulnar variance (**b**)

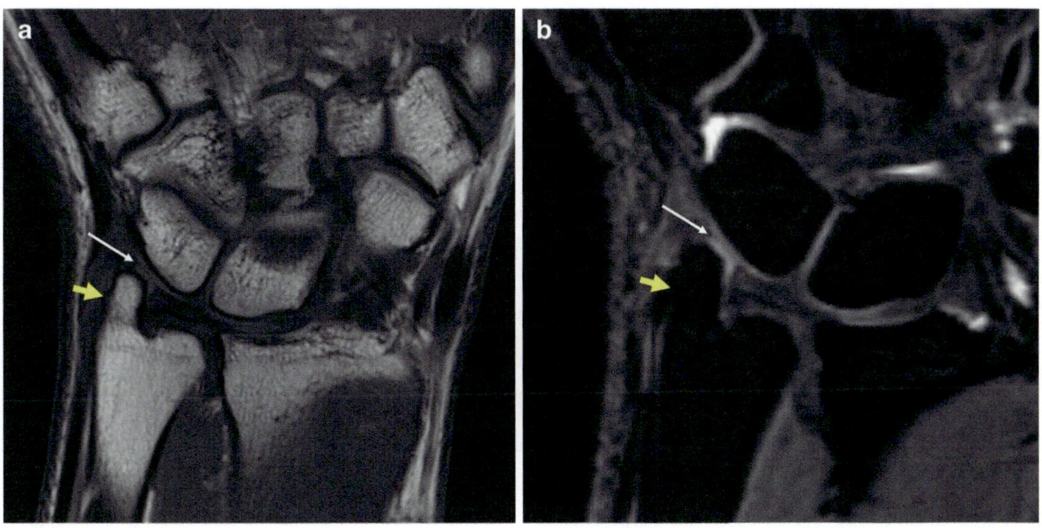

Fig. 27 Elongated or prominent ulnar styloid. Coronal T1-w (**a**) and fat-suppressed T1*-w (**b**) showing the increased (8 mm) length of the styloid (short arrows). The opposing articular surfaces of the styloid tip and the triquetrum are shown (thin arrow)

edema is present at the proximal pole of the hamate in patients with a type II lunate, especially in the absence of trauma (Malik et al. 1999). The corrugated appearance of the volar lunate surface as depicted on sagittal MR images is an additional normal variant (Fig. 29c). This may be due to the insertion of the radiolunotriquetral and short radiolunate ligaments or the penetration of multiple nutrient vessels (Berger and Landsmeer 1990). Lunate bipartition is a rare

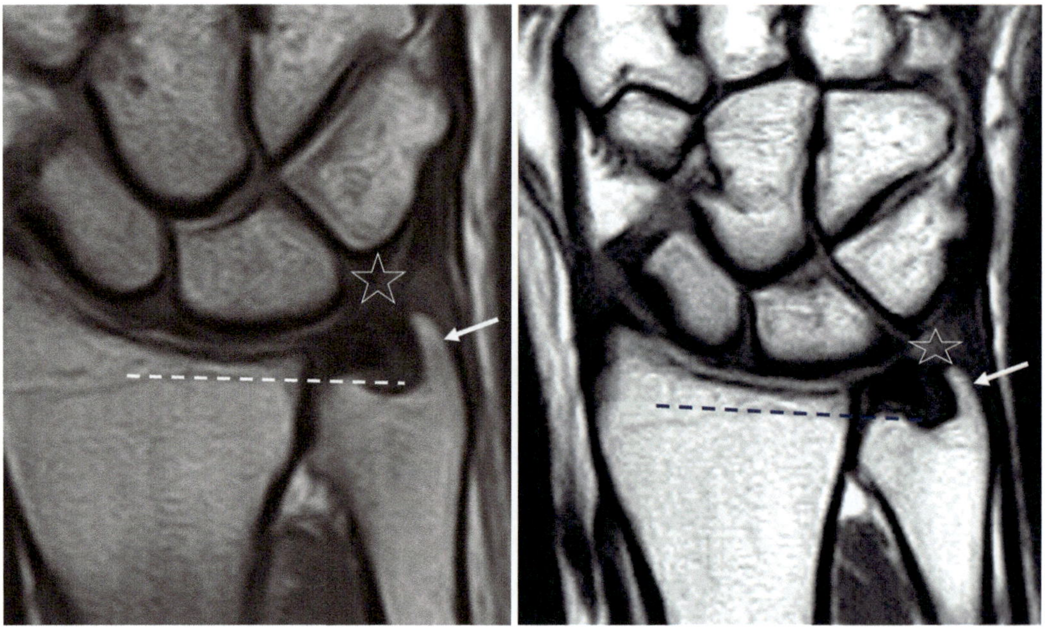

Fig. 28 Elongated or prominent ulnar styloid in two different patients. Coronal T1-w MR images showing the elongated process (arrows). The coexistence of minor ulnar variance (dashed lines), increased distance is shown between the tip of the process and the triquetrum (open star), and thus, the risk of ulnocarpal impaction syndrome is minimized

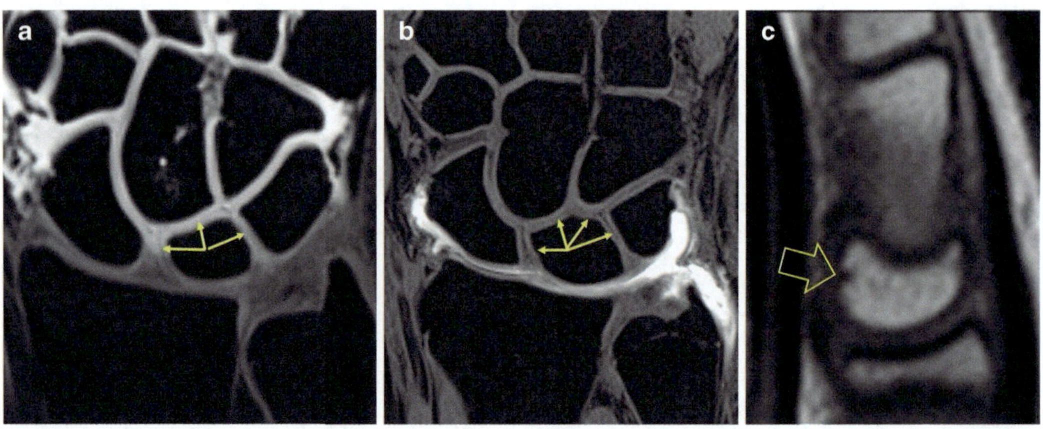

Fig. 29 Coronal fat-suppressed T1-w 3D gradient echo MR arthrographic images showing (arrows) type I lunate which articulates with scaphoid, capitate, and triquetrum (**a**) and type II lunate which articulates in addition to the hamate bone (**b**). Sagittal T1-w MR image showing the corrugated appearance of the volar lunate irregular surface (arrow) (**c**)

variant and MR imaging can differentiate this from lunate fracture and post-traumatic pseudoarthrosis (Akahane et al. 2002). The presence of hyaline cartilage detected between the articulation of the two ossicles on cartilage-specific sequences is diagnostic.

5.3.1.4 Scaphoid

Bipartite carpal scaphoid is a very rare developmental variant in which the scaphoid appears as two distinct bony fragments, one proximal and one distal, also known as "naviculare carpi secundarium radiale" and "ulnare," respectively (Freyschmidt and Brossmann 2011). Patients are usually asymptomatic. The following criteria of bipartite scaphoid are commonly encountered (Chang et al. 2015): bilateral presentation of this anomaly, absence of history or signs of previous injury, distinct space between the ossicles with round edges at the joint surfaces, equal size and similar bone density of each bony fragment, hyaline cartilage detected between the articulation of the two ossicles, and absence of degenerative changes between both parts and the radius. Congenital aplasia or hypoplasia of the scaphoid bone is very rare (Patankar 1998). It may be encountered either as an isolated finding or in association with anomalies of the thumbray, the wrist, the distal radius, and hypoplasia of the thenar and forearm muscles. Six types of scaphoid hypoplasia, ranging from mild hypoplasia of the thumb (type 1) to a four-fingered hand with hypoplastic radius (type 6), have been described (Davison 1962). MRI is inferior to X-rays, which can reliably reveal the spectrum of the above-mentioned osseous abnormalities. A rare variant is a bony outgrowth on the radial aspect of the middle third of the bone (Fig. 30). Proper diagnosis requires the absence of previous trauma or history of repetitive trauma.

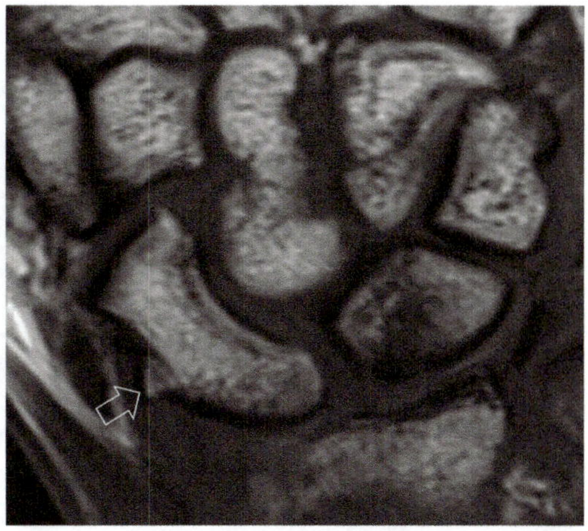

Fig. 30 Coronal T1-w MR image showing bony outgrowth on the mid-radial surface of the scaphoid bone in a patient who did not have any history of fracture or injury

5.3.1.5 Hamate

The hook of the hamate, also known as "hamulus," represents the radial border of the carpal tunnel and the ulnar border of the Guyon's canal. The hook is the insertion site of retinacula, tendons, and ligaments. An elongated hook is very rare and no distinct definition exists regarding its length (Fig. 31) (Davis 2017). Despite no published studies, it is reasonable to consider association between an elongated hook and Guyon's canal syndrome as well as with an increased risk for fractures, particularly in golfers. Bipartite hamulus is a rare variant and can be associated with Guyon's canal syndrome (Davis 2017). Recognition of a bipartite hamulus is important when planning open or endoscopic carpal tunnel release in order to avoid any injury to the ulnar neurovascular bundle (Chow et al. 2005).

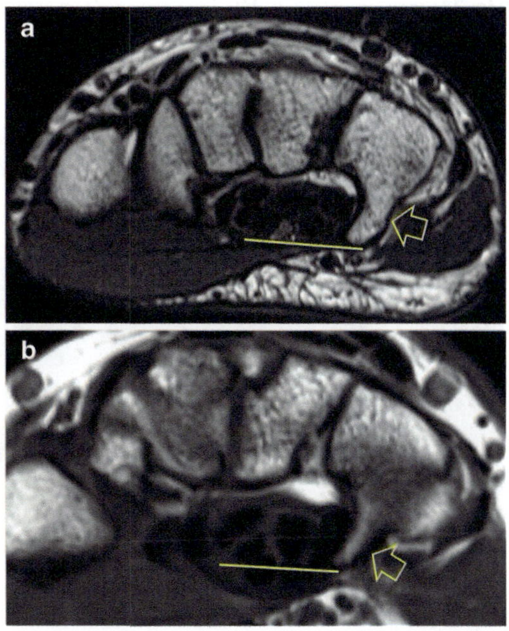

Fig. 31 Axial T1-w MR images. (**a**) An elongated hook of the hamate is shown. Its tip extends up the most palmar border of the carpal tunnel (arrow). (**b**) A normal sized hook crosses at the tip level the distal row of the flexor tendons (arrow)

5.3.1.6 Accessory Ossicles

Accessory ossicles of the wrist derive from unfused secondary ossification centers which are separate from the underlying bone. In selected cases, a previous trauma may have predisposed to

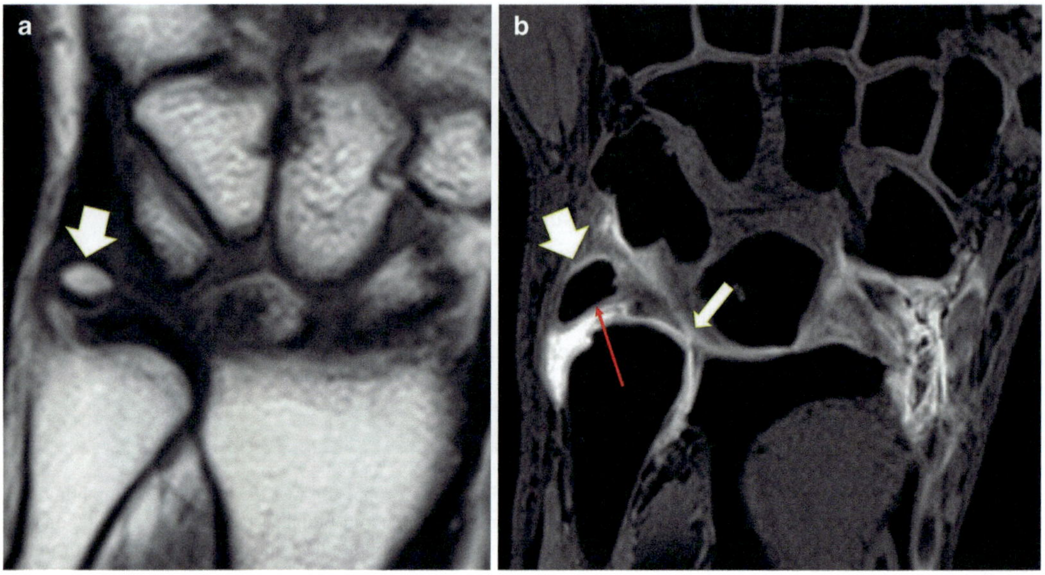

Fig. 32 (**a**) Coronal T1-w MR image showing a lunula (arrow). (**b**) Coronal fat-suppressed 3D T1-w gradient echo arthrographic MR image in a 24-year-old male patient with ulnar side pain, showing a TFC tear (arrow). A nonossified ulnar styloid ossification center is also shown (thick arrow) covered with articular cartilage (thin long arrow)

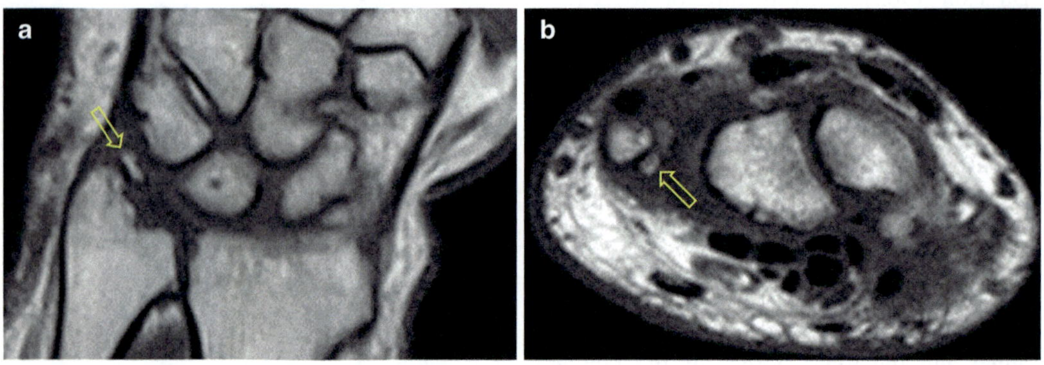

Fig. 33 Coronal (**a**) and axial (**b**) T1-w MR images showing an os triangulare (arrows) located between the ulnal styloid, lunate, and triquetrum

their appearance (Koehler and Zimmer 1993). Over 20 accessory bones may be encountered in the wrist. They frequently appear as incidental findings on wrist radiographs associated with little clinical significance. Their recognition is based on knowledge of their typical location, and radiologists should be aware to differentiate them from previous fractures. In MRI, the most valuable sequences for their depiction are the T1-w. The *lunula* is an accessory ossicle embedded in the meniscal homologue of the TFCC (Fig. 32a). The *persistent ulnar styloid ossicle* is the result of a failure of the ulna styloid ossification center to unite with the ulna (Fig. 32b). The *os triangulare* is located distal to the ulnar fovea and radially to the styloid process (Fig. 33). The *carpal boss*, also known as "*os styloideum*," is a bony excrescence varying in size which is located at the dorsal aspect of the wrist at the level of the carpometacarpal joints. It may be completely isolated, but in most cases it likely coalesces with the base of the second or third metacarpal bone

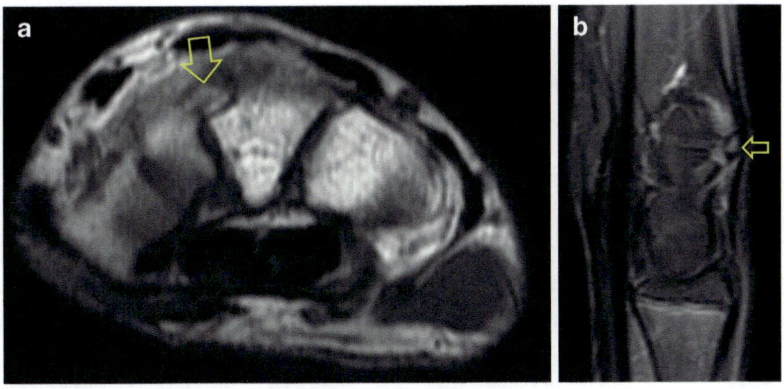

Fig. 34 Carpal boss. Axial T1-w (**a**) and sagittal fat-suppressed PD-w (**b**) MR images showing an os styloideum (arrows). Bone marrow edema in the os is in keeping with the symptoms of the patient

and even rarely with the capitate or the trapezoid (Conway et al. 1985). Patients with carpal boss are usually asymptomatic. However, in selected cases, pain and limitation of motion of the affected hand may be present (Conway et al. 1985). Bone marrow edemas depicted on MR images are strongly related with symptomatic os styloideum (Fig. 34). MRI can reliably demonstrate the morphologic variability of carpal boss as well as associated the soft tissue abnormalities (Mespreuve et al. 2017). CT may contribute to the preoperative planning due the thin sections it can provide (Park et al. 2008). Although the initial therapeutic approach is conservative, surgical treatment may be required in cases of failure. However, the wide excision of the carpal boss may lead to progressive joint instability (Park et al. 2008). The *trapezium secundarium* lies at the superomedial aspect of the trapezium.

5.3.1.7 Coalitions

Carpal coalition or carpal synostosis is a congenital osseous, fibrous, or cartilaginous fusion of wrist bones (Mellado et al. 2003). Idiopathic coalitions involve adjacent bones in the same carpal row. In syndrome-related coalitions, bones in adjacent rows may be engaged (Timins 1999a). Idiopathic coalitions have a general prevalence approximately 0.1%, are mostly bilateral, and most commonly encountered in black individuals with a female predilection (Delaney and Eswar 1992). The commonest isolated carpal fusion is the lunotriquetral, which has been classified into three types (Fig. 35). In the majority of cases, they are asymptomatic, but in a few partial (type 1) cases they may be painful (Simmons and McKenzie 1985). Scapholunate joint space diastasis may be normally observed in patients with a lunotriquetral coalition (Metz et al. 1993). The capitohamate, although infrequent, is the second commonest type of isolated coalition (Fig. 36). The pisiform-hamate and triquetrum-hamate coalitions are very rare (Fig. 37). Plain radiographs and MR images, including both T1-w and gradient echo sequences, can reliably distinguish partial or complete fusion and fibrous or cartilaginous fusion.

5.3.1.8 Congenital Absence or Hypoplasia of Carpal Bones

Extremely rare cases of bilateral and asymmetrical lunate hypoplasia without clinical symptoms as well as unilateral lunate hypoplasia associated with congenital scaphoid absence have been reported (Kobayashi et al. 1991). A rare congenital absence of the triquetrum accompanied by wrist pain and weakness of grip has been reported (Kao et al. 1996). Hypoplasia of the scaphoid bone should not be confused with a race compilation of scaphoid absorption following a previous fracture (Fig. 38).

5.3.2 Ligaments and Muscles

The central and the volar parts of the scapholunate ligament are usually of intermediate signal intensity, which should not be mistaken for

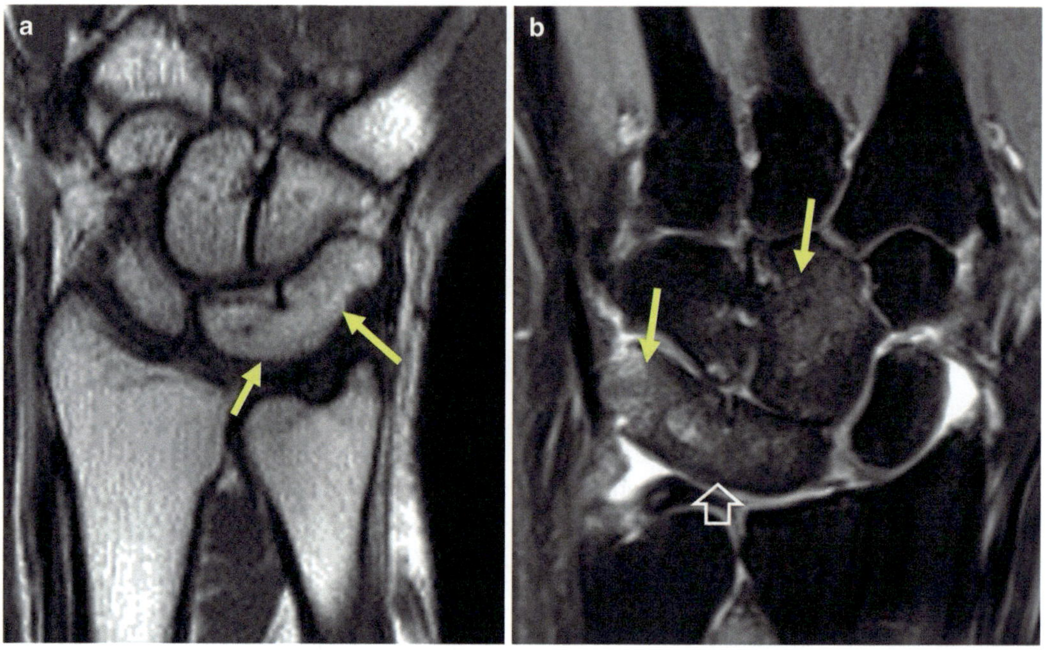

Fig. 35 (**a**) Coronal T1-w MR image showing lunotriquetral coalition (arrows). (**b**) Coronal fat-suppressed PD-w MR image in a patient with inflammatory arthritis of the wrist showing lunotriquetral coalition (open arrow) and joint effusion and bone marrow edema (arrows)

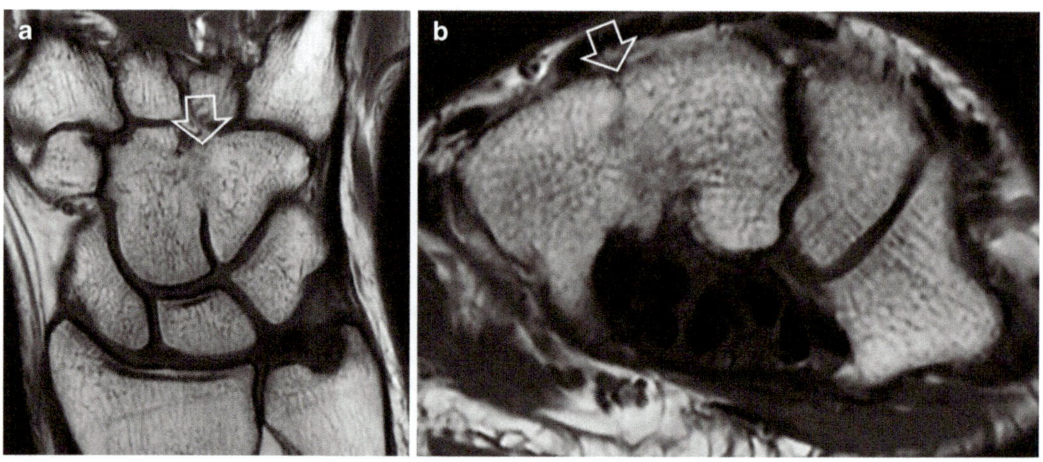

Fig. 36 Coronal (**a**) and axial (**b**) T1-w images show the capitohamate coalition (arrows)

degenerative change or tear. However, this signal should not be as bright as joint fluid on fluid-sensitive sequences (Smith 1994). The volar part of the ligament may also demonstrate a striated appearance. Both the shape and the signal intensity of the central part of both ligaments can be altered depending upon the wrist being in ulnar or radial deviation (Smith 1994; Smith and Snearly 1994).

The extrinsic ligaments of the wrist originate from the radius or the ulna and extend to the carpal and the metacarpal bones or even to the retinacula and tendons. They are best seen in MR imaging by utilizing 3D gradient echo sequences, with or without arthrography, in all planes (Fig. 39). Due to their inherent low signal-to-noise ratio, the thin section gradient echo images may result in striated rather than uniform low signal intensity of the ligaments. Although variants relating to the morphology and course of the ligaments may exist, there are no known pitfalls in this connection. Variants of the dorsal radiocarpal ligaments have been described according to the ligament appearance and its insertions: the ligament may present a single broadband, a branched appearance with separate triquetroscaphoid and triquetrotrapezial fascicles, complete separation of the triquetroscaphoid and the triquetrotrapezial fascicles, and a variant with the triquetrotrapezial fascicle being larger than the triquetroscaphoid. The radiotriquetral ligament may originate from a single ligament and can arise from the distal radius right next to Lister's tubercle or may have dual origin from the styloid process of the radius and Lister's tubercle.

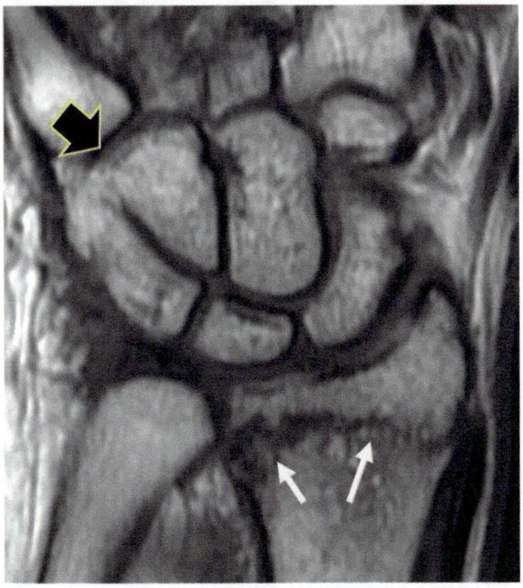

Fig. 37 Coronal T1-w MR image showing triquetrohamate coalition (thick arrow). A recent fracture of the distal radius is shown (arrows)

Muscle variants in the wrist are often incidental findings. The importance of the anomalous muscles lies in the fact that they can have clinical relevance when they are seen as unexplained mass-like lesions or when they result in compressive neuropathies (Pfirrmann and Zanetti 2005; Timins 1999b). An accessory *abductor digiti minimi* muscle is seen in about 24% of all wrists. It is usually asymptomatic but may cause compressive ulnar neuropathy. This muscle lies on the ulnar and palmar sides of the wrist and is usually seen as a fusiform mass lateral and anterior to the pisiform bone in close proximity to Guyon's canal on axial MR images (Fig. 40) (Rixey et al. 2021).

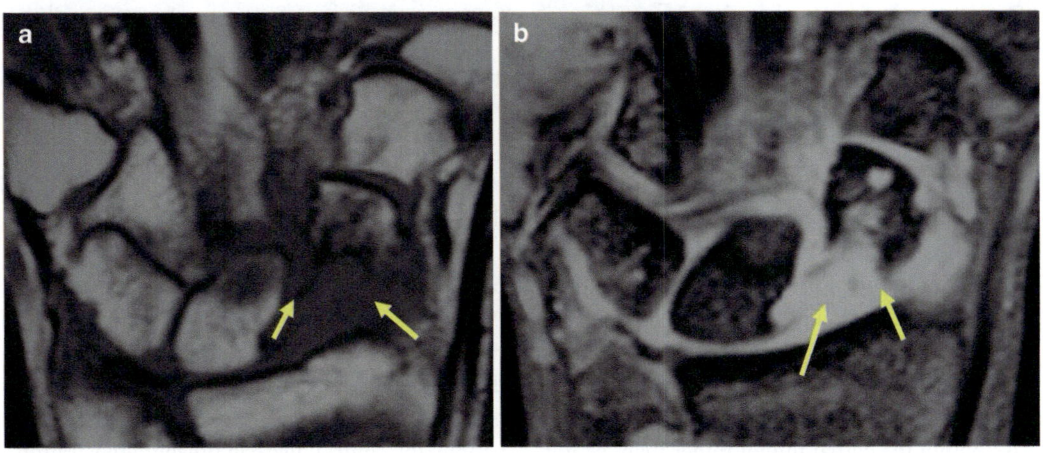

Fig. 38 Coronal T1-w (**a**) and fat-suppressed PD-w (**b**) MR images showing proximal scaphoid bone absorption following a previous fracture (arrows)

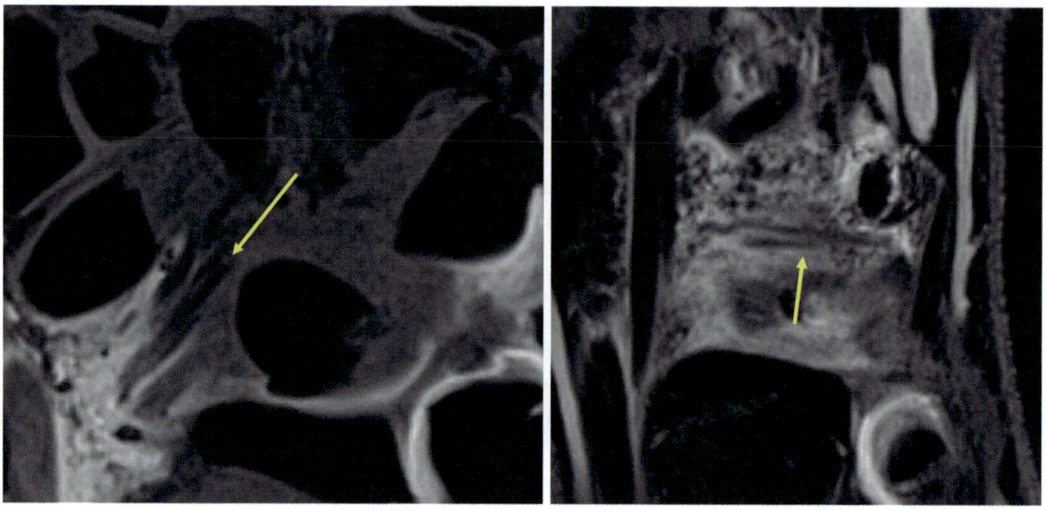

Fig. 39 Coronal T1-w MR arthrographic images demonstrate the striated appearance of the extrinsic ligaments in two different patients (arrows)

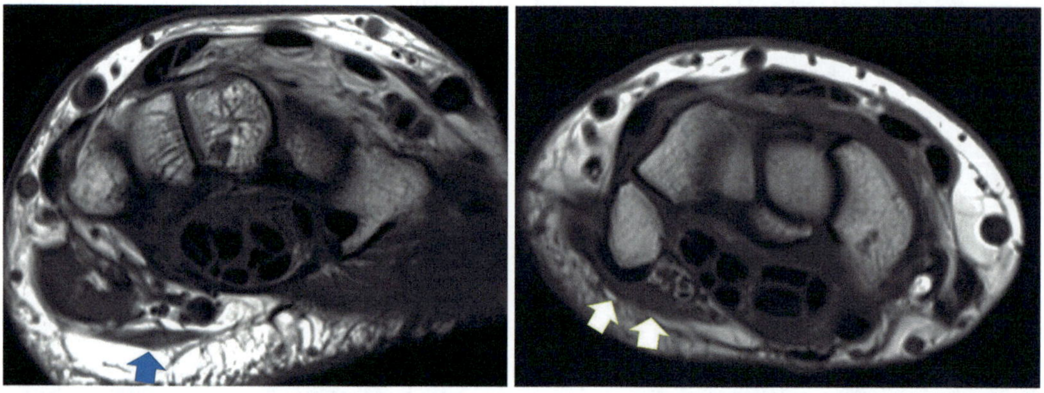

Fig. 40 Axial T1-w MR images in two patients, showing the various appearances of the accessory abductor digiti minimi muscle (arrows) in close proximity to the ulnar neurovascular bundle

The *extensor digitorum brevis manus* muscle is seen on approximately 1–3% of all wrists. It is located on the dorsal aspect of the wrist, within the 4th extensor tendon compartment and ulnarly to the extensor tendon of the index finger and can be mistaken clinically for a ganglion cyst (Fig. 41) (Rodríguez-Niedenführ et al. 2002). In about 22% of individuals, the *lumbrical* muscles arise within the carpal tunnel rather than, as normally expected, from the flexor tendons outside the tunnel (Pfirrmann and Zanetti 2005; Timins 1999b). Less frequently identified accessory muscles of the wrist include the *accessory flexor digitorum superficialis*, the *palmaris longus*, and the *flexor carpi ulnaris muscle* (Timins 1999b).

5.3.3 Triangular Fibrocartilage

An insertion of the disc over the entire length of the ulnar styloid process to its distal tip or along the ulnar head is a variant of the ulnar attachment (Fig. 42) (Zlatkin et al. 1989). In older people, the central disc can present fenestrations, which may be erroneously considered as tears. The ulnomeniscal homologue, located at the ulnar aspect of the radiocarpal joint between the triquetrum and the ulnar styloid, may have an

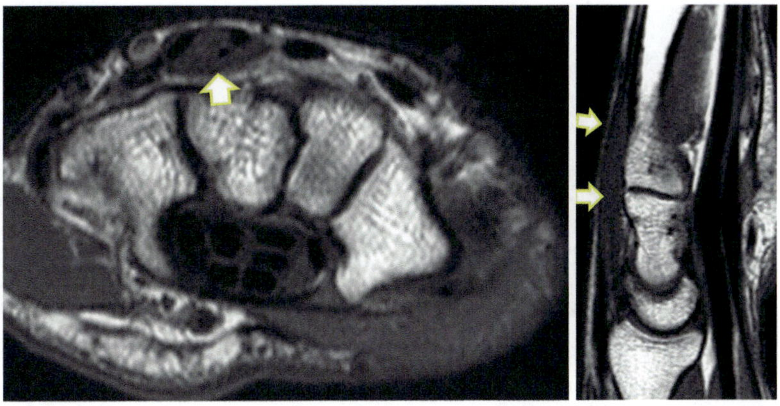

Fig. 41 Axial (left) and sagittal (right) T1-w MR images showing the accessory extensor digitorum brevis manus muscle (arrows)

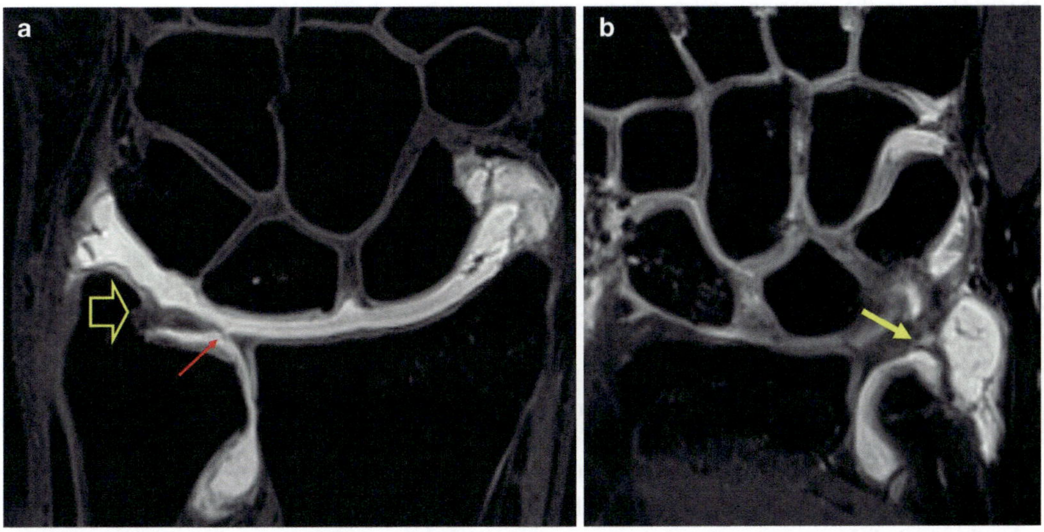

Fig. 42 Coronal fat-suppressed 3D T1-w MR arthrographic images. (**a**) The insertion of the disc covers the entire length of the ulnar styloid process (open arrow). A tear of the disc is shown on the radial aspect (arrow) allowing contrast migration to the distal radioulnar joint. (**b**) An opening of the ulnomeniscal homologue to the prestyloid recess (arrow) represents a normal variant

opening to the prestyloid recess which can be wide, narrow, or even absent (Fig. 42) (Buck et al. 2009). The prestyloid recess separates the ulnomeniscal homologue from the fibrocartilage and shows variations in shape, saccular being the more common (Stein et al. 2011; Zlatkin and Rosner 2004).

5.3.4 Nerves and Arteries

The median nerve at the distal boundary of the carpal tunnel usually splits into two or three distinct branches. A bifid median nerve bifurcates before or within the carpal tunnel and is a variant seen in 18% of wrists (Figs. 16 and 43) (Dag et al. 2022). These nerves are more prone to compression in the carpal tunnel since their cross-sectional area is proportionally larger than the single nerves. Normally, the median artery regresses after the eighth week of intrauterine life. In up to 15% of individuals, the median artery persists in adults. Persistent median artery usually originates from the ulnar artery and lies palmarly or radially to the median nerve in the tunnel. This variant may result in compression of

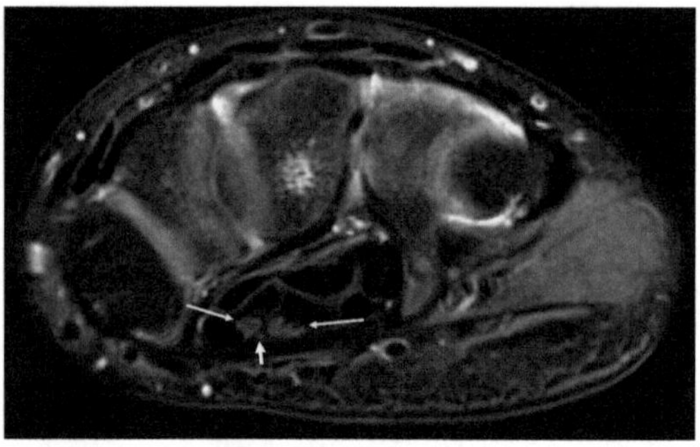

Fig. 43 Axial fat-suppressed intermediate weighted MR image showing a bifid median nerve (arrows) and a persistent median artery (short arrow)

the median or the anterior interosseous nerve. Accurate depiction is feasible using MR imaging (Fig. 43) (Dag et al. 2022).

6 Conclusion

Deep knowledge of the anatomy and the physical principles of MR imaging matched with a proper acquisition technique can lead to the depiction and accurate interpretation of pitfalls and artifacts. Variants of the normal anatomy are often encountered in the wrist and less frequently in the hand. Awareness of the normal anatomy as well as of the variants can help in distinguishing findings without any clinical significance from those related to pathology.

References

Akahane M, Ono H, Sada M, Saitoh M (2002) Bilateral bipartite lunate: a case report. J Hand Surg Am 27:355–359

Ali AH, Qenawy OK, Saleh WR, Ali AM, Abdul Monem ES, Omar NN (2022) Radio-carpal wrist MR arthrography: comparison of ultrasound with fluoroscopy and palpation-guided injections. Skeletal Radiol 51:765–775

Andreisek G, Kilgus M, Burg D, Saupe N, Crook DW, Meyer V, Marincek B, Weishaupt D (2005) MRI of the intrinsic muscles of the hand: spectrum of imaging findings and clinical correlation. AJR Am J Roentgenol 185:930–939

Andreisek G, Duc SR, Froehlich JM, Hodler J, Weishaupt D (2007) MR arthrography of the shoulder, hip, and wrist: evaluation of contrast dynamics and image quality with increasing injection-to-imaging time. AJR Am J Roentgenol 188:1081–1088

Bateni CP, Bartolotta RJ, Richardson ML, Mulcahy H, Allan CH (2013) Imaging key wrist ligaments: what the surgeon needs the radiologist to know. AJR Am J Roentgenol 200:1089–1095

Berger RA, Landsmeer JM (1990) The palmar radiocarpal ligaments: a study of adult and fetal human wrist joints. J Hand Surg Am 15:847–854

Block KT, Uecker M, Frahm J (2008) Suppression of MRI truncation artifacts using total variation constrained data extrapolation. Int J Biomed Imaging 2008:184123

Buck FM, Gheno R, Nico MAC, Haghighi P, Trudell DJ, Resnick D (2009) Ulnomeniscal homologue of the wrist: correlation of anatomic and MR imaging findings. Radiology 253:771–779

Burns JE, Tanaka T, Ueno T, Nakamura T, Yoshioka H (2011) Pitfalls that may mimic injuries of the triangular fibrocartilage and proximal intrinsic wrist ligaments at MR imaging. Radiographics 31:63–78

Cerezal L, del Piñal F, Abascal F, García-Valtuille R, Pereda T, Canga A (2002) Imaging findings in ulnar-sided wrist impaction syndromes. Radiographics 22:105–121

Cerezal L, Abascal F, García-Valtuille R, Del Piñal F (2005) Wrist MR arthrography: how, why, when. Radiol Clin North Am 43:709–731, viii

Chang AC, Leonello DT, Webb JM (2015) Congenital bipartite scaphoid. J Hand Surg Eur Vol 40:537–538

Chang EY, Bencardino JT, French CN (2024) SSR white paper: guidelines for utilization and performance of direct MR arthrography. Skeletal Radiol 53:209–244

Choi JY, Kang HS, Hong SH, Lee JW, Kim NR, Jun WS, Moon SG, Choi JA (2008) Optimization of the contrast mixture ratio for simultaneous direct MR and CT arthrography: an in vitro study. Korean J Radiol 9:520–525

Chow JCY, Weiss MA, Gu Y (2005) Anatomic variations of the hook of hamate and the relationship to carpal tunnel syndrome. J Hand Surg Am 30:1242–1247

Conway WF, Destouet JM, Gilula LA, Bellinghausen HW, Weeks PM (1985) The carpal boss: an overview of radiographic evaluation. Radiology 156:29–31

Dag F, Dirim Mete B, Gursoy M, Uluc ME (2022) Variations ignored in routine wrist MRI reports: prevalence of the median nerve anatomical variations and persistent median artery. Acta Radiol 63:76–83

Dallaudière B, Meyer P, Larbi A, Moinard M, Moreau-Durieux M-H, Poussange N, Pelé E, Pesquer L (2015) Magnetic resonance arthrography of the wrist with axial traction: An iconographic review. Diagn Interv Imaging 96:1307–1312

Davis DL (2017) Hook of the hamate: The spectrum of often missed pathologic findings. AJR Am J Roentgenol 209:1110–1118

Davison EP (1962) Congenital hypoplasia of the carpal scaphoid bone. J Bone Joint Surg Br 44-B:816–827

Del Grande F, Santini F, Herzka DA, Aro MR, Dean CW, Gold GE, Carrino JA (2014) Fat-suppression techniques for 3-T MR imaging of the musculoskeletal system. Radiographics 34:217–233

Delaney TJ, Eswar S (1992) Carpal coalitions. J Hand Surg Am 17:28–31

Ehman EC, Felmlee JP, Frick MA (2015) Imaging of the proximal and distal radioulnar joints. Magn Reson Imaging Clin N Am 23:417–425

Elentuck D, Palmer WE (2004) Direct magnetic resonance arthrography. Eur Radiol 14:1956–1967

ESSR (2016) ESSR guidelines for MR imaging of sports injuries [WWW Document]. URL https://www.essr.org/content-essr/uploads/2016/10/ESSR-MRI-Protocols-Wrist.pdf

Fleming JL 2nd, Dodd L, Helms CA (2005) Prominent vascular remnants in the calcaneus simulating a lesion on MRI of the ankle: findings in 67 patients with cadaveric correlation. AJR Am J Roentgenol 185:1449–1452

Freyschmidt J, Brossmann J (2011) Koehler/Zimmer's borderlands of normal and early pathological findings in skeletal radiography. Thieme Medical, Stuttgart

Gilula LA, Weeks PM (1978) Post-traumatic ligamentous instabilities of the wrist. Radiology 129:641–651

Hauger O, Chung CB, Lektrakul N, Botte MJ, Trudell D, Boutin RD, Resnick D (2000) Pulley system in the fingers: normal anatomy and simulated lesions in cadavers at MR imaging, CT, and US with and without contrast material distention of the tendon sheath. Radiology 217:201–212

Hersh B, D'Auria J, Scott M, Fowler JR (2019) A comparison of Ultrasound and MRI measurements of the cross-sectional area of the median nerve at the wrist. Hand (N Y) 14:746–750

Imaeda T, Nakamura R, Shionoya K, Makino N (1996) Ulnar impaction syndrome: MR imaging findings. Radiology 201:495–500

Kao SD, Watson HK, Fong D (1996) Congenital triquetral absence: a case report of an asymptomatic wrist. J Hand Surg Am 21:314–316

Karantanas A, Dailiana Z, Malizos K (2007) The role of MR imaging in scaphoid disorders. Eur Radiol 17:2860–2871

Kobayashi H, Kosakai Y, Usui M, Ishii S (1991) Bilateral deficiency of ossification of the lunate bone. A case report. J Bone Joint Surg Am 73:1255–1256

Koehler A, Zimmer E (1993) Borderlands of normal and early pathologic findings in skeletal radiography. Thieme Verlag, New York

Kreuz PC, Steinwachs M, Angele P (2018) Single-dose local anesthetics exhibit a type-, dose-, and time-dependent chondrotoxic effect on chondrocytes and cartilage: a systematic review of the current literature. Knee Surg Sports Traumatol Arthrosc 26:819–830

Lenkinski RE, Rofsky NM (2024) Contrast media-driven anthropogenic gadolinium: Knowns and unknowns. Radiology 311:e240020

Malik AM, Schweitzer ME, Culp RW, Osterman LA, Manton G (1999) MR imaging of the type II lunate bone: frequency, extent, and associated findings. AJR Am J Roentgenol 173:335–338

Malone WJ, Snowden R, Alvi F, Klena JC (2010) Pitfalls of wrist MR imaging. Magn Reson Imaging Clin N Am 18:643–662

Mellado JM, Calmet J, Domènech S, Saurí A (2003) Clinically significant skeletal variations of the shoulder and the wrist: role of MR imaging. Eur Radiol 13:1735–1743

Mespreuve M, De Smet L, De Cuyper K, Waked K, Vanhoenacker F (2017) MRI diagnosis of carpal boss and comparison with radiography. Acta Radiol 58:1245–1251

Metz VM, Schimmerl SM, Gilula LA, Viegas SF, Saffar P (1993) Wide scapholunate joint space in lunotriquetral coalition: a normal variant? Radiology 188:557–559

Morelli JN, Runge VM, Ai F, Attenberger U, Vu L, Schmeets SH, Nitz WR, Kirsch JE (2011) An image-based approach to understanding the physics of MR artifacts. Radiographics 31:849–866

Moser T, Dosch J-C, Moussaoui A, Buy X, Gangi A, Dietemann J-L (2008) Multidetector CT arthrography of the wrist joint: how to do it. Radiographics 28:787–800; quiz 911

Omoumi P, Mercier GA, Lecouvet F, Simoni P, Vande Berg BC (2009) CT arthrography, MR arthrography, PET, and scintigraphy in osteoarthritis. Radiol Clin North Am 47:595–615

Park MJ, Namdari S, Weiss A-P (2008) The carpal boss: review of diagnosis and treatment. J Hand Surg Am 33:446–449

Patankar H (1998) Bilateral congenital aplasia of the scaphoid. J Hand Surg Br 23:817–819

Patel RP, McGill K, Motamedi D, Morgan T (2023) Ultrasound-guided interventions of the upper extremity joints. Skeletal Radiol 52:897–909

Petchprapa CN, Vaswani D (2019) MRI of the fingers: An update. AJR Am J Roentgenol 213:534–548

Pfirrmann CWA, Zanetti M (2005) Variants, pitfalls and asymptomatic findings in wrist and hand imaging. Eur J Radiol 56:286–295

Plotkin B, Sampath SC, Sampath SC, Motamedi K (2016) MR Imaging and US of the wrist tendons. Radiographics 36:1688–1700

Rastogi AK, Davis KW, Ross A, Rosas HG (2016) Fundamentals of joint injection. AJR Am J Roentgenol 207:484–494

Rixey A, Wenger D, Baffour F, Kakar S, McKenzie G (2021) Accessory abductor digiti minimi muscle, less muscular than thought: an update on prevalence, morphology, and review of the literature. Skeletal Radiol 50:1687–1695

Rodríguez-Niedenführ M, Vázquez T, Golanó P, Parkin I, Sañudo JR (2002) Extensor digitorum brevis manus: anatomical, radiological and clinical relevance. A review. Clin Anat 15:286–292

Sagerman SD, Hauck RM, Palmer AK (1995) Lunate morphology: can it be predicted with routine x-ray films? J Hand Surg Am 20:38–41

Simmons BP, McKenzie WD (1985) Symptomatic carpal coalition. J Hand Surg Am 10:190–193

Smith DK (1994) Scapholunate interosseous ligament of the wrist: MR appearances in asymptomatic volunteers and arthrographically normal wrists. Radiology 192:217–221

Smith DK, Snearly WN (1994) Lunotriquetral interosseous ligament of the wrist: MR appearances in asymptomatic volunteers and arthrographically normal wrists. Radiology 191:199–202

Smith J, Rizzo M, Sayeed YA, Finnoff JT (2011) Sonographically guided distal radioulnar joint injection: technique and validation in a cadaveric model. J Ultrasound Med 30:1587–1592

Stein JM, Cook TS, Simonson S, Kim W (2011) Normal and variant anatomy of the wrist and hand on MR imaging. Magn Reson Imaging Clin N Am 19:595–608; ix

Taljanovic MS, Karantanas A, Griffith JF, DeSilva GL, Rieke JD, Sheppard JE (2012) Imaging and treatment of scaphoid fractures and their complications. Semin Musculoskelet Radiol 16:159–173

Timins ME (1999a) Osseous anatomic variants of the wrist: findings on MR imaging. AJR Am J Roentgenol 173:339–344

Timins ME (1999b) Muscular anatomic variants of the wrist and hand: findings on MR imaging. AJR Am J Roentgenol 172:1397–1401

Tolat AR, Sanderson PL, De Smet L, Stanley JK (1992) The gymnast's wrist: acquired positive ulnar variance following chronic epiphyseal injury. J Hand Surg Br 17:678–681

Ugas MA, Huynh BH, Fox MG, Patrie JT, Gaskin CM (2014) MR arthrography: impact of steroids, local anesthetics, and iodinated contrast material on gadolinium signal intensity in phantoms at 1.5 and 3.0 T. Radiology 272:475–483

Vassa R, Garg A, Omar IM (2020) Magnetic resonance imaging of the wrist and hand. Pol J Radiol 85:e461–e488

Yilmaz A, Bozer C, Uluçam E, Taşkinalp O (2009) An anomaly of flexor muscles of the fifth (little) finger of the hand: an anatomical case report. Clinics (Sao Paulo) 64:1133–1135

Zanetti M, Hodler J, Gilula LA (1998) Assessment of dorsal or ventral intercalated segmental instability configurations of the wrist: reliability of sagittal MR images. Radiology 206:339–345

Zanetti M, Saupe N, Nagy L (2007) Role of MR imaging in chronic wrist pain. Eur Radiol 17:927–938

Zlatkin MB, Rosner J (2004) MR imaging of ligaments and triangular fibrocartilage complex of the wrist. Magn Reson Imaging. Clin N Am 12:301–331, vi–vii

Zlatkin MB, Chao PC, Osterman AL, Schnall MD, Dalinka MK, Kressel HY (1989) Chronic wrist pain: evaluation with highresolution MR imaging. Radiology 173:723–729

Nuclear Medicine Imaging of the Hand and Wrist

Anbalagan Kannivelu, Godwin Jeeva, and Wilfred C. G. Peh

Contents

Abstract

Bone scintigraphy is the most common and oldest nuclear medicine technique being used to evaluate the musculoskeletal system, including the hands and wrists. Because of their widespread availability and better resolution over the last few decades, advanced imaging choices such as computed tomography (CT) and magnetic resonance imaging have replaced many nuclear medicine techniques as first line investigations. However, triphasic bone scintigraphy remains the investigation of choice in a few unique indications such as reflex sympathetic dystrophy. Recently, single photon emission computed tomography/CT and positron-emission tomography/CT have revolutionized nuclear medicine imaging because of three-dimensional imaging ability and better anatomical correlation that enable accurate interpretation of equivocal findings. Increasing availability of advanced hybrid scanners and invention of new tracers will enable nuclear medicine techniques to regain the lost turf in musculoskeletal imaging.

Abbreviations

[^{18}F]-FDG	[^{18}F]-Fluorodeoxyglucose
[^{18}F]-NaF	[^{18}F]-Sodium fluoride
^{111}In/In-111	Indium-111

A. Kannivelu (✉) · W. C. G. Peh
Department of Diagnostic Radiology, Khoo Teck Puat Hospital, Singapore, Republic of Singapore
e-mail: dranbukan@gmail.com; wilfred.peh@gmail.com

G. Jeeva
Gemini Scans, Vadapalani, Chennai, India
e-mail: godwinjeeva@gmail.com

Med Radiol Diagn Imaging (2025)

https://doi.org/10.1007/174_2025_608,
Published Online: 24 August 2025

^{18}F/F-18	Fluorine-18
^{67}Ga/Ga-67	Gallium-67
^{99m}Tc/Tc-99m	Technetium-99m
^{99m}Tc-MDP	^{99m}Tc-methyl diphosphonate
CT	Computed tomography
MBq	Megabecquerel
mCi	Millicurie
MRI	Magnetic resonance imaging
PET	Positron-emission tomography
SPECT	Single photon emission computed tomography

1 Introduction

Bone scintigraphy is a useful imaging technique that complements radiographic examination of the hands and wrists in certain clinical indications. It can help in the evaluation of avascular necrosis of the scaphoid, occult fractures, reflex sympathetic dystrophy, and arthritis. Sometimes, Technetium-99m (^{99m}Tc)-labelled leukocytes and Gallium-67 (^{67}Ga) scintigraphy can be used to diagnose infection in the hands and wrists. Due to rapid recent advances in the development of new positron-emission tomography (PET) tracers and their widespread availability, PET/computed tomography (CT) has also become useful for the evaluation of various pathologies of musculoskeletal system, including the hands and wrists.

2 Bone Scintigraphy

2.1 Technique

Bone scintigraphy is the primary nuclear medicine imaging technique using radioactive tracers to evaluate distribution of active bone formation and destruction in the skeleton. Bone scintigraphy is highly sensitive and detects metabolic abnormality, which happens in the bones before morphological changes can be identified on radiographs. The radiotracers most used for performing bone scan are ^{99m}Tc-labelled radiopharmaceuticals, such as ^{99m}Tc-methyl diphosphonate (^{99m}Tc-MDP), ^{99m}Tc-hydroxymethylene diphosphonate (^{99m}Tc-HMDP), and ^{99m}Tc-hydroxyethylene diphosphonate (^{99m}Tc-HDP). Tc-99m decays by isomeric transition with emission of 140.5 keV gamma rays per decay and a half-life of 6.02 h. In adults, 555–740 MBq of ^{99m}Tc MDP (15–20 mCi) is intravenously administered for the procedure. These tracers attach to the bone matrix by chemisorption in proportion to hyperemia and osteoblastic activity.

The preferred approach for the evaluation of the hands and wrists is by three-phase bone scintigraphy including blood flow, blood pool, and delayed bone phases rather than single-phase delayed bone scan (Fig. 1). The angiographic phase images are obtained in the first minute after injection at 1–3 s per frame, intermediate blood pool phase images are obtained at 3–5 min per frame within 10–15 min, and delayed bone scan is usually obtained after 3 h. Sometimes, four-phase bone scintigraphy is performed with an additional scan around 24 h, to differentiate osteomyelitis from cellulitis (Streek et al. 1998; Van den Wyngaert et al. 2016).

The hybrid imaging technique single photon emission computed tomography (SPECT)/CT has become widely available and can be utilized as an additional technique in bone scintigraphy for evaluation of the hands and wrists. Anatomical information of the CT images adds value to metabolic information of SPECT and provides three-dimensional (3D) imaging with accurate localization of abnormal increased tracer uptake. SPECT/CT improves the specificity of bone scintigraphy by clarifying equivocal findings and reducing false-positives (Kannivelu et al. 2021).

2.2 Normal Variants and Pitfalls

Bone scintigraphy is not sensitive for small and purely lytic lesions without bone reaction. Bone scintigraphy has limited specificity because of accumulation of tracer at locations of degenerative changes, stress-associated changes, soft tissue inflammation, and physiological extraosseous uptake. Proper positioning of both hands in a near-symmetrical position is essential to obtain

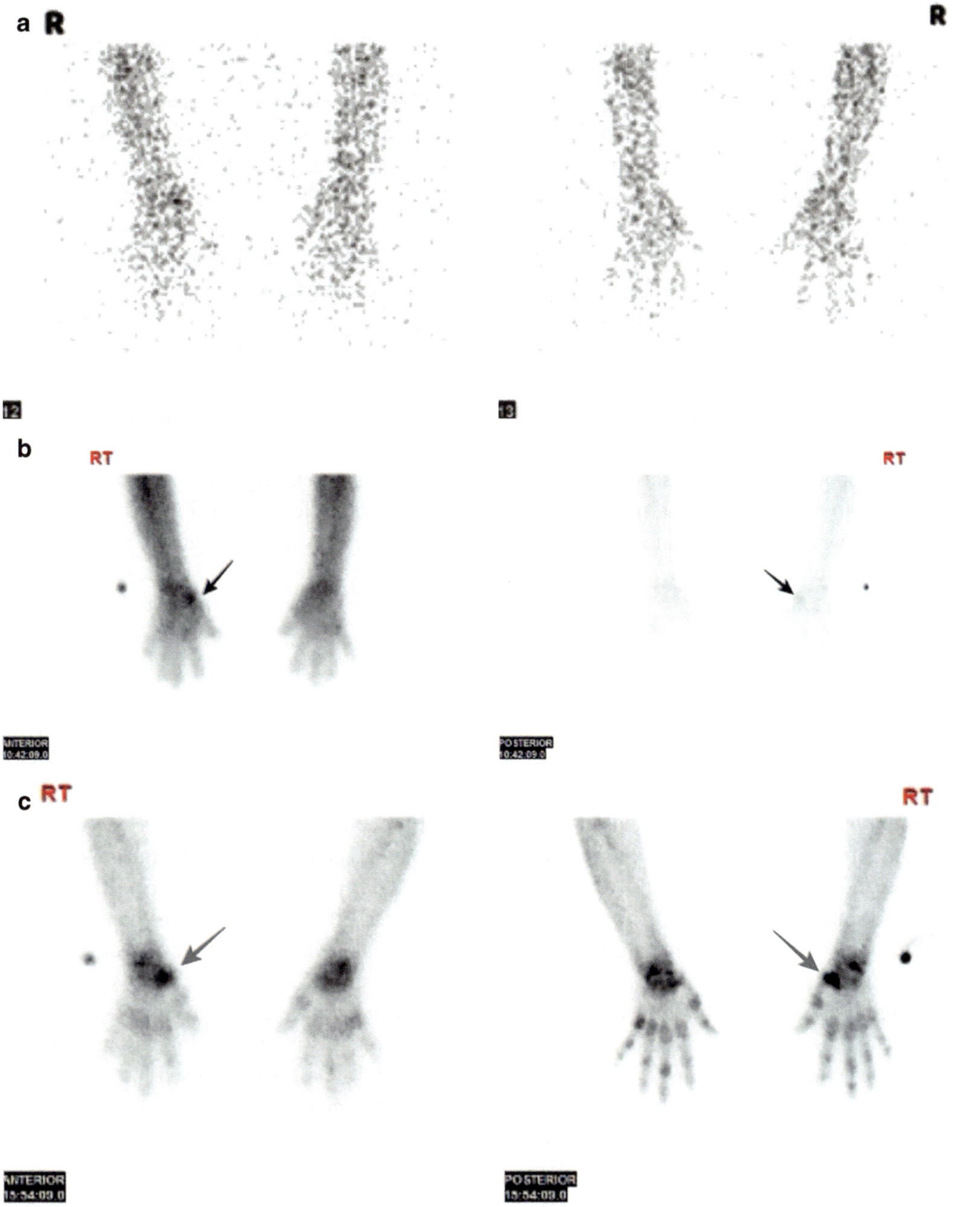

Fig. 1 Triphasic bone scintigraphy was performed for a patient presenting with non-specific right wrist pain. (**a**) Blood flow images showed mildly increased asymmetric tracer distribution to right forearm, wrist, and hand. (**b**) Blood pool images show focal increased tracer accumulation in the radial aspect of the right wrist (black arrows). (**c**) Delayed bone scan images show more intense tracer localization in the right 1st carpometacarpal joint (grey arrows) amidst the background degenerative changes of both wrist joints and small joints of both hands. These findings were suggestive active inflammation in that joint and confirmed the clinical diagnosis of seronegative inflammatory arthritis

good images which are comparable. Tracer should be injected away from both hands and wrists and if possible in the lower limb veins, to avoid confusion between vascular and osseous tracer activity. Prior radiotherapy may reduce the tracer uptake because of matrix loss and prior instrumentation may increase the tracer uptake due to reactive changes.

Extraosseous increased tracer uptake seen in enthesopathy, myositis, and heterotopic bone formation after trauma may obscure the bones. Bone scintigraphy performed immediately after radiotherapy and chemotherapy can result in increased tracer uptake due to false-positive osteoblastic reaction and it is called "flare response." Knowledge about normal variants and pitfalls due to physiological changes and prior intervention is essential to correctly interpret the true abnormal lesions in bone scintigraphy (Gnanasegaran et al. 2009).

3 Other Techniques: Infection Imaging

Radiopharmaceuticals such as Gallium-67, Technetium-99m or Indium-111 are used for the assessment of osteomyelitis and soft tissue infections. Even though they are currently not primary modalities for investigation of infection, they add value when other imaging results are equivocal. ^{67}Ga-citrate scintigraphy was an old nuclear medicine imaging choice and widely used the early 1970s to mid-1980s. The physical half-life of ^{67}Ga is 78 h. After administering 150–250 MBq of ^{67}Ga-citrate, imaging is done at few time points between 17 and 72 h. The usual administered dose is 150–220 MBq, up to 330 MBq in larger patients. ^{67}Ga scintigraphy is usually reserved for chronic infections.

^{99m}Tc-labelled leukocyte scintigraphy is preferred for acute infection and inflammation. ^{99m}Tc-labelled leukocyte imaging is performed within 4 h after the injection of radiotracers. The scans performed for infection imaging are often compared and interpreted together with bone scintigraphy or sulphur colloid marrow imaging to increase diagnostic accuracy. Incongruous lesions with more uptake in infection imaging are highly suspicious for focus of infection or inflammation (Seabold et al. 1997; Love and Palestro 2004; Kannivelu et al. 2021).

4 Positron-Emission Tomography

PET/CT is extensively used for oncological imaging and staging for various cancers due to its increasing availability, high resolution, improvement in the time of procedure, and cost efficiency. It is evolving into a single stop imaging technique for evaluation of local extension, regional spread, and distant metastases for various malignancies. Two most widely used PET tracers for skeletal imaging are [^{18}F]-Fluorodeoxyglucose ([^{18}F]-FDG) and [^{18}F]-sodium fluoride ([^{18}F]-NaF). The physical half-life of ^{18}F is 110 min, and it reaches a plateau of accumulation around 45 min. The routine dose of [^{18}F]-FDG is 370–740 MBq and the scan is performed after 1–2 h to achieve a good tumor-to-background ratio. Compared to [^{18}F]-FDG, the uptake of [^{18}F]-NaF is more specific to bones and has similar pharmacokinetics to ^{99m}Tc-MDP. The routine dose of [^{18}F]-NaF is 185–370 MBq and the scan is done approximately1 h after injection. In few specific clinical situations, special tracers are used. For example, in neuroendocrine tumors, Gallium-68 (^{68}Ga)-DOTA-peptide is used and in metastatic prostate cancers, and ^{68}Ga-PSMA is used for whole-body imaging (Kannivelu and Peh 2024).

5 Nuclear Medicine Techniques for Specific Clinical Conditions in the Hand and Wrist

Nuclear medicine imaging is very useful in few clinical scenarios where conventional radiographs and advanced imaging techniques such as

CT and magnetic resonance imaging (MRI) are equivocal for establishing the diagnoses. Correct selection between bone scintigraphy and PET/CT, tailored imaging protocols, and awareness about the various pattern of tracer uptake and their limitations will help to make accurate diagnoses for further management.

5.1 Trauma and Complications

Radiographs are usually the first imaging modality performed for the evaluation of suspected fractures and assessment of osseous alignment of the hands and wrists. CT plays an important role in preoperative planning for complex fractures and dislocations. MRI is the primary imaging modality for diagnosis of occult fractures and soft tissue injuries of the hands and wrists in the event of trauma (Balzer et al. 2021). Before the era of MRI, triphasic bone scintigraphy was used to identify fractures, which are not conspicuous on radiographs. In an acute fracture, abnormal localization of tracer is seen on all the three phases of bone scintigraphy. Nuclear medicine imaging is also helpful in the examination of subsequent complications of trauma such as post-traumatic arthritis, hardware loosening, periprosthetic fracture, and infection (Streek et al. 1998).

The scaphoid is the most common carpal bone to be fractured and second only to distal radius fracture among the injuries of wrist. Scaphoid fracture occurs often after a fall on an outstretched hand and patients classically present with pain in the anatomical snuff box. Almost two-thirds of fractures occur across the waist of scaphoid and about half are transversely oriented. Approximately one-third of the fractures of the middle third and most of the fractures of the proximal pole are associated with non-union and osteonecrosis. Bone scintigraphy can be performed for occult fractures where the patient is symptomatic and radiographs are negative even after 2 weeks (Holder et al. 1995).

A systematic review and meta-analysis conducted by Yin et al. (2010) for comparison of the diagnostic performance of bone scintigraphy, MRI, and CT for suspected scaphoid fractures included 26 studies. The pooled sensitivity and specificity were, respectively, 97% and 89% for bone scintigraphy, 96% and 99% for MRI, and 93% and 99% for CT. They concluded that bone scintigraphy was comparable to MRI in sensitivity, but less specific due to false-positive uptake in bone bruise, soft tissue injury, and inflammation of the adjacent joints (Yin et al. 2010).

Patients with reflex sympathetic dystrophy (RSD), which is also known as complex regional pain syndrome type I, often present with pain, swelling, tenderness, vasomotor disturbances, dystrophic skin changes, and motor abnormalities. Not all patients present with the classical symptoms of RSD. Patchy demineralization, juxta-articular and subchondral lysis of the bones with or without soft tissue swelling can be seen on radiographs. Bone scintigraphy shows increased tracer distribution in the blood flow phases and increased periarticular uptake in multiple joints in the delayed phase images (Fig. 2). For bone scintigraphy, the reported sensitivity ranges from 60% to 96%, with a specificity of 92%. Bone scintigraphy is the cornerstone of imaging for RSD, especially when the radiographs are negative (Streek et al. 1998). The diagnosis of RSD can be confused by co-existing pathologies such as arthritis and diabetic neuropathy. Steroids are the mainstay of the treatment for RSD and it can be detrimental to other pathologies. Hence, confirmation of RSD is necessary before initiating steroid treatment.

In a prospective study conducted by Shehab et al. (2005), triphasic bone scintigraphy was performed for 20 consecutive patients referred for RSD with suspicious clinical symptoms. Steroids and physiotherapy were given to nine patients who had positive scan findings. All the seven patients for whom complete follow-up was available showed significant clinical improvement with reduced pain and improved range of motion.

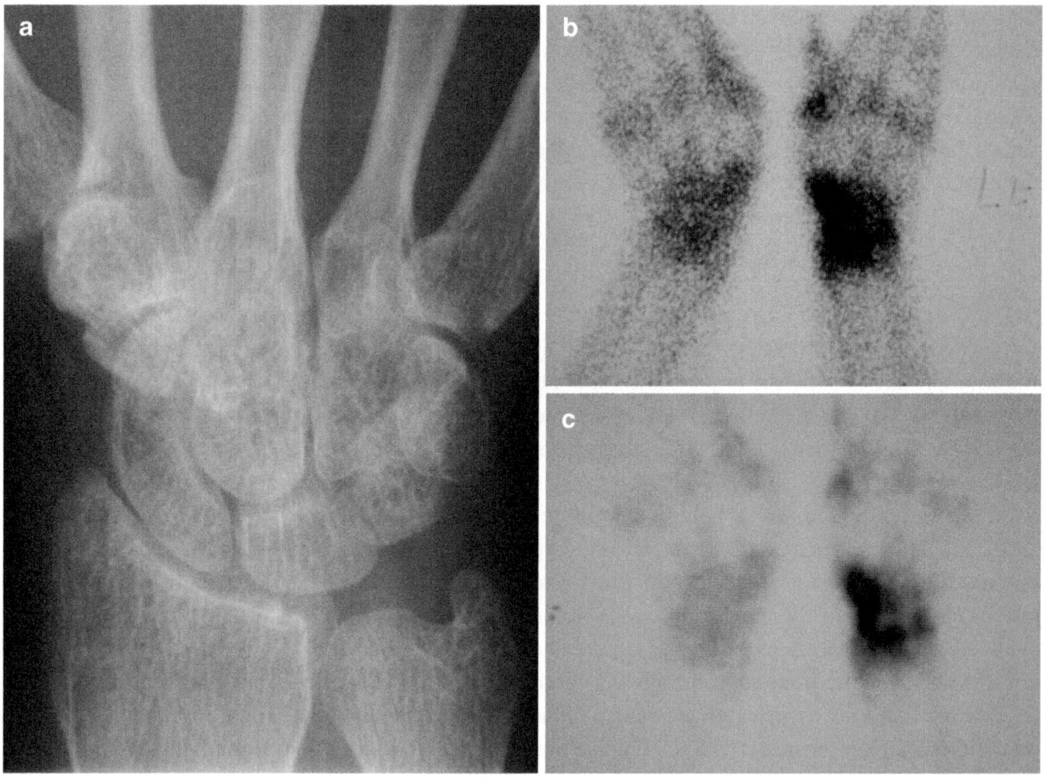

Fig. 2 Patient with reflex sympathetic dystrophy secondary to wrist injury. (**a**) Anteroposterior radiograph shows mild generalized osteoporosis. Triphasic bone scintigraphic (**b**) blood pool and (**c**) delayed bone scan images show markedly increased intense isotope uptake in the carpal bones. (Reproduced with permission from Quek and Peh (2002))

For the remaining 11 patients, the final diagnoses were osteoarthritis 6, healing fracture 2, inflammatory arthritis 1, lymphedema 1, and carpal tunnel syndrome 1. Steroids were not given to these patients except for one who had inflammatory arthritis. None of these patients developed contractures and trophic skin changes of long-standing untreated RSD. This study established the diagnostic role of triphasic bone scintigraphy in RSD and more importantly, its significant impact on the clinical management (Shehab et al. 2005).

5.2 Arthritis

In recent years, nuclear medicine imaging has been widely used to characterize and diagnose inflammatory and infectious arthritis. Rheumatoid arthritis is a chronic persistent inflammatory synovitis caused by increased neovascularity, increased capillary permeability, and exudation of plasma proteins into the synovial stroma, leading to cartilage destruction, bone erosion, and joint destruction. Bone scintigraphy is relatively more sensitive and reflects disease activity better than clinical and radiographical evaluation. In the early or acute stage of arthritis, triphasic bone scintigraphy shows increased blood pool activity, with or without increased periarticular increased uptake. In the advanced stage or treated disease, reduced tracer uptake is seen in bone scintigraphy, with joint deformity on radiographs. Continued increased tracer uptake in the chronic stages is suspicious for persistent subclinical synovitis. Bone scintigraphy can also identify tenosynovitis and bursitis associated with rheumatoid arthritis.

Hybrid SPECT/CT increases specificity further in clinical practice by combining the anatomical information of CT with tracer activity of SPECT, permitting better characterization of equivocal lesions in small joints (Rosado-de-Castro et al. 2014; Choi and Kim 2017). Similarly, in [^{18}F]-FDG PET/CT, increased [^{18}F]-FDG is seen in the joints involved in rheumatoid arthritis because of synovitis and pannus formation. Palmer et al. (1995) compared [^{18}F]-FDG PET/CT and MRI for 12 patients with rheumatoid arthritis under anti-inflammatory treatment and found that both modalities were strongly correlated with clinical findings in the wrists and these techniques permitted quantification of joint inflammation (Palmer et al. 1995). Abdelhafez et al. (2022) conducted a prospective study for the evaluation of total body [^{18}F]-FDG PET/CT in patients with autoimmune arthritis and concluded that there was high concordance of PET/CT findings with joint-by-joint rheumatological evaluation, moderate-to-strong correlation with outcome measures, and that [^{18}F]-FDG PET/CT had the ability to potentially detect subclinical disease activity which accounted for approximately 20% of the joints involved (Abdelhafez et al. 2022).

In osteoarthritis, increased tracer uptake seen in bone scintigraphy is related to the rate of subchondral bone turnover and growing and remodeling osteophytes. Pattern of tracer uptake in SPECT is helpful to differentiate rheumatoid arthritis, which shows preferential central tracer uptake, from osteoarthritis which shows eccentric tracer uptake in the joints. Uptake in SPECT matches the areas of marrow edema and destruction on MRI (Ostendorf et al. 2006). Quantitative measurements based on modern methods of iterative SPECT/CT reconstructed images can potentially overcome the subjective bias of visual analysis. Patients with rheumatoid arthritis consistently show higher frequency and intensity of tracer uptake based on standardized uptake value (SUV) measurements than osteoarthritis, and it is likely associated with higher bone turnover. In addition, relative highest SUV uptake in proximal interphalangeal joints, metacarpophalangeal joints, and wrist joints can distinguish rheumatic arthritis from other conditions such as fibromyalgia and osteoarthritis (Lim et al. 2022) (Fig. 3).

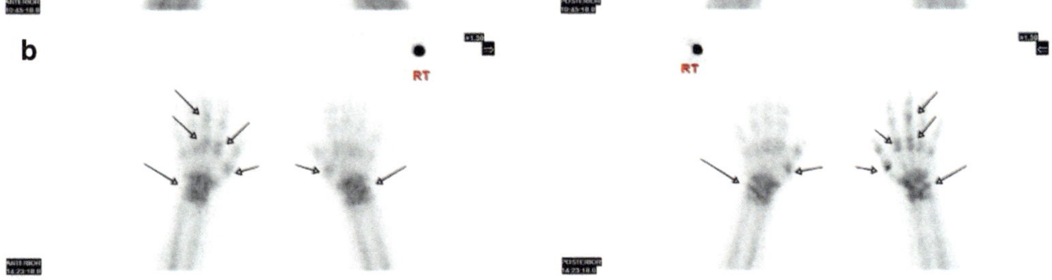

Fig. 3 Patient with clinical suspicion of rheumatoid arthritis. Triphasic bone scintigraphic (**a**) blood pool images show mildly increased tracer accumulation in both wrists, more on the left. (**b**) Delayed bone scan images show relatively more intense tracer uptake in both wrists (L > R), metacarpophalangeal joints (bilateral 1st and left 2nd and 3rd) and left middle finger proximal interphalangeal joint (black open arrows) with sparing of distal interphalangeal joints. Joint involvement pattern was consistent with rheumatoid arthritis

5.3 Infection

Infection of the hand and wrist may occur as a result of trauma, laceration, contiguous spread, penetrating injury, or by hematogenous spread. Three-phase or four-phase bone scintigraphy is useful in differentiating soft tissue infection from osteomyelitis. The sensitivity of triphasic bone scintigraphy is high, ranging from 76% to 100%, but specificity is only 45%. Normal bone scintigraphy almost completely excludes active infection because of its high negative predictive value (Sambri et al. 2021). ^{67}Ga and ^{99m}Tc- or ^{111}In-labelled leukocyte scintigraphy is sometimes used for the assessment of infection of the hand and wrist. Radiolabeled leukocyte scintigraphy has higher specificity than bone scintigraphy for the evaluation of appendicular musculoskeletal system infection and is helpful in the presence of previous surgery or fractures. Hybrid fusion imaging techniques such as SPECT/CT discriminate the soft tissue and bone infection better by providing additional morphological information (Streek et al. 1998; Sambri et al. 2021).

5.4 Malignancy

Bone scintigraphy remains the primary imaging modality for the initial evaluation and assessment of treatment response of bone metastases. For the detection of bone metastases, bone scintigraphy has sensitivity of 78% and specificity of 48%. Additional SPECT/CT improves both sensitivity and specificity to 87% and 91%, respectively (O'Sullivan 2015). However, metastases to bones of the hands are rare, with a reported incidence of just 0.1%. It is associated with a poor prognosis with median survival of 5–6 months, because they are often overlooked initially due to rarity of the condition (Morris et al. 2017). Most of the tumors and tumor-like swellings in the hand and wrist are usually benign. Malignancy accounts for less than 10% of the tumors in hand and wrist, of which majority arise from the skin and soft tissue (Fig. 4). Bone scintigraphy is used for staging in proven malignancies of the hand and wrist (Thomas et al. 2011).

Bone tumors of the hand and wrist can be broadly classified into cartilaginous and osseous lesions. The most common benign cartilaginous tumors are enchondroma, osteochondroma, chondroblastoma, and chondromyxoid fibroma. The most common primary cartilaginous tumor, enchondroma, is frequently found in the medullary portion of tubular bones of the hands. They are mostly asymptomatic. If pain is present, patients should be evaluated for pathological fracture or malignant transformation. Ollier's disease and Maffuci's syndrome are associated with multiple enchondromas with more propensity to undergo sarcomatous transformation. Bone scintigraphy shows mild to moderately increased tracer uptake in benign tumors and moderate to intensely increased tracer uptake in malignant tumors, with significant overlap. If the tracer uptake in bone scintigraphy is more intense and present as ring-like or donut-shaped pattern of increased activity localized to the peripheral portion of the tumor, it suggests that the lesion is more likely to be malignant (Giudici et al. 1993; Streek et al. 1998).

Among the osseous lesions, frequently seen bone islands or enostosis demonstrate normal to mildly increased tracer uptake on bone scintigraphy. Osteoid osteoma is a benign osteoblastic tumor that typically presents with night pain which is classically relieved by aspirin and other nonsteroidal anti-inflammatory drugs. Bone scintigraphy shows increased uptake within the lesion, which may take the form of a "double density." Cystic tumors such as unicameral and aneurysmal bone cysts usually show increased uptake in the periphery. If they

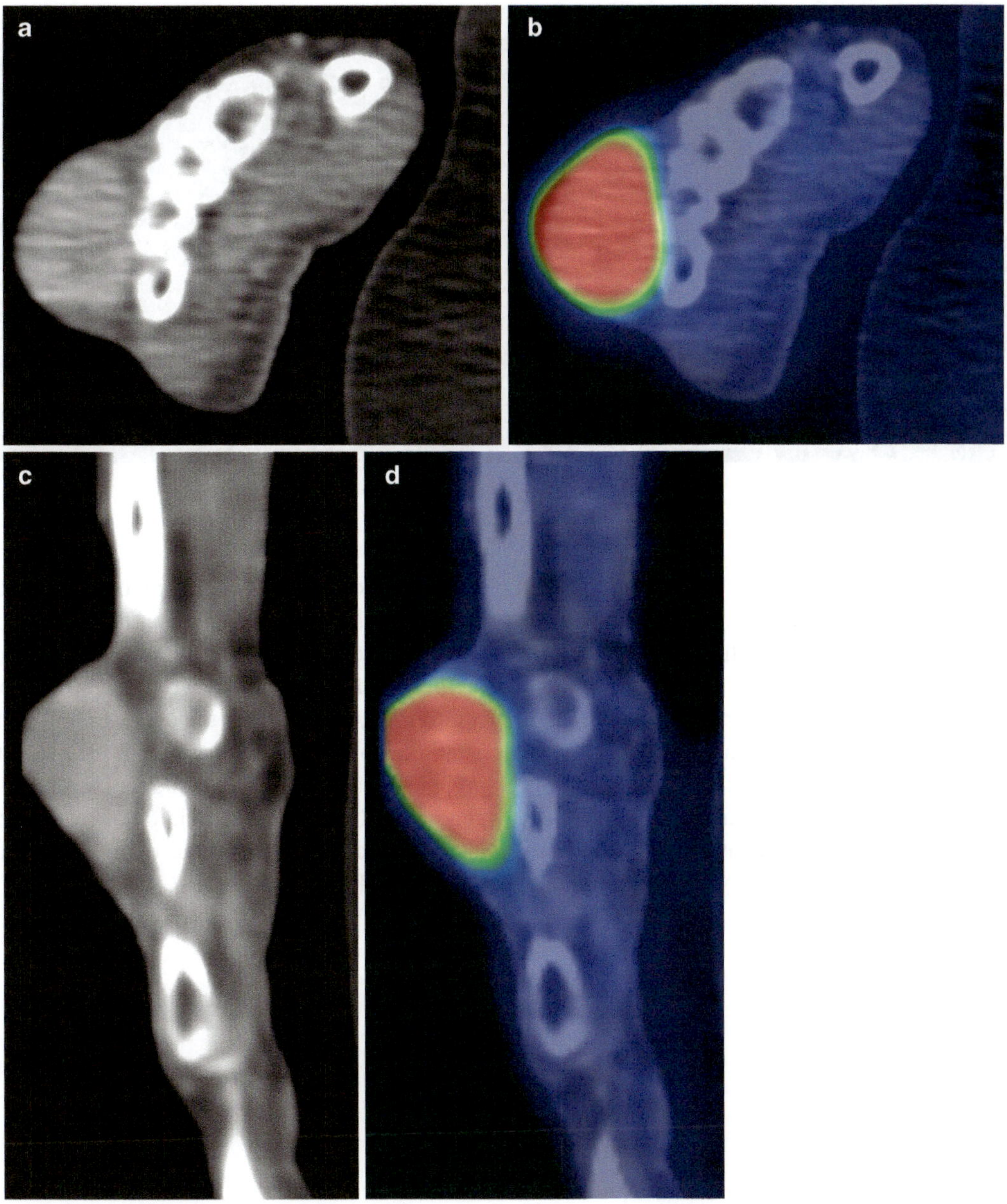

Fig. 4 Patient presenting with swelling in the dorsum of the right wrist. Axial (**a**) CT and (**b**) fusion and sagittal (**c**) CT and (**d**) fusion PET/CT images show a dense intensely FDG-avid soft tissue dense mass at the ulnar aspect of the dorsum of the wrist. Histological diagnosis was soft tissue sarcoma. (**e**) Axial T1-W MR image shows an infiltrating soft tissue tumor with encasement of the adjacent extensor tendons (white arrows)

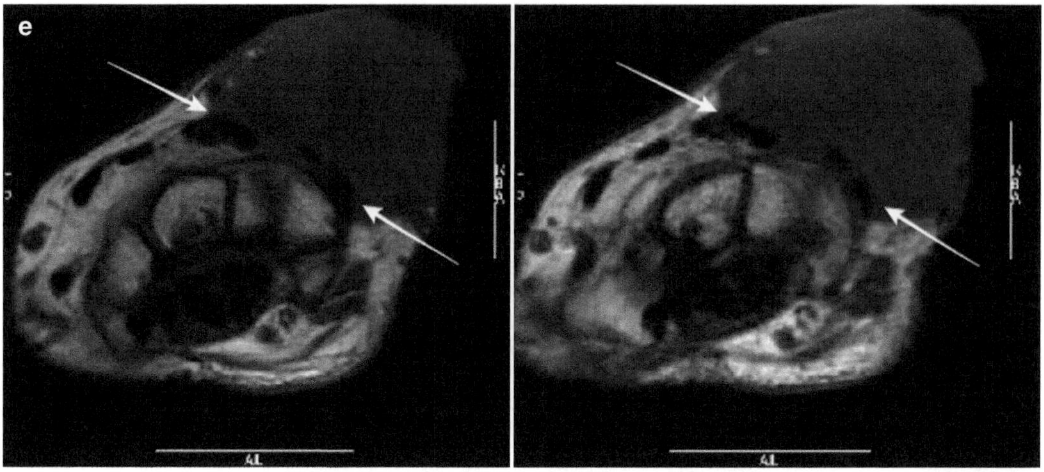

Fig. 4 (continued)

present with pathological fracture, the uptake is variable and more diffuse. Giant cell tumors can be seen in the distal radius and phalanges of the hands. Three-phase bone scintigraphy shows increased tracer distribution in the blood flow and blood pool phases, with a donut appearance of tracer uptake in delayed bone scan, with intense uptake along periphery and decreased uptake in the central part. Bone scintigraphy can also identify hypertrophic osteoarthropathy or lymphedema associated with primary malignancies elsewhere. Rarely, osteosarcoma and Ewing's sarcoma can arise from the bones of the hand and wrist (Fig. 5). Bone scintigraphy is useful for the evaluation of metastatic lesions and not very useful for evaluating the local extent for malignant lesions in general as there is overestimation of tumor size in the adjacent bones or the entire extremity (Streek et al. 1998) (Fig. 6).

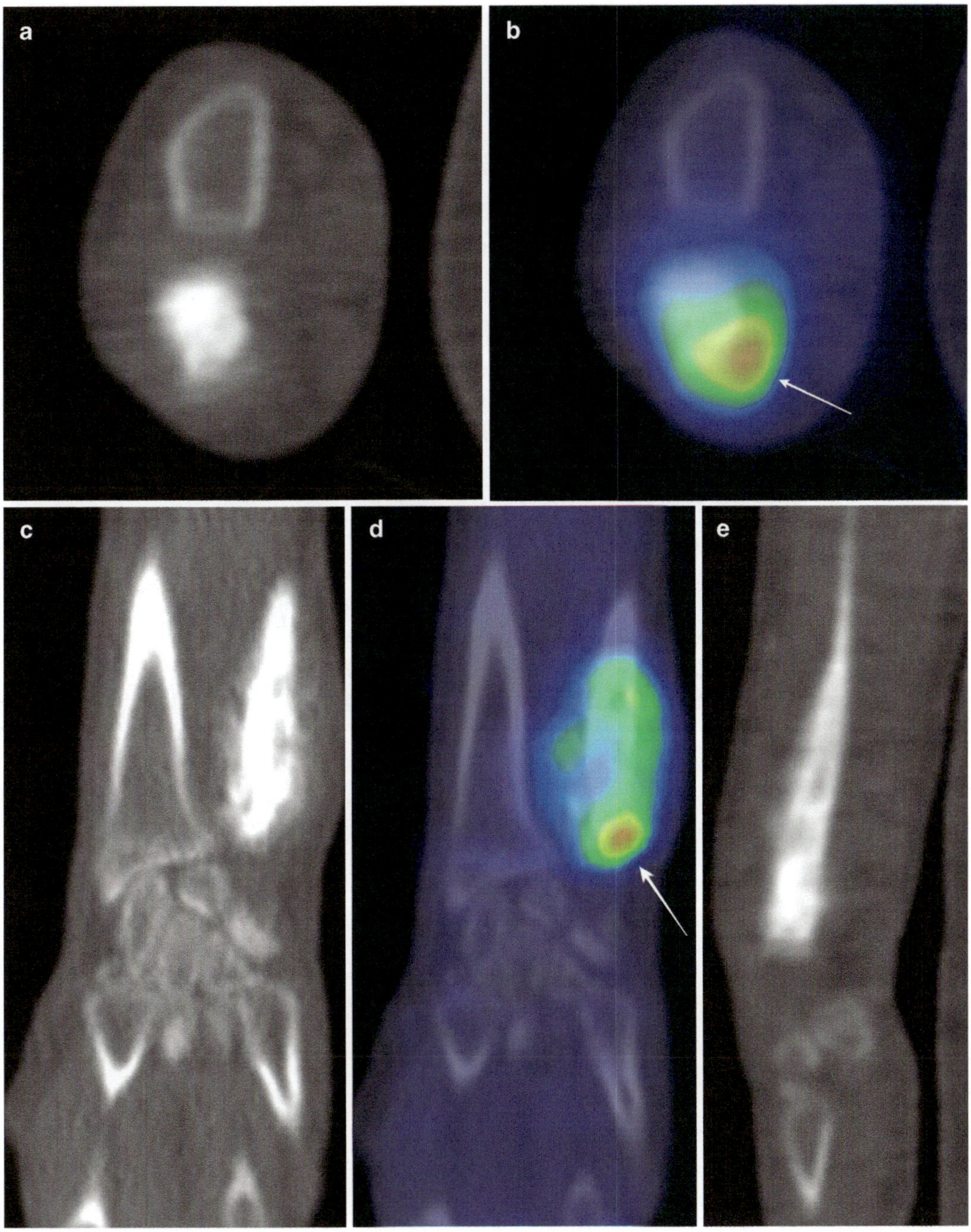

Fig. 5 Patient presenting with a slow-growing hard tumor in the right wrist. Axial (**a**) CT and (**b**) fusion, coronal (**c**) CT and (**d**) fusion and sagittal (**e**) CT and (**f**) fusion PET/CT images show a mixed lytic-sclerotic lesion in the distal ulna with a permeative pattern of destruction and sunburst periosteal reaction. There is increased FDG uptake which is marked in the inferior aspect (white arrows). Biopsy was performed in the most metabolically active location shown on PET/CT and diagnosis of osteosarcoma was established. (**g**) Volume rendered surface 3D-reconstructed CT image shows the location and extension of the malignant tumor in distal ulna (black arrows)

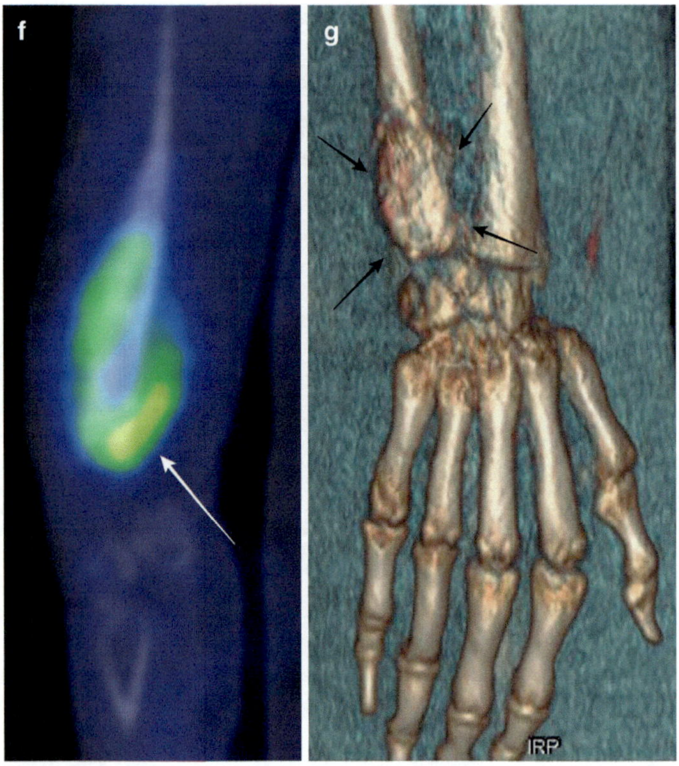

Fig. 5 (continued)

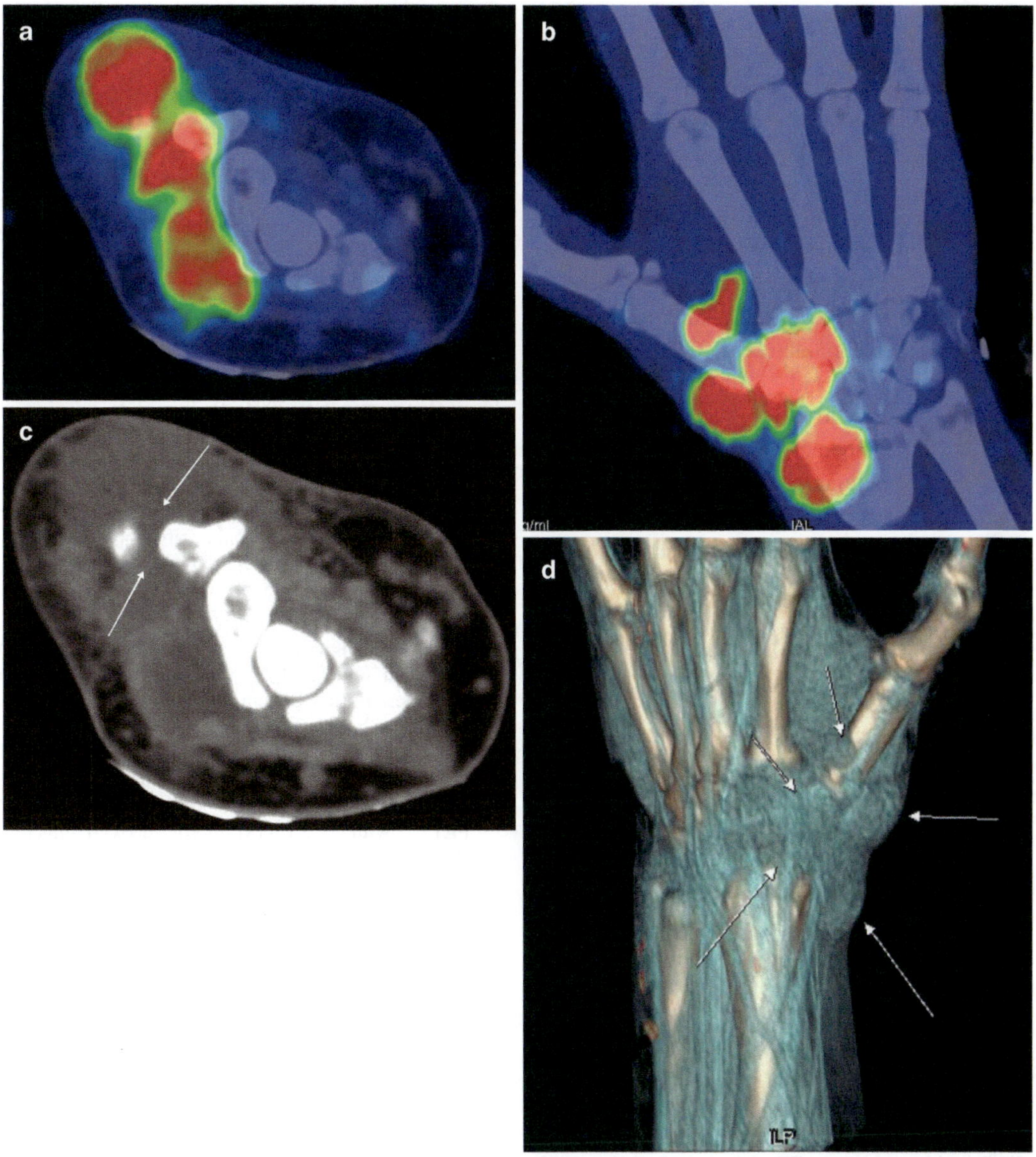

Fig. 6 Patient presenting with swelling in the radial aspect of the left wrist. (**a**) Axial and (**b**) coronal fusion PET/CT images show a dense irregular soft tissue lesion with intense FDG uptake which resulted in blooming of metabolic activity projected over adjacent bones, with overestimation of the primary tumor. (**c**) Axial and (**d**) volume-rendered surface 3D-reconstructed CT images show the soft tissue tumor insinuating between the bones (white arrows), clearly without bone destruction. Histology revealed malignant round cell tumor

6 Conclusion

Bone scintigraphy is the most used and relevant primary nuclear medicine imaging technique for the evaluation of the hand and wrist, even in the present era of modern imaging modalities. It remains the modality of choice for the diagnosis of few specific clinical conditions such as reflex sympathetic dystrophy and autoimmune arthritis. Proper clinical history and examination combined with correct choice of imaging aids in correct diagnosis and subsequent clinical management. Hybrid imaging techniques such as SPECT/CT provide accurate anatomical correlation and semiquantitative measurements of uptake and assist in the follow-up to differentiate treatment response and failures. PET/CT has revolutionized nuclear medicine imaging and recently, is used more often in autoimmune arthritis such as rheumatoid arthritis and psoriatic arthritis for initial diagnosis and further management.

References

Abdelhafez Y, Raychaudhuri SP, Mazza D et al (2022) Total-body 18F-FDG PET/CT in autoimmune inflammatory arthritis at ultra-low dose: initial observations. J Nucl Med 63:1579–1585. https://doi.org/10.2967/jnumed.121.263774

Balzer A, Patel A, Palisch A (2021) Wrist and hand trauma imaging. Clin Sports Med 40:625–639. https://doi.org/10.1016/j.csm.2021.05.003

Choi YY, Kim JY (2017) Nuclear medicine imaging in rheumatic diseases. J Rheum Dis 24:4–13. https://doi.org/10.4078/jrd.2017.24.1.4

Giudici MA, Moser RP, Kransdorf MJ (1993) Cartilaginous bone tumors. Radiol Clin North Am 31:237–259

Gnanasegaran G, Cook G, Adamson K, Fogelman I (2009) Patterns, variants, artifacts, and pitfalls in conventional radionuclide bone imaging and SPECT/CT. Semin Nucl Med 39:380–395. https://doi.org/10.1053/j.semnuclmed.2009.07.003

Holder LE, Mulligan ME, Gillespie TE (1995) Diagnosis of scaphoid fractures: the role of nuclear medicine. J Nucl Med 36:48–50

Kannivelu A, Peh WCG (2024) Nuclear medicine imaging of the hip and bony pelvis. In: Davies M, Botchu R, Iyengar KP (eds) Imaging of the hip and bony pelvis. Medical radiology. Springer, Cham. https://doi.org/10.1007/174_2024_490

Kannivelu A, Tong AKT, Loke KSH, Ng DCE (2021) Nuclear medicine imaging of spinal infection. In: Ladeb MF, Peh WCG (eds) Imaging of spinal infection. Medical radiology. Springer, Cham. https://doi.org/10.1007/978-3-030-70459-9_5

Lim CH, Kim HS, Lee KA et al (2022) Clinical significance of quantitative bone SPECT/CT in the evaluation of hand and wrist pain in patients with rheumatic disease. Sci Rep 12:1–8. https://doi.org/10.1038/s41598-021-03874-9

Love C, Palestro CJ (2004) Radionuclide imaging of infection. J Nucl Med Technol 32:47–59

Morris G, Evans S, Stevenson J et al (2017) Bone metastases of the hand. Ann R Coll Surg Engl 99:563–567. https://doi.org/10.1308/rcsann.2017.0096

O'Sullivan GJ (2015) Imaging of bone metastasis: an update. World J Radiol 7:202–211. https://doi.org/10.4329/wjr.v7.i8.202

Ostendorf B, Scherer A, Wirrwar A et al (2006) High-resolution multipinhole single-photon-emission computed tomography in experimental and human arthritis. Arthritis Rheum 54:1096–1104. https://doi.org/10.1002/art.21732

Palmer WE, Rosenthal DI, Schoenberg OI et al (1995) Quantification of inflammation in the wrist with gadolinium-enhanced MR imaging and PET with 2-[F-18]-fluoro-2-deoxy-D-glucose. Radiology 196:647–655. https://doi.org/10.1148/radiology.196.3.7644624

Quek ST, Peh WCG (2002) Radiology of osteoporosis. Semin Musculoskelet Radiol 6(3):197–206. https://doi.org/10.1055/s-2002-36717

Rosado-de-Castro PH, de Souza SAL, Alexandre D et al (2014) Rheumatoid arthritis: nuclear medicine state-of-the-art imaging. World J Orthop 5:312–318. https://doi.org/10.5312/wjo.v5.i3.312

Sambri A, Spinnato P, Tedeschi S et al (2021) Bone and joint infections: the role of imaging in tailoring diagnosis to improve patients' care. J Pers Med 11:1317. https://doi.org/10.3390/jpm11121317

Seabold JE, Palestro CJ, Brown ML et al (1997) Procedure guideline for gallium scintigraphy in inflammation. Society of Nuclear Medicine. J Nucl Med 38:994–997

Shehab D, Elgazzar A, Collier BD et al (2005) Impact of three-phase bone scintigraphy on the diagnosis and treatment of complex regional pain syndrome type I or reflex sympathetic dystrophy. Med Princ Pract 15:46–51. https://doi.org/10.1159/000089385

Streek PV, Carretta RF, Weiland FL, Shelton DK (1998) Upper extremity radionuclide bone imaging: the wrist and hand. Semin Nucl Med 28:14–24. https://doi.org/10.1016/S0001-2998(98)80016-0

Thomas BP, Sasi K, Pallapati SCR et al (2011) Malignant tumours of the hand and wrist. Indian J Plast Surg 44:337–347. https://doi.org/10.4103/0970-0358.85355

Van den Wyngaert T, Strobel K, Kampen WU et al (2016) The EANM practice guidelines for bone scintigraphy. Eur J Nucl Med Mol Imaging 43:1723–1738. https://doi.org/10.1007/s00259-016-3415-4

Yin ZG, Zhang JB, Kan SL, Wang XG (2010) Diagnosing suspected scaphoid fractures: a systematic review and meta-analysis. Clin Orthop Relat Res 468:723–734. https://doi.org/10.1007/s11999-009-1081-6

Ultrasound Imaging Techniques and Procedures

Neha Nischal, Gaurav Kant Sharma, René de Gautard, Giorgio Tamborrini, Stefan Mariacher, Paresh Sonsale, and Rajesh Botchu

Contents

N. Nischal (✉)
Department of Radiology, Holy Family Hospital, New Delhi, India

G. K. Sharma
JISPI, Jaipur, India

R. de Gautard
CIM SA Cabinet Imagerie Medicale, Geneva, Switzerland

G. Tamborrini
Rheumaklinik, Universitäts-Spital Zürich, Zürich, Switzerland

S. Mariacher
Chefarzt und stv. Vorsitzender der Klinikleitung, aarReha Schinznach, Schinznach-Bad, Switzerland

Abstract

The role of ultrasound (US) in the assessment of musculoskeletal disorders is persistently increasing. Recent developments in hardware and software of US equipments and in particular use of small-size, high-frequency transducers have allowed accurate assessment of a wide variety of hand and wrist disorders.

1 Introduction

The role of ultrasound (US) in the assessment of musculoskeletal disorders is persistently increasing (Van Holsbeeck and Introcaso 2001; McNally 2004; Brasseur and Tardieu 2006; Bianchi and Martinoli 2007; Adler 2024). Recent developments in hardware and software of US equipments and in particular use of small-size, high-frequency transducers have allowed accurate assessment of a wide variety of hand and wrist disorders. The main advantages of US are its low cost, readiness, noninvasivity and possibility to perform a dynamic examination. Certain pathologies such as snapping of the ten-

P. Sonsale
Department of Orthopedics, University Hospitals Birmingham NHS Foundation Trust, Birmingham, UK

R. Botchu
Department of Musculoskeletal Radiology, Royal Orthopedic Hospital, Birmingham, UK

Med Radiol Diagn Imaging (2025)
https://doi.org/10.1007/174_2025_611,
Published Online: 18 October 2025

dons can only be appreciated on dynamic scanning, which may remain undiagnosed in static MR images (Mak et al. 2019). The main disadvantage is the impossibility to detect and assess deep structures, located behind bones. The cortex of bones however can be assessed impressively by US leading to identification of radiographically occult fractures (Botchu and Bianchi 2014; Nischal and Bianchi 2023). In addition, US is a highly operator-dependent technique and has a long learning curve.

US has been used in the assessment of wrist and hand traumatic, degenerative and infective disorders, as well as in evaluating local masses (Read et al. 1996; Ferrara and Marcelis 1997; Bianchi et al. 1999, 2001, 2003; Teefey et al. 2000; Milbradt et al. 1990; Chiou et al. 2001; Moschilla and Breidahl 2002; Botchu and Bhatt 2012). Additional studies have stressed its role in the evaluation of inflammatory arthritis (Koski 1992; Grassi et al. 1993; Di Matteo et al. 2020). Quantification of inflammation and of structural damage is mandatory in the assessment, management and monitoring of rheumatoid arthritis (RA).

Without appropriate treatment (e.g. DMARD's, biologics), RA inflammation can progress and result in joint dysfunction and deformity. An early diagnosis can lead to early instauration of a successful treatment. Standard radiographs have an important role to identify changes such as osteopenia, joint space reduction or erosions in patients with advanced arthritis. US is a useful tool in the assessment and follow-up of early to established RA (Wakefield et al. 2000; Szkudlarek et al. 2004a, b; D'Agostino et al. 2016) and can efficiently guide local procedures such as aspiration of effusions or therapeutic injection (Karim et al. 2001). It enhances safety with more accurate needle placement while avoiding inadvertent injury to nearby structures (Raza 2003; Cunnington et al. 2010). US-guided injections for tenosynovitis are reported to be less painful with better response in terms of reduced power Doppler signals (Gutierrez et al. 2016).

In RA US can detect different pathologic changes including synovitis, cartilage and bone changes, tenosynovitis and tendon tears, bursitis, rheumatoid nodules or secondary nerve entrapment (e.g. carpal tunnel syndrome). Clinical studies have shown that US is as effective or even more effective in detecting inflammatory changes as clinical examination. Sensitivity and specificity of US in assessment of joint changes in RA is comparable to MR imaging (Backhaus et al. 1999, 2002; Szkudlarek et al. 2004a, b; Scheel et al. 2006). Power Doppler and Colour Doppler US detects active synovial inflammation associated with hypervascularization and neoangiogenesis. In the presence of an active synovitis, there is an increase in signal activity, which is correlated to the degree of inflammatory activity. Therefore, the use of colour and power Doppler US facilitates a differentiation between active and inactive synovitis. Furthermore, numerous studies have shown a good correlation between activity of synovitis at power Doppler and inflammatory changes evident at MRI and at histopathology studies (Walther et al. 2001; Terslev et al. 2003). Echo-contrast-enhanced US has shown an improvement in the measurement of synovial thickness and activity of synovial processes in patients with rheumatoid arthritis and allows better differentiation between effusion and synovial proliferation (Goldberg et al. 1994; Blomley et al. 2001). Microvascular flow imaging (MVFI) or superb microvascular imaging (SMI) has been shown to be better than power Doppler and as sensitive as contrast-enhanced US for detection of active synovitis (Platzgummer et al. 2009; Yu et al. 2018; Diao et al. 2022). This technique allows visualization of low-velocity flow in microvessels without administration of contrast (Fig. 1).

Besides assessment of the synovium, US can evaluate pathological changes of cartilages and bones if performed using high-resolution ultrasound probes. Bone erosions are a pathophysiological hallmark of RA. US can provide a more accurate and comprehensive assessment of bone erosions than plain radiography. The size of erosions can be monitored to evaluate disease progression.

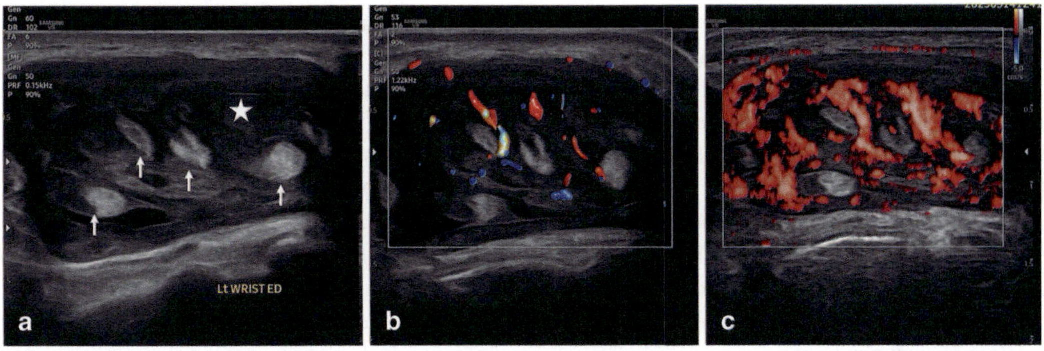

Fig. 1 Transverse sonograms at the dorsal aspect of wrist in a patient with rheumatoid arthritis. (**a**) Greyscale image shows extensive hypoechoic synovial proliferation (*star*) affecting the fourth extensor compartment tendons (*arrows*). (**b**) Colour doppler image shows moderate vascularity. (**c**) Microvascular flow imaging (MVFI) reveals intense vascular signals

Another benefit of ultrasound is its capability to evaluate post-operative patients with hardware, providing real-time imaging without interference from metal implants. This makes it valuable for assessing soft tissue healing, detecting infections and identifying potential hardware impingement (Guillin et al. 2012).

Accurate knowledge of the normal anatomy, technique of US examination and of the US appearance of the hand and wrist are definite prerequisites for a successful US examination. The target of this chapter is to present the technique of the US examination and the normal US anatomy of the hand and wrist.

2 Technique of Examination and Normal US Appearance

Before starting the US examination, any previous imaging studies and blood tests, if available, are reviewed. Every effort must be made to obtain a recent radiographic examination, in at least two perpendicular views, since this allows a good analysis of joints and bones and is complementary to US that permits an excellent assessment of most soft tissues.

A brief clinical evaluation is always obtained since it helps in pointing the attention of the examiner to a specific area, thus shortening the time of examination and allowing a more detailed local assessment. The patient is asked for duration of symptoms, type and rhythm of pain (mechanic or inflammatory), presence of tingling, numbness or morning stiffness. If pain is the main symptom, its location and modification during muscle contraction or joint movements can often orient toward the correct diagnosis. In De Quervain tenosynovitis, for example, a sharp, acute pain located over the radial styloid and worsened by ulnar deviation of the wrist with the thumb flexed is highly suggestive of the diagnosis. The distribution of peripheral tingling can indicate the injured nerve (radial, ulnar or median). A brief regional physical examination including assessment of any local or diffuse swelling, warmth or redness follows. The joint range of motion and local tenderness are also briefly assessed.

Schematically, there are two main kinds of performing a US examination of the wrist and hand. A *focused examination* generally performed in patients suffering from disorders affecting the periarticular tissues and a *systemic examination* mostly directed to the joints.

The first is a shorter examination concentrated on a specific region, selected by the sonologist according to the data available from the physician's US request, type of symptoms and results of the brief clinical examination described earlier. For instance, in a patient presenting with a painless lump at the dorsum of the wrist suspected to be a ganglion by the referring physician, the US examination can be limited to the dorsal aspect of the wrist. A time-consuming, detailed examination of all metacarpophalangeal and interphalangeal joints is not necessary and useless in such a patient.

The second type of US examination is a more time-consuming, systematic examination usually obtained only in patients with a clinical suspicion or diagnosis of systemic arthritis. In both cases, a scrupulous technique of realization of the US examination, including images obtained in several planes and dynamic test, must be deployed (Creteur and Peetrons 2000; Middleton et al. 2001; Lee and Healy 2005; Tagliafico et al. 2007).

For didactic purposes, we first describe the basic anatomy of the main structures amenable to US assessment followed by description of the US technique of examination and of the normal US anatomy. We will follow an anatomic pattern, starting with the dorsal aspect of the wrist and the hand followed by the palmar aspect.

For optimal US examination of the wrist and hand, the patient can either sit facing the examiner with the forearm resting on the examination bed or can lie down on the examination bed with the limb under investigation towards the examiner. The latter position is especially preferred while doing US-guided interventions to reduce the risk of a vasovagal syncope. We routinely start the examination by scanning the dorsal aspect of the wrist followed by the hand through transverse and sagittal sonograms. Then, the patient is asked to supinate the hand that now lies on its dorsal aspect, to allow examination of its palmar aspect. Again transverse sonograms are followed by longitudinal images. Colour Doppler is routinely obtained. Dynamic scanning allows identification of each extensor and flexor tendon of the fingers and, most importantly, allows optimal judgement of tendons' gliding and eventual impingement inside osteofibrous tunnels. This is very useful in judging the presence of tendon adhesions.

Application of variable pressure with the transducer permits obtaining additional data. A firm pressure helps in eliciting local pain and thus in focalizing the examination. It also assists in judging consistency of masses facilitating for example the diagnosis of soft tissue lipoma. On the contrary, large amount of gel must be used in assessing fluid collections in order to lessen local pressure through the probe and avoid inadvertent displacement of the fluid that can result in a negative examination. In assessing presence of vessels with colour Doppler, excessive pressure can result in squeezing of vessels resulting in impossibility to accurately detect local hypervascular changes. In testing the permeability of subcutaneous veins, colour Doppler is obtained during squeezing of the soft tissues distal to the site of examination performed with the contralateral hand of the examiner. This allows a temporary increase in venous blood velocity and its easier detection at colour Doppler. On the contrary, blocking the venous drainage at the forearm causes dilatation of the distal vein and results in stagnation of blood inside venous masses.

As previously discussed, palpation under US guidance can be realized through the transducer when a large mass is evaluated. When the mass is small, US-guided palpation is better performed by using an opened paper clip. Once placed between the transducer and the skin, this can be followed under real-time scanning thanks to its typical posterior comet tail artefact. This technique works well in cutaneous marking of soft tissue foreign bodies as well as in accurate localization of small neuromas.

3 Dorsal Aspect

US allows an accurate evaluation of the dorsal aspect of wrist and hand (Figs. 2, 3, 4, 5, 6, 7, 8, 9, 10, 11, 12, 13, 14, and 15). Accessory muscles

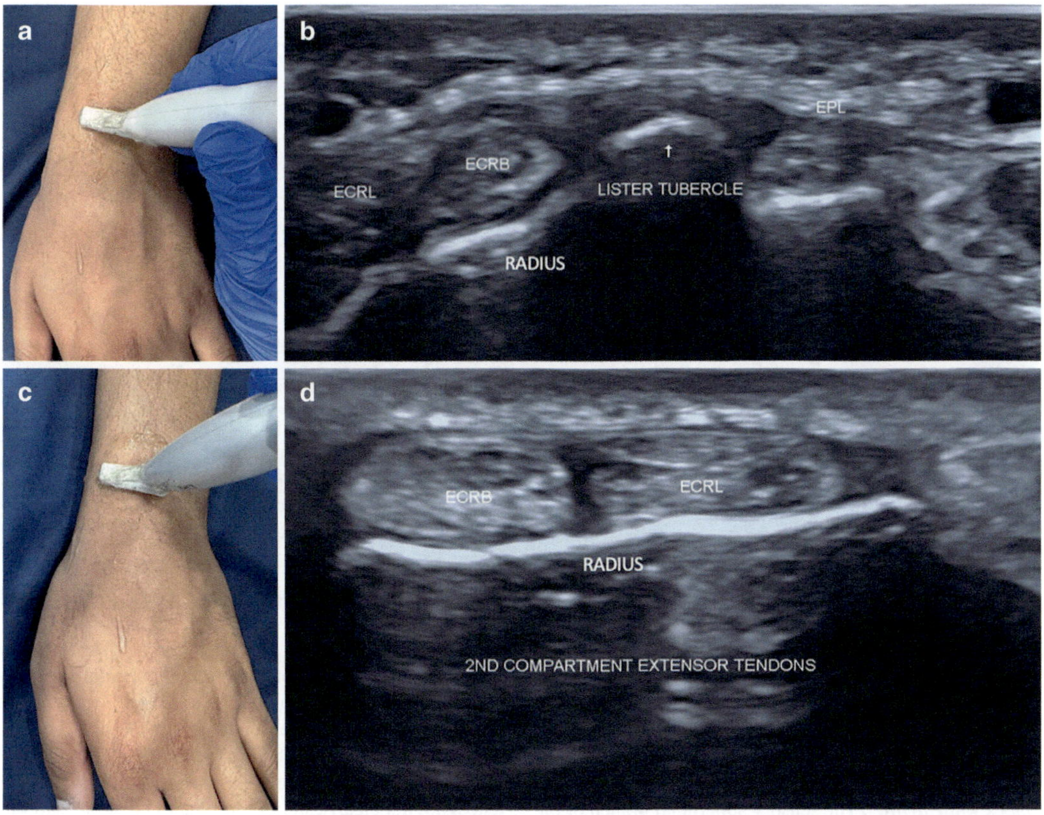

Fig. 2 Dorsal aspect. (**a**, **c**) Probe positioning for transverse examination. (**b**) Sonogram obtained as shown in **a**. US shows the Lister's tubercle (*small white arrow*) as the most prominent bony landmark on the dorsal aspect of distal radius dividing the second extensor compartment (ECRL, ECRB) on the radial aspect from the third compartment (EPL) on the ulnar aspect. (**d**) Sonogram obtained as shown in **c**. US better depicts the compact echogenic morphology of the second extensor compartment tendons with the ECRB on the radial and ECRL on the ulnar aspect

can be found at the dorsal face of the wrist (Muncibì et al. 2008) as anatomic variants mimicking local tumours. They show at US the typical internal muscle structure made by alternating hypoechoic (muscle fibres) and hyperechoic (fibroadipose septa) bands. Dynamic examination during resisted contraction shows contraction of the accessory muscle thus confirming the diagnosis.

Located under the skin and subcutaneous tissues, a thin fascia covers the extensor tendons (ET). These tendons take origin from the myotendinous junctions, located in the forearm at different levels for each muscle, run distally between the joint plane and the subcutaneous tissue, to finally insert into the bone of the wrist and hand. Since all ET change their course before joining their insertion, they are prone to instability during changes of position of the wrist and hand joints. To avoid instability, the ET run inside fibro-osseous tunnels. These are made by the surface of bones covered by periosteum (the floor) and by superficial fibrous bands named retinaculae (the ceiling). To further increase tendon stability, the bone surface is not flat but made by grooves, sulci or protuberances. A synovial sheath composed by a visceral and parietal layer, gliding one over the other, surrounds the tendons and reduces local frictions during gliding. The visceral layer is adherent to the tendon and moves with it, while the parietal layer is lax and

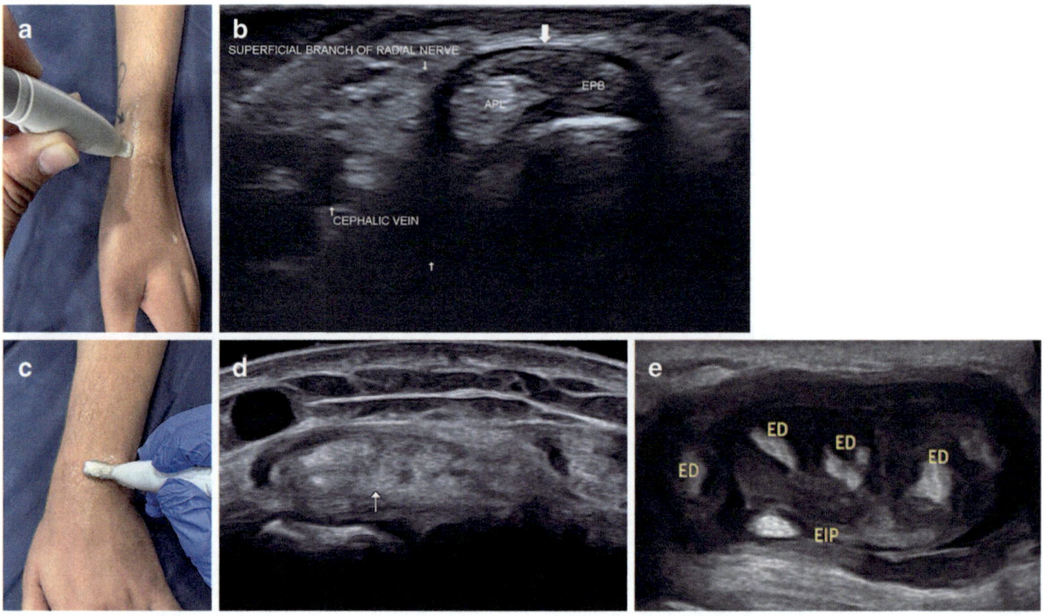

Fig. 3 Dorsal aspect. (**a**) Probe positioning for transverse examination to evaluate the first extensor compartment with forearm in mid-pronation or the "karate-chop" position. (**b**) Sonogram obtained as shown in **a**. US shows the first extensor compartment tendons (APL, EPB) on the radial styloid with the overlying thin extensor retinaculum (*block white arrow*). The sensory superficial branch of the radial nerve and cephalic vein lie in close relation to this compartment and these structures are at risk of injury while performing interventions for de Quervain's tenosynovitis. (**c**) Probe positioning for transverse examination to evaluate the fourth extensor compartment (**d**) Sonogram obtained as shown in **c**. US shows the EDs with the EIP (*white arrow*). (**e**) US image from a patient with extensive tenosynovitis clearly shows the four ED tendons superficial to the EIP tendon

blends with the retinacula and other peritendinous structures. The layers are separated by a thin amount of synovial fluid.

At the level of the distal radius and wrist, the twelve ET run inside six tunnels. The tunnels are numbered from the most radial to the most ulnar. The first tunnel is located over the radial styloid while the sixth is found at the level of the cubital head. The Lister's tubercle is the most prominent bony landmark on the dorsal aspect of distal radius which separates the radially placed second compartment tendons from the third compartment tendon, the extensor pollicis longus (EPL) lying toward the ulnar aspect of the tubercle. Table 1 resumes the arrangement of the tendons inside the six tunnels.

US shows the ET as hyperechoic, homogeneous structures showing a typical fibrillar structure in the longitudinal sonograms. The borders of normal tendons are regular and well defined. The normal synovial sheath and the tiny amount of fluid contained inside it can't be detected even if high-resolution transducers are used. Retinacula are imaged at US as hyper or hypoechoic structures depending on the incidence of the US bean. They present different thicknesses depending on the fibro-osseous tunnel examined. The retinaculum of the fourth compartment is the thickest and, since it appears mostly hypoechoic, can simulate an effusion to unexperienced examiners (Robertson et al. 2007). The mean value of thickness of the retinacula in other tunnels is around 0.3–0.5 mm. The fourth compartment consists of four ED tendons and one EIP tendon which runs deep to the ED tendons (Yammine 2015). The EIP is commonly employed for tendon transfer to restore function in cases of injuries to other ETs. In case of suspicion of mild thickening of retinacula, the contralateral side can be scanned to improve diagnostic confidence.

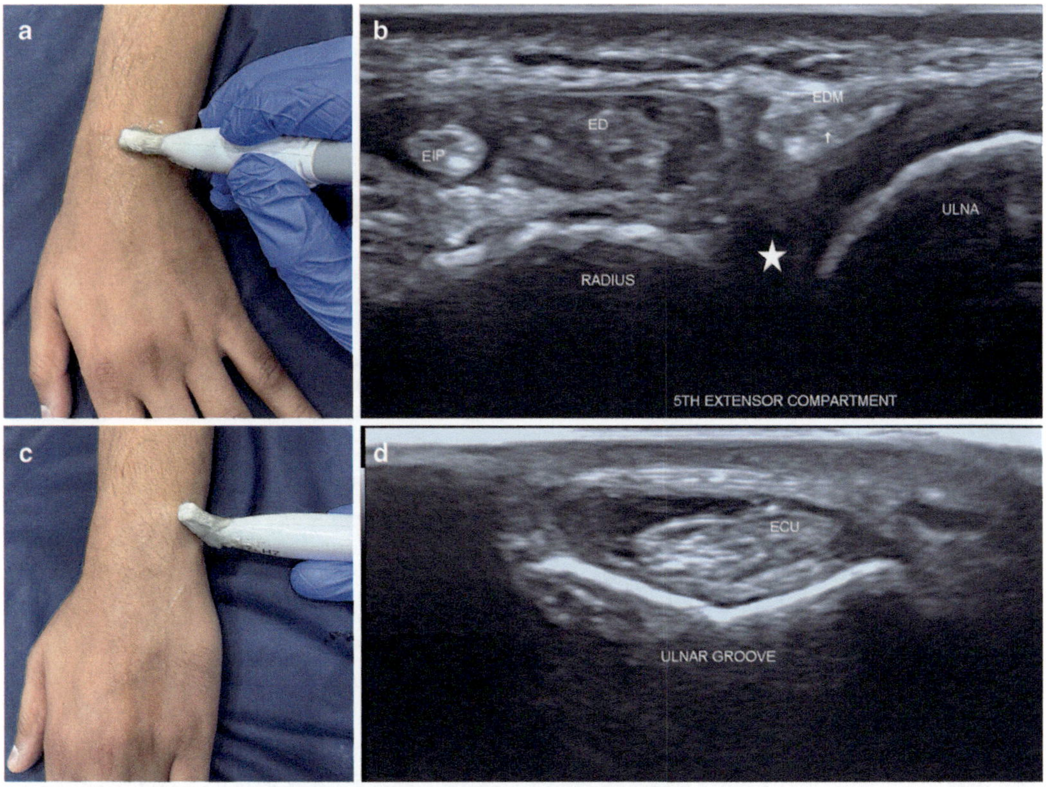

Fig. 4 Dorsal aspect. (**a**, **c**) Probe positioning for transverse examination to evaluate the fifth and sixth extensor compartments. (**b**) Sonogram obtained as shown in **a**. US shows the fifth extensor compartment tendon (EDM) overlying the distal radio-ulnar joint (*star*). (**d**) Sonogram obtained as shown in **c**. US shows the sixth extensor compartment tendon (ECU) lying within the ulnar groove. This tendon is covered by the extensor retinaculum as well as its own sub-sheath, pathology of which may lead to ECU instability

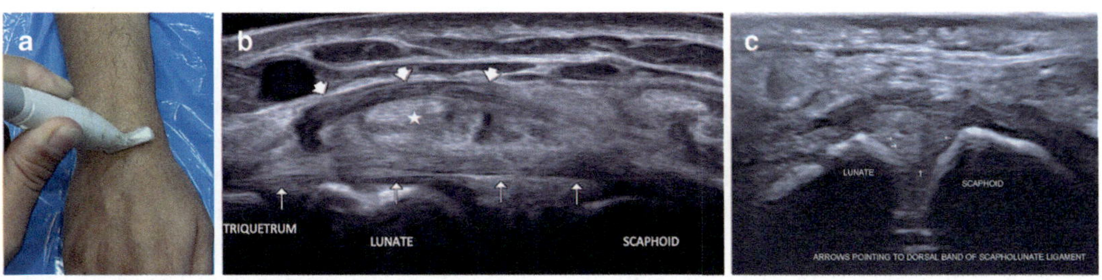

Fig. 5 Dorsal aspect. (**a**) Probe positioning for transverse examination just distal to the distal end of radius. (**b**) Sonogram obtained as shown in **a**. US shows the dorsal carpal ligaments (*thin arrows*) with the overlying fourth extensor compartment tendons (*star*). Note that normally the retinaculum of this compartment is thicker than that of others (*bold arrows*). (**c**) US shows the dorsal component of the scapho-lunate ligament (*small white arrows*) between the scaphoid and lunate bones

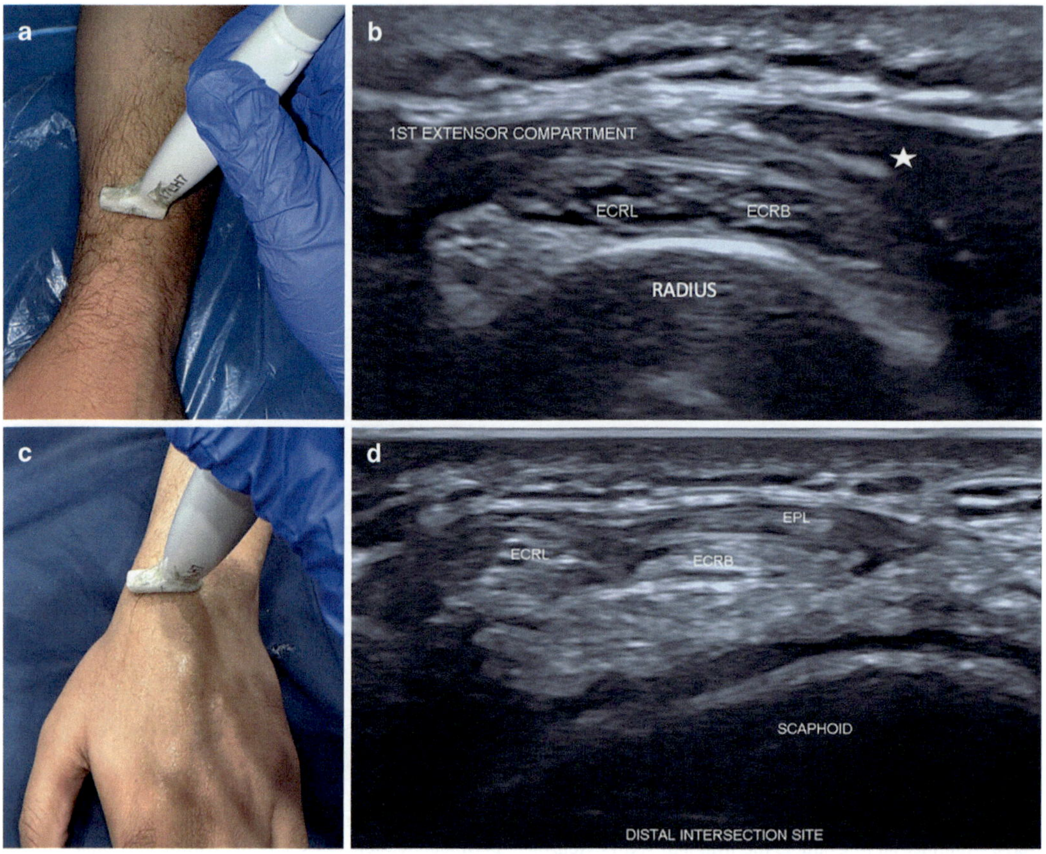

Fig. 6 Dorsal aspect. (**a**, **c**) Probe positioning for transverse examination to evaluate the proximal and distal intersections. (**b**) Sonogram obtained as shown in **a**. US shows the myotendinous junction(*star*) of first extensor compartment tendons crossing over the second compartment tendons (ECRL, ECRB). (**d**) Sonogram obtained as shown in **c**. US shows the third extensor compartment tendon (EPL) crossing over the second compartment tendons (ECRL, ECRB). Repeated friction at these sites can lead to intersection syndromes causing pain and discomfort in these areas

In normal conditions, colour or power Doppler does not allow detecting the normal vascularization of tendons, sheath or retinacula. Any Doppler signals inside these structures must be retained as pathologic. Axial images allow a good analysis of details of different ET. To give an example, the APL is almost always made by multiple thin tendons rather than by a single tendon (De Maeseneer et al. 2009). This normal variation seems to facilitate impingement inside the first osteofibrous tunnel.

Deep to the ET of the third compartment, located close to the lateral aspect of the Lister's tubercle, the distal sensitive branch of the posterior interosseous nerve can be seen running from the forearm to the dorsal aspect of the wrist. At its distal portion, the normal nerve can present a bulbous swelling (Acrel's ganglion) that must not be interpreted as a pathologic neuroma or as evidence of chronic compression. The origin of this fusiform swelling is unknown. Histologically, it is made by normal peripheral nerve structures without any neuronal cell bodies (Tubbs et al. 2007). The term pseudoganglion seems then more appropriate than that of ganglion. In younger subjects, a small artery (distal anterior interosseous artery) can be detected running close to the nerve.

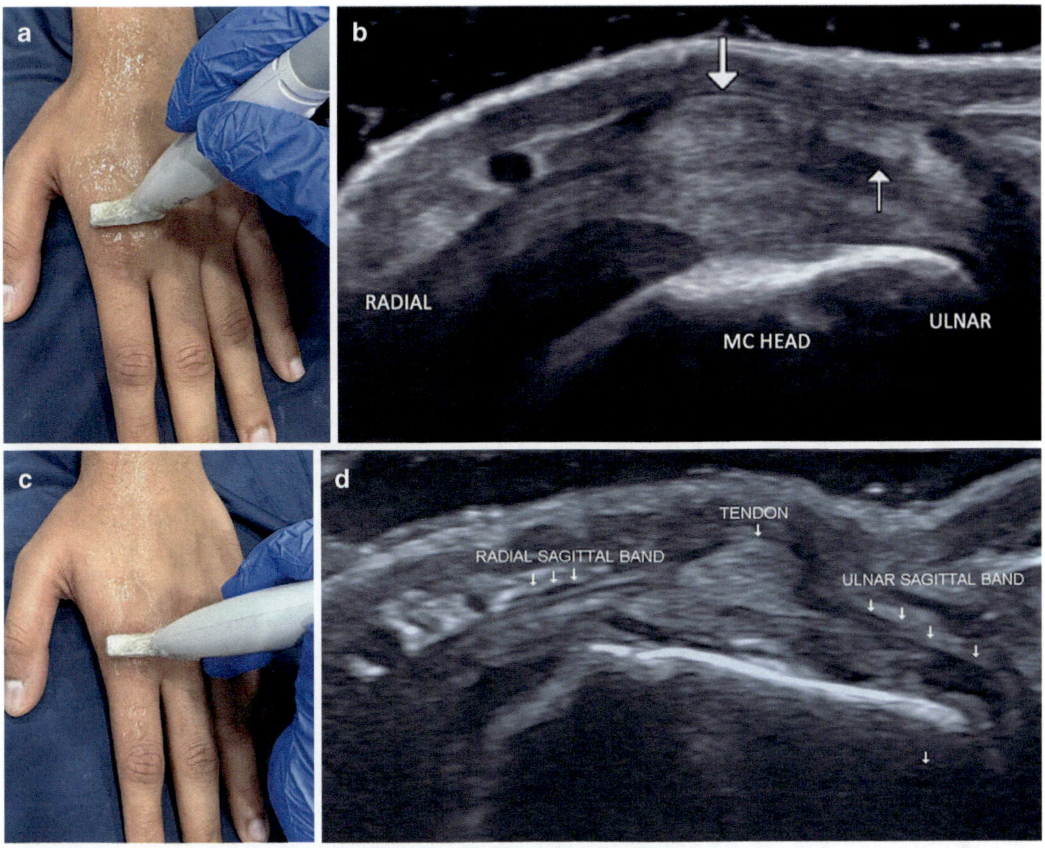

Fig. 7 Dorsal aspect. (**a**, **c**) Probe positioning for transverse examination. (**b**) Sonogram obtained as shown in **a**. US shows the EIP tendon (*small white arrow*) lying medial to the ED tendon (*big white arrow*) at the level of second metacarpal head (*MC head*). (**d**) Sonogram obtained as shown in **c**. US shows the radial and ulnar sagittal bands (*short white arrows*) extending from the ED tendon of the respective fingers

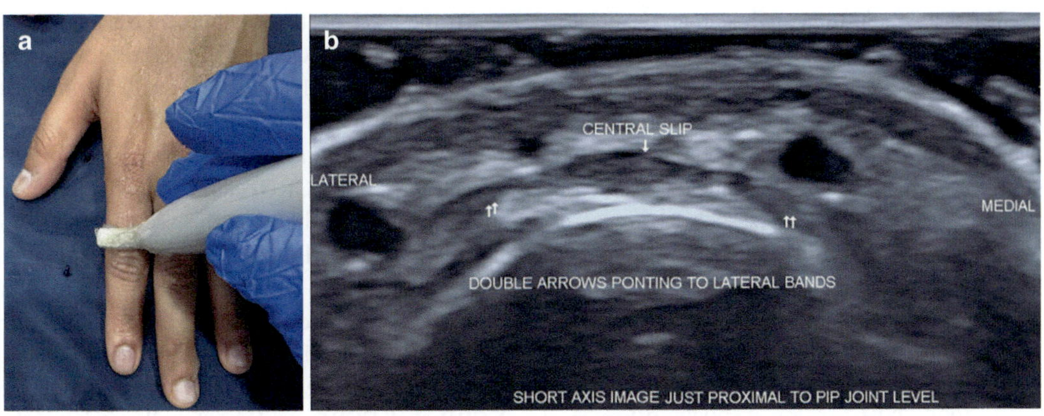

Fig. 8 Dorsal aspect. (**a**) Probe positioning for transverse examination just proximal to the PIP joint. (**b**) Sonogram obtained as shown in **a**. US shows the central slip of extensor tendon (*single white arrow*) and the lateral slips on either side (*double white arrows*)

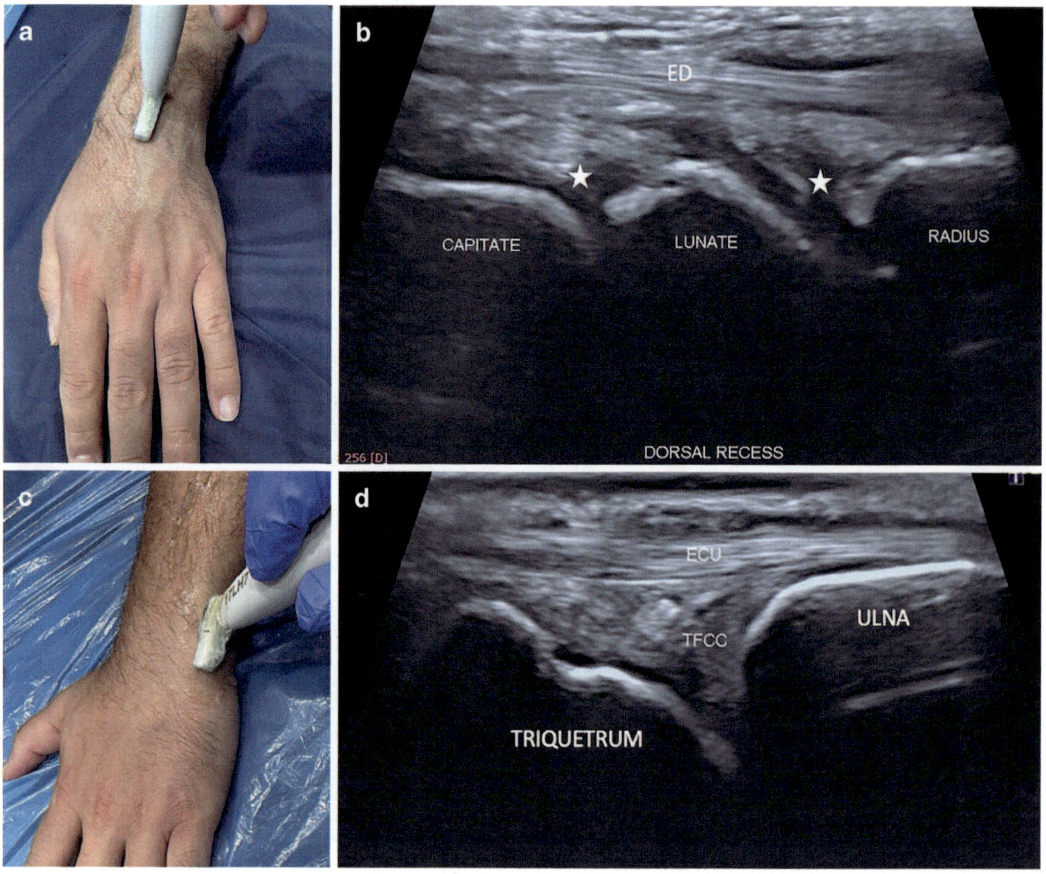

Fig. 9 Dorsal aspect. (**a**, **c**) Probe positioning for longitudinal examination. (**b**) Sonogram obtained as shown in **a**. US shows the dorsal joint recesses at the wrist (*stars*) with overlying ED tendon. (**d**) Sonogram obtained as shown in **c**. US shows the ECU tendon in long axis with underlying triangular fibrocartilage complex (TFCC)

The distal radio-ulnar, radiocarpal, mediocarpal and carpo-metacarpal joints can be well imaged and changes related to degenerative, inflammatory or erosive arthropathy detected. US can efficiently guide intraarticular injections (Lohman et al. 2007) under real-time control. This helps in avoiding injury to adjacent structures such as nerves and vessels and in confirming the correct site of injection. US allows detection and assessment of several extrinsic articular ligaments as well as of the dorsal scapho-lunate ligament (Griffith et al. 2001; Jacobson et al. 2002; Finlay et al. 2004; Boutry et al. 2005; Taljanovic et al. 2008; Bihan et al. 2009; Renoux et al. 2009).

At the level of the dorsum of the hand and of the fingers, the ET can be followed till their distal insertion by US. The EPB is one of the thinnest tendons and inserts into the base of the proximal phalanx of the thumb. The two extensor carpi tendons (ECRL and ECRB) can be followed till their insertion into the base of the second and third metacarpals. The EPL has a more complex course. At the distal radius, it reflects on the medial aspect of the Lister's tubercle, a bony ridge separating the third and the second compartment of the ET. Then, it points to the base of the thumb and overlies the ECRB and ECRL tendons. Finally, it joins the EPB at the level of the head of the first metacarpal

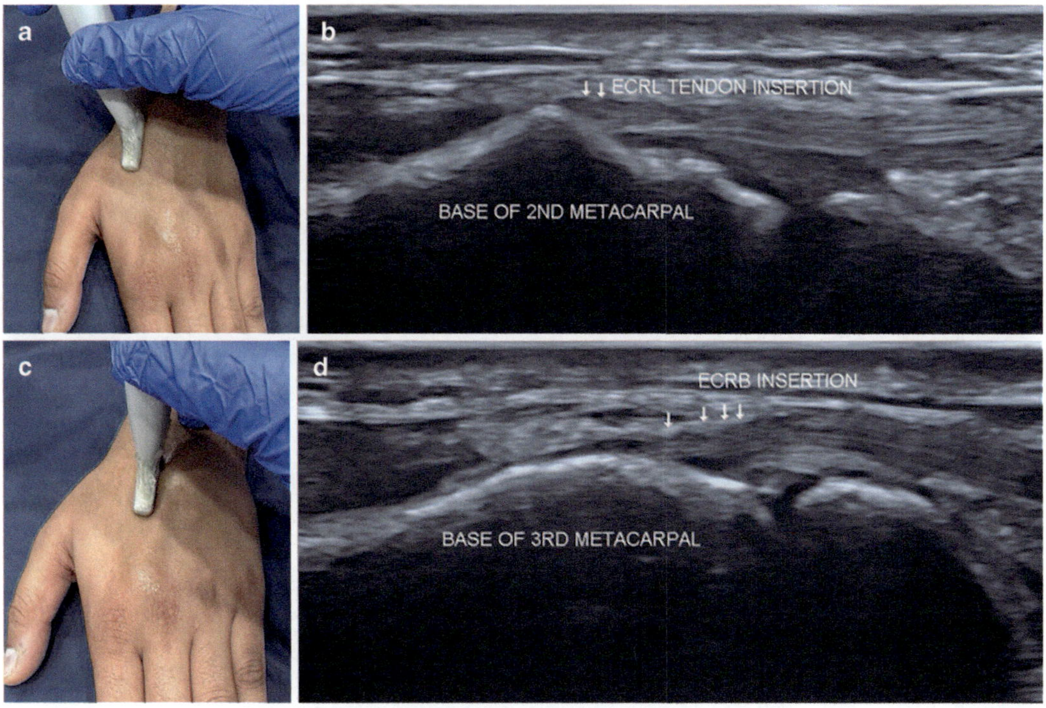

Fig. 10 Dorsal aspect. (**a**, **c**) Probe positioning for longitudinal examination. (**b**) Sonogram obtained as shown in **a**. US shows the insertion of ECRL tendon (*double white arrows*) at the base of second metacarpal. (**d**) Sonogram obtained as shown in **c**. US shows the insertion of ECRB tendon (*white arrows*) at the base of third metacarpal

to then insert into the base of the distal phalanx of the thumb. The EPL is then subject to local friction at two levels: at the Lister tubercle and when it crosses with the two extensor carpi tendons, the latter being termed as the "distal intersection" (De Maeseneer et al. 2005).

The index has two extensor tendons, the communis and the indicis proprius, which runs medial to the communis. They have similar size and course. The EIP can be harvested and used as a tendon graft in several surgical procedures. The extensor digitorum communis tendons present a high variable organization at the dorsum of the hand related to presence of the so-called tendinous junctions. These are thin tendons directed obliquely and joining adjacent ET. The dorsal interossei muscles can be seen appreciated lying among the hyperechoic metatarsals.

At the level of the metacarpophalangeal joints, the ET are retained over the dorsal aspect of the joint by the radial and ulnar sagittal bands, thin ligaments that prevent palmar displacement of the tendons during flexion of the fingers. These bands appear as thin hyperechoic laminae covering the tendons and inserting into the periphery of the capsule. At the level of the proximal phalanx, the ET of the 2–5 fingers split into a central band and two lateral bands. The central band inserts into the base of the middle phalanx while the lateral bands join into the midline to insert into the base of distal phalanx. The ET are well assessed by US at the level of the metacarpophalangeal (MCP) joint. Their distal splitting is sometimes difficult to be appreciated at transverse images. Longitudinal images allow visualization of the insertion of the central band as well as of the distal insertion into the distal phalanx.

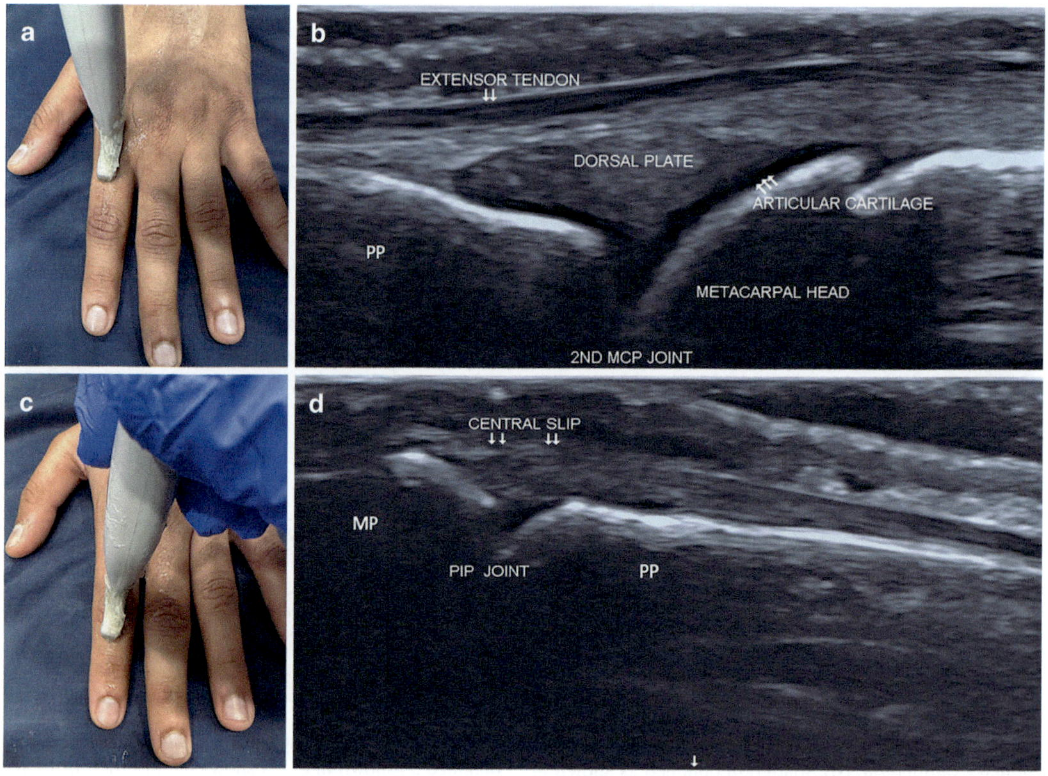

Fig. 11 Dorsal aspect. (**a**, **c**) Probe positioning for longitudinal examination. (**b**) Sonogram obtained as shown in **a**. US shows the insertion of dorsal plate at the level of MCP joint. The articular cartilage is visualized as a smooth anechoic area over the metacarpal head (*small white arrows*). (**d**) Sonogram obtained as shown in **c**. US shows the insertion of central slip of the extensor tendon (*white arrows*) at the base of middle phalanx (MP). PP—proximal phalanx

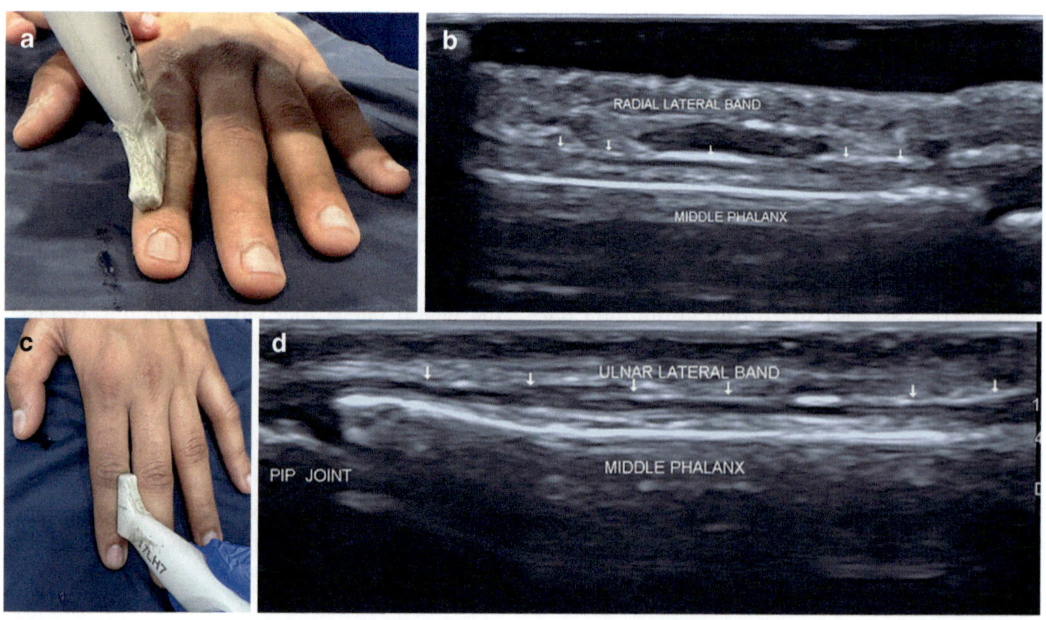

Fig. 12 Dorsal aspect. (**a**, **c**) Probe positioning for longitudinal examination. (**b**, **d**) Sonograms obtained as shown in (**a**, **c**) US show the radial lateral band (*small white arrows in* **b**) and ulnar lateral band (*small white arrows in* **d**) at the level of middle phalanx

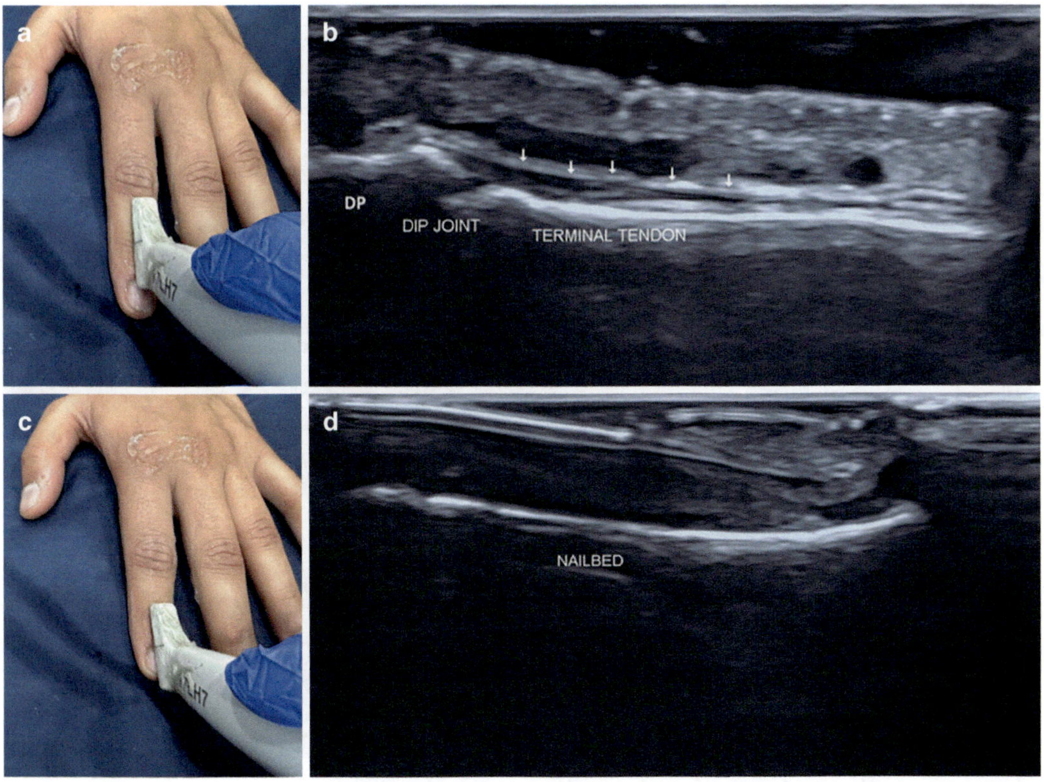

Fig. 13 Dorsal aspect. (**a**, **c**) Probe positioning for longitudinal examination. (**b**) Sonogram obtained as shown in **a**. US shows the insertion of terminal tendon (*small white arrows*) at the base of distal phalanx (DP). (**d**) Sonogram obtained as shown in **c**. US shows the nail bed at the distal phalanx

Details of the insertion of the intrinsic muscles are not detected at US.

The metacarpophalangeal and interphalangeal joints can be imaged in the sagittal and axial plane. US allows an accurate assessment of erosive articular changes (McNally 2008). The cartilage of the metacarpal and phalangeal head can be judged by using a dorsal and palmar approach in the extended and flexed joint while the cartilage of the bases of the phalanges is not detectable at US. US examination performed during gentle stress of the fingers' joints can help in judging the capsulo-ligamentous complex. This is most often performed at the level of the MCP of the thumb in the evaluation of tears of the ulnar collateral ligament.

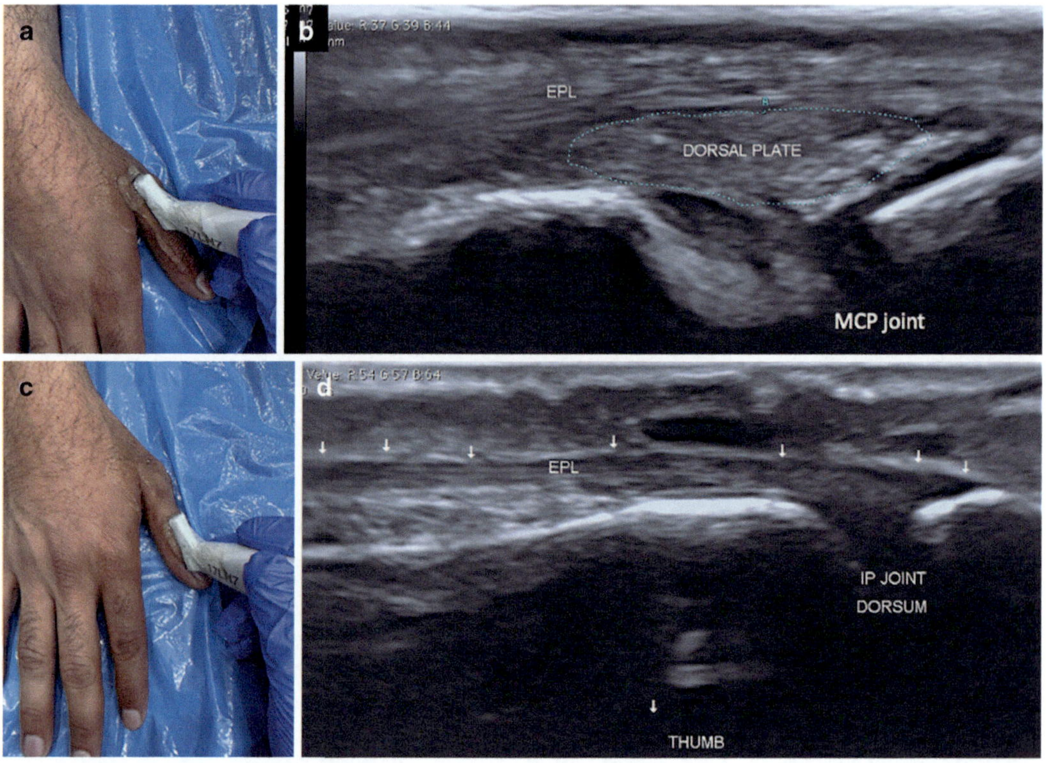

Fig. 14 Dorsal aspect. (**a**, **c**) Probe positioning for longitudinal examination. (**b**) Sonogram obtained as shown in **a**. US shows the dorsal plate at the metacarpophalangeal (MCP) joint of the thumb with overlying EPL tendon. (**d**) Sonogram obtained as shown in **c**. US shows the insertion of EPL tendon (*short white arrows*) at the base of distal phalanx (DP) of thumb. PP—proximal phalanx

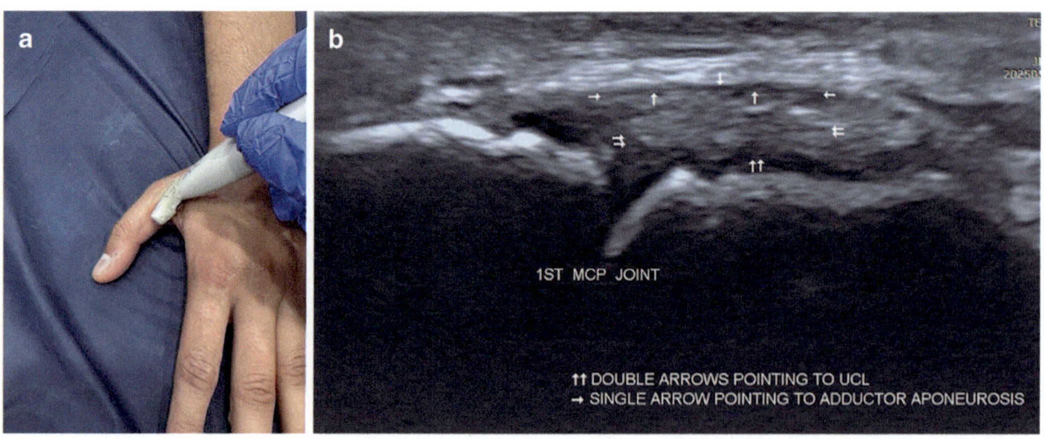

Fig. 15 Dorsal aspect. (**a**) Probe positioning for longitudinal examination at the ulnar aspect of MCP joint of the thumb. (**b**) Sonogram obtained as shown in **a**. US shows the aponeurosis of the adductor pollicis brevis muscle (*single white arrow*) overlying the ulnar collateral ligament (UCL) marked by double white arrows

Table 1 Extensor tendons

1 Tunnel = abductor pollicis longus (APL), extensor pollicis brevis (EPB)
2 Tunnel = extensor carpi radialis longus (ECRL), extensor carpi radialis brevis (ECRB)
3 Tunnel = extensor pollicis longus (EPL)
4 Tunnel = extensor digitorum communis (ED) and extensor indicis proprius (EIP)
5 Tunnel = extensor digiti minimi (EDM)
6 Tunnel = extensor carpi ulnaris (ECU)

4 Palmar Aspect

The palmar aspect of the wrist houses several tendons, nerves and vessels (Figs. 16, 17, 18, 19, 20, 21, 22, 23, 24, 25, 26, 27, 28, and 29). Abbreviations for these structures are listed in Table 2. The most superficial and thinnest tendon is the PG that runs in the midline of the wrist within the subcutaneous tissue. The PG presents

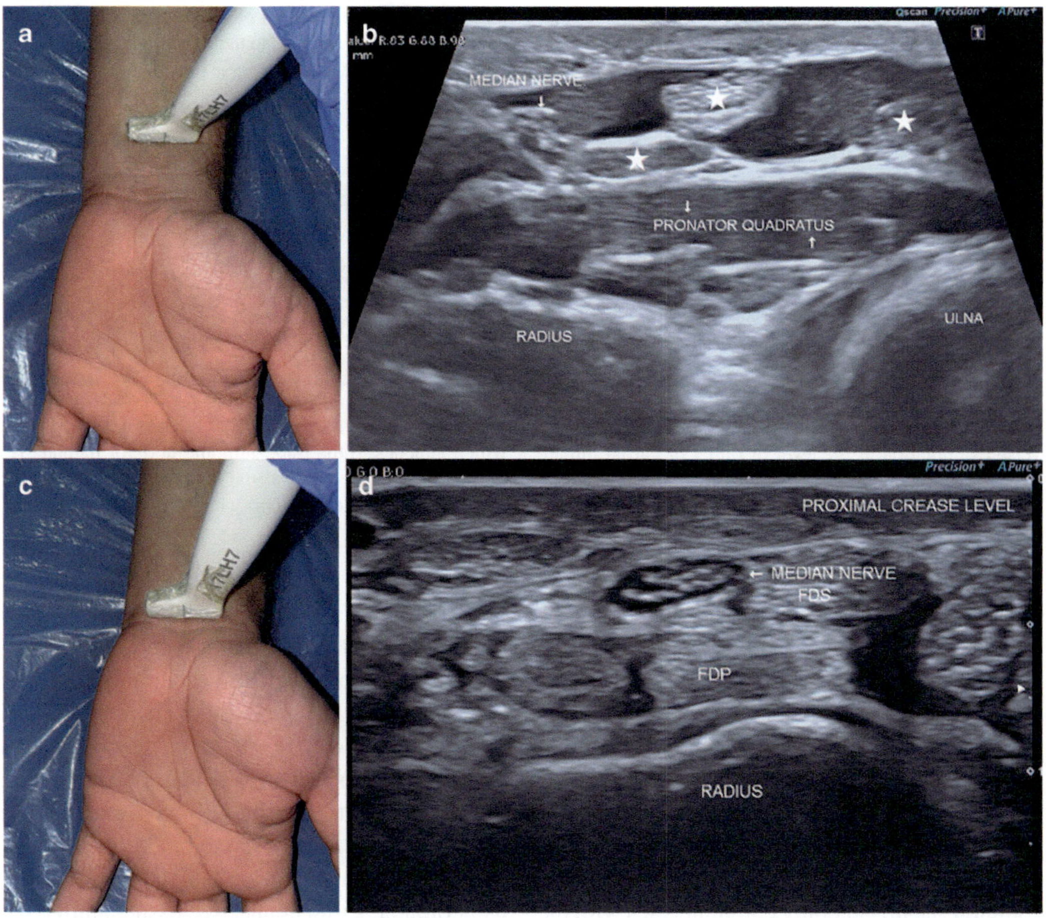

Fig. 16 Palmar aspect. (**a**, **c**) Probe positioning for transverse examination. (**b**) Sonogram obtained as shown in **a**. US shows the transversely oriented pronator quadratus muscle in distal forearm with the overlying myotendinous junctions of flexor tendons (*stars*) and the median nerve (*short white arrow*). (**d**) Sonogram obtained as shown in **c**. US shows the honeycomb appearance of the median nerve (*short white arrow*) and the compact echogenic appearance of flexor tendons (FDS, FDP) just before they enter the carpal tunnel

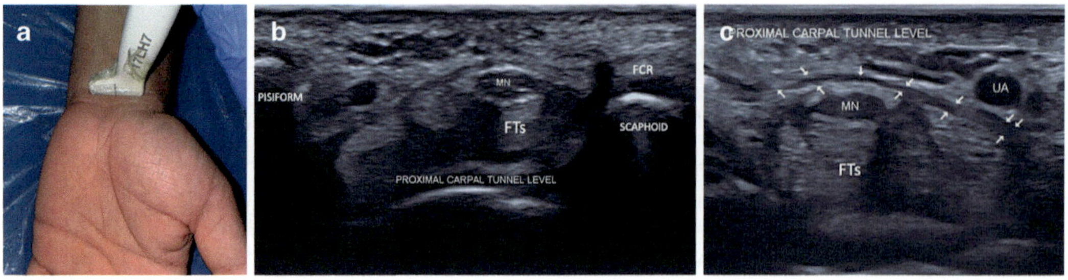

Fig. 17 Palmar aspect. (**a**) Probe positioning for transverse examination at the level of inlet of carpal tunnel. (**b**, **c**) Sonograms obtained as shown in **a**. US shows the median nerve(MN) and the flexor tendons (FTs) traversing underneath the transverse carpal ligament or the flexor retinaculum (short white arrows in **c**) which attaches to the scaphoid and pisiform bones. The ulnar artery (UA) lies outside the carpal tunnel. Note that normally there is no major vascular structure within the carpal tunnel. The flexor carpi radialis (FCR) tendon overlies the scaphoid bone. The flexor carpi ulnaris tendon has already attached to the pisiform bone and is thus not seen at this level in a transverse image

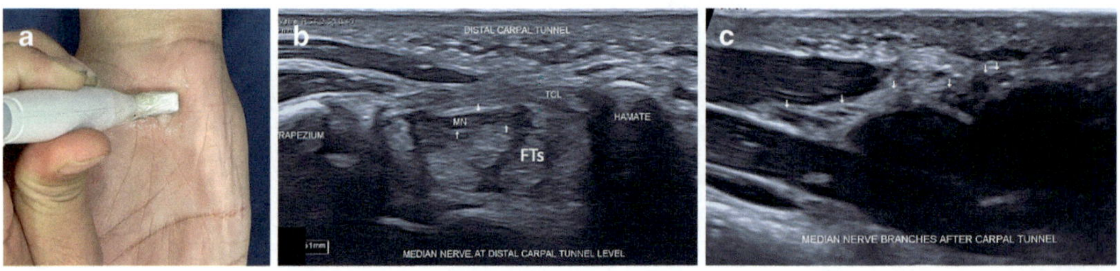

Fig. 18 Palmar aspect. (**a**) Probe positioning for transverse examination at the level of outlet of carpal tunnel. (**b**) Sonogram obtained as shown in **a**. US shows the median nerve(MN) and the flexor tendons (FTs) traversing underneath the transverse carpal ligament(TCL) which attaches to the trapezium and hook of hamate. (**c**) Sonogram obtained just distal to the outlet shows the median nerve branches (*short white arrows*)

a high anatomic variability. It can be absent or be replaced by a muscle (palmaris inversus).

In a deeper position, the flexor tendons of the fingers (FDS, FDP, FPL) run inside the carpal tunnel (CT), a fibro-osseous tunnel made by the carpal bones (the floor) and a palmar thick ligament, the transverse carpal ligament (TCL) (the ceiling). Inside the CT, the tendons are surrounded by a common synovial sheath enveloping the FDS and FDP of the 2–5 fingers. This common sheath generally communicates with the digital sheath of the fifth finger. The 2–4 fingers have separate digital sheaths. The FPL has a separate long sheath extending from the CT to the proximal phalanx of the thumb.

The FCR, a strong tendon surrounded by its own synovial sheath, runs in a lateral channel, separated from the CT by a vertical retinacular septum (Luong et al. 2014). In its distal portion, the FCR overlies the tubercle of the scaphoid and reflects over the palmar aspect of scapho-trapezio-trapezoid joint to deepen and reach its distal insertion into the base of the 2nd and 3rd metacarpals. The FCU is a straight tendon located at the medial aspect of the anterior face of the wrist that inserts into the proximal pole of the pisiform. Since it has a straight course this tendon is not surrounded by a synovial sheath but by its peritenon, a thin connective tissue lamina that facilitates its gliding.

Besides several tendons, the CT houses also the MN, a flat nerve located just under the TCL at the radial aspect of the tunnel. The nerve has a close relation with the FDP and FDS of the index. It innervates the muscles of the thenar eminence as well as the 1st and 2nd lumbrical muscles. The

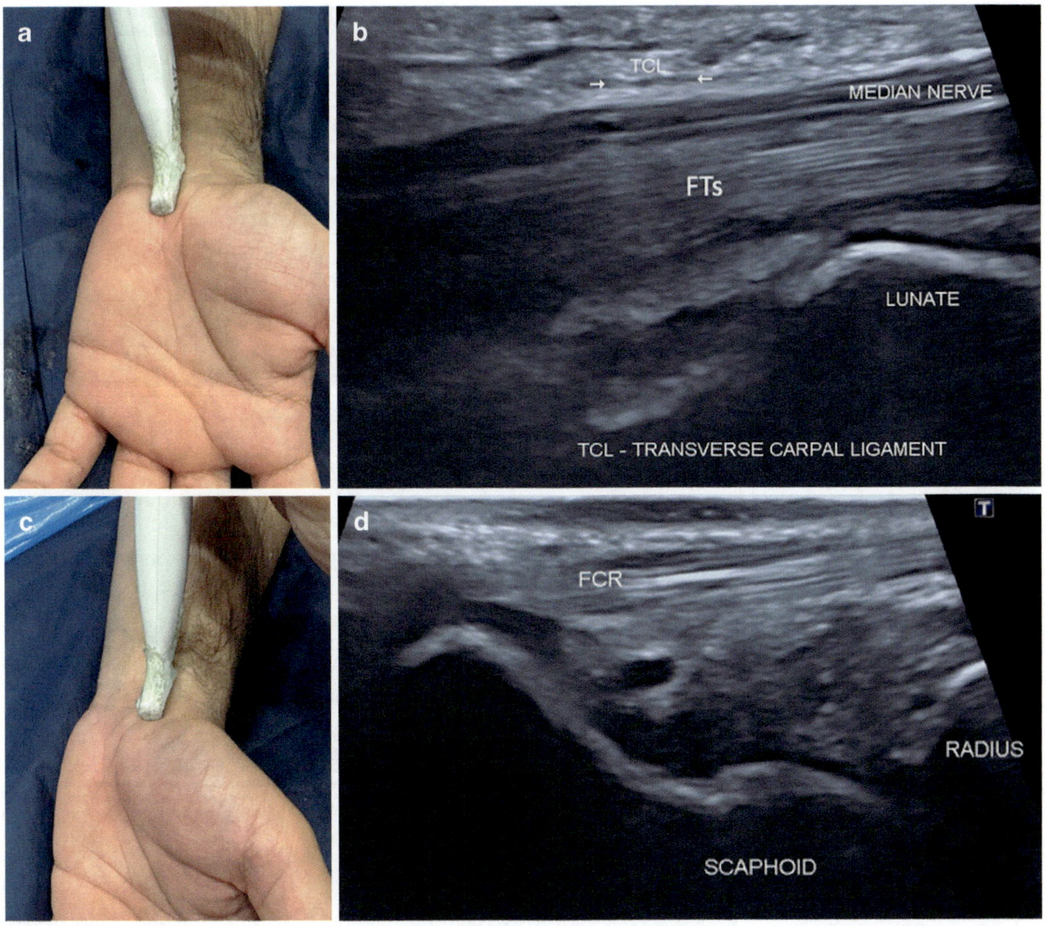

Fig. 19 Palmar aspect. (**a**, **c**) Probe positioning for longitudinal examination. (**b**) Sonogram obtained as shown in **a**. US shows the median nerve traversing over the flexor tendons (FTs) as they pass underneath the transverse carpal ligament (TCL). (**d**) Sonogram obtained as shown in **c**. US shows the flexor carpi radialis (FCR) tendon passing over the scaphoid. Distally it courses in close relation to the scapho-trapezio-trapezoid (STT) joint, pathologies of which can lead to tenosynovitis of the FCR

MN is responsible for sensitivity of the first three fingers and radial aspect of the fourth finger. US along with clinical evaluation and nerve conduction studies plays a crucial role in evaluating patients with carpal tunnel syndrome (CTS). It is also a robust tool for investigating potential causes of failed decompression in post-operative patients (Botchu et al. 2012). Details of its anatomy and anatomic variations will be discussed in more detail in "Nerve Entrapment Syndromes".

The Guyon's tunnel is a small fibro-osseous tunnel located medial to the CT extending from the level of pisiform till the hook of hamate. It is delimited by the TCL (floor) and the lateral aspect of the pisiform (the medial wall) and the palmar carpal ligament (the roof) in its proximal part. The tunnel houses, embedded by fat, the UN and the UAr surrounded by several UVe. The nerve is located between the artery and the pisiform. At a variable level inside the tunnel or immediately distal to it, the UN splits in one motor branch and one or two sensitive branches (Nischal and Bianchi 2023; Saran et al. 2025). A more detailed description of the Guyon's anat-

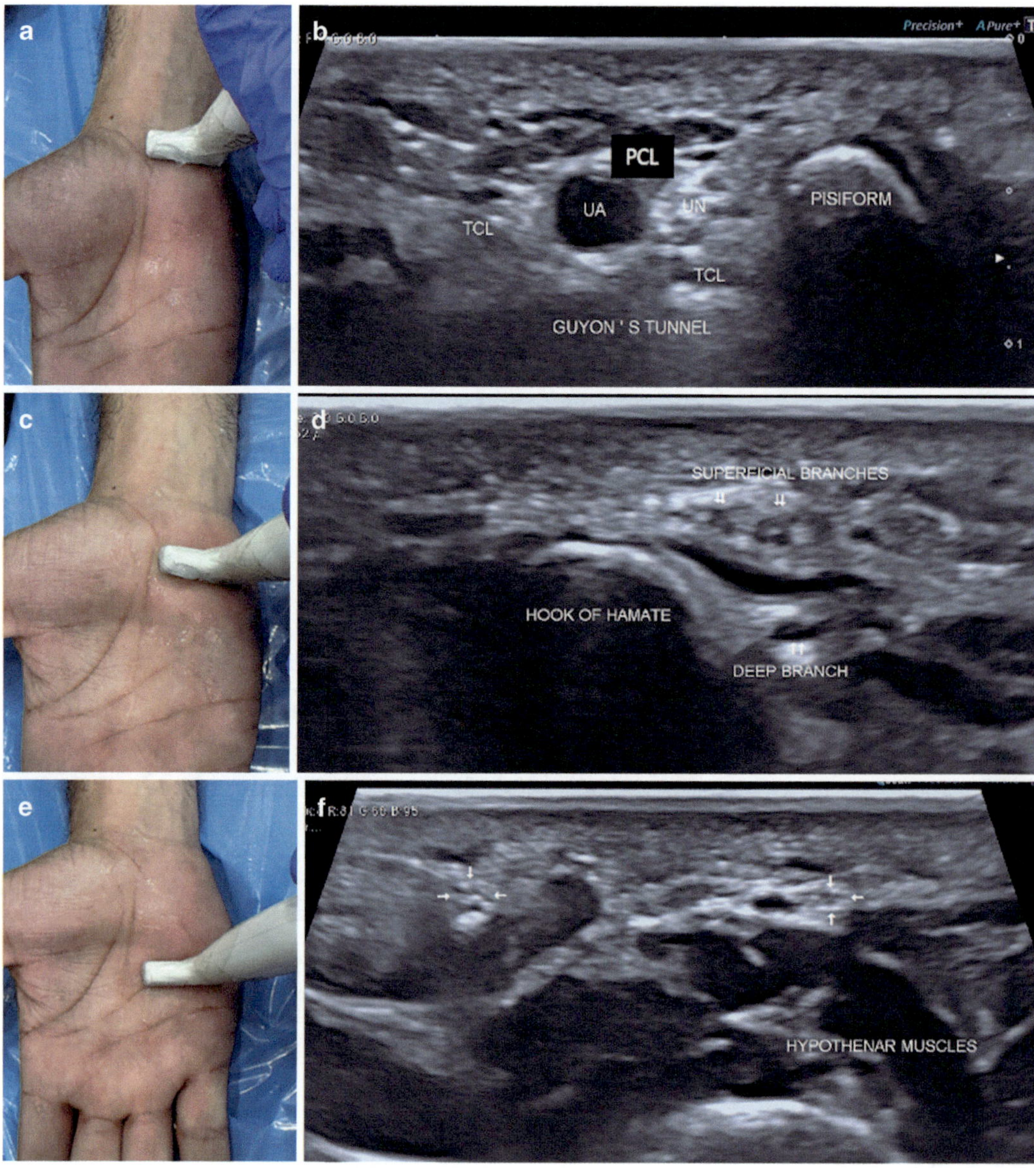

Fig. 20 Palmar aspect. (**a**, **c**, **e**) Probe positioning for transverse examination. (**b**) Sonogram obtained as shown in **a**. US shows the ulnar nerve(UN) along with the ulnar artery (UA) traversing the Guyon's canal. The transverse carpal ligament (TCL) forms the floor and the palmar carpal ligament (PCL) form the roof of the canal. (**d**) Sonogram obtained as shown in **c**. US shows the superficial and deep branches of the ulnar nerve at the level of hook of hamate. (**f**) Sonogram obtained as shown in **e**. US shows the digital branches of the ulnar nerve (*arrows*) overlying the hypothenar muscles

omy will be presented in "Nerve Entrapment Syndromes". The UN is responsible for sensitivity of the fifth finger and medial aspect of the fourth finger.

At the radial aspect of the wrist, the RAr is found running deep to the superficial fascia surrounded by satellite veins. The artery has close relation with the distal part of the sensitive branch of the RN. At the palm of the hand, the FDS and the FDP of the 2–5 fingers run together to join at the base of the fingers. Their synovial sheaths are not detectable even when high-frequency transducers are used. The FDP, located just inferior to the FDS, give insertion

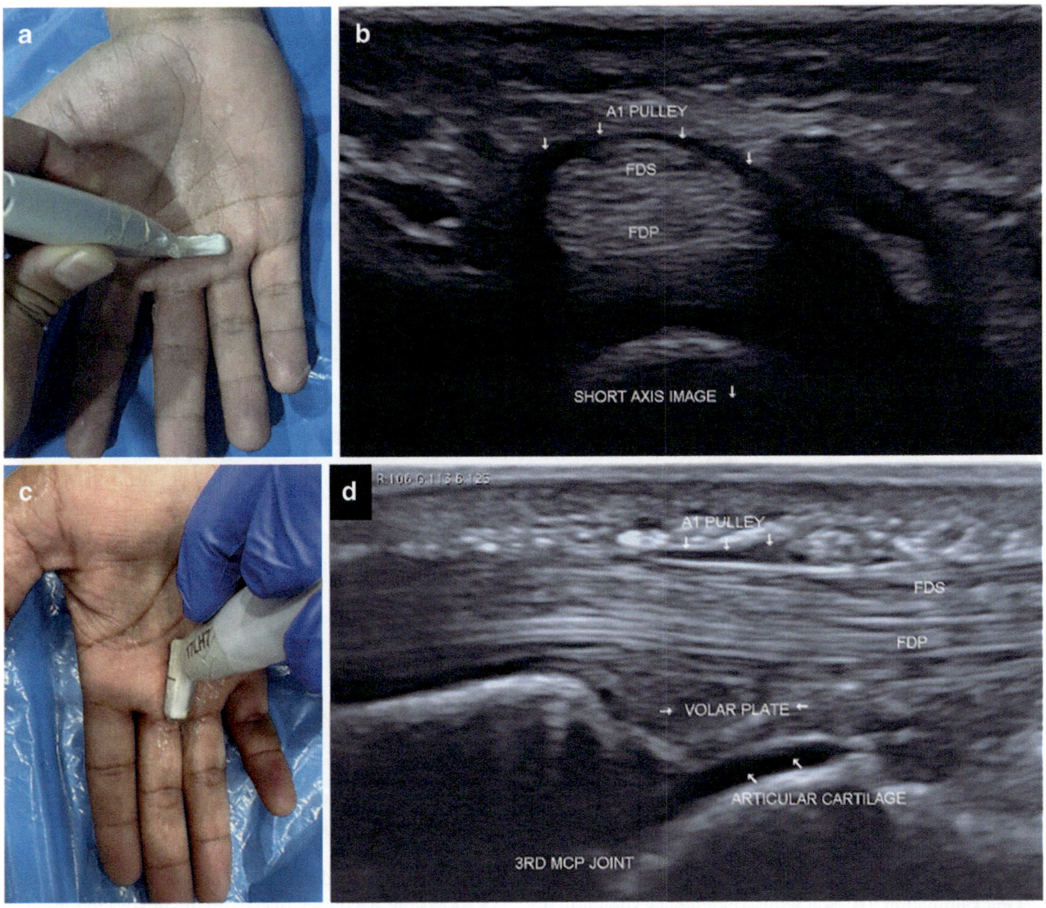

Fig. 21 Palmar aspect. (**a**, **c**) Probe positioning for transverse and longitudinal examination respectively. (**b**) Sonogram obtained as shown in **a**. US shows the A1 annular pulley (short white arrows) over the flexor tendons (FDS and FDP) at the level of metacarpal head. (**d**) Sonogram obtained as shown in **c**. US shows the volar plate at the level of MCP joint with anechoic smooth articular cartilage overlying the head of metacarpal. The FDS and FDP tendons seen in long axis with the overlying A1 pulley

to the lumbrical muscles. The vessels and the branches of the MN and UN run together located among the lumbrical muscles and the FDS surrounded by fat. More deeply are located the palmar interossei muscles.

Utilization of high-frequency probes allows an optimal assessment of the anatomy of the flexor tendons at the fingers. Transverse images show splitting of the FDS at the level of the proximal phalanx. The two tendinous laminae are located from proximal to distal: first superior, then lateral and medial and finally, inferior to the FDP tendon. They insert into the base of the middle phalanx. The FDP presents typically a triangular aspect with the base inferior in proximal scans and superior in more distal images. A frequent anatomic variation is bifidity of the FDP at the level of the distal part of the middle phalanx. This must not be interpreted as a posttraumatic longitudinal split. Longitudinal images are best suited to evaluate the tendons dynamically. When performed at the level of the MCP joint during flexion of the distal interphalangeal (DIP) joint, they show selective movements of the FDP tendon. Simultaneous flexion of the proximal interphalangeal (PIP) joint allows concomitant movements of the FDS tendon. The insertion of the two FDS hemitendons can be imaged at the level of the intermediate phalanx by displacing the transducer medially and laterally. The insertion of the FDP into the base of the distal

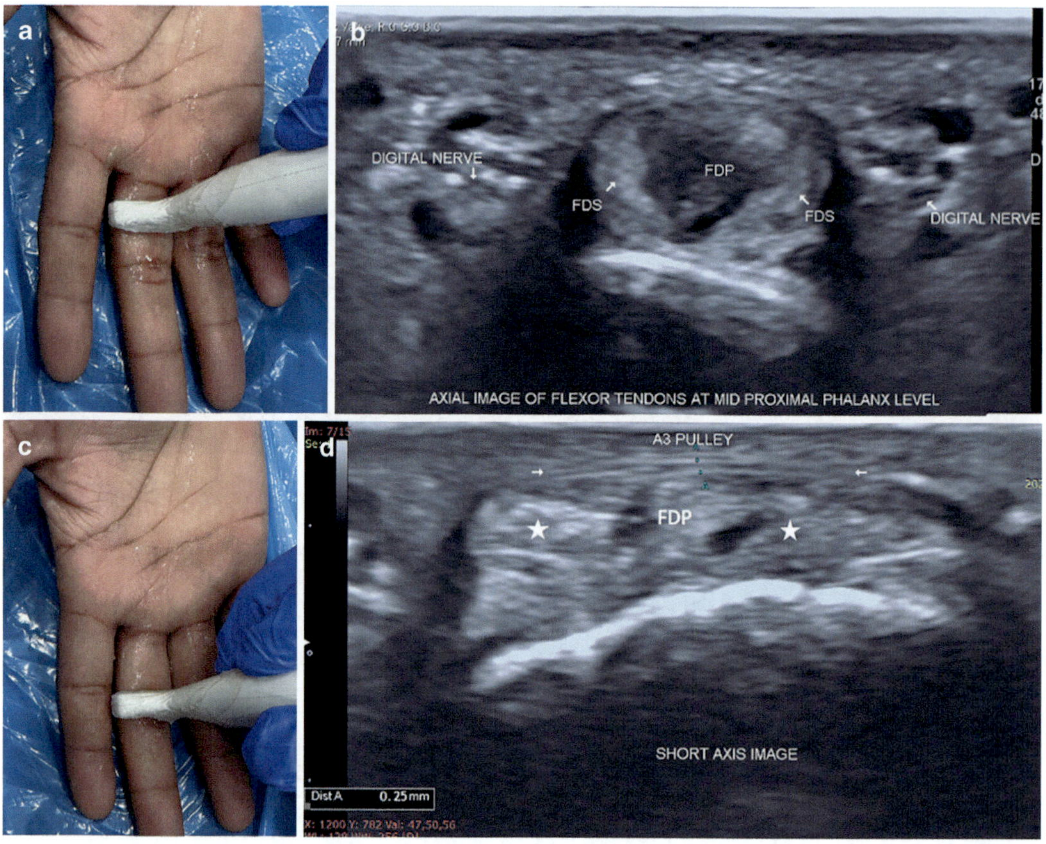

Fig. 22 Palmar aspect. (**a**, **c**) Probe positioning for transverse examination. (**b**) Sonogram obtained as shown in **a**. US shows the split of the FDS tendon with the slips in a lateral position relative to the FDP tendon at the level of proximal phalanx. (**d**) Sonogram obtained as shown in **c**. US shows the A3 pulley overlying the flexor tendons. The two tendinous slips of FDS tendon (star) seen going beneath the FDP tendon

phalanx is readily evident on sagittal images obtained over the distal phalanx.

A variety of pulleys (annular and cruciform) retain the flexor tendons against the palmar aspect of the phalanges thus preventing palmar instability during flexion (Bodner et al. 1999; Martinoli et al. 2000). Annular pulleys are quite rigid and are the main structures that prevent tendons bowstringing during flexion. They are numbered from 1 to 5 from proximal to distal. The A2 and A4 pulleys located, respectively, at the base of P1 and mid part of P2 are functionally the most important. The A1, A3 and A5 pulleys are located at the level of MCP, PIP and DIP joints respectively. The annular pulleys are visualized as thin hyperechoic structures in longitudinal images. They show a normal thickening of their insertion in transverse images. The cruciform pulleys are more lax and located among the annular pulleys. They are numbered C1, C2 and C3 and situated in between A2-A3, A3-A4 and A4-A5 pulleys respectively. They can be visualized at US only when a significant amount of fluid is present inside the tendon sheath and are otherwise not imaged routinely.

The different joints of the fingers can be examined by sagittal and axial sonograms. The palmar plates are well depicted as hyperechoic structures,

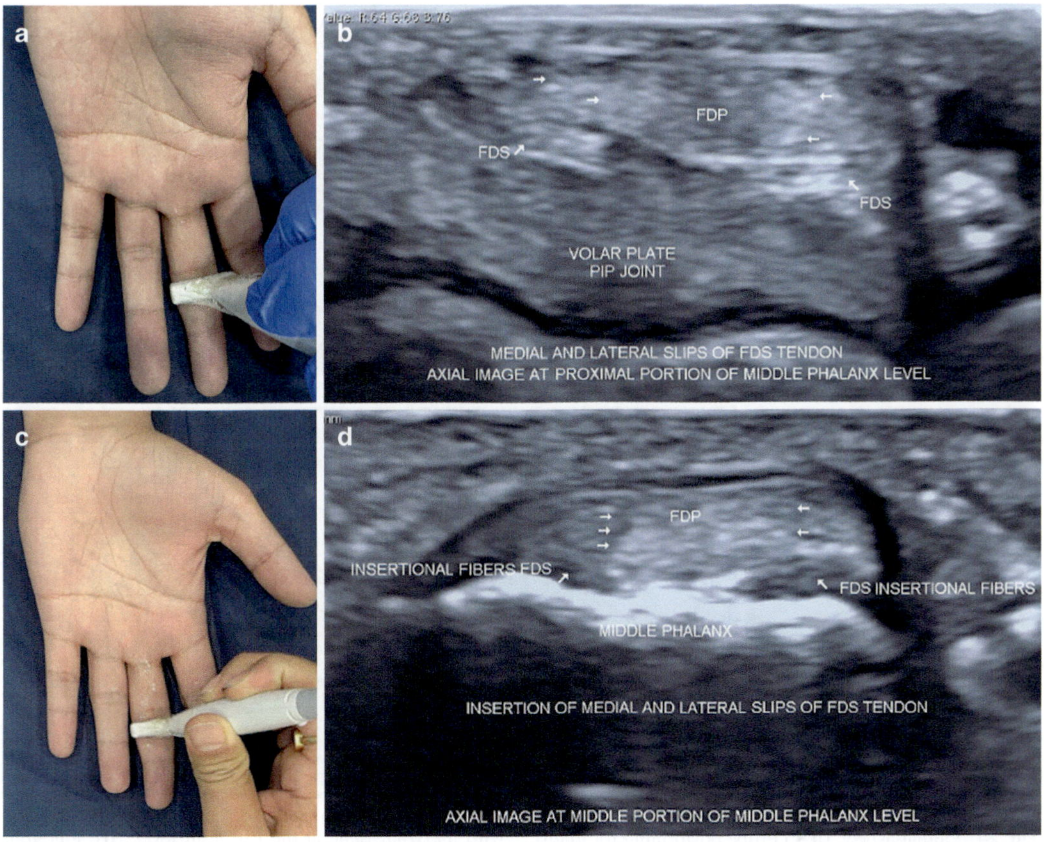

Fig. 23 Palmar aspect. (**a**, **c**) Probe positioning for transverse examination. (**b**) Sonogram obtained as shown in **a**. US shows the split of the FDS tendon with the slips deep to the FDP tendon. The echogenic volar plate is seen at this level. (**d**) Sonogram obtained as shown in **c**. US shows the fibres of FDS tendon inserting at the mid part of middle phalanx

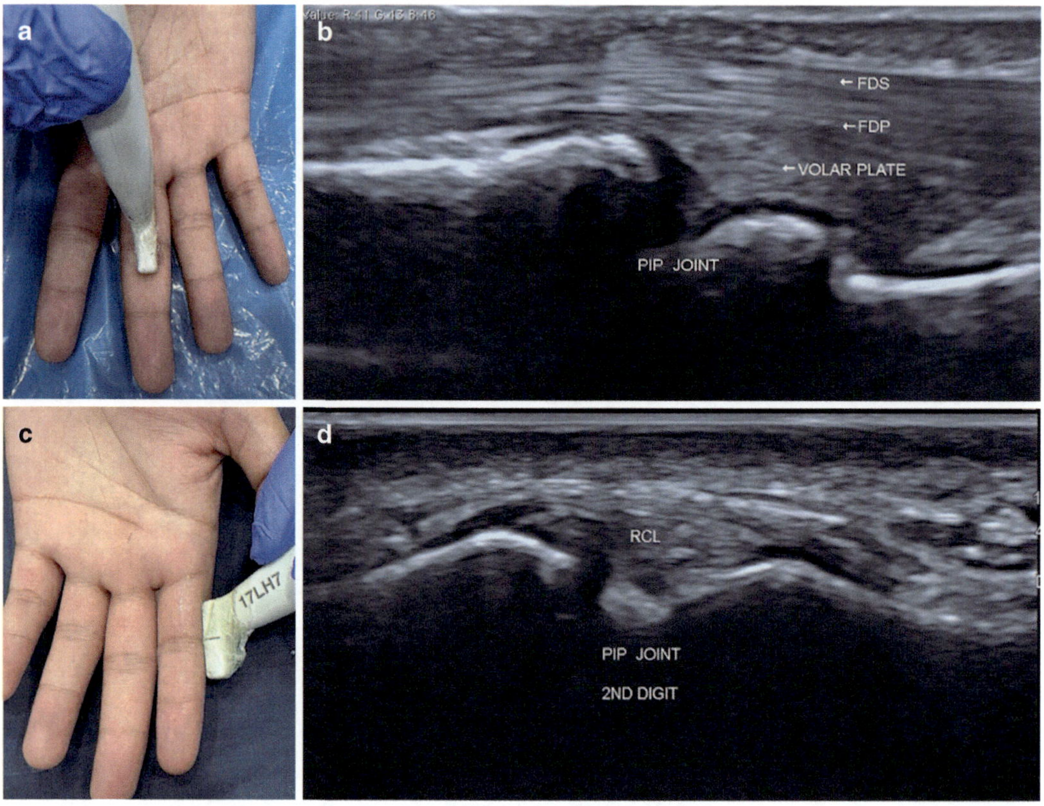

Fig. 24 Palmar aspect. (**a**, **c**) Probe positioning for longitudinal examination. (**b**) Sonogram obtained as shown in **a**. US shows the flexor tendons (FDS, FDP) in long axis with the volar plate at the PIP joint level. (**d**) Sonogram obtained as shown in **c**. US shows the radial collateral ligament (RCL) at the level of PIP joint of index finger

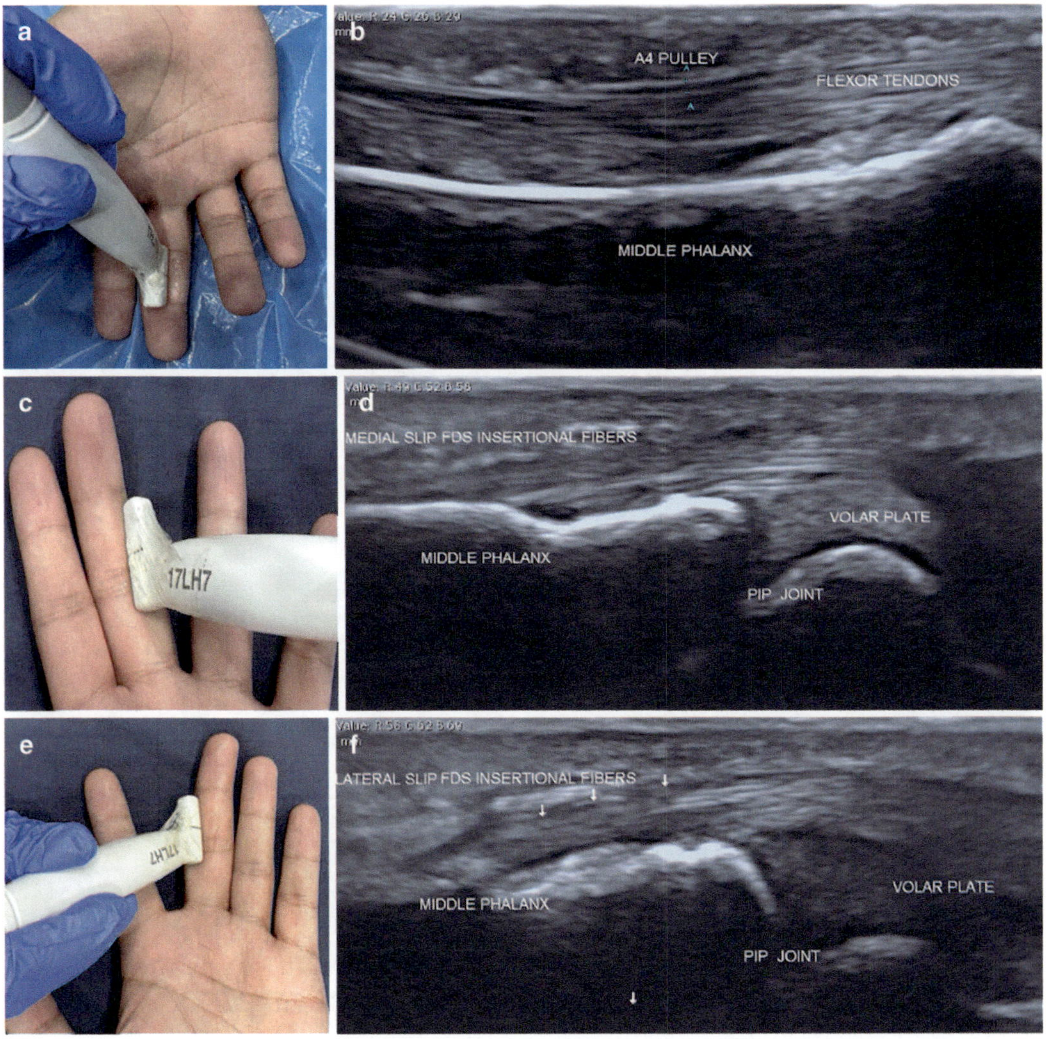

Fig. 25 Palmar aspect. (**a**, **c**, **e**) Probe positioning for longitudinal examination. (**b**) Sonogram obtained as shown in **a**. US shows the A4 pulley at the level of shaft of middle phalanx overlying the flexor. (**d**, **f**) Sonograms obtained as shown in **c**, **e** US shows the insertional medial and lateral fibres of the FDS tendons

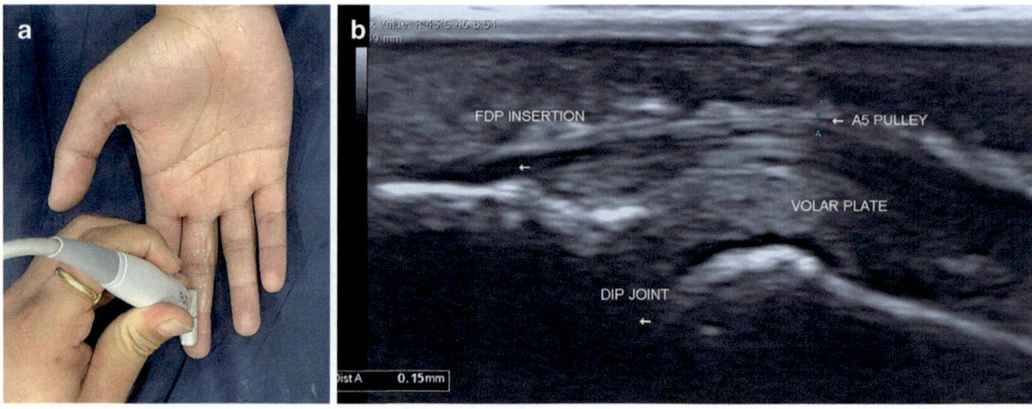

Fig. 26 Palmar aspect. (**a**) Probe positioning for longitudinal examination. (**b**) Sonogram obtained as shown in **a**. US shows the insertion of FDP tendon at the base of distal phalanx

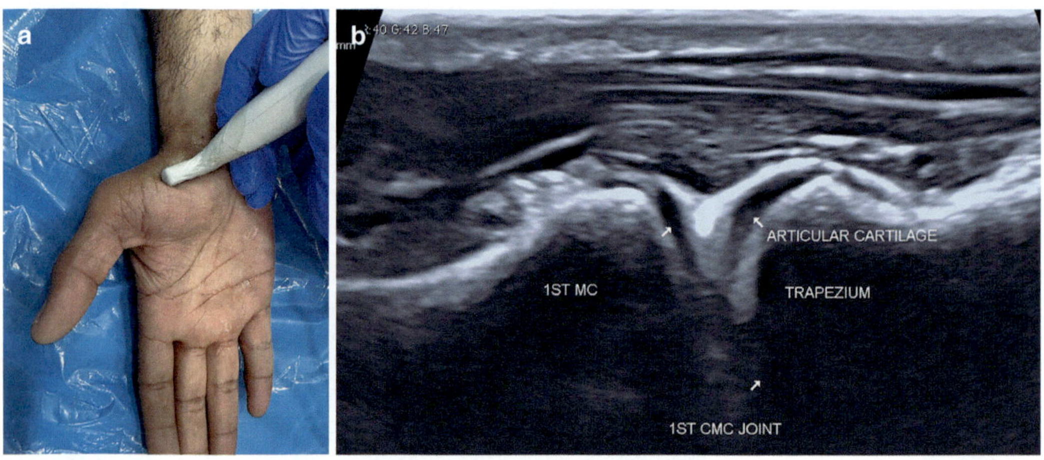

Fig. 27 Palmar aspect. (**a**) Probe positioning for longitudinal examination. (**b**) Sonogram obtained as shown in **a**. US shows the carpo-metacarpal (CMC) joint of the thumb

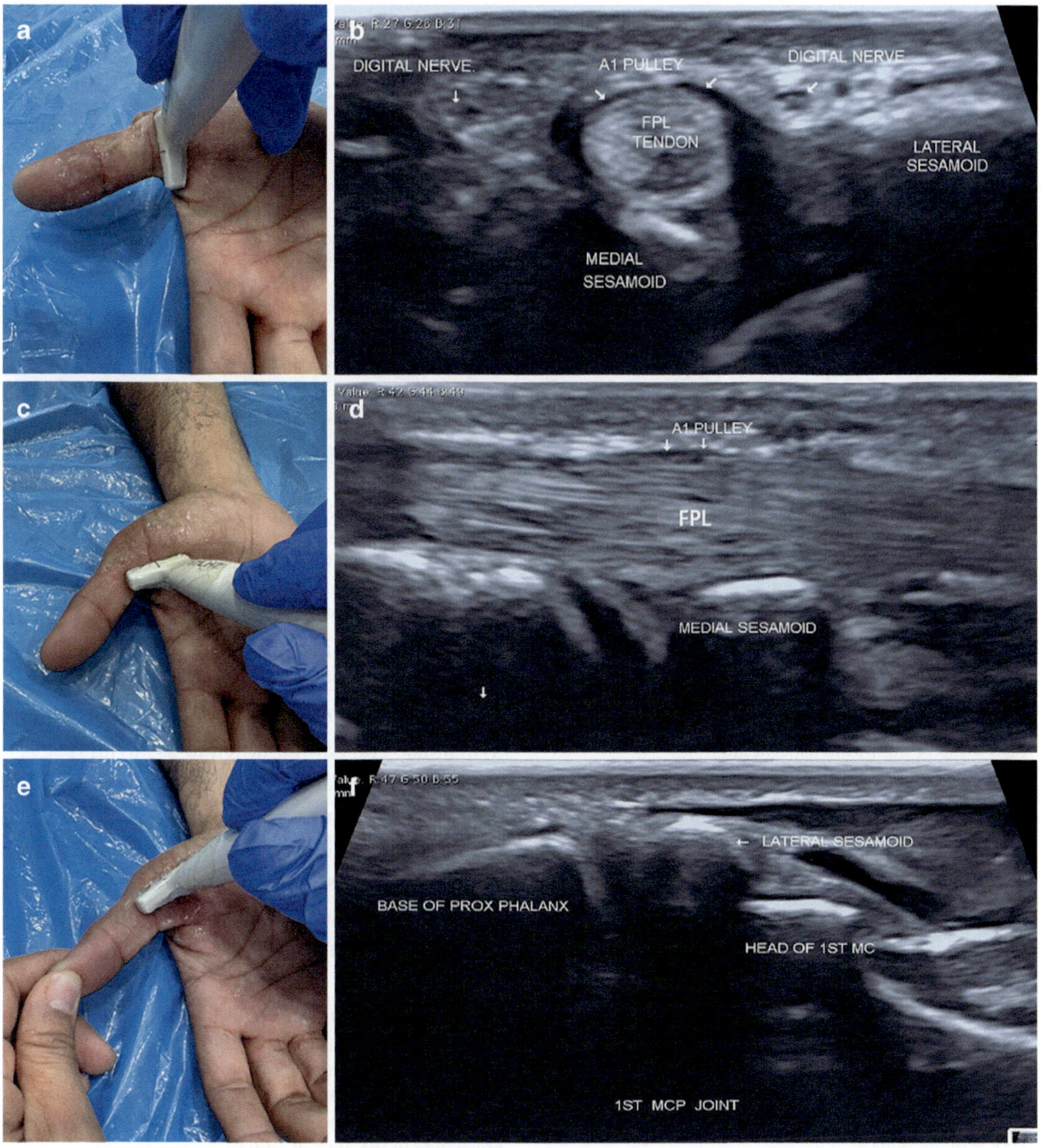

Fig. 28 Palmar aspect. (**a**, **c**, **e**) Probe positioning for examination of the thumb. (**b**) Sonogram obtained in transverse axis as shown in **a**. US shows the A1 pulley overlying the flexor pollicis longus (FPL) tendon. (**d**, **f**) Sonograms obtained in longitudinal axis as shown in **c**, **e**. US shows the medial and lateral sesamoid bones in relation to the head of thumb metacarpal

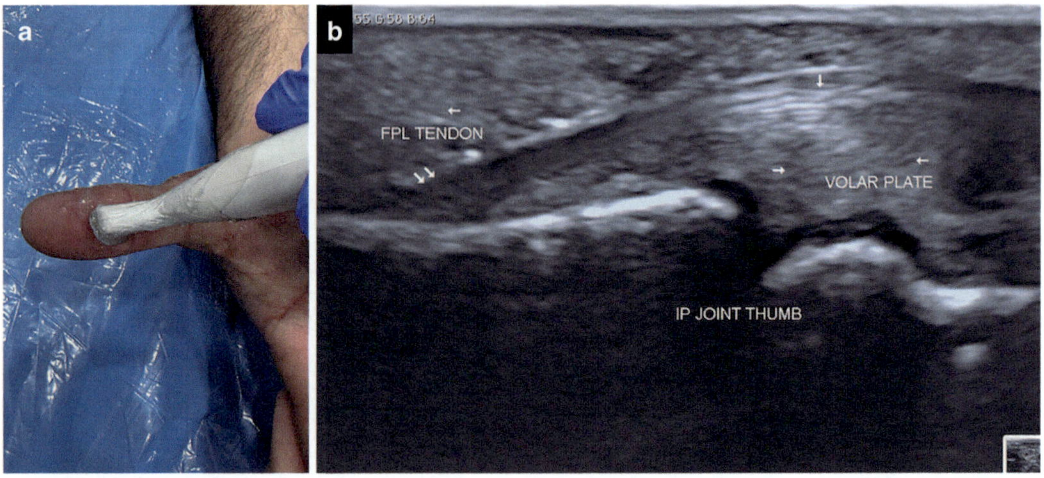

Fig. 29 Palmar aspect. (**a**) Probe positioning for longitudinal examination. (**b**) Sonogram obtained as shown in **a**. US shows the insertion of FPL tendon at the distal phalanx of thumb. The volar plate at the interphalangeal joint is labelled

Table 2 Anatomic structures of the palmar aspect of the wrist

Flexor tendons
PG = palmaris gracilis
FDS = flexor digitorum superficialis
FDP = flexor digitorum profundus
FPL = flexor pollicis longus
FCR = flexor carpi radialis
FCU = flexor carpi ulnaris
Nerves
MN = median nerve
UN = ulnar nerve
RN = radial nerve
Vessels
RAr = radial artery
RVe = radial veins
UAr = ulnar artery
UVe = ulnar veins

with homogeneous internal appearance, inserting into the base of the phalanges. Examination performed during gentle hyperextension of the examined joint can help in analysis of local tears or avulsions. The palmar articular synovial recess is readily evident and must be analysed for local effusion or synovial hypertrophy. Axial sonograms of the digital soft tissues allow assessment of the digital vessels and nerves till the level of the distal interphalangeal joint if high-frequency transducers are used.

Acknowledgement We would like to thank the authors of the previous edition Dr. Stefano Bianchi, Dr. René de Gautard, Dr. Giorgio Tamborrini and Dr. Stefan Mariacher for their contribution. We would also like to acknowledge Dr. Amit Thakur and Dr. Meet Radadia for their valuable assistance in the current edition.

Appendix A. Key Points

Advantages of Ultrasound in Wrist and Hand Assessment

- Ready available
- Noninvasive
- Inexpensive
- Patient-friendly
- Dynamic
- High resolution

Disadvantages of Ultrasound in Wrist and Hand Assessment

- Long learning curve
- Operator dependent
- Partial assessment of cartilages, ligaments and bones

Operator Requisites for US Examination in Wrist and Hand Assessment

- Perfect knowledge of the normal anatomy and anatomic variants
- Clinical knowledge of the main disorders affecting the wrist and hand
- Use of accurate and standardized technique of examination

Basic Principles of US Technique of Examination in Wrist and Hand Assessment

- Perform a basic clinical examination of the affected area and review other imaging studies before starting the US examination
- Focus the examination on the basis of clinical findings
- Analyse the structures using multiple planes of scanning
- Perform dynamic examination and colour Doppler examination
- Bilateral examination if required

References

Adler RS (2024) What is the place of ultrasound in MSK imaging? Skeletal Radiol 53(9):1699–1709. https://doi.org/10.1007/s00256-024-04642-2

Backhaus M, Kamradt T, Sandrock D et al (1999) Arthritis of the finger joints: a comprehensive approach comparing conventional radiography, scintigraphy, ultrasound, and contrast-enhanced magnetic resonance imaging. Arthritis Rheum 42:1232–1245

Backhaus M, Burmester G-R, Sandrock D et al (2002) Prospective two-year follow-up study comparing novel and conventional imaging procedures in patients with arthritic finger joints. Ann Rheum Dis 61:895–904

Bianchi S, Martinoli C (2007) Ultrasound of the musculoskeletal system. Springer, Heidelberg

Bianchi S, Martinoli C, Abdelwahab IF (1999) High-frequency ultrasound examination of the wrist and hand. Skeletal Radiol 28:121–129

Bianchi S, Martinoli C, Sureda D et al (2001) Ultrasound of the hand. Eur J Ultrasound 14:29–34

Bianchi S, Martinoli C, Montet X et al (2003) Wrist and hand ultrasound. Radiologe 43:831–840

Bihan M, Pesquer L, Meyer P et al (2009) High resolution sonography of the dorsal radiocarpal and intercarpal ligaments: findings in healthy subjects with anatomic correlation to cadaveric wrists. J Radiol 90:813–817

Blomley MJ, Cooke JC, Unger EC et al (2001) Microbubble contrast agents: a new era in ultrasound. BMJ 322:1222–1225

Bodner G, Rudish A, Gabl M et al (1999) Diagnosis of digital flexor tendon annular pulley disruption: comparison of high frequency ultrasound and MRI. Ultraschall Med 20:131–136

Botchu R, Bhatt R (2012) USG of mass in hand and wrist. J Dr NTR Univ Health Sci 1(3):148. https://doi.org/10.4103/2277-8632.102437

Botchu R, Bianchi S (2014) Sonography of trapezial ridge fractures. J Clin Ultrasound 42(4):241–244. https://doi.org/10.1002/jcu.22083

Botchu R, Khan A, Jeyapalan K (2012) Pictorial essay: role of ultrasound in failed carpal tunnel decompression. Indian J Radiol Imaging 22(01):31–34. https://doi.org/10.4103/0971-3026.95401

Boutry N, Lapegue F, Masi L et al (2005) Ultrasonographic evaluation of normal extrinsic and intrinsic carpal ligaments: preliminary experience. Skeletal Radiol 34:513–521

Brasseur J-L, Tardieu M (2006) Echographie de l'appareil locomoteur. Masson, Paris

Chiou HJ, Chou YH, Chang CY (2001) Ultrasonography of the wrist. Can Assoc Radiol J 5:302–311

Creteur V, Peetrons P (2000) Ultrasonography of the wrist and the hand. J Radiol 81:346–352

Cunnington J, Marshall N, Hide G et al (2010) A randomized, double-blind, controlled study of ultrasound-guided corticosteroid injection into the joint of patients with inflammatory arthritis. Arthritis Rheum 62(7):1862–1869. https://doi.org/10.1002/art.27448

D'Agostino MA, Wakefield RJ, Berner-Hammer H et al (2016) Value of ultrasonography as a marker of early response to abatacept in patients with rheumatoid arthritis and an inadequate response to methotrexate: results from the APPRAISE study. Ann Rheum Dis 75(10):1763–1769. https://doi.org/10.1136/annrheumdis-2015-207709

De Maeseneer M, Marcelis S, Osteaux M et al (2005) Sonography of a rupture of the tendon of the extensor pollicis longus muscle: initial clinical experience and correlation with findings at cadaveric dissection. AJR Am J Roentgenol 184:175–179

De Maeseneer M, Marcelis S, Jager T et al (2009) Spectrum of normal and pathologic findings in the region of the first extensor compartment of the wrist: sonographic findings and correlations with dissections. J Ultrasound Med 28:779–786

Di Matteo A, Mankia K, Azukizawa M, Wakefield RJ (2020) The role of musculoskeletal ultrasound in the rheumatoid arthritis continuum. Curr Rheumatol Rep 22(8):41. https://doi.org/10.1007/s11926-020-00911-w

Diao XH, Shen Y, Chen L et al (2022) Superb microvascular imaging is as sensitive as contrast-enhanced ultrasound for detecting synovial vascularity in rheumatoid arthritis. Quant Imaging Med Surg 12(5):2866–2876. https://doi.org/10.21037/qims-21-859

Ferrara MA, Marcelis S (1997) Ultrasound examination of the wrist. J Belg Radiol 80:78–80

Finlay K, Lee R, Friedman L (2004) Ultrasound of intrinsic wrist ligament and triangular fibrocartilage injuries. Skeletal Radiol 33:85–90

Goldberg BB, Liu JB, Forsberg F (1994) Ultrasound contrast agents: a review. Ultrasound Med Biol 20:319–333

Grassi W, Tittarelli E, Pirani O et al (1993) Ultrasound examination of metacarpophalangeal joints in rheumatoid arthritis. Scand J Rheumatol 22:243–247

Griffith JF, Chan DP, Ho PC et al (2001) Sonography of the normal scapholunate ligament and scapholunate joint space. J Clin Ultrasound 29:223–229

Guillin R, Botchu R, Bianchi S (2012) Sonography of orthopedic hardware impingement of the extremities. J Ultrasound Med 31(9):1457–1463. https://doi.org/10.7863/jum.2012.31.9.1457

Gutierrez M, Di Matteo A, Rosemffet M et al (2016) Short-term efficacy to conventional blind injection versus ultrasound-guided injection of local corticosteroids in tenosynovitis in patients with inflammatory chronic arthritis: a randomized comparative study. Joint Bone Spine 83(2):161–166. https://doi.org/10.1016/j.jbspin.2015.04.017

Jacobson JA, Oh E, Propeck T et al (2002) Sonography of the scapholunate ligament in four cadaveric wrists: correlation with MR arthrography and anatomy. AJR Am J Roentgenol 179:523–527

Karim Z, Wakefield RJ, Conaghan PG et al (2001) The impact of ultrasonography on diagnosis and management of patients with musculoskeletal conditions. Arthritis Rheum 44:2932–2933

Koski JM (1992) Ultrasonography in the detection of effusion in the radiocarpal and midcarpal joints. Scand J Rheumatol 21:79–81

Lee JC, Healy JC (2005) Normal sonographic anatomy of the wrist and hand. Radiographics 25:1577–1590

Lohman M, Vasenius J, Nieminen O (2007) Ultrasound guidance for puncture and injection in the radiocarpal joint. Acta Radiol 48:744–747

Luong DH, Smith J, Bianchi S (2014) Flexor carpi radialis tendon ultrasound pictorial essay. Skeletal Radiol 43(6):745–760. https://doi.org/10.1007/s00256-014-1846-1

Mak D, James S, Botchu R (2019) Dynamic ultrasound assessment of extensor compartment 1 of the wrist-snapping thumb. Sonography 6(3):134–136. https://doi.org/10.1002/sono.12190

Martinoli C, Bianchi S, Derchi L et al (2000) Sonographic evaluation of digital annular pulleys tears. Skeletal Radiol 29:387–391

McNally E (2004) Practical musculoskeletal ultrasound. Elsevier, Amsterdam

McNally EG (2008) Ultrasound of the small joints of the hands and feet: current status. Skeletal Radiol 37:99–113

Middleton WD, Teefey SA, Boyer MI (2001) Hand and wrist sonography. Ultrasound Q 17:21–36

Milbradt H, Calleja Cancho E, Qaiyumi SA et al (1990) Sonography of the wrist and the hand. Radiologe 30:360–365

Moschilla G, Breidahl W (2002) Sonography of the finger. AJR 178:1451–1457

Muncibì F, Carulli C, Paez DC et al (2008) A case of bilateral extensor digitorum brevis manus. Chir Organi Mov 92:133–135

Nischal N, Bianchi S (2023) Ultrasound of the hook of hamate region: pictorial review. J Ultrasound Med 42(2):497–512. https://doi.org/10.1002/jum.16031

Platzgummer H, Schueller G, Grisar J, Weber M, Schueller-Weidekamm C (2009) Quantification of synovitis in Rheumatoid Arthritis: do we really need quantitative measurement of contrast-enhanced ultrasound? Eur J Radiol 71(2):237–241. https://doi.org/10.1016/j.ejrad.2009.03.044

Raza K (2003) Ultrasound guidance allows accurate needle placement and aspiration from small joints in patients with early inflammatory arthritis. Rheumatology 42(8):976–979. https://doi.org/10.1093/rheumatology/keg269

Read JW, Conolly WB, Lanzetta M et al (1996) Diagnostic ultrasound of the hand and wrist. J Hand Surg 21:1004–1010

Renoux J, Zeitoun-Eiss D, Brasseur JL (2009) Ultrasonographic study of wrist ligaments: review and new perspectives. Semin Musculoskelet Radiol 13:55–65

Robertson BL, Jamadar DA, Jacobson JA et al (2007) Extensor retinaculum of the wrist: sonographic characterization and pseudotenosynovitis appearance. AJR Am J Roentgenol 188:198–202

Saran S, Reddy PS, Shirodkar K, Shah AB, Agarwal A, Shah A, Iyengar KP, Botchu R (2025) Unveiling Guyon's canal: insights into clinical anatomy, pathology, and imaging. Diagnostics (Basel) 15(5):592

Scheel AK, Hermann KG, Ohrndorf S et al (2006) Prospective long term follow-up imaging study comparing radiography, ultrasonography and magnetic resonance imaging in rheumatoid arthritis finger joints. Ann Rheum Dis 65:595–600

Szkudlarek M, Narvestad E, Klarlund M et al (2004a) Ultrasonography of the metatarsophalangeal joints in rheumatoid arthritis: comparison with magnetic resonance imaging, conventional radiography, and clinical examination. Arthritis Rheum 50:2103–2112

Szkudlarek M, Narvestad E, Court-Payen M et al (2004b) Ultrasonography of the RA finger joints is more sensitive than conventional radiography for detection of erosions without loss of specificity, with MRI as a reference method. Ann Rheum Dis 63:82–83

Tagliafico A, Rubino M, Autuori A et al (2007) Wrist and hand ultrasound. Semin Musculoskelet Radiol 11:95–104

Taljanovic MS, Sheppard JE, Jones MD et al (2008) Sonography and sonoarthrography of the scapholunate and lunotriquetral ligaments and triangular fibrocartilage disk: initial experience and correlation with arthrography and magnetic resonance arthrography. J Ultrasound Med 27:179–191

Teefey SA, Middleton WD, Boyer MI (2000) Sonography of the hand and wrist. Semin Ultrasound CT MR 21:192–204

Terslev L, Torp-Pedersen S, Savnik A et al (2003) Doppler ultrasound and magnetic resonance imaging of synovial inflammation of the hand in rheumatoid arthritis: a comparative study. Arthritis Rheum 48:2434–2441

Tubbs RS, Stetler W, Kelly DR et al (2007) Acrel's ganglion. Surg Radiol Anat 29:379–381

Van Holsbeeck M, Introcaso JH (2001) Musculoskeletal ultrasound, 2nd edn. Mosby Co, St Louis

Wakefield RJ, Gibbon WW, Conaghan PG et al (2000) The value of sonography in the detection of bone erosions in patients with rheumatoid arthritis. Arthritis Rheum 43:2762–2770

Walther M, Harms H, Krenn V et al (2001) Correlation of power Doppler sonography with vascularity of the synovial tissue of the knee joint in patients with osteoarthritis and rheumatoid arthritis. Arthritis Rheum 44:331–829

Yammine K (2015) The prevalence of the extensor indicis tendon and its variants: a systematic review and meta-analysis. Surg Radiol Anat 37:247–254

Yu X, Li Z, Ren M, Xi J, Wu J, Ji Y (2018) Superb microvascular imaging (SMI) for evaluating hand joint lesions in patients with rheumatoid arthritis in clinical remission. Rheumatol Int 38(10):1885–1890. https://doi.org/10.1007/s00296-018-4112-3

Interventions of the Hand and Wrist

Sonal Saran, Saavi Reddy Pellakuru, Ankit B. Shah, Feiran Wu, and Rajesh Botchu

Contents

S. Saran (✉)
Department of Diagnostic and Intervention Radiology, AIIMS Rishikesh, Uttarakhand, India

S. R. Pellakuru
Department of Radiology, Apollo Institute of Medical Sciences and Research, Hyderabad, India

A. B. Shah
Department of Radiology, Eclat Imaging Centre, Mumbai, India

F. Wu
Birmingham Hand Centre, Queen Elizabeth Hospital, University Hospitals Birmingham NHS Foundation Trust, Birmingham, UK

R. Botchu
Department of Musculoskeletal Radiology, Royal Orthopedic Hospital, Birmingham, UK

Med Radiol Diagn Imaging (2025)
https://doi.org/10.1007/174_2025_561,
Published Online: 18 February 2025

Abstract

Interventional procedures for the wrist and hand have become essential tools in the management of a variety of musculoskeletal conditions, including tendinopathies, joint disorders, and soft tissue pathologies. Advancements in imaging modalities—ultrasound, fluoroscopy, computed tomography (CT), and magnetic resonance imaging (MRI)—have improved procedural accuracy, safety, and patient outcomes. Ultrasound remains the most versatile tool, facilitating dynamic, real-time imaging for guided injections, aspirations, and barbotage. Fluoroscopy offers the advantage of visualizing contrast dispersion for confirming joint access, while CT provides unmatched detail for complex bone biopsies. MRI, though limited by availability and cost, holds the potential for precision targeting in soft tissue interventions. Adherence to sterile techniques, proper patient selection, and thorough preprocedural evaluation are vital to minimizing risks. Comprehensive patient education, informed consent, and realistic outcome expectations further ensure procedural success. Emerging technologies, including robotics and enhanced imaging systems, are poised to advance the precision and scope of interventions, paving the way for more effective, minimally invasive treatments. As the field evolves, ongoing research and innovation will continue to refine techniques, expand applications, and improve patient outcomes, solidifying the role of interventional procedures as a cornerstone of wrist and hand musculoskeletal care.

1 Background

Wrist and hand complaints are prevalent in the general population, with incidence ranging from 10% to 20% annually depending on the condition and demographic factors and represent a frequent indication for interventional radiology procedures. For example, studies have shown that carpal tunnel syndrome (CTS) has an incidence of approximately 3.5 per 1000 person-years (Atroshi et al. 1999), while the incidence of hand osteoarthritis increases with age, affecting up to 20% of individuals over 55 years (Kloppenburg and Kwok 2011). In addition, tendinopathies and soft tissue injuries are also frequent contributors to wrist and hand pain (Walker-Bone et al. 2003).

The wrist and hand region are characterized by intricate and highly specialized anatomy, which necessitates a comprehensive understanding of both anatomical structures and procedural techniques to ensure the accurate and safe performance of any interventions. This region comprises multiple critical joints, including the radio-carpal joint (RCJ), distal radio-ulnar joint (DRUJ), intercarpal joints, scaphotrapeziotrapezoid (STT) joint, and the carpometacarpal joints (CMCJ), with particular importance given to the first carpometacarpal joint (1st CMCJ) due to its common involvement in conditions like osteoarthritis. Additionally, the metacarpophalangeal (MCP) joints (1st–5th) and the interphalangeal (IP) joints (1st–5th) are key articulations in hand function and mobility. Surrounding these joints are essential supporting structures, such as the flexor and extensor tendons, ligaments, and pulleys, which are vital for movement and stability (Chim 2017). Moreover, the neurovascular elements traversing this region further contribute to its complexity and are critical considerations during interventions. Given this intricate anatomy, the wrist and hand frequently require image guidance for diagnostic and therapeutic procedures, which ensures the necessary precision to avoid complications and optimize clinical outcomes.

This chapter provides a comprehensive overview of the imaging modalities employed in wrist and hand interventions, detailing the techniques specific to each modality. It addresses key procedural considerations, including the selection of appropriate hardware, such as needles and injectable agents, as well as essential patient preparation protocols to ensure safe and effective outcomes. A thorough discussion of the indications and contraindications for various interventions will be included, offering clinicians a clear understanding of when and how to perform these procedures.

2 Imaging Modalities and Techniques

The wrist and hand, being relatively superficial anatomical regions, are particularly well suited for image-guided interventions using ultrasonography. Ultrasound has become the preferred modality for many wrist and hand procedures due to its real-time visualization, accessibility, and superior ability to clearly delineate soft tissue structures such as tendons, ligaments, nerves, and fluid collections. Its non-ionizing nature, dynamic imaging capability, and cost-effectiveness further enhance its utility, making it a highly efficient and patient-friendly option (Colio et al. 2016; Orlandi et al. 2014).

Traditionally, fluoroscopy was a widely utilized imaging modality, particularly for interventions targeting bony structures and joint spaces, such as the RCJ, DRUJ, intercarpal joints, and MCP joints. Its reliability and ability to provide clear, real-time visualization of joint spaces make it an effective and practical choice for these procedures. In particular, injections into the RCJ and DRUJ were commonly performed under fluoroscopic guidance, given the precision required to access these small and complex joint spaces (Chopra et al. 2016).

However, with advancements in ultrasound technology and operator expertise, the majority of other wrist and hand interventions—especially those involving the soft tissues—are now primarily performed using ultrasound guidance. This shift is driven by the numerous advantages of ultrasound, including its non-ionizing nature, which eliminates radiation exposure, and its ability to provide dynamic imaging. This allows clinicians to evaluate and guide needle placement in relation to soft tissue structures in real time.

2.1 Ultrasound

Ultrasound-guided interventions in the wrist and hand can be broadly classified into direct and indirect methods. The direct method utilizes a dynamic, free-hand approach to advance the needle under continuous real-time ultrasound guidance. This technique ensures optimal accuracy in needle placement, allowing clinicians to make immediate adjustments based on live imaging feedback. Conversely, the indirect method involves an initial ultrasound examination to localize the target in two planes. The skin entry point is marked, and the procedure is performed without real-time ultrasound guidance. While less dynamic, the indirect method remains advantageous in settings where real-time imaging is impractical.

Real-time ultrasound-guided procedures can be further categorized into in-plane and out-of-plane techniques. The in-plane technique, where the needle is advanced parallel to the ultrasound transducer, is typically preferred as it enables visualization of the entire needle length during advancement. This visibility minimizes the risk of complications and ensures precise placement. In contrast, the out-of-plane technique involves advancing the needle perpendicular to the long axis of the transducer. While the entire needle is not continuously visualized, this approach is particularly useful for superficial interventions where a shorter and more direct needle path is sufficient (Fig. 1) (Patel et al. 2023).

Before performing ultrasound-guided interventions in the wrist and hand region, several factors must be considered. A 10 MHz or higher high-frequency linear-array probe is recommended to ensure optimal image resolution. Given the small anatomical areas involved, a small footprint probe, such as a hockey stick probe, can be particularly advantageous for improved maneuverability and access. It is essential to ensure that both the operator and the patient are in a comfortable position to facilitate a smooth and precise procedure. Additionally, a good “gel stand-off” between the probe and the patient’s skin can enhance the visualization of superficial structures and needle, improving accuracy during the intervention (Fig. 2) (Chopra et al. 2016).

Common ultrasound-guided interventions around the wrist and hand include joint injections into the RCJ, DRUJ, 1st CMCJ, and STT joint. Ultrasound is also frequently employed for tendon sheath injections, such as in the first extensor

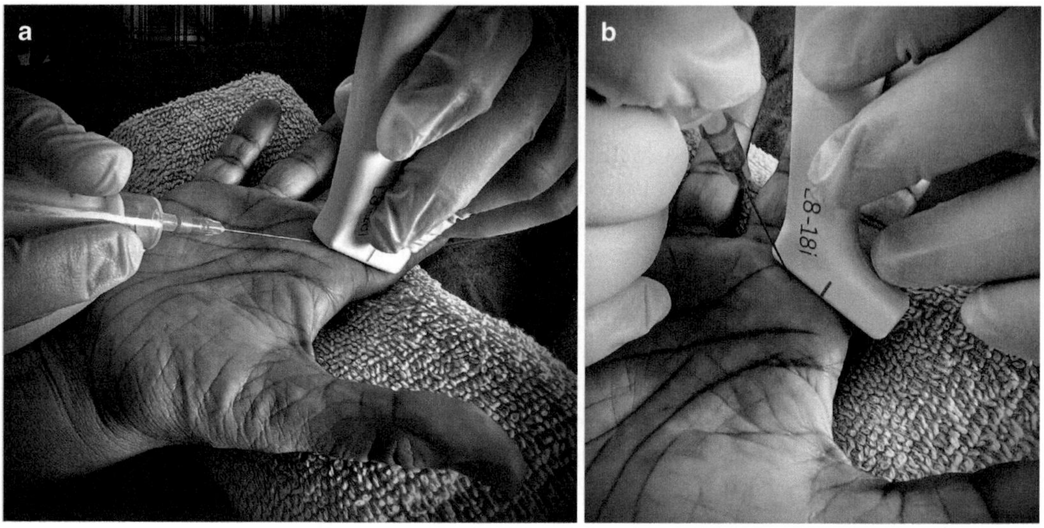

Fig. 1 (**a**) The in-plane technique, where the needle is advanced parallel to the ultrasound transducer, enables visualization of the entire needle length during advancement. (**b**) The out-of-plane technique advancing the needle perpendicular to the long axis of the transducer, in which the full needle is not continuously visualized

compartment for patients with De Quervain's tenosynovitis. In addition, ultrasound is widely used for carpal tunnel injections in cases of CTS, pulley release in the trigger finger, and aspiration of ganglion cysts. It can serve as a valuable tool for guiding biopsies of synovium and soft tissue tumors around the wrist and hand or targeting the soft tissue component of bone tumors in this region (Chopra et al. 2016).

2.2 Fluoroscopy

Fluoroscopy is an effective modality for performing various interventions in the wrist and hand, particularly joint injections into the RCJ, DRUJ, 1st CMCJ, and STT joint. A key advantage of fluoroscopy over ultrasound is the real-time visualization of contrast dispersion within the joint, allowing for documentation and confirmation of accurate injection placement (Chopra et al. 2016).

Additionally, fluoroscopy offers a hands-free approach, enabling the practitioner to operate with both hands unobstructed, unlike ultrasound-guided procedures where one hand is required to hold the probe. This freedom facilitates smoother equipment handling and transfers between the patient and the sterile field, enhancing procedural efficiency.

2.3 Others

Computed tomography (CT) guidance, while effective for specific procedures, involves tradeoffs such as ionizing radiation exposure and higher costs. CT is primarily used for bone biopsies and ablative procedures targeting osseous lesions, where its detailed imaging of bony structures is essential. However, its role in routine wrist and hand interventions, particularly those involving soft tissues, is limited. The precise bone imaging offered by CT is generally unnecessary for such procedures, making it less ideal. CT is typically reserved for complex cases requiring precise bone access, where its superior anatomical detail and cross-sectional imaging ensure accurate targeting and procedural success (Bansal et al. 2021).

Magnetic resonance imaging (MRI) is a more recent addition to musculoskeletal intervention guidance. With its superior contrast resolution, MRI allows for detailed visualization of soft tissues without ionizing radiation, making it ideal for targeting inflamed or pathological areas,

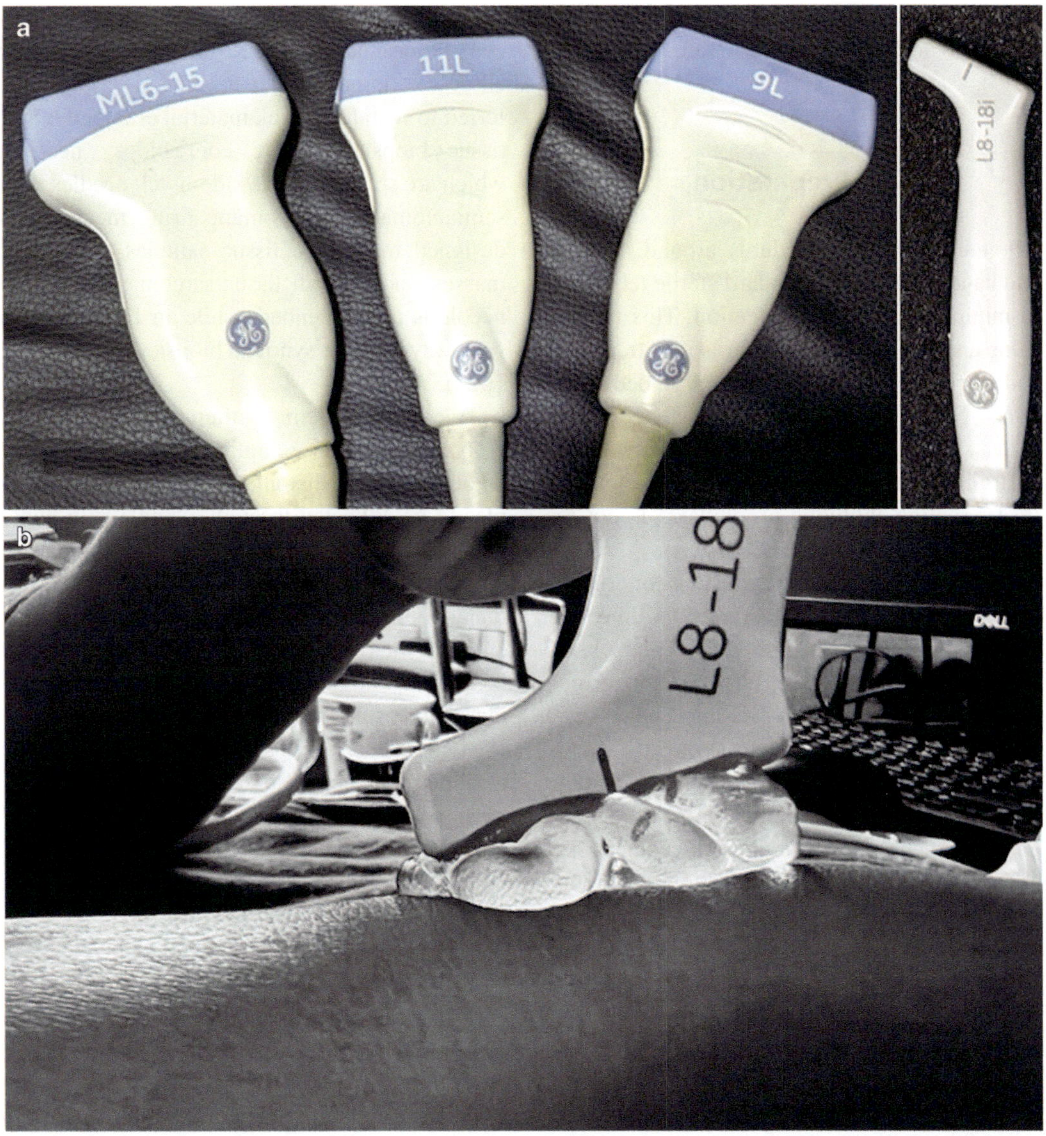

Fig. 2 (**a**) Different types of high-frequency ultrasound probes used for performing ultrasound-guided interventions in the wrist and hand region. (**b**) "Gel stand-off" between the probe and the patient's skin can enhance the visualization of superficial structures and the needle, improving accuracy during the intervention

potentially improving therapeutic outcomes (Smith et al. 2008). However, MRI-guided interventions remain limited due to the scarcity of MR-compatible hardware and the specialized expertise required, limiting widespread adoption in routine practice.

Integrating robotic devices and needle guides into image-guided interventions represents a significant advancement, offering enhanced precision and efficiency. These technologies improve needle placement accuracy, particularly in cases requiring complex three-dimensional angulation while reducing procedural time and radiation exposure during CT or fluoroscopy-guided procedures. Once the optimal path is determined through imaging, needle guides can be attached to ultrasound probes or robotic devices to stabilize needle angulation based on preprocedural CT or MRI planning. This combination of robotics and imaging enables accurate access to challenging targets, enhancing procedural safety and efficacy (Cleary et al. 2006; Kassamali and Ladak 2015).

3 Patient Preparation

All interventional procedures around the wrist and hand must follow standard sterile techniques to minimize the risk of infection. This includes using a sterile cover for the ultrasound transducer and sterile gel during ultrasound-guided procedures. Since these interventions are performed under sterile conditions and do not involve the gastrointestinal, genitourinary, or respiratory tracts, routine antibiotic prophylaxis is not recommended (Chehab et al. 2018).

Periprocedural laboratory testing for coagulation parameters, such as prothrombin time (PT), partial thromboplastin time (PTT), and platelet count, is typically unnecessary, except for biopsies or ablative treatments. Testing is reserved for patients at higher bleeding risk, such as those with hematological malignancies, those undergoing chemotherapy, or patients on oral anticoagulants. In such cases, evaluating bleeding risk is essential to prevent complications (Foremny et al. 2015).

Written informed consent is usually required for higher-risk procedures like biopsies or ablative treatments. Formal written consent may not be mandatory for less invasive procedures, such as corticosteroid injections for pain management. However, patients must still be fully informed about potential side effects, including the possibility of a "steroid flare" (a temporary increase in pain post injection), fat necrosis, and fluctuations in blood glucose levels, particularly in diabetic patients. The patient's positioning will be addressed in detail in the following sections.

4 Hardware

For delivering local anesthetic agents to the skin and subcutaneous tissues and for most joint injections in the wrist and hand, hypodermic needles with a gauge size of 23–25G and a length of 1.5–2 cm are typically used. For aspirating viscous fluids, such as those from ganglion cysts or abscesses, larger-caliber needles (18G) are preferred to withdraw thick material efficiently. Soft tissue biopsies require core biopsy needles, which are spring-loaded, side-notch needles with semiautomatic or automatic firing mechanisms designed to capture tissue samples. For larger masses, such as soft tissue sarcomas, a 14–16G needle is recommended, while an 18G needle is generally used for synovial biopsies (Bansal et al. 2021).

A coaxial system is often employed during biopsies to reduce complications. This involves an outer cannula that allows multiple tissue samples to be collected through a single skin puncture, minimizing trauma. The outer cannula can also be used to embolize the biopsy tract with materials like gel foam, glue, or coils when vascular lesions are involved, helping to prevent bleeding and other complications. Trephine needles, such as the Jamshidi needle, are commonly used for bone biopsies. These needles are designed to penetrate bone and obtain core samples, making them ideal for collecting high-quality biopsy material from bony lesions (Bansal et al. 2021).

5 Injectables

5.1 Local Anesthetics (LA)

Local anesthetics (LAs) are commonly used to provide immediate and short-term pain relief, depending on the agent administered. Frequently used LAs include lidocaine, bupivacaine, and ropivacaine, each differing in onset and duration of action. With its rapid onset (typically within 1 min), lidocaine provides effective anesthesia for 2–3 h, making it ideal for numbing the skin and underlying tissues before minor procedures or interventions. In contrast, bupivacaine has a slower onset, taking up to 30 min, but provides prolonged pain relief lasting 10–12 h. This extended duration makes bupivacaine particularly suitable for intra-articular injections, where it is often combined with corticosteroids to enhance both immediate and sustained pain relief. The typical volume for this anesthetic–corticosteroid mixture is 1–2 mL for most joints in the wrist and hand (MacMahon et al. 2009).

However, intra-articular injections of LAs carry a risk of chondrolysis, which can be compounded when corticosteroids are co-administered (Jayaram et al. 2019). Among the available agents, ropivacaine, especially at concentrations ≤0.5%, has been shown to have the lowest chondrotoxicity, making it a safer option for intra-articular use when joint preservation is a priority.

5.2 Steroids

Steroids, potent anti-inflammatory agents, are widely used to relieve pain in inflammatory and degenerative musculoskeletal conditions, offering primarily palliative relief. As they do not address the underlying cause of pain, their effects are often short-lived. Steroids are classified into two types: (1) steroid esters (e.g., triamcinolone acetonide and methylprednisolone acetate), formulated as insoluble particulate preparations, and (2) steroid salts (e.g., dexamethasone and betamethasone), formulated as soluble preparations (MacMahon et al. 2009; Rastogi et al. 2016; Shah et al. 2019).

Steroid esters provide prolonged effects due to the slow absorption of particulates, making them preferable for intra-articular and bursal injections. They are often combined with LAs to offer immediate pain relief alongside their extended anti-inflammatory action. In contrast, steroid salts act more quickly but have a shorter duration of effect, making them ideal for superficial injections where they pose a lower risk of complications such as skin atrophy, depigmentation, and fat necrosis (MacMahon et al. 2009; Shah et al. 2019).

It is critical to avoid injecting steroids directly into tendons as they impair connective tissue formation and increase the risk of tendon rupture (Gialanella and Prometti 2011). Common side effects of steroid injections include post-injection flares, characterized by increased local inflammation lasting 2–3 days, cartilage damage, hypopigmentation of skin, and blood glucose fluctuations. A minimum interval of six weeks is recommended for repeat injections, with a maximum of three injections per year to minimize potential adverse effects (Louis 2008).

5.3 Autologous Blood and Platelet-Rich Plasma (PRP)

Autologous blood injections have been used to treat tendinopathies due to their regenerative potential. Blood is rich in growth factors that promote collagen deposition and granulation tissue formation, which mature and strengthen the tendon during recovery. A more advanced approach involves platelet-rich plasma (PRP) derived through centrifugation of autologous blood. PRP contains high concentrations of platelets, which release growth factors and cytokines that support cellular proliferation, angiogenesis, and collagen synthesis while inhibiting catabolic processes. This regenerative potential makes PRP a promising treatment for chronic tendinopathies, acute tendon tears, and cartilage repair via intra-articular injection (Mariani and Pulsatelli 2020; Le et al. 2018).

Certain precautions are necessary before administering PRP injections. Patients taking anticoagulants, nonsteroidal anti-inflammatory drugs (NSAIDs), or corticosteroids require careful evaluation as these medications can impair platelet function and reduce treatment efficacy. PRP is generally indicated for partial-thickness tendon tears and early osteoarthritis but is ineffective for complete tendon ruptures or advanced osteoarthritis. Patient expectations must be managed as PRP therapy does not typically provide immediate pain relief, and multiple sessions may be required for optimal results. Outcomes can also vary based on the condition being treated. Post injection, patients should be advised to avoid strenuous activities to allow proper tissue regeneration and healing (Mariani and Pulsatelli 2020; Le et al. 2018).

5.4 Normal Saline

Isotonic saline, containing 0.9% sodium chloride in water, is commonly used in percutaneous irrigation to treat calcific tendinosis by dissolving intratendinous calcifications, helping to alleviate pain and improve function. This procedure, known as barbotage, is frequently performed to address calcific tendinopathies. Traditionally, a single-needle technique was used for both saline injection and aspiration of calcific material. However, recent advancements have introduced a dual-needle technique, which enhances efficiency by enabling continuous lavage through separate channels for injection and aspiration (Sconfienza et al. 2012).

6 Ultrasound-Guided Interventions

6.1 Radio-Carpal Joint Injection

The radio-carpal joint (RCJ) is a synovial joint formed by the distal end of the radius and the articular disc of the distal radio-ulnar joint (proximally) and the scaphoid, lunate, and triquetrum (distally). It facilitates flexion, extension, radial deviation, and ulnar deviation of the wrist. The synovial capsule surrounds the joint, making it accessible for intra-articular injections. Common pathologies include osteoarthritis, rheumatoid arthritis (RA), post-traumatic arthritis, and gout. Inflammatory or degenerative conditions lead to pain, stiffness, and reduced wrist function. Persistent wrist pain unresponsive to conservative treatment in cases of osteoarthritis, inflammatory arthritis, and crystalline arthropathies is the most common indication for injection (Lohman et al. 2007).

To perform the procedure, the patient can be seated or supine, with the hand resting on a flat surface and palm facing down. The wrist is positioned in slight flexion using a rolled towel or small pad under the volar surface of the wrist to optimize joint accessibility. We place a high-frequency linear transducer (10–15 MHz) in a longitudinal or transverse orientation over the dorsal wrist, centered on the RCJ joint. The distal radius and carpal bone are identified, with the joint space appearing as a hypoechoic gap and the probe adjusted to visualize the joint clearly. The in-plane approach, which is the often preferred one, is used, with the needle inserted parallel to the probe (placed transversely or longitudinally) for continuous visualization of the needle shaft and tip. Insert the needle from the dorsal aspect of the wrist, slightly proximal to the joint line, angling it toward the hypoechoic joint space. If the probe is placed longitudinally, the needle can be advanced from the cauda-cranial, and if the probe is placed transversely, the needle is generally advanced from the radial to ulnar direction. Under ultrasound guidance, advance the needle into the joint space between the radius and the lunate or scaphoid. Slowly inject the solution while ensuring no resistance or extravasation (Fig. 3). Maintain patient comfort by explaining each step and minimizing wrist movement during the procedure. Ensure the injectate delivery does not infiltrate surrounding tendons or ligaments. In the out-of-plane approach, the needle is inserted perpendicular to the probe, with the needle tip visible as a hyperechoic dot.

6.2 Distal Radio-Ulnar Joint (DRUJ) Injection

The distal radio-ulnar joint (DRUJ) is formed by the ulnar notch of the distal radius and the head of the ulna. It allows forearm pronation and supination by facilitating the rotation of the radius around the ulna. The joint is supported by the triangular fibrocartilage complex (TFCC), which acts as a stabilizer and cushions the joint. TFCC also separates this joint from the RCJ. The synovial capsule encloses the joint, making it accessible for injection. Common joint conditions include inflammatory arthritis (e.g., RA), osteoarthritis, TFCC injury, and post-traumatic arthritis. These conditions lead to pain, instability, and restricted motion in the DRUJ. Persistent pain and/or swelling localized to the DRUJ that is unresponsive to conservative management is the

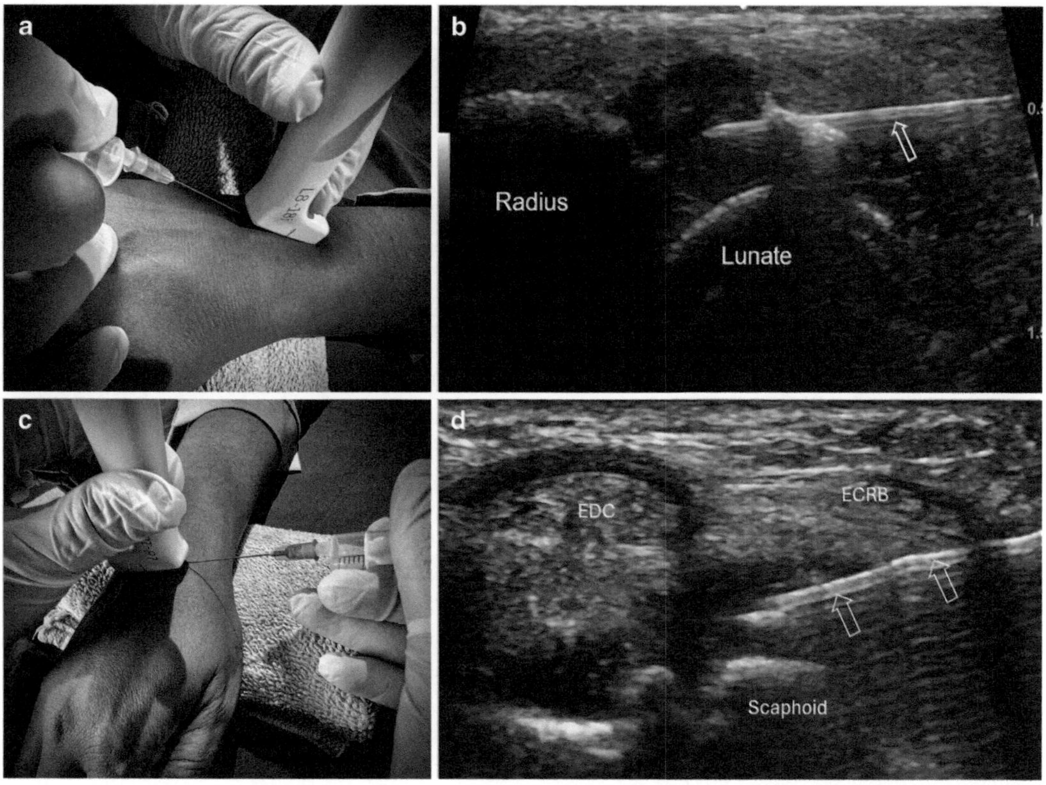

Fig. 3 (**a**) Needle and transducer position for long-axis, in-plane technique (craniocaudal). (**b**) Ultrasound image demonstrating long-axis view of radio-carpal joint with in-plane needle placement (arrow). (**c**) Needle and transducer position for short-axis, in-plane technique (radial to ulnar direction). (**d**) Ultrasound image demonstrating short-axis view of radio-carpal joint with in-plane needle placement (arrows). The needle is placed radial to the extensor compartment 4. ECRB, extensor carpi radialis brevis tendon; EDC, extensor digitorum communis

most common indication for injection. Diagnostic injection to confirm the DRUJ as the source of pain and therapeutic management for inflammatory arthritis, osteoarthritis, or TFCC-related synovitis are other indications (Smith et al. 2011).

The patient is seated or supine, with the forearm resting on a flat surface and palm facing either down or in neutral rotation (thumb pointing upward). Ensure the wrist is in a comfortable and relaxed position. Place a high-frequency linear transducer transversely over the dorsal wrist, centered over the DRUJ. Identify the distal ulna and radius, with the joint space appearing as a hypoechoic gap between the two bony structures. Adjust the probe to optimize the visualization of the joint space while minimizing anisotropy. The probe can be rotated to a longitudinal orientation depending upon needle approach and operator preference. Insert the needle parallel to the probe (placed transversely or longitudinally) for continuous visualization of the needle shaft and tip. If the probe is placed transversely, the needle is generally approached from the radial side. If the probe is placed longitudinally, the needle is generally approached from the wrist toward the forearm. Insert the needle slightly proximal to the joint space and confirm intra-articular placement by observing fluid spread within the joint or mild distension of the capsule on injection. Slowly inject the solution, ensuring no resistance or extravasation into surrounding tissues (Fig. 4). Avoid excessive probe pressure to prevent compression of the joint space, which can make the injection more difficult.

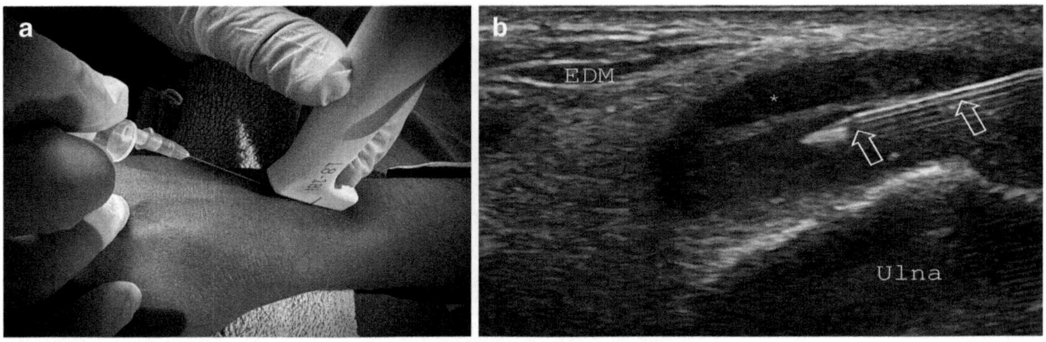

Fig. 4 (**a**) Needle and transducer position for long-axis, in-plane technique for DRUJ injection. (**b**) Long-axis ultrasound image demonstrating mild distension of DRUJ (*) with in-plane needle placement (arrows)—distal to proximal approach. EDM, extensor digiti minimi

6.3 First CMCJ Injection

The 1st CMCJ is a saddle-shaped joint formed by the trapezium and the base of the first metacarpal. It provides a wide range of thumb motion, including flexion, extension, abduction, adduction, and opposition. The joint is stabilized by several ligaments, including the anterior oblique ligament, a critical structure in preventing subluxation. Degenerative or inflammatory changes commonly affect the 1st CMCJ due to repetitive stress and its crucial role in thumb function. Osteoarthritis is the most frequent pathology, leading to joint pain, stiffness, and deformity (e.g., "squaring" of the thumb base). Synovitis or tenosynovitis associated with inflammatory arthropathies (e.g., RA) can also affect the joint. Persistent pain unresponsive to conservative measures (rest, splinting, NSAIDs) is the most common indication for injection. Diagnostic confirmation of pain origin in the 1st CMCJ is another indication (Gharib et al. 2024).

The patient is seated or supine, with the hand resting on a flat surface and palm facing up or semiprone. Ensure the thumb is relaxed in slight abduction to expose the joint adequately. Position a high-frequency linear transducer in a longitudinal orientation over the 1st CMCJ, visualizing the trapezium and the base of the first metacarpal. Ensure the joint space is identified as a hypoechoic gap between the bony surfaces. Adjust the probe to achieve a clear joint image while minimizing anisotropy. The needle is advanced parallel to the probe (through thenar eminence), allowing real-time visualization of the needle shaft and tip as it enters the joint (Fig. 5). Use a small amount of local anesthetic to minimize patient discomfort during the procedure. Avoid injecting into surrounding tendons or soft tissues to prevent complications. Ensure the injectate spreads evenly within the joint space to optimize therapeutic effects.

6.4 STT Joint Injection

The scaphotrapeziotrapezoid (STT) joint is a synovial joint formed by the distal scaphoid, trapezium, and trapezoid bones. Located on the radial aspect of the wrist, it stabilizes the radial wrist column during grip and pinch activities. The joint is supported by ligaments and surrounded by a thin synovial capsule. Osteoarthritis is the most common condition affecting the STT joint due to chronic mechanical stress. Synovitis or degenerative changes lead to pain, stiffness, and reduced thumb or wrist function. Persistent radial wrist pain localized to the STT joint, typically exacerbated by wrist radial and ulnar deviation and unresponsive to conservative treatment, is the most common indication for injection (Chopra et al. 2016).

The patient is seated or supine, with the hand resting on a flat surface and palm facing upward.

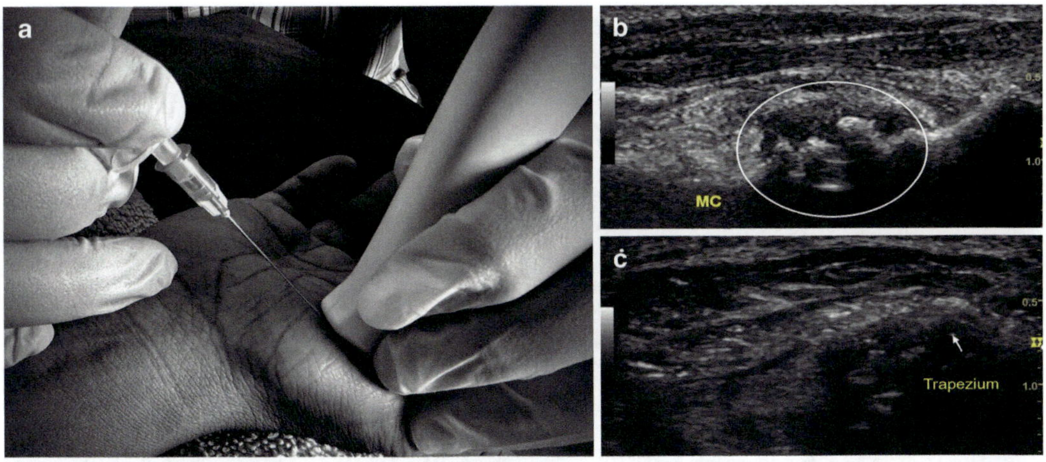

Fig. 5 (**a**) Needle and transducer position through the thenar eminence for long-axis, in-plane technique for injection of the 1st CMCJ. (**b**) Long-axis ultrasound image showing degenerative changes in the 1st CMCJ (circle). (**c**) Arrow shows the needle. MC, metacarpal

Place a high-frequency linear transducer longitudinally over the radial aspect of the wrist, aligned with the first metacarpal, and move proximally to locate the STT joint. Identify the scaphoid, trapezium, and trapezoid bones, with the STT joint appearing as a narrow hypoechoic space between them. Adjust the probe angle to optimize visualization and minimize anisotropy. Insert the needle parallel to the probe (from thenar eminence) for continuous visualization of the shaft and tip. Reassure the patient and minimize wrist movement during the procedure for optimal comfort.

6.5 Metacarpophalangeal (MCP) and Interphalangeal (IP) Joint Injections

MCP joints are synovial hinge joints between the metacarpal heads and the proximal phalanges. They allow flexion, extension, and limited abduction and adduction. IP joints are also hinge joints that allow flexion and extension. These joints are stabilized by collateral ligaments and the volar plate, enclosed by a thin synovial capsule. Degenerative changes such as osteoarthritis (especially in the distal IP joints) lead to pain, stiffness, and bony enlargement from osteophyte formation (e.g., Heberden's or Bouchard's nodes). Inflammatory conditions like RA result in synovitis, pain, swelling, and deformity, predominantly in MCP and proximal IP joints. Traumatic injuries may also cause capsular or ligamentous damage with secondary pain and stiffness. Persistent joint pain due to osteoarthritis or inflammatory arthritis, unresponsive to conservative measures, is a common indication for injection (Patel et al. 2023).

The patient is seated, with the hand resting on a flat surface and the palm facing up in a comfortable, relaxed position. The affected finger(s) should be extended and supported to provide easy access to the joint. For the MCP joint, place the probe longitudinally over the volar aspect of the MCP joint and identify the metacarpal head and the base of the proximal phalanx, with the joint space appearing as a hypoechoic gap. For IP joints, position the probe longitudinally over the volar aspect of the affected IP joint. The needle is inserted parallel to the probe (craniocaudal or caudocranial) for real-time visualization of the needle shaft and tip (Figs. 6 and 7). An out-of-plane approach can also be preferred due to the limited space available where the needle is inserted perpendicular to the probe, with the tip appearing as a hyperechoic dot.

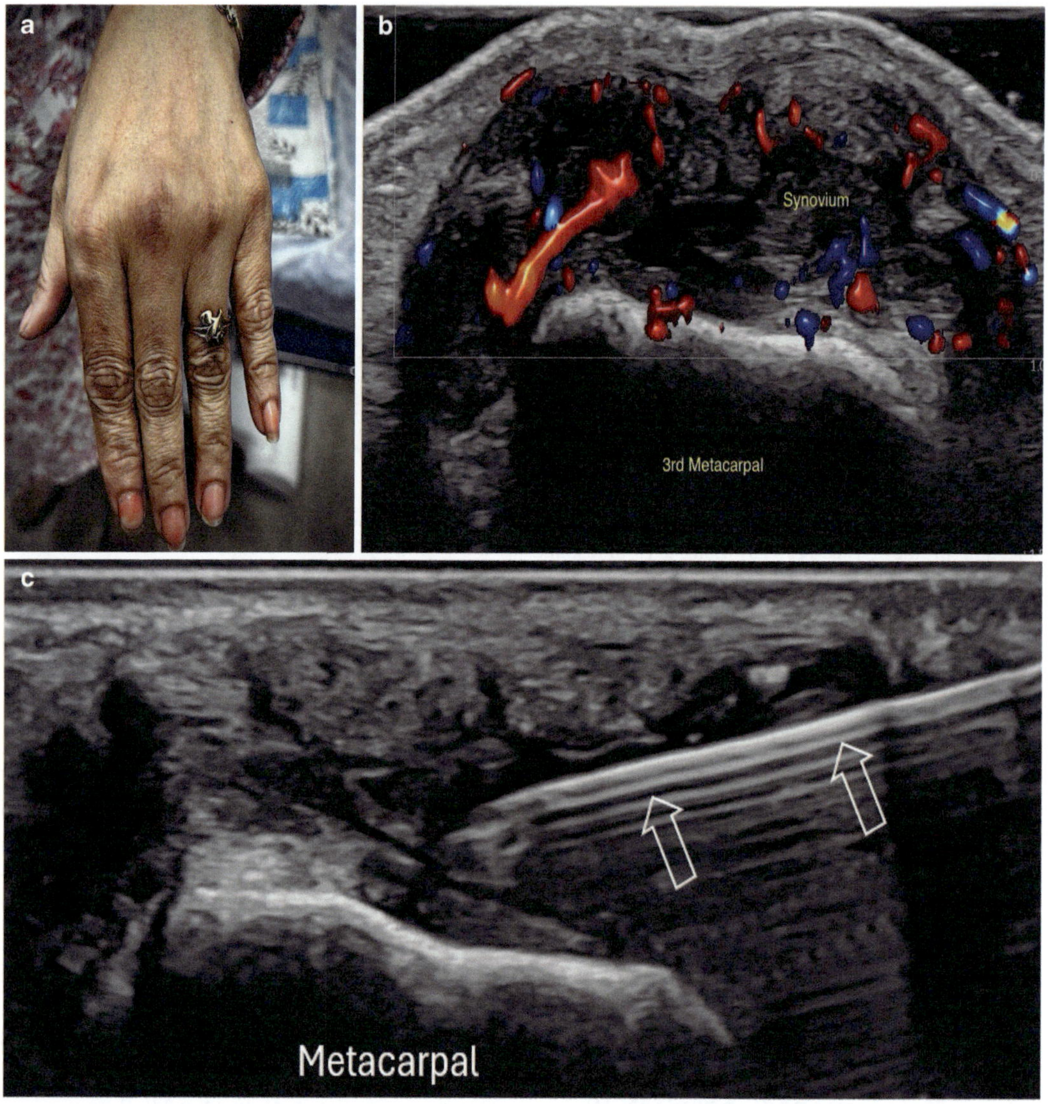

Fig. 6 (**a**) A 46-year-old woman with swelling in the third MCP joint. (**b**) Ultrasound image in short-axis view showing hypertrophied synovium with increased internal vascularity. (**c**) Ultrasound-guided injection in the MCP joint by in-plane technique. Arrows showing needle

6.6 Extensor Tendon Sheath Injection

The extensor tendons in the wrist and hand are surrounded by synovial sheaths that reduce friction and facilitate smooth tendon gliding. On the dorsal aspect, there are six compartments that house different extensor tendons responsible for the extension of the wrist and fingers. Of particular importance is the first extensor compartment, which contains abductor pollicis longus (APL) and extensor pollicis brevis (EPB) tendons, and this compartment gets commonly affected by inflammation often due to repetitive thumb motion leading to De Quervain's tenosynovitis (McDermott et al. 2012). Another condition affecting the dorsal wrist and distal forearm is intersection syndrome, where the second exten-

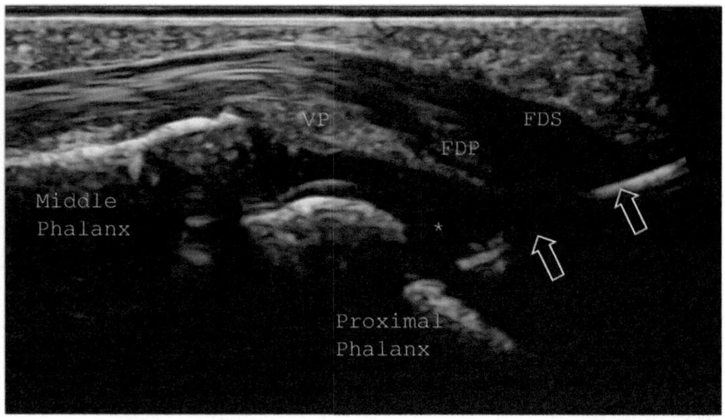

Fig. 7 Ultrasound image demonstrating needle position (arrows) for long-axis, in-plane approach for proximal interphalangeal joint injection—caudocranial direction. *Joint effusion. VP, volar plate; FDP, flexor digitorum profundus tendon; FDS, flexor digitorum superficialis tendon

sor compartment tendons are irritated by the crossing of the first compartment tendons. Extensor carpi ulnaris, a tendon located in the sixth extensor compartment, is one of the most common tendons affected by RA and is prone to subluxation/dislocation due to a shallow ulnar styloid process groove, disruption of the ECU sub-sheath through trauma, or synovitis from the underlying DRUJ. These conditions, when becoming unresponsive to conservative measures, demand injections.

The patient is seated or supine, with the wrist resting on a flat surface and the palm facing down or in a semi-prone position. The patient can be asked to hold a towel roll. Place the probe longitudinally or transversely over the affected tendon. Identify the fibrillar tendon surrounded by a hyperechoic sheath. The fluid within the sheath may indicate tenosynovitis. Ensure continuous visualization of the needle shaft and tip during advancement. For De Quervain's tenosynovitis, the needle is advanced from radially, angling toward the hypoechoic sheath around the APL and EPB tendons (Fig. 8). Commonly, there will be one or more septa between or within these tendons (the APL tendon can be in two or more slips), and a separate injection into each subcompartment is necessary.

Use minimal probe pressure to avoid compressing the sheath. Maintain real-time visualization of the needle tip to prevent inadvertent tendon injury. Inject slowly to minimize patient discomfort and confirm sheath distension. Tendon injury or rupture can occur if the injectate is placed intratendinously instead of in the sheath.

6.7 Flexor Tendon Sheath Injection

Flexor tendon sheaths are tubular synovial structures encasing the flexor tendons. They extend from the wrist to the fingers, with the fingers containing pulleys (A1–A5, C1–C3) to stabilize tendon motion. The A1 pulley, located at the MCP joint, is involved in stenosing tenosynovitis (trigger finger), which leads to impaired tendon gliding, and the finger becomes locked in flexion. Flexor carpi radialis is another tendon that is intricately related to the STT joint and is often affected by tenosynovitis. The flexor carpi ulnaris tendon, though not surrounded by a synovial sheath, is often affected by calcific tendinosis. The radial and ulnar bursa are two important bursae on the volar aspect of the wrist that can be involved in inflammatory arthritis or infection. Persistent pain, swelling, or triggering of the digit unresponsive to conservative measures necessitates injection (Tunçez et al. 2023).

The patient is seated, with the hand supinated and resting on a flat surface. The affected finger or wrist should be fully extended and relaxed. For the trigger finger, place the probe longitudinally over the volar aspect of the MCP joint and identify the flexor tendon and its surrounding hypoechoic sheath. The A1 pulley appears as a

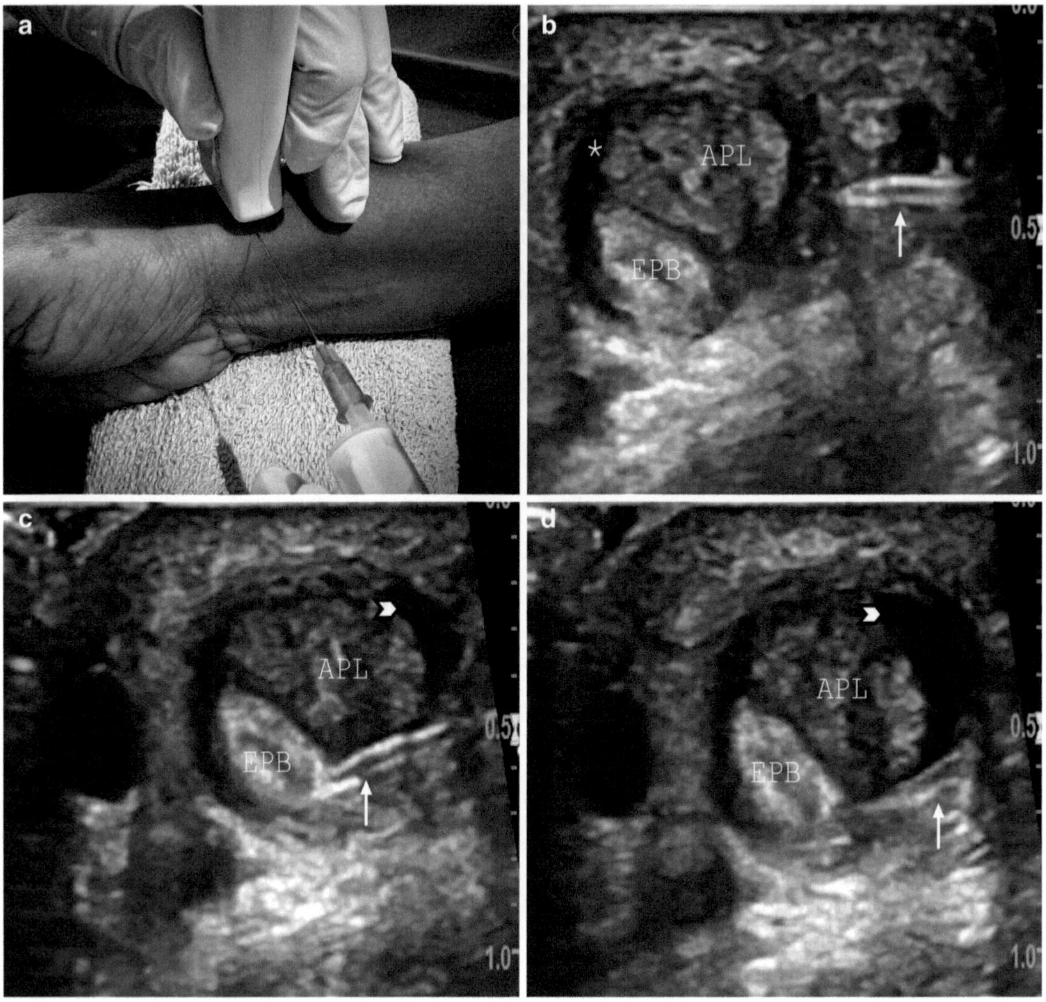

Fig. 8 (**a**) Needle and transducer position for short-axis, in-plane technique of first extensor compartment injection. (**b**) Short-axis ultrasound view of De Quervain's tenosynovitis and needle (arrow) approaching it (* thickened overlying extensor retinaculum). (**c**, **d**) Needle tip (arrow) in the compartment with the delivery of the injectate (arrowhead) into the tendon sheath. APL, abductor pollicis longus; EPB, extensor pollicis brevis

hypoechoic band over the tendon. The needle is advanced parallel to the probe for real-time visualization, often longitudinally from the craniocaudal or caudocranial direction. Insert the needle at a shallow angle to the skin, aiming toward the flexor tendon sheath. Advance the needle under ultrasound guidance, ensuring it remains in the hypoechoic sheath without penetrating the tendon. Confirm correct needle placement by observing fluid spread around the tendon, causing sheath distension (Figs. 9 and 10).

6.8 Carpal Tunnel Injections

The carpal tunnel is a fibro-osseous canal located at the volar wrist. The roof is formed by a transverse carpal ligament (flexor retinaculum), and the carpal bones form the floor. Its contents include the median nerve and nine tendons (four flexor digitorum superficialis, four flexor digitorum profundus, and flexor pollicis longus). The median nerve lies superficial and slightly radial within the tunnel, just deep into the flexor reti-

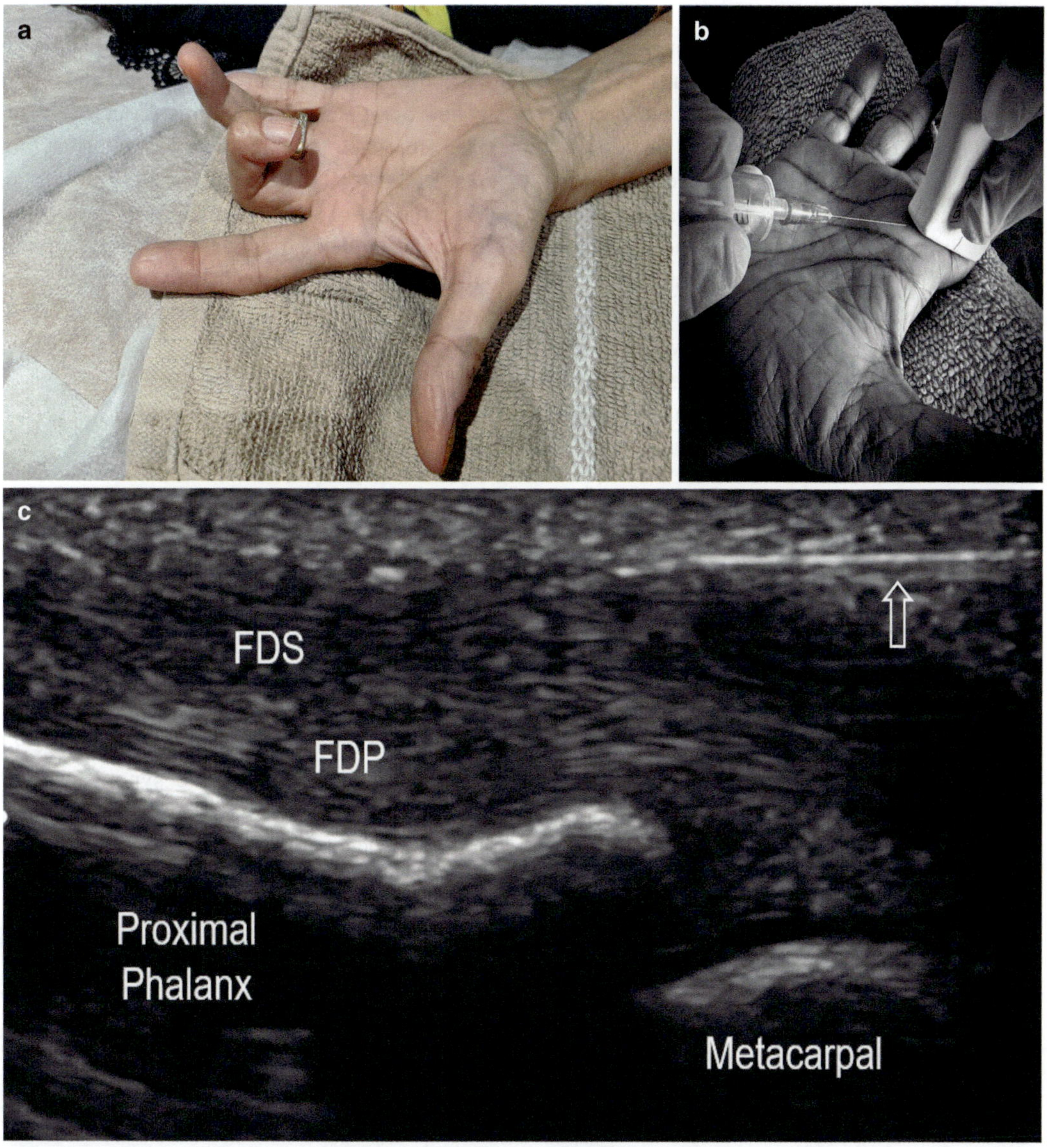

Fig. 9 A 73-year-old woman with a locked trigger finger and a history of RA. (**a**) Clinical picture showing a locked 3rd digit. (**b**) Needle and transducer position for long-axis, in-plane technique of ultrasound-guided release of trigger finger. (**c**) Long-axis ultrasound view demonstrating needle approach (arrow) for A1 pulley release. FDS, flexor digitorum superficialis tendon; FDP, flexor digitorum profundus tendon

naculum. CTS is caused by compression of the median nerve within the carpal tunnel, which is most commonly idiopathic but can also be due to hypothyroidism, pregnancy, or caused by a space-occupying lesion in the tunnel. The patient often presents with pain, paresthesia, and weakness in the median nerve distribution (thumb, index, middle, and radial half of the ring finger). Persistent symptoms of CTS despite conservative management (splints, NSAIDs) are an indication for injection. Sometimes, space-occupying lesions in the tunnel, like a ganglion cyst, demand aspiration. Persistent symptoms post-carpal tunnel release are another indication (Kumar et al. 2023).

The patient is seated or supine, with the arm resting on a flat surface, the wrist in slight dorsiflexion, and the palm facing upward. Place the probe transversely over the volar wrist crease. Identify key landmarks like the median nerve that appears as a hyperechoic oval structure superficial to the tendons. Also, the ulnar nerve and artery should be identified. The needle is advanced parallel to the probe at a shallow angle, allowing continuous visualization. Insert the needle from the ulnar or radial side, avoiding direct contact with the median nerve. Place the tip either superficial or deep to the median nerve and slowly inject the solution. Manipulate the needle to inject all around the nerve without directly penetrating it (Fig. 11). Advise the patient to monitor for improvement of symptoms and report any new or worsening symptoms. Effective injections can reduce inflammation and relieve symptoms for several weeks to months, aiding in symptom control and functional recovery. Thread ultrasound-guided carpal tunnel release is a minimally invasive procedure that uses a thread and ultrasound guidance to treat CTS (Kumar et al. 2023).

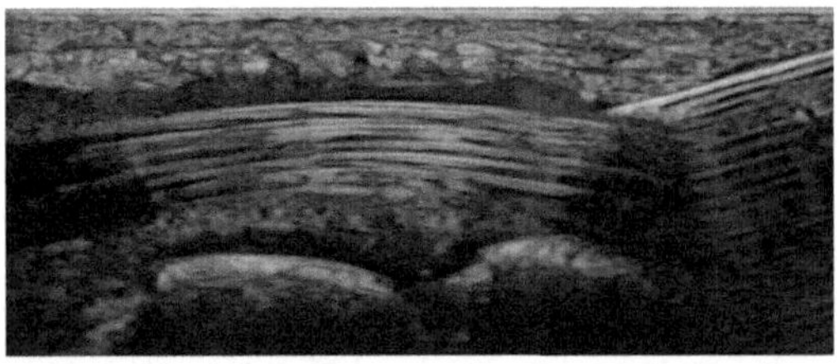

Fig. 10 A 33-year-old woman with a locked trigger finger. Long-axis ultrasound view demonstrating needle approach for A1 pulley release and injection in the flexor tendon sheath

6.9 Ganglion Cyst Aspiration

Ganglion cysts are fluid-filled sacs arising from the synovium of a joint or tendon sheath. Common locations around the wrist and hand include the dorsal wrist, where it most frequently originates from the scapholunate ligament, the volar wrist associated with the RCJ or STT joint, and in fingers in relation to the flexor tendon sheath and pulleys. It is caused by leakage of synovial fluid into a herniated synovial sac or capsular defect as a result of repetitive microtrauma or degenerative changes in the joint.

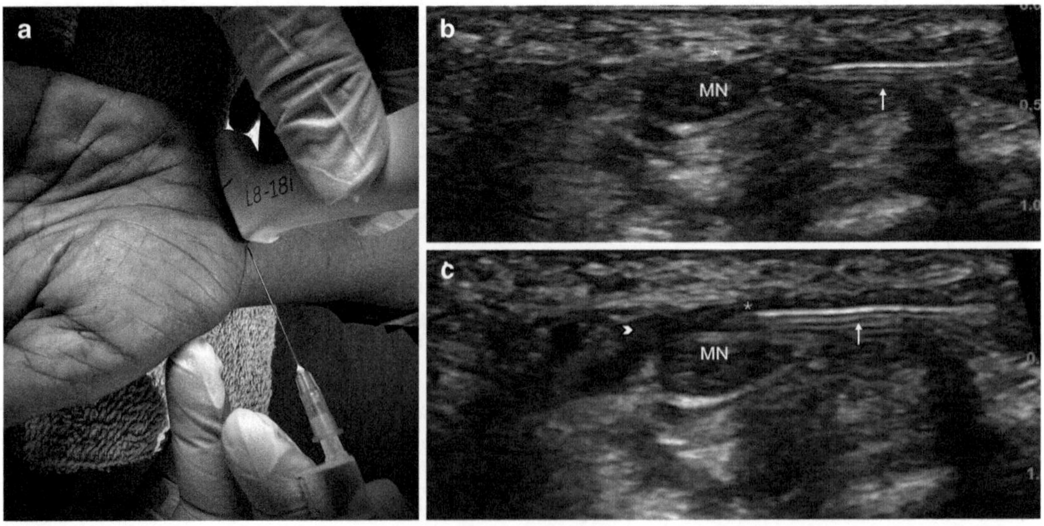

Fig. 11 (**a**) Needle and transducer position for short-axis, in-plane technique of ultrasound-guided carpal tunnel injection. (**b**, **c**) Short-axis ultrasound images illustrating the approach of needle (arrow) for delivery of perineural injection (arrowhead) around the median nerve. * Thickened overlying flexor retinaculum. MN, median nerve

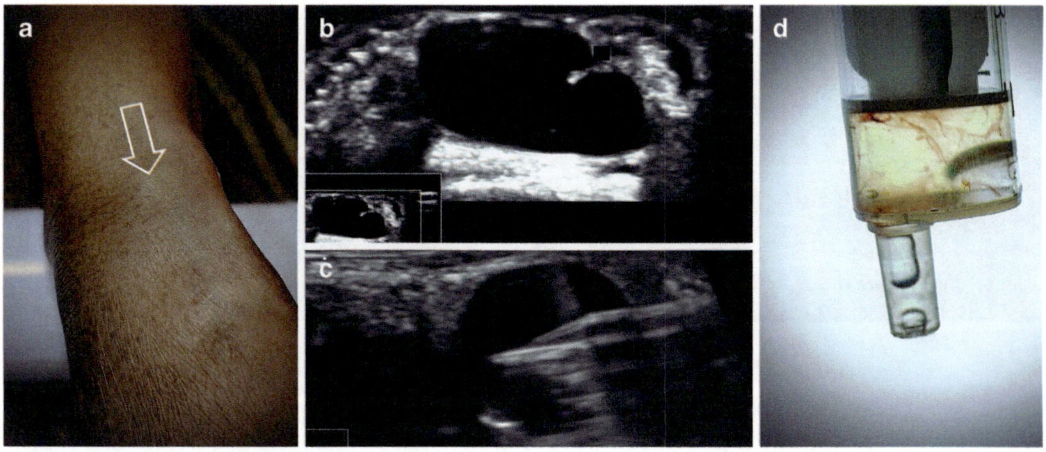

Fig. 12 (**a**) A 61-year-old woman with swelling along the radial aspect of her right wrist (arrow). (**b**) Ultrasound image showing a well-defined cystic lesion. (**c**) In-plane technique for ultrasound-guided aspiration of ganglion cyst. (**d**) Aspirated gelatinous material

Asymptomatic and small ganglion cysts can be left alone, whereas symptomatic ganglion cysts causing pain or cosmetic concerns demand aspiration and injection (Saboeiro and Sofka 2008; Zeidenberg et al. 2016).

Position the patient based on cyst location. For the dorsal wrist, the hand is pronated on a flat surface, and for the volar wrist, the hand is supinated with slight dorsiflexion. Place a high-frequency probe over the ganglion cyst to confirm its size, shape, and depth. Visualize adjacent structures such as tendons, vessels, and nerves. Use an 18–22-gauge needle attached to a 5–10 mL syringe. A thicker needle is often needed for ganglion cysts due to its thick gelatinous contents. Insert the needle at a shallow angle to the skin, targeting the cyst under ultrasound guidance. Avoid penetrating adjacent structures (e.g., tendons, vessels). Advance the needle into the cyst and apply gentle suction to withdraw the gelatinous fluid (Fig. 12). Post-aspiration injection is optional, and it involves injecting a small amount of corticosteroid (e.g., 0.5–1 mL of triamcinolone) into the cyst cavity to reduce recurrence risk. Avoid corticosteroid injection in cases of suspected infection or prior ruptured cyst. Aspiration often provides symptomatic relief but may require repeated procedures or surgical excision for definitive treatment.

6.10 Diagnostic Fluid Aspiration and Synovial Biopsy

Effusion in the small joints of the hand and wrist and bursae can occur secondary to inflammatory (e.g., RA), infectious (e.g., septic or tubercular arthritis), or degenerative (e.g., osteoarthritis) processes. Sometimes, there is minimal effusion but exuberant synovial thickening, which requires a synovial biopsy to identify the cause. The patient and probe position depends upon the location. For aspiration, a 22–25-gauge needle attached to a 5–10 mL syringe is used. A thick needle may be required in cases of complex collection. Gently aspirate fluid into the syringe for laboratory analysis (e.g., Gram stain, culture, cytology, and crystals). For the synovial biopsy, first, identify the region with maximum synovial thickening. Use an 18 G semiautomated (preferred) or automated biopsy needle under ultrasound guidance to target the thickened synovium. Insert the needle under ultrasound guidance into the thickened synovium, avoiding critical structures like tendons, nerves, and vessels. Obtain 2–3 tissue cores for histopathology, microbiology, and molecular studies if needed (e.g., PCR for tuberculosis) (Figs. 13 and 14). Post biopsy, pressure must be applied to the site to minimize bleeding (Kelly et al. 2015).

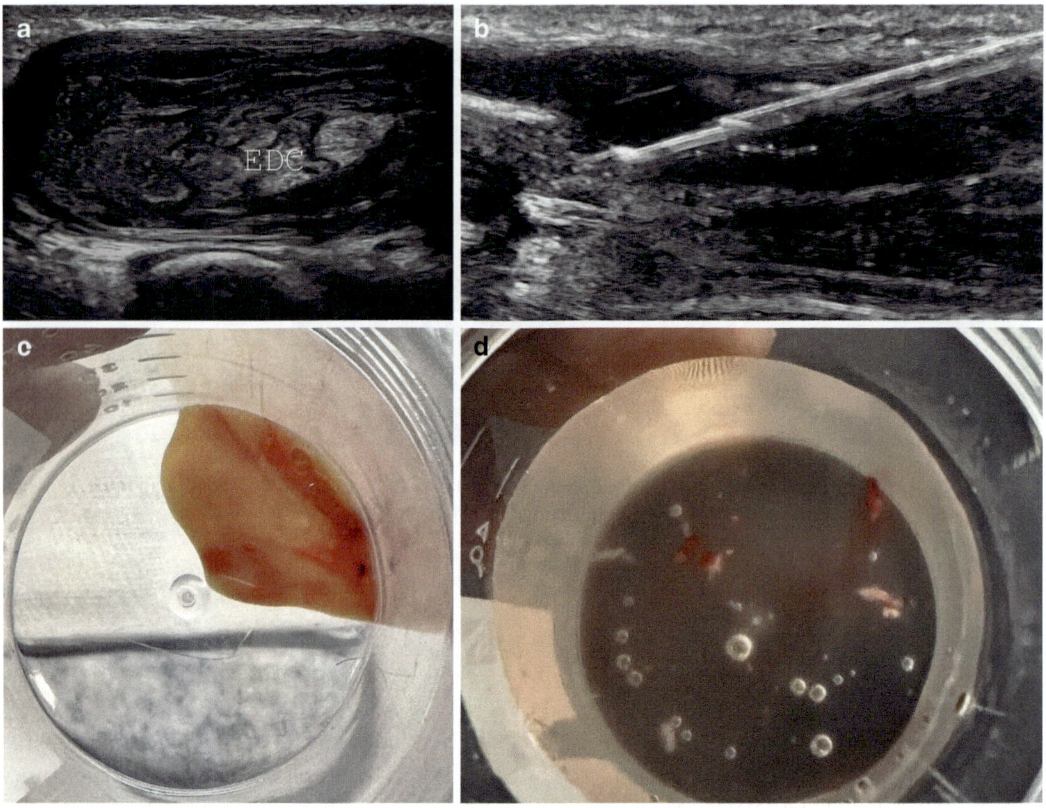

Fig. 13 (**a**) Ultrasound of a 36-year-old man with wrist swelling shows tenosynovitis of the extensor digitorum communis (EDC) tendon sheath. (**b**) Ultrasound-guided aspiration of collection and synovial biopsy were performed. (**c**) Aspirated pus. (**d**) Synovial biopsy cores

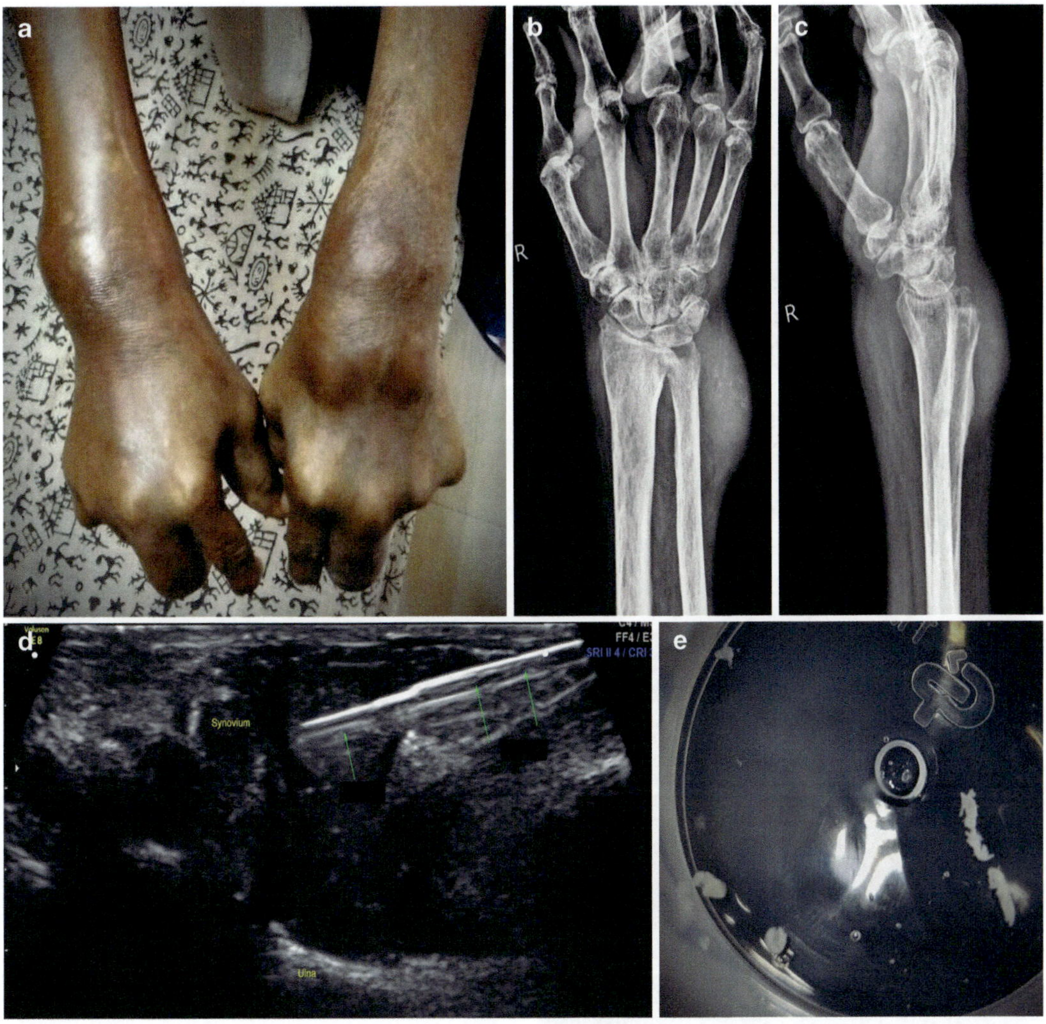

Fig. 14 (**a**) A 53-year-old woman with bilateral wrist swelling. (**b**, **c**) Radiograph showing soft tissue swelling surrounding wrist joint with periarticular osteopenia in the bones associated with erosions and loss of joint spaces. (**d**) Ultrasound-guided biopsy from the hypertrophied synovium. (**e**) Sample obtained revealed caseating granulomatous inflammation, suggesting mycobacterial etiology

7 Fluoroscopy-Guided Interventions

Fluoroscopy is an effective modality for performing various interventions in the wrist and hand, particularly joint injections into the RCJ, DRUJ, 1st CMCJ, and STT joint. A key advantage of fluoroscopy over ultrasound is the real-time visualization of contrast dispersion within the joint, allowing for documentation and confirmation of accurate injection placement. For RCJ and DRUJ, the patient's hand is positioned prone on the fluoroscopy table, and the target joint is identified on the radiographic image. Adjust the fluoroscopy unit to achieve a true posteroanterior (PA) or lateral view of the wrist to clearly visualize the joint space. The site on the skin is marked with the help of a metal wire or needle, followed by sterilizing the skin. Under continuous fluoroscopic guidance, insert a 22- to 25-gauge needle toward the target joint. Advance the needle cautiously until its tip is within the joint space, confirming placement fluoroscopically by a small amount of contrast injection. Observe for appropriate spread of the contrast within the joint without extravasation. Now, slowly inject the therapeutic agent into the joint. Gently withdraw the needle and apply a sterile dressing to the injection site. Monitor the patient briefly for any immediate reactions (e.g., allergic reaction or vasovagal syncope). Provide postprocedure instructions, including rest for the injected joint and any signs to report, such as increasing pain, swelling, or redness. The same process can be followed for 1st CMCJ, STT, and other small joints of the hand (Figs. 15, 16, 17, 18, and 19) (Chopra et al. 2016).

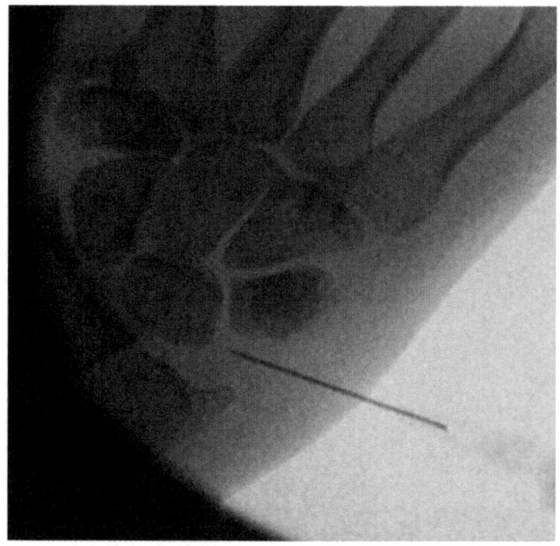

Fig. 16 The fluoroscopic image of the hand demonstrates needle placement into the ulnocarpal joint

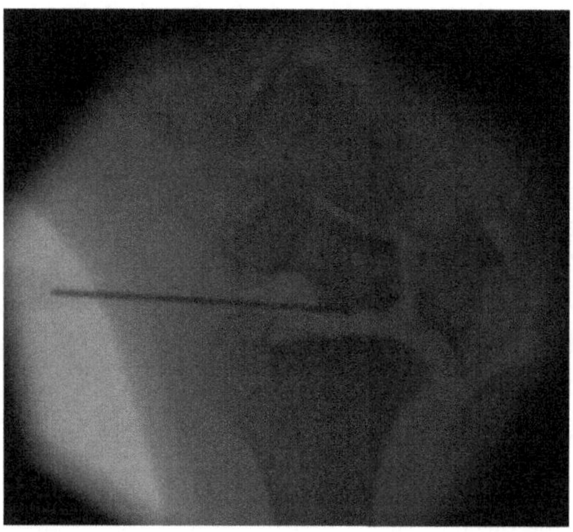

Fig. 15 Fluoroscopy-guided injection of the radio-carpal joint

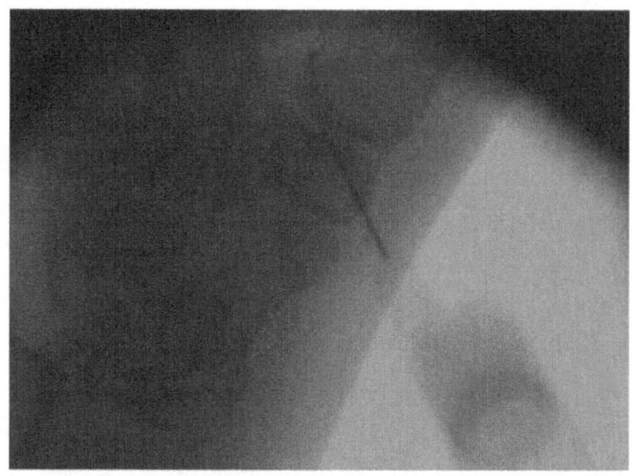

Fig. 17 The fluoroscopic image of the hand demonstrates needle placement into the first carpometacarpal joint

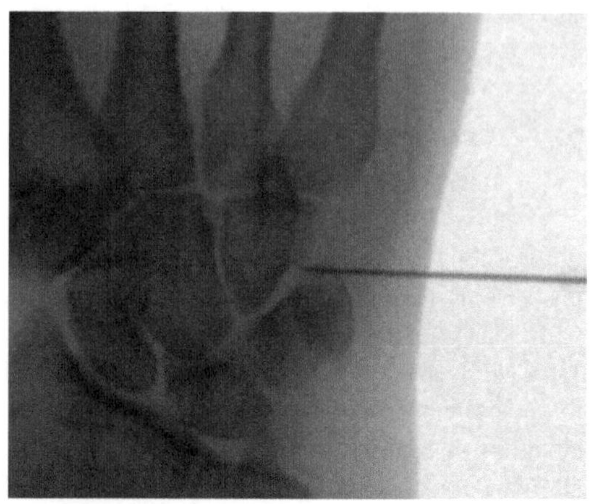

Fig. 18 Fluoroscopy-guided injection of the pisotriquetral joint

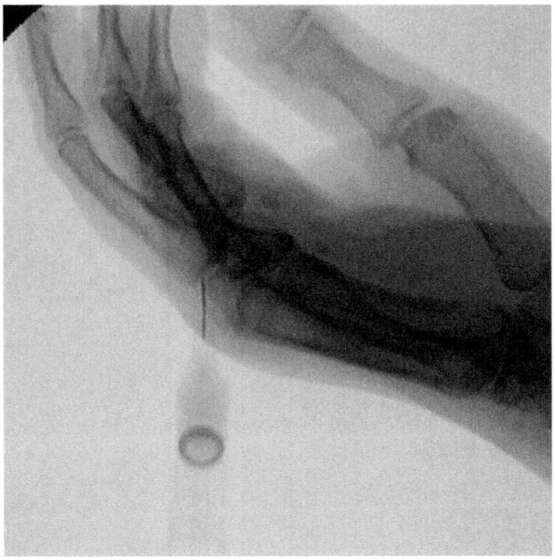

Fig. 19 The lateral fluoroscopic image of the hand demonstrates needle placement into the third metacarpophalangeal joint

8 CT-Guided Interventions

CT guidance plays a significant role in advanced musculoskeletal interventions, particularly when targeting osseous lesions in the wrist and hand. While not commonly employed for routine procedures, CT's precision is indispensable in certain complex cases. Advanced CT units with real-time fluoroscopy-like capabilities enhance procedural accuracy. Trephine biopsy needles are commonly used for bone biopsies and for advancing radiofrequency ablation (RFA) or cryoablation probes for ablative procedures. The patient is positioned based on lesion location (e.g., prone, supine, or lateral). The wrist and hand are immobilized using supports or sandbags. Local anesthesia is typically used. Sedation may be considered for prolonged or complex procedures. A preprocedural CT scan is performed to identify the exact location and dimensions of the lesion. The imaging helps determine the safest and most direct path to the target while avoiding critical structures such as neurovascular bundles and tendons. After marking the skin entry point, the biopsy or ablation needle is advanced incrementally. If targeting a deeply located lesion or dense cortical bone, a bone trocar or drill may be used to facilitate penetration. For biopsies, tissue samples are collected using a core biopsy technique. For ablation, the probe is positioned within the lesion, and energy (e.g., RF or cryogenic) is delivered to ablate the tissue (Figs. 20, 21, 22, 23 and 24). A final CT scan is performed to confirm the procedure's success and ensure no complications, such as hematoma or probe misplacement. The patient is observed for a short period for immediate postprocedural complications. Instructions for wound care and activity restrictions are provided. CT-guided interventions in the wrist and hand are invaluable in specific scenarios requiring precise bone access or complex anatomical navigation. However, its routine use for soft tissue or less demanding procedures is limited due to its cost, radiation exposure, and the availability of alternative imaging modalities better suited for such purposes (Kurup and Callstrom 2010; Filippiadis et al. 2022).

9 Conclusion

Interventional procedures around the wrist and hand offer effective therapeutic options for managing a wide range of musculoskeletal conditions, from tendinopathies to joint inflammation and cartilage injuries. Advances in imaging modalities such as ultrasound, fluoroscopy, CT, and MRI have significantly improved the precision and safety of these interventions, allowing for tailored approaches that minimize complications and optimize outcomes. Techniques like ultrasound-guided barbotage for calcific tendinosis and platelet-rich plasma (PRP) injections for tendinopathy and early osteoarthritis exemplify the progress in regenerative therapies. Similarly, innovations in procedural techniques, such as the dual-needle approach for lavage and coaxial systems for biopsies, have enhanced efficiency and reduced procedural risks.

Despite these advancements, the success of these interventions depends on adherence to sterile techniques, appropriate patient selection, and comprehensive preprocedural planning, including evaluation of anticoagulant use and other comorbidities. Patient education and informed

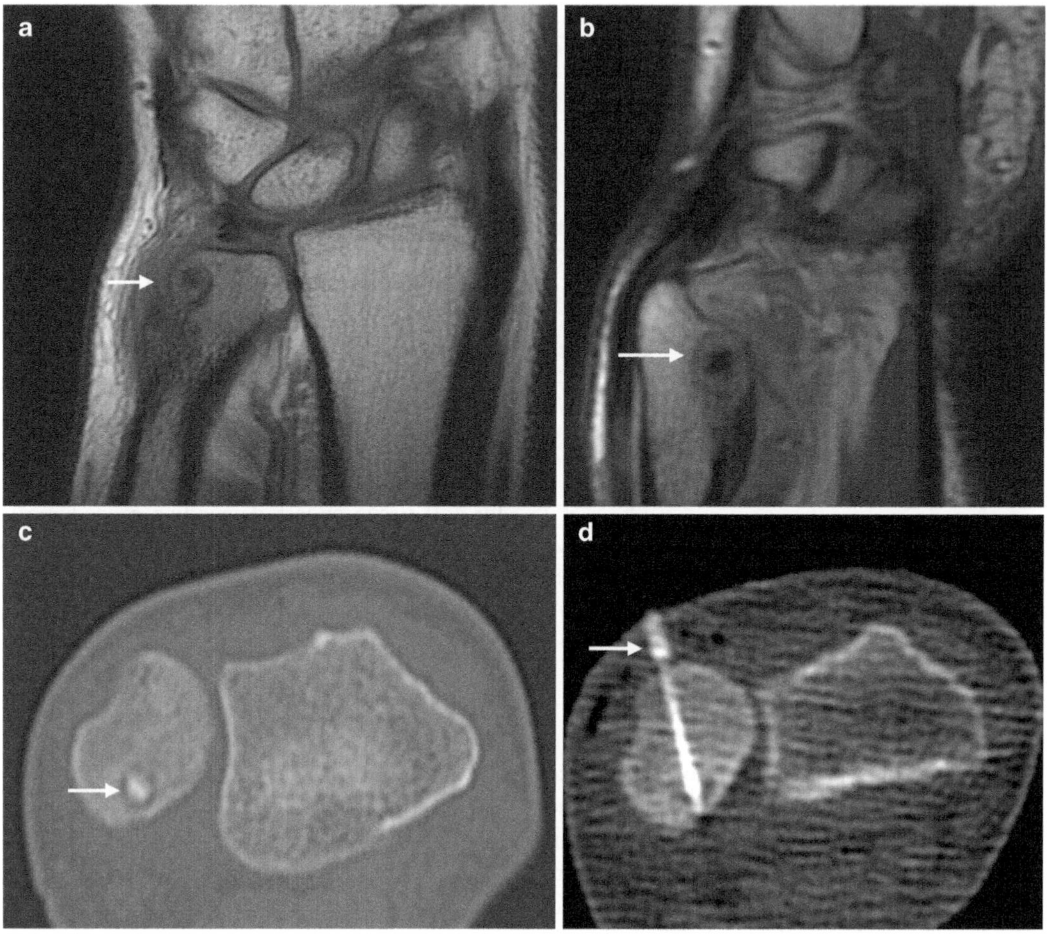

Fig. 20 (**a**, **b**) Coronal and sagittal PD MRI images of the wrist showing an osteoid osteoma in the distal ulna (arrow). (**c**) Axial image of a noncontrast CT scan illustrating the osteoid osteoma (arrow). (**d**) Axial CT image demonstrating radiofrequency ablation with needle (arrow) placement within nidus

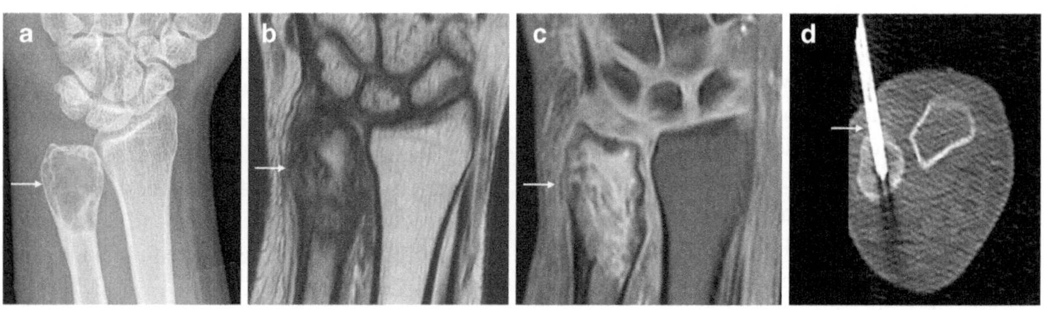

Fig. 21 (**a**) Radiographs showing a mildly expansile lucent lesion in the distal ulna. (**b**, **c**) The lesion shows heterogeneous signal on T1 (**b**) and STIR (**c**) MRI images. (**d**) Axial section of noncontrast CT demonstrating placement of biopsy needle (arrow) within the lesion

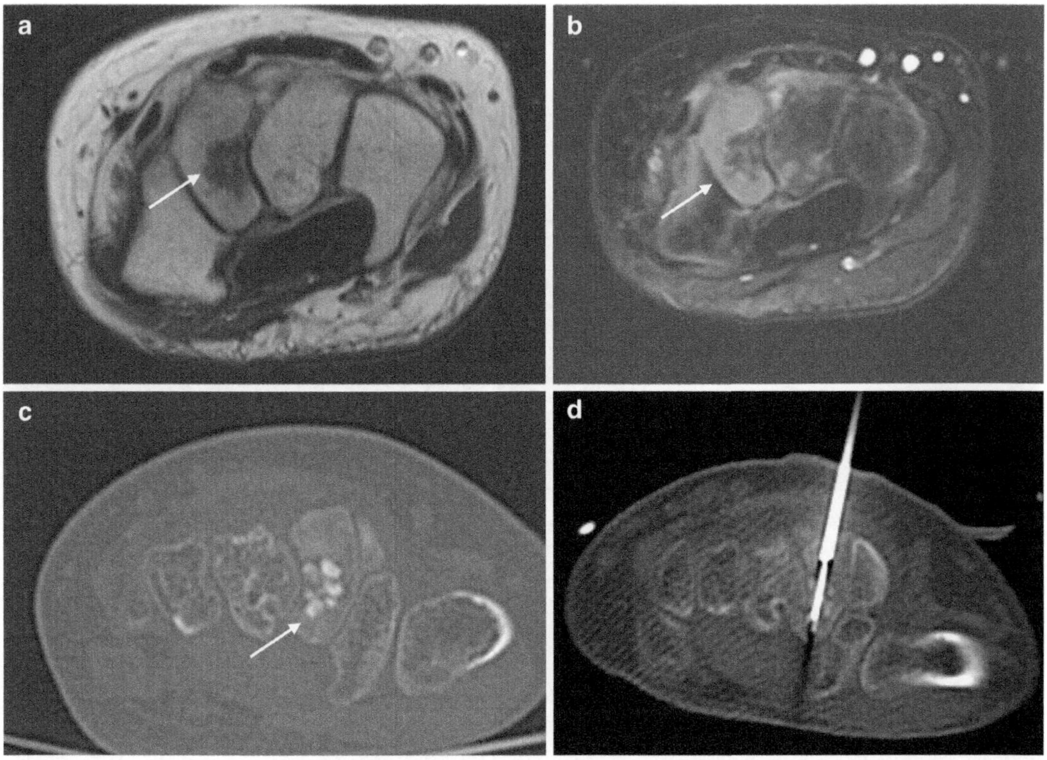

Fig. 22 Axial T1W (**a**) and STIR (**b**) MR images and CT (**c**) of the wrist show an osteoid osteoma in the trapezoid (arrow). (**d**) Axial CT image showing the placement of the radiofrequency ablation needle (arrow) within the lesion

consent remain central to setting realistic expectations and ensuring compliance with postprocedural care. As imaging and therapeutic technologies continue to evolve, the scope and efficacy of wrist and hand interventions will expand, offering new opportunities for minimally invasive, targeted treatments. Future innovations, including robotic assistance and improved biological therapies, promise even greater precision and effectiveness in addressing complex musculoskeletal conditions.

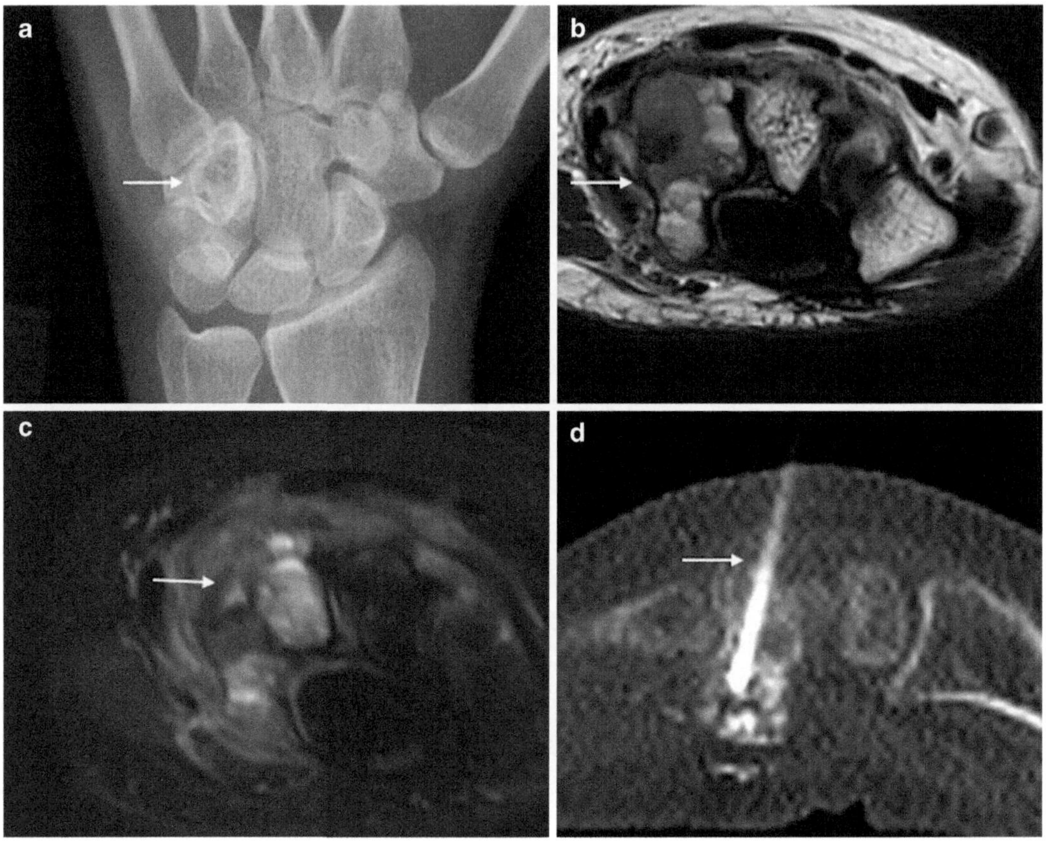

Fig. 23 Radiograph of the wrist (**a**), T2W (**b**), and STIR (**c**) images showing an aneurysmal bone cyst within the hamate with fluid-fluid levels. (**d**) Axial section of non-contrast CT demonstrating placement of needle (arrow) for injection of sclerosing agent into the lesion; note the contrast medium within the aneurysmal bone cyst

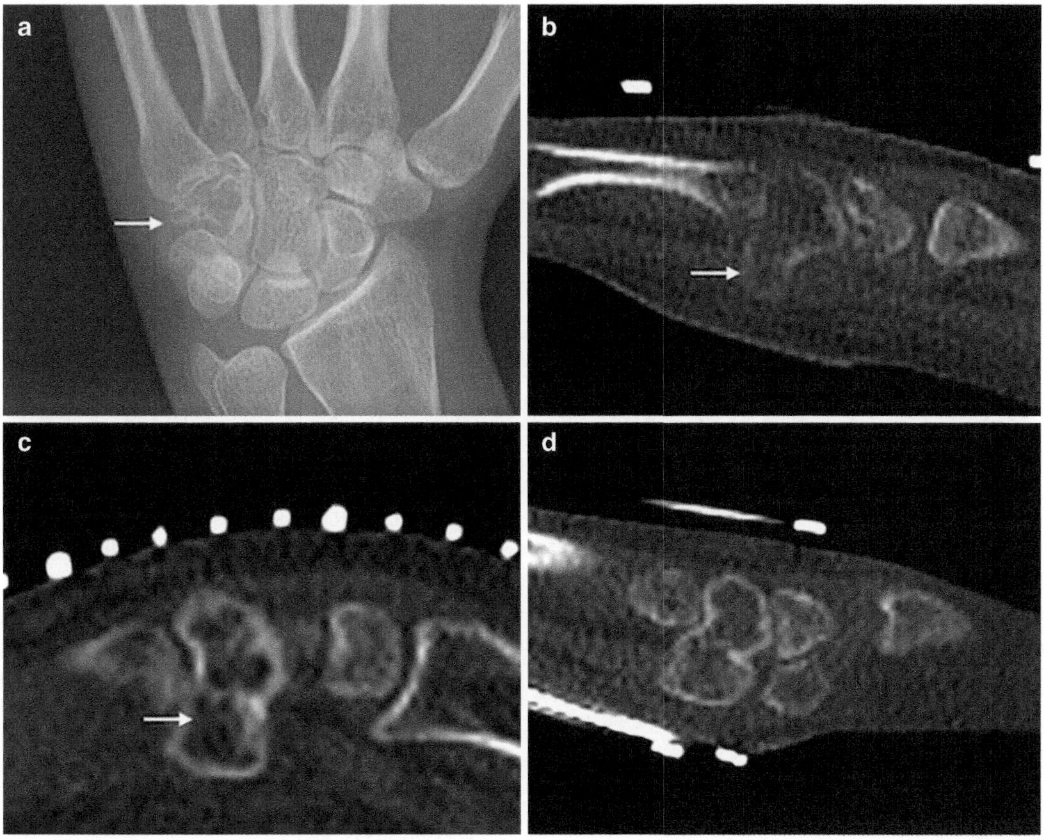

Fig. 24 Radiograph (**a**) and sagittal noncontrast CT of the wrist (**b**) show a lytic lesion within the hamate, suggesting an aneurysmal bone cyst (arrow). (**c**, **d**) Sagittal CT section showing post-sclerotherapy consolidation of the lesion in the hamate

References

Atroshi I, Gummesson C, Johnsson R, Ornstein E, Ranstam J, Rosén I (1999) Prevalence of carpal tunnel syndrome in a general population. JAMA 282(2):153–158

Bansal A, Goyal A, Gamanagatti S, Srivastava DN, Manhas V (2021) Current updates in image-guided musculoskeletal interventions. J Clin Orthop Trauma 22:101601

Chehab MA, Thakor AS, Tulin-Silver S, Connolly BL, Cahill AM, Ward TJ, Padia SA, Kohi MP, Midia M, Chaudry G, Gemmete JJ, Mitchell JW, Brody L, Crowley JJ, Heran MKS, Weinstein JL, Nikolic B, Dariushnia SR, Tam AL, Venkatesan AM (2018) Adult and pediatric antibiotic prophylaxis during vascular and IR procedures: a society of interventional radiology practice parameter update endorsed by the Cardiovascular and Interventional Radiological Society of Europe and the Canadian Association for Interventional Radiology. J Vasc Interv Radiol 29(11):1483–1501.e2

Chim H (2017) Hand and wrist anatomy and biomechanics: a comprehensive guide. Plast Reconstr Surg 140(4):865

Chopra A, Rowbotham EL, Grainger AJ (2016) Radiological intervention of the hand and wrist. Br J Radiol 89(1057):20150373

Cleary K, Melzer A, Watson V, Kronreif G, Stoianovici D (2006) Interventional robotic systems: applications and technology state-of-the-art. Minim Invasive Ther Allied Technol 15(2):101–113

Colio SW, Smith J, Pourcho AM (2016) Ultrasound-guided interventional procedures of the wrist and hand: anatomy, indications, and techniques. Phys Med Rehabil Clin N Am 27(3):589–605

Filippiadis D, Stefanou D, Mazioti A, Foti L, Tsochatzis A, Kelekis N, Kelekis A (2022) Computed tomography guided radiofrequency ablation of osteoid osteoma in children: a single center's experience. Skeletal Radiol 51(4):855–861

Foremny GB, Pretell-Mazzini J, Jose J, Subhawong TK (2015) Risk of bleeding associated with interventional musculoskeletal radiology procedures. A comprehensive review of the literature. Skeletal Radiol 44(5):619–627

Gharib M, Cleland T, Enriquez R, Kasitinon D, Konda C, Schaaf S, Song A, Williams R, Özçakar L, Jain NB (2024) Ultrasound-guided first carpometacarpal joint injection technique. Am J Phys Med Rehabil 103(11):e171

Gialanella B, Prometti P (2011) Effects of corticosteroids injection in rotator cuff tears. Pain Med 12(10):1559–1565

Jayaram P, Kennedy DJ, Yeh P, Dragoo J (2019) Chondrotoxic effects of local anesthetics on human knee articular cartilage: a systematic review. PM R 11(4):379–400

Kassamali RH, Ladak B (2015) The role of robotics in interventional radiology: current status. Quant Imaging Med Surg 5(3):340–343

Kelly S, Humby F, Filer A, Ng N, Di Cicco M, Hands RE, Rocher V, Bombardieri M, D'Agostino MA, McInnes IB, Buckley CD, Taylor PC, Pitzalis C (2015) Ultrasound-guided synovial biopsy: a safe, well-tolerated and reliable technique for obtaining high-quality synovial tissue from both large and small joints in early arthritis patients. Ann Rheum Dis 74(3):611–617

Kloppenburg M, Kwok WY (2011) Hand osteoarthritis—a heterogeneous disorder. Nat Rev Rheumatol 8(1):22–31

Kumar N, Chandan SK, Jalan D, Sinha S, Jaiswal B, Singh DK (2023) Ultrasound-guided interventions in primary carpal tunnel syndrome: perineural injection to thread carpal tunnel release. Br J Radiol 96(1150):20230552

Kurup AN, Callstrom MR (2010) Image-guided percutaneous ablation of bone and soft tissue tumors. Semin Interv Radiol 27(3):276–284

Le ADK, Enweze L, DeBaun MR, Dragoo JL (2018) Current clinical recommendations for use of platelet-rich plasma. Curr Rev Musculoskelet Med 11(4):624–634

Lohman M, Vasenius J, Nieminen O (2007) Ultrasound guidance for puncture and injection in the radiocarpal joint. Acta Radiol 48(7):744–747

Louis LJ (2008) Musculoskeletal ultrasound intervention: principles and advances. Radiol Clin North Am 46(3):515–533, vi

MacMahon PJ, Eustace SJ, Kavanagh EC (2009) Injectable corticosteroid and local anesthetic preparations: a review for radiologists. Radiology 252(3):647–661

Mariani E, Pulsatelli L (2020) Platelet concentrates in musculoskeletal medicine. Int J Mol Sci 21(4):1328

McDermott JD, Ilyas AM, Nazarian LN, Leinberry CF (2012) Ultrasound-guided injections for de Quervain's tenosynovitis. Clin Orthop Relat Res 470(7):1925–1931

Orlandi D, Corazza A, Silvestri E, Serafini G, Savarino EV, Garlaschi G, Mauri G, Cimmino MA, Sconfienza LM (2014) Ultrasound-guided procedures around the wrist and hand: how to do. Eur J Radiol 83(7):1231–1238

Patel RP, McGill K, Motamedi D, Morgan T (2023) Ultrasound-guided interventions of the upper extremity joints. Skeletal Radiol 52(5):897–909

Rastogi AK, Davis KW, Ross A, Rosas HG (2016) Fundamentals of joint injection. AJR Am J Roentgenol 207(3):484–494

Saboeiro GR, Sofka CM (2008) Ultrasound-guided ganglion cyst aspiration. HSS J 4(2):161–163

Sconfienza LM, Bandirali M, Serafini G, Lacelli F, Aliprandi A, Di Leo G, Sardanelli F (2012) Rotator cuff calcific tendinitis: does warm saline solution improve the short-term outcome of double-needle US-guided treatment? Radiology 262(2):560–566

Shah A, Mak D, Davies AM, James SL, Botchu R (2019) Musculoskeletal corticosteroid administration: current concepts. Can Assoc Radiol J 70(1):29–36

Smith KA, Carrino JA, Carrino J (2008) MRI-guided interventions of the musculoskeletal system. J Magn Reson Imaging 27(2):339–346

Smith J, Rizzo M, Sayeed YA, Finnoff JT (2011) Sonographically guided distal radioulnar joint injection: technique and validation in a cadaveric model. J Ultrasound Med 30(11):1587–1592

Tunçez M, Turan K, Aydin ÖD, Çetin Tunçez H (2023) Ultrasound guided versus blinded injection in trigger finger treatment: a prospective controlled study. J Orthop Surg Res 18(1):459

Walker-Bone KE, Palmer KT, Reading I, Cooper C (2003) Soft-tissue rheumatic disorders of the neck and upper limb: prevalence and risk factors. Semin Arthritis Rheum 33(3):185–203

Zeidenberg J, Aronowitz JG, Landy DC, Owens PW, Jose J (2016) Ultrasound-guided aspiration of wrist ganglions: a follow-up survey of patient satisfaction and outcomes. Acta Radiol 57(4):481–486

Congenital and Developmental Abnormalities

Neha Nischal, Saavi Reddy Pellakuru, Rajesh Botchu, Emily J. Stenhouse, James J. R. Kirkpatrick, and Greg J. Irwin

Contents

N. Nischal (✉)
Department of Radiology, Holy Family Hospital, New Delhi, India

S. R. Pellakuru
Department of Radiology, Apollo Institute of Medical Sciences, Hyderabad, India

R. Botchu
Department of Musculoskeletal Radiology, Royal Orthopedic Hospital, Birmingham, UK

E. J. Stenhouse
Royal Hospital for Sick Children, Glasgow, UK

J. J. R. Kirkpatrick
Canniesburn Plastic Surgery Unit, Glasgow Royal Infirmary and Royal Hospital for Sick Children, Glasgow, UK

G. J. Irwin
Diagnostic Imaging, Royal Hospital for Sick Children, Glasgow, UK

Med Radiol Diagn Imaging (2025)
https://doi.org/10.1007/174_2025_596,
Published Online: 26 September 2025

Abstract

Congenital hand differences (CHD) have been estimated to occur in 10% of children born with congenital abnormalities. CHD can be classified according to their predominant abnormality using the Swanson classification. Failure of differentiation represents the most common group. Associated (nonlimb) abnormalities are common, and it is important to identify those CHD requiring systemic evaluation. Radiology is important in the diagnosis and management of CHD with plain films providing the mainstay of imaging postnatally. The management of CHD should be within a multidisciplinary environment.

1 Introduction

Of the 1–2% of newborns born with congenital defects, 10% are born with upper limb malformations (McCarroll 2000). The incidence is higher in boys, with pre- and post-term births, with multiple pregnancies and with increased maternal age (Giele et al. 2001). Congenital hand abnormalities are now commonly described as congenital hand differences (CHD). The majority (60%) of CHD has an unknown etiology, but genetic factors may be attributable in 20% and environmental teratogens in 20% (Netscher and Baumholtz 2007). The embryologic limb bud can be seen at 4 weeks after fertilization, and the existing fetal limb structures continue to grow and develop for 8 weeks after fertilization. Most CHD are thought to arise during this 4-week interval (Kozin 2003; Oberg et al. 2010).

CHD vary widely in their functional and aesthetic implications. Associated (nonlimb) abnormalities are also common, up to 26.7% in some series (De Smet 2002). It is important to identify those CHD which require further systemic evaluation and to differentiate them from isolated CHD. For example, radial deficiency occurs commonly in a number of syndromes such as the VACTERL association (vertebral abnormalities, ano-rectal and cardiac abnormalities, tracheo-esophageal fistula, esophageal atresia, renal defects, radial dysplasia, and lower limb abnormalities) (Stoll et al. 2010).

Management must always be conducted in a multidisciplinary environment, involving surgeons, physiotherapists, orthotists, pediatricians, prosthetists, psychologists, anesthetists, geneticists, and radiologists. The purpose of this review is to provide an illustrated classification of congenital hand differences for radiologists, which will also be of interest to the other members of the multidisciplinary team.

2 Imaging

CHD may be demonstrated by antenatal ultrasound particularly late in the first trimester and in the middle of the second trimester of pregnancy (Rypens et al. 2006; Edwards and Hui 2018) (Fig. 1). Three-dimensional ultrasound may be helpful in defining the abnormality more clearly (Ploeckinger-Ulm et al. 1996; Leung 2021). Prenatal classification and characterization may help to identify fetuses that would benefit from more complete prenatal cardiac and karyotypic workup.

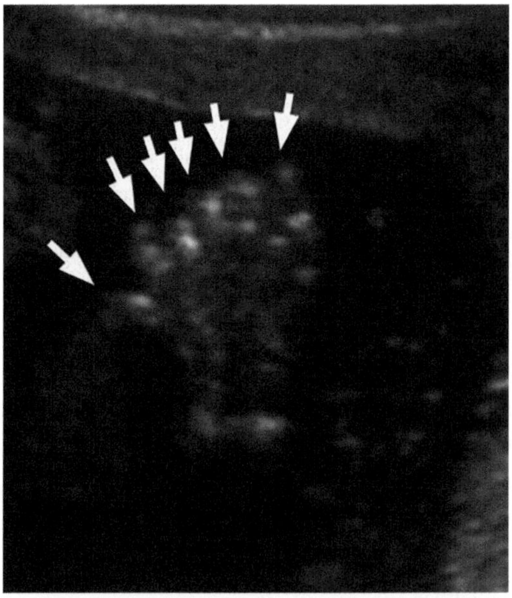

Fig. 1 2D Ultrasound image of a fetal hand of a fetus in the second trimester with trisomy 13 and post-axial polydactyly. (Image courtesy of Dr Françoise Rypens)

Postnatally, plain films provide the mainstay of imaging, with ultrasound and magnetic resonance imaging (MRI) providing useful additional characterization in a minority of cases, principally in the clarification of the nature of masses and other causes of overgrowth (Winfeld and Otero 2016).

3 Classification

The most widely accepted classification of CHD was proposed by Frantz and O'Rahilly and presented by Swanson (Frantz and O'Rahilly 1961; Swanson 1976). This was subsequently modified by the International Federation of Societies for Surgery of the Hand (IFSSH) in 1983 (Swanson et al. 1983), and further modified by the Japanese Society of Surgery of the Hand (JSSH) in 2000 (Ogino 2000). In 2014, the IFSSH adopted the Oberg, Manske, and Tonkin (OMT) classification as the preferred system (Oberg et al. 2010). This system was based on the knowledge of errors in the developmental axes or genetic/molecular pathways and was last updated in 2020.

The major categories of the Swanson classification are listed in Table 1 and are subsequently discussed for the ease of understanding.

The seven categories differentiate the CHD according to the predominant abnormality, and further define the abnormality according to the nature of the embryonic failure during development. Group II (failure of differentiation) represents the most common group (Laub 2021).

Table 1 Abbreviated embryologic classification of CHD

1	Failure of formation
2	Failure of differentiation
3	Duplication
4	Overgrowth
5	Undergrowth
6	Constriction ring syndrome
7	Generalized skeletal abnormalities

Adapted from Swanson (1976)

4 Failure of Formation

Failure of formation of parts can be divided into transverse and longitudinal subgroups. Transverse deficiencies occur when growth stops abruptly, resulting in a "congenital amputation" and a shortened or truncated limb. Longitudinal deficiencies occur when structures are hypoplastic or absent along a longitudinal axis of the limb, resulting in abnormal formation and function biased down one "side" of the limb (either the radial or ulnar sides, or "centrally" between the two) (Kozin 2004). In reality, most CHD within this group are mixed to some degree.

4.1 Transverse

This is defined according to the bone segment at which the growth arrest occurs (Van Heest 1996; Klaritsch 2024). The most common transverse deficiency occurs at the junction of the proximal and middle thirds of the forearm (Fig. 2).

These anomalies are usually unilateral, sporadic, and are rarely associated with other anom-

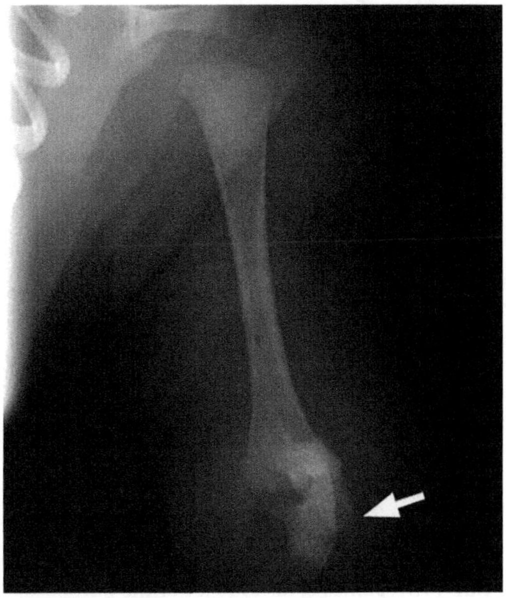

Fig. 2 Commonest level of transverse growth arrest at proximal radius and ulna (*arrow*)

alies. Rudimentary "nubbins" or dimpling may be found at the distal end of the congenital amputation (Kozin 2003). This should not be confused with constriction ring syndrome which may also manifest as an "amputation" but requires the presence of a constriction ring either affecting the involved extremity or elsewhere (Wiedrich 1998; Demetri et al. 2021).

4.2 Longitudinal

In this group, the radial, central, or ulnar side of the limb is abnormal. They may very rarely be characterized by absence of one or more "segments" ("forearm" vs. "upper arm" vs "both") of the upper limb (phocomelia), such as those defects attributed to maternal exposure to thalidomide. For example, when both segments are missing ("complete phocomelia"), the hand is attached directly to the shoulder (Rypens et al. 2006).

4.2.1 Radial

Radial dysplasia is the most common longitudinal deficiency and occurs when structures on the radial side of the arm fail to develop properly. It is frequently bilateral (40–60%) with a male:female ratio of 3:2 (Van Heest 1996). It has been described as "an abnormal hand joined to a poor limb by a bad wrist" (Flatt 1994) (Fig. 3).

Radial deficiency can range from mild hypoplasia to complete absence of the radius and thumb (the commonest type) (Fig. 4). The child presents with a hand that is radially deviated at the wrist. In the hand, the thumb is almost always affected and the fingers frequently have limited motion and function, the severity of which decreases from the radial to the ulnar side (James et al. 2004; Gandhi et al. 2019). The ulna is also usually shortened and bowed and may need later osteotomy (Fig. 5a, b).

A classification scheme has been described by Bayne and Klug for radial deficiency with proposed modifications by James et al. (Bayne and Klug 1987; James et al. 1999). For the purposes of imaging, it is useful to divide the deficiency into components and describe the characteristics of each component (James et al. 1999; Kozin 2003).

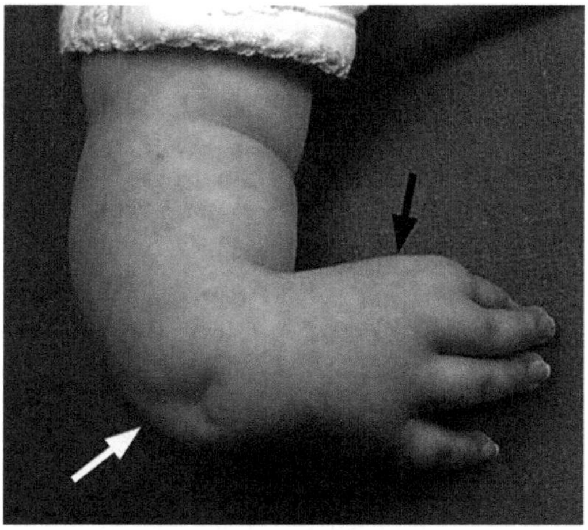

Fig. 3 Radial dysplasia displays an array of upper limb differences, the most striking of which are usually the radially deviated wrist (*white arrow*), absent thumb (*black arrow*), shortened forearm, and stiff elbow

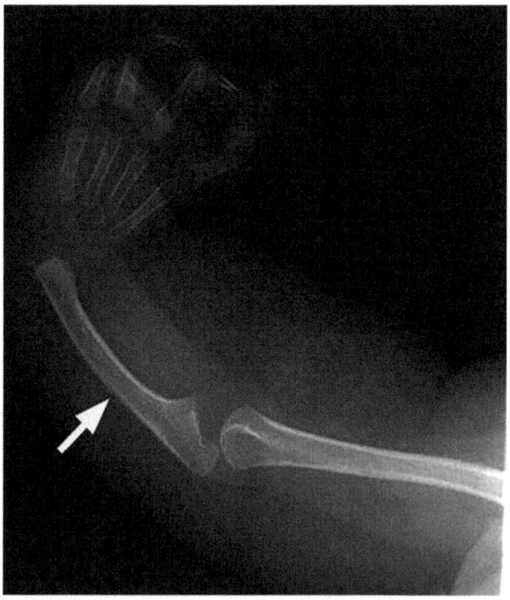

Fig. 4 Radial dysplasia has a spectrum of abnormalities of the radius, the commonest being complete absence of the radius. In such cases, the ulna (*arrow*) is relatively hypoplastic also

1. Thumb:
   I. Absent
   II. Hypoplastic
2. Carpal bones:
   I. Normal
   II. Absent

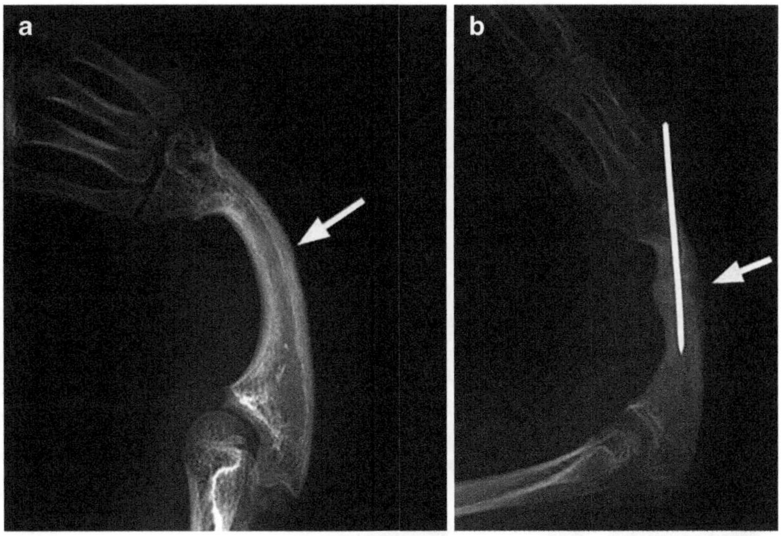

Fig. 5 (**a**, **b**) In radial dysplasia the ulna is frequently bowed, and may require correction as in this case which had been centralized 10 years previously. The osteotomy site (*arrow*) is secured with a large K-wire, removed at 6 weeks (**a**) pre-op (**b**) post-op

III. Hypoplastic
IV. Coalition

(Nb: Ossification centers of the carpal bones appear at a variety of ages ranging from 2 months for the capitate and hamate, to 4 years for the scaphoid, trapezium, and trapezoid.)

3. Distal radius
   I. Normal
   II. >2 mm shorter than ulna
   III. Absent physis
   IV. Absent
4. Proximal radius:
   I. Normal
   II. Radioulnar synostosis
   III. Radial head dislocation
   IV. Hypoplastic
   V. Absent

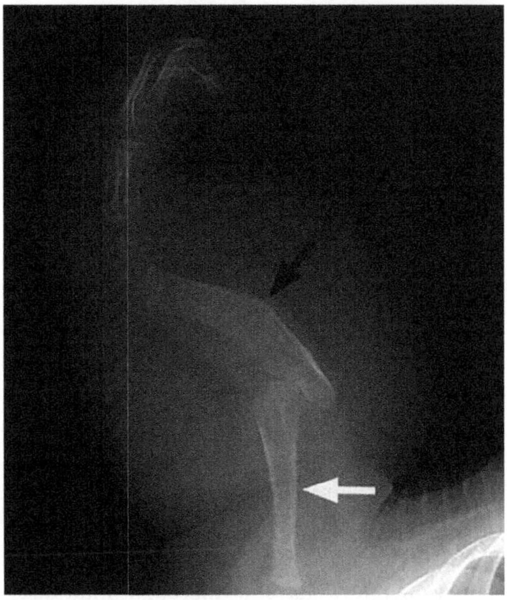

Fig. 6 Radial dysplasia with severe hypoplasia of the ulna (*black arrow*) and humerus (*white arrow*), both of which are shorter than the hand itself

The elbows are commonly stiff, and the abnormal features frequently extend further proximally (Fig. 6). Recently Goldfarb and colleagues (Goldfarb et al. 2005) proposed a further subtype of proximal radial longitudinal deficiency, involving an abnormal glenoid, an absent proximal humerus (with the distal humerus articulating with the ulna), and radial-sided hand abnormalities.

Treatment involves straightening (centralization) of the wrist, currently achieved by initial distraction (Fig. 7a) followed by centralization (Fig. 7b) (both of which require perioperative fluoroscopic screening), and later pollicization (shortening and rotation of the index ray on its neurovascular pedicle to the position of the thumb, with tendon and intrinsic muscle rebalancing to create a "thumb" from the index finger).

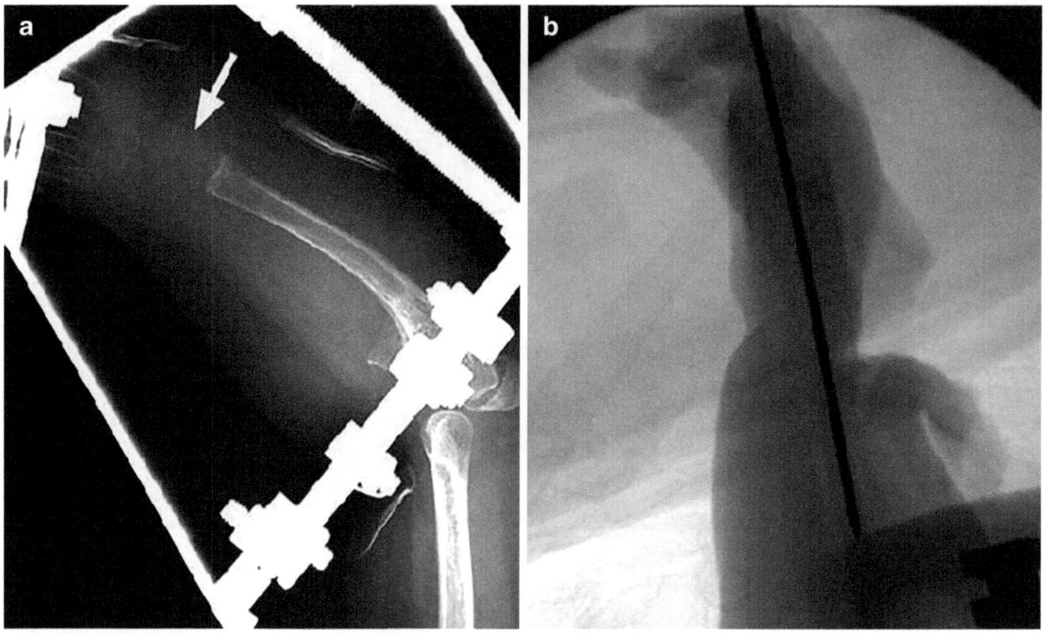

Fig. 7 Treatment of the radially deviated wrist is best achieved by (**a**) initial gradual lengthening of the soft tissues using an external distraction frame to bring the hand in line (*arrow*) over the end of the ulna, followed by (**b**) removal of the frame and formal centralization, with tendon transfers and temporary axial K-wire fixation, requiring intraoperative fluoroscopy

Importantly, radial longitudinal deficiencies often present as part of a syndrome. Associations include hematological conditions (e.g., thrombocytopenia-absent radius syndrome and Fanconi's anemia), cardiac anomalies (e.g., Holt Oram syndrome), the VACTERL syndrome (see Sect. 1), and craniofacial syndromes (e.g., Nager and Duane syndromes) (Lourie and Lins 1998; Goldfarb et al. 2006).

Children with radial longitudinal deficiencies should therefore have a thorough multidisciplinary evaluation at the time of presentation to exclude associated abnormalities, understanding that some of these may not be immediately apparent (e.g., Fanconi's anemia has a median age of onset of 7 years of age) (Kozin 2003).

4.2.2 Central

This involves deficiencies of the central part of the hand and is also known descriptively as "cleft hand," with traditional terms such as "split hand" or "lobster claw hand" having been rightly dropped because of their potentially emotive nature. Two types of cleft hand have been described, formerly known as "typical" and "atypical." Although they may appear similar morphologically, they both have major clinical differences and probably different embryological derivations (Miura and Suzuki 1984; Ogino 1990).

The typical cleft hand (now known as "true" cleft hand) has a deep V-shaped defect (Fig. 8a, b). Most commonly, the phalanges are missing. The metacarpals may be absent or malpositioned (Fig. 9), but are rarely hypoplastic. Joints at the site of the cleft can be very complex (Fig. 10), (Barsky 1964; Ogino 1990). This type of deficiency is often bilateral, and is usually inherited. There may be syndactyly of the ring-small or thumb-index web space, and associated foot involvement is common (Fig. 11). True central dysplasia is also associated with cleft lip and pal-

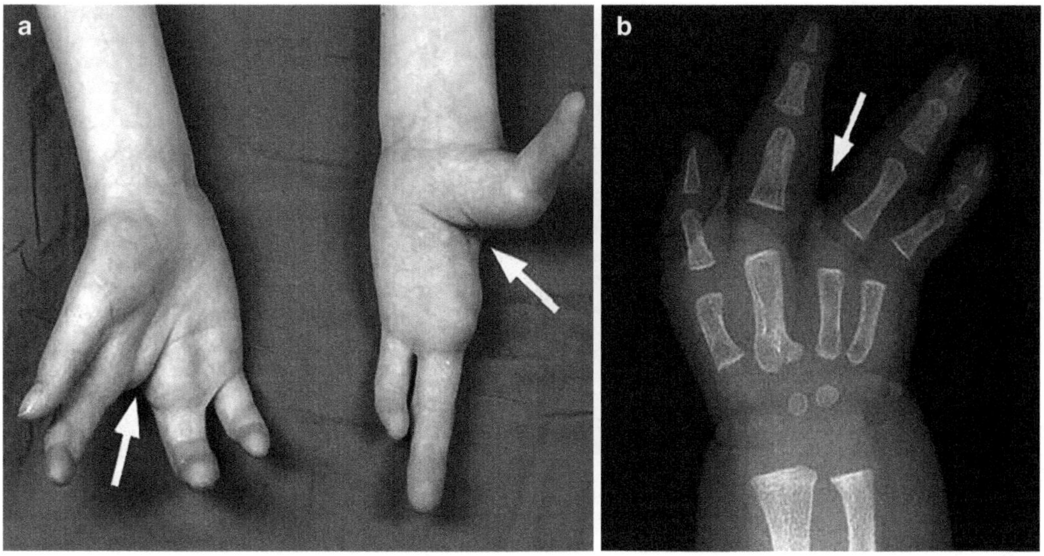

Fig. 8 (**a**) True cleft hand is usually bilateral, with V-shaped clefts (*arrows*), though the severity may differ between the two hands as in this case. (**b**) True clefts are usually centered on an absent third ray (*arrow*)

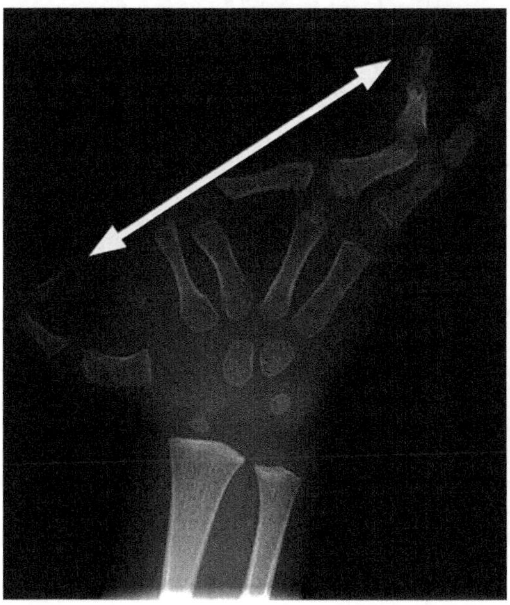

Fig. 9 In true cleft hand, a wide spectrum of severity is seen, in which transverse metacarpals can cause progressive widening of the cleft (*arrow*)

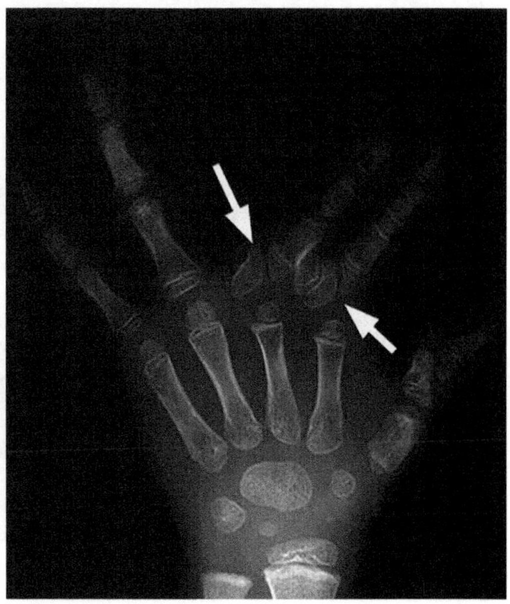

Fig. 10 This unusual variant demonstrates the complex joints (*arrows*) which can exist in cleft hands, requiring vigilance during surgical corrections

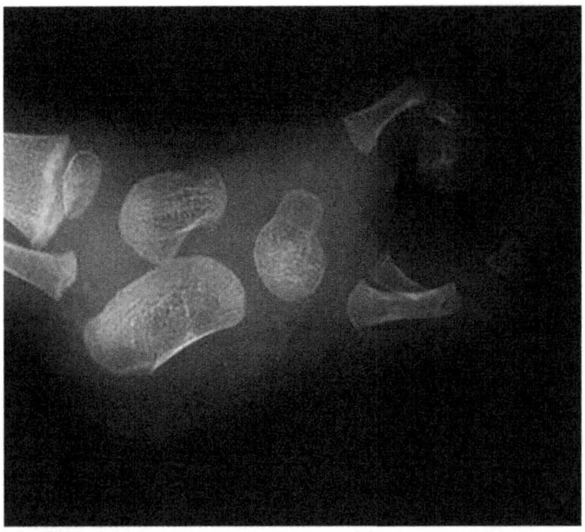

Fig. 11 Foot involvement is common in true cleft hand patients

ate but not Poland syndrome (Miura and Suzuki 1984; Ogino 1990, 2021).

Atypical cleft hand has a shallower, U-shaped central defect that involves the central three digits (index, long, and ring) (Fig. 12a), (Kozin 2003). It is a form of symbrachydactyly (shortened and webbed digits) that can vary in degree from the "short finger type" (Fig. 12b), to absence of the central three digits (Fig. 12a), to a monodactylous type (thumb only, no fingers) (Fig. 12c, d), to complete absence of all digits, with only very rudimentary "nubbins" (peromelic type) (Fig. 12e) (Özdemir et al. 2019a, b).

Atypical cleft hand is usually unilateral and sporadic. It is not associated with lower limb malformations or cleft lip and palate (Miura and

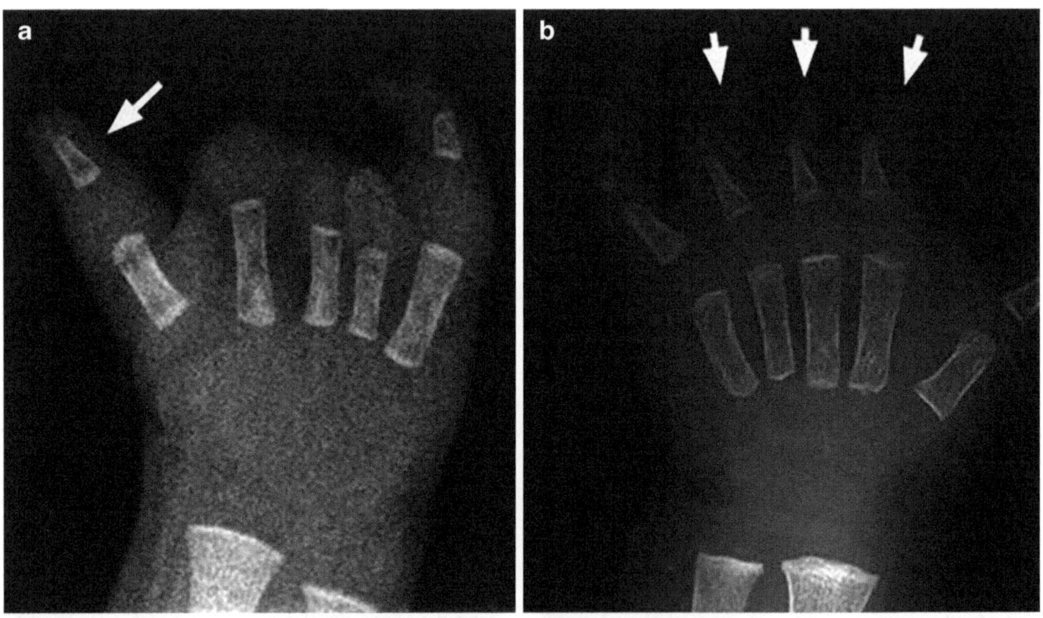

Fig. 12 Symbrachydactyly subtypes. (**a**) Atypical cleft hand also known as "U-shaped cleft hand type" with absence of the central three digits, leaving only the thumb (*arrow*) and little finger, both of which are hypoplastic in this case. (**b**) Short finger type, with proximal phalanges and reasonable soft tissue envelopes distally (*arrows*) of the central three digits, which could be amenable to augmentation with bone grafts. (**c**) Monodactylous type, in which only the thumb remains (*white arrow*), but potentially useful soft tissue envelopes to the index and little fingers (*black arrows*). (**d**) Monodactylous type, with only the thumb, and no distal soft tissue. Function would be greatly improved by free toe transfers, or even custom-made prostheses. (**e**) Peromelic type, with severe attenuation at metacarpal level (*arrow* denotes proximal palmar crease)

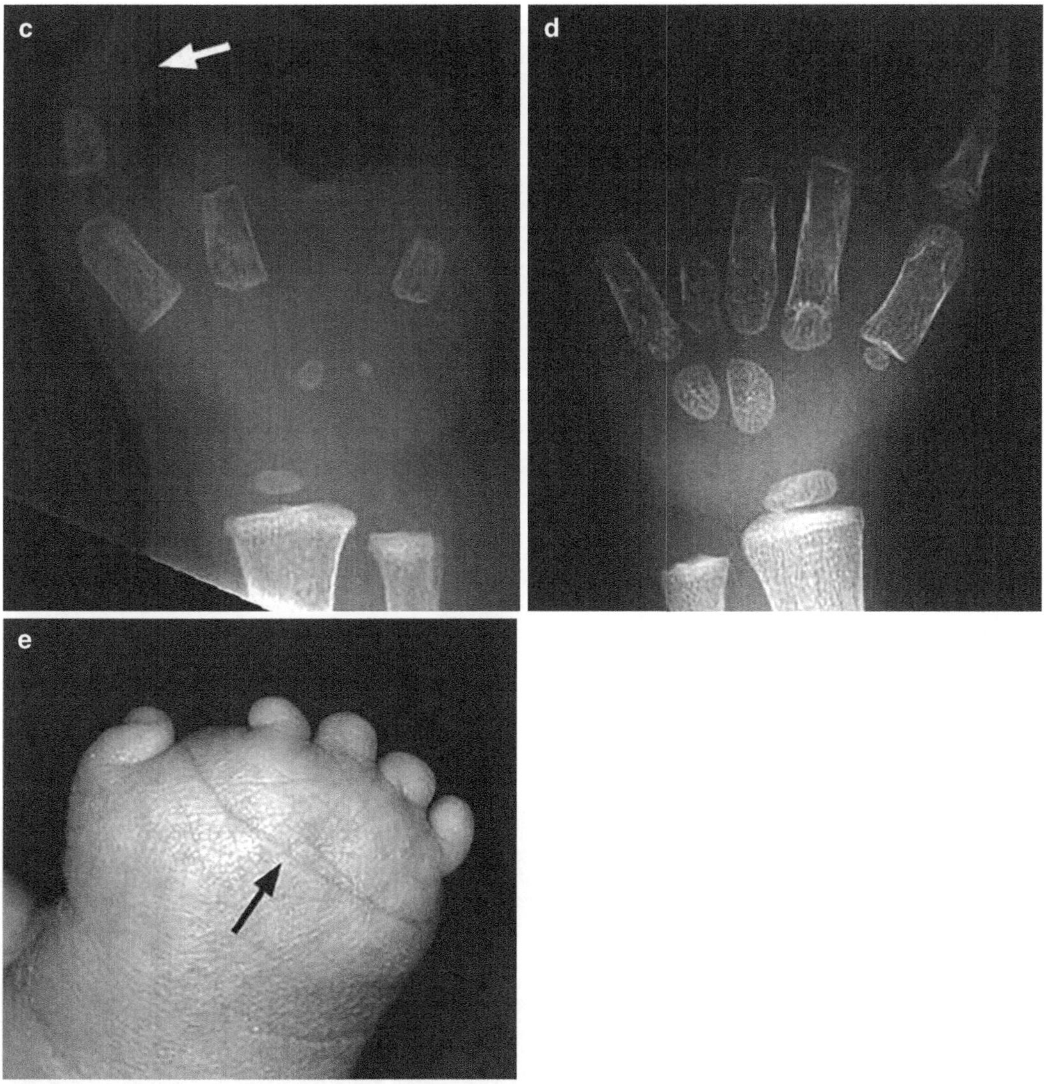

Fig. 12 (continued)

Suzuki 1984; Ogino 1990) but is associated with Poland syndrome (Fig. 13) (Ireland et al. 1976). The degree of hand deficiency in Poland syndrome does not correlate with that of the chest wall deformity; therefore, clinical evaluation of the chest wall is required with all cases of symbrachydactyly (Kozin 2003).

4.2.3 Ulnar

This represents a spectrum of abnormalities along the ulnar surface of the upper limb. It is far less common than radial and central longitudinal deficiency (Miller et al. 1986) (Figs. 14a, b, 15, and 16a, b).

Radial-sided hand anomalies may co-exist with ulnar longitudinal deficiency, and hand abnormalities are present in 68–100% of cases (Miller et al. 1986). Ulnar longitudinal deficiency may be associated with other musculoskeletal anomalies (e.g., scoliosis), but it is not associated with the visceral and hematopoietic disorders seen in radial deficiencies (Özdemir et al. 2019a, b).

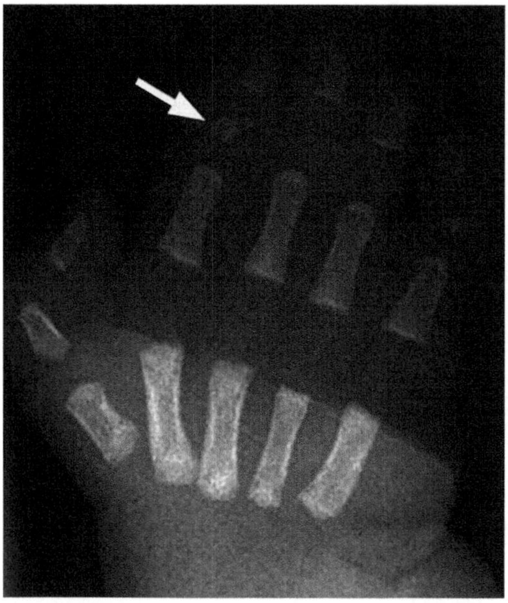

Fig. 13 Poland's syndrome with shortened digits due mostly to attenuation or absence of the middle phalanges (*arrow*), syndactylies, and global hypoplasia of the hand, in association with other upper limb and chest deformities

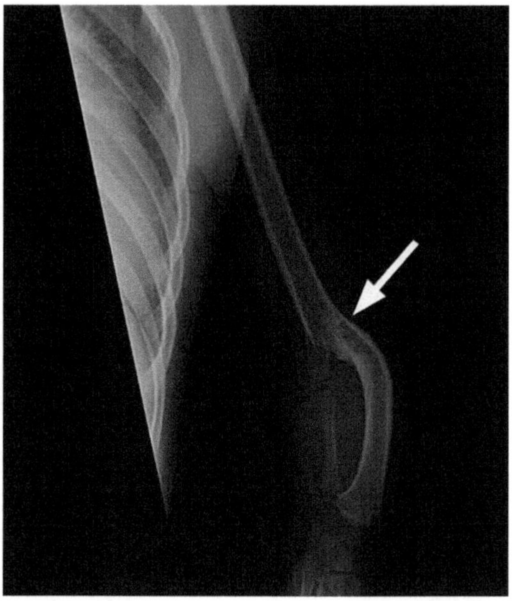

Fig. 15 Radiohumeral synostosis (*arrow*) can be seen in ulnar dysplasia

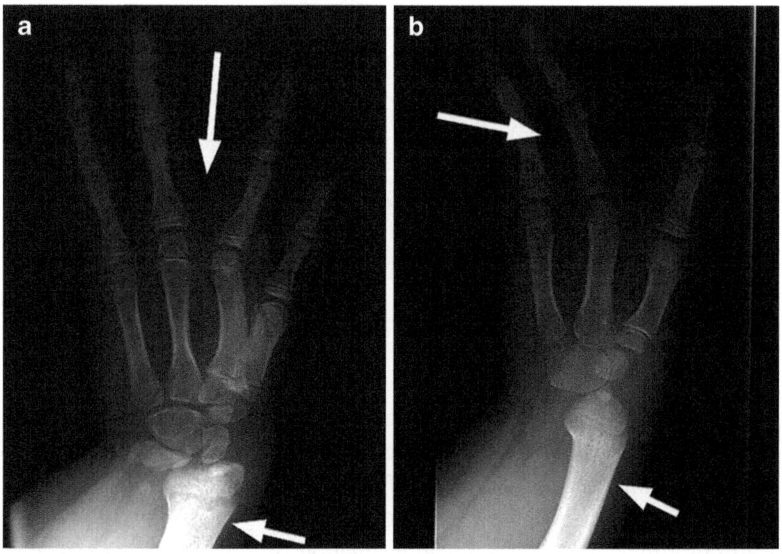

Fig. 14 (**a**, **b**) Ulnar dysplasia has deficiencies of the ulnar side of the upper limb, with partial or complete absence of the ulna, commonly with the radius providing a one-bone forearm (*short arrows*), loss of ulnar digits, ulnar deviation at the wrist, and syndactylies (*long arrows*)

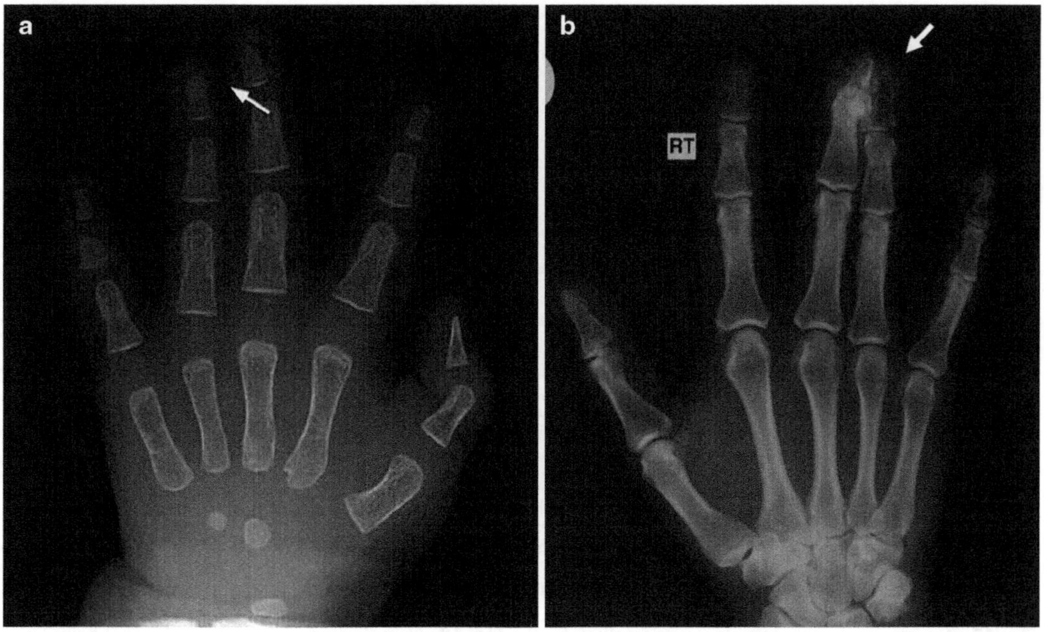

Fig. 16 Syndactyly. (**a**) Simple, complete syndactyly with soft tissue union only, distal-to-distal interphalangeal joint (*arrow*). (**b**) Complex syndactyly with bony union which is usually at the distal phalangeal level (*arrow*), and requires earlier release than simple syndactyly as bony deformities can occur quickly with growth

5 Failure of Differentiation

5.1 Syndactyly

Syndactyly is one of the most common hand anomalies and results from incomplete separation of two or more adjacent digits. It has an incidence of 1:2000 live births (Flatt 1994). The anomaly can be sporadic or familial (a family history is present in 10–40% of cases), and it may be associated with other syndromes including Poland syndrome and craniosynostoses such as Apert's syndrome (Fig. 17) (Kozin 2001).

It is classified as "complete" if it reaches the distal interphalangeal joint (Fig. 16a), "incomplete" if proximal to this joint, "simple" if it involves only skin and soft tissue, and "complex" if there is a bony fusion (usually distal) (Fig. 16b) (Van Heest 1996; Sonal and Sean 2023). Any combination of web spaces may be involved, but the commonest is an isolated third web-space involvement (between the ring and middle fingers). Syndactyly can also be classified as "complicated" if it occurs in association with other abnormalities in the affected area, such as duplication (Fig. 18). Syndactyly should be differentiated from "acrosyndactyly" (distal fusion with a proximal fenestration) which occurs in association with constriction ring syndrome (see Sect. 9) (Adu and Annan 2008).

Radiographs may indicate that separation of syndactyly is not always appropriate (Fig. 19a, b).

5.2 Arthrogryposis

This term has been used to describe conditions that present with congenital joint contractures (Mennen et al. 2005). This clinical entity has also been described by Sheldon as amyoplasia (Sheldon 1932) and most affected children (84%) present with involvement of all four limbs (Sells et al. 1996).

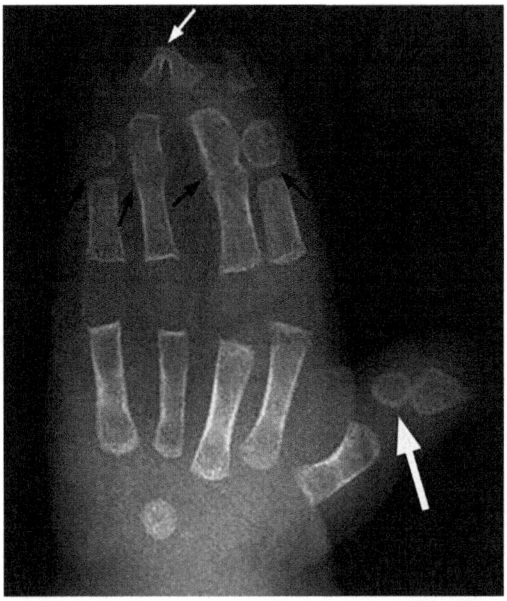

Fig. 17 Apert's hand with complex syndactyly (*short white arrow*), poorly developed or absent proximal interphalangeal joints ("symphalangism" (*black arrows*)), and a shortened deviated thumb caused by a delta phalanx (*large white arrow*)

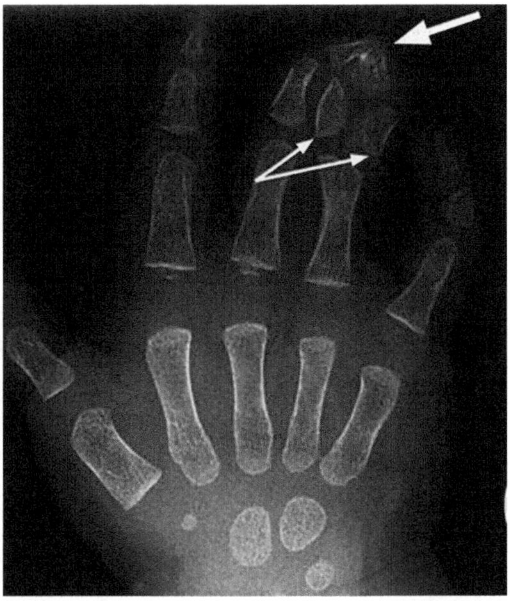

Fig. 18 Complicated syndactyly, with distal bony union (*large arrow*) and unusual duplication of the middle phalanx (*small arrows*)

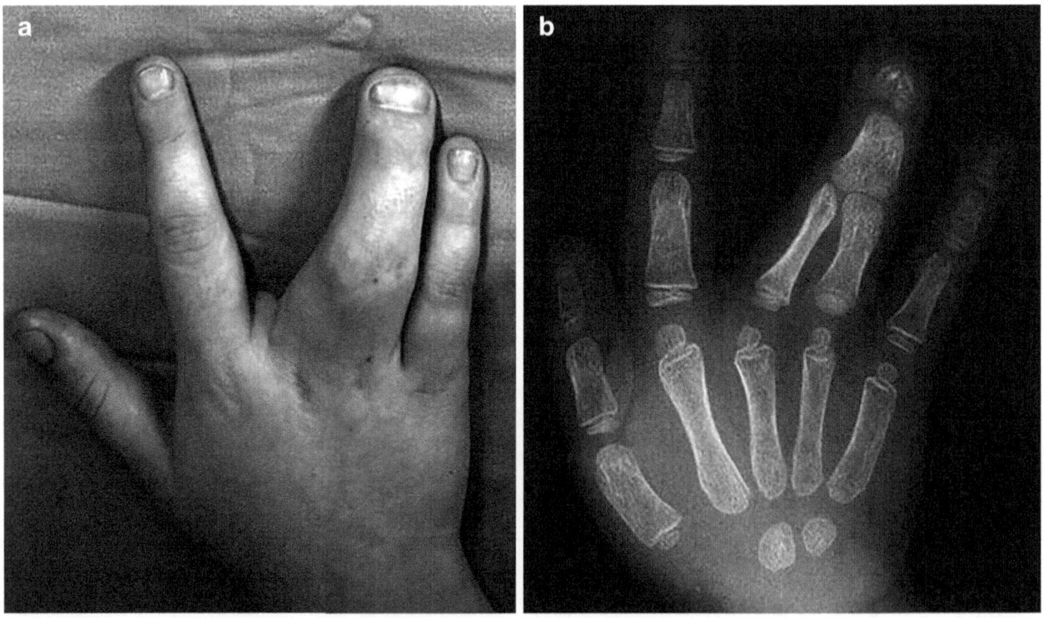

Fig. 19 Clinical photograph of the patient's hand (**a**) with visible deformity, possibly with an underlying syndactyly. Syndactyly release is sometimes contraindicated, as X-rays (**b**) may reveal that the fingers work better together than if they were separated

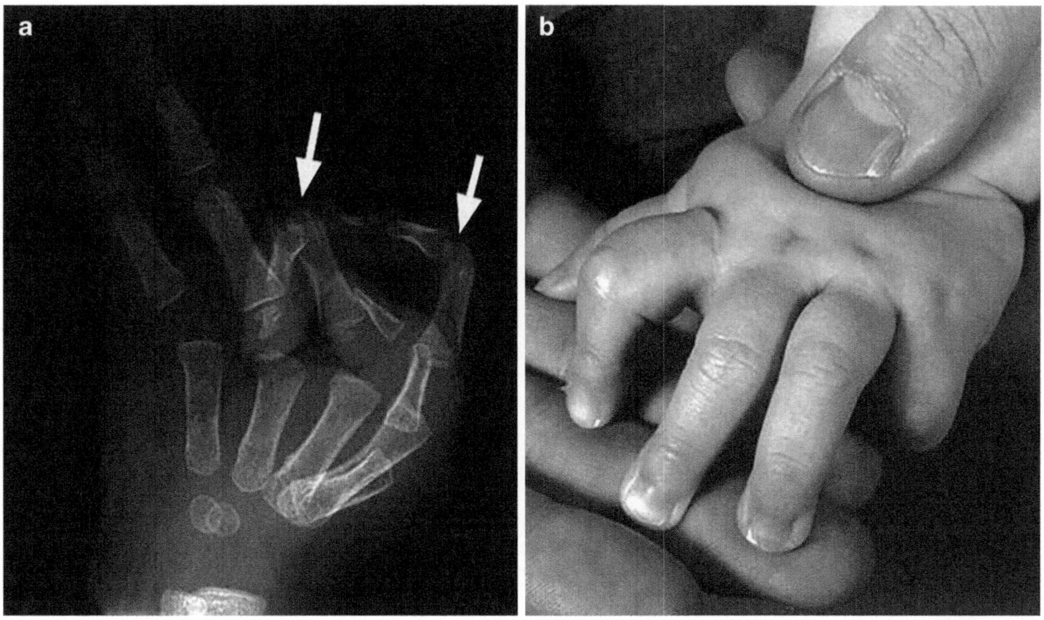

Fig. 20 Arthrogryposis is frequently associated (**a**) with multiple camptodactylies (*arrows*), sometimes affecting all digits (**b**)

The contractures are thought to be the end result of decreased intrauterine movement by the fetus which may occur because of neuropathies, myopathies, abnormal connective tissue, or decreased intrauterine space (Skaria et al. 2019). It is a sporadic condition with an incidence of 1 in 10,000 live births (Hall 1997) (Fig. 20a, b).

5.3 Camptodactyly

This is a painless flexion contracture of the proximal interphalangeal joint (PIPJ) that usually affects the little finger and may be progressive (Kloc et al. 2023). It is not related to trauma and is estimated to affect just under 1% of the population to some degree (Smith and Kaplan 1968) (Fig. 21). A classification system has been described by Benson with three main types (Benson et al. 1994). Type I presents in infancy and is frequently confined to one or both little fingers, with approximately equal sex incidence. Type II presents in adolescence with females being affected more commonly than males. The deformity worsens with the adolescent growth spurt. Type III is more severe and usually affects multiple digits in both hands (Koman et al. 1990), and may be associated with chromosomal disorders and skeletal abnormalities. Most structures

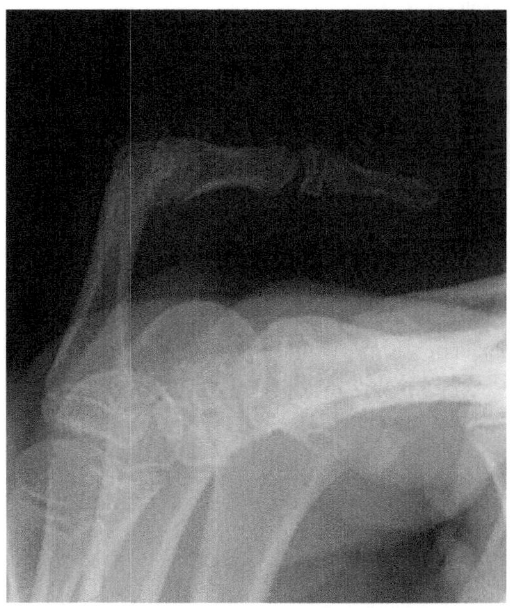

Fig. 21 Camptodactyly most commonly involves the little fingers, with stretching exercises and splintage forming the mainstay of treatment, with surgery often yielding disappointing results

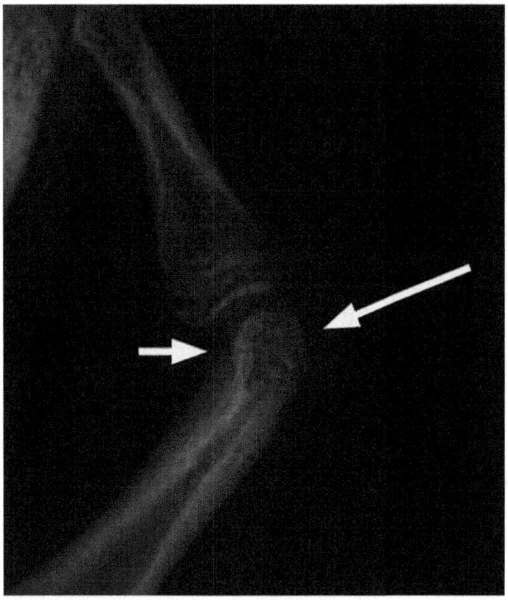

Fig. 22 Bony changes in camptodactyly: chisel-shaped head of proximal phalanx (*long arrow*), indentation of the neck of the proximal phalanx (*short arrow*), and widening of the base of the middle phalanx augur a poor surgical result

within the finger have been implicated, although abnormalities of the intrinsic lumbrical muscles of the superficial flexor tendon are not uncommon operative findings (Favril et al. 2019).

Plain radiograph assessment is vital, as the presence of classical bony changes around the joint predicts a very poor surgical outcome. These bony changes include flattening of the head of the proximal phalanx, widening of the base of the middle phalanx, and an indentation at the neck of the proximal phalanx (Ty and James 2009) (Fig. 22).

5.4 Clinodactyly

This refers to an abnormal deviation of a finger in the coronal or radioulnar plane which typically affects the middle phalanx of the little finger. The finger deviation is usually directed radially. Minor angulation of <10° is so common that it may be regarded as a normal variant (Banda and Yaish 2023).

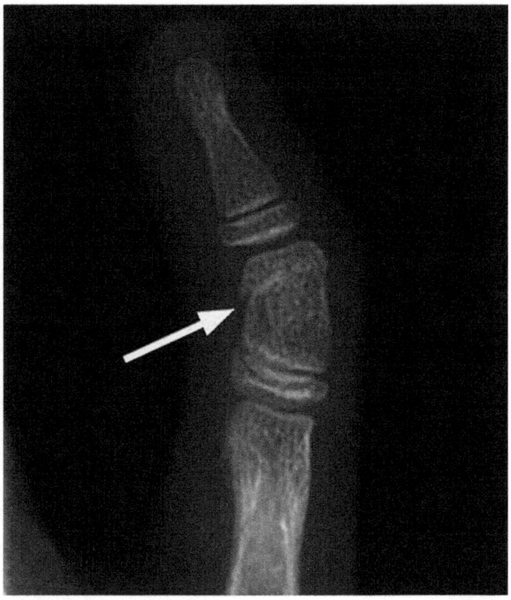

Fig. 23 Clinodactyly showing abnormal C-shaped epiphysis of middle phalanx (*arrow*)

Familial clinodactyly with an autosomal dominant pattern of inheritance usually presents bilaterally, and it is not associated with genetic syndromes. Clinodactyly may also be associated with syndromic and genetic conditions, most notably Down syndrome, in which the prevalence has been estimated at 35–79% (Flatt 1994).

The deformity is caused by an abnormally shaped middle phalanx, which may be triangular (a "delta" phalanx) or trapezoidal because of a C-shaped epiphysis (Jones 1964, Norat et al. 2008) (Fig. 23). Serial plain radiographs can be useful for objective monitoring of the angle of deviation. If progression occurs despite non-operative treatments (principally night splintage), surgery in the form of a wedge osteotomy may be required (Fig. 24a, b).

Delta phalanges can occur elsewhere in the hand and are frequently seen in the thumbs of Apert's patients, where they can cause marked deviation (Fig. 25) and often require surgery.

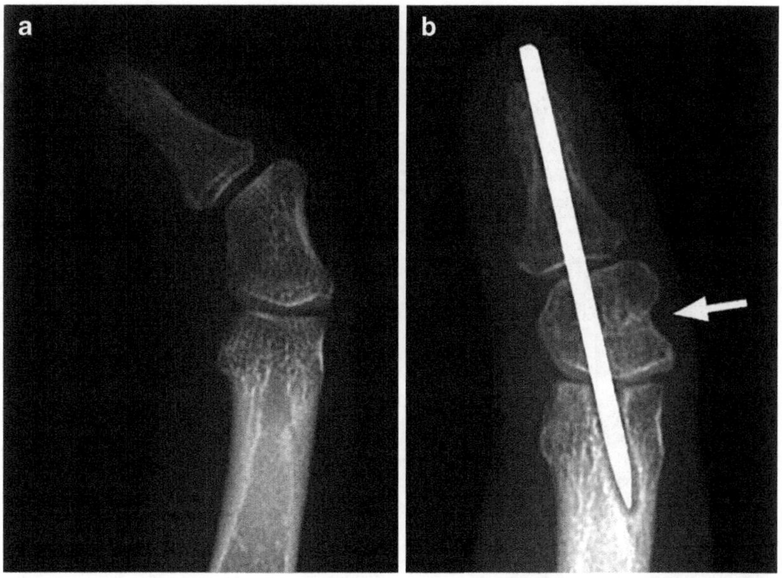

Fig. 24 Clinodactyly showing (**a**) a delta phalanx with fused epiphysis, treated by (**b**) a closing wedge osteotomy (*arrow*) and temporary K-wire

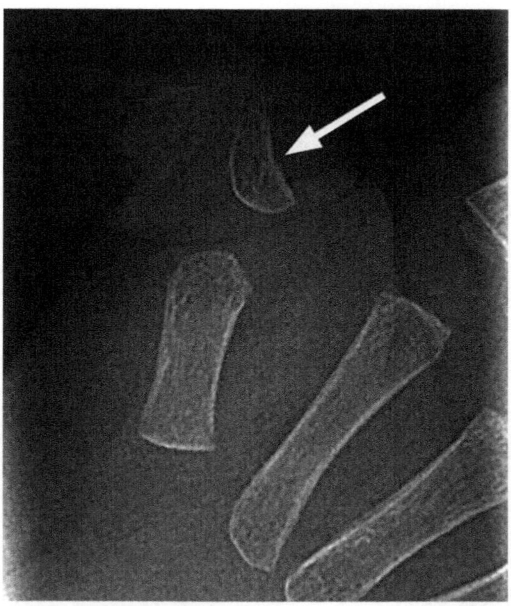

Fig. 25 Apert's thumb delta phalanx (*arrow*), which usually requires surgical correction

5.5 Congenital Thumb Flexion Deformities

Trigger and clasped thumbs are the two main causes of congenital flexion deformities of the thumb, with flexion, respectively, at the interphalangeal and metacarpophalangeal joints. In trigger thumbs, a thickening in the flexor tendon may be felt at the A1 pulley level (clinically at the level of the metacarpophalangeal level).

In clasped thumbs, there is a wide spectrum of differences, starting with attenuation then absence of the extensors, and progressing to flexion contractures with global thumb hypoplasias. Clinical evaluation usually suffices, though ultrasound may be useful in assessment of the tendons to aid in treatment planning. Hypoplastic extensors in a clasp thumb may respond to simple splintage, whereas aplasias require tendon transfer.

6 Duplication

This probably results from splitting of the original embryonic part rather than a true duplication (Van Heest 1996). Polydactyly may be "preaxial" (radial, i.e., thumb), post-axial (ulnar, i.e., little finger), or central (Bubshait 2022).

6.1 Post-axial Polydactyly

Duplications involving the ulnar aspect of the hand are more common in patients of African descent. The incidence is reported as 1 in 1339 live births in Caucasians and 1 in 143 live births

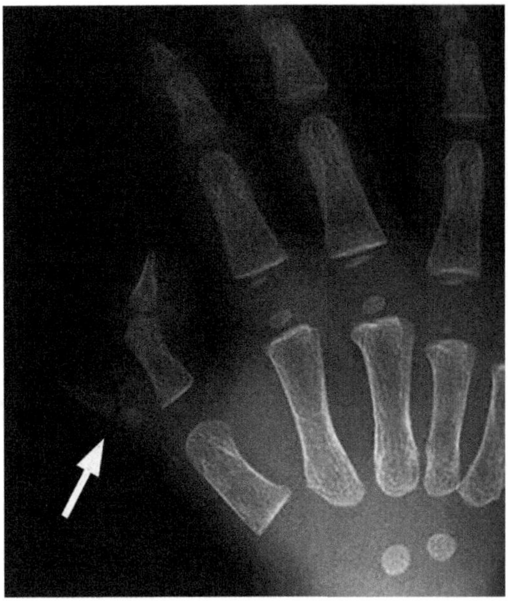

Fig. 26 Rudimentary radial duplicate (*arrow*)

in African Americans (Watson and Hennrikus 1997).

Although it is commonly an isolated finding with autosomal dominant transmission and a favorable prognosis, it may also be associated with various syndromes. The presence of post-axial polydactyly in Caucasians is more suggestive of an underlying syndrome and merits systemic evaluation. Syndromes include trisomy 13, Meckel-Gruber syndrome, Bardet-Biedl syndrome, Smith-Lemli-Opitz syndrome, short rib-polydactyly syndromes, and Ellis-van Creveld syndrome (Lachman 2007).

Accessory digits may be well developed or rudimentary (Fig. 26) (Watson and Hennrikus 1997).

Commonly the digit is rudimentary and held by a soft tissue bridge requiring only a simple excision (Fig. 27a), though there can be bony

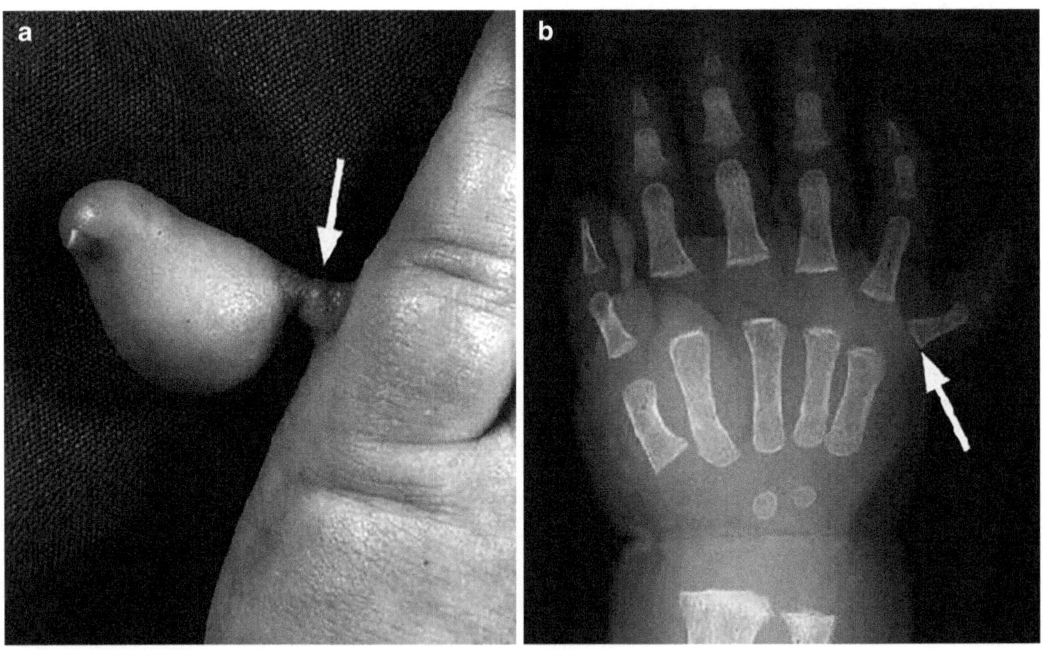

Fig. 27 Ulnar duplication is based on the Stelling classification. (**a**) *Type 1* skin bridge only (*arrow*) requiring only simple excision. (**b**) *Type 2* strong bony attachment, requiring preservation and reinsertion of the ulnar collateral ligament from accessory digit to fifth finger (position of insertion marked with *arrow*). *Type 3* is complete duplication of metacarpal

attachments at proximal phalangeal or metacarpal level (Fig. 27b), requiring more involved surgery.

6.2 Pre-axial Polydactyly

Although it is less common than post-axial polydactyly, it is more common in Caucasians and particularly in Orientals. The incidence is 1 in every 3000 live births in the white population (Graham and Ress 1998). Duplication alone is usually unilateral and sporadic; however, if one of the duplicates is a triphalangeal thumb (Fig. 28a, b), a possible syndromic association should be considered (Rypens et al. 2006), and this can be inherited in an autosomal dominant pattern.

Thumb duplications are classified according to the level of duplication, and Wassel's classification is the most widely used and accepted (Fig. 29a–d). The most common type [Wassel type IV (Fig. 30a)] involves a duplicated proximal and distal phalanx sharing a common metacarpal articulation (Watt and Chung 2009).

Treatment usually involves creation of one good thumb out of the two duplicates, particularly if they are of a fairly even size match, (i.e., amalgamation rather than excision) (Fig. 30b) and therefore plain radiographs are vital for surgical planning.

6.3 Central Polydactyly

This includes duplications that involve the index, middle, or ring fingers and is often accompanied by syndactyly and cleft hand (Graham and Ress 1998; Comer et al. 2018).

6.4 Mirror-Hand and Mirror-Hand Spectrum

Duplication of the ulna, absence of the radius and thumb, and duplication of the ring and small fingers about a common central finger characterize this exceedingly rare deformity. Only six cases of true mirror hand have been described in the literature (Watt and Chung 2009).

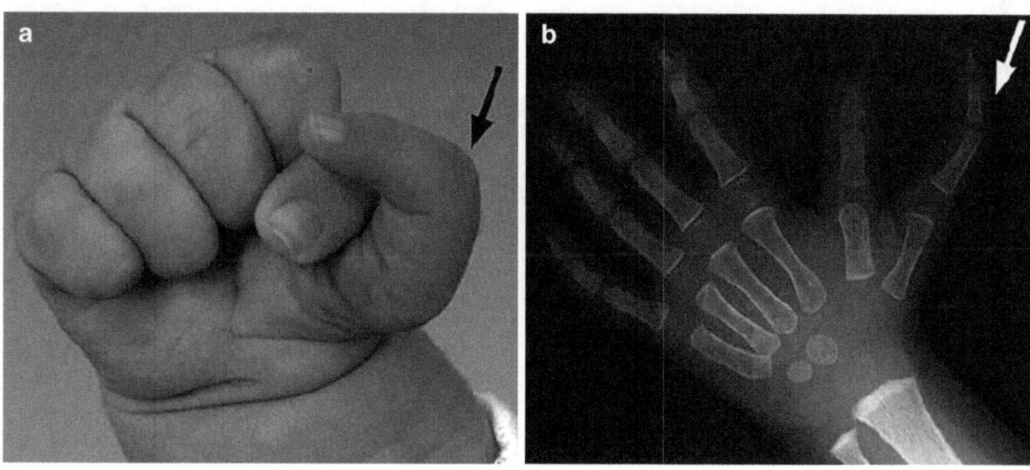

Fig. 28 Clinical photograph (**a**) and radiograph (**b**) of triphalangeal thumb (arrow)

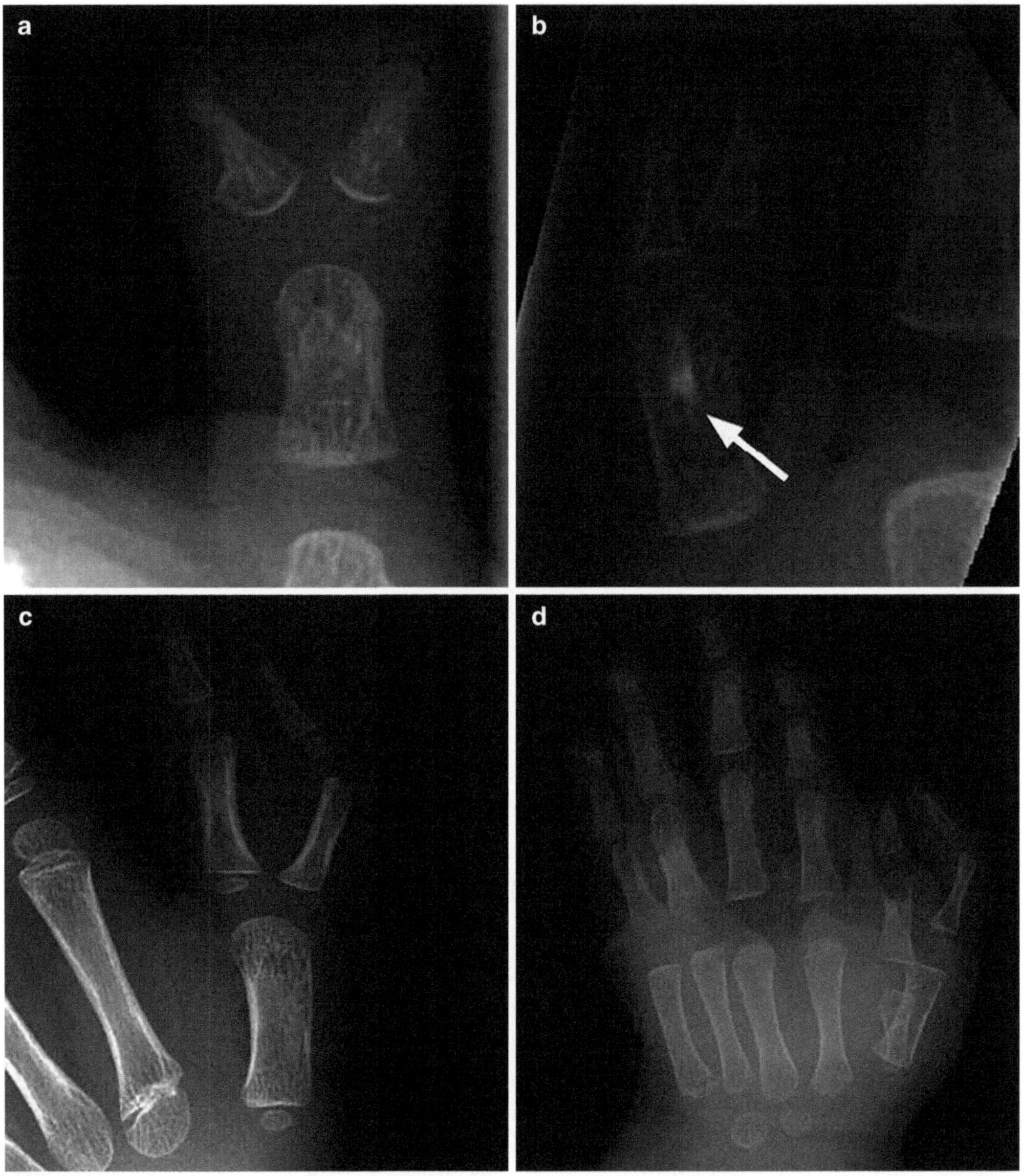

Fig. 29 The Wassel classification divides radial duplication into seven subtypes. (**a**) *Type 2* duplicated distal phalanx. (**b**) *Type 3* bifid proximal phalanx. (**c**) *Type 4* duplicated proximal phalanx. (**d**) *Type 6* duplicated metacarpal. *Type 1* is a bifid distal phalanx, *type 5* is a bifid metacarpal, and any duplication with a triphalangeal element is classified as a Wassel *type 7*

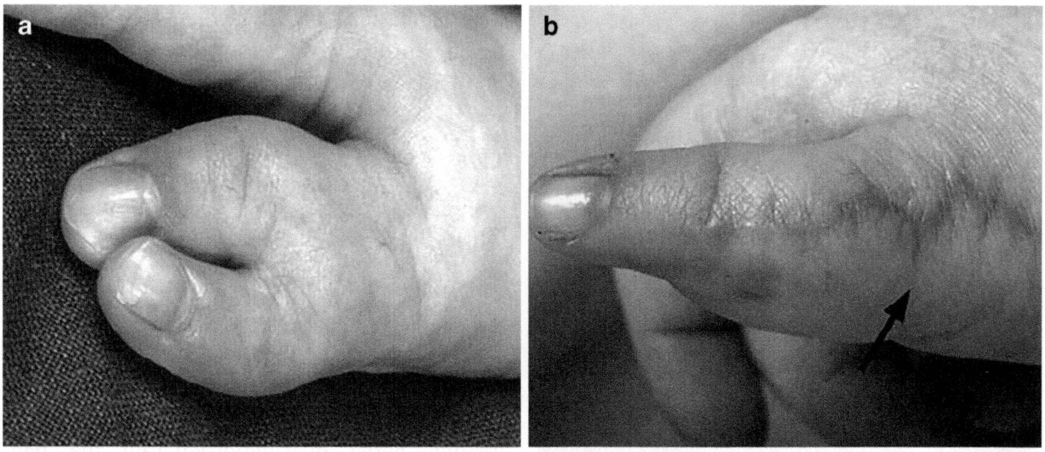

Fig. 30 Wassel 4 duplication at the metacarpophalangeal level is the commonest subtype (50%). (**a**) Well-matched duplicates, which would require skeletal amalgamation. (**b**) Post-amalgamation procedure of Wassel 4 duplication in which the radial duplicate was relatively hypoplastic, but which still requires preservation of soft tissues (*arrow*) from radial duplicate (radial collateral ligament, thenar muscle insertions, and almost all of the skin), and reinsertion into the dominant ulnar duplicate. Only the hypoplastic skeleton, pulp, and nail complex has been discarded

7 Overgrowth Conditions

These account for a small proportion of CHD and the region affected ranges from the entire limb, forearm, hand, or digit. Overgrowth syndromes, which may involve the hand, include nerve territory orientated macrodactyly, lipomatous overgrowth, Proteus syndrome (Fig. 31), hemihypertrophy, Maffucci syndrome, Ollier disease (Fig. 32), Parkes Weber syndrome, Klippel-Trenaunay syndrome, and CLOVE syndrome (capillary malformations (C), lipomatous overgrowth of the trunk or extremities (LO), vascular malformations (V), epidermal nevi (E)), and generalized skeletal abnormalities (Sapp et al. 2007).

In such cases, ultrasound and MRI can be very useful in clarifying the nature and soft tissue origin of the overgrowth (Figs. 33a–c, 34a, b, and 35a, b). The typical MRI features of lipofibroma-

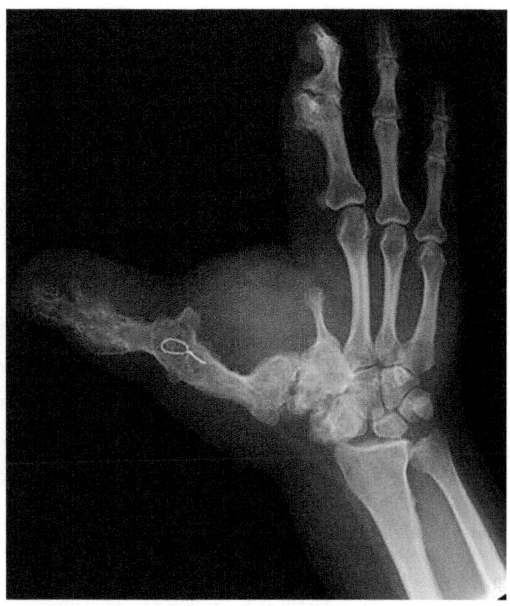

Fig. 31 Proteus syndrome

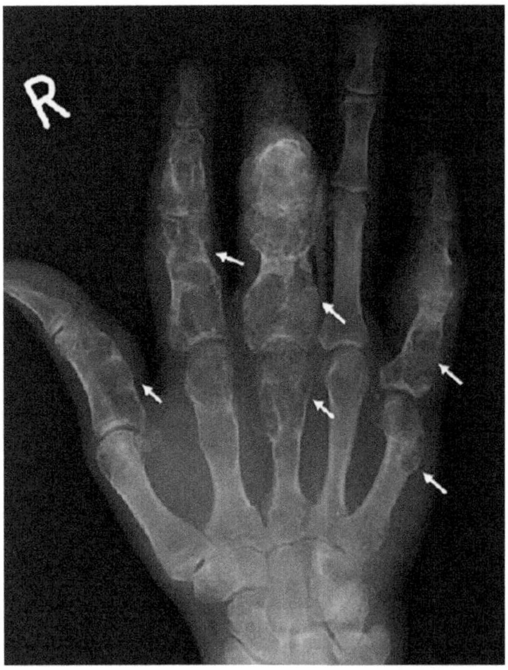

Fig. 32 Ollier's disease—multiple enchondromas (*arrows*)

tous hamartoma of the median nerve are illustrated (Fig. 36a–c).

7.1 Nerve Territory Oriented Macrodactyly and Lipomatous Macrodactyly

This is the most common overgrowth condition presenting to a hand surgeon. It is usually unilateral with a male predominance and no familial inheritance (Carty et al. 2009). The lipomatous overgrowth may correspond with the ulnar or median nerve distribution within the hand (Fig. 37a–d). The affected nerves within the palm are characteristically grossly enlarged and compression neuropathies are common. The intrinsic muscles, joints, periarticular structures, and skeletal parts are enlarged but blood vessels are of normal size. This latter fact is of great importance as the relative ischemia in this condition can lead to difficulties in healing post surgery.

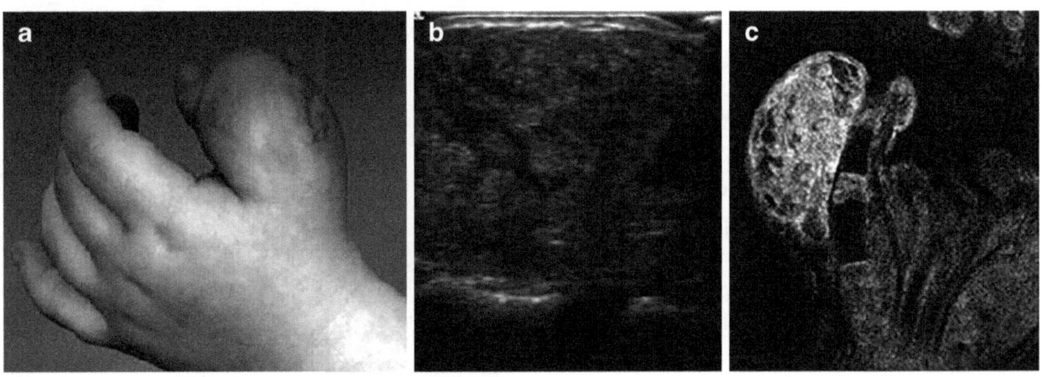

Fig. 33 (**a**) Large soft tissue mass on dorsum of thumb of an 18-month-old boy. Rapid growth raises possibility of malignant change, meriting initial urgent radiological investigation. Plain XR revealed no bony changes or calcification. This proved to be a benign lipoblastoma. (**b**) Ultrasound shows superficial heterogeneous soft tissue mass. (**c**) Coronal T1 fat saturated sequence post contrast shows avid enhancement in the lipoblastoma adjacent to the thumb

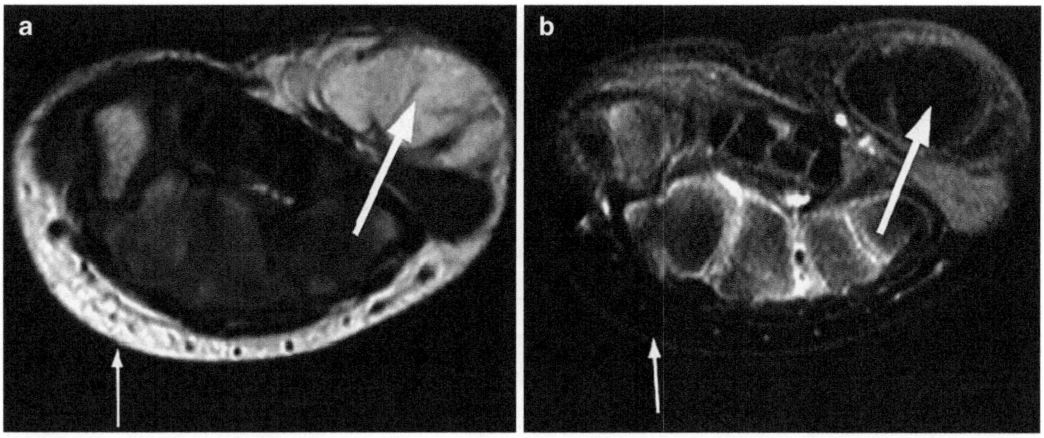

Fig. 34 MR of right hand. (**a**) On the T1 sequence, the mass in the hypothenar eminence (*large arrow*) has the same signal as fat (*small arrow*). (**b**) On the T2 fat saturated sequence, both fat and the mass saturate out, confirming the fatty nature of the mass

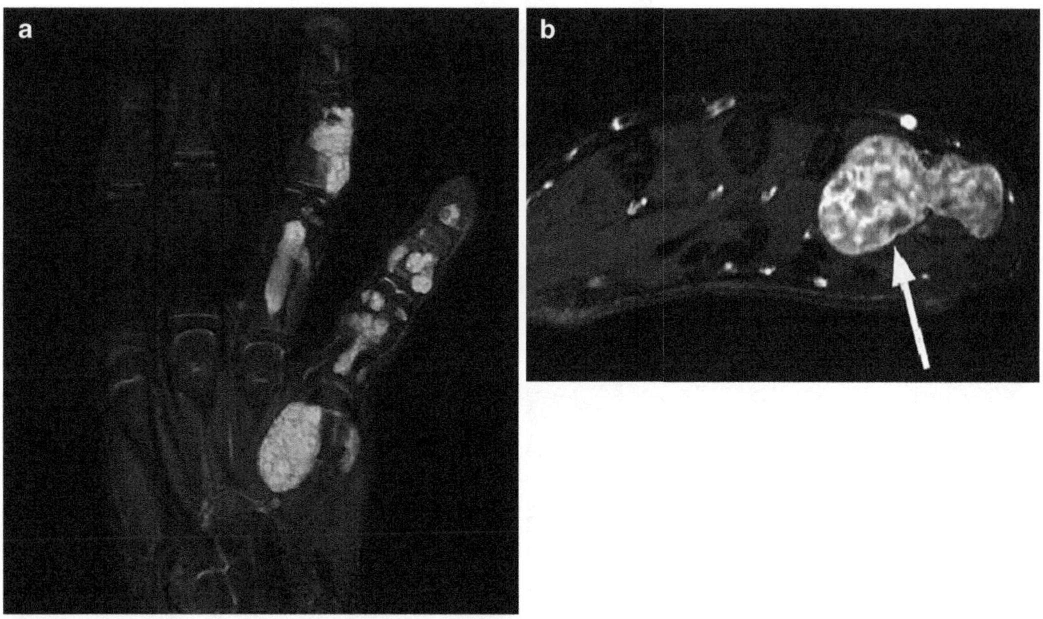

Fig. 35 Ollier's disease MRI. (**a**) T2 fat saturated coronal image shows the distribution of the high signal enchondromata (**b**) T1 fat saturated axial image post contrast shows a typical mottled chondroid type enhancement pattern in one lesion (*arrow*)

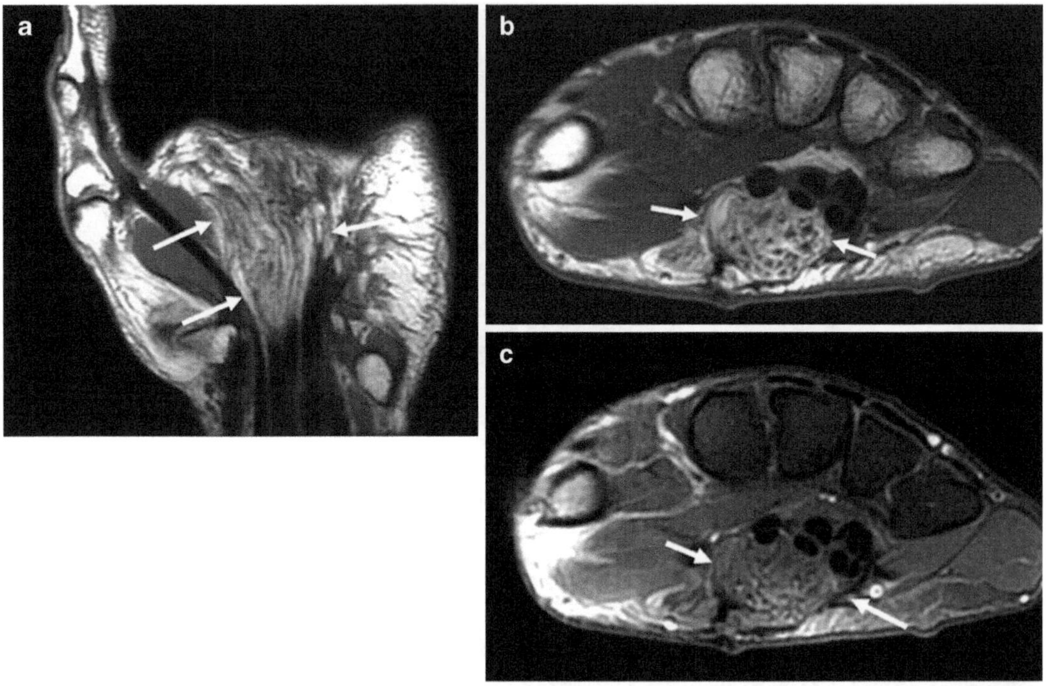

Fig. 36 Lipofibromatous hamartoma of the median nerve. (**a**) Coronal T1 shows high signal mass in the carpal tunnel (*arrows*). (**b**) Axial T1 sequence again shows the mass infiltrating the median nerve (*arrows*). (**c**) Axial STIR image shows suppression of the fat signal within the mass confirming the diagnosis (*arrows*)

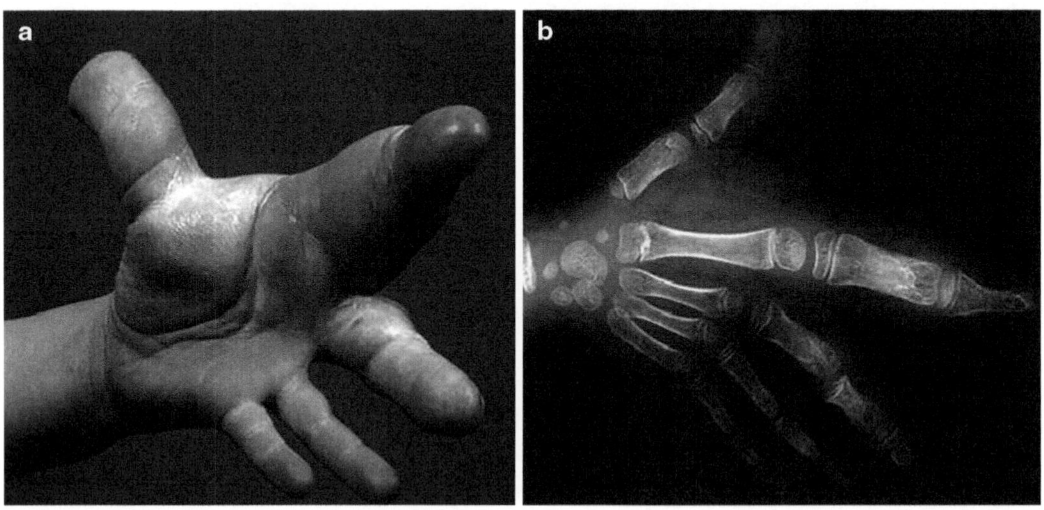

Fig. 37 Nerve-orientated macrodactyly following the median nerve distribution in a child (**a**, **b**) and in an adult (**c**, **d**)

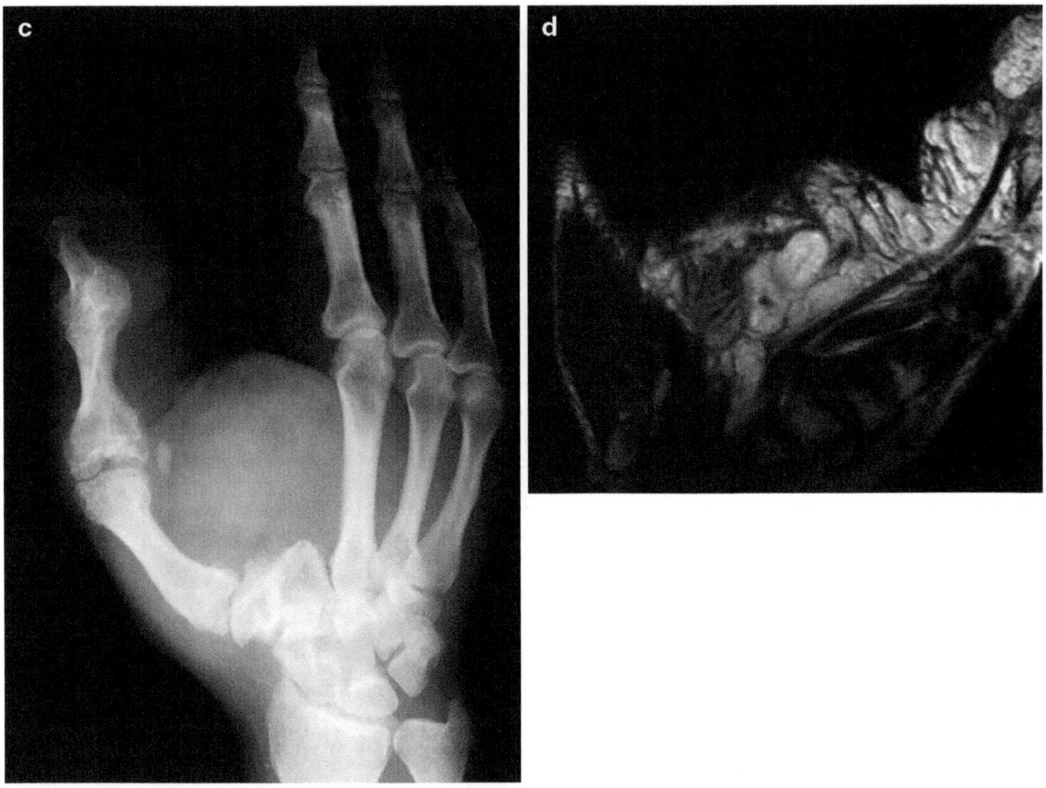

Fig. 37 (continued)

8 Undergrowth Including Hypoplastic Thumb

This results from complete formation of the part during the embryonic period but incomplete growth and development during the fetal period (Van Heest 1996; França 2013).

This group consists largely of the spectrum of hypoplasia of the thumb which can occur as an isolated entity, or more commonly in association with radial deficiencies. It is frequently bilateral and is often found in association with other hand differences, including multiple other short digits, duplicated thumbs, and a number of syndromes (Netscher and Baumholtz 2007).

The classification of thumb hypoplasia by (Blauth 1967) is useful in treatment planning, with less severe types requiring either no surgery or augmentation procedures (such as tendon transfers, ligament reconstruction and web-space deepening), whereas more severe forms (Fig. 38)

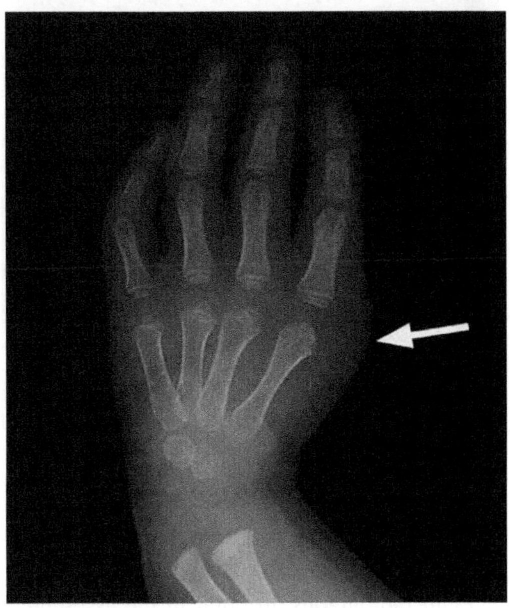

Fig. 38 Total aplasia of the thumb (Blauth grade 5)

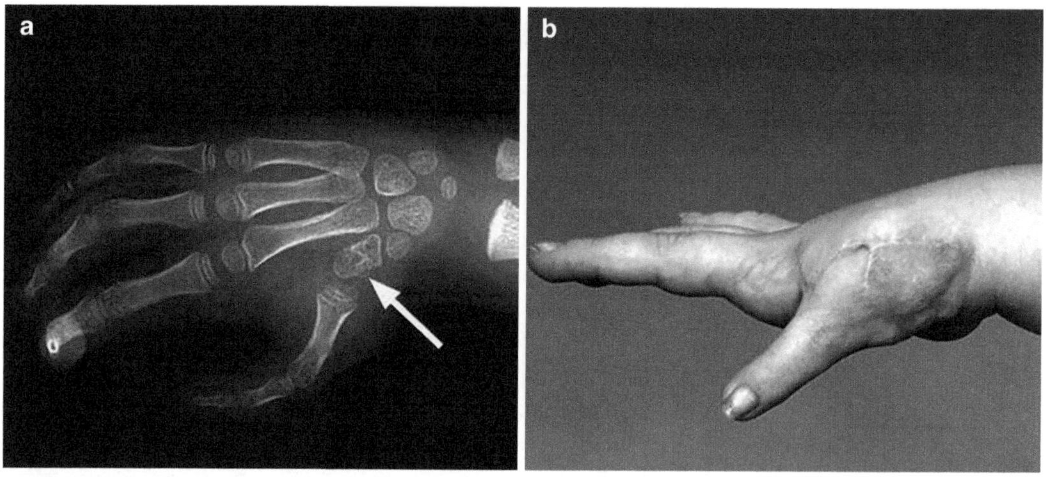

Fig. 39 Pollicization of index finger for patient in Fig. 38 with aplasia of the thumb. (**a**) Neo trapezium(arrow) created by head of index metacarpal. (**b**) Pollicization in such cases greatly upgrades the function of the hand

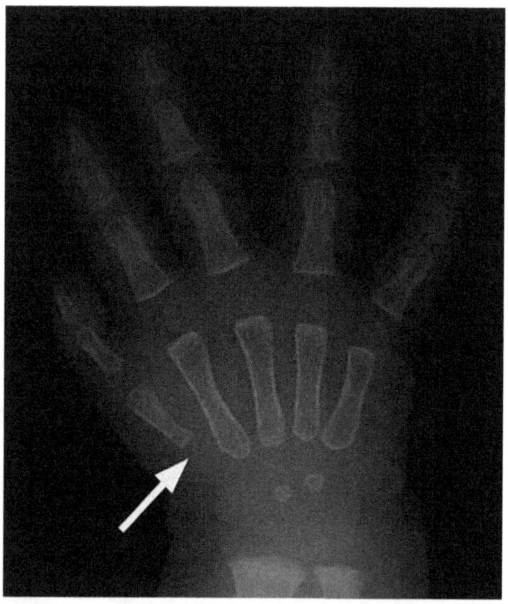

Fig. 40 A poorly developed basal joint in thumb hypoplasia (Blauth grade 3c) makes it very difficult to augment it into a useful thumb, though free metatarsophalangeal joint transfer from the foot has been used

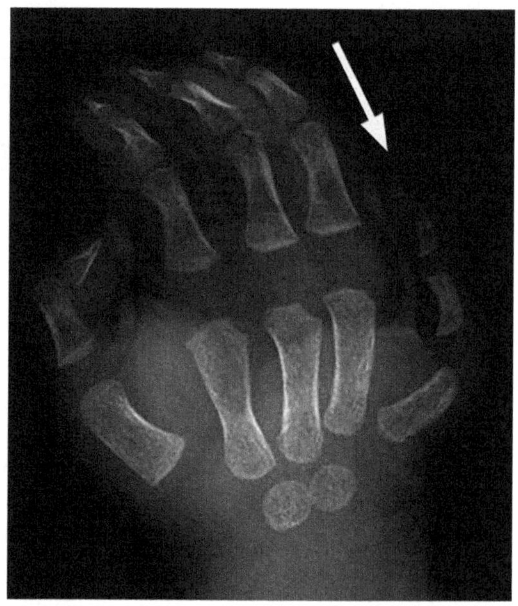

Fig. 41 Little finger hypoplasia. The marked attenuation of the fifth ray makes it difficult to augment, and was therefore treated in this case by ray amputation

require the creation of a new thumb by pollicization of the adjacent index finger (Fig. 39a, b).

Plain radiographs are vital in the assessment of the hypoplastic thumb, as the absence of a well-formed thumb basal joint (Fig. 40) indicates that augmentation procedures would be unlikely to produce a useful thumb and requires a pollicization of the index finger, with removal of the poorly developed original thumb.

Hypoplasia of the fingers most commonly affects the index and little fingers with the middle phalanx being the most commonly affected bone (Fig. 41). This CHD is frequently inherited in an autosomal dominant pattern, and is associated with numerous congenital syndromes including Treacher Collins, Apert, Poland, Cornelia de Lange, and Bloom syndromes (Flatt 1994).

9 Constriction Ring Syndrome

This is a rare condition where the fetus may become entangled in the amniotic membrane although the exact etiology remains controversial. It had been postulated that early amniotic rupture leads to the development of fibrous bands, which entangle the digits and limbs leading to intrauterine amputations and malformations (Torpin 1965; Bernal and Oeltjen 2009). It has also been described as amniotic band syndrome. Prenatal risk factors include prematurity, low birth weight, maternal drug exposure, maternal illness, or trauma during pregnancy (Kawamura and Chung 2009). The reported incidence is 1 in 15,000 live births. There is no sex predilection and 60% have an abnormal antenatal history (Foulkes and Reinker 1994).

The abnormalities are characteristically asymmetric, and the most common findings include distal ring constrictions (Fig. 42a–c), intrauterine amputations (Fig. 43a–d), and acrosyndactyly (distal fusion of digits with a proximal fenestration that communicates the dorsal side with the volar side) (Fig. 44). The fingers may be truncated, a small cleft remains at the site of the web space, and lower limb constriction bands and talipes deformities may be seen (Kozin 2003; Wiedrich 1998; Foulkes and Reinker 1994). These features are not typically present with syndactyly resulting from inheritable and sporadic causes.

Interpretation of plain radiographs can be difficult in the more severe forms, in which the digits can be entwined and fused (Figs. 45a, b and 46a, b).

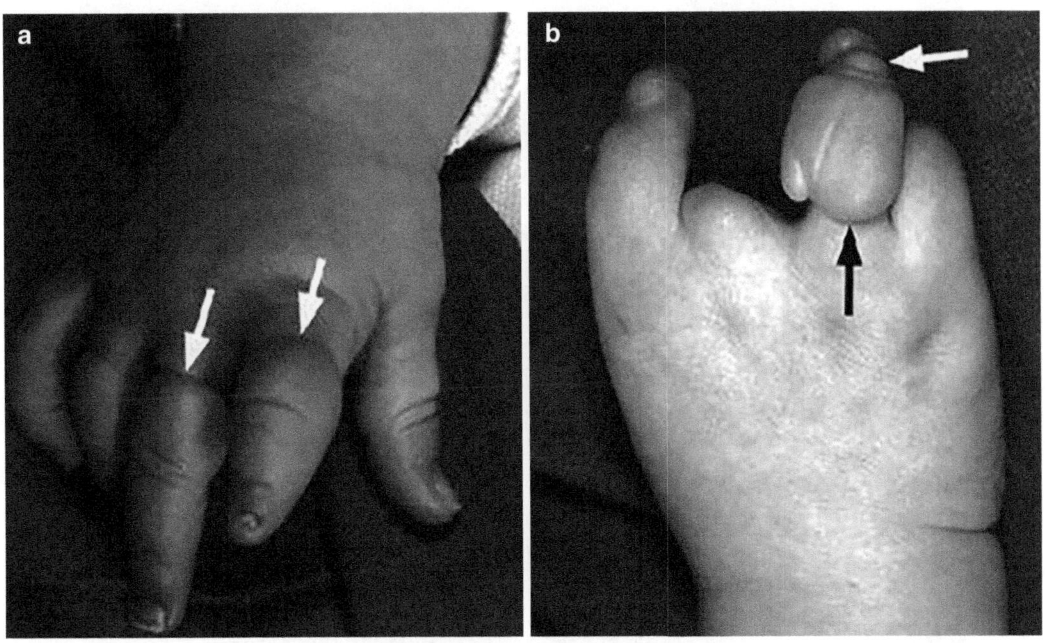

Fig. 42 Ring constriction syndrome. (**a**) Tight constrictions (*arrows*) with distal lymphedema, needs relatively urgent release. (**b**) Marked distal lymphedema, with rings at two levels on the same digit (*arrows*), plus autoamputations. (**c**) XR confirms involvement of all digits to varying degrees

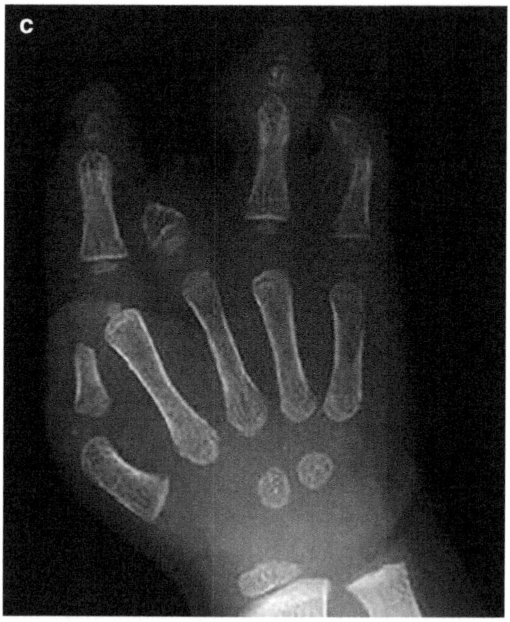

Fig. 42 (continued)

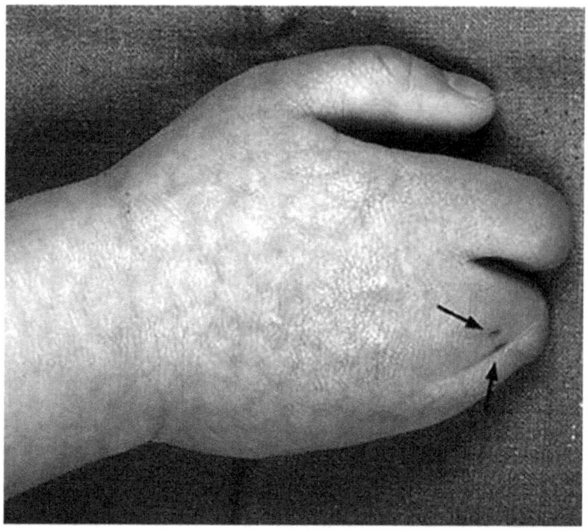

Fig. 44 Ring constriction syndrome with acrosyndactyly, and proximal fenestrations (*arrows*)

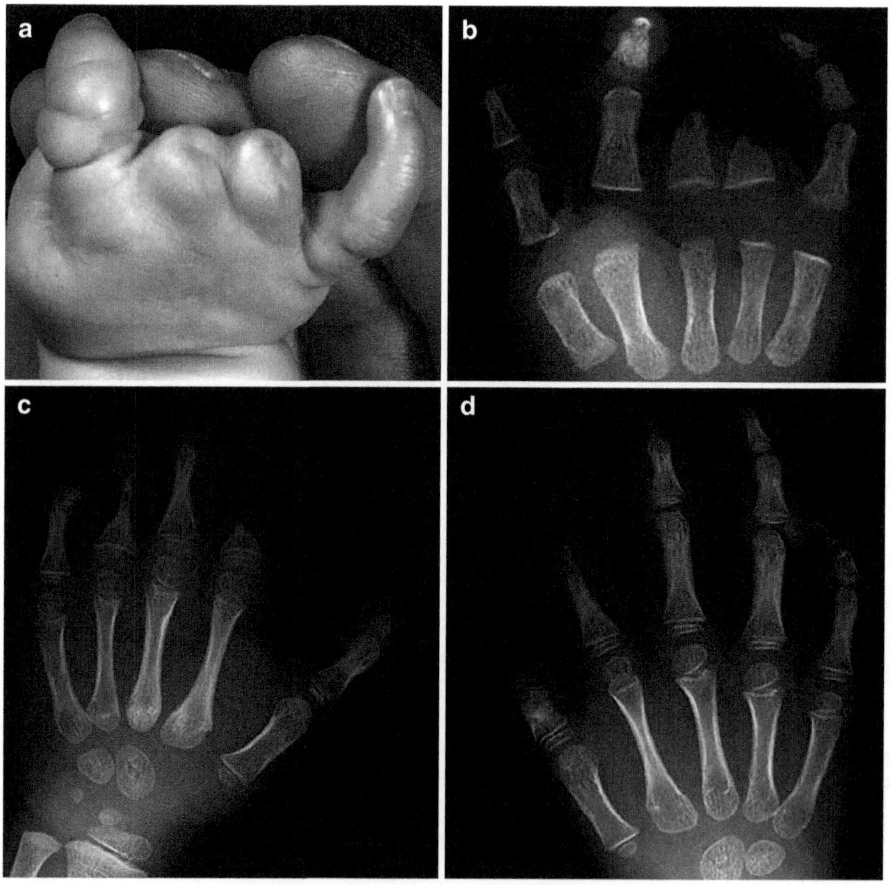

Fig. 43 (**a, b**) Autoamputations. (**c, d**) Bilateral asymmetrical involvement

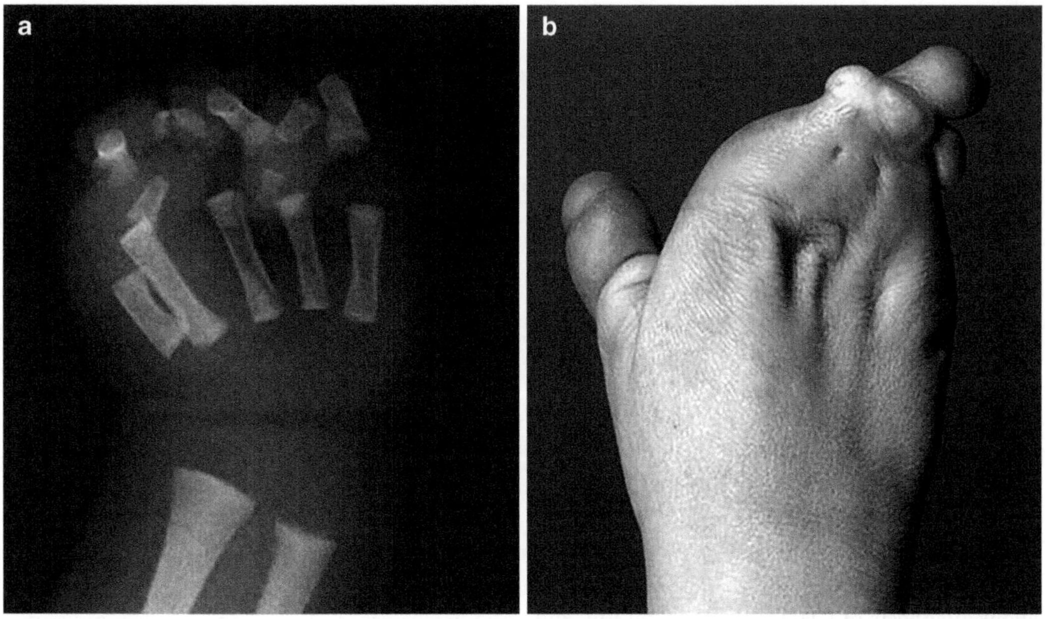

Fig. 45 (**a**, **b**) Ring constriction with complex arrangement of acrosyndactylies, necessitating very early release to prevent intractable bony deformities

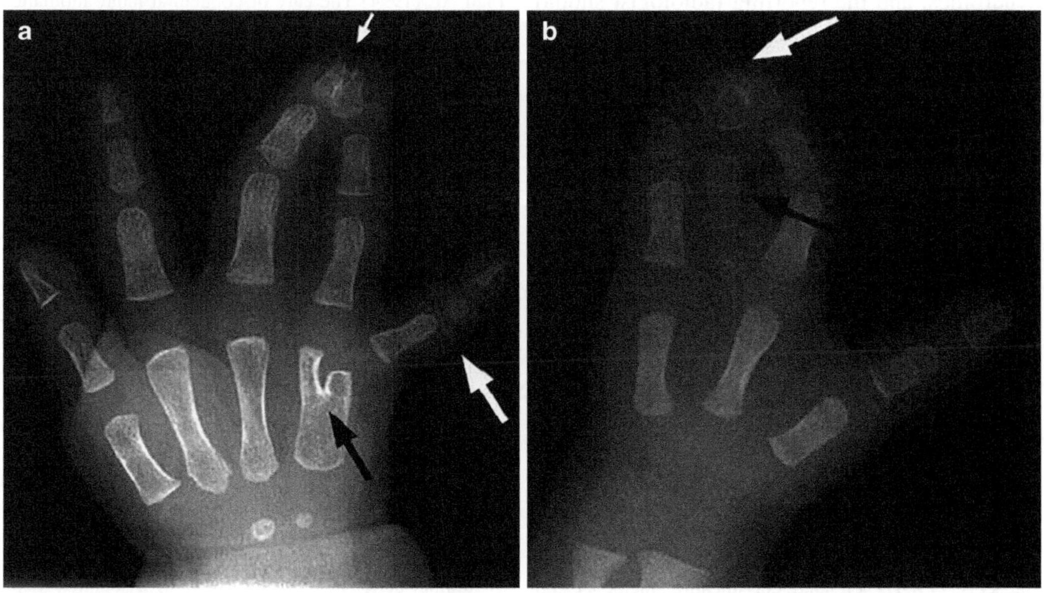

Fig. 46 Difficulties of classification. (**a**) Elements of syndactyly (*small white arrow*), hypoplasia (*large white arrow*), and bony synostosis (*black arrow*) in same hand. (**b**) Central duplication (*black arrow*), failure of formation (missing rays), and complex syndactylies (*white arrow*) in same hand

10 Summary

While the classification of CHD presented is broadly and most commonly used in clinical practice, it has many limitations, not least that some differences could comfortably be placed in several groups (e.g., Fig. 46a, b).

Radiology is vital for the assessment, treatment planning, and follow-up of all but the mildest cases of CHD, with plain films remaining the main imaging modality. Ultrasound and MRI are reserved for specific indications. Ultrasound can be extremely helpful in the assessment of tendons, and in the clarification of the nature of isolated swellings. MRI may provide additional information in selected cases, and is particularly important in the management of more complex overgrowth syndromes. Obstetric ultrasound now allows diagnosis of CHD earlier in fetal life, and advances in this modality will continue to raise the possibility of novel management opportunities and present new dilemmas.

Several CHD are associated with systemic syndromes, and the reporting radiologist should be aware of these to highlight the need for further evaluation.

The management of CHD must be within a multidisciplinary environment with a team able to deal with all of the complex issues presented by this challenging group of patients.

Acknowledgment We would like to acknowledge the contribution of the authors from the first edition.

References

Adu EJ, Annan C (2008) Congenital constriction ring syndrome of the limbs: a prospective study of 16 cases. Afr J Paediatr Surg 5(2):79–83

Banda DN, Yaish AM (2023) Clinodactyly. In: StatPearls [Internet]. StatPearls Publishing

Barsky AJ (1964) Cleft hand: classification, incidence and treatment. Review of the literature and report of nineteen cases. J Bone Joint Surg Am 46:1707–1720

Bayne LG, Klug MS (1987) Long-term review of the surgical treatment of radial deficiencies. J Hand Surg Am 12(2):169–179

Benson LS, Waters PM, Kamil NI, Simmons BP, Upton J III (1994) Camptodactyly: classification and results of nonoperative treatment. J Pediatr Orthop 14(6):814–819

Bernal E, Oeltjen JC (2009) Constriction ring syndrome. J Craniofac Surg 20(4):1018–1020

Blauth W (1967) Der hypoplastische daumen. Archiv für orthopädische und Unfall-Chirurgie, mit besonderer Berücksichtigung der Frakturenlehre und der orthopädisch-chirurgischen Technik 62:225–246

Bubshait DK (2022) A review of polydactyly and its inheritance: connecting the dots. Medicine 101(50):e32060

Carty MJ, Taghinia A, Upton J (2009) Overgrowth conditions: a diagnostic and therapeutic conundrum. Hand Clin 25(2):229–245

Comer GC, Potter M, Ladd AL (2018) Polydactyly of the hand. J Am Acad Orthop Surg 26(3):75–82

De Smet L (2002) Classification for congenital anomalies of the hand: the IFSSH classification and the JSSH modification. Genet Couns 13(3):331–338

Demetri LR, Starcevich AG, Manske MC, James MA (2021) Clinical manifestations of constriction band syndrome. JBJS. 10–2106

Edwards L, Hui L (2018) First and second trimester screening for fetal structural anomalies. Semin Fetal Neonatal Med 23(2):102–111. WB Saunders

Favril A, Vanhoenacker F, Goubau Y, Jager T (2019) Camptodactyly resulting from anatomical variation of lumbrical muscles: imaging findings. Skeletal Radiol 48(12):2009–2014

Flatt AE (1994) The care of congenital hand anomalies. In: The care of congenital hand anomalies. Quality Medical Pub., Inc, St. Louis, pp x–466

Foulkes GD, Reinker K (1994) Congenital constriction band syndrome: a seventy-year experience. J Pediatr Orthop 14(2):242–248

França EN (2013) Congenital deformities of the upper limbs. Part III: overgrowth; undergrowth; Streeter and others. Rev Bras Ortop 48(2):121–125

Frantz CH, O'Rahilly R (1961) Congenital skeletal limb deficiencies. JBJS 43(8):1202–1224

Gandhi M, Rac MW, McKinney J, Society for Maternal-Fetal Medicine (SMFM) (2019) Radial ray malformation. Am J Obstet Gynecol 221(6):B16–B18

Giele H, Giele C, Bower C, Allison M (2001) The incidence and epidemiology of congenital upper limb anomalies: a total population study. J Hand Surg Am 26(4):628–634

Goldfarb CA, Manske PR, Busa R, Mills J, Carter P, Ezaki M (2005) Upper-extremity phocomelia reexamined: a longitudinal dysplasia. JBJS 87(12):2639–2648

Goldfarb CA, Wall L, Manske PR (2006) Radial longitudinal deficiency: the incidence of associated medical and musculoskeletal conditions. J Hand Surg Am 31(7):1176–1182

Graham TJ, Ress AM (1998) Finger polydactyly. Hand Clin 14(1):49–64

Hall JG (1997) Arthrogryposis multiplex congenita: etiology, genetics, classification, diagnostic approach, and general aspects. J Pediatr Orthop B 6(3):159–166

Ireland DC, Takayama N, Flatt AE (1976) Poland's syndrome: a review of forty three cases. J Bone Joint Surg Am 58:52–58
James MA, McCarroll HR Jr, Manske PR (1999) The spectrum of radial longitudinal deficiency: a modified classification. J Hand Surg Am 24(6):1145–1155
James MA, Green HD, McCarroll HR Jr et al (2004) The association of radial deficiency with thumb hypoplasia. J Bone Joint Surg Am 86A(10):2196–2205
Jones GB (1964) Delta phalanx. J Bone Joint Surg Br 46:226–228
Kawamura K, Chung KC (2009) Constriction band syndrome. Hand Clin 25(2):257–264
Klaritsch P (2024) Transverse limb deficiency of the upper extremities. Ultraschall Med-Eur J Ultrasound 45(03):220–231
Kloc J, Dzula B, Varga I, Klein M, Steno B (2023) Camptodactyly: from embryological basis to surgical treatment. Medicina 59(5):966
Koman LA, Toby EB, Poehling GG (1990) Congenital flexion deformities of the proximal interphalangeal joint in children: a subgroup of camptodactyly. J Hand Surg Am 15(4):582–586
Kozin SH (2001) Syndactyly. J Am Soc Surg Hand 1:1–13
Kozin SH (2003) Upper-extremity congenital anomalies. JBJS 85(8):1564–1576
Kozin SH (2004) Pediatric hand surgery. In: Beredjiklian PK, Bozentka DJ (eds) Review of hand surgery. Saunders, Philadelphia, pp 223–245
Lourie GM, Lins RE (1998) Radial longitudinal deficiency. A review and update. Hand Clin 14:85–99
Ploeckinger-Ulm B, Ulm MR, Lee A, Kratochwil A, Bernaschek G (1996) Antenatal depiction of fetal diagnosis with three-dimensional ultrasonography. Am J Obstet Gynaecol 175:571–574
Lachman RS (2007) Taybi and Lachman's radiology of syndromes, metabolic disorders and skeletal dysplasias, 5th edn. Mosby, St Louis
Laub DR (2021) Incidence and prevalence of congenital anomalies of the upper limb. In: Congenital anomalies of the upper extremity: etiology and management. Springer, Cham, pp 37–40
Leung KY (2021) Applications of advanced ultrasound technology in obstetrics. Diagnostics 11(7):1217
McCarroll HR (2000) Congenital anomalies: a 25-year overview. J Hand Surg Am 25(6):1007–1037
Mennen U, Van Heest AN, Ezaki MB, Tonkin M, Gericke G (2005) Arthrogryposis multiplex congenita. J Hand Surg 30(5):468–474
Miller JK, Wenner SM, Kruger LM (1986) Ulnar deficiency. J Hand Surg Am 11(6):822–829
Miura T, Suzuki M (1984) Clinical differences between typical and atypical cleft hand. J Hand Surg 9(3):311–315
Netscher DT, Baumholtz MA (2007) Treatment of congenital upper extremity problems. Plast Reconstr Surg 119(5):101e–129e
Norat F, Dreant N, Lebreton E, Magalon G (2008) Clinodactylies: delta phalanx and Kirner deformity. Chir Main 27:S165–S173
Oberg KC, Feenstra JM, Manske PR, Tonkin MA (2010) Developmental biology and classification of congenital anomalies of the hand and upper extremity. J Hand Surg Am 35(12):2066–2076
Ogino T (1990) Cleft hand. Hand Clin 6(4):661–671
Ogino T (2000) Modified IFSSH classification. J Japan Soc Surg Hand 17:353–365
Ogino T (2021) Central deficiency (cleft hand). In: Congenital anomalies of the upper extremity: etiology and management. Springer, Cham, pp 255–280
Özdemir M, Kavak RP, Karacif O, Selek Y (2019a) Atypical cleft hand with complex syndactyly: an unusual form of hand oligodactyly. Radiol Case Rep 14(11):1407–1409
Özdemir M, Turan A, Kavak RP (2019b) Ulnar hemimelia: a report of four cases. Skeletal Radiol 48:1137–1143
Rypens F, Dubois J, Garel L, Fournet JC, Michaud JL, Grignon A (2006) Obstetric US: watch the fetal hands. Radiographics 26(3):811–829
Sapp JC, Turner JT, van de Kamp JM, van Dijk FS, Lowry RB, Biesecker LG (2007) Newly delineated syndrome of congenital lipomatous overgrowth, vascular malformations, and epidermal nevi (CLOVE syndrome) in seven patients. Am J Med Genet A 143(24):2944–2958
Sells JM, Jaffe KM, Hall JG (1996) Amyoplasia, the most common type of arthrogryposis: the potential for good outcome. Pediatrics 97(2):225–231
Sheldon W (1932) Amyoplasia congenital. Arch Dis Child 7:117–136
Skaria P, Dahl A, Ahmed A (2019) Arthrogryposis multiplex congenita in utero: radiologic and pathologic findings. J Matern Fetal Neonatal Med 32(3):502–511
Smith RJ, Kaplan EB (1968) Camptodactyly and similar atraumatic flexion deformities of the proximal interphalangeal joints of the fingers: a study of thirty-one cases. JBJS 50(6):1187–1249
Sonal M, Sean T (2023) Syndactyly in the pediatric population: a review of the literature. Cureus 15(3):e36118
Stoll C, Alembik Y, Dott B, Roth MP (2010) Associated malformations in patients with limb reduction deficiencies. Eur J Med Genet 53(5):286–290
Swanson AB (1976) A classification for congenital limb malformations. J Hand Surg Am 1(1):8–22
Swanson AB, Swanson GD, Tada K (1983) A classification for congenital limb malformation. J Hand Surg Am 8(5):693–702
Torpin R (1965) Amniochorionic mesoblastic fibrous strings and amnionic bands: associated constricting fetal malformations or fetal death. Am J Obstet Gynecol 91(1):65–75
Ty JM, James MA (2009) Failure of differentiation: part II (arthrogryposis, camptodactyly, clinodactyly, madelung deformity, trigger finger, and trigger thumb). Hand Clin 25(2):195–213
Van Heest AE (1996) Congenital disorders of the hand and upper extremity. Paediatr Clin North Am 43(5):1113–1133

Watson BT, Hennrikus WL (1997) Postaxial type-B polydactyly. Prevalence and treatment. J Bone Joint Surg Am 79(1):65–68

Watt AJ, Chung KC (2009) Duplication. Hand Clin 25(2):215–227

Wiedrich TA (1998) Congenital constriction band syndrome. Hand Clin 14(1):29–38

Winfeld MJ, Otero H (2016) Radiographic assessment of congenital malformations of the upper extremity. Pediatr Radiol 46:1454

Hand Trauma

Anand Kirwadi, Siddharth Thaker, Nikhil A. Kotnis, and Andrew Dunn

Contents

A. Kirwadi (✉)
Department of Radiology, Manchester Royal Infirmary, Manchester, UK
e-mail: anand.kirwadi@nhs.net

S. Thaker
Department of Radiology, Leicester Royal Infirmary, Leicester, UK

N. A. Kotnis
Department of Radiology, Northern General Hospital, Sheffield Teaching Hospitals NHS Foundation Trust, Sheffield, UK

A. Dunn
The OrthTeam Centre, Didsbury, Manchester, UK

Med Radiol Diagn Imaging (2025)
https://doi.org/10.1007/174_2025_620,
Published Online: 18 October 2025

Abstract

Hand injuries account for a large proportion of all injuries presenting to emergency departments. Avulsion injuries of the FDP tendons are a common sporting injury. Bowstringing of the flexor tendons is an important imaging sign of multiple annular pulley injuries. Mallet finger is the most common closed tendon injury in a sportsman. Rupture of the volar plate is a common complication of hyperextension injury. Imaging plays a crucial role in the management of collateral ligament injuries. The extensor mechanism of the fingers is extremely intricate. Understanding relevant anatomy is quintessential for diagnosing and treating extensor mechanism injuries. Intra-articular metacarpal base fractures are commonly missed on initial presentation, and pronated oblique radiographs help demonstrate the severity of this injury. Imaging evaluation of sports-related injuries of the hand should begin with radiographs. Ultrasound and magnetic resonance imaging play a vital role in diagnoses of soft tissue injuries. CT may be useful in understanding complex bony injuries.

1 Introduction

Traumatic hand injuries account for a large proportion of the workload of all emergency departments. Of a study of 50,272 patients, Angermann and Lohmann found that hand and wrist injuries made up 28.6% of all injuries (Angermann and Lohmann 1993). Of these, 87% involved the hand. Hill et al. found that the majority of isolated cases of hand and wrist injuries arise from either a fall or sports-related injury (Hill et al. 1998).

In this chapter, we describe the most common traumatic soft tissue and bone injuries to the hand. We pay attention to the anatomy and mechanism of injury as this is fundamental to understanding and recognising patterns of injury on imaging. We also briefly mention some of the key management options that are important to be aware of whilst assessing the imaging of these injuries.

2 Volar Soft Tissue Injuries

2.1 Flexor Tendons

First described by Von Zander in 1891, avulsion injuries of the flexor tendon are common injuries in athletes. However, flexor tendon injuries are not as common as injuries to the extensor apparatus (Clavero et al. 2002).

The flexor mechanism of the digits comprises two tendons: the flexor digitorum superficialis (FDS) that inserts on the midportion of the middle phalanx and the flexor digitorum profundus (FDP) that inserts on the volar aspect of the base of the distal phalanx. At the metacarpal head, the FDS splits and passes round the FDP tendon forming a ring aperture through which the FDP passes to become the more superficial tendon at the level of the proximal phalanx shaft (Clavero et al. 2002). These tendons run underneath the annular (A1–A5) and cruciform (C1–C3) pulleys lined by a synovial sheath that provides lubrication and nutrition. The vincula, which also provide blood supply to the tendons, connect the tendon to the synovial sheath (Hunter 1984).

Based on the mechanism of injury, these can be classified as open or closed injuries. For further discussion, we will concentrate on closed injuries. Open injuries are common due to lacerations. Closed injuries commonly occur when the finger is forcibly extended during maximum contraction of the profundus muscle—when a player is attempting to make a tackle and the ring finger slips off of the opposing player's shorts or jersey, hence the name "Jersey finger" (Aronowitz and Leddy 1998). Although it can occur in any finger, the ring finger is the most commonly involved finger accounting for 75% cases (Hong 2005). McMaster in 1933 showed that the tendon was the strongest link in the musculotendinous chain and that rupture most commonly occurs at the bony insertion (McMaster 1933). When the tendon ruptures from its insertion, it may or may not avulse a bone fragment of variable size. Rarely, the closed traumatic rupture of the FDP tendon can happen along its origin at the lumbricals (Germann and Stanley 2024).

Table 1 Leddy and Packer classification of closed FDP injuries (Leddy and Packer 1977)

Type I	Retraction of the tendon into the palm with disruption of the vincular system resulting in loss of blood supply to the tendon
Type II	Most common type. Tendon retracts to the level of PIP joint, being held by the intact long vinculum preserving some blood supply
Type III	Large bony fragment that gets held in place by the A4 pulley
Type IV (Buscemi and Page 1987)	Tendon rupture with attached bony fragment and concomitant separate intra-articular fracture fragment

The most reliable finding is a complete loss of active flexion at the Distal Interphalangeal (DIP) joint (Buscemi and Page 1987). Because pain and swelling often mask the inability to flex the DIP joint (DIPJ), it is not uncommon for this injury to be missed initially and go untreated (Aronowitz and Leddy 1998).

Treatment and prognosis are influenced by several of the following factors: the level to which the tendon retracts, the remaining blood supply to the tendon, the length of time between injury and treatment, and the presence and size of a bony avulsion fragment (Aronowitz and Leddy 1998). Based on the level of retraction and presence of bony fragment, Leddy and Packer have classified this injury into three main types (Table 1).

Buscemi et al., after describing four cases of FDP tendon injuries, have suggested that avulsion of the FDP tendon with a separate intra-articular fracture of the base of the distal phalanx should be classified as a Type IV injury in the Leddy and Packer classification (Buscemi and Page 1987).

Radiographs may show an avulsed bone fragment from the distal phalanx. Severe comminution of the distal phalanx precludes accurate restoration of the articular surface and is important to note as it is a contra-indication to early FDP re-insertion (Jebson 1998).

At ultrasound, normal tendons are echogenic in the hand and wrist compared to muscle. They also show a typical fibrillar echotexture, which reflects their histological structure of longitudinally oriented bundles of collagen fibres

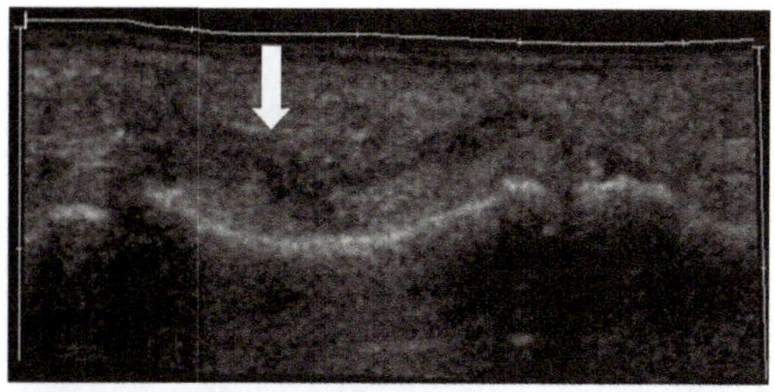

Fig. 1 Ultrasound of the finger using a linear probe in longitudinal plane showing empty FDP tendon sheath (*arrow*). DIPJ and PIPJ are on the *left* and *right* side of the image, respectively

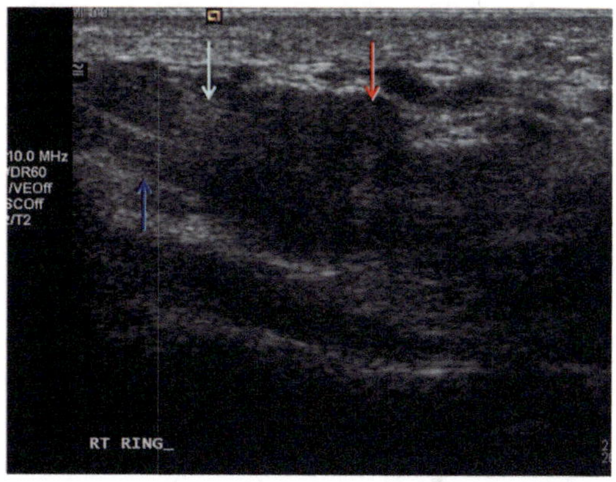

Fig. 2 Ultrasound of the ring finger using (different patient to Fig. 1) a high-frequency linear probe showing FDS rupture (*Red arrow*—at torn end), FDS (*Green arrow*) lying superficial to the FDS (*Blue arrow*)

(Jeyapalan et al. 2008). In cases of tendon rupture, discontinuity with a gap in the flexor tendon may be seen. The gap may be filled with disorganised, echogenic fibrinous material (Jeyapalan et al. 2008). In the presence of tendon rupture, discontinuity of the flexor tendon is seen with the gap at the rupture site (Figs. 1 and 2). In some patients, the tendon remains in continuity but is attenuated with subtle loss of fibrillar pattern due to partial division. These tendons may show less excursion than tendons in the neighbouring fingers on dynamic ultrasound assessment (Jeyapalan et al. 2008).

On all magnetic resonance (MR) sequences, the flexor tendons appear as low-signal-intensity structures. In general, T1-W images provide good anatomical detail, while T2-W images are useful in assessment of inflammatory change that

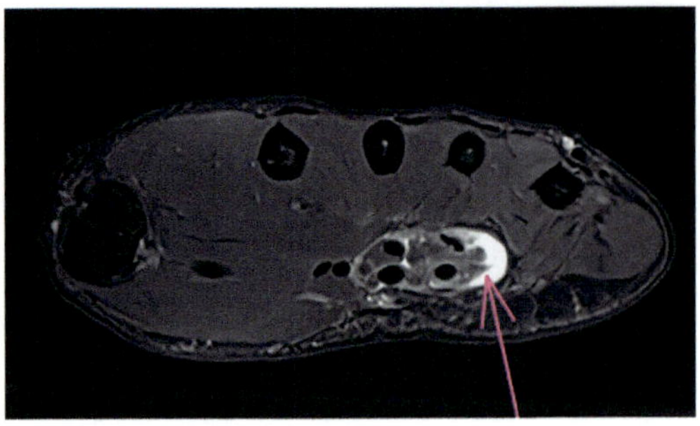

Fig. 3 Axial MR PDFS image showing complete full thickness tear of the little finger FDS and FDP tendons with fluid filling the tendon sheath (pin arrow)

is associated with most pathological conditions (Clavero et al. 2002). Magnetic resonance imaging provides a non-invasive method to identify the site of tear, the degree of retraction of the torn fibres and other associated soft tissue injuries (Peterson and Bancroft 2006). In the presence of trauma, the associated oedema, haematoma and fibrosis compromise the tendon image quality and a tendon rupture is unlikely to be identified (Beltran et al. 1987). On MR imaging, the degree of proximal retraction, fluid within the tendon sheath and surrounding soft tissue injury can be assessed (Fig. 3).

Based on the current literature review, there is a general consensus that prompt reinsertion of an acute FDP avulsion injury is the preferred choice of treatment. In chronic injuries, the patient may be asymptomatic as they adapt by passively assisting DIPJ flexion and do not require any further treatment (Aronowitz and Leddy 1998; Jebson 1998). If there is instability of the DIPJ with weakness of pinch or recurrent dorsal dislocations, joint arthrodesis or tenodesis should be considered (Aronowitz and Leddy 1998).

2.2 Annular Pulleys

Normal finger flexion is a complex fine motor action that requires the integrity and orchestration of a number of delicate structures that are centred around the flexor tendon system (Hauger et al. 2000). The flexor tendon sheath pulley system is of paramount biomechanical importance in flexion, not only for accurate tracking of the tendon but also to maintain the apposition of tendon and bone across the joint and provide a fulcrum to elicit flexion and extension (Lin et al. 1989). Doyle and Blythe in 1975 originally defined a pulley system of four annular and three cruciate pulleys. In 1981, Kleinhert and Broudy defined an additional fifth pulley arising distal to the fourth annular pulley.

In recent years, the number of people involved in climbing sports has increased exponentially as a result of easy and readily available access to artificial rock-climbing walls and indoor rock climbing facilities. The annular pulley injuries are caused by climbing techniques where the entire body weight is placed on one or two fingerholds, especially in overhung wall climbs. These techniques place high forces on the proximal interphalangeal (PIP) joint and the digital pulley system, resulting in finger injuries known as climber's finger (Klauser et al. 1999). The ring and middle fingers are most commonly affected, as they are most often used in climbing and are diagnosed in up to 30% of climbers with finger injuries (Le Viet et al. 1996). Injury to the pulley system can result in loss of strength and decreased range of motion within the affected finger, bowstringing of the FDP tendon and fixed flexion contracture of the PIP joint (PIPJ). Pain and soft tissue swelling can make clinical evaluation a difficult and limited exercise. Many studies have claimed that bowstringing of the FDP tendon across the PIPJ with resisted flexion of the fingertips is diagnostic of A2 pulley rupture. However, in a laboratory study of 21 cadaveric fingers by Marco et al. (1998), isolated or even combined rupture of A2 and A4 pulley did not result in detectable bowstringing. Rupture of at least three pulleys was required to produce obvious bowstringing in this study. Early recognition of the injury and appropriate treatment are important in avoiding complications like fixed flexion contractures (Bollen 1990).

The A2 and A4 annular pulleys, located at the proximal third of the proximal phalanx and middle phalanges, respectively, are the broader and the most functionally important annular pulleys (Lin et al. 1989). Experimental studies performed by Marco et al. (1998) showed that the A4 pulley is predisposed to rupture first when the hand is in the crimp grip. The A2 pulley usually fails from its distal to its proximal edge, whereas the A4 pulley tears from its proximal to its distal edge (Marco et al. 1998). It is important to accurately differentiate the complete from incomplete tears, as decision for operative versus non-operative management depends on this vital finding.

Various studies have been published advocating the use of ultrasound (Klauser et al. 1999, 2002; Martinoli et al. 2000; Hauger et al. 2000; Fontes et al. 2024), computed topography (CT) (Le Viet et al. 1996) and MR (Hauger et al. 2000; Klauser et al. 2002). An inability to directly delineate the pulleys along with the exposure to ionising radiation and relatively higher cost in comparison to ultrasound makes CT an unsuitable modality for diagnosing pulley injuries.

The magnetic resonance imaging (MRI) criteria for identifying pulley injuries include direct signs such as disrupted A2 and A4 pulleys (Hauger et al. 2000) or indirect signs like bowstringing (appreciated as increased tendon–phalangeal (TP) distance) or fluid in between the phalanx and tendon (Gabl et al. 1998). The MR has been the most accurate modality for imaging in the diagnosis of A4 lesions (Hauger et al. 2000). However, the expense, length of the examination and lack of real-time assessment are some of the drawbacks of MR examination. Along with annual pulley tears, increased TP distance, excess fluid in the tendon sheath and changes in the surrounding soft tissues can be assessed accurately on MR imaging (Fig. 4a, b).

Dynamic assessment gives ultrasound an advantage in the evaluation of pulley injuries. Ultrasound can demonstrate visualisation of fluid between the tendon and phalanx and allows assessment of the gliding ability of the tendons. Ultrasound demonstrated a sensitivity of 98%, specificity of 100%, a positive predictive value of 100% and a negative predictive value of 97% for the detection of finger pulley injuries (Klauser et al. 2002). Martinoli et al. (2000) demonstrated that examination in the longitudinal plane alone was sufficient as transverse sonograms added no significant information. Hauger et al. (2000) have suggested using TP distance measurements following a study performed using a cadaveric model (see Fig. 5a–c). A TP distance of greater than 1.0 mm was indicative of pulley system injury. An increase of the TP distance with forced flexion less than 3.0 mm was considered a sign of incomplete A2 pulley rupture, while a distance greater than 3.0 mm was considered a sign of complete rupture. Further increase in the TP distance to more than 5.0 mm was used as a sign for complete combined rupture of A2 and A3 pulley. An increase of TP distance equal to or greater than 2.5 mm was used as a sign for complete rupture of A4 pulley. Maximal active forced flexion during dynamic ultrasound examination is the most important factor for assessment of TP distance and detection of finger pulley injuries (Klauser et al. 2002).

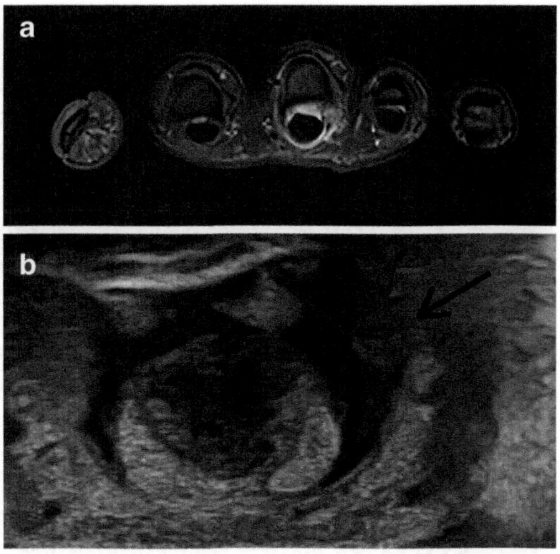

Fig. 4 (**a**) Axial PDFS image showing high-grade partial thickness tear of the A2 pulley of the middle finger with increased TP distance, small trace of fluid and surrounding soft tissue oedema. (**b**) Corresponding magnified US image showing the same A″ tear along the ulnar aspect

Indications for non-operative or operative treatment are based on the clinical finding of bowstringing, functional disability, persistent pain, failure of non-operative treatment and on the amount of bowstringing of the involved flexor tendons (Gabl et al. 1998). Incomplete tears are normally treated conservatively, while complete tears are treated surgically. The treatment of complete tears with surgery has been controversial. In

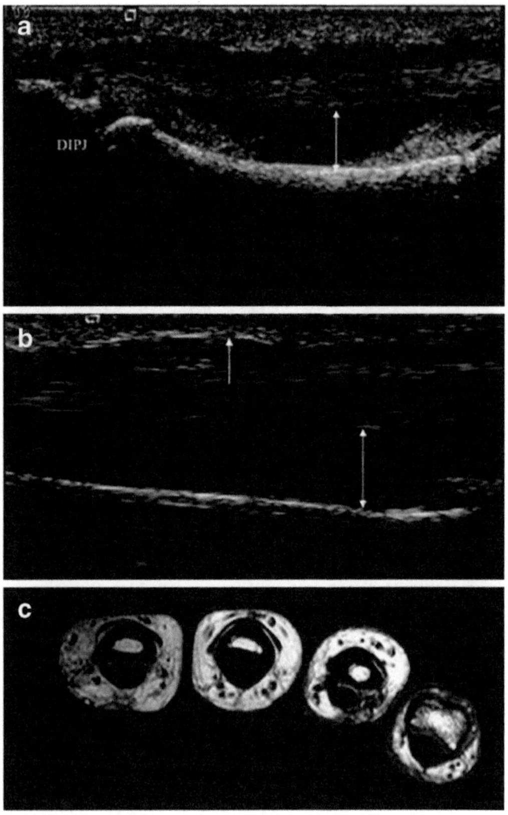

Fig. 5 (**a**, **b**) Both images taken in the same patient show increased tendo-phalangeal distance (*double arrow heads*) over the middle and proximal phalanges, respectively, indicating rupture of the A2 and A4 pulleys. *Arrow* in **b** shows the ruptured A2 pulley. (**c**) Axial MR image shows increased tendo-phalangeal distance (*double arrow heads*) due to chronic rupture of the A2 pulley

a study conducted by Gabl et al. (1998), complete ruptures were treated with surgery after non-operative treatment had failed. In the same study, functional outcome after non-operative and operative therapy was equal. Diagnosis and treatment at an early stage will prevent the progression of lesions and decrease the risk of long-term complications that are associated with fixed finger contracture (Hauger et al. 2000).

2.3 Volar Plate

Volar plate (VP) injury results as a consequence of hyperextension injury to the PIPJ. There may or may not be an associated intra-articular fracture

Table 2 Eaton classification of VP injuries (Eaton 1971)

Type 1	No fracture or dislocation
Type 2	Dorsal dislocation without fracture
Type 3 stable	Fracture–dislocation with <40% PIP joint surface
Type 3 unstable	Fracture–dislocation with >40% PIP joint surface

(Yoong et al. 2010). Even when present, the fracture can be easily overlooked resulting in significant instability of the PIPJ (Nance Jr et al. 1979).

The VP is a multi-layered condensation of dense fibrocartilaginous tissue that lies between the flexor tendons and the PIPJ capsule. The VP attaches firmly only at the critical corner of the middle phalanx base, without strong insertion centrally. Proximally, the VP blends directly with the periosteum rather than direct insertion into the bone (Williams et al. 1998). Its important functions at the PIPJ level include providing stability against hyperextension, acting as a meniscus at the PIPJ, forming part of the intracavitary lining of the PIPJ and providing a smooth gliding surface for the flexor tendon (Williams et al. 1998).

The most common mechanism of injury is forced or sudden hyperextension at the PIPJ (Phair et al. 1989). The diagnosis of VP injury is usually made clinically, with tenderness over the volar aspect of the PIPJ, pain on passive hyperextension and instability with loss of pinch power (Nance Jr et al. 1979). The commonly used classifications are shown in Tables 2 and 3 below.

Along with AP and lateral views of the involved PIPJ, oblique views can also be helpful. In a study of 58 cases conducted by Nance Jr. et al., 65% of the fractures were best seen on the lateral view, while most of the others were best appreciated on the oblique projection (Nance Jr et al. 1979). Subtle dorsal subluxation can be identified by observing a V-shaped gap between the articular surfaces of the PIP joint—'V' sign. On ultrasound examination, the VP is seen as a wedge-shaped structure of intermediate echogenicity interposed between the flexor tendon and underlying PIPJ (Yoong et al. 2010). The complex three-layered collagen fibres running in different orientations (Williams et al. 1998) probably account for its mixed echogenic appearance

Table 3 Stability-based classification (Keifhaber and Stern 1998)

Stable	<30% articular surface
Tenuous	30–50% articular surface
Unstable	>50% articular surface

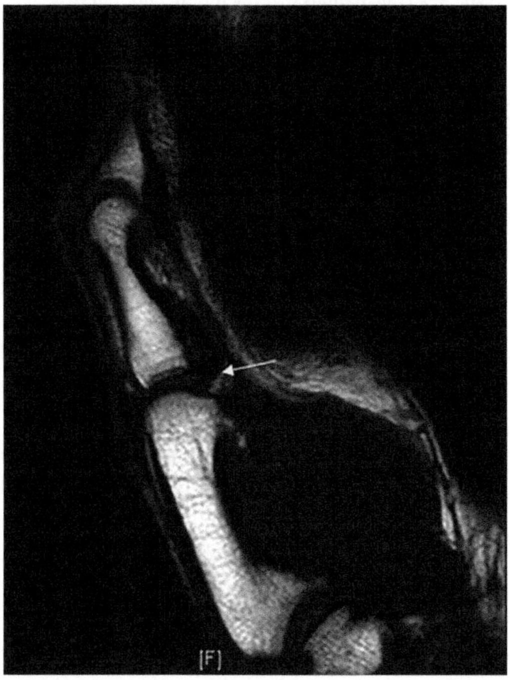

Fig. 6 Sagittal T1 W MR image of the thumb showing chronic type 1 volar plate injury (*White arrow*)

on ultrasound. The VP is best seen in the sagittal plane and is of low signal on all MRI sequences (Fig. 6) (Yoong et al. 2010). To the best of our knowledge, there are currently no studies comparing the efficacy of ultrasound or MRI for diagnosing VP injuries. More recently dynamic evaluation of the interphalangeal joint volar plate motion has been attempted to understand the complex interaction of the VP with PIP joint and aiding in evaluation of the VP (Lutter et al. 2023).

There is a consensus that the stable injuries involving less than 30% of articular surface are treated conservatively either by splinting with extension-block or neighbour strapping. Various studies (Phair et al. 1989; Gaine et al. 1998) have shown favourable results with early active and passive mobilisation rather than splinting. Unstable injuries involving >50% of articular surface are treated surgically with open reduction and internal fixation using various techniques or palmar plate arthroplasty, with later being preferred (Keifhaber and Stern 1998). The tenuous fractures involving 30–50% of articular surface can be treated conservatively, if the articular surface congruity can be maintained with 30° flexion; if not they are best managed operatively (Keifhaber and Stern 1998).

3 Extensor Mechanism Injuries

3.1 Anatomy

The anatomy and function of the extensor mechanism of the hand comprise of a complex set of interlinked muscles, tendons and ligaments that are intricately coordinated to bring about the fine movements of the digits. The extensor mechanism of the hand can be divided into eight zones to aide in the evaluation and treatment of acute injuries (Kleinhert and Verdan 1983). The even-numbered zones are over bones, with the odd-numbered zones over the joints. Owing to the lesser number of the phalanges in the thumb, the numbering system is slightly different.

The extrinsic and intrinsic muscles of the hand make up the extensor mechanism. Zone VIII, containing the musculotendinous junctions of the extrinsic muscles, is the most proximal zone. In zone VII, the extensor tendons are contained within the extensor retinaculum over the wrist joint. In zone VI, the tendons of the middle, ring and little finger are connected by juncturae tendinum. These interconnections must be considered when evaluating extensor tendon injuries (Newport 1997). In zone V, the extensor tendons are located centrally and are stabilised over the dorsum of the metacarpal head by the extensor hood. The sagittal bands (SB) are the main components of the extensor hood, which starts at the VP and has a dorsal tendinous point of insertion, gliding with the extensor system as the digit moves (Clavero et al. 2002). Distal to metacarpophalangeal (MCP) joint, the extensor mechanism becomes more complicated as the extrinsic and intrinsic muscles blend into the dorsal apparatus.

The extrinsic extensor tendons divide into central and lateral slips with the central slip inserting into the dorsal aspect of the base of middle phalanx. The intrinsic muscles contribute to form the lateral slips to form conjoint tendons, which converge distally to form the terminal tendon that inserts on the base of the distal phalanx (Kleinhert and Verdan 1983). The intrinsic tendons are directed volar to the axis of MCP joint (MCPJ), flexing this joint and directing dorsal to the axis of PIPJ and DIPJs, extending these joints (Newport 1997).

On MR images, the normal extensor apparatus appears as low-signal structures at the expected locations, axial and sagittal planes being most useful (Clavero et al. 2002).

3.2 Mallet Injury (Zone 1)

Disruption of the terminal extensor tendon at the DIPJ, caused by sudden forced flexion of the extended finger, results in extension lag deformity at the DIPJ called mallet finger. Other terms like 'baseball finger' and 'drop finger' have been used to describe this. This terminal extensor tendon can rupture at or near its insertion into the distal phalanx (soft tissue mallet injury) or can avulse a bony fragment from the base of distal phalanx (bony mallet injury) (Handoll and Vaghela 2004). As a result of this injury, the DIPJ cannot be actively extended. A mallet finger may be open but is more often a closed injury (Rockwell et al. 2000). It is the most common closed tendon injury in sports persons (Posner 1977) and can occur either after a direct blow to the DIPJ or a relatively minor trauma to the fingertip. The middle finger is most often involved, followed by the little finger (Stark et al. 1962). Doyle has classified this injury into four types as follows (Table 4).

Table 4 Doyle classification of mallet injuries (Doyle 1999)

Type 1	Closed or blunt trauma, with or without avulsion fracture (most commonest type)
Type 2	Rupture of the tendon near or at the DIP joint
Type 3	Open, with deep abrasion of the tissues
Type 4	Trans-epiphyseal fracture in children, fractures involving a large part of the joint surface

The patient may present with swelling and bruising over the DIPJ. This being a rarely painful condition, patients frequently seek help late in the course of the event (Perron et al. 2001). Also, the extensor lag at the DIPJ may not appear for several days. Patients rarely complain of functional disability because there are relatively few activities which require full digital extension (Brzezienski and Schneider 1995). On clinical examination, apart from the fixed flexion deformity, the patient will be unable to actively extend the DIPJ. However, the deformity is correctable by passive extension.

Plain radiographs are routinely performed to exclude bony involvement (Fig. 7). Ultrasound may demonstrate: discontinuity of the extensor tendon with partial or complete tear; avulsion fracture; no real-time movements of the extensor tendon; and fluid in the region of the extensor tendon insertion (Kleinbaum et al. 2005). These findings can be used to differentiate traumatic mallet finger from others caused by fixed flexion deformity. In cases with no bone avulsion on plain film, sagittal MR images can be used to assess for terminal extensor tendon injuries and thus can be used to decide treatment (Clavero et al. 2002; Tabbal et al. 2009).

The most common type of mallet injury, closed type 1 injuries are generally managed conservatively with hyperextension splint for around 6–8 weeks. This is followed by further 4 weeks of splinting at night. Surgical treatment is usually reserved for open injuries, DIPJ instability/subluxation or a large (>30%) displaced articular fracture fragment. A cadaveric study conducted by Hussain et al. concluded that palmar subluxation of a DIPJ without pre-existing arthritic deformity is expected when more than one half of the dorsal articular surface is injured (Hussain et al. 2008).

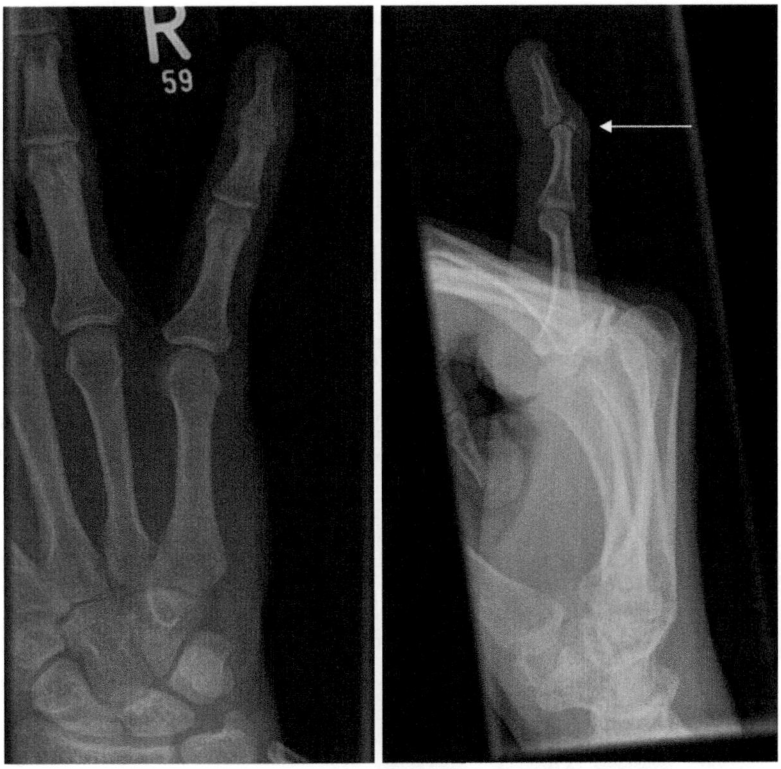

Fig. 7 AP and lateral radiographs of right little finger. Lateral radiograph demonstrates avulsion fracture (*white arrow*) at the site of extensor tendon insertion into the base of the terminal phalanx, usually seen in closed traumatic extensor tendon disruption with avulsion fracture (type 1)

3.3 Boutonniere Deformity (Zone III Injury)

A boutonniere deformity occurs as a result of an injury to the central slip at or near its insertion at the base of the middle phalanx. The term *boutonniere* is derived from the French for 'buttonhole', as the head of the proximal phalanx can pass through the defect in the extensor mechanism (Aronowitz and Leddy 1998). Most of these are caused by an unrecognised volar lateral dislocation of the PIPJ or less commonly by a blow to the dorsal aspect of the middle phalanx that forces the PIPJ into flexion while the finger is being actively extended (Aronowitz and Leddy 1998; Perron et al. 2001). This injury can either be open or closed, and the central slip may avulse with or without a bony fragment.

The patient usually presents with pain and swelling with maximal tenderness at the PIPJ. The classic boutonniere deformity is rarely seen in the acute phase (Aronowitz and Leddy 1998). In the early acute phase, active extension is retained by the normally orientated lateral slips; but the head of the proximal phalanx eventually goes through the central slip, resulting in migration of the lateral slips palmar to the PIPJ, which flexes the PIPJ and hyperextends the DIPJ resulting in the classic boutonniere deformity (Griffin et al. 2012). The above-described deformity usually occurs 1–2 weeks after the initial injury (Hart et al. 1993).

Burton has described three stages of the boutonniere deformity (Table 5).

The Elson test, which demonstrates rigidity of the DIPJ during attempted PIP extension from a flexed position, has been shown to reliably diagnose an early central slip injury. However, the drawbacks of this test are it will not demonstrate partial rupture of the central slip and may be impeded by pain (Elson 1986). Initially, plain radiographs are obtained to evaluate for an avulsion fracture at the base of the middle phalanx (Fig. 8). In equivocal cases, where clinical evaluation is difficult owing to pain and swelling, MRI can be an effective method for detecting central

Table 5 Stages of the boutonniere deformity (Burotn 1982)

Stage 1	Dynamic imbalance, fully correctable passively
Stage 2	Extensor mechanism contracture, not passively correctable but does not involve the joint structure
Stage 3	Fixed contracture with joint changes involving collateral ligament, volar plate scarring and intra-articular adhesions

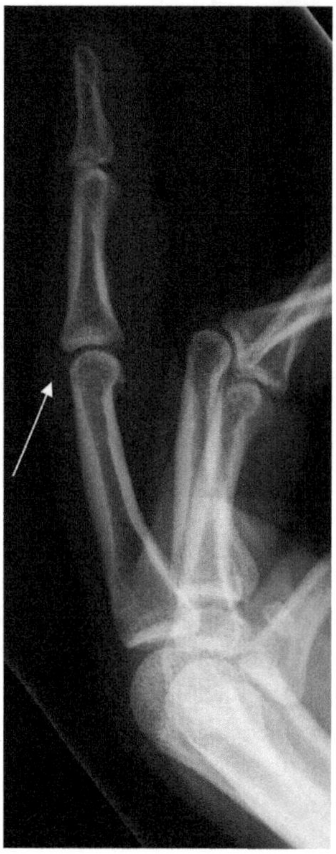

Fig. 8 Lateral radiograph showing a subtle avulsion fracture (*white arrow*) with associated soft tissue swelling at the base of the left middle finger intermediate phalanx

slip lesions (Clavero et al. 2002). Magnetic resonance imaging can also provide valuable information about associated VP and ligamentous lesions of the PIPJ. To the best of our knowledge, there are no current studies available comparing the efficiency of clinical examination, ultrasound or MRI in diagnosing the central slip injuries.

Treatment of central slip injuries remains highly controversial. Generally these are treated closed with extension splinting of the PIPJs for 4–6 weeks followed by 2 weeks of night time splinting (Aronowitz and Leddy 1998). Surgical treatment is implemented when (1) displaced avulsion fracture, (2) axial and lateral instability of the PIPJ associated with loss of active or passive extension of the joint and (3) failed conservative treatment (Griffin et al. 2012). However, surgical reconstruction is the treatment of choice for a chronic symptomatic boutonniere deformity (Aronowitz and Leddy 1998).

It is important to differentiate between a boutonniere and a pseudo-boutonniere deformity so that appropriate treatment plan can be implemented. Although the appearances may be similar, their aetiology is different. The pseudo-boutonniere deformity results from a PIPJ VP injury due to PIPJ hyperextension and resulting in PIPJ flexion contracture, rather than an injury to the central slip (Hong 2005). Typically, the flexion contracture of the PIPJ is fixed, and passive extension is not possible (Aronowitz and Leddy 1998). In a pseudo-boutonniere deformity, radiographs may slow calcification along the volar lateral aspect of the proximal phalanx. These injuries are managed conservatively by dynamic splinting, if the flexion contracture is less than 45° and surgical release may be needed to restore extension if the PIP flexion contracture is more than 45° (Aronowitz and Leddy 1998).

3.4 Boxer's Knuckle (Zone V Injury)

The extensor hood at the MCPJ is a retinacular system comprising the sagittal, oblique and transverse bands that stabilise the extensor tendon at the dorsal aspect of the MCPJ and keeps the tendon in place during flexion and extension. The SB is the most important structure of the extensor hood; this composes of a superficial and deep layer forming a tunnel through which the extensor tendon passes through (Kichouh et al. 2011). Sagittal band ruptures referred to as 'Boxer's

Table 6 Rayan and Murray classification of sagittal band injuries (Rayan and Murray 1994)

Type I	Mild injury with no instability
Type II	Moderate injury with extensor tendon subluxation
Type III	Severe injury with tendon dislocation

Knuckle' can occur spontaneously, secondary to trauma or can be associated with synovial disorders like rheumatoid arthritis (Kichouh et al. 2011). Congenitally absent or lax SBs have been previously reported (Inoue and Tamura 1996). The most commonly injured finger is the middle finger, and the most frequently involved SB is the radial with ulnar instability (Rayan and Murray 1994). It has been thought that underlying normal ulnar inclination of the index and middle finger may predispose them to radial band disruption (Lopez-Ben et al. 2003). However, ruptures of the ulnar SB resulting in radial instability have also been reported in the literature. Patients commonly present with pain, swelling, loss of full extension and subluxation of the extensor tendon. Rayan and Murray classified SB injuries into three types as shown in Table 6.

However, the overlying soft tissue swelling and pain can make clinical assessment difficult to diagnose tendon subluxation (Lopez-Ben et al. 2003). As a result, accurate diagnosis of SB rupture may be difficult without imaging. Advantages of ultrasound over MRI include dynamic assessment, cost-effectiveness and easy availability.

Various studies have been published describing the use of ultrasound and MRI for diagnosing SB injuries. The SB is best seen in the axial plane with the MCP in slight flexion, appearing as a linear hypoechoic structure. Focal hyperechoic thickening of the SB or disappearance of the normal architecture of the SB can be demonstrated in patients with extensor hood injuries (Kichouh et al. 2011). Dynamic ultrasound with the fingers alternatively extended and then flexed in a clenched fist enables excellent visualisation of extensor tendon subluxation and dislocation at the MCPJ (Fig. 9) (Lopez-Ben et al. 2003; Fenech 2023).

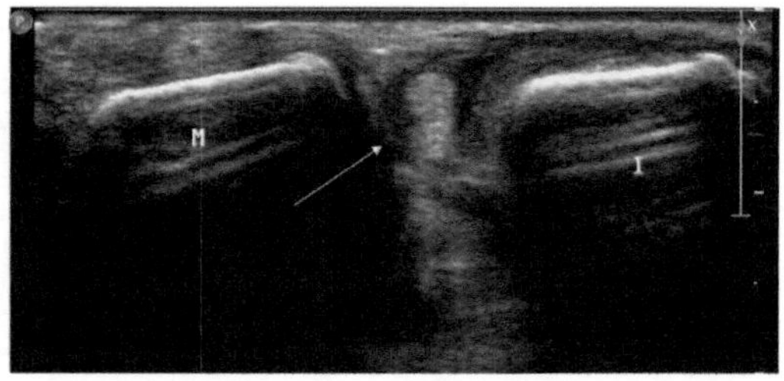

Fig. 9 Ultrasound image at MCPJ level shows subluxation of the index finger (I) extensor tendon (*white arrow*), secondary to extensor hood injury (not shown in this image)

On MRI, the SB is depicted as uniform low-signal intensity structure on all sequences. The T2W sequences are more accurate than T1W or post-contrast T1W sequences, and post-contrast imaging does not improve the sensitivity in depicting the SB (Drape et al. 1994). The MR findings in acute injuries include morphologic and signal intensity changes, together with poor definition, focal discontinuity and focal thickening (Clavero et al. 2002). Magnetic resonance imaging of MCPJs in different kinematic positions has also been found useful in diagnosing SB injuries (Lopez-Ben et al. 2003). The role of oblique and transverse bands is not well known currently, and these are also difficult to demonstrate on ultrasound and MRI (Kichouh et al. 2011). MR imaging can accurately assess thickening, partial or full thickness tears of the sagittal bands (Fig. 10a, b).

Like other extensor mechanism injuries, the treatment of SB injuries also remains highly controversial. Ritts et al. advocate conservative treatment with splinting of the MCPJ in extension, while Hame and Melone Jr. concluded that direct surgical repair with realignment of the central tendon is highly successful (Ritts et al. 1985; Hame and Melone Jr 2000). These will need to be treated as open infected injuries if the extensor mechanism or the SB injury is secondary to human bites with surgical debridement, intravenous antibiotics and splinting (Matzon and Bozentka 2010).

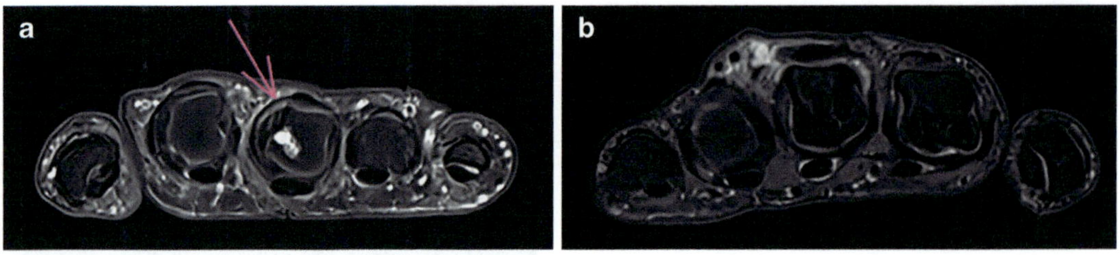

Fig. 10 (**a**) Axial PDFS image shows chronic thickening of the radial sagittal band of the middle finger in a elite boxer. (**b**) Axial PDFS image demonstrating full thickness tear of the ulnar sagittal band of the middle finger in

4 Collateral Ligament Injuries

4.1 Ulnar Collateral Ligament of the Thumb

The ulnar and radial collateral ligaments are primary stabilisers of the thumb MCPJ against radial and ulnar stress, respectively. Injury to these structures may result in joint instability, leading to significant disability and pain (Tang 2011). A correct early diagnosis influences management decisions and treatment outcomes (Sollerman et al. 1991). The thumb MCPJ is stabilised by static and dynamic stabilisers (Tsiouri et al. 2009). The static restraints include the VP, the dorsal capsule and the ulnar and radial collateral ligaments. The extrinsic and intrinsic muscles of the thumb make up the dynamic stabilisers. The ulnar collateral ligament (UCL) comprises a proper and an accessory ligament (Tsiouri et al. 2009). In flexion, the proper collateral ligament is taut, while the accessory collateral ligament is taut in extension.

Two acronyms are commonly used to describe UCL injuries, Gamekeeper's thumb and Skier's thumb. Gamekeeper's thumb was first reported by Campbell in 1955 to describe chronic attritional attenuation of the UCL in Scottish gamekeepers, secondary to strain induced on the first Web space (Campbell 1955). The Skier's thumb is used to describe acute injuries where the thumb is forced into abduction and hyperextension against the ski pole (Gerber et al. 1981). Thumb UCL injuries are the second most common skiing-related injury, after medial collateral ligament injury of the knee (Tsiouri et al. 2009).

Injury to the UCL is caused by sudden excessive valgus stress on the thumb MCPJ. Although this was attributed to the straps of the ski pole initially, later studies have showed that the incidence of the injury remained the same even with new pole designs without a strap (Derkash et al. 1987). In approximately 90% of cases, the thumb UCL avulses from the base of the proximal phalanx (Coyle Jr 2003). Although less frequent, it can avulse from proximal attachment or tear in the midsubstance. In 1962, Stener described a lesion in which the distal end of the avulsed UCL is displaced superficial to the adductor aponeurosis and is prevented from reapproximation to its anatomic insertion site (Stener 1962). Avulsion of UCL can be accompanied by more than one bony avulsion fragment with failure of the ligament bone complex at the site of the ligament–bone interface and also within the bone itself (Giele and Martin 2003; Weintraub et al. 2020).

Patients with acute injuries present with pain, swelling and reduced range of motion. Chronic presentations include deformity and loss of strength in particular pinching or grasping. On examination, tenderness to palpation will be present at the site of injury. A palpable mass on the medial side may represent the superficially displaced end of the UCL, suggestive of a Stener lesion. However, the absence of a palpable mass does not definitively rule out a Stener lesion (Heyman et al. 1993).

Evaluation of joint stability is the most important part of examination. The primary aim is to determine whether the injury is incomplete (Grade 1 or 2) or complete (Grade 3) (Tang 2011). Current consensus include testing the joint

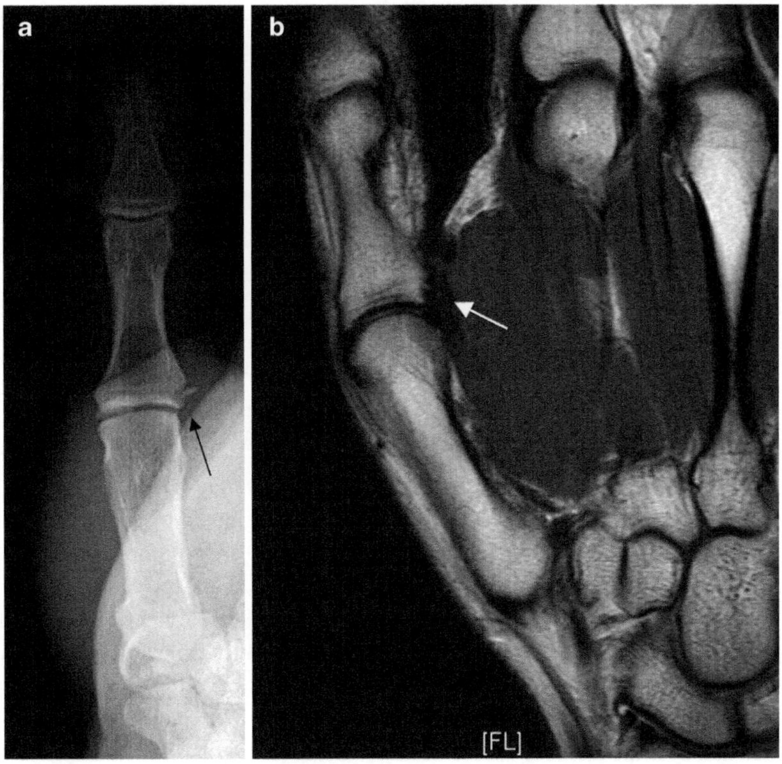

Fig. 11 (**a**, **b**) Plain radiograph AP view (**a**) and Coronal T1W MRI (**b**) showing bony avulsion fracture (*arrow*) at the site of UCL insertion

in zero degrees of extension and 30° flexion to evaluate accessory and proper collateral ligament components, respectively. Instability is defined as radial deviation of the proximal phalanx on the metacarpal head of >30–35° (Heyman et al. 1993). Stress examination demonstrating a firm end-point indicates an incomplete tear, whilst opening of the MCPJ without a firm end-point indicates a complete tear (Patel et al. 2010).

Plain radiographs are routinely performed to rule out a fracture or subluxation (Fig. 11a). Previously, stress radiography, ultrasound and MR with or without arthrography have been used to assess thumb UCL injuries. In addition to the discrepancies concerning the performance and interpretation of stress radiographs, the most significant drawback is their inability to direct the treatment because they do not differentiate between a non-displaced tear and a Stener lesion (Green and Rowlan 1984). In a study conducted by Harper et al. comparing the efficacy of stress radiography versus MR examination with and without arthrography, the overall sensitivity of stress radiography was found to be only 64% (Harper et al. 1996).

Ultrasound is useful in detecting partial and complete tears of the thumb UCL and has shown promising results in differentiating between complete tears and Stener lesions (Schnur et al. 2002). The normal thumb UCL appears as a hyperechoic structure spanning the ulnar side of the first MCPJ. Displaced UCL tears appear as a retracted, folded-on-itself structure which is displaced proximal and superficial to the adductor aponeurosis, creating the appearance of a 'yo–yo on a string' on coronal MRI scans (Ebrahim et al. 2006). The positive predictive value for ultrasound in identifying UCL tears is very high (87.5% Schnur et al. and 94% Jones et al.). However, the specificity varies between 83% for displaced ruptures and 91% for non-displaced ruptures (Hergan et al. 1995). Inexpensive and easy availability along with good overall comparable results with MR make ultrasound an attractive tool for evaluation of UCL tears. The primary disadvantage of ultrasound is that it is operator dependent. Ultrasound has been recommended to be used only in the 1st week after injury, as scarring may decrease accuracy of the method (Hergan et al. 1997).

Excellent soft tissue characterisation makes MR examination a very good modality to use in UCL injuries (Fig. 8b). The sensitivity and specificity have been shown to be 100% (Harper et al. 1996; Hergan et al. 1995). Thus, MR plays a vital role in making management plans for patients with UCL tears. Cost-effectiveness and availability remain the major deterrents for using MR as the primary modality in diagnosing UCL tears. Various pitfalls as described by Hergan et al. (1997) can cause misinterpretation between displaced and non-displaced UCL tears which can have serious implications on patient recovery. Hence, MR examination has been advocated when a non-displaced UCL tear is suspected by ultrasound (Hergan et al. 1997).

Conservative versus surgical management of UCL tears has been controversial and extensively debated over the last four to five decades. Grade 1 and 2 tears are managed conservatively. Surgery is indicated in the following instances: a Stener lesion is suspected; a displaced avulsion fracture exists, where there is an acute, grossly unstable joint; in symptomatic chronic injury; and in cases of volar subluxation seen on radiographs (Smith 1977). Surgical treatment has been widely accepted as treatment of choice for Grade 3 UCL tears.

4.2 Radial Collateral Ligament

Injuries of radial collateral ligament (RCL) comprise 10%–14% of the collateral ligament injuries to the thumb MCPJ (Coyle Jr 2003). These have been referred to as "reverse gamekeeper's thumb" (Cooney et al. 1990).

The RCL originates dorsally on the lateral condyle of the metacarpal head and extends in a distal and palmar direction to insert into the lateral tubercle of the proximal phalanx. (Edelstein et al. 2008). Like UCL, the RCL also consists of proper and accessory collateral ligaments which act as static restraints when MCPJ is in flexion and extension, respectively.

Injuries of the RCL result from forced and sudden adduction of the MCPJ which can occur from a fall or during sports when a ball or player strikes the thumb. Acutely, the patient presents with pain, stiffness, swelling and deformity. In the chronic situation, once the swelling and pain has subsided, patients present with persistent pain with activities that require a radial-sided force such as closing a door (Edelstein et al. 2008).

It is important to identify partial from complete RCL tears as complete tears are treated surgically, while partial tears are treated conservatively. Radial stress test and drawer tests may be used to assess for RCL injury. A recent study by Coyle Jr. found proximal tears (55%) are commoner than distal (29%) or midsubstance tears (16%) (Coyle Jr 2003). This can be explained by the fact that the distal width of the RCL insertion is equal to or wider than the RCL origin at the metacarpal (Lyons et al. 1998). Complete RCL tear can result in both static and dynamic instability (Edelstein et al. 2008). Although there are several classification systems for UCL injuries, there are no specific ones for the RCL injuries. A generalised classification is used instead. Grade 1: Small incomplete tear, Grade 2: larger but still incomplete tear and Grade 3: complete tear.

Conventional radiographs are obtained to assess for avulsion fractures and subluxation. Volar subluxation of the phalanx >3 mm is much more common with RCL injury than with the UCL injury (Tang 2011) as RCL is a primary support preventing volar subluxation. Stress dynamic fluoroscopy may also aid in evaluation of instability. Because of the high correlation between stress examination and operative findings, arthrography, ultrasonography (Fig. 12) or MRI are usually not needed (Edelstein et al. 2008).

On the basis of the current available literature, RCL and UCL injuries can be managed in a similar manner (Patel et al. 2010). Generally, Grade 1 and 2 injuries are treated conservatively, while treatment of Grade 3 injuries remains controversial. Various surgical methods have been described in the literature for Grade 3 injuries and no general agreement is present.

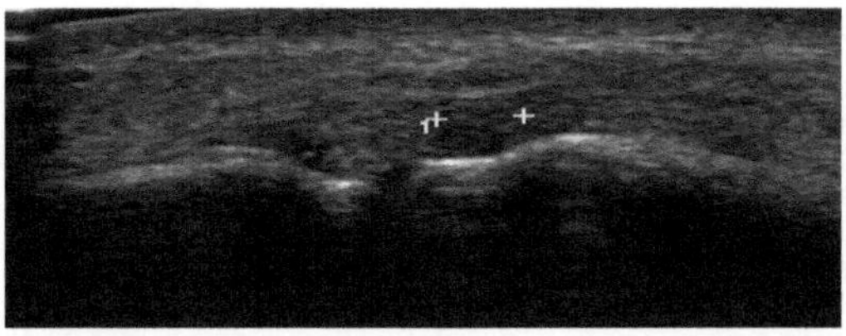

Fig. 12 Longitudinal ultrasound image showing rupture of radial collateral ligament

Table 7 Gedda classification of Bennett fractures (Gedda 1954, cited by Carlsen and Moran (2009))

Type 1	Large single ulnar fragment and metacarpal base subluxation
Type 2	Impaction fracture without metacarpal base subluxation
Type 3	Small ulnar avulsion fragment with metacarpal dislocation

5 Fractures

Among the injuries sustained during sporting activities in the general population, it is fractures of the upper limb that predominate. The vast number of patients attending emergency department due to these injuries reflects this. In a retrospective study conducted by Aitken and Court-Brown looking at nearly 6000 fractures, 24% of them occurred in hand and 22.4% of these were sporting injuries. The thumb and the little fingers were most commonly involved fingers accounting for up to 57.3% (Aitken and Court-Brown 2008). Metacarpal fractures of the thumb and little fingers are discussed below.

5.1 Thumb Fractures

The thumb provides up to 40% of hand function (Carlsen and Moran 2009). Injuries to the thumb are predominantly fractures of the proximal phalanx or the metacarpal and ligamentous injuries around the MCPJ. Ligamentous injuries have been discussed in detail along with other soft tissue injuries of the hand. Thumb fractures are found to occur most commonly in children and the elderly (Stanton et al. 2007).

Thumb metacarpal base fractures form an important subset and will be discussed further.

5.1.1 Bennett Fracture

In 1882, Edward Hallaran Bennett first described the fracture involving the base of the thumb metacarpal. However, a Bennett fracture now refers to a two-part intra-articular fracture or dislocation involving the base of the thumb metacarpal (Rettig 2004). The mechanism of injury is classically an axial load to the flexed and adducted thumb (Hong 2005). The volar–ulnar fragment is held in place by its ligamentous attachment to the trapezium, known as the anterior oblique ligament, also described as the beak ligament (Bettinger et al. 1999). As a result of the injury, the remainder of the first metacarpal shaft subluxes in a dorsal, proximal and radial direction due to the pull of the abductor pollicis longus, extensor pollicis longus, extensor pollicis brevis and the adductor pollicis longus (Carlsen and Moran 2009). Gedda in 1954 has classified Bennett fractures as follows (Table 7).

Following clinical examination, a radiographic evaluation forms an integral part of the initial clinical assessment (Fig. 13a). True antero–posterior and lateral views can be obtained with the Robert's and Bett's view, respectively, to look for fracture displacement and joint congruency (Carlsen and Moran 2009). In subtle undisplaced cases, MR imaging can demonstrate the undispaced fracture and associated capsular ligamentous injury (Fig. 13b). These fractures are unstable and should be promptly referred to a hand surgeon for appropriate management. Closed reduction with percutaneous pin fixation is recommended if the fragment is less than 25% of the articular surface and if the fragment is larger than 25% of articular surface, and those irreducible by closed techniques should be opened, reduced and internally fixed (Weinstein and Hanel 2002).

5.1.2 Rolando Fracture

This was first described by Silvio Rolando in 1910, a Y-pattern fracture of the thumb metacarpal base (Fig. 14). Currently, this eponym is used widely for any comminuted intra-articular fracture of the thumb metacarpal base (Hong 2005).

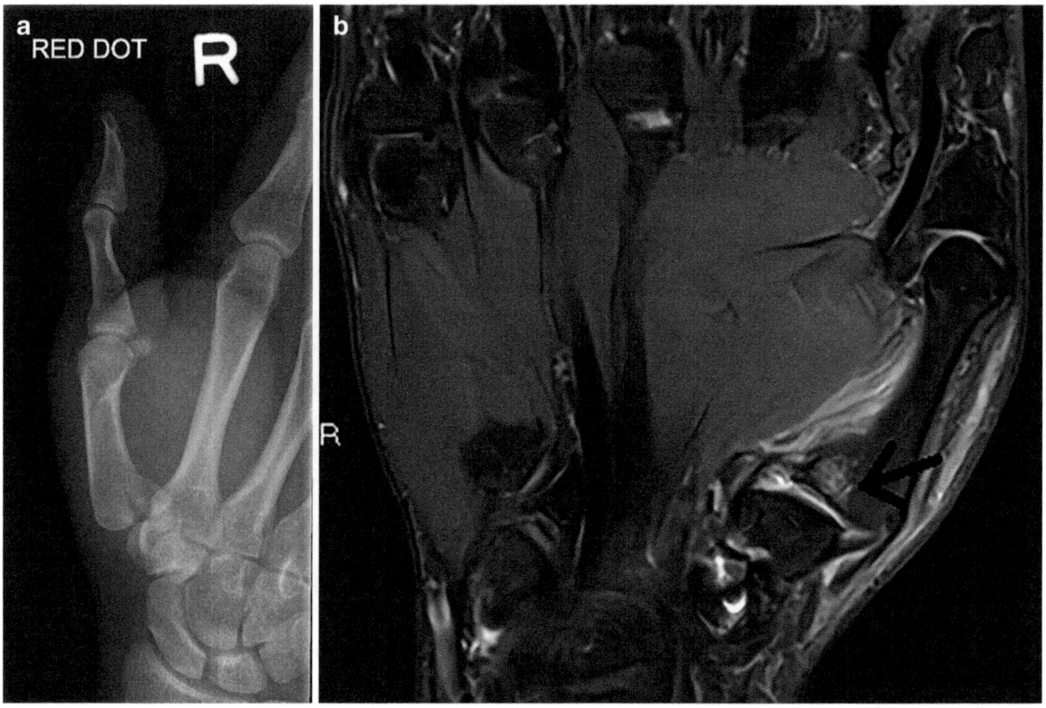

Fig. 13 (**a**) Lateral radiograph of thumb showing fractures of the metacarpal base (Bennett fracture type 1) and proximal phalanx shaft. (**b**) Coronal PDFS MR image demonstrates fracture of the metacarpal base (black arrow) and capsuloligamentous sprain

These are similar in location and aetiology to Bennett fracture (Hong 2005). This fracture pattern is considerably more difficult to treat and has a worse prognosis than that of the Bennett fracture (Carlsen and Moran 2009). When there are two large fragments without considerable comminution, open reduction and internal fixation can be successful. For markedly comminuted fractures, distraction and reliance on ligamentous reduction of the fragments may be necessary (Carlsen and Moran 2009).

5.2 Boxer's Fracture

The most common fracture of the hand is fracture of the little finger metacarpal, accounting for up to 50% of all metacarpal fractures and 20% of all fractures of the hand (Lee and Jupiter 2000). A fracture to the little finger metacarpal neck is referred to as boxer's fracture. These result from incorrect technique in swinging a fist that puts an oblique force applied to the smallest, weakest metacarpal (Walsh 2004). The fracture occurs just below the metacarpal head and is normally displaced in a volar direction (Fig. 15). It is important to assess for malrotation by examining the direction of the fingers in flexion (Hong 2005). Apex volar angulation of up to 40° is acceptable and can be treated conservatively with immobilisation in a gutter splint with ring and little finger MCPJs in a 90° flexed position (Hong 2005). Fractures that are markedly comminuted or angulated may need open reduction and internal fixation (Peterson and Bancroft 2006).

5.3 Intra-articular Fractures and Dislocations of the Carpometacarpal Joints

Intra-articular metacarpal base fractures are high-energy injuries that are often missed on initial presentation (Liaw et al. 1995). These

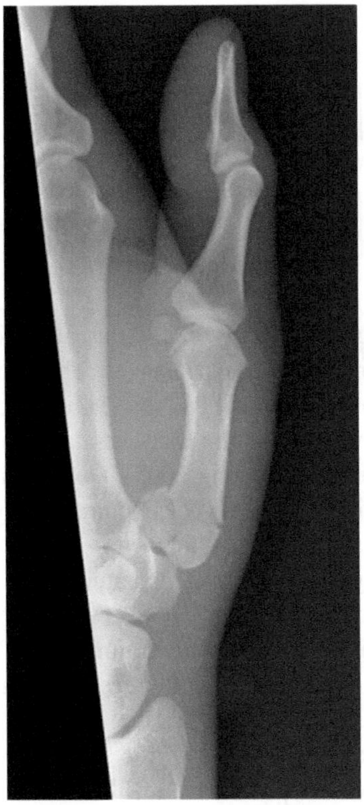

Fig. 14 Rolando fracture of the metacarpal base on a lateral radiograph of the thumb

are associated with carpometacarpal (CMC) dislocations and most commonly occur in the ring and little fingers.

The mechanism of injury involves axial load transmission through the fourth metacarpal onto the carpal bones (Cain et al. 1987). The ring and little finger CMC joints being modified saddle joints allow considerable movement in the antero–posterior plane that predisposes these joints to dislocation (Liaw et al. 1995). At a certain stage when the ring finger metacarpal is unable to dissipate the force, a fracture occurs resulting in shortening of the ring finger metacarpal. The axial load is then transferred to the little finger metacarpal causing the little finger CMC joint injury (Liaw et al. 1995). The degree of the little finger metacarpal flexion determines the type and degree of hamate injury (Cain et al. 1987). Flexion of the metacarpal during impact may cause dorsal dislocation of the little finger metacarpal base, dorsal CMC ligament disruption and hamate fracture. In the little finger, the ECU, FCU and abductor digiti minimi tendon exert deforming forces on the fracture fragments (Weinstein and Hanel 2002). Cain et al. in 1987 have classified the combined ring

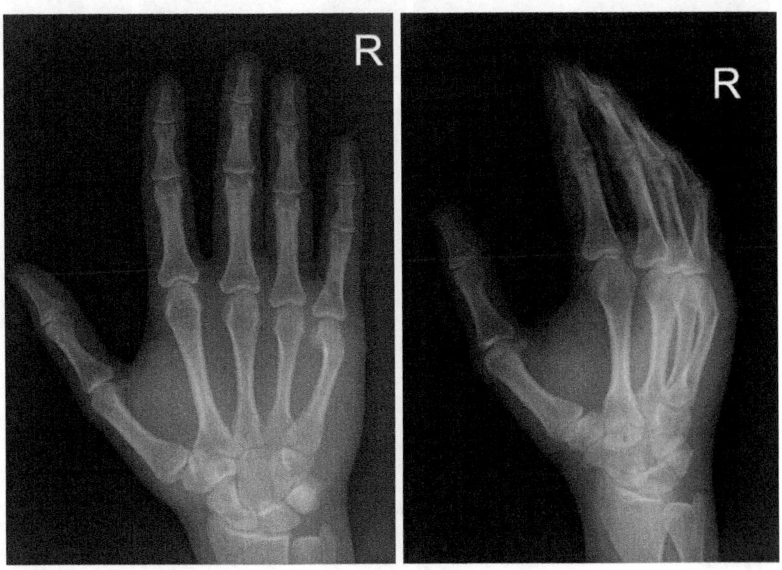

Fig. 15 AP and oblique radiographs showing little finger metacarpal neck fracture (Boxer's fracture) with volar angulation

and little finger metacarpal fracture and little finger CMC joint injury into three categories as follows (see Table 8).

The routine AP and lateral radiographs of the hand may not reveal the full extent of the ring and little finger CMC joints (Fig. 16), and a CT scan may be needed to demonstrate the full extent of the injury (Fig. 17). The 45° pronated oblique and 15° pronated oblique views are helpful in assessing the severity of this injury (Liaw et al. 1995).

The treatments of these injuries depend on the severity and stability of the CMC joints. Type 1 stable injuries treated conservatively. Closed reduction and percutaneous pinning can be used to treat unstable type 1 injuries (Cain et al. 1987). Type 2 and 3 injuries are potentially unstable and will require open reduction and internal fixation (Liaw et al. 1995).

Table 8 Cain et al. classification of intra-articular fractures and dislocations of carpometacarpal joints (Cain et al. 1987)

Type	Characteristic Features
1A	Subluxation or dislocation of the little finger metacarpal base without hamate fracture
1B	Type 1A + small dorsal rim hamate avulsion fracture
2	Dorsal hamate comminution is present
3	Coronal splitting of the hamate

5.4 Phalangeal Fractures

Phalangeal fractures can occur at head, neck, shaft or base of the phalanges. There are many variations of these involving various locations. Shaft fractures can be transverse, oblique, spiral or comminuted (Hong 2005). Displacement and angulation of phalangeal fractures result from a combination of two main factors: the mechanism of injury and the deforming nature of the fracture (Peterson and Bancroft 2006). A direct blow can result in transverse or comminuted fracture, while a twisting injury often results in an oblique or spiral fracture (Lee and Jupiter 2000).

Condylar fractures of the head of proximal phalanx are typically the result of axial loading. London described three types of Condylar frac-

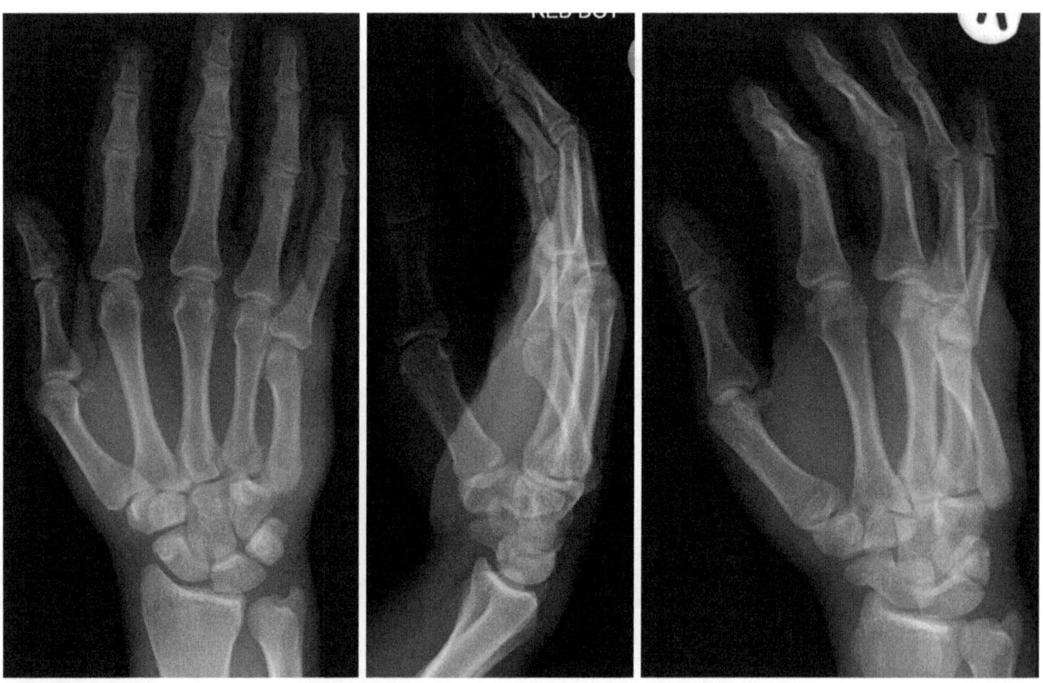

Fig. 16 AP, lateral and oblique radiographs of the right hand showing little finger CMC joint dislocation. Note hamate fracture (seen on CT—Fig. 14) is not visible on these plain films

tures that influence prognosis and management: a type I stable, undisplaced unicondylar fracture; a type II unstable, displaced, unicondylar; and type III comminuted bicondylar fracture (London 1971).

Along with standard AP and lateral radiographs, CT can provide further information that may assist the surgeons in management.

Oblique or spiral fractures may be associated with malrotation. No malrotation is acceptable for phalangeal fractures, because this leads to overlap and malalignment of the digit (Peterson and Bancroft 2006). Acceptable reduction is less than 6 mm of shortening, less than 15° of angulation and with no rotational deformity (Lee and Jupiter 2000).

Non-displaced fractures are treated conservatively, while displaced and malrotated fractures should be reduced; closed at first, but then surgically if needed (Hong 2005). For condylar fractures, London types II and III are treated surgically and stable type I injuries are managed conservatively (Stern 2005).

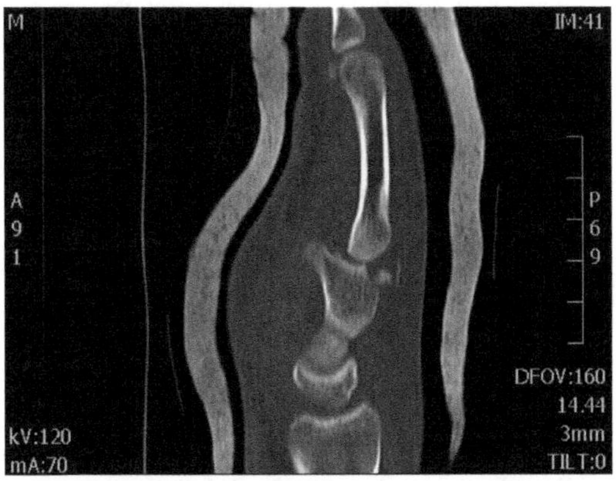

Fig. 17 Sagittal CT image shows little finger CMC joint subluxation with rim fracture of the hamate (Cain et al. type 1B CMC joint injury)

5.5 Interphalangeal Joint Dislocations

Interphalangeal (IP) dislocations are common injuries in athletes. These injuries usually result from significant force and may result in ligamentous injury or tear. Most IP joint dislocations involve the PIPJ (Morgan and Slowman 2001). The PIPJ is susceptible especially to forced abnormal motion produced in ball sports and in sports resulting in axial loading of the digit (Morgan and Slowman 2001). Most IP joint dislocations are dorsal, with dorsal dislocation of the middle phalanx and disruption of the VP (Fig. 18) (Hong 2005).

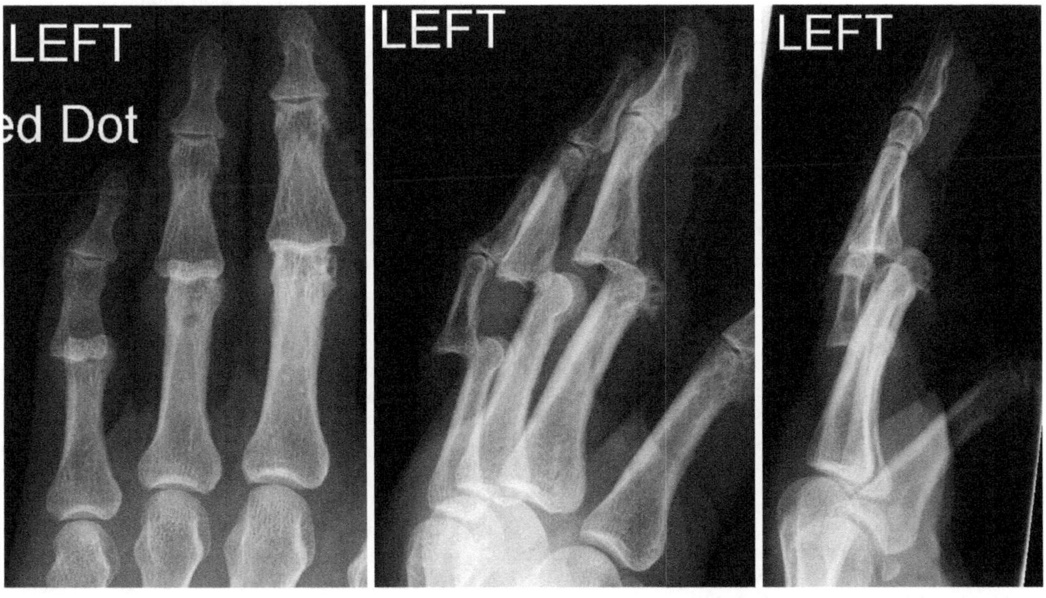

Fig. 18 AP, oblique and lateral radiographs of the middle, ring and little fingers showing dorsal dislocation of the proximal interphalangeal joints

6 Conclusion

This chapter has described the most common soft tissue and bone injuries to the hand. We have related the anatomy and mechanism of these injuries to the imaging assessment. We have also discussed factors that influence management decisions which enable a more thorough imaging assessment.

Acknowledgments The authors wish to sincerely thank Dr. David Moore, Dr. Steven L. J. James and Dr. Andrew J. Grainger for providing some of the images used in this chapter.

References

Aitken S, Court-Brown CM (2008) The epidemiology of sports-related fractures of the hand. Injury 39:1377–1383

Angermann P, Lohmann M (1993) Injuries to the hand and wrist. A study of 50,272 injuries. J Hand Surg Br 18(5):642–644

Aronowitz ER, Leddy JP (1998) Closed tendon injuries of the hand and wrist in athletes. Clin Sports Med 17:449–467

Beltran J, Noto AM, Herman LJ, Lubbers LM (1987) Tendons: high field strength surface coil MR imaging. Radiology 162:735–740

Bettinger PC, Linscheid RL, Berger RA, Cooney WP III, An KN (1999) An anatomic study of the stabilizing ligaments of the trapezium and trapeziometacarpal joint. J Hand Surg 24(4):786–798

Bollen (1990) Injury to the A2 pulley in rock climbers. J Hand Surg Br 15(2):268–270

Brzezienski MA, Schneider LH (1995) Extensor tendons injuries at the distal interphalangeal joint. Hand Clin 11:373–386

Burotn RI (1982) Extensor tendon-late reconstruction. In: Green DP (ed) Operative hand surgey. Churchill Livingstone, New York, p 2073

Buscemi MJ, Page BJ (1987) Flexor digitorum profundus avulsions with associated distal phalanx fractures: a report of four cases and review of the literature. Am J Sports Med 15:366–370

Cain JE, Shepler TR, Wilson MR (1987) Hamatometacarpal fracture-dislocation: classification and treatment. J Hand Surg 12(5 Pt 1):762–767

Campbell CS (1955) Gamekeeper's thumb. J Bone Joint Surg Br 37:148–149

Carlsen BT, Moran SL (2009) Thumb trauma: Bennett fractures, rolando fractures, and ulnar collateral ligament injuries. J Hand Surg Am 34(5):945–952

Clavero JA, Alomar X, Monill JM, Esplugas M, Golano P, Mendoza M, Salvador A (2002) MR imaging of ligament and tendon injuries of the fingers. Radiographics 22:237–256

Cooney WP, Arnold D, Grace J (1990) Collateral ligament injury of the thumb. Adv Orthop Surg 13:235–248

Coyle MP Jr (2003) Grade III radial collateral ligament injuries of the thumb metacarpophalangeal joint: treatment by soft tissue advancement and bony reattachment. J Hand Surg Am 28(1):14–20

Derkash RS, Matyas JR, Weaver JK et al (1987) Acute surgical repair of the skier's thumb. Clin Orthop Relat Res 216:29–33

Doyle JR (1999) Extensor tendons—acute injuries. In: Geen DP, Hotchkiss RN, Pederson WC (eds) Green's operative hand surgery, 4th edn. Churchill Livingstone, Edinburgh, pp 1950–1986

Drape JL, Dubert T, Silbermann O, Thelen P, Thivet A, Benacerraf R (1994) Acute trauma of the extensor hood of the metacarpophalangeal joint: MR imaging evaluation. Radiology 192:469–476

Eaton RG (1971) Joint injuries of hand. Charles C. Thomas, Springfield

Ebrahim SF, De Maeseneer M, Jager T, Marcelis S, Jamadar DA, Jacobson JA (2006) US diagnosis of UCL tears of the thumb and stener lesions: technique, pattern-based approach, and differential diagnosis. Radiographics 26:1007–1020

Edelstein DM, Kardashian G, Lee SK (2008) Radial collateral ligament injuries of the thumb. J Hand Surg 33A:760–770

Elson RA (1986) Rupture of the central slip of the extensor hood of the finger. A test for early diagnosis. J Bone Joint Surg Br 68(2):229–231

Fenech M (2023) Boxer's knuckle: sonographic anatomy and assessment of sagittal band tears of the dorsal hood. Australas J Ultrasound Med 26(4):216–229

Fontes T, Sebastião M, Saraiva F (2024) Ultrasound features of a pulley strain in a sport climber: a discussion based on a case report. J Ultrasound 27(2):425–428

Gabl M, Rangger C, Lutz M, Fink C, Rudisch A, Pechlaner S (1998) Disruption of the finger flexor pulley system in elite rock climbers. Am J Sports Med 26:651–655

Gaine WJ, Beardsmore J, Fahmy N (1998) Early active mobilisation of volar plate avulsion fractures. Injury 29:589–591

Gerber C, Senn E, Matter P (1981) Skier's thumb: surgical treatment of recent injuries to the ulnar collateral ligament of the thumb's metacarpophalangeal joint. Am J Sports Med 9:171–177

Germann AM, Stanley SS (2024) Not a Jersey finger – a case of a closed traumatic rupture of the small finger flexor digitorum profundus tendon at the lumbrical origin. Eplasty 24:e57. PMID: 39474003; PMCID: PMC11520356

Giele H, Martin J (2003) The two-level ulnar collateral ligament injury of the metacarpophalangeal joint of the thumb. J Hand Surg 28B:92–93

Green DP, Rowlan SA (1984) Fractures and dislocations in the hand. In: Rockwood CA Jr, Green DP (eds) Fractures in adults, 2nd edn. JB Lippincott, Philadelphia, pp 388–394

Griffin M, Hindocha S, Jordan D, Saleh M, Khan W (2012) Management of extensor tendon injuries. Open Orthop J 6(Suppl 1:M4):36–42

Hame SL, Melone CP Jr (2000) Boxer's knuckle in the professional athlete. Am J Sports Med 28:879882

Handoll HHG, Vaghela M (2004) Interventions for treating mallet finger injuries. Cochran Database Syst Reviews 2004, Issue 3. Art. No.: CD004574.

Harper MT, Chandnani VP, Spaeth J, Santangelo JR, Providence BC, Bagg MA (1996) Gamekeeper thumb: diagnosis of ulnar collateral ligament injury using magnetic resonance imaging, magnetic resonance arthrography and stress radiography. J Magn Reson Imaging 6(2):322–328

Hart RG, Uehara DT, Kutz JE (1993) Extensor tendon injuries of the hand. Emerg Med Clin North Am 11(3):637–649

Hauger O, Chung CB et al (2000) Pulley system in the fingers: normal anatomy and simulated lesions in cadavers at MR imaging, CT and US with and without contrast material distention of the tendon sheath. Radiology 217:201–212

Hergan K, Mittler C, Oser W (1995) Ulnar collateral ligament: differentiation of displaced and nondisplaced tears with US and MR imaging. Radiology 194:65–71

Hergan K, Mittler C, Oser W (1997) Pitfalls in sonography of the gamekeeper's thumb. Eur Radiol 7:65–69

Heyman P, Gelberman RH, Duncan K, Hipp JA (1993) Injuries of the ulnar collateral ligament of the thumb metacarpophalangeal joint: biomechanical and prospective clinical studies on the usefulness of valgus stress testing. Clin Orthop Relat Res 292:165–171

Hill C, Riaz M, Mozzam A, Brennen ND (1998) A regional audit of hand and wrist injuries. J Hand Surg (Br Eur) 23B(2):196–200

Hong E (2005) Hand injuries in sports medicine. Prim Care 32:91–103

Hunter JM (1984) Anatomy of the flexor tendons: pulley, vincular, synovial, and vascular structures. In: Spinner M (ed) Kaplan's functional and surgical anatomy of the hand, 3rd edn. Lippincott, Philadelphia, pp 65–92

Hussain SN, Dietz JF, Kalainov DM, Lautenschlager EP (2008) A biomechanical study of distal interphalangeal joint subluxation after mallet fracture injury. J Hand Surg 33A:26–30

Inoue G, Tamura Y (1996) Dislocation of the extensor tendons over the metacarpophalangeal joints. J Hand Surg [Am] 21:464–469

Jebson PJL (1998) Flexor digitorum profundus tendon avulsions. Oper Tech Orthop 8:63–66

Jeyapalan K, Bisson MA, Dias JJ, Griffin Y, Bhatt R (2008) The role of ultrasound in the management of flexor tendon injuries. J Hand Surg (Eur) 33E(4):430–434

Keifhaber TR, Stern PJ (1998) Fracture dislocations of the proximal interphalangeal joint. J Hand Surg Am 23:368–380

Kichouh M, De Maesenner M, Jager T, Marcelis S, Van Hedent E, Van Roy P, De Mey J (2011) Ultrasound findings in injuries of dorsal extensor hood: correlation with MR and follow-up findings. Eur J Radiol 77:249–253

Klauser A, Bodner G, Frauscher F, Gabl M, Xur Nedden D (1999) Finger injuries in extreme rock climbers assessment of high-resolution ultrasonography. Am J Sports Med 27:733–737

Klauser A, Frauscher F, Bodner G, Halpern E, Schoke MF, Springer P, Gable M, Judamaier W, Nedden D (2002) Finger pulley injuries in extreme rock climbers: depiction with dynamic US. Radiology 222:755–761

Kleinbaum Y, Heyman Z, Ganel A, Blankstein A (2005) Sonographic imaging of mallet finger. Ultraschall Med 26(3):223–226

Kleinhert HE, Verdan C (1983) Report of the committee on tendon injuries. J Hand Surg [Am] 8(5 pt 2):794–798

Le Viet D, Rousselin B, Roulot E, Lantieri L, Godefroy D (1996) Diagnosis of digital pulley rupture by computed tomography. Hand Surg 21A:245–248

Leddy JP, Packer JW (1977) Avulsion of the profundus tendon insertion in athletes. J Hand Surg [Am] 2:66–69

Lee SG, Jupiter JB (2000) Phalangeal and metacarpal fractures of the hand. Hand Clin 16:323–332

Liaw Y, Kalnins G, Kirsh G, Meakin I (1995) Combined fourth and fifth metacarpal fracture and fifth carpometacarpal joint dislocation. J Hand Surg (Br Eur) 20B(2):249–252

Lin GT, Amadio PC, An KN, Cooney WP (1989) Functional anatomy of the human digital flexor pulley system. J Hand Surg Am 14:949–956

London PS (1971) Sprains and fractures involving the interphalangeal joints. Hand 3:155–158

Lopez-Ben R, Lee DH, Nicolodi DJ (2003) Boxer knuckle (injury of the extensor hood with extensor tendon subluxation): diagnosis with dynamic us—report of three cases. Radiology 228:642–646

Lutter C, Kuerten S, Geppert C, Mittelmeier W, Klinder A, Söder S, Römer F, Uder M, Janka R, Bayer T (2023) Dynamic study of the finger interphalangeal joint volar plate-motion analysis with magnetic resonance cinematography and histologic comparison. Skeletal Radiol 52(8):1493–1501

Lyons RP, Kozin SH, Failla JM (1998) The anatomy of the radial side of the thumb: static restraints in preventing subluxation and rotation after injury. Am J Orthop 27:759–763

Marco RA, Sharkey NA, Smith TS, Zissimos AG (1998) Pathomechanics of closed rupture of the flexor tendon pulleys in rock climbers. J Bone Joint Surg Am 80:1012–1019

Martinoli C, Bianchi S, Nebiolo M, Dechi LE, Garcia JF (2000) Sonographic evaluation of digital annular pulley tears. Skeletal Radiol 29:387–391

Matzon JL, Bozentka DJ (2010) Extensor tendon injuries. J Hand Surg 35A:854–861

McMaster PE (1933) Tendon and muscle ruptures: clinical and experimental studies on the causes and location of subcutaneous ruptures. J Bone Joint Surg 15:705

Morgan WJ, Slowman LS (2001) Acute hand and wrist injuries in athletes: evaluation and management. J Am Acad Orthop Surg 9:389–400

Nance EP Jr, Kaye JJ, Milek MA (1979) Volar plate fractures. Radiology 133:61–64

Newport ML (1997) Extensor tendon injuries in the hand. J Am Acad Orthop Surg 5:59–66

Patel S, Potty A, Taylor EJ, Sorene ED (2010) Collateral ligament injuries of the metacarpophalangeal joint of the thumb: a treatment algorithm. Strateg Trauma Limb Reconstr 5:1–10

Perron AD, Brady WJ, Keats TE, Hersh RE (2001) Orthopaedic pitfalls in the emergency department: closed tendon injuries of the hand. Am J Emerg Med 19:76–80

Peterson JJ, Bancroft LW (2006) Injuries of the fingers and thumb in the athlete. Clin Sports Med 25:527–542

Phair IC, Quinton DN, Allen MJ (1989) The conservative management of volar avulsion fractures of the PIP joint. J Hand Surg Br 14:168–170

Posner MA (1977) Injuries to the hand and wrist in athletes. Orthop Clin North Am 8:593–618

Rayan GM, Murray D (1994) Classification and treatment of closed sagittal band injuries. J Hand Surg 19A:590–594

Rettig AC (2004) Athletic injuries of the wrist and hand. Part II: overuse injuries of the wrist and traumatic injuries to the hand. Am J Sports Med 32:262–273

Ritts GD, Wood MB, Engber WD (1985) Nonoperative treatment of traumatic dislocations of the extensor digitorum tendons in patients without rheumatoid disorders. J Hand Surg 10A:714–716

Rockwell WB, Butler PN, Byrne BA (2000) Extensor tendon: anatomy, injury, and reconstruction. Plast Reconstr Surg 106:1592–1603

Schnur DP, DeLone FX, McClellan MR, Bonavita J, Witham RS (2002) Ultrasound: a powerful tool in the diagnosis of ulnar collateral ligament injuries of the thumb. Ann Plast Surg 49:19–23

Smith RJ (1977) Post-traumatic instability of the metacarpophalangeal joint of the thumb. J Bone Joint Surg Am 59-A:14–21

Sollerman C, Abrahamso SO, Lundborg G, Adalbert K (1991) Functional splinting versus plaster cast for ruptures of the ulnar collateral ligament of the thumb. Acta Orthop Scand 62:524–526

Stanton JS, Dias JJ, Burke FD (2007) Fractures of the tubular bones of the hand. J Hand Surg 32E:626–636

Stark HH, Boyes JH, Wilson JN (1962) Mallet finger. J Bone Joint Surg Am 44(6):1061–1068

Stener B (1962) Displacement of the ruptured ulnar collateral ligament of the metacarpo-phalangeal joint of the thumb. J Bone Joint Surg (Br) 44-B:869–879

Stern PJ (2005) Fractures of the metacarpals and phalanges. In: Green DP (ed) Green's operative hand surgery, 5th edn. Elsevier Churchill Livingstone, Philadelphia

Tabbal GN, Bastidas N, Sharma S (2009) Closed mallet thumb injury: a review of the literature and case study of the use of magnetic resonance imaging in deciding treatment. Plast Reconstr Surg 124(1):222–226

Tang P (2011) Collateral ligament injuries of the thumb metacarpophalangeal joint. J Am Acad Orthop Surg 19:287–296

Tsiouri C, Hayton MJ, Baratz M (2009) Injury to the ulnar collateral ligament of the thumb. Hand 4:12–18

Walsh JJ (2004) Fractures of the hand and carpal navicular bone in athletes. South Med J 97:762–765

Weinstein LP, Hanel DP (2002) Metacarpal fractures. J Am Soc Surg Hand 2:168–180

Weintraub MD, Hansford BG, Stilwill SE, Allen H, Leake RL, Hanrahan CJ, Chan BY, Soltanolkotabi M, Kobes P, Mills MK (2020) Avulsion injuries of the hand and wrist. Radiographics 40(1):163–180

Williams EH, McCarthy E, Bickel KD (1998) The histologic anatomy of the volar plate. J Hand Surg Am 23A:805–810

Yoong P, Goodwin RW, Chojnowski A (2010) Phalangeal fractures of the hand. Clin Radiol 65:773–780

Wrist Instability

Shashank Chapala, Shubham Arora, Milko C. de Jonge, G. J. Streekstra, M. Maas, Kapil Shirodkar, and Rajesh Botchu

Contents

S. Chapala (✉)
Department of Radiology, AIG Hospital, Hyderabad, India

S. Arora
Department of Radiology, Lady Hardinge Medical College, New Delhi, India

M. C. de Jonge
Department of Radiology, St. Andotonius Hospital Midden-Nederland, Utrecht, Netherlands

G. J. Streekstra
Department of Biomedical Engineering and Physics, Academic Medical Center, Amsterdam, The Netherlands

M. Maas
Radiology Room C1-120, Meibergdreef, Amsterdam, The Netherlands

K. Shirodkar
Department of Radiology, Royal Lancaster Infirmary, Lancaster, UK

R. Botchu
Department of Radiology, Royal Orthopedic Hospital, Birmingham, UK

Med Radiol Diagn Imaging (2025)
https://doi.org/10.1007/174_2025_618,
Published Online: 26 October 2025

Abstract

The painful clunking, unstable wrist has been an area of specific interest for clinicians and radiologists for many years. This chapter aims to focus on the unstable wrist, reviewing the clinical problem, exploring current hypotheses, critically evaluating radiological tools in aiding the clinician, and illustrating the integrative views of the authors based on their fundamental research and clinical practice. This chapter cannot provide a complete overview as this is a controversial area with an extremely extensive literature.

Abbreviations

CH	Capitohamate
CL	Capitolunate
CT	Capitotrapezoid
DIC	Dorsal intercarpal
DISI	Dorsal intercalated segment instability
DRT	Dorsal radiotriquetral
LRL	Long radiolunate (aka radiolunotriquetral)
LTD	Lunotriquetral dissociation
LTIL	Lunotriquetral interosseous ligament
RL	Radiolunate
RS	Radioscaphoid
RSC	Radioscaphocapitate
RSL	Radioscapholunate ligament
SC	Scaphocapitate
SL	Scapholunate
SLD	Scapholunate dissociation
SLIL	Scapholunate interossesous ligament
SRL	Short radiolunate
STT	Scaphotrapeziotrapezoid
TH	Triquetrohamate
THC	Triquetro-hamate-capitate
UC	Ulnocapitate
UL	Ulnolunate
VISI	Volar intercalated segment instability

1 Introduction

Carpal instability is a problem of unknown extent, of which sparse literature suggests an incidence of 2.6% in adults (Mink van der Molen 1997). The lack of reliable data relating to incidence is partly due to the lack of consensus relating to diagnosis and terminology and also the result of differences between ways in which carpal instability is classified (Kobayashi et al. 1997). The wrist has a complex anatomy involving 15 bones comprising the radius and ulna, carpal bones, and metacarpal bases. However, the biomechanical principles governing carpal kinematics and instability remain poorly understood.

2 Anatomy

The wrist is a complex structure comprising multiple joints formed by the carpal bones, which are organized into proximal and distal rows (Fig. 1). The proximal row includes the scaphoid, lunate, triquetrum articulating with the distal ends of the radius and ulna. The distal row consists of the trapezium, trapezoid, capitate, and hamate. Gilula first arc is smooth curve outlining proximal convexities of scaphoid, lunate, triquetrum whereas second arc lines the distal convex surface of same carpals, third arc outlines proximal curvatures of capitate and hamate (Fig. 2).

Additionally, the pisiform, a sesamoid bone serves as an attachment point to flexor carpi ulnaris tendon (Herzberg 2008). With the exception of flexor carpi ulnaris on the pisiform, none of the tendons that move the wrist inserts onto carpal bones. This means stabilization of the carpal bones is almost entirely passive, movements being dependent on the shapes of the articulations between bones and their passive stabilization by a complicated series of intrinsic ligaments.

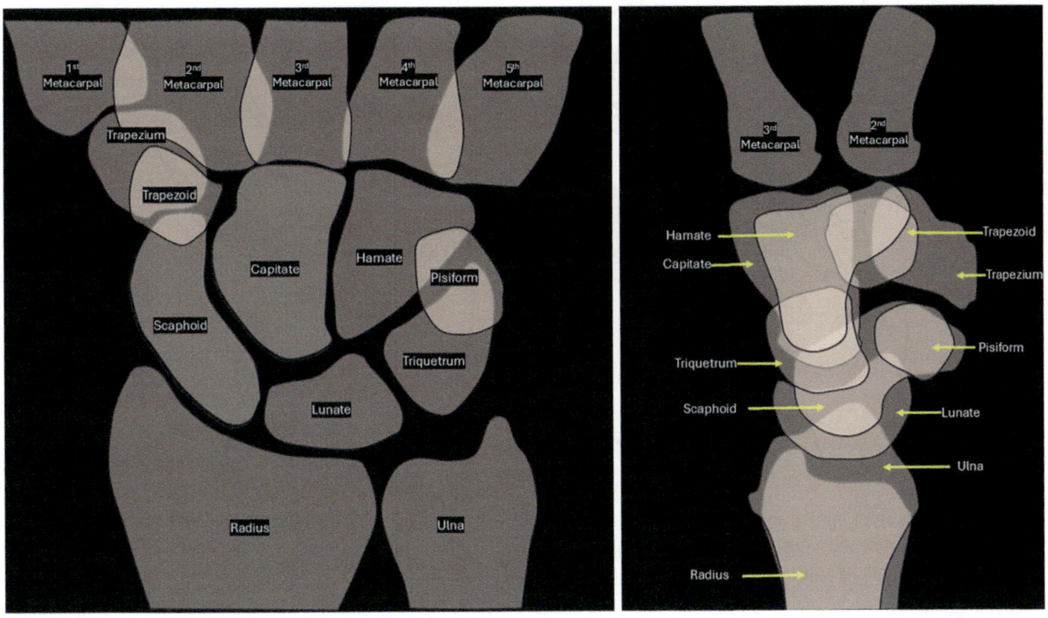

Fig. 1 Schematic representation of wrist joint bones in AP and coronal view

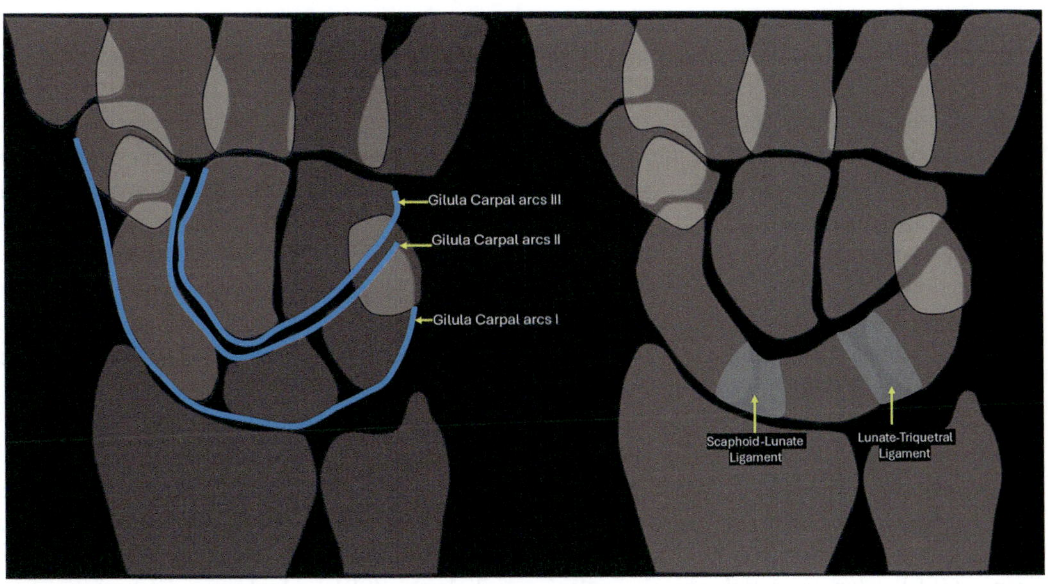

Fig. 2 Schematic representation of Gilula carpal arcs, SL, LT ligaments

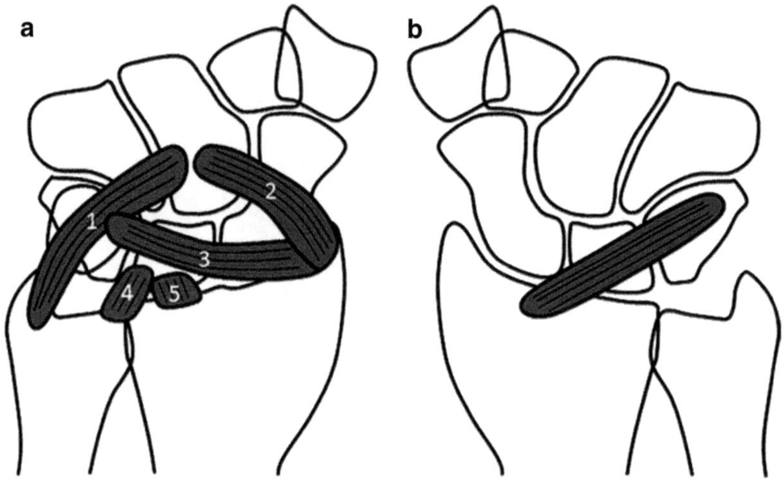

Fig. 3 Diagram showing the major extrinsic ligaments of the wrist. (**a**) Volar showing 1 = ulnotriquetralcapitate, 2 = radioscaphoidcapitate, 3 = radiolunatetriquetral, 4 = ulnolunate, 5 = radiolunate. (**b**) Dorsal showing the radiotriquetral ligament which also has an attachment to the lunate

The radiocarpal joint partly includes distal articular surface of the radius and the convex surfaces of scapholunate bones. The midcarpal joint is defined by several areas: the scaphotrapeziotrapezoid (STT) and scaphocapitate spaces laterally, the lunocapitate space centrally, and the triquetral-hamate space medially (Moritomo et al. 2007). Most ligaments of the wrist are located within the joint capsule, with exceptions being the transverse carpal ligament and the pisohamate, pisometacarpal ligaments, which attach to the pisiform.

Wrist ligaments fall into two groups: the extrinsic ligaments linking the radius or ulna to the carpal bones and the intrinsic ligaments running between carpal bones. The two most important intrinsic ligaments lie in the proximal carpal row, between the scaphoid and lunate (scapholunate) and between the lunate and triquetral (lunatetriquetral) bones. Scapholunate interosseous ligament (SLIL), lunotriquetral interosseous ligament (LTIL), midcarpal ligaments, and the interosseous ligaments of the distal carpal row. Among the midcarpal ligaments, the triquetro-hamate-capitate (THC) and scaphocapitate (SC) ligaments are critical, forming the arcuate ligament that spans the midcarpal joint. The volar aspect of the wrist lacks a distinct capsular ligament connecting the lunate and capitate, an area known as the space of Poirier, which is relatively weak. The interosseous ligaments of the distal carpal row play a key role in protecting the contents of the carpal tunnel (Garcia-Elias et al. 1989). The dorsal component of the SL and the volar component of the LT ligaments are the thickest and most important components for stabilization (Cerezal et al. 2012). The lunate attachments of the two ligaments are stronger than the scaphoid and triquetral attachments which means injury will tend to occur at the scaphoid attachment of the SL ligament and at the triquetral attachment of the LT ligament.

Extrinsic ligaments are divided into palmar and dorsal groups. Important palmar extrinsic radiocarpal and ulnocarpal ligaments include the radioscaphocapitate (RSC), radioscaphoid (RS), long radiolunate (LRL)/radiolunotriquetral, short radiolunate (SRL), ulnolunate (UL), ulnotriquetral (UT), ulnocapitate (UC), and ligaments. The RSC and LRL ligaments are visible on standard MR imaging. Dorsal radiotriquetral (DRT) ligament, a broad fan-shaped structure connecting the dorsal radius and triquetrum (Berger 1997) (Figs. 3 and 4).

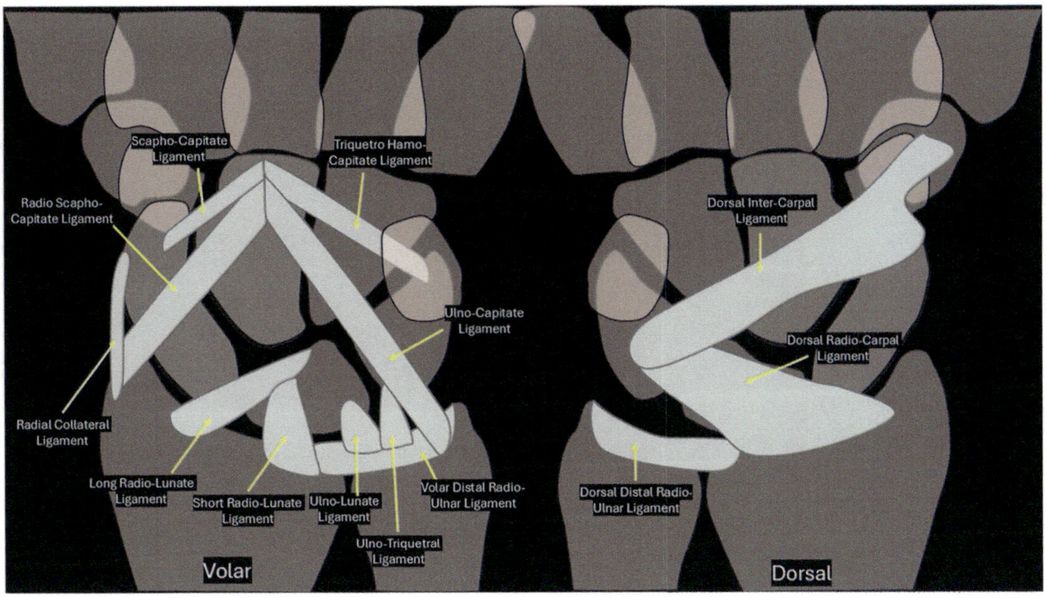

Fig. 4 Schematic representation of ligaments wrist on Volar, Dorsal aspect

3 The Clinical Problem

The classical presentation of carpal instability is a patient presenting with reduced range of motion and wrist pain and mechanical symptoms, usually a clunk. Such a presentation requires the clinician to establish the cause of the mechanical symptoms by identifying the site of instability.

A clunk is described as a low-pitched dull sound, caused by sudden subluxation or reduction of a partially dislocated carpal bone (Gilula et al. 2002). Various types are described. The origin may be from a particular carpal row with disruption of the SL ligament within the proximal carpal row the most frequently described entity (Amadio 1991). LT instability is a less frequently encountered pattern of proximal carpal row instability. In the authors' experience, midcarpal laxity or instability (MCI) is the most frequently encountered cause of the clunking wrist in daily practice.

The most frequently used and widely recognized system for the classification of carpal instability is the MAYO classification. This system identifies four categories of instability (Dobyns 1998).

Type I:	Carpal instability dissociative (CID), representing instability occurring within a carpal row with S-L or L-T intercarpal ligament disruption as examples.
Type II:	Carpal instability non-dissociative (CIND), described as carpal instability between rows. This falls into three broad groups: instability between the radius and proximal carpal row, instability between the proximal and distal carpal rows, or a combination of the two.
Type III:	Carpal instability complex (CIC), a combination of types I and II.
Type IV:	Adaptive carpal instability (CIA), in which abnormal carpal kinematics result from trauma such as a distal radial malunion, or congenital dysplasia.

The reality is frequently more complex than this apparently simple classification suggests and the clinical situation is rarely clear. Because of this imaging assessment is commonly required.

3.1 Carpal Instability Dissociative (CID)

CID involves misalignment between bones of the same carpal row. This can affect the proximal row, with examples including scapholunate dis-

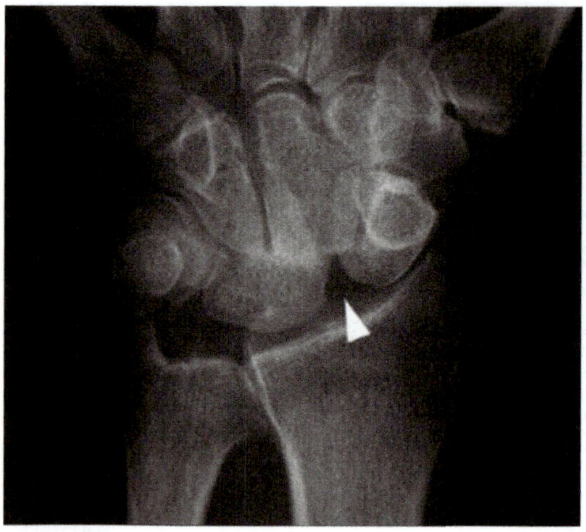

Fig. 5 Scapholunate dissociation. There is widening of the scapholunate interval (*arrowhead*) and the resulting flexion of the scaphoid results in overlapping of the body and distal pole of the scaphoid giving the signet-ring sign

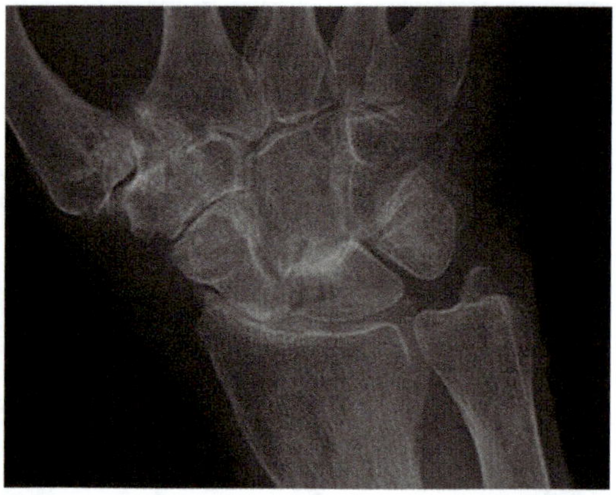

Fig. 6 Scapoholunate advanced collapse (SLAC). Long-standing scapholunate dissociation has resulted in osteoarthritis with joint space loss and sclerosis at the midcarpal and radioscaphoid joints

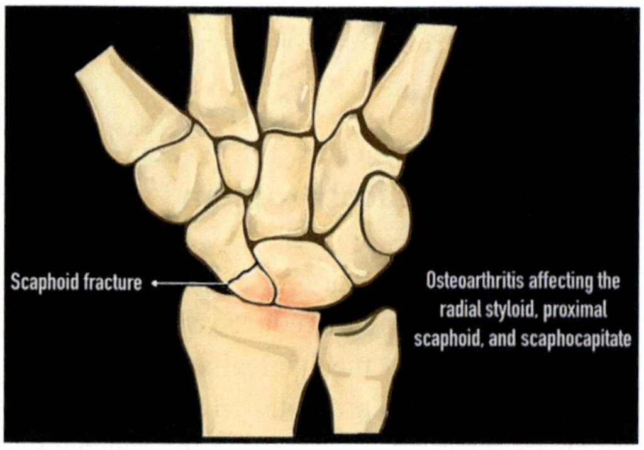

Fig. 7 Schematic representation of radiocarpal osteoarthritis

sociation (SLD), scaphoid fracture, Kienböck's disease, lunotriquetral dissociation or the distal row such as axial carpal dislocations. SLD is the most common CID pattern, often resulting from an injury causing wrist hyperextension and ulnar deviation, leading to static carpal collapse with volar flexion of the scaphoid and dorsal tilt of the lunate.

Scapholunate Dissociation (SLD): Disruption of the connection between the scaphoid and lunate (Fig. 5). It can occur as an isolated injury or associated with distal radial or displaced scaphoid fractures. An advanced stage, rotary subluxation of the scaphoid, involves failure of ligaments at both ends of the scaphoid, causing it to collapse into flexion and pronation (Watson et al. 1997). If scaphoid stabilizers (palmar RSC, SC, and anterolateral STT ligaments) also fail, permanent carpal misalignment results, leading to a DISI deformity (volar tilt of the scaphoid and dorsal tilt of the lunate). Chronic SLD can progress to scapholunate advanced collapse (SLAC), marked by degenerative changes, severe radioscaphoid space narrowing, and proximal capitate migration between the scaphoid and lunate.

In long-standing, often missed, SL lesions a Scapho-Lunate-Advanced-Collapse (SLAC) (Fig. 6) wrist will develop, although it is unknown how fast this may occur. Depending on the stage of the disease the radiograph will show the SL dissociation combined with osteoarthritis typically at the radioscaphoid and/or the midcarpal joints (Fig. 7). Radiologists need to detect and recognize early SL ligament lesions, in order to prevent this often devastating condition.

Clinical diagnosis of SLD is confirmed with a positive scaphoid shift test (Watson et al. 1988). Imaging shows a widened and irregular SL gap (>4.5 mm), lack of parallel alignment of scapholunate bones on coronal images, fluid accumulation surrounding torn or an absent ligament, in sagittal section images appearance of DISI should raise suspicion of SLD (Linscheid et al. 1972).

Lunotriquetral Dissociation (LTD): LTD can result from trauma/ulnocarpal abutment, often associated with TFCC (triangular fibrocartilage complex lesions) (Shin et al. 2001). It typically occurs from a fall on an outstretched hand with external arm rotation, forearm supination, and wrist extension with radial deviation. This leads to slight dorsal lunate translation due to scaphoid flexion (via an intact SLIL), causing a VISI deformity. MRI accuracy for detecting LTIL tears is about 50%, with fluid accumulation serving as an indirect sign, scapholunate angle in VISI deformity <30°, and capitolunate angle >30° (normal capitolunate angle <30°, normal scapholunate angle 30–60°) (Figs. 8 and 9).

The classic signs described on PA and lateral radiographs of the wrist are the dorsal intercalated segmental instability (DISI) and volar intercalated segmental instability (VISI) pattern (Gilula et al. 2002). It must be remembered that these are not diagnoses as such; they are merely signs reflecting underlying pathology although they are also seen in healthy individuals (then sometimes referred to as DISI or VISI configuration (Metz et al. 1997)).

A DISI deformity is characterized by dorsal tilting of the lunate compared to the scaphoid. This will result in an increased scapho-lunate (SL) angle, generally above 60–80° (there is some variation in the normal values given in the literature) (Fig. 10). A DISI pattern is classically described in patients with lesions of the SL ligament (Fig. 11) while a VISI pattern is classically described in patients with lesions of the LT liga-

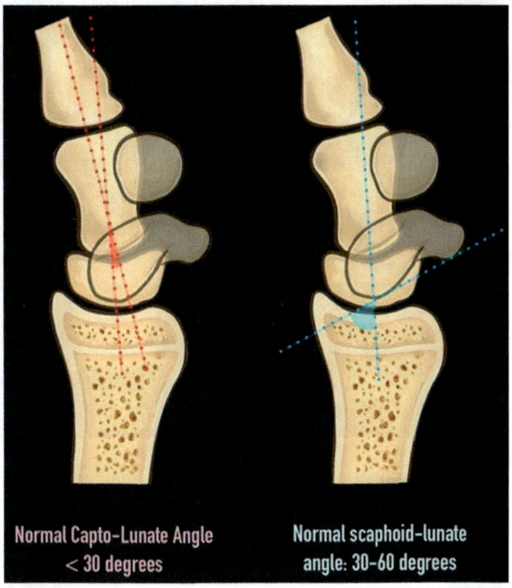

Fig. 8 Schematic representation of normal Captolunate, Scapholunate angles

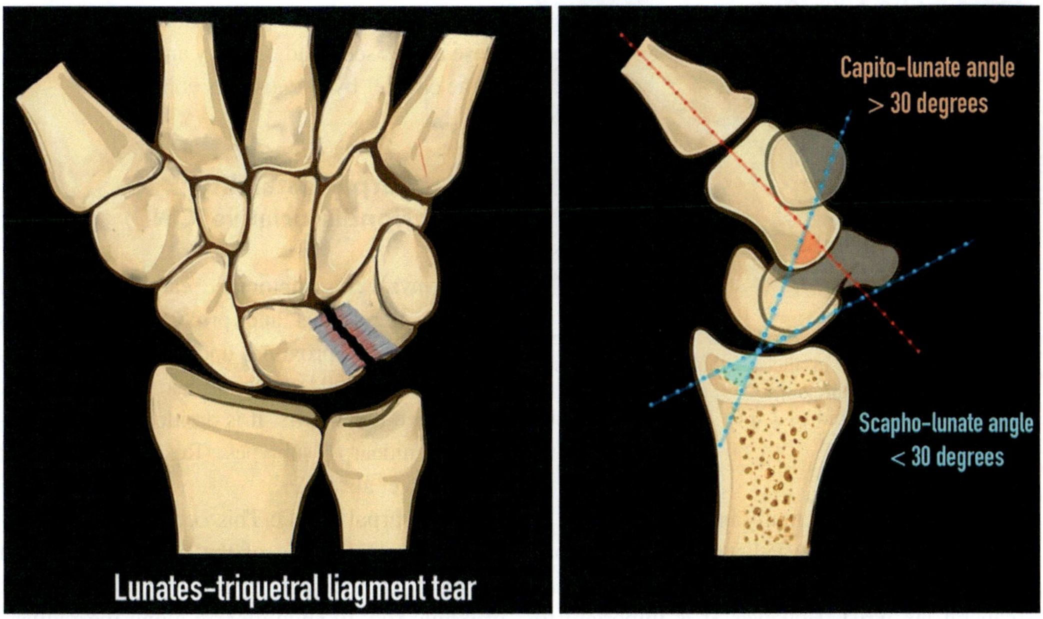

Fig. 9 Schematic representation of LT ligament tear

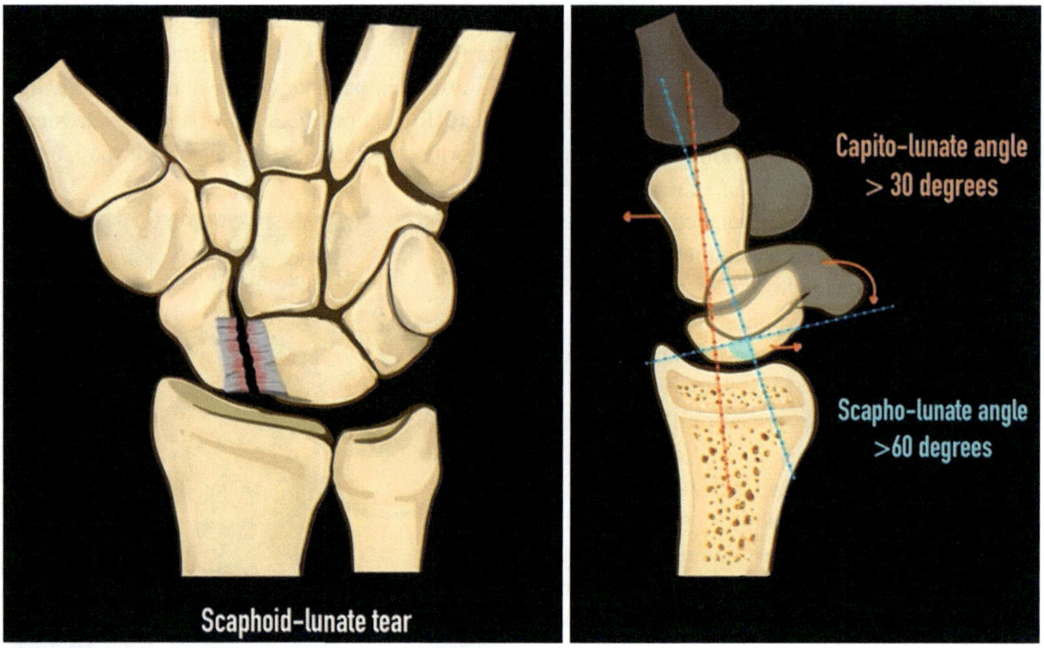

Fig. 10 Schematic representation of SL ligament tear

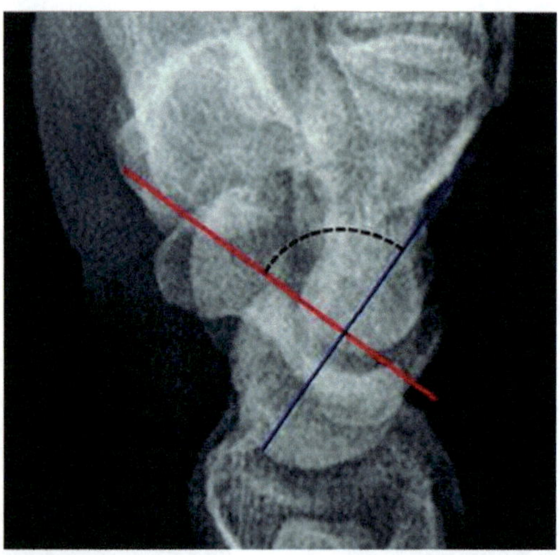

Fig. 11 DISI deformity on lateral wrist radiograph. There is an increase in the scapholunate angle (see "Radiography and Arthrography") (*dotted line*) between the axis of the scaphoid (*red line*) and the axis of the lunate (*blue line*)

ment however this is actually infrequently seen in LT ligament lesions. A VISI stance is much more frequently encountered in midcarpal instability or a general lax wrist. However, it is important to realize that both are also seen in patients with intact SL and LT ligaments who have other injured ligaments (Dobyns 1998). A VISI deformity is identified when there is volar tilting of the lunate compared to the scaphoid resulting in a decreased scapho-lunate angle. Generally, this is described as below 30° although again numbers vary in the literature. For details of methods of measuring these angles see "Radiography and Arthrography" in the chapter by Davies, this volume.

3.2 Carpal Instability Nondissociative (CIND)

CIND involves symptomatic carpal dysfunction between the radius and proximal row carpals or between the proximal and distal carpal rows (Wright et al. 1994), without disruption within or in between these rows. It is divided into radiocarpal and midcarpal subtypes. (Resnick et al. 2006; Linscheid et al. 1972).

Radiocarpal CIND: This occurs due to insufficiency or disruption of the obliquely oriented extrinsic radiocarpal ligaments, allowing the proximal row to slide ulnarly along the radius's sloped articular surface (Rayhack et al. 1987;

Backhouse 1986). It is associated with conditions like rheumatoid arthritis, Madelung's deformity, distal ulna surgical excision, or injury (Cooney et al. 1980). Common forms of CIND include ulnar translocation, radial translocation, and pure radiocarpal dislocation.

Ulnar Translocation: Here, part or all of the proximal carpal row shifts ulnarly along the radius's distal surface. This may result from wrist hyperextension, pronation and ulnar deviation during injury. Taleisnik described two types (Backhouse 1986): Type I, where the entire carpus, including the scaphoid, shifts ulnarly due to RS and RSC ligament failure, widening the radial styloid-scaphoid distance; and Type II, where the scaphoid and radius stay aligned, but other carpal bones move ulnarly, increasing the scapholunate interval (Resnick et al. 2006).

Midcarpal Instability Nondissociative (MCI)/ Midcarpal Instability: MCI involves dysfunction of both radiocarpal and midcarpal joints, with the midcarpal joint being primarily affected. Key stabilizers include the THC, dorsolateral STT, and RSC ligaments. Four types exist: palmar, dorsal, combined, and extrinsic.

In palmar MCI, the proximal row flexes volarly, causing a VISI pattern due to failure of midcarpal-crossing intrinsic ligaments, especially the THC ligament, with additional dorsal radiocarpal ligament insufficiency. Dorsal MCI, seen in young patients with hypermobile wrists, features dorsal capitate subluxation and dorsal tilting of the scaphoid and lunate, associated with an additional volar RSC ligament failure. Combined MCI shows exaggerated dorsal MCI with additional dorsal subluxation of scaphoid, lunate, and capitate. Extrinsic MCI stems from a malunited distal radius fracture, causing dorsal tilting of the articular surface and subsequent lunate dorsal tilt.

3.3 Carpal Instability Complex (CIC)

CIC occurs when carpal misalignment involves both within-row (CID features) and between-proximal and distal row (CIND features) disruptions. Five CIC groups are recognized:

(1) Dorsal perilunate dislocation (lesser arc injury). (2) Dorsal perilunate fracture-dislocation (greater arc injury). (3) Palmar perilunate dislocation (lesser or greater arc injury). (4) Axial dislocation. (5) Isolated carpal bone dislocation

Lesser arc injuries are pure ligamentous, while greater arc injuries involve trans osseous injuries with carpal fractures around the lunate. The first two groups involve lunate-centered derangements (lesser and greater arc injuries, respectively). The third group, palmar perilunate dislocation, results from a different mechanism causing distal row displacement relative to the lunate. The fourth and fifth groups are non-perilunate dislocations from high-energy trauma.

Dorsal Perilunate Dislocation (Lesser Arc Injury): This common injury involves dorsal displacement of the carpus while the lunate remains in the radius's lunate fossa, as a pure dislocation without fracture. Mayfield et al. outlined four stages of progressive perilunate instability (Mayfield et al. 1980):

- Stage I: Hyperextension forces the distal row to extend, pulling the scaphoid via the scapho-trapeziocapitate ligament, opening the space of Poirier. The lunate's limited extension, constrained by the SRL, may lead to SLIL failure, starting dorsally, defining SLD (Moritomo et al. 2007).
- Stage II: The scaphoid-capitate complex dislocates dorsally relative to the lunate, with the RSC ligament limiting translation (Garcia-Elias et al. 1989) as the distal row and dissociated proximal row follow dorsally, widening the space of Poirier.
- Stage III: Persistent hyperextension may extend the triquetrum via the THC ligament, tearing the LTIL or causing triquetrum avulsion. Complete LTIL disruption tears the LRL's ulnar expansions, leaving the SRL (Schuind et al. 1992) and volar UL ligaments as lunate stabilizers.
- Stage IV: The dorsally displaced capitate, pulled by the intact RSC (Garcia-Elias et al. 1989) proximally and volarly into the radiocarpal

space, pushing the lunate volarly through the space of Poirier, resulting in lunate dislocation as end stage of dorsal perilunate dislocation.

Dorsal Perilunate Fracture-Dislocation (Greater Arc Injury): This involves perilunate dislocation with fractures of the either scaphoid, hamate, capitate or triquetrum. The only true greater arc injury is a trans-scaphoid, transtriquetral, transcapitate and transhamate perilunate fracture-dislocation. Other forms include bone avulsions, ligament ruptures and additional fractures, with trans-scaphoid perilunate dislocation being the most common.

3.4 Carpal Instability Adaptive (CIA)

CIA arises from extracarpal pathology rather than intracarpal issues (1). Examples include malunion of a distal radial fracture causing proximal row adaptation to abnormal radial tilt; Madelung's deformity with volar radius tilt and dorsally subluxed ulna, leading to proximal row changes (Taleisnik and Watson 1984).

For diagnosing CIA it requires ruling out significant intracarpal ligament injury to distinguish it from extrinsic MCI, though similarities exist due to similar extracarpal pathologies. Treatment focuses on correcting the malunion (Carlsen and Shin 2008).

4 Imaging

4.1 Conventional Radiography

The primary imaging modality for wrist problems in general and specifically for patients with an unstable wrist is conventional radiography. It is recommended that both wrists are imaged enabling comparison; this can only be done if standardized techniques are used. Although this standardized technique is well described in the literature (Gilula et al. 2002; Peh and Gilula 1994), awareness of such standardization among radiographers and clinicians is often lacking. Training of radiology technicians and radiographers in how to achieve optimal and reproducible images should be part of the clinical responsibility of the supervising radiologist. The measurement of specific angles that are extensively described in the literature with respect to carpal instabilities can only be done reliably on these standardized images (Gilula et al. 2002). Ideally, the technician should be part of the team dealing with wrist pathologies.

Although the use of conventional PA and lateral radiographs is widely adopted, the value of additional views is questionable and debated in the literature and among clinicians. Several additional views (instability series and/or stress views) are described; PA views with maximal ulnar and maximal radial deviation, and AP clenched fist views are among the ones most commonly used (Gilula et al. 2002; Peh and Gilula 1994; De Filippo et al. 2006; Metz et al. 1997). In some cases up to 15 different additional views to analyze the wrist of a single patient are described (Metz et al. 1997). However, the literature on standardization of technique and reproducibility of these additional views is very limited. Although these views are described as being advantageous for analyzing wrist instability in the authors' opinion they hold significant limitations. Too many variables are introduced, for instance the maximum ulnar or radial deviation differs enormously between patients and within the same patient at different time points. Furthermore, these views have not been tested in a healthy population with no established normal parameters. An additional problem is that views with maximal ulnar and radial deviation only provide information on the endpoints of deviation and lack information on the whole pathway of the movement (see section on 4D imaging, White 2019). One also has to be aware of the normal movement patterns of the carpals and their projection on the radiographs in normal situations. In maximal radial deviation, the projection of the scaphoid and lunate is completely different compared to views in maximal ulnar deviation. If the radiologist is unaware of this phenomenon, adequate interpretation of these views is difficult.

4.2 Other Imaging Modalities

4.2.1 MR Imaging and CT

The aim with cross-sectional imaging modalities is to identify the nature and extent of ligamentous disruption and to identify any associated abnormality such as articular cartilage damage. As discussed above, the conventional radiographic signs only develop later after injury and direct visualization of the ligaments is required to diagnose their disruption. If primary ligament repair is planned this has to be undertaken early or there is a high risk of nonhealing (Garcia-Elias and Geissler 2005; Lindau 2010).

The sensitivity of MRI for SL ligament tear detection is reported as between 37 and 95% (Johnstone et al. 1997; Manton et al. 2001; Zlatkin et al. 1989). Using non-arthrographic 3T MRI the sensitivity is better for complete tears than for partial tears and the sensitivity and specificity for SL lesions is higher than for LT lesions. Sensitivity is considerably improved by the use of MR arthrography but this turns a non-invasive investigation into one with intra-articular injections in at least 1 or 2 compartments (radiocarpal and midcarpal joints). Sensitivity is reported as between 62% and 100% (Braun et al. 2003; Meier et al. 2002; Schmitt et al. 2003). It is not uncommon to have normal degenerative perforations in the membranous component of the intrinsic ligaments which means that the passage of contrast on MR arthrography between the radiocarpal and midcarpal joints is not in itself evidence of a symptomatic or significant ligament injury. Although 3T conventional MRI shows good sensitivity to intrinsic ligament disruption, arthrographic contrast still seems to improve sensitivity (Magee 2009). There are no comparative studies between 1.5 and 3T regarding lesions of the SL and/or LT ligament (Saupe 2009; Schmid et al. 2005; Stehling et al. 2009). In the authors' experience 3T non-arthrographic studies provide adequate demonstration of the morphology of the important intrinsic wrist ligaments (Figs. 12 and 13). When this is combined with functional assessment using videofluoroscopy MR arthrography is rarely needed.

Coronal and axial imaging provides the best means of assessing the intrinsic wrist ligaments. Full-thickness ligament disruption is seen as non-visualization, or a full-thickness defect in the ligament (Figs. 14 and 15). Partial ligament disruption may be appreciated as a focal discontinuity in a component of the ligament (Fig. 16).

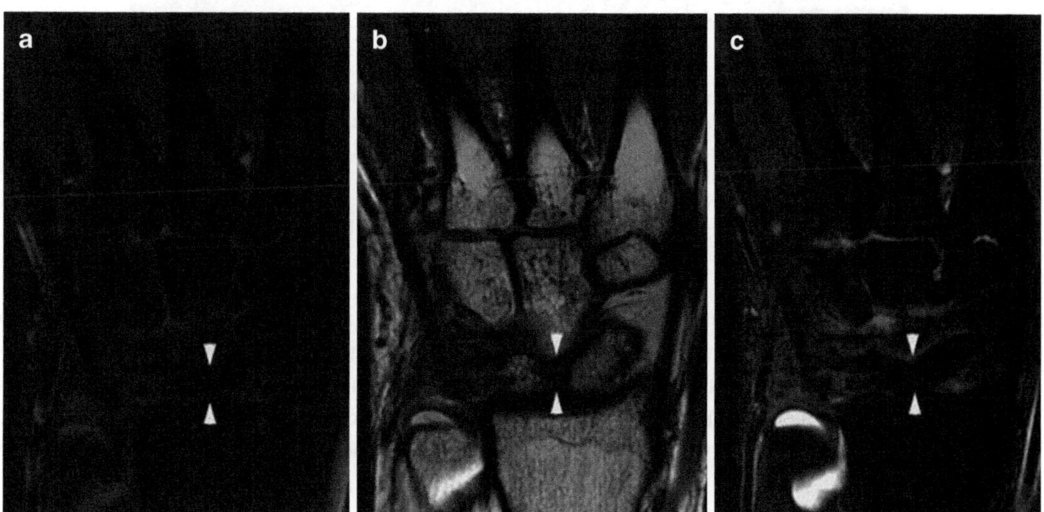

Fig. 12 Coronal 3T images (2 mm, dedicated wrist coil) on T1 FS (**a**), PD (**b**) and T2 FS (**c**) the dorsal, functionally most important, component of the scapho-lunate intrinsic ligament (SLIL) is seen. The separate fibers are well delineated (*arrowheads*)

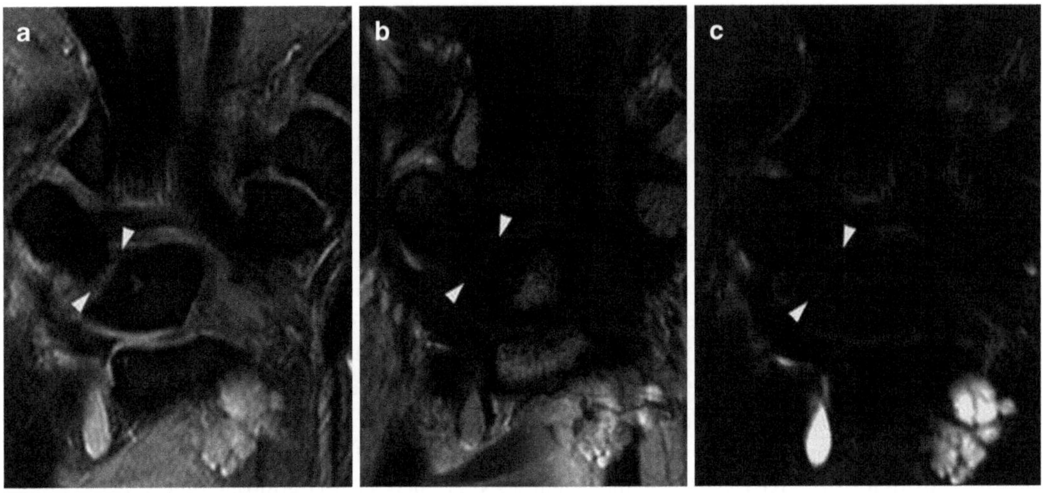

Fig. 13 Coronal 3T images (2 mm, dedicated wrist coil) On T1 FS (**a**), PD (**b**) and T2 FS (**c**) the functionally most important volar component of the luno-triquetral intrinsic ligament (LTIL) is seen and separate fibers are well delineated (*arrowheads*)

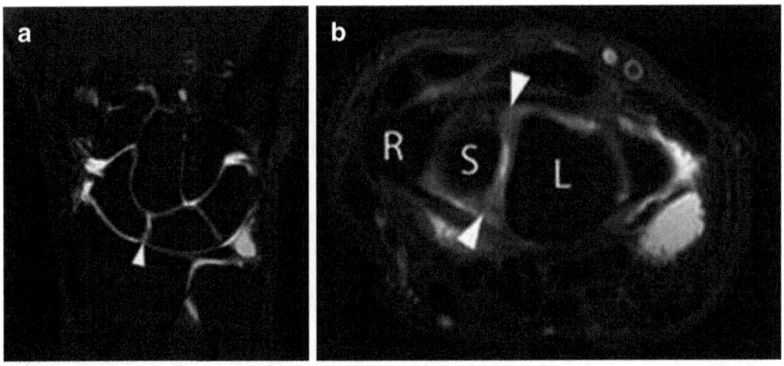

Fig. 14 Full-thickness tear of scapholunate ligament. (**a**) Coronal T1 fat-suppressed image from MR arthrogram. Only the radial carpal joint was injected with gadolinium, but contrast passes freely through the scapholunate interval into the midcarpal joint as a result of a scapholunate ligament tear (*arrowhead*). Note also contrast is seen in the distal radioulnar joint as a result of a triangular fibrocartilage complex tear. This coronal section only shows the tear in the membranous portion of the ligament. (**b**) Axial T1 image from MR arthrogram. The proximal scaphoid (S) and lunate (L) are demonstrated with complete disruption of the volar and dorsal components of the scapholunate ligament arrowheads. R = radial styloid. (Figure supplied by Dr AJ Grainger, Leeds, UK)

High signal intensity can be seen in the ligament of fat-saturated images. However, it should be noted that discontinuities in the membranous portion of the ligament may not be significant if the volar and dorsal components of the ligament are intact (Fig. 17).

MRI is the imaging modality of choice for the evaluation of the extrinsic ligaments of the wrist. The palmar scapho-capitate and triquetro-hamo-capitate ligaments, together often called the arcuate ligament are the most important ones to identify in patients with palmar midcarpal instability. The visualization of the arcuate ligament is described in cadavers using conventional MR imaging as well as with MR arthrography (Theumann et al. 2003; Chang et al. 2007); however clinical descriptions of its use are rare.

CT on its own is of less value in the diagnosis of carpal instability. However, combined with an arthrographic injection demonstration of the intrinsic ligaments can be achieved and there is literature comparing MR imaging and MR arthrography versus CT arthrography in which the latter is more sensitive especially for partial injuries to the intrinsic ligaments (Schmid et al. 2005; Moser et al. 2007). CT can be useful to assess the later stages of the disease (SLAC wrist), especially to determine the amount of cartilage damage. In the preoperative planning of salvage procedures, such as proximal row carpectomy or four-corner fusion, Lunate-Capitate-Triquetrum-Hamate (LCTH) arthrodesis, CT scanning provides essential additional information for the hand surgeon.

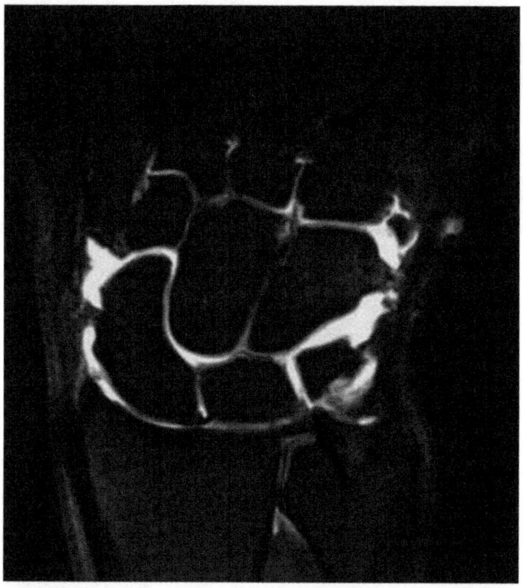

Fig. 15 Tear of lunate-triquetral ligament. Coronal T1 fat-suppressed MR arthrographic image. There is diastasis of the lunate-triquetral joint with disruption of the lunate-triquetral ligament (*arrow*)

4.2.2 Cineradiography

The drawback of cross-sectional imaging (as with radiographs) is the static nature of these modalities. Since instability is essentially a dynamic problem, dynamic imaging modalities such as cineradiography and fluoroscopy are particularly suited for its investigation (Protas and Jackson 1980). Both wrists can easily be examined, at relatively little cost and in a minimum amount of time compared to an MRI study. Examining both wrists offers the advantage that the examiner has a good idea of the movement pattern of the non-injured wrist and this can be compared with the injured wrist. The images obtained can be easily stored in PACS for reviewing and for demonstration to the clinician. A standardized protocol has to be performed which should be developed after discussion with the hand surgeon. Different stress tests can be performed, although the Watson test (clinical test for

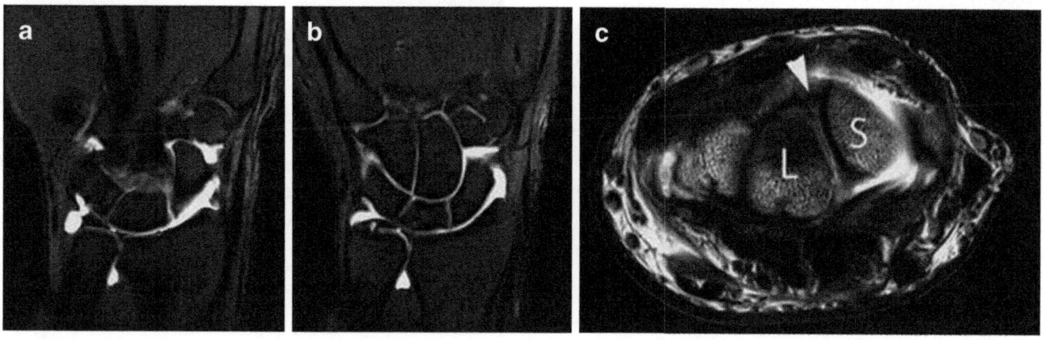

Fig. 16 Incomplete tear of scapholunate ligament. (**a**) Coronal T1 fat-suppressed MR arthrographic image through the volar aspect of the scapholunate joint shows disruption of the scapholunate ligament. (**b**) An adjacent coronal section from the same series showing the scapholunate ligament is intact more dorsally. (**c**) Axial T1MR arthrographic image through the proximal scapholunate joint (S = Scaphoid, L = Lunate) confirms the volar scapholunate ligament disruption with an intact dorsal component (*arrowhead*). Note A and B also show a full-thickness perforation of the triangular fibrocartilage with passage of contrast into the distal radioulnar joint. (Figure supplied by Dr AJ Grainger, Leeds, UK)

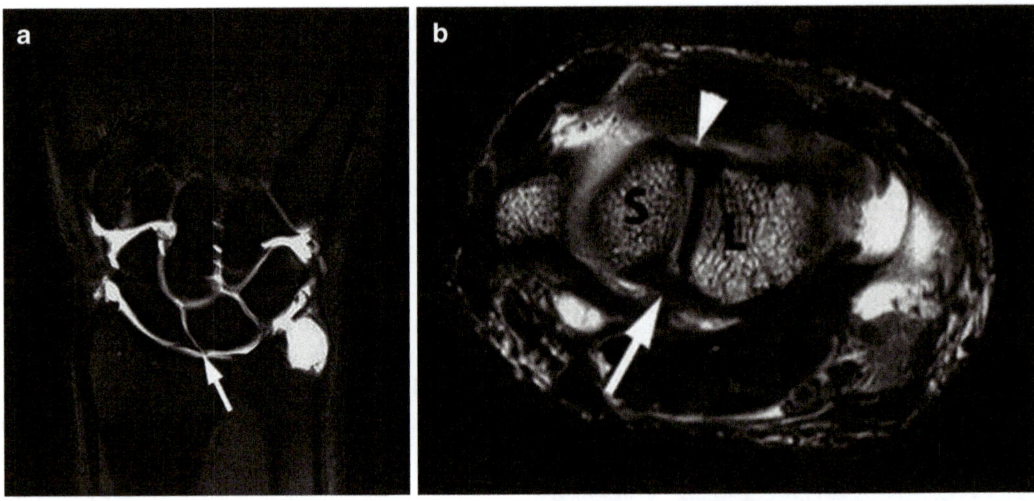

Fig. 17 Perforation of membranous component of scapholunate ligament. (**a**) Coronal T1 fat-suppressed MR arthrographic image through the scapholunate joint shows a perforation in the ligament with contrast communicating through the ligament into the midcarpal joint (*arrow*). (**b**) Axial T1 MR arthrographic image through the proximal scapholunate joint shows the important fibrous components of the ligament on the volar (*arrow*) and dorsal (*arrowhead*) aspects of the joint are intact. S = Scaphoid, L = Lunate

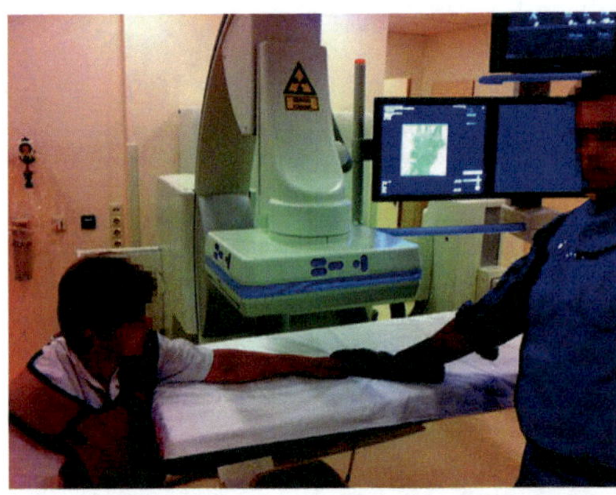

Fig. 18 Undertaking a cineradiographic examination of the wrist. The patient is seated at the end of the fluoroscopy table at the left side of the examiner. Both wear lead protection. The examiner wears protective lead gloves. The monitors are right in front of the examiner to evaluate the movement patterns in close detail

scapho-lunate instability) is difficult to perform due to technical reasons (lead gloves worn by the examiner). In order to perform a fluoroscopic examination one has to understand the normal kinematic movements of the wrist. Normal kinematics are extensively described in several (experimental) studies (Arimitsu et al. 2008; Kaufmann et al. 2006). A routine assessment of the non-injured wrist also helps understanding these normal kinematic patterns.

It is important to position the patient well during fluoroscopy (Fig. 18). The arm rests with the elbow on the fluoroscopy table to eliminate as much muscle action of the upper and lower arm on the hand (Fig. 19). Our protocol consists of: PA and lateral view with radial and ulnar deviation (Fig. 20), lateral view with palmar and dorsal flexion (Fig. 21), lateral view with anterior and posterior drawer test (Fig. 22), and finally the Lichtman test (Fig. 23).

There are surprisingly few studies that deal with the diagnostic accuracy of cineradiography for SL lesions. A study by Kwon and Baek (2008), using a cutoff point of a 2 mm scapholunate gap at fluoroscopy, mentioned a maximum sensitivity of 95% (Kwon and Baek 2008). In an unpublished study by the authors a

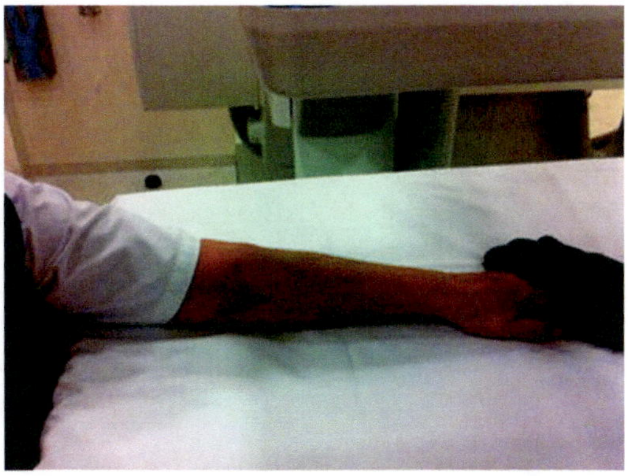

Fig. 19 Arm positioning. The elbow of the patient rests on the fluoroscopy table to eliminate forces exerted on the hand

sensitivity of 95% was found. In the authors' opinion the most appropriate imaging modality after plain films in cases of SL instability should be a fluoroscopic examination of the wrist because of the aforementioned advantages.

In midcarpal instability the Lichtman test is, in our opinion the most important stress test to perform, both clinically as well as using cine-radiography (Lichtman et al. 1981, 1993). In this test the thumb of the investigator is placed over the distal carpal row. With palmar translation of the carpus the proximal carpal row will move in flexion and with axial loading the

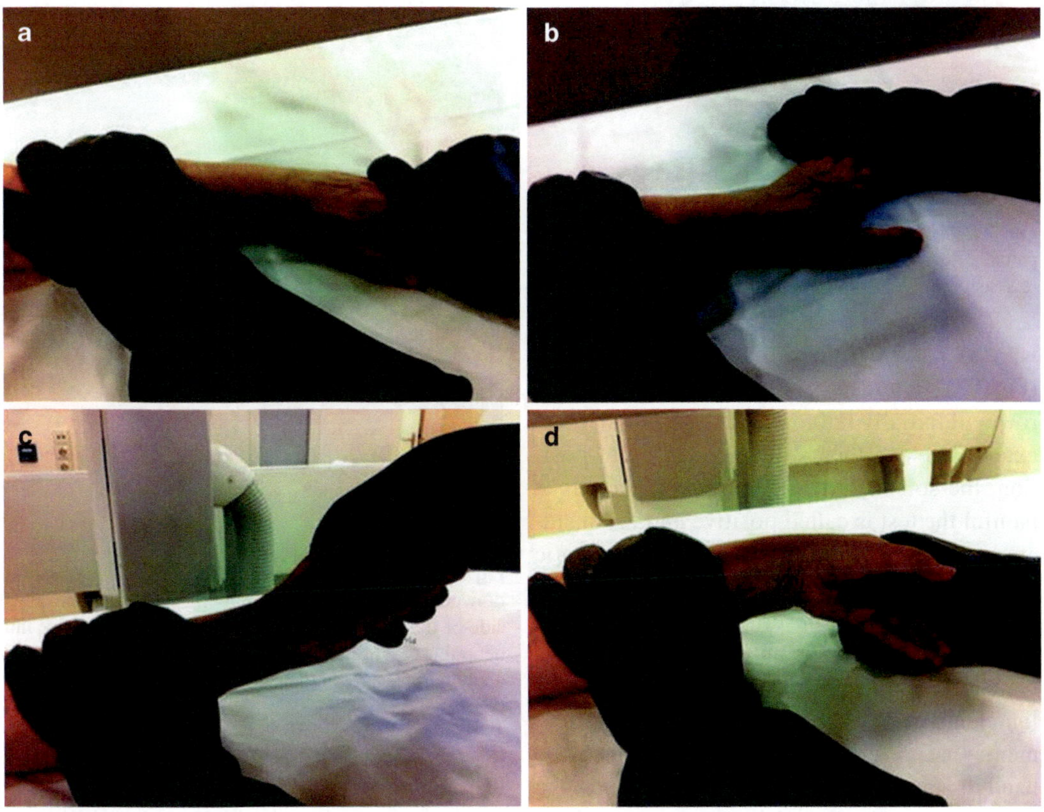

Fig. 20 The movements of the hand during the beginning of the examination. (**a**) PA view with radial deviation; (**b**) PA view with ulnar deviation; (**c**) lateral view with radial deviation; (**d**) lateral view with ulnar deviation

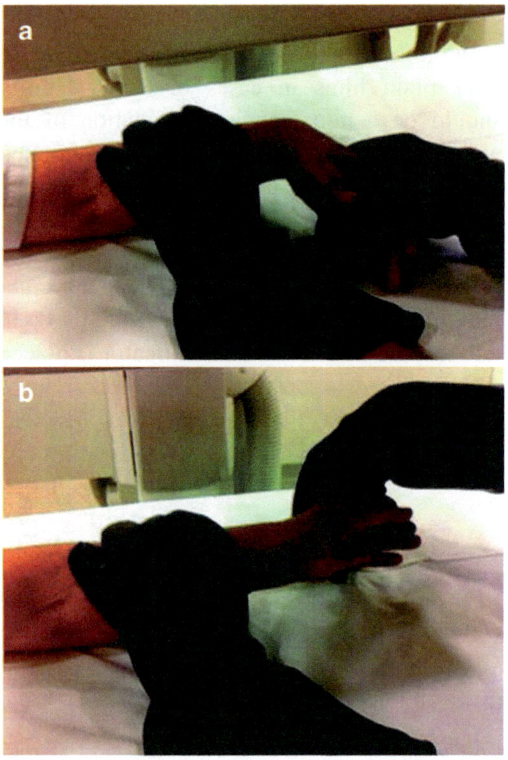

Fig. 21 Additional movements. (**a**) Lateral view with palmar flexion; (**b**) lateral view with dorsal flexion (extension)

wrist is moved from radial to ulnar deviation (Fig. 23). In midcarpal instability the proximal row will initially fail to translocate radially and extend but will then suddenly snap into position, the so-called "catch-up clunk". If this is painful the test is called positive and is considered a diagnostic indicator of a symptomatic midcarpal instability. The anterior and posterior drawer tests as described by Garcia-Elias are also important. The anterior drawing test is aimed at demonstrating laxity of the palmar ligaments especially the scaphotrapezial ligament; the posterior drawer test, in which the hand is translated dorsally compared to the wrist stresses the dorsal ligaments, especially the dorsal scaphotriquetral ligament. It is this test which is felt to be the most important test to demonstrate dorsal midcarpal instability.

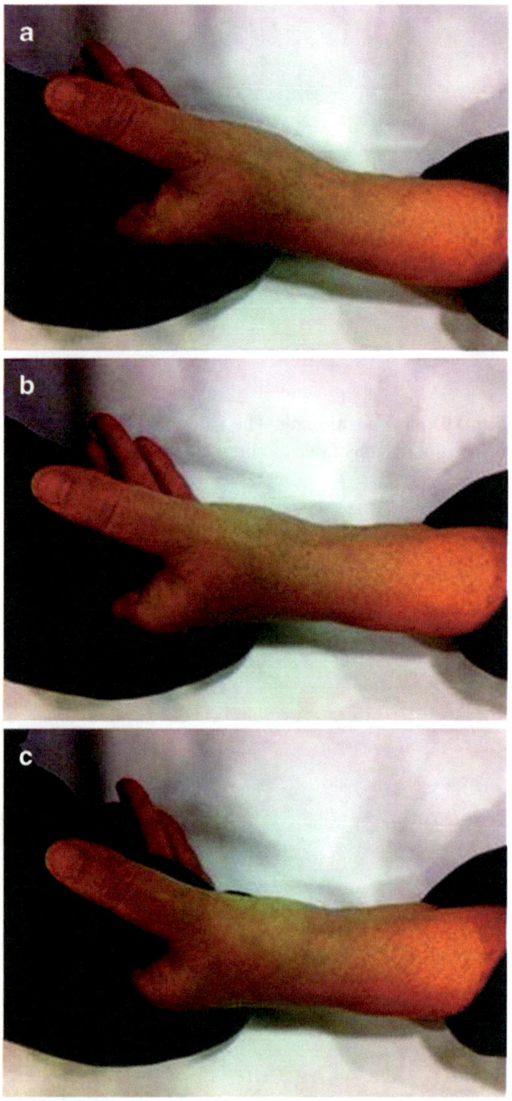

Fig. 22 Additional movements-drawer test. (**a**) Anterior drawer test is performed by applying pressure at the dorsal side of the hand. (**b**) The hand is then brought back into neutral. (**c**) The posterior drawer test is performed by applying pressure on the palmar side of the hand

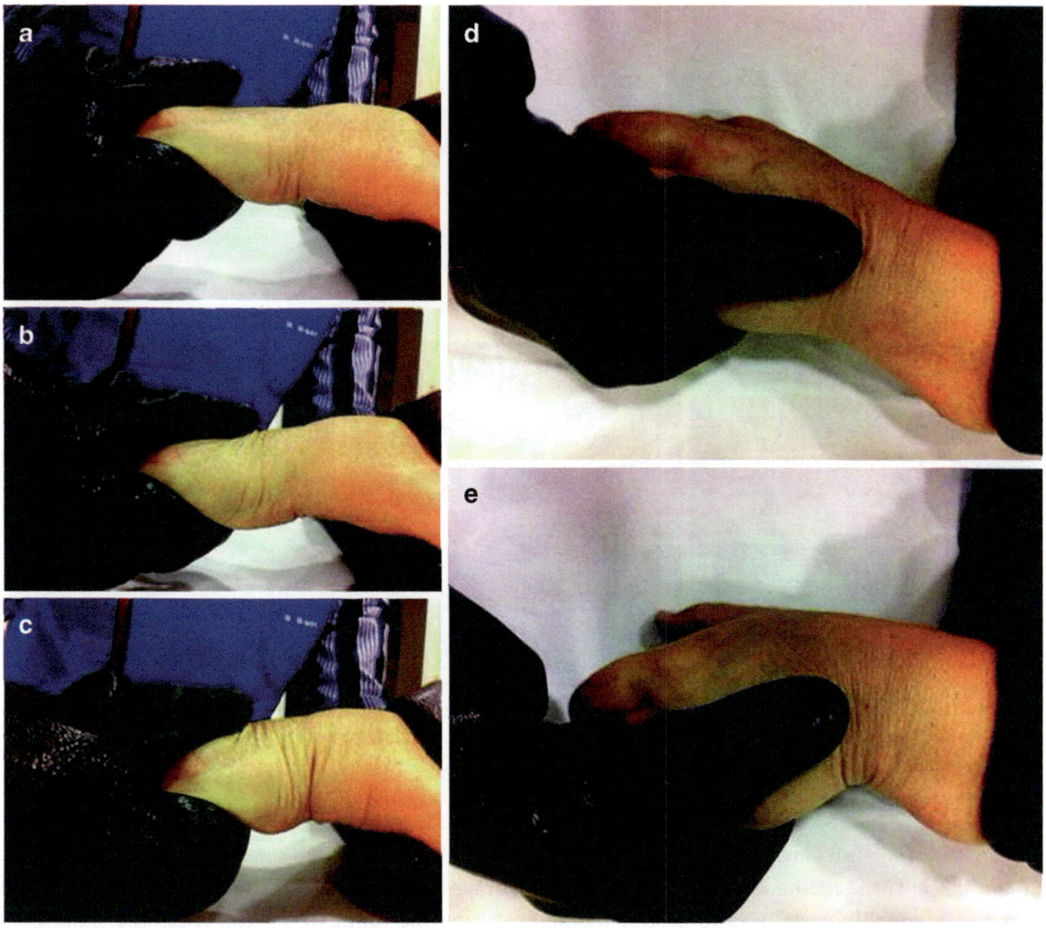

Fig. 23 The Lichtman or midcarpal shift test. (**a**) Initially the hand is in neutral position. (**b**) Dorsal pressure is applied. (**c–e**) Axial loading is then given and the hand is moved from radial to ulnar deviation

5 Understanding of Wrist Biomechanics by 4D Imaging

As discussed above, analysis of motion patterns of the carpal bones is often useful in diagnosis of instability patterns. Analysis of the complete motion trajectory of the carpal bones has been shown to be particular beneficial when no diagnostic signs are found in radiographs and stress views at maximal radial or ulnar deviation also show no abnormalities (Protas and Jackson 1980; Braunstein et al. 1985; Obermann 1996; Schmitt et al. 2006).

For the past 30 years cineradiography has been the instrument to image these instability patterns. New developments in detecting motion patterns of carpal bones are devoted to 4D imaging of carpal kinematics. Four-dimensional imaging provides for visualization and quantification of motion patterns of each individual carpal bone in 3D space (Carelsen et al. 2009; Crisco et al. 1999; Snel et al. 2000). Four-dimensional imaging methods are divided into quasi-dynamic CT-imaging of the wrist using multiple static poses of the hand (Crisco et al. 1999; Snel et al. 2000) and also true dynamic 4D imaging of car-

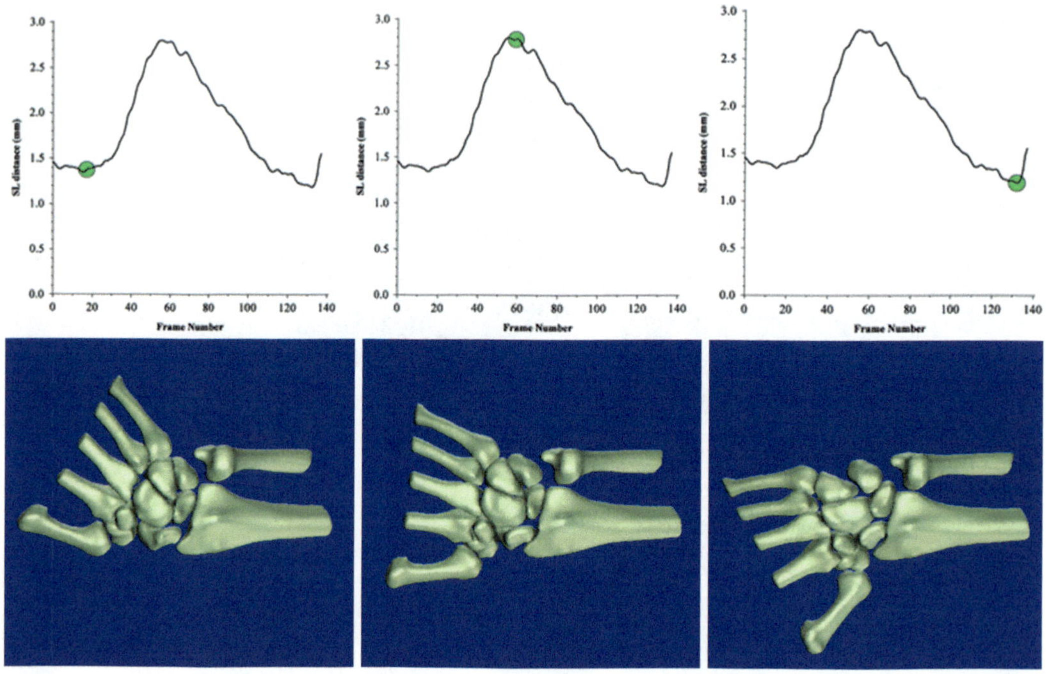

Fig. 24 Three time frames of a 4D image sequence of moving wrist bones in a patient with SL-dissociation. The image sequence shows widening and narrowing of the gap between the scaphoid and lunate (SL-distance) as a function of the hand position

pal bones during movement of the hand (Carelsen et al. 2009). These methods have advantage that they are potentially easier to interpret than cineradiography that uses 2D projections of the bone anatomy for each time frame. In 4D imaging the full 3D geometry of each carpal bone is available in each time frame. This also allows quantitative analysis of motion patterns in terms of translations and rotations of each individual bone as a function of time.

Currently, 4D imaging of the wrist joint is primarily used for basic research on joint biomechanics (Foumani et al. 2010a, b; Moojen et al. 2002, 2003; Moore et al. 2007; Streekstra et al. 2010) but has the potential to be used for clinical evaluation true 3D carpal instability patterns. An example of this potential is the detection of 3D motion pattern in a patient with SL dissociation. The motion pattern demonstrated reveals that widening of the bone gap between the scaphoid and lunate is not observed at maximal radial or ulnar deviation but at an intermediate of the hand during the range of motion (Fig. 16). This is in agreement with qualitative cineradiographic observations of carpal motion through radial-ulnar deviation (Snel et al. 2000). The added value of 4D imaging is the quantitative nature of the observation in terms of translations and rotations of carpal bones that may help to develop more objective parameters to diagnose instability patterns of joints (Fig. 24).

Another example of the possible usefulness of the 4D approach in diagnosing wrist problems is the detection of joint space width as a representation of cartilage thickness over the entire joint surface area as a function of hand position (Fig. 25). In patients with SL-dissociation the joint space seems to be reduced over the entire joint surface compared to healthy volunteers (Foumani et al. 2010a, b).

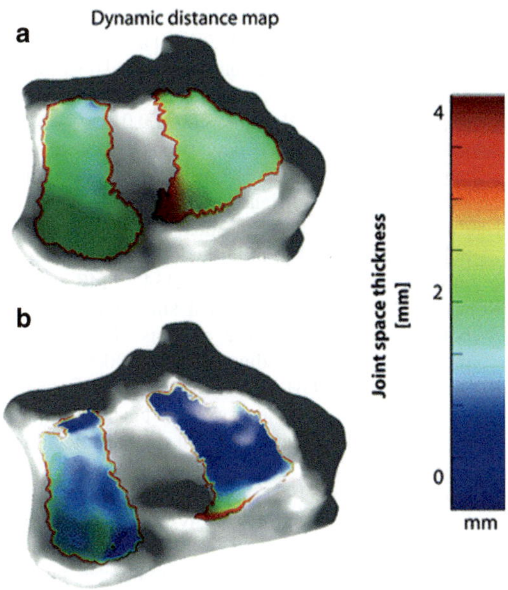

Fig. 25 Dynamic distance maps showing reduced minimal distance between adjacent joint surfaces in a follow-up acquisition of patients and healthy volunteers. (**a**) Healthy Volunteers. (**b**) Patients with scapholunate dissociation

6 Treatment and Clinical Perspective

One of the key purposes of non-invasive diagnostics is the triage between a conservative or invasive (arthroscopy or arthrotomy) therapeutic approach. In our setting cineradiography aids in tailoring the appropriate treatment for the specific patient with chronic undiagnosed wrist pain (CUWP), making the choice between surgical and physical therapy easier.

Fundamental research has shown that chronic wrist pain, without any morphological anatomical substrate detected by state-of-the-art diagnostic tools, could be controlled by non-surgical therapeutic strategies, such as adaptations in motor control (Smeulders et al. 2001). In a comparative study, Smeulders et al. 2001 found a significant difference in fluency of motion between patients and controls. They concluded that disturbance of fine motor control in CUWP may be a contributing factor to chronic wrist pain. A second case-control study in patients with CUWP compared to healthy volunteers described a significant difference in fluency of movement between the two groups (Smeulders et al. 2002). This difference was strikingly found in the unaffected wrist, in which the authors hypothesized that chronic wrist pain is maintained by persistent abnormal cerebral motor function.

Since instability of the wrist is a possible cause for unilateral wrist pain, undiagnosed with standard radiography, MRI or CT, the cause of this may also be due to persistent abnormal motor function. This has led to the development of a specialized training regime for this CUWP patient group (Videler et al. 1998). This exercise program tackles unstable wrists combining central cerebral focused motor re-education and muscle strengthen coordination. The use of cine radiography as a triage modality may be a beneficial, cost-effective manner of managing patients with pain in the chronic unstable wrist. In excluding other causes of wrist pain, and a positive finding of midcarpal instability, cineradiography can play a pivotal role.

Treatment details for carpal instability exceed this overview's scope and depend on factors like arthritis presence, injury chronicity, tissue quality, and deformity reducibility. For acute injuries with good soft tissue quality and reducible deformity, treatment aims to restore normal anatomy through ligament repair, carpal angle correction, and reconstruction. In cases with poor soft tissue quality, ligament reconstruction or salvage procedures like intercarpal or total wrist arthrodesis are considered.

Note: TFCC injuries subtopic has been covered in ulnar side wrist joint pain topic

Acknowledgments We would like to thank M. Foumani MD and Mrs. M.R.W. Evers-van Bavel for their help in preparing the manuscript.

References

Amadio PC (1991) Carpal kinematics and instability: a clinical and anatomic primer. Clin Anat 4(1):1–12

Arimitsu S et al (2008) Analysis of radiocarpal and midcarpal motion in stable and unstable rheumatoid wrists using 3-dimensional computed tomography. J Hand Surg 33(2):189–197

Backhouse K (1986) The wrist by Julio Taleisnik. 442 pages. Illustrations. Index. Bibliography. £80. Churchill Livingstone, New York, Edinburgh, London and Melbourne. 1985 ISBN 0-443-08134-4. J Hand Surg 11:483. https://doi.org/10.1016/0266-7681_86_90195-6

Berger RA (1997) The ligaments of the wrist. A current overview of anatomy with considerations of their potential functions. Hand Clin 13:63–82

Braun H et al (2003) Direct MR arthrography of the wrist-value in detecting complete and partial defects of intrinsic ligaments and the TFCC in comparison with arthroscopy. Rofo 175(11):1515–1524

Braunstein EM et al (1985) Fluoroscopic and arthrographic evaluation of carpal instability. AJR Am J Roentgenol 144(6):1259–1262

Carelsen B et al (2009) Detection of in vivo dynamic 3-D motion patterns in the wrist joint. IEEE Trans Biomed Eng 56(4):1236–1244

Carlsen BT, Shin AY (2008) Wrist instability. Scand J Surg 97:324–332. https://doi.org/10.1177/145749690809700409

Cerezal L et al (2012) MR and CT arthrography of the wrist. Semin Musculoskelet Radiol 16(1):27–41

Chang W et al (2007) Arcuate ligament of the wrist: normal MR appearance and its relationship to palmar midcarpal instability: a cadaveric study. Skeletal Radiol 36(7):641–645

Cooney WP, Dobyns JH, Linscheid RL (1980) Complications of Colles' fractures. J Bone Joint Surg Am 62:613–619

Crisco JJ, McGovern RD, Wolfe SW (1999) Noninvasive technique for measuring in vivo three-dimensional carpal bone kinematics. J Orthop Res 17(1):96–100

De Filippo M et al (2006) Pathogenesis and evolution of carpal instability: imaging and topography. Acta Biomed 77(3):168–180

Dobyns JH (1998) Classification of carpal instability. In: Cooney WP, Linscheid RL (eds) The wrist: diagnosis and operative treatment. Mosby, St. Louis, pp 490–500

Foumani M et al (2010a) In vivo dynamic and static three-dimensional joint space distance maps in the radiocarpal joint. In: 11th triennial congress of the international federation of societies for surgery of the hand, Seoul, Korea

Foumani M et al (2010b) The effect of tendon loading on in vitro carpal kinematics of the wrist joint. J Biomech 43(9):1799–1805

Garcia-Elias M, Geissler WB (2005) Carpal instability. In: Green DP et al (eds) Green's operative hand surgery. Elsevier Churchill Livingstone, Philadelphia, pp 535–604

Garcia-Elias M, Dobyns JH, Cooney WP, Linscheid RL (1989) Traumatic axial dislocations of the carpus. J Hand Surg 14:446–457. https://doi.org/10.1016/s0363-5023(89)80003-6

Gilula LA et al (2002) Wrist: terminology and definitions. J Bone Joint Surg Am 84-A(Suppl 1):1–73

Herzberg G (2008) Perilunate and axial carpal dislocations and fracture–dislocations. J Hand Surg 33:1659–1668. https://doi.org/10.1016/j.jhsa.2008.09.013

Johnstone DJ et al (1997) A comparison of magnetic resonance imaging and arthroscopy in the investigation of chronic wrist pain. J Hand Surg 22(6):714–718

Kaufmann RA et al (2006) Kinematics of the midcarpal and radiocarpal joint in flexion and extension: an in vitro study. J Hand Surg 31(7):1142–1148

Kobayashi M et al (1997) Normal kinematics of carpal bones: a three-dimensional analysis of carpal bone motion relative to the radius. J Biomech 30(8):787–793

Kwon BC, Baek GH (2008) Fluoroscopic diagnosis of scapholunate interosseous ligament injuries in distal radius fractures. Clin Orthop Relat Res 466(4):969–976

Lichtman DM et al (1981) Ulnar midcarpal instability-clinical and laboratory analysis. J Hand Surg 6(5):515–523

Lichtman DM et al (1993) Palmar midcarpal instability: results of surgical reconstruction. J Hand Surg 18(2):307–315

Lindau T (2010) Arthroscopic management of scapholunate dissociation. In: Del Pinal F, Mathoulin C (eds) Arthroscopic management of distal radius fractures. Springer, Berlin, pp 99–108

Linscheid RL, Dobyns JH, Beabout JW, Bryan RS (1972) Traumatic instability of the wrist. Diagnosis, classification, and pathomechanics. J Bone Joint Surg Am 54:1612–1632

Magee T (2009) Comparison of 3-T MRI and arthroscopy of intrinsic wrist ligament and TFCC tears. AJR Am J Roentgenol 192(1):80–85

Manton GL et al (2001) Partial interosseous ligament tears of the wrist: difficulty in utilizing either primary or secondary MRI signs. J Comput Assist Tomogr 25(5):671–676

Mayfield JK, Johnson RP, Kilcoyne RK (1980) Carpal dislocations: pathomechanics and progressive perilunar instability. J Hand Surg 5:226–241. https://doi.org/10.1016/s0363-5023(80)80007-4

Meier R et al (2002) Scapholunate ligament tears in MR arthrography compared with wrist arthroscopy. Handchir Mikrochir Plast Chir 34(6):381–385

Metz VM, Metz-Schimmerl SM, Yin Y (1997) Ligamentous instabilities of the wrist. Eur J Radiol 25(2):104–111

Mink van der Molen AB (1997) Carpale letsels, onderzoek naar de verzuimaspecten ten gevolge van carpale letsels in Nederland 1990–1993—(Carpal injuries, research of work-related absence due to carpal injuries in the Netherlands 1990–1993). Thesis, Rijksuniversity Groningen

Moojen TM et al (2002) Scaphoid kinematics in vivo. J Hand Surg 27(6):1003–1010

Moojen TM et al (2003) In vivo analysis of carpal kinematics and comparative review of the literature. J Hand Surg 28(1):81–87

Moore DC et al (2007) A digital database of wrist bone anatomy and carpal kinematics. J Biomech 40(11):2537–2542

Moritomo H, Apergis EP, Herzberg G, Werner FW, Wolfe SW, Garcia-Elias M (2007) 2007 IFSSH committee report of wrist biomechanics committee: biomechanics of the so-called dart-throwing motion of the wrist. J Hand Surg 32:1447–1453. https://doi.org/10.1016/j.jhsa.2007.08.014

Moser T et al (2007) Wrist ligament tears: evaluation of MRI and combined MDCT and MR arthrography. AJR Am J Roentgenol 188(5):1278–1286

Obermann WR (1996) Wrist injuries: pitfalls in conventional imaging. Eur J Radiol 22(1):11–21

Peh W, Gilula LA (1994) Imaging of the wrist—a customized approach. Curr Orthop 8:23–31

Protas JM, Jackson WT (1980) Evaluating carpal instabilities with fluoroscopy. AJR Am J Roentgenol 135(1):137–140

Rayhack JM, Linscheid RL, Dobyns JH, Smith JH (1987) Posttraumatic ulnar translation of the carpus. J Hand Surg 12:180–189. https://doi.org/10.1016/s0363-5023(87)80268-x

Resnick D, Kang HS, Pretterklieber ML (2006) Internal Derangements of Joints (2nd ed.). Saunders; Elsevier

Saupe N (2009) 3-Tesla high-resolution MR imaging of the wrist. Semin Musculoskelet Radiol 13(1):29–38

Schmid MR et al (2005) Interosseous ligament tears of the wrist: comparison of multi-detector row CT arthrography and MR imaging. Radiology 237(3):1008–1013

Schmitt R et al (2003) Direct MR arthrography of the wrist in comparison with arthroscopy: a prospective study on 125 patients. Rofo 175(7):911–919

Schmitt R et al (2006) Carpal instability. Eur Radiol 16(10):2161–2178

Schuind FA, Linscheid RL, An KN, Chao EY (1992) A normal data base of posteroanterior roentgenographic measurements of the wrist. J Bone Joint Surg Am 74:1418–1429

Shin AY, Weinstein LP, Berger RA, Bishop AT (2001) Treatment of isolated injuries of the lunotriquetral ligament. A comparison of arthrodesis, ligament reconstruction and ligament repair. J Bone Joint Surg Br 83:1023–1028. https://doi.org/10.1302/0301-620x.83b7.11413

Smeulders MJ, Kreulen M, Bos KE (2001) Fine motor assessment in chronic wrist pain: the role of adapted motor control. Clin Rehabil 15(2):133–141

Smeulders MJ et al (2002) Motor control impairment of the contralateral wrist in patients with unilateral chronic wrist pain. Am J Phys Med Rehabil/Assoc Acad Physiatrists 81(3):177–181

Snel JG et al (2000) Quantitative in vivo analysis of the kinematics of carpal bones from three-dimensional CT images using a deformable surface model and a three-dimensional matching technique. Med Phys 27(9):2037–2047

Stehling C et al (2009) Three-tesla magnetic resonance imaging of the wrist: diagnostic performance compared to 1.5-T. J Comput Assist Tomogr 33(6):934–939

Streekstra GJ et al (2010) 4D-Imaging of voluntary joint motion from biplane fluoroscopy images. In: 96th annual meeting of the radiological society of North America (RSNA), Chicago

Taleisnik J, Watson HK (1984) Midcarpal instability caused by malunited fractures of the distal radius. J Hand Surg 9:350–357. https://doi.org/10.1016/s0363-5023(84)80222-1

Theumann NH et al (2003) Extrinsic carpal ligaments: normal MR arthrographic appearance in cadavers. Radiology 226(1):171–179

Videler AJ, Kreulen M, Brandsma W (1998) An exercise program for patients with chronic, undiagnosed wrist pain. Physiopraxis 7(11):10–13

Watson HK, Ashmead D, Makhlouf MV (1988) Examination of the scaphoid. J Hand Surg 13:657–660. https://doi.org/10.1016/s0363-5023(88)80118-7

Watson HK, Weinzweig J, Zeppieri J (1997) The natural progression of scaphoid instability. Hand Clin 13:39–49

White J, Couzens G, Jeffery C (2019) The use of 4D-CT in assessing wrist kinematics and pathology. Bone Joint J 101-B(11):1325–1330. https://doi.org/10.1302/0301-620X.101B11.BJJ-2019-0361.R1

Wright TW, Dobyns JH, Linscheid RL, Macksoud W, Siegert J (1994) Carpal instability non-dissociative. J Hand Surg Br 19:763–773. https://doi.org/10.1016/0266-7681(94)90255-0

Zlatkin MB et al (1989) Chronic wrist pain: evaluation with high-resolution MR imaging. Radiology 173(3):723–729

Ulnar-Sided Wrist Pain

Eelin Tan, Chern Yue Glen Ong,
Adriel Guang Wei Goh, and Ankit Tandon

Contents

E. Tan (✉) · C. Y. G. Ong
Diagnostic Radiology, Tan Tock Seng Hospital, Singapore, Singapore

A. G. W. Goh
Department of Radiology, Sengkang General Hospital, Singapore, Singapore

A. Tandon
Diagnostic Radiology, Tan Tock Seng Hospital, Singapore, Singapore

Lee Kong Chian School of Medicine, Nanyang Technological University, Singapore, Singapore

Med Radiol Diagn Imaging (2025)
https://doi.org/10.1007/174_2025_580,
Published Online: 26 April 2025

Abstract

Ulnar-sided wrist pain has been likened to lower back pain as it is relatively common, has a wide differential and is challenging to both diagnose and treat. This chapter provides an overview of the relevant anatomy and presents a comprehensive list of pathologies with a focus on the MRI findings.

1 Introduction

Ulnar-sided wrist pathologies can be divided into three categories: patients with (i) pain only, (ii) pain with instability or (iii) pain with arthritis (Brogan et al. 2019). The four most important domains to assess are distal radioulnar joint (DRUJ) bony alignment, triangular fibrocartilage complex (TFCC) status, cartilage quality and extensor carpi ulnaris (ECU) tendon stability (Kakar and Garcia-Elias 2016). A detailed history, systematic physical examination and provocative tests can usually help narrow the differential (Brogan et al. 2019; Cohen-Tanugi and Gaston 2021; DaSilva et al. 2017). Imaging, particularly magnetic resonance imaging (MRI) and magnetic resonance arthrography (MRA), plays an integral role in the diagnosis of ulnar-sided wrist pain, albeit with some limitations. Arthroscopy remains the gold standard for the confirmation of TFCC injuries, carpal instability and degenerative wrist disease (Selvin et al. 2021).

2 Distal Radioulnar Joint and Triangular Fibrocartilage Complex

2.1 Anatomy and Imaging

The DRUJ is the articulation between the concave sigmoid notch of the radius and convex lateral surface of the ulnar head called the ulnar seat (af Ekenstam and Hagert 1985). DRUJ motion is primarily rotational, whereby the radiocarpal unit rotates around a fixed ulna, to allow forearm supination-pronation (Kleinman 2007). The DRUJ has intrinsic translational dorsal and palmar instability (Kleinman 2007) due to lack of osseous constraints as the radius of the sigmoid notch is about 1.5 times greater than the radius of the ulnar seat (af Ekenstam and Hagert 1985), and there is minimal contact between the sigmoid notch and ulnar seat at the extremes of pronation-supination (af Ekenstam and Hagert 1985). DRUJ stability is therefore primarily afforded by soft tissues restraints.

The primary soft tissue stabilizer of the DRUJ is the TFCC (Kleinman 2007). The TFCC consists of the articular disc, dorsal and volar distal radioulnar ligaments (DRULs), ulnar collateral ligament (UCL), ulnomeniscal homologue (UMH) and ECU tendon sheath (Palmer and Werner 1981) (Fig. 1). Secondary extrinsic stabilizers include the ECU tendon as it crosses the ulnar head, semi-rigid sixth extensor compartment, pronator quadratus muscle and interosseous membrane (Kleinman 2007).

The central fibrocartilaginous disc articulates with the ulnar pole (af Ekenstam and Hagert 1985) and its principle role is load transmission from the carpus to the ulna (Kleinman 2007). At its radial aspect, the articular disc has a broad attachment to the hyaline cartilage of the sigmoid notch (Yoshioka and Burns 2012).

The dorsal and volar DRULs play the biggest role in DRUJ stability (af Ekenstam and Hagert 1985). The DRULs are peripheral thickenings of the articular disc at its dorsal- and volar-most aspects (Ishii et al. 1998). Both ligaments have superficial and deep layers that originate from the ulnar rim of the radius via direct bony entheses (Yoshioka and Burns 2012). The deep fibres are believed to have a more significant stabilizing effect compared to the superficial fibres (Kleinman 2007). The superficial and deep layers split from each other about halfway between the radial sigmoid notch and ulnar styloid (Ishii et al. 1998). The superficial layers unite at the ulnar-most portion of the disc to insert at an acute angle onto the ulnar styloid (Ishii et al. 1998) and is termed the distal (styloid) lamina. The styloid lamina inserts onto cartilage at the ulnar styloid tip. The deep layers insert at an obtuse angle onto the fovea (af Ekenstam and Hagert 1985) and is termed the proximal (foveal) lamina.

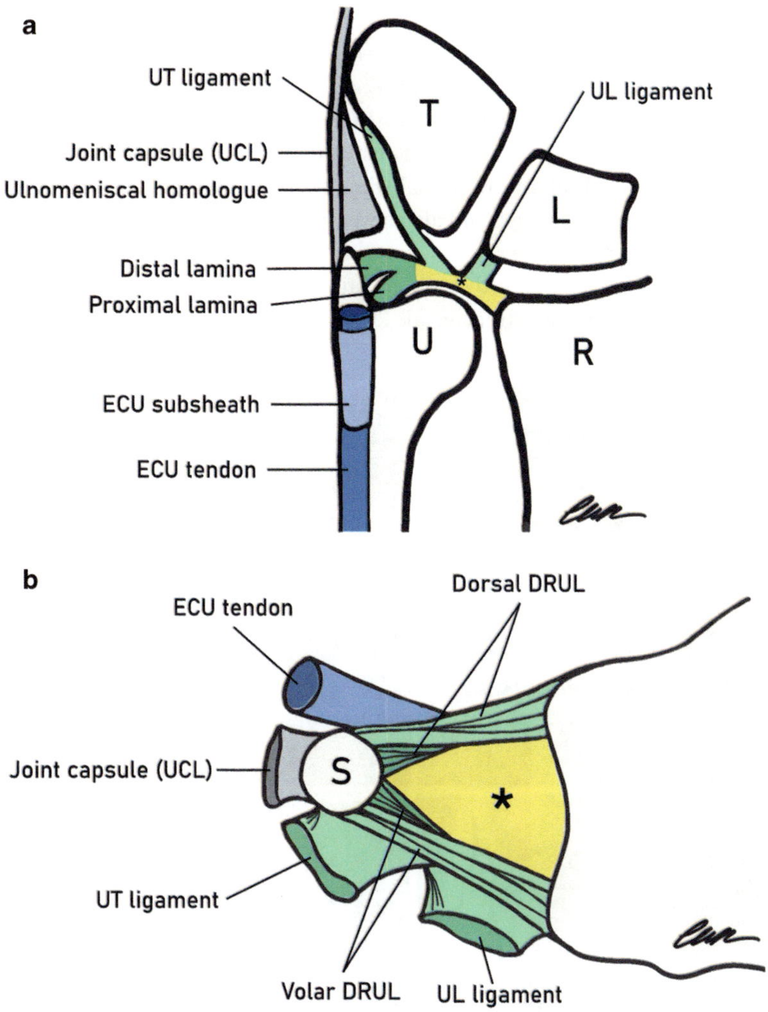

Fig. 1 2D illustrations of the TFCC from (**a**) dorsal and (**b**) top-down perspectives. The dorsal and volar distal radioulnar ligaments (DRUL) are thickenings at the periphery of the articular disc (*). Superficial fibres of the DRUL (**b**, lighter green) form the distal lamina and insert onto the styloid, while the deep fibres (**b**, darker green) form the proximal lamina and insert onto the fovea. The ulnotriquetral (UT) and ulnolunate (UL) ligaments blend with the volar DRUL proximally. The ulnar joint capsule or ulnar collateral ligament (UCL) and ulnomeniscal homologue are in grey. The extensor carpi ulnaris (ECU) tendon and its subsheath are in blue. L = Lunate. R = Radius. S=Ulnar styloid. T = Triquetrum. U=Ulna. (Illustrations by Alana Lee)

The UCL is essentially the ulnar capsule and cannot be separately identified on anatomic dissections or MRI (Buck et al. 2009; Ishii et al. 1998; Theumann et al. 2003). Some authors propose referring to the ulnar joint capsule/UCL, ECU tendon sheath and collateral component of the UMH as the ulnar collateral ligament complex as these structures are inseparable (Buck et al. 2009).

Many also consider the volar ulnocarpal ligaments (ulnolunate [UL] and ulnotriquetral [UT] ligaments) part of the TFCC (Flores et al. 2023; Yoshioka and Burns 2012) even though these were not included by Palmer and Werner. The UL and UT ligaments blend with the volar DRUL proximally and attach onto the volar aspects of the lunate and triquetrum distally.

At our institution, we perform proton density, proton density fat-suppressed, T2-weighted fat-suppressed and 3D gradient-echo pulse sequences for routine wrist MRI. Images can be optimized with appropriate coil selection, use of contiguous thin sections and higher magnetic field strength (Yoshioka and Burns 2012). MRI has high accuracy for detecting TFCC tears (Magee 2009; Potter et al. 1997; Zhao et al. 2024b) but has lower sensitivity for peripheral tears compared to central and radial-sided lesions (Haims et al. 2002; Oneson et al. 1997). On MRI, the central disc is biconcave and returns uniformly low signal (Fig. 2). The peripheral laminae are best assessed on the coronal plane and normally return intermediate signal with a striated pattern (Ng et al. 2019; Yoshioka and Burns 2012) (Fig. 2).

The two laminae are separated by intervening high signal *ligamentum subcruentum* (Ishii et al. 1998; Yoshioka and Burns 2012; Zhao et al. 2024a), which can be confounding (Fig. 2). At the disc level, the DRULs are best assessed on the sagittal plane and return low signal (Fig. 2). The volar radiocarpal ligaments are also best assessed on the sagittal plane (Fig. 2).

Direct MRA can improve diagnostic accuracy of TFCC lesions (Boer et al. 2018; Omar et al. 2019; Petsatodis et al. 2019). Single-compartment (radiocarpal) MRA is the most common technique for the wrist (Fig. 3). Addition of DRUJ injection for double-compartment MRA can be considered when there is suspicion of a partial tear of the proximal TFCC (Rastogi et al. 2016; Yoshioka and Burns 2012) (Fig. 3). Some advocate axial traction during MRA to further increase joint width (Dallaudière et al. 2015; Lee et al. 2016).

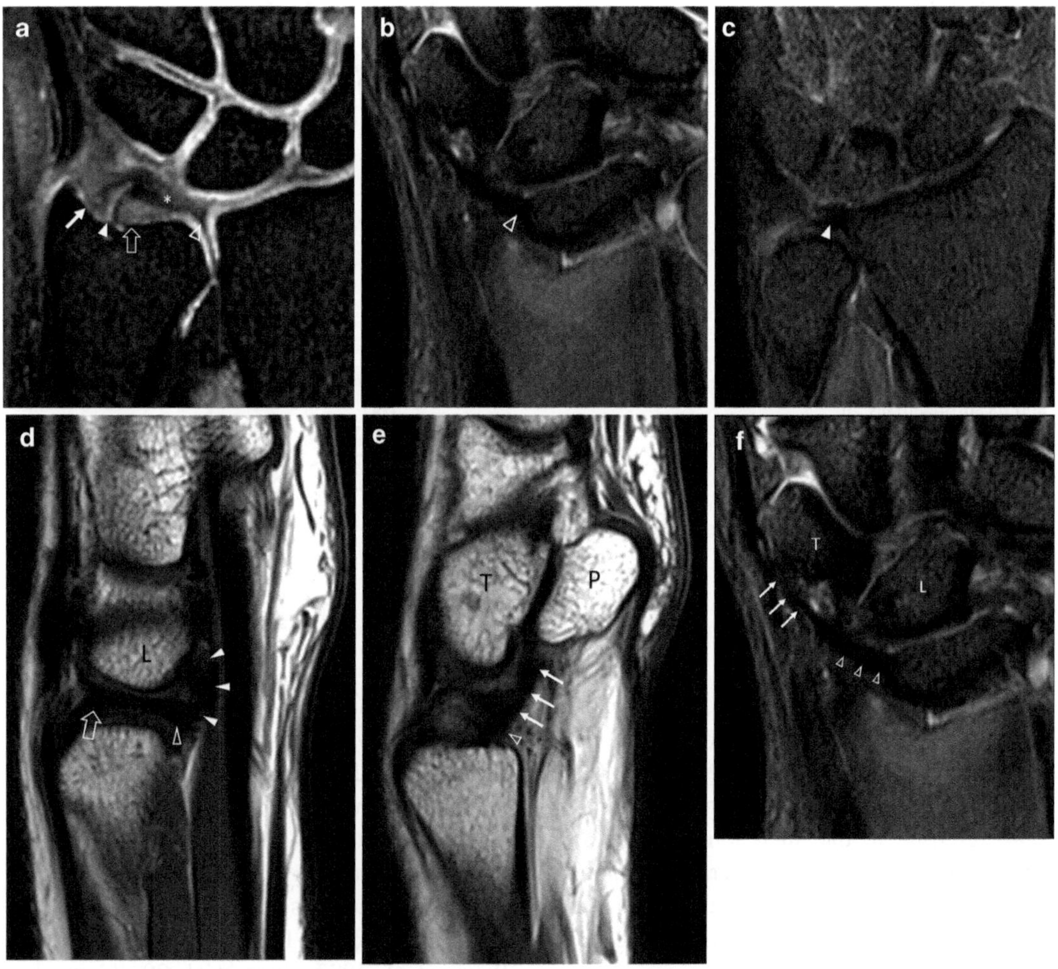

Fig. 2 Normal TFCC anatomy on MRI. (**a**) Coronal 3D DESS image: Distal lamina (arrow) inserts onto the cartilage of the ulnar styloid. Proximal lamina (empty arrow) inserts onto the fovea. Normal intervening high signal *ligamentum subcruentum* (arrowhead). Note the intermediate signal intensity and striated appearance of the peripheral laminae. Articular disc (*) shows uniform low signal intensity. Radial attachment (empty arrowhead) inserts into the cartilage of the sigmoid notch. (**b**, **c**) Coronal PD FS images: Volar DRUL (empty arrowhead) and dorsal DRUL (arrowhead) attach directly to the bone of the sigmoid notch. (**d**) Sagittal PD image: Ulnolunate ligament (arrowheads) blends with the volar DRUL (empty arrowhead) proximally and attaches to the volar aspect of the lunate (L) distally. Dorsal DRUL (empty arrow) is marked. (**e**) Sagittal PD and (**f**) coronal PD FS images: Ulnotriquetral ligament (arrows) blends with the volar DRUL (empty arrowheads) proximally and attaches to the volar aspect of the triquetrum (T) distally. Pisiform (P). Lunate (L)

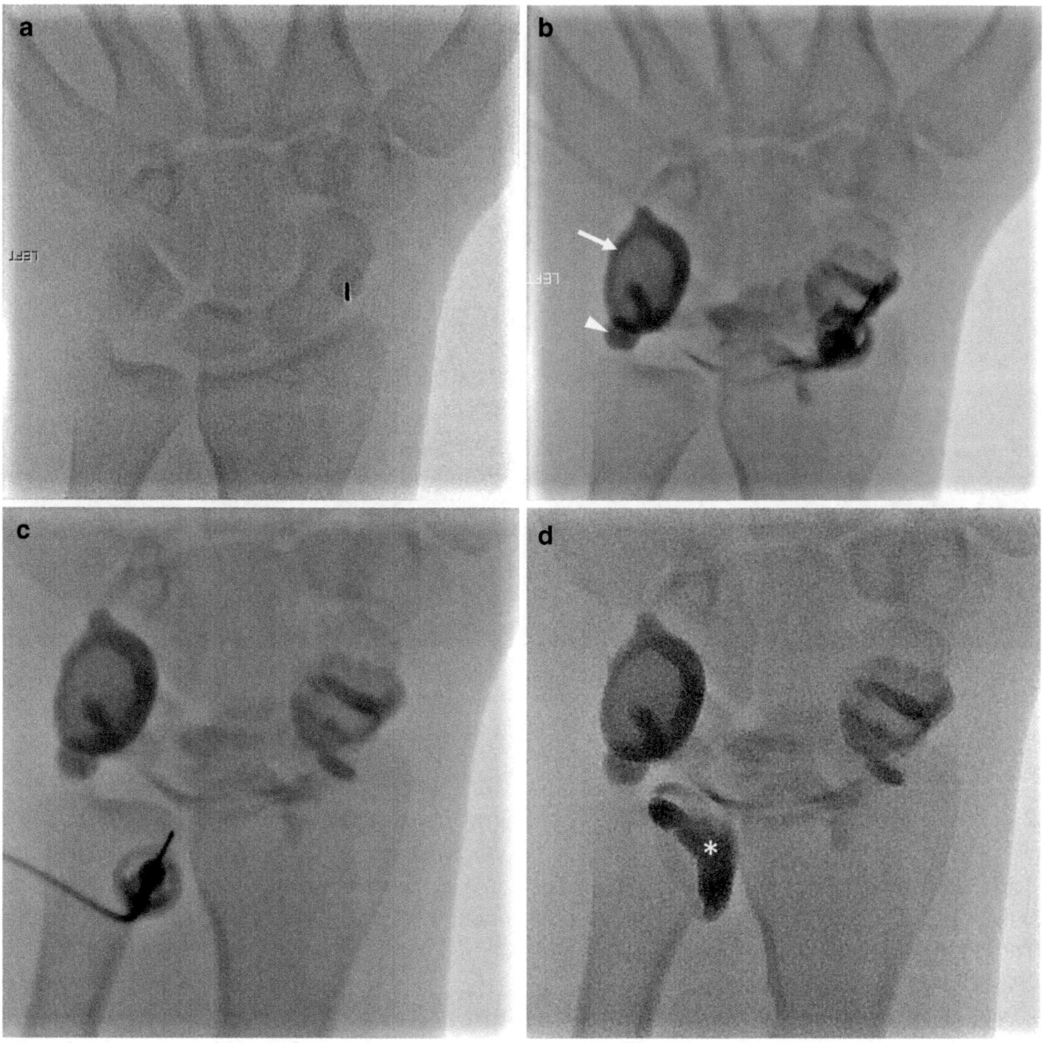

Fig. 3 Fluoroscopic-guided injections and normal TFCC anatomy on double-compartment MRA. (**a**) Radiocarpal joint injection: needle tip is positioned over the proximal cortex of the mid-scaphoid to target the radioscaphoid recess. (**b**) Resultant normal radiocarpal arthrogram with opacification of the prestyloid recess (arrowhead) and pisotriquetral recess (arrow). (**c**) DRUJ injection: needle tip is positioned over the radial-most aspect of the ulnar head (ulnar seat). (**d**) Resultant normal DRUJ (*) arthrogram. (**e**, **f**) Coronal T1W FS images from double-compartment MRA show contrast outlining the distal lamina (arrow), proximal lamina (empty arrow), radial attachment (arrowhead), articular disc (*) and ulnomeniscal homologue (empty arrowhead). No contrast leakage into the midcarpal joint

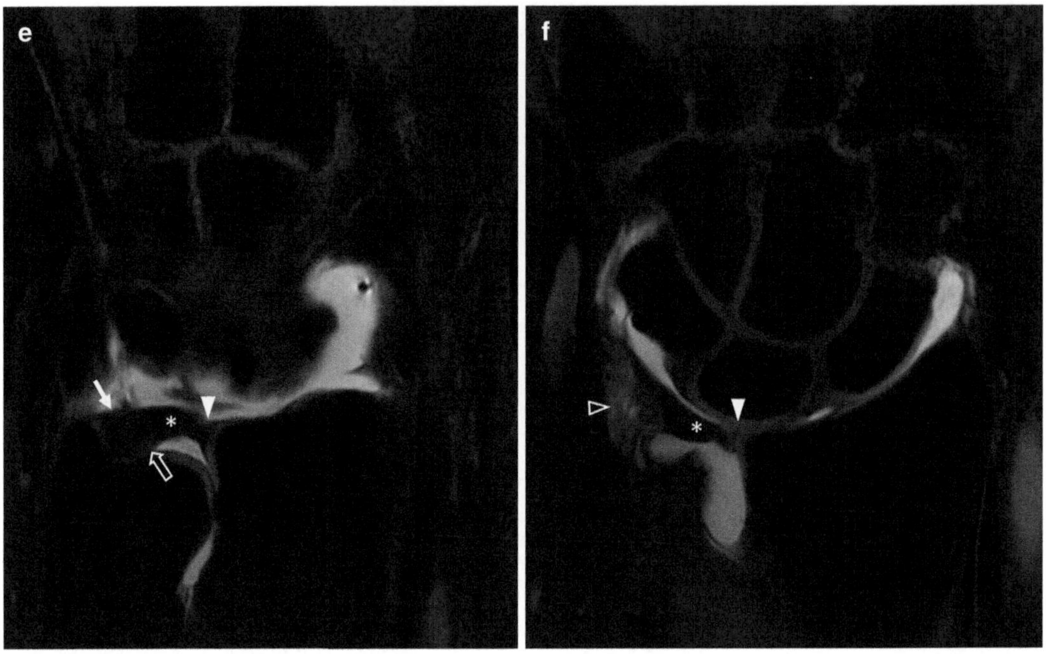

Fig. 3 (continued)

2.2 TFCC Injuries

TFCC injuries are often implicated in ulnar-sided symptoms. The Palmer classification divides TFCC lesions into traumatic (class 1) and degenerative (class 2) types (Palmer 1989).

Traumatic lesions are assigned Palmer class 1A to 1D based on tear location (Table 1). Combined traumatic tears are not uncommon. The Atzei classification for peripheral TFCC tears further stratifies Palmer class 1B lesions, incorporates clinical, radiologic and arthroscopic findings and considers healing potential in providing treatment recommendations (Atzei 2009) (Table 2). Some TFCC injuries such as bucket handle and dorsal peripheral tears do not fit into either classification system (Abe et al. 2016; Estrella et al. 2007; Zhan et al. 2020). Direct MRI signs of peripheral tears include signal alteration on fluid-sensitive sequences, fibre discontinuity, scarring (thickened and wavy appearance) and retraction (Hur et al. 2024) (Fig. 4). Chronic peripheral injuries can be associated with ganglion cysts. Articular disc perforation usually occurs in a paracentral location near the radial attachment and can be differentiated from radial avulsions by residual rim of articular disc (Fig. 4). Intermediate signal in the articular disc not reaching the articular surface is related to degeneration and should not be mistaken for perforation (Burns et al. 2011) (Fig. 4). On MRA, contrast leak confirms a full-thickness tear, while contrast imbibition provides greater confidence in diagnosing non-communicating partial tears (Fig. 4).

Degenerative lesions are related to ulnocarpal abutment syndrome and assigned Palmer class 2A to 2E based on severity and extent (Table 1). Positive ulnar variance increases load across the ulnocarpal joint and predisposes to ulnar impaction (Palmer 1989). On MRI, TFC wear manifests as thinning of the articular disc, while perforation is seen as a full-thickness gap. The proximal lunotriquetral ligament (LTL) should be assessed for degenerative tear.

Table 1 Palmer classification of TFCC injuries (Palmer 1989)

Class I: Traumatic		Comments
1A	Central perforation	Usually paracentral within 2–3 mm of the radial attachment with residual rim of articular disc.
1B	Ulnar avulsion With ulnar styloid fracture Without ulnar styloid fracture	Further classified by Atzei (Table 2). May have DRUJ instability, particularly if foveal lamina is torn.
1C	Distal avulsion	Distal avulsion of the volar ulnocarpal ligament(s). May have associated LTL tear and/or ulnar carpal instability.
1D	Radial avulsion With sigmoid notch fracture Without sigmoid notch fracture	No residual rim of articular disc at radial side.
Class 2: Degenerative		Comments
2A	TFC wear	Ulnocarpal abutment syndrome
2B	TFC wear + Lunate and/or ulnar chondromalacia	
2C	TFC perforation + Lunate and/or ulnar chondromalacia	
2D	TFC perforation + Lunate and/or ulnar chondromalacia + LT ligament perforation	
2E	TFC perforation + Lunate and/or ulnar chondromalacia + LT ligament perforation + Ulnocarpal arthritis	

Subchondral marrow oedema and cystic changes at the ulnar head, proximal lunate and/or radial triquetrum usually indicate underlying full-thickness chondrosis (Fig. 5); however, isolated subchondral oedema at the radial aspect of the proximal lunate can occasionally be a false positive finding (Bordalo-Rodrigues et al. 2005). MRI and MRA are insensitive for partial-thickness chondral lesions (Haims et al. 2004; Mutimer et al. 2008). Due to these limitations, arthroscopy remains the gold standard for assessing chondromalacia at the wrist (Selvin et al. 2021).

2.3 DRUJ Instability

DRUJ instability is commonly related to TFCC injuries. DRUJ dislocations are usually traumatic and part of complex forearm fracture-dislocations. The mechanism of injury is hyperpronation in dorsal DRUJ dislocation and hypersupination in volar DRUJ dislocation (Sharma et al. 2011). Dorsal dislocation is often obvious as the wrist is locked in painful pronation with dorsal prominence of the ulnar head.

DRUJ congruency can be assessed on radiographs; however, obtaining a true lateral view is tricky, which has led to some institutions using a support device (Larsen et al. 1990; Nakamura et al. 1995; Yang et al. 1997). Criteria for a true lateral view include interposition of the volar cortex of the pisiform between the volar cortices of the distal scaphoid tubercle and capitate head (Yang et al. 1997) and complete superimposition of the lunate, proximal scaphoid pole and triquetrum (Mino et al. 1983) (Fig. 6). On a true lateral view, the distal radius and ulna overlap. A good posterior-anterior (PA) radiograph shows collinearity of the long axis of the third metacarpal, capitate and radius and minimal overlap of the distal radius and ulna at the DRUJ (Fig. 6). In volar dislocation, there is superimposition of the distal ulna over the radius on PA view and the distal ulna projects volar to the radius on the lateral view (Fig. 6). In dorsal dislocation, a widened DRUJ is seen on the PA view and the distal ulna projects dorsal to the radius on the lateral view.

Table 2 Atzei's comprehensive classification of TFCC peripheral tears and associated ulnar styloid fractures (Atzei 2009; Atzei and Luchetti 2011)

		Class 0	Class 1	Class 2	Class 3	Class 4	Class 5
		Isolated styloid fracture	Distal peripheral tear	Complete peripheral tear	Proximal peripheral tear	Non-repairable TFCC tear	DRUJ arthritis
Clinical findings	DRUJ ballotement test	Negative	Slight laxity (hard endpoint)	Mild to severe laxity (soft endpoint)			Variable
Radiographic findings	Ulnar styloid	Fracture	Intact or fracture	Intact or fracture	Intact or fracture	Intact	
Arthroscopic findings	Distal TFCC[a]	Intact	Tear	Tear	Intact	Tear with significant defect (4A) or poor healing potential (4B)	Variable
	Proximal TFCC[b]	Intact	Intact	Tear	Tear (class 3) or avulsion fracture (class 3A)	Tear with significant defect (4A) or poor healing potential (4B)	Variable
	DRUJ cartilage	Preserved					Defect
Suggested treatment		Splinting	Repair: TFCC suture	Repair: Foveal refixation or excision for floating styloid[c]	Repair: Foveal refixation (class 3) or styloid fixation (class 3A)	Tendon graft reconstruction	Salvage: Arthroplasty or joint replacement

[a]Assessed on radiocarpal arthroscopy
[b]Assessed with hook test or DRUJ arthroscopy
[c]Floating styloid refers to a basilar ulnar styloid fracture with few ligamentous attachments

Cross-sectional imaging can better assess DRUJ alignment but is confounded by normal translational motion at the DRUJ during rotation, whereby the ulna moves more palmar in supination and more dorsal in pronation (King et al. 1986). Methods for assessing DRUJ displacement include the radioulnar line method, epicentre method, congruency method, radioulnar ratio and subluxation ratio (Lo et al. 2001; Mino et al. 1983; Park and Kim 2008; Wechsler et al. 1987). Although there is no consensus on the best method and normal values change depending on wrist position, studies suggest reliability of the epicentre method and subluxation ratio (Park and Kim 2008; Wijffels et al. 2016). These methods are best assessed on computed tomography (CT) but can be extrapolated to MRI. We prefer the epicentre method as it is not affected by rotational position (Fig. 7).

2.4 DRUJ Osteoarthritis

DRUJ osteoarthritis can be primary or secondary. Secondary forms are commonly post-traumatic and related to distal radial fracture malunions (Minami et al. 2005). Concomitant ulnocarpal abutment syndrome is often present (Minami et al. 2005).

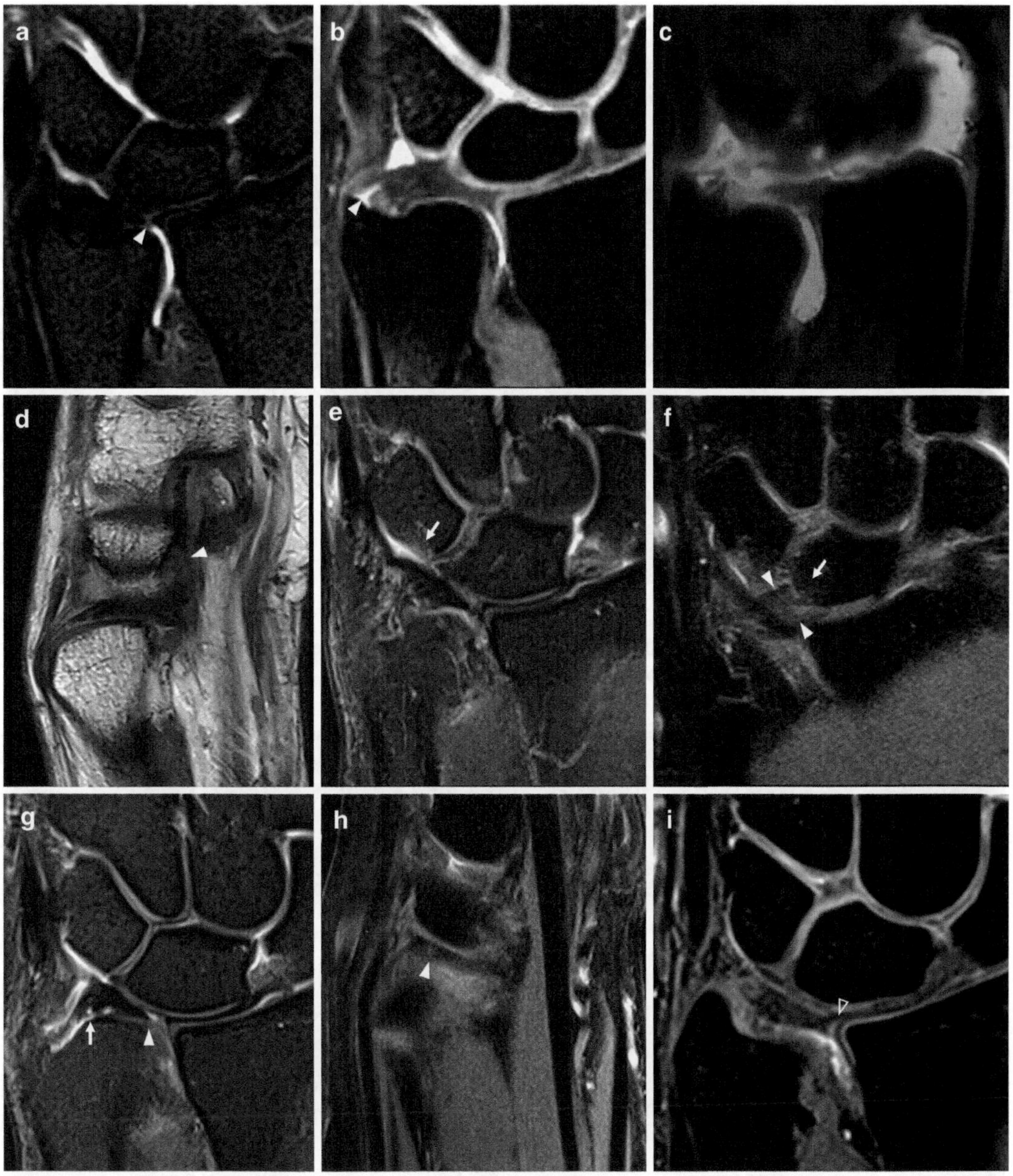

Fig. 4 Traumatic TFCC lesions and pitfall. (**a**) Coronal T2W FS image shows central perforation (arrowhead); Palmer 1A. (**b**) Coronal 3D DESS image shows intrasubstance partial tear of the styloid attachment (arrowhead); Palmer 1B. (**c**) Coronal T1W FS image from single-compartment (radiocarpal) MRA shows avulsions of the styloid and foveal attachments with retraction of the disc and contrast leak into the DRUJ; Palmer 1B. (**d**) Sagittal PD and (**e**) coronal T2W FS images show partial tear of the distal ulnotriquetral ligament (arrowhead) with marrow oedema at the triquetral attachment (arrow); Palmer 1C. (**f**) Coronal T2W FS image shows partial tear of the distal ulnolunate ligament (arrowheads) with marrow oedema at the lunate attachment (arrow); Palmer 1C. (**g**) Coronal T2W FS image shows radial avulsion (arrowhead), as well as avulsion and retraction of the foveal attachment (arrow); combined Palmer 1D and 1B. (**h**) Sagittal PD FS image shows small tear in the dorsal distal radioulnar ligament (arrowhead). (**i**) Coronal 3D DESS: Pitfall—Intermediate signal in the articular disc not reaching the articular surface related to degeneration (empty arrowhead) should not be mistaken for perforation

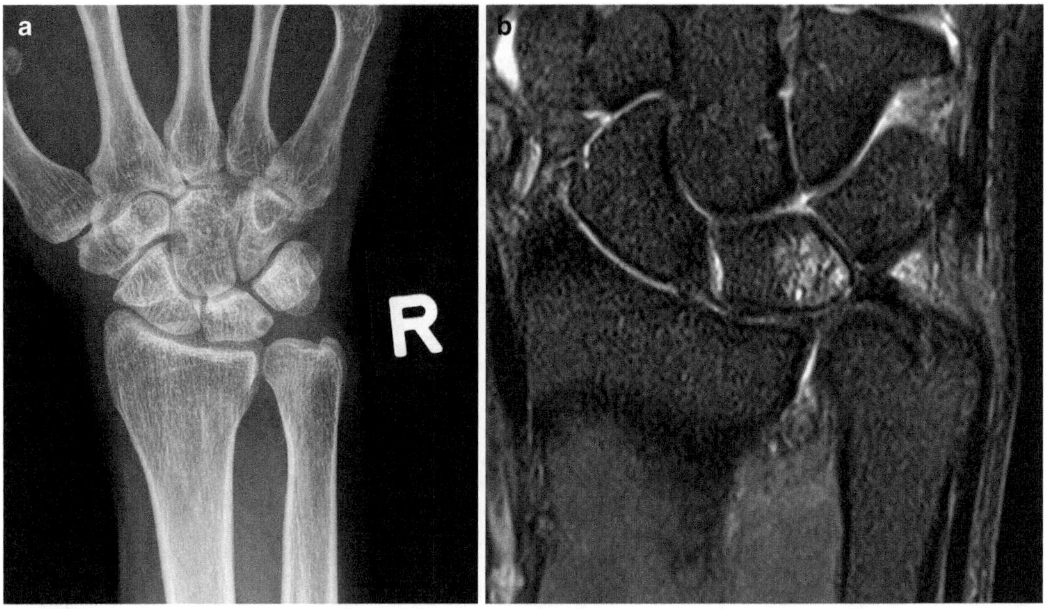

Fig. 5 Ulnocarpal abutment syndrome. (**a**) PA radiograph of the right wrist shows subchondral cyst at the ulnar side of the proximal lunate. (**b**) Coronal T2W FS image of the same patient shows TFC perforation and lunate chondromalacia with subchondral changes; Palmer 2C

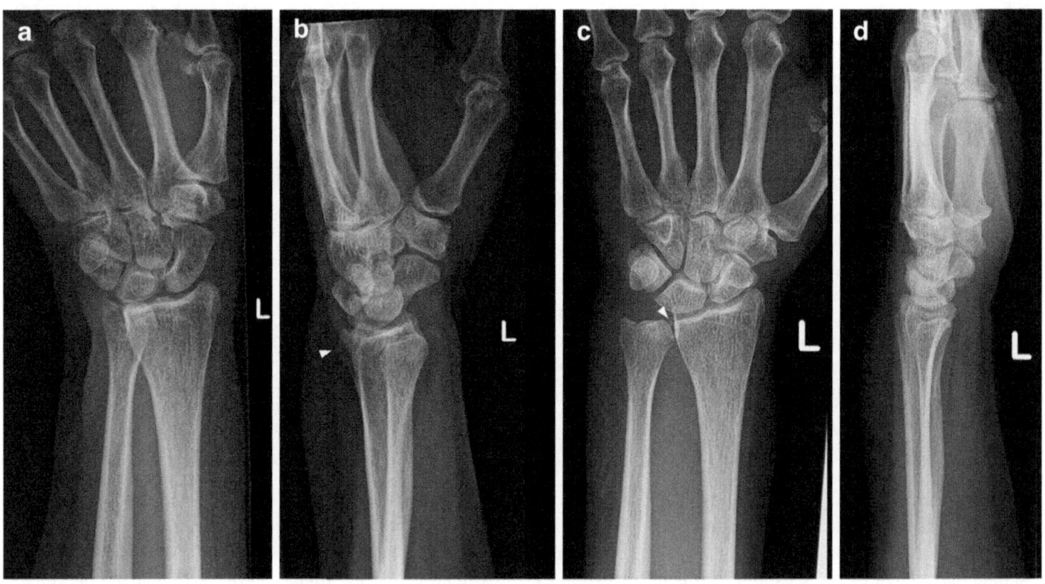

Fig. 6 Radiographic and CT assessment of DRUJ congruency. (**a**, **b**) Volar DRUJ dislocation. (**a**) Frontal view of the left wrist shows abnormal overlap of the distal radius and ulnar. (**b**) Lateral view is suboptimal as the pisiform is projected dorsal to the scaphoid; nevertheless, there is volar displacement of the distal ulna in relation to the radius. Tiny bony density dorsal to the distal radius is probably a chip fracture (arrowhead). (**c**, **d**) Restoration of DRUJ congruency following manipulation and reduction. (**c**) Frontal and (**d**) lateral views shows restoration of DRUJ congruency. This lateral view is technically adequate (volar cortices of the pisiform bone and scaphoid are overlapping). Tiny chip fracture is projected over the DRUJ (arrowhead)

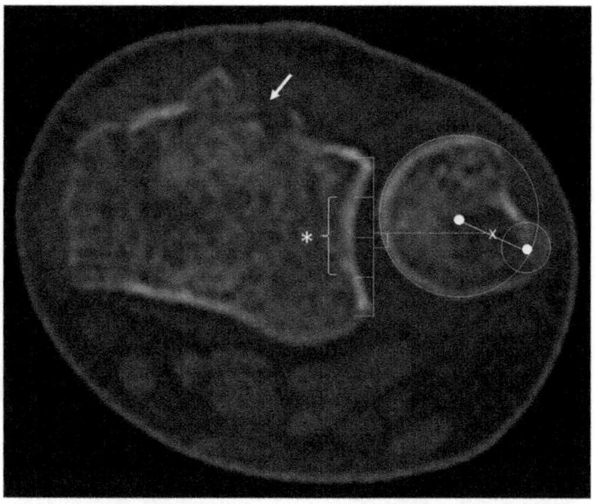

Fig. 7 Epicentre method for assessment of DRUJ congruency on axial non-contrast CT of the wrist. The centre of rotation of the DRUJ is the midpoint (x) between the centre of the ulnar head and centre of the ulnar styloid. A perpendicular line drawn from the chord of the sigmoid notch to the centre of rotation of the DRUJ falling within the middle half of the sigmoid notch (*) is considered normal (Wechsler et al. 1987). Distal radius fracture involving Lister's tubercle can be seen on this image

3 Extensor Carpi Ulnaris Tendon

3.1 Anatomy and Imaging

The ECU has two muscle bellies, one originating from the lateral epicondyle of the humerus via the common extensor tendon and the other from the dorsal border of the ulnar shaft. The muscle inserts as a single tendon onto the dorsal aspect of the fifth metacarpal base. It is common to see increased signal within the central substance of the ECU tendon at the level of the ulnar styloid on short and long TE pulse sequences in the axial plane (ECU pseudolesion) (Ali et al. 2015; Timins et al. 1996) (Fig. 8). This is related to normal inter-tendinous ground substance between the two distal heads (Ali et al. 2015), and patients are often asymptomatic (Kuntz et al. 2015). MRI signal increases with increasing amounts of mucoid material (mucoid degeneration) (Ali et al. 2015).

Within the sixth extensor compartment at the level of the distal ulna, the tendon is enclosed by a fibro-osseous tunnel formed by the ulnar groove and ECU subsheath (Omokawa et al. 2021; Taleisnik et al. 1984). The ECU subsheath lies deep to the extensor retinaculum and attaches to the periosteum at the margins of the ulnar groove (Omokawa et al. 2021) (Fig. 8). This arrangement allows unrestricted rotation of the radius and ulna at the DRUJ (Allende and Le Viet 2005). Distal extension of the ECU subsheath connects the ulnar styloid process and superficial fibres of the DRULs (Omokawa et al. 2021).

It is important to note normal physiologic medial subluxation of the ECU tendon over the ulnar styloid during supination (Lee et al. 2009; Pfirrmann et al. 2001; Taleisnik et al. 1984). Ulnar deviation and flexion of the wrist further increases ECU tendon displacement (Lee et al. 2009). The upper limit for physiologic displacement has been reported as 5 mm or 50% tendon displacement beyond the apex of the ulnar border of the ulnar groove (Lee et al. 2009). The *linea juguta*, a longitudinal sling of collagen fibres, tightens during extreme supination to prevent further medial and palmar displacement of the ECU tendon (Taleisnik et al. 1984).

Ultrasound provides excellent assessment of the ECU muscle and tendon (Fig. 8). The ultrasound operator can extend the scan coverage to interrogate anywhere from the muscle down to the distal tendon insertion. In addition, tendon stability can be readily evaluated via dynamic manoeuvres. The main strength of MRI is the ability to provide a global assessment of the wrist and exclude other ulnar-sided conditions that may present in similar fashion.

3.2 ECU Tendinopathy and Instability

Like all tendons, the ECU tendon is liable to tendinopathy, tenosynovitis, rupture (tear) and instability. Aetiologies of repetitive stress and trauma are commonly encountered in practice. Inflammatory conditions such as rheumatoid arthritis and gout can also be culprit. Shallower and shorter ulnar grooves may predispose to ECU subluxation, while negative ulnar variance may predispose to ECU subluxation and tendinopathy (Chang et al. 2014).

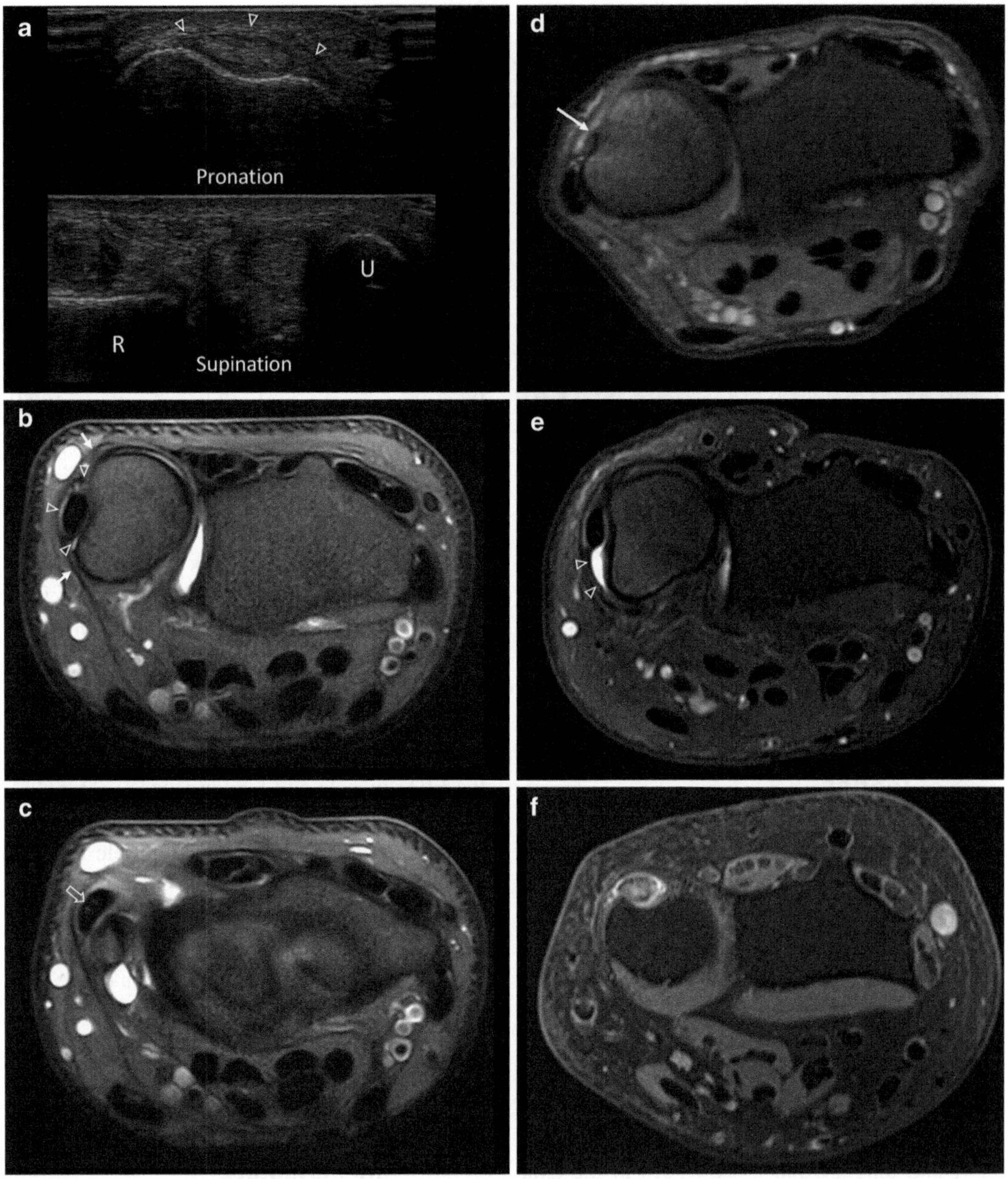

Fig. 8 Normal and pathologic ECU tendon and subsheath. (**a**) Transverse ultrasound images show normal ECU tendon within the ulnar groove on pronation. The subsheath is superficial to the tendon (empty arrowheads). On supination, the tendon moves towards the ulnar side of the groove. R = Radius. U=Ulna. (**b**, **c**) Normal ECU tendon and subsheath on axial PD FS images. (**b**) ECU subsheath surrounds the tendon and attaches to the periosteum at the margins of the ulnar groove (empty arrowheads). The subsheath is located just deep to the low signal supratendinous part of the extensor retinaculum (arrows). (**c**) At the level of the ulnar styloid, focal intermediate signal within the central part of the tendon reflects normal intertendinous ground substance (empty arrow). (**d**) Axial PD FS image shows subsheath tear with medial and palmar dislocation of the ECU tendon from the ulnar groove. Also note the shallow ulnar groove (arrow). (**e**) Axial PS FS image shows periosteal stripping at the ulnar insertion of the subsheath with formation of a false pouch (empty arrowheads); Inoue & Tamura type C. ECU tendon remains within the ulnar groove on this static image. (**f**) Axial PD FS image shows ECU tenosynovitis and tendinosis. The latter manifests as tendon enlargement and signal increase involving the full thickness of the tendon

ECU tendinopathy can be constrained (intact subsheath) or unconstrained (torn or attenuated subsheath) (Garcia-Elias 2015). Constrained ECU tendinopathies include ECU tendinosis and stenosing tenovaginitis (Garcia-Elias 2015). Unconstrained tendinopathies can be traumatic subsheath tears, which are commonly associated with racket and batting/stick sports, or pathologic subsheath tears secondary to rheumatoid tenosynovitis (Allende and Le Viet 2005; Garcia-Elias 2015; Inoue and Tamura 2001). Inoue and Tamura grouped subsheath tears into three types: type A tears occur at the ulnar side of the subsheath and the tendon can relocate back into the ulnar groove on pronation; type B tears occur at the radial side and the tendon can overlie the subsheath preventing healing; and type C tears consist of periosteal stripping at the ulnar insertion forming a false pouch (Fig. 8) (Inoue and Tamura 2001).

MRI features of subsheath injuries include abnormal medial and palmar subluxation of the ECU tendon from the ulnar groove, fragmented, thickened and/or lax appearance of the subsheath and peritendinous oedema (Fig. 8). Chronic ECU instability is often associated with persistent tenosynovitis. ECU tendinosis is characterized by diffuse tendon signal increase and tendon enlargement on MRI (Fig. 8) and can be accompanied by longitudinal splits or tendon rupture if chronic and severe.

4 Carpus

4.1 Kienböck Disease

Kienböck disease refers to osteonecrosis of the lunate bone. Its aetiology and natural history remain elusive (Lutsky and Beredjiklian 2012). Possible predisposing factors include anatomic variants (lunate morphology, negative ulnar variance, decreased radial inclination), certain vascular patterns and repetitive microtrauma (Lee 1963; Lutsky and Beredjiklian 2012). The Lichtman osseous classification assesses the lunate bone (bone density and morphology) and carpal alignment on radiographs (Lichtman et al. 2010) (Table 3). Stage IIIC for complete coronal split of the lunate is a proposed addition to the

Table 3 Radiographic and MRI classification of Kienböck disease

(a) Lichtman osseous classification (Lichtman et al. 2010)	
Stage	Radiographic findings
I	Normal lunate density and shape; changes visible on MRI only (MRI stage I)
II	Change in lunate density (sclerotic and lytic) with normal shape
IIIA	Lunate sclerosis and collapse without changes in carpal alignment
IIIB	Lunate sclerosis and collapse with carpal collapse and fixed scaphoid palmar flexion (cortical ring sign on PA view)
IIIC[a]	Complete coronal split of the lunate regardless of lunate or wrist morphology
IV	Lunate collapse with radiocarpal or midcarpal degenerative changes (Kienböck disease advanced collapse)

(b) Bone marrow viability and perfusion on MRI (Schmitt et al. 1997)			
Stage	Fluid sensitive	T1 weighted	Post-contrast
Normal	No marrow oedema	Fatty marrow signal	No enhancement
I-Ischemia	Proximal lunate or diffuse marrow oedema	Proximal lunate or diffuse hypointensity	Enhancement in areas of marrow oedema
II-Partial necrosis	Inhomogeneous marrow oedema	Proximal lunate hypointensity	Inhomogeneous enhancement (non-enhancing proximal lunate, enhancing reparative zone and viable distal lunate)
III-Complete necrosis	Diffuse hypointensity	Diffuse hypointensity	No enhancement

[a]Proposed addition by Lichtman et al. in 2010

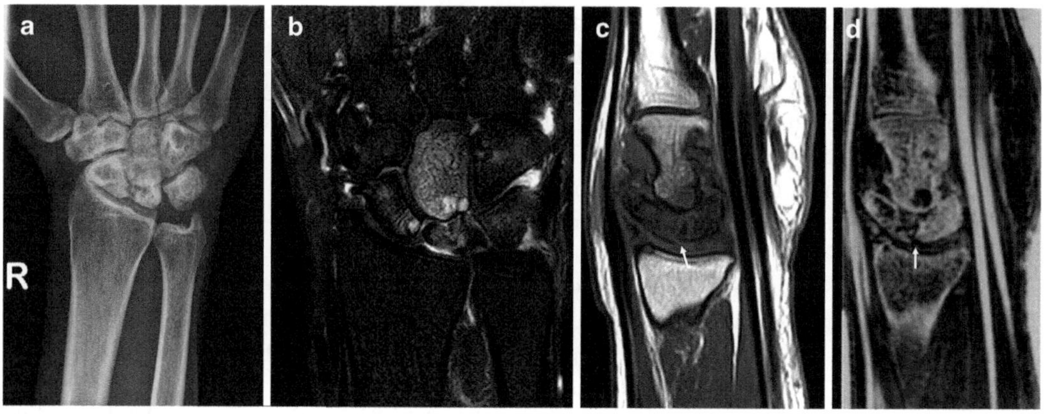

Fig. 9 Kienböck disease advanced collapse. (**a**) PA radiograph of the right wrist shows increased density and abnormal orientation of the lunate with disruption of carpal arcs I and II. (**b**) Coronal T2W FS image shows oedema-like signal and partial collapse of the lunate, as well as midcarpal degenerative changes at the scaphoid and capitate. (**c**) Sagittal T1W image through the lunate shows reduced T1w signal of the lunate and cortical step proximally (arrow). (**d**) Sagittal zero echo-time CT-like image through the lunate clearly demonstrates coronal split of the lunate (arrow)

original classification (Lichtman et al. 2010). Stage IV disease has been termed Kienböck disease advanced collapse by some authors (Lichtman et al. 2010) (Fig. 9). Bone marrow viability and perfusion are assessed on contrast-enhanced MRI (Schmitt et al. 1997) (Table 3). The Bain and Begg arthroscopic classification assesses chondral integrity based on the number of non-functional articular surfaces at the lunate and adjacent articulations (Bain and Begg 2006). Treatment depends on the information provided by all three classification systems (Lichtman et al. 2017).

4.2 Lunotriquetral Instability

Similar to the scapholunate ligament (SLL), the LTL is a C-shaped ligament with continuous dorsal, proximal and volar components (Ritt et al. 1998). The volar and dorsal components are true ligaments, while the proximal (membranous) component is fibrocartilaginous. The volar LTL is the thickest and strongest (Ritt et al. 1998). The lunate is kept in place by the flexion moment exerted by the scaphoid via the SLL and opposing extension moment exerted by the triquetrum via the LTL (Shin et al. 2000).

LTL tears can be traumatic, degenerative (see Sect. 2.2) or secondary to inflammatory arthritis (Shin et al. 2000). Degenerative proximal tears are often asymptomatic. Lunotriquetral instability can be predynamic (partial tear with no radiographic abnormality), dynamic (partial or complete tear with radiographic abnormality only under stress) or static (fixed carpal collapse with volar intercalated segmental instability [VISI]) (Shin et al. 2000). Clenched fist views can reveal dynamic instability. VISI manifests as volar flexion of the lunate and scaphoid with reduced scapholunate angle <30° and increased capitolunate angle >30° (Linscheid et al. 1972). Development of VISI requires concomitant extrinsic ligament injury, most often of the dorsal radiocarpal and dorsal intercarpal ligaments (Tanaka et al. 2008).

On MRI, the dorsal and volar components are best assessed on axial and axial oblique images. Isotropic 3D DESS pulse sequences allow multiplanar reconstruction along the true axial plane ligaments (Eladawi et al. 2022). The volar LTL is thicker with striated pattern (Fig. 10). The proximal component is best evaluated on the coronal plane and has a variety of shapes and signal intensities, most commonly triangle-shaped and with linear raised signal transversing the distal surface (Smith and Snearly 1994; Yoshioka et al.

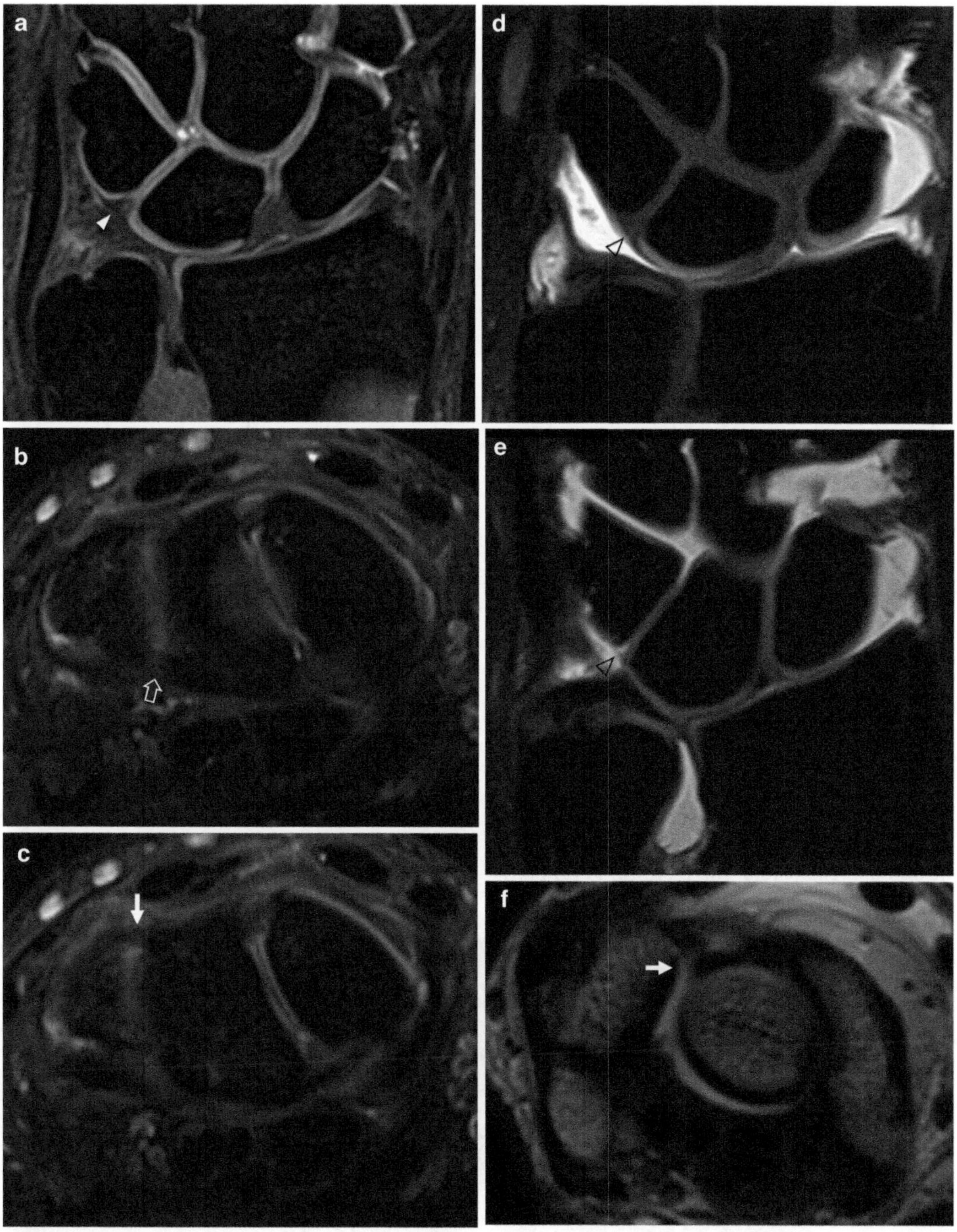

Fig. 10 Normal and injured LTL. (**a–c**) Normal LTL on MRI. (**a**) Coronal 3D gradient-echo image shows triangle-shaped proximal LTL (arrowhead). (**b**, **c**) Consecutive axial PD FS images show the thicker striated volar LTL (empty arrow) and thinner dorsal component (arrow). (**d**) Normal LTL on MRA. Coronal T1W FS image from single-compartment (radiocarpal) MRA shows intact proximal LTL (open arrowhead) and no contrast leakage into the midcarpal joint or DRUJ. (**e**) LTL tear on MRA. Coronal T1W FS image from single-compartment (radiocarpal) MRA shows full-thickness tear in the membranous LTL (empty arrowhead) with contrast leakage into the midcarpal joint. (**f**) LTL tear on MRA in another patient. Axial T1W image from single-compartment (radiocarpal) MRA shows full-thickness tear in the dorsal LTL (arrow) with contrast leakage into the midcarpal joint

2006). Complete tears manifest as abnormal ligament morphology to the point of complete absence of the ligament or fluid signal through the full thickness of the ligament (Tanaka et al. 2008) (Fig. 10). Partially altered ligament morphology with fluid signal through only a portion of the ligament suggests partial tear (Tanaka et al. 2008); however, MRI is insensitive for partial tears (sensitivity 30–63%) (De Santis et al. 2021; Eladawi et al. 2022; Manton et al. 2001; Moser et al. 2007). CT arthrography has been found to be more accurate than MRI and MRA for partial tear detection (Moser et al. 2007). LT step-off is a highly specific secondary sign for LTL disruption (Manton et al. 2001; Ringler 2013). Chronic LTL disruption can lead to hamate arthrosis lunotriquetral ligament tear (HALT) syndrome (Harley et al. 2004). Arthroscopy is the gold standard in assessing intrinsic ligaments tears and carpal instability (Selvin et al. 2021).

4.3 Pisotriquetral Joint Disorders

The pisiform bone is a sesamoid bone that lies within the flexor carpi ulnaris (FCU) tendon and articulates with the triquetrum. Considerable motion occurs at the pisotriquetral joint during flexion and extension. The pisiform is primarily stabilized by the FCU tendon, pisohamate (PHL), pisometacarpal (PML) and pisotriquetral ulnar (PTUL) ligaments (Moraux et al. 2014). The PHL attaches to the hamate hook, while the PML attaches to the fourth and fifth metacarpal bases. The PTUL is a thickening of the joint capsule at the ulnar side and is difficult to separate from the extensor retinaculum on MRI.

Traumatic pisiform dislocation is rare but can occur following direct trauma or forceful FCU contraction (Immermann 1948). The latter will result in proximal dislocation. On lateral or semi-supinated oblique views, pisiform dislocation can be suspected when pisotriquetral joint space exceeds 4 mm and when displacement of the pisiform in relation to the triquetrum exceeds 15% of the joint surface (Blum et al. 2006; Vasilas et al. 1960). Ligamentous injuries are best appreciated on MRI.

The pisotriquetral joint is subject to the same diseases as any other synovial joint, for example, osteoarthritis, chondromalacia, synovitis (Fig. 11), synovial cyst formation, osteochondromatosis (Fig. 11) and rheumatologic disorders. Ultrasound-guided or fluoroscopic-guided injection of local anaesthetic with or without steroids can confirm the diagnosis of pisotriquetral joint dysfunction (Miller and Bis 2022; Pessis et al. 2006).

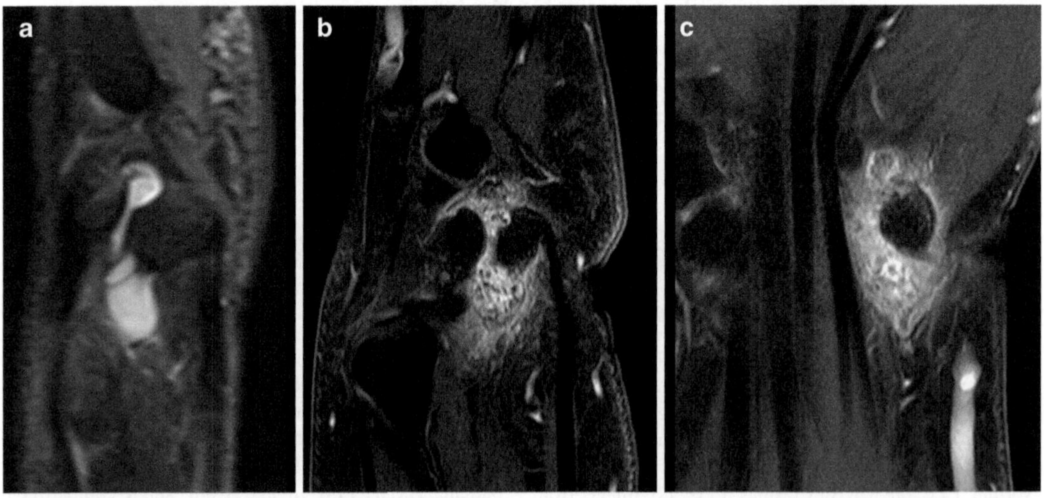

Fig. 11 Pisotriquetral joint disorders. (**a**) Sagittal TIRM image shows large effusion of unknown aetiology at the pisotriquetral joint. (**b**, **c**) Post-contrast T1W FS images in the (**b**) sagittal and (**c**) coronal planes show multiple tiny loose bodies of relatively uniform size distending the pisotriquetral joint suggestive of primary synovial chondromatosis

4.4 Lunotriquetral Coalition (Fibrocartilaginous Type)

Lunotriquetral coalition is the most frequent type of carpal coalition and is most commonly classified into four types (Minnaar 1952). Fibrocartilaginous lunotriquetral coalition (Minnaar type 1) is an extremely rare cause ulnar-sided wrist pain resulting from pseudarthrosis or post-traumatic disruption (Mespreuve et al. 2015; van Schoonhoven et al. 2001).

5 Other Pathologies

5.1 Fractures

Fractures of the ulnar styloid, triquetrum, pisiform, hook of the hamate and 4th or 5th metacarpal bases produce ulnar-sided pain. A fall on an outstretched hand is the most common mechanism of injury. Hook of hamate fractures can occur in racket and batting sports from a direct blow or as a fatigue fracture (Tian and Goldfarb 2021). Fatigue fracture of the pisiform has been documented in volleyball players (Israeli et al. 1982). Some of these fractures, particularly impacted fractures and osteochondral fractures of the carpal bones, can be occult on standard wrist radiographs and are at risk of delayed diagnosis (Pinto et al. 2018). Special views such as the carpal tunnel view (Fig. 12) and semi-supinated oblique view allow better visualization of the hamate, pisiform and pisotriquetral joint. Cross-sectional imaging readily demonstrates these fractures (Fig. 12), with MRI having a higher sensitivity than CT (Mallee et al. 2015; Sahu et al. 2023). Dual-energy CT improves acute fracture detection by depicting bone marrow oedema and is especially useful in the emergency setting (Ali et al. 2018; Müller et al. 2020).

Hamate hook fractures are prone to non-union, and ulnar nerve irritation and flexor tendon injuries are occasionally associated with pisiform and hamate fractures (Blum et al. 2006; Tian and Goldfarb 2021). In the chronic setting, ulnar styloid non-union can cause symptoms as a result of symptomatic pseudarthrosis (Fig. 12), carpal abutment or impinging the ECU subsheath (Hauck et al. 1996).

5.2 Impaction Syndromes

Ulnocarpal abutment syndrome related to overloading across the ulnocarpal joint is discussed in Sect. 2.2.

Ulnar styloid impaction syndrome results from an elongated ulnar styloid impacting on the triquetrum. The ulnar styloid is elongated when its length exceeds 6 mm (Biyani et al. 1990; van Der Heijden et al. 2005). Patients with this syndrome have average styloid process lengths just over 7 mm (Bain and Bidwell 2006; Topper et al. 1997). The ulnar styloid process index and ulnar styloid-capitate ratio can also be used to evaluate for a long ulnar styloid (Garcia-Elias 1987; van Der Heijden et al. 2005). The syndrome can also result from styloid process malunion (Giachino et al. 2007). Radiographic signs of impaction include sclerosis, subchondral cysts and flattening, in addition to chondromalacia, subchondral changes and synovitis on MRI (Fig. 13). Dynamic impingement can be documented on fluoroscopy (Bain and Bidwell 2006).

Ulnar impingement syndrome is caused by a shortened distal ulna impinging on the distal radius proximal to the sigmoid notch. Ulnar shortening is most often the result of surgical excision (e.g. Darrach procedure for DRUJ osteoarthritis) but can also be from post-traumatic growth arrest or de novo negative ulnar variance (Bell et al. 1985). Ulnar shortening leads to radioulnar convergence (Sauerbier et al. 2003), which is asymptomatic in most (McKee and Richards 1996), but can lead to painful bone-on-bone contact or pseudarthrosis (Bell et al. 1985). Distal radius scalloping at the point of impaction is a late radiographic finding (Bell et al. 1985; Cerezal et al. 2002). Reproduction of pain on stress-loaded radiographs (Lees and Scheker 1997) and MRI showing subchondral changes at

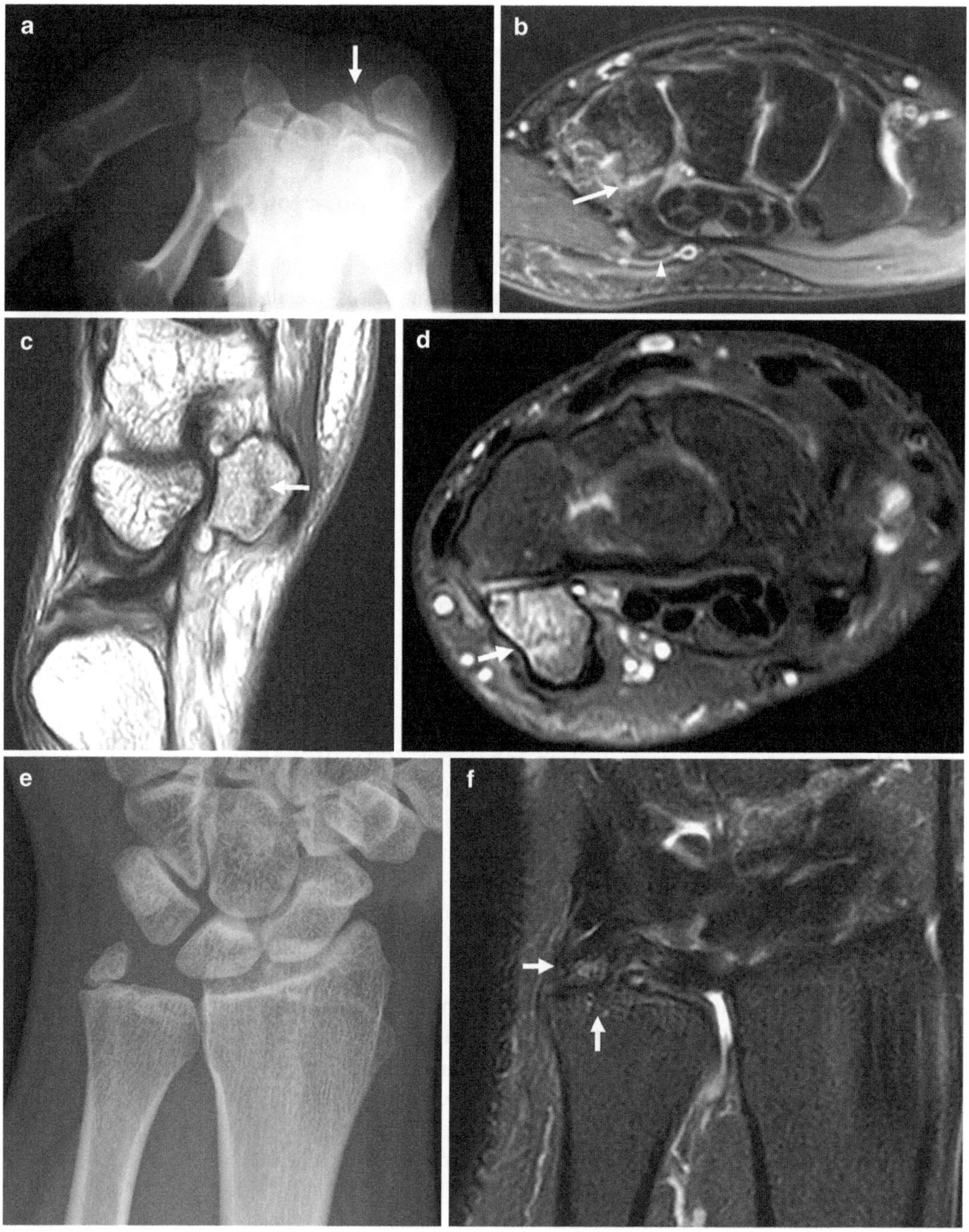

Fig. 12 Fractures. (**a**, **b**) Radiographically occult hook of hamate fracture. (**a**) Carpal tunnel view of the wrist did not demonstrate any fracture, including at the hook of the hamate (arrow). (**b**) Axial PD FS image shows non-displaced hamate hook fracture indenting on the superficial branch of the ulnar nerve (arrowhead). (**c**) Sagittal PD and (**d**) axial PD FS images show non-displaced pisiform fracture (arrow) associated with marrow oedema and small reactive effusion at the pisotriquetral joint. (**e**, **f**) Ulnar styloid non-union with symptomatic pseudarthrosis. (**e**) PA radiograph of the wrist shows chronic ulnar styloid non-union. (**f**) Coronal PD FS image shows marrow oedema across the pseudarthrosis

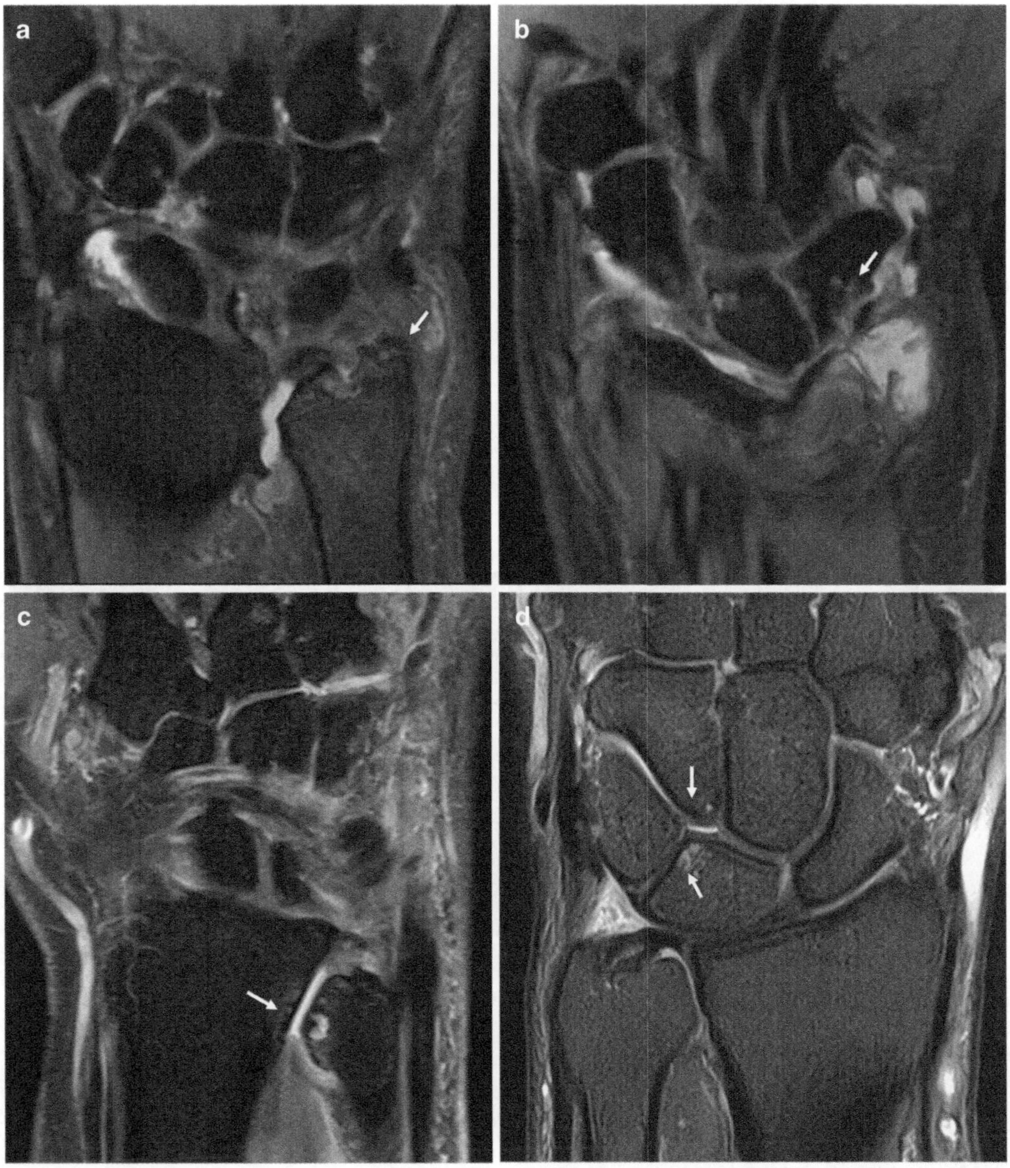

Fig. 13 Impaction syndromes at the wrist. (**a, b**) Ulnar styloid impaction syndrome secondary to ulnar styloid malunion. Coronal PD FS images show hypertrophic malunion of the ulnar styloid, subchondral cystic changes at the tip of the styloid process and proximal triquetrum (arrows), and surrounding synovitis. (**c**) Ulnar impingement syndrome related to negative ulnar variance. Coronal PD FS image shows negative ulnar variance and subchondral cysts at the ulnar seat. Subchondral oedema at the distal radius proximal to the sigmoid notch suggests impaction at this location (arrow). (**d**) Hamatolunate impaction syndrome. Coronal PD FS image shows type II lunate morphology, as well as subchondral changes at the accessory medial facet at the distal lunate and proximal hamate (arrows)

the site of impaction (Fig. 13) can help confirm the diagnosis at an earlier stage.

Hamatolunate impaction syndrome occurs in the setting of type II lunate morphology, defined an accessory medial facet at the distal lunate articulating with the hamate (Viegas 1990). This anatomic variant is extremely common (range: 46–73%) (Burgess 1990; Malik et al. 1999; Viegas et al. 1993) and predisposes to hamate chondromalacia, which can be inferred from subchondral marrow oedema at the at the proximal pole of the hamate (Fig. 13). Hamate chondromalacia can occasionally occur with type I lunate morphology (Malik et al. 1999) and LT instability.

5.3 Other Tendinopathies

Extensor digiti minimi (EDM) tenosynovitis is associated with repetitive activities like handwriting (Meraj et al. 2017). Vaughan-Jackson syndrome describes sequential attritional rupture of the extensor tendons starting at the ulnar side related to DRUJ arthrosis (Vaughan-Jackson 1948). This rare syndrome usually occurs secondary to rheumatoid arthritis at the DRUJ but has also been reported with primary DRUJ osteoarthritis, ulnar impingement syndrome (Figs. 13 and 14) and Kienböck disease (Dawood and Mahmood 2021; Low et al. 2023; Mazhar and Rambani 2011).

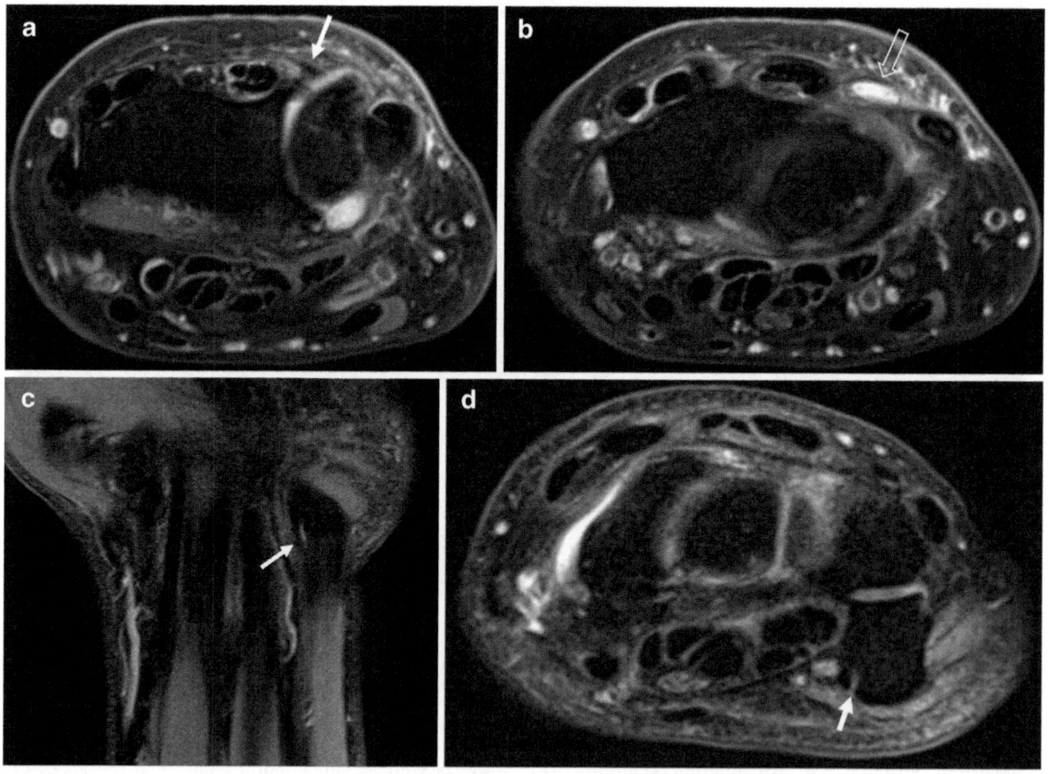

Fig. 14 EDM and FCU tendinopathies. (**a, b**) Attritional rupture of the EDM tendon secondary to DRUJ osteoarthritis. (**a**) Axial PD FS image at the level of the DRUJ shows prominent dorsal osteophyte impinging the EDM tendon, which is attenuated (arrow). (**b**) More distally, there is rupture of the EDM tendon at the level of the proximal carpal row with empty tendon sheath (empty arrow). (**c, d**) Interstitial split tear of the FCU tendon. (**c**) Coronal and (**d**) axial PD FS images show interstitial split tear of the FCU tendon at the pisiform insertion

The FCU tendon is subject to calcific tendinitis, tendinosis, paratenonitis (due to lack of tendon sheath) and tear (Fig. 14). FCU tendinopathy is rare and usually encountered in the setting of racket sports and golf (Blum et al. 2006).

5.4 Guyon Canal Syndrome

The ulnar nerve divides into its two terminal branches, the deep motor branch and superficial branch, within Guyon canal at the wrist. The deep (motor) branch supplies all the hypothenar and interossei muscles, 3rd and 4th lumbricals and adductor pollicis (Atkins et al. 2009). The deep (motor) branches also variably supply the opponens pollicis and flexor pollicis brevis (Atkins et al. 2009; Gil et al. 2016). The superficial branch is a mixed nerve, providing motor innervation to the palmaris brevis and sensory innervation to the hypothenar eminence and volar medial one and a half fingers.

Guyon canal is a fibro-osseous tunnel of about 4 cm long bounded by the pisiform on the ulnar side and hamate hook on the radial side and can be divided into three zones. Zone 1 is the area proximal to the ulnar nerve bifurcation, zone 2 surrounds the deep motor branch, and zone 3 surrounds the superficial branch (Gross and Gelberman 1985). Compression within zone 1 produces mixed motor and sensory deficits, compression within zone 2 causes weakness, and compression within zone 3 causes sensory symptoms.

Ganglia (Fig. 15) and hook of hamate fractures are the common causes of entrapment in zones 1 and 2, while accessory muscles (Fig. 15) and ulnar artery thrombosis are common in zone 3 (Earp et al. 2014). Other causes include repetitive trauma, prolonged compression from cycling (handlebar palsy) (Capitani and Beer 2002) and peripheral nerve sheath tumours (Fig. 15). MRI can identify space-occupying lesions within the canal, signal and morphologic changes of the nerve and any denervation changes.

5.5 Hypothenar Hammer Syndrome

Hypothenar hammer syndrome describes symptomatic digital ischemia secondary to ulnar artery thrombosis or aneurysm typically from repetitive striking of the hamate hook against the superficial ulnar artery (Yuen et al. 2011). Pre-existing fibromuscular dysplasia probably predisposes to this condition (Ferris et al. 2000). The diagnosis can be confirmed on Doppler ultrasound. CT, MR or catheter angiography are usually required for treatment planning (Yuen et al. 2011). The disease can manifest as corkscrew configuration, wall thickening, aneurysm (Fig. 16) or segmental occlusion of the superficial ulnar artery adjacent to the hamate hook (Blum et al. 2006). Embolic occlusion of the palmar arches and digital arteries is common (Marie et al. 2007).

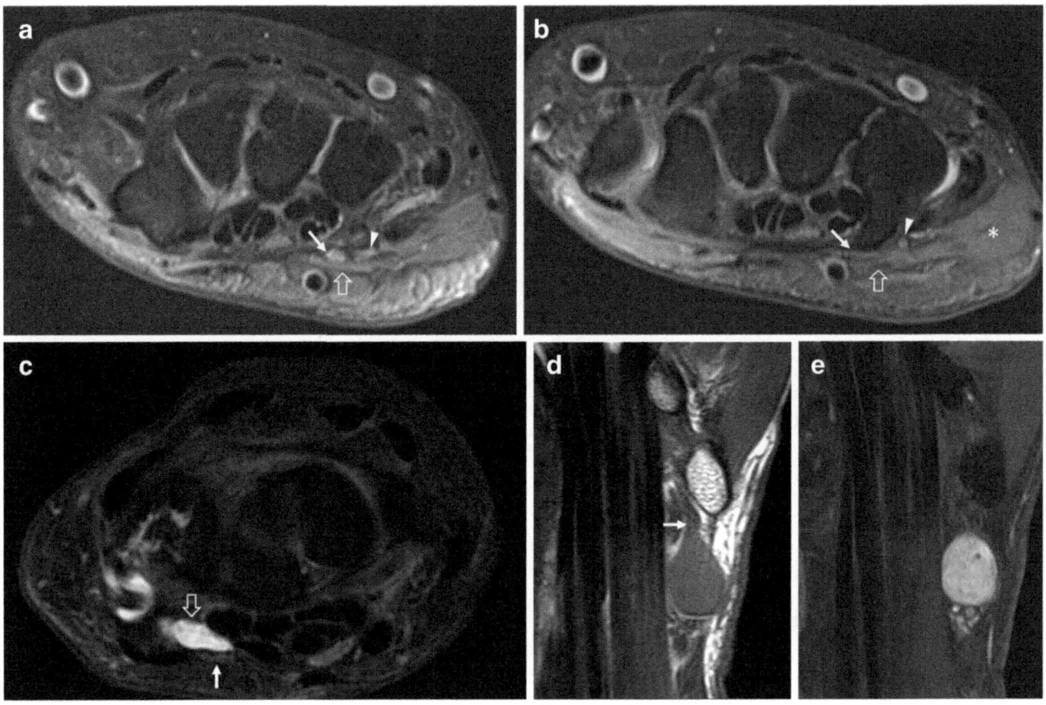

Fig. 15 Ulnar nerve entrapment and peripheral nerve sheath tumour. (**a**, **b**) Axial PD FS images show accessory abductor digiti minimi muscle slip (empty arrow) compressing the superficial branch of the ulnar nerve (arrow) at the level of the hamate hook. Deep branch of the ulnar nerve (arrowhead) and abductor digiti minimi muscle (*) are also marked. (**c**) Axial PD FS image shows ganglion cyst (empty arrow) in Guyon canal compressing the ulnar nerve (arrow). (**d**) Coronal T1W and (**e**) coronal post-contrast T1W FS images show an enhancing oval mass just proximal to Guyon canal in continuity with the ulnar nerve (arrow), consistent with a peripheral nerve sheath tumour

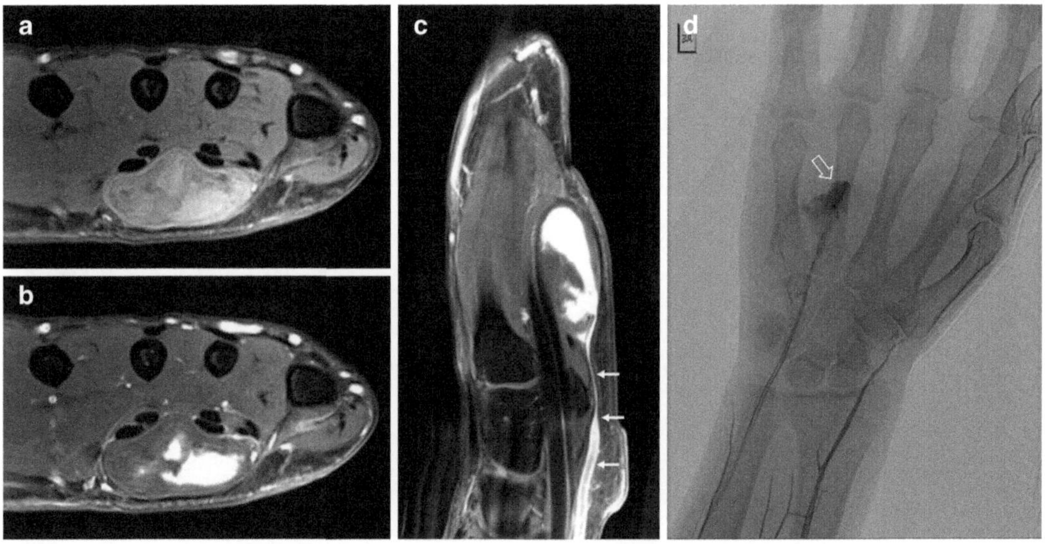

Fig. 16 Hypothenar hammer syndrome. (**a**) Axial T1W FS, (**b**) axial post-contrast T1W FS and (**c**) coronal post-contrast T1W FS images demonstrate a partially enhancing mass in the palm of the hand continuous with the superficial ulnar artery (arrows) just distal to Guyon canal, which was suspicious for a partially thrombosed aneurysm. (**d**) Catheter angiography confirmed the aneurysm at the superficial palmar arch (empty arrow)

6 Summary

For easy reference, the many causes of ulnar-sided wrist pain are summarized in Table 4 and potential pitfalls on MRI are highlighted in Table 5.

Table 4 Causes of ulnar-sided wrist pain

Category	Causes
Fractures	Fractures of the ulnar styloid, hamate hook, triquetrum, pisiform, 4th or 5th metacarpal base, etc.
TFCC	Traumatic tears
	Degenerative tears (ulnocarpal abutment syndrome)
DRUJ	DRUJ instability
	DRUJ arthritis
Carpus	Kienböck disease
	Lunotriquetral instability
	Pisotriquetral dislocation and arthropathy
	Lunotriquetral coalition (fibrocartilaginous type)
Impaction syndromes	Ulnocarpal abutment syndrome
	Ulnar styloid impaction syndrome
	Ulnar impingement syndrome
	Hamatolunate impingement syndrome
Tendon	ECU tendinopathy and instability
	FCU tendinopathy
	EDM tenosynovitis and attritional rupture
Ulnar nerve	Guyon canal syndrome
	Ulnar nerve PNST
Vascular	Hypothenar hammer syndrome

Table 5 Pitfalls on MRI

	Pitfall
Articular disc	Radial attachment to the hyaline cartilage of the sigmoid notch should not be mistaken for radial-sided tear.
	Intermediate signal in the disc not reaching the articular surface is related to degeneration and should not be mistaken for perforation.
TFCC peripheral attachments	High signal ligamentum subcruentum between the two laminae should not be mistaken for a tear.
	Styloid lamina inserts onto intermediate signal dense cartilage at the ulnar styloid tip and should not be mistaken for a tear.
DRUJ	Overcalling DRUJ subluxation. Distal ulna normally moves more palmar in supination and more dorsal in pronation. We recommend epicentre method to assess DRUJ displacement on axial images.
ECU tendon	Increased signal within the central substance of the tendon (ECU pseudolesion) is related to inter-tendinous ground substance or mucoid degeneration, whereas signal abnormality in ECU tendinosis is diffuse.
	Overcalling ECU subluxation. Supination causes physiologic medial and palmar subluxation of the tendon. Upper limit of physiologic displacement is 5 mm or 50% beyond the apex of the ulnar border of the ulnar groove.
LTL	Normal variations in shape and signal intensity of the proximal component should not be mistaken for tears.

References

Abe Y, Moriya A, Tominaga Y, Yoshida K (2016) Dorsal tear of triangular fibrocartilage complex: clinical features and treatment. J Wrist Surg 5:042–046

af Ekenstam F, Hagert CG (1985) Anatomical studies on the geometry and stability of the distal radio ulnar joint. Scand J Plast Reconstr Surg 19:17–25. https://doi.org/10.3109/02844318509052861

Ali S, Cunningham R, Amin M, Popoff S, Mohamed F, Barbe M (2015) The Extensor Carpi Ulnaris pseudolesion: evaluation with microCT, histology, and MRI. Skeletal Radiol 44:1735–1743. https://doi.org/10.1007/s00256-015-2224-3

Ali IT, Wong WD, Liang T, Khosa F, Mian M, Jalal S, Nicolaou S (2018) Clinical utility of dual-energy CT analysis of bone marrow edema in acute wrist fractures. Am J Roentgenol 210:842–847. https://doi.org/10.2214/AJR.17.18673

Allende C, Le Viet D (2005) Extensor carpi ulnaris problems at the wrist–classification, surgical treatment and results. J Hand Surg 30:265–272

Atkins SE, Logan B, McGrouther DA (2009) The deep (motor) branch of the ulnar nerve: a detailed examination of its course and the clinical significance of its damage. J Hand Surg Eur Vol 34:47–57. https://doi.org/10.1177/1753193408097489

Atzei A (2009) New trends in arthroscopic management of type 1-B TFCC injuries with DRUJ instability. J Hand Surg Eur Vol 34:582–591. https://doi.org/10.1177/1753193409100120

Atzei A, Luchetti R (2011) Foveal TFCC tear classification and treatment. Hand Clin 27:263–272. https://doi.org/10.1016/j.hcl.2011.05.014

Bain GI, Begg M (2006) Arthroscopic assessment and classification of Kienbock's disease. Tech Hand Up Extrem Surg 10:8–13. https://doi.org/10.1097/00130911-200603000-00003

Bain GI, Bidwell TA (2006) Arthroscopic excision of ulnar styloid in stylocarpal impaction. Arthroscopy 22:677.e1–677.e3. https://doi.org/10.1016/j.arthro.2006.04.083

Bell MJ, Hill RJ, McMurtry RY (1985) Ulnar impingement syndrome. J Bone Joint Surg Br 67:126–129. https://doi.org/10.1302/0301-620X.67B1.3968131

Biyani A, Mehara A, Bhan S (1990) Morphological variations of the ulnar styloid process. J Hand Surg 15:352–354. https://doi.org/10.1016/0266-7681_90_90018-y

Blum A, Zabel J-P, Kohlmann R, Batch T, Barbara K, Zhu X, Dautel G, Dap F (2006) Pathologic conditions of the hypothenar eminence: evaluation with multidetector CT and MR imaging. Radiographics 26:1021–1044. https://doi.org/10.1148/rg.264055114

Boer BC, Vestering M, van Raak SM, van Kooten EO, Huis in 't Veld R, Vochteloo AJH (2018) MR arthrography is slightly more accurate than conventional MRI in detecting TFCC lesions of the wrist. Eur J Orthop Surg Traumatol 28:1549–1553. https://doi.org/10.1007/s00590-018-2215-x

Bordalo-Rodrigues M, Schweitzer M, Bergin D, Culp R, Barakat MS (2005) Lunate chondromalacia: evaluation of routine MRI sequences. Am J Roentgenol 184:1464–1469. https://doi.org/10.2214/ajr.184.5.01841464

Brogan DM, Berger RA, Kakar S (2019) Ulnar-sided wrist pain: a critical analysis review. JBJS Rev 7:e1. https://doi.org/10.2106/JBJS.RVW.17.00207

Buck FM, Gheno R, Nico MAC, Haghighi P, Trudell DJ, Resnick D (2009) Ulnomeniscal homologue of the wrist: correlation of anatomic and MR imaging findings. Radiology 253:771–779. https://doi.org/10.1148/radiol.2533090743

Burgess RC (1990) Anatomic variations of the midcarpal joint. J Hand Surg 15:129–131

Burns JE, Tanaka T, Ueno T, Nakamura T, Yoshioka H (2011) Pitfalls that may mimic injuries of the triangular fibrocartilage and proximal intrinsic wrist ligaments at MR imaging. Radiographics 31:63–78

Capitani D, Beer S (2002) Handlebar palsy—a compression syndrome of the deep terminal (motor) branch of the ulnar nerve in biking. J Neurol 249:1441–1445. https://doi.org/10.1007/s00415-002-0864-4

Cerezal L, del Piñal F, Abascal F, García-Valtuille R, Pereda T, Canga A (2002) Imaging findings in ulnar-sided wrist impaction syndromes. Radiographics 22:105–121

Chang CY, Huang AJ, Bredella MA, Kattapuram SV, Torriani M (2014) Association between distal ulnar morphology and extensor carpi ulnaris tendon pathology. Skeletal Radiol 43:793–800

Cohen-Tanugi S, Gaston RG (2021) Examination of ulnar-sided wrist pain. Hand Clin 37:467–475. https://doi.org/10.1016/j.hcl.2021.06.002

Dallaudière B, Meyer P, Larbi A, Moinard M, Moreau-Durieux M-H, Poussange N, Pelé E, Pesquer L (2015) Magnetic resonance arthrography of the wrist with axial traction: an iconographic review. Diagn Interv Imaging, Imaging of the hand and fingers 96:1307–1312. https://doi.org/10.1016/j.diii.2014.11.028

DaSilva MF, Goodman AD, Gil JA, Akelman E (2017) Evaluation of ulnar-sided wrist pain. J Am Acad Orthop Surg 25:e150–e156. https://doi.org/10.5435/JAAOS-D-16-00407

Dawood AA, Mahmood HM (2021) Vaughan Jackson syndrome due to distal radioulnar joint osteoarthritis: a case report. J Musculoskelet Res 24:2150014. https://doi.org/10.1142/S0218957721500147

De Santis S, Cozzolino R, Luchetti R, Cazzoletti L (2021) Comparison between MRI and arthroscopy of the wrist for the assessment of posttraumatic lesions of intrinsic ligaments and the triangular fibrocartilage complex. J Wrist Surg 11:28–34. https://doi.org/10.1055/s-0041-1729757

Earp BE, Floyd WE, Louie D, Koris M, Protomastro P (2014) Ulnar nerve entrapment at the wrist. J Am Acad Orthop Surg 22:699–706

Eladawi S, Balamoody S, Amerasekera S, Choudhary S (2022) 3T MRI of wrist ligaments and TFCC using true plane oblique 3D T2 Dual Echo Steady State (DESS) – a study of diagnostic accuracy. Br J Radiol 95:20210019. https://doi.org/10.1259/bjr.20210019

Estrella EP, Hung L-K, Ho P-C, Tse WL (2007) Arthroscopic repair of triangular fibrocartilage complex tears. Arthroscopy 23:729–737.e1

Ferris BL, Taylor LM, Oyama K, McLafferty RB, Edwards JM, Moneta GL, Porter JM (2000) Hypothenar hammer syndrome: proposed etiology. J Vasc Surg 31:104–113. https://doi.org/10.1016/S0741-5214(00)70072-3

Flores DV, Umpire DF, Rakhra KS, Jibri Z, Belmar GAS (2023) Distal radioulnar joint: normal anatomy, imaging of common disorders, and injury classification. Radiographics 43:e220109. https://doi.org/10.1148/rg.220109

Garcia-Elias M (1987) Dorsal fractures of the triquetrum—avulsion or compression fractures? J Hand Surg 12:266–268

Garcia-Elias M (2015) Tendinopathies of the extensor carpi ulnaris. Handchir Mikrochir Plast Chir 47:312–315. https://doi.org/10.1055/s-0035-1559720

Giachino AA, McIntyre AI, Guy KJ, Conway AF (2007) Ulnar styloid triquetral impaction. Hand Surg 12:123–134

Gil YC, Shin KJ, Lee SH, Koh KS, Song WC (2016) Anatomy of the deep branch of the ulnar nerve. J Hand Surg Eur Vol 41:843–847. https://doi.org/10.1177/1753193415622188

Gross MS, Gelberman RH (1985) The anatomy of the distal ulnar tunnel. Clin Orthop (196):238–247

Haims AH, Schweitzer ME, Morrison WB, Deely D, Lange R, Osterman AL, Bednar JM, Taras JS, Culp RW (2002) Limitations of MR imaging in the diagnosis of peripheral tears of the triangular fibrocartilage of the wrist. Am J Roentgenol 178:419–422. https://doi.org/10.2214/ajr.178.2.1780419

Haims AH, Moore AE, Schweitzer ME, Morrison WB, Deely D, Culp RW, Forman HP (2004) MRI in the diagnosis of cartilage injury in the wrist. Am J Roentgenol 182:1267–1270. https://doi.org/10.2214/ajr.182.5.1821267

Harley BJ, Werner FW, Boles SD, Palmer AK (2004) Arthroscopic resection of arthrosis of the proximal hamate: a clinical and biomechanical study. J Hand Surg 29:661–667. https://doi.org/10.1016/j.jhsa.2004.04.016

Hauck RM, Skahen J, Palmer AK (1996) Classification and treatment of ulnar styloid nonunion. J Hand Surg 21:418–422. https://doi.org/10.1016/S0363-5023(96)80355-8

Hur Y, Ahn JM, Kim HJ, Jeon Y, Kang Y, Gong HS (2024) Peripheral tear of the triangular fibrocartilage complex: diagnostic accuracy of magnetic resonance imaging and diagnostic performance of the primary and secondary signs. Skeletal Radiol 53:1153–1163. https://doi.org/10.1007/s00256-023-04517-y

Immermann EW (1948) Dislocation of the pisiform. J Bone Joint Surg Am 30:489

Inoue G, Tamura Y (2001) Surgical treatment for recurrent dislocation of the extensor carpi ulnaris tendon. J Hand Surg 26:556–559. https://doi.org/10.1054/jhsb.2001.0615

Ishii S, Palmer AK, Werner FW, Short WH, Fortino MD (1998) An anatomic study of the ligamentous structure of the triangular fibrocartilage complex. J Hand Surg 23:977–985. https://doi.org/10.1016/S0363-5023(98)80003-8

Israeli A, Engel J, Ganel A (1982) Possible fatigue fracture of the pisiform bone in volleyball players. Int J Sports Med 3:56–57

Kakar S, Garcia-Elias M (2016) The "four-leaf clover" treatment algorithm: a practical approach to manage disorders of the distal radioulnar joint. J Hand Surg 41:551–564. https://doi.org/10.1016/j.jhsa.2016.01.005

King GJ, McMurtry RY, Rubenstein JD, Gertzbein SD (1986) Kinematics of the distal radioulnar joint. J Hand Surg 11:798–804. https://doi.org/10.1016/s0363-5023(86)80225-8

Kleinman WB (2007) Stability of the distal radioulna joint: biomechanics, pathophysiology, physical diagnosis, and restoration of function what we have learned in 25 years. J Hand Surg 32:1086–1106. https://doi.org/10.1016/j.jhsa.2007.06.014

Kuntz MT, Janssen SJ, Ring D (2015) Incidental signal changes in the extensor carpi ulnaris on MRI. Hand (NY) 10:750–755. https://doi.org/10.1007/s11552-015-9764-9

Larsen CF, Stigsby B, Mathiesen FK, Lindequist S (1990) Radiography of the wrist: a new device for standardized radiographs. Acta Radiol 31:459–462

Lee MLH (1963) The intraosseus arterial pattern of the carpal lunate bone and its relation to avascular necrosis. Acta Orthop Scand 33:43–55

Lee KS, Ablove RH, Singh S, De Smet AA, Haaland B, Fine JP (2009) Ultrasound imaging of normal displacement of the extensor carpi ulnaris tendon within the ulnar groove in 12 forearm–wrist positions. Am J Roentgenol 193:651–655. https://doi.org/10.2214/AJR.08.1725

Lee RKL, Griffith JF, Ng AWH, Nung RCH, Yeung DKW (2016) Wrist traction during MR arthrography improves detection of triangular fibrocartilage complex and intrinsic ligament tears and visibility of articular cartilage. AJR Am J Roentgenol 206:155–161. https://doi.org/10.2214/AJR.15.14948

Lees VC, Scheker LR (1997) The radiological demonstration of dynamic ulnar impingement. J Hand Surg 22:448–450

Lichtman DM, Lesley NE, Simmons SP (2010) The classification and treatment of Kienböck's disease: the state of the art and a look at the future. J Hand Surg Eur Vol 35:549–554. https://doi.org/10.1177/1753193410374690

Lichtman DM, Pientka WF II, Bain GI (2017) Kienböck disease: a new algorithm for the 21st century. J Wrist Surg 6:002–010

Linscheid RL, Dobyns JH, Beabout JW, Bryan RS (1972) Traumatic instability of the wrist: diagnosis, classification, and pathomechanics. JBJS 54:1612–1632

Lo IK, MacDermid JC, Bennett JD, Bogoch E, King GJ (2001) The radioulnar ratio: a new method of quantifying distal radioulnar joint subluxation. J Hand Surg 26:236–243. https://doi.org/10.1053/jhsu.2001.22908

Low YX, Goh AGW, Quek ST (2023) Extensor tendon rupture in ulnar impingement syndrome: a case report. J Phys Med Rehabil 5:1–5. https://doi.org/10.33696/rehabilitation.5.033

Lutsky K, Beredjiklian PK (2012) Kienböck disease. J Hand Surg 37:1942–1952. https://doi.org/10.1016/j.jhsa.2012.06.029

Magee T (2009) Comparison of 3-T MRI and arthroscopy of intrinsic wrist ligament and TFCC tears. Am J Roentgenol 192:80–85. https://doi.org/10.2214/AJR.08.1089

Malik AM, Schweitzer ME, Culp RW, Osterman LA, Manton G (1999) MR imaging of the type II lunate bone: frequency, extent, and associated findings. AJR Am J Roentgenol 173:335–338

Mallee WH, Wang J, Poolman RW, Kloen P, Maas M, de Vet HCW, Doornberg JN (2015) Computed tomography versus magnetic resonance imaging versus bone scintigraphy for clinically suspected scaphoid fractures in patients with negative plain radiographs. Cochrane Database Syst Rev 2015:CD010023. https://doi.org/10.1002/14651858.CD010023.pub2

Manton GL, Schweitzer ME, Weishaupt D, Morrison WB, Osterman AL, Culp RW, Shabshin N (2001) Partial interosseous ligament tears of the wrist: difficulty in utilizing either primary or secondary MRI signs. J Comput Assist Tomogr 25:671–676

Marie I, Hervé F, Primard E, Cailleux N, Levesque H (2007) Long-term follow-up of hypothenar hammer syndrome: a series of 47 patients. Medicine (Baltimore) 86:334–343. https://doi.org/10.1097/MD.0b013e31815c95d3

Mazhar T, Rambani R (2011) Vaughan-Jackson-like syndrome as an unusual presentation of Kienböck's disease: a case report. J Med Case Rep 5:325. https://doi.org/10.1186/1752-1947-5-325

McKee MD, Richards RR (1996) Dynamic radio-ulnar convergence after the darrach procedure. J Bone Joint Surg Br 78-B:413–418. https://doi.org/10.1302/0301-620X.78B3.0780413

Meraj S, Gyftopoulos S, Nellans K, Walz D, Brown MS (2017) MRI of the extensor tendons of the wrist. Am J Roentgenol 209:1093–1102. https://doi.org/10.2214/AJR.17.17791

Mespreuve M, Vanhoenacker F, Verstraete K (2015) Lunotriquetral coalition, a normal variant that may rarely cause ulnar sided wrist pain. JBR-BTR 98:72–78. https://doi.org/10.5334/jbr-btr.769

Miller TT, Bis G (2022) Ultrasound-guided injection of the pisotriquetral joint: technique and case series. Skeletal Radiol 51:1687–1694. https://doi.org/10.1007/s00256-022-03992-z

Minami A, Iwasaki N, Ishikawa J, Suenaga N, Yasuda K, Kato H (2005) Treatments of osteoarthritis of the distal radioulnar joint: long-term results of three procedures. Hand Surg 10:243–248

Minnaar AD (1952) Congenital fusion of the lunate and triquetral bones in the South African Bantu. J Bone Joint Surg Br 34:45–48

Mino DE, Palmer AK, Levinsohn EM (1983) The role of radiography and computerized tomography in the diagnosis of subluxation and dislocation of the distal radioulnar joint. J Hand Surg 8:23–31. https://doi.org/10.1016/S0363-5023(83)80046-X

Moraux A, Lefebvre G, Pansini V, Aucourt J, Vandenbussche L, Demondion X, Cotten A (2014) Pisotriquetral joint disorders: an under-recognized cause of ulnar side wrist pain. Skeletal Radiol 43:761–773. https://doi.org/10.1007/s00256-014-1848-z

Moser T, Dosch J-C, Moussaoui A, Dietemann J-L (2007) Wrist ligament tears: evaluation of MRI and combined MDCT and MR arthrography. Am J Roentgenol 188:1278–1286. https://doi.org/10.2214/AJR.06.0288

Müller FC, Gosvig KK, Børgesen H, Gade JS, Brejnebøl M, Rodell A, Nèmery M, Boesen M (2020) Dual-energy CT for suspected radiographically negative wrist fractures: a prospective diagnostic test accuracy study. Radiology 296:596–602. https://doi.org/10.1148/radiol.2020192701

Mutimer J, Green J, Field J (2008) Comparison of MRI and wrist arthroscopy for assessment of wrist cartilage. J Hand Surg Eur Vol 33:380–382. https://doi.org/10.1177/1753193408090395

Nakamura R, Horii E, Imaeda T, Tsunoda K, Nakao E (1995) Distal radioulnar joint subluxation and dislocation diagnosed by standard roentgenography. Skeletal Radiol 24:91–94. https://doi.org/10.1007/BF00198067

Ng AW, Tong CS, Hung EH, Griffith JF, Tse WL, Wong CW, Mak MC, Ho PC (2019) Top-ten tips for imaging the triangular fibrocartilaginous complex. Semin Musculoskelet Radiol. Thieme Medical Publishers 23:436–443

Omar NN, Mahmoud MK, Saleh WR, Almallah HG, Qenawy OK, Mourad AF, Abdul Monem ES (2019) MR arthrography versus conventional MRI and diagnostic arthroscope in patients with chronic wrist pain. Eur J Radiol Open 6:265–274. https://doi.org/10.1016/j.ejro.2019.06.003

Omokawa S, Gumpangseth T, Komutrattananont P, Inchai C, Mahakkanukrauh P (2021) Anatomical study of stabilizing structures of the extensor carpi ulnaris tendon around the wrist. J Hand Surg 46:930.e1–930.e9. https://doi.org/10.1016/j.jhsa.2021.02.008

Oneson SR, Timins ME, Scales LM, Erickson SJ, Chamoy L (1997) MR imaging diagnosis of triangular fibrocartilage pathology with arthroscopic correlation. AJR Am J Roentgenol 168:1513–1518. https://doi.org/10.2214/ajr.168.6.9168716

Palmer AK (1989) Triangular fibrocartilage complex lesions: a classification. J Hand Surg 14:594–606. https://doi.org/10.1016/0363-5023(89)90174-3

Palmer AK, Werner FW (1981) The triangular fibrocartilage complex of the wrist—anatomy and function. J Hand Surg 6:153–162. https://doi.org/10.1016/s0363-5023(81)80170-0

Park MJ, Kim JP (2008) Reliability and normal values of various computed tomography methods for quantifying distal radioulnar joint translation. J Bone Joint Surg Am 90:145. https://doi.org/10.2106/JBJS.F.01603

Pessis E, Drapé J-L, Bach F, Feydy A, Guerini H, Chevrot A (2006) Direct arthrography of the pisotriquetral joint. Am J Roentgenol 186:800–804. https://doi.org/10.2214/AJR.04.1640

Petsatodis E, Pilavaki M, Kalogera A, Drevelegas A, Agathangelidis F, Ditsios K (2019) Comparison between conventional MRI and MR arthrography in the diagnosis of triangular fibrocartilage tears and correlation with arthroscopic findings. Injury 50:1464–1469. https://doi.org/10.1016/j.injury.2019.07.032

Pfirrmann CW, Theumann NH, Chung CB, Botte MJ, Trudell DJ, Resnick D (2001) What happens to the triangular fibrocartilage complex during pronation and supination of the forearm? Analysis of its morphology and diagnostic assessment with MR arthrography. Skeletal Radiol 30:677–685. https://doi.org/10.1007/s002560100429

Pinto A, Berritto D, Russo A, Riccitiello F, Caruso M, Paola Belfiore M, Roberto Papapietro V, Carotti M, Pinto F, Giovagnoni A, Romano L, Grassi R (2018) Traumatic fractures in adults: missed diagnosis on plain radiographs in the Emergency Department. Acta Biomed 89:111–123. https://doi.org/10.23750/abm.v89i1-S.7015

Potter HG, Asnis-Ernberg L, Weiland AJ, Hotchkiss RN, Peterson MG, McCORMACK RR (1997) The utility of high-resolution magnetic resonance imaging in the evaluation of the triangular fibrocartilage complex of the wrist. J Bone Joint Surg Am 79:1675–1684

Rastogi AK, Davis KW, Ross A, Rosas HG (2016) Fundamentals of joint injection. AJR Am J Roentgenol 207:484–494. https://doi.org/10.2214/AJR.16.16243

Ringler MD (2013) MRI of wrist ligaments. J Hand Surg 38:2034–2046

Ritt MJPF, Bishop AT, Berger RA, Linscheid RL, Berglund LJ, An K-N (1998) Lunotriquetral ligament properties: a comparison of three anatomic subregions. J Hand Surg 23:425–431. https://doi.org/10.1016/S0363-5023(05)80460-5

Sahu A, Kuek DK, MacCormick A, Gozzard C, Ninan T, Fullilove S, Suresh P (2023) Prospective comparison of magnetic resonance imaging and computed tomography in diagnosing occult scaphoid fractures. Acta Radiol 1987(64):201–207. https://doi.org/10.1177/02841851211064595

Sauerbier M, Berger R, Fujita M, Hahn M (2003) Radioulnar convergence after distal ulnar resection: mechanical performance of two commonly used soft tissue stabilizing procedures. Acta Orthop Scand 74:420–428

Schmitt R, Heinze A, Fellner F, Obletter N, Strühn R, Bautz W (1997) Imaging and staging of avascular osteonecroses at the wrist and hand. Eur J Radiol 25:92–103. https://doi.org/10.1016/S0720-048X(97)00065-X

Selvin O, Tandioy-Delgado FA, Mathew P (2021) Wrist arthroscopy: indications, portal anatomy and therapeutic advances. Orthop Trauma 35:234–248. https://doi.org/10.1016/j.mporth.2021.06.002

Sharma A, Kumar A, Singh P (2011) Anatomical study of the distal end of cadaveric human ulnae: a clinical consideration for the management of distal radioulnar joint injuries. Singapore Med J 52:673–676

Shin AY, Battaglia MJ, Bishop AT (2000) Lunotriquetral instability: diagnosis and treatment. J Am Acad Orthop Surg 8:170–179. https://doi.org/10.5435/00124635-200005000-00004

Smith DK, Snearly WN (1994) Lunotriquetral interosseous ligament of the wrist: MR appearances in asymptomatic volunteers and arthrographically normal wrists. Radiology 191:199–202

Taleisnik J, Gelberman RH, Miller BW, Szabo RM (1984) The extensor retinaculum of the wrist. J Hand Surg 9:495–501. https://doi.org/10.1016/s0363-5023(84)80100-8

Tanaka T, Ogino S, Yoshioka H (2008) Ligamentous injuries of the wrist. Semin Musculoskelet Radiol. © Thieme Medical Publishers 12:359–377

Theumann NH, Pfirrmann CWA, Antonio GE, Chung CB, Gilula LA, Trudell DJ, Resnick D (2003) Extrinsic carpal ligaments: normal MR arthrographic appearance in cadavers. Radiology 226:171–179. https://doi.org/10.1148/radiol.2261011715

Tian A, Goldfarb CA (2021) Hook of hamate fractures. Hand Clin 37:545–552. https://doi.org/10.1016/j.hcl.2021.06.013

Timins ME, O'Connell SE, Erickson SJ, Oneson SR (1996) MR imaging of the wrist: normal findings that may simulate disease. Radiographics 16:987–995

Topper SM, Wood MB, Ruby LK (1997) Ulnar styloid impaction syndrome. J Hand Surg 22:699–704. https://doi.org/10.1016/S0363-5023(97)80131-1

van Der Heijden B, Groot S, Schuurman AH (2005) Evaluation of ulnar styloid length. J Hand Surg 30:954–959. https://doi.org/10.1016/j.jhsa.2005.05.007

van Schoonhoven J, Prommersberger K-J, Schmitt R (2001) Traumatic disruption of a fibrocartilage lunate-triquetral coalition—a case report and review of the literature. Hand Surg 06:103–108. https://doi.org/10.1142/S0218810401000497

Vasilas A, Grieco RV, Bartone NF (1960) Roentgen aspects of injuries to the pisiform bone and pisotriquetral joint. J Bone Joint Surg Am 42:1317–1328

Vaughan-Jackson OJ (1948) Rupture of extensor tendons by attrition at the inferior radio-ulnar joint; report of two cases. J Bone Joint Surg Br 30B:528–530

Viegas SF (1990) The lunatohamate articulation of the midcarpal joint. Arthroscopy 6:5–10

Viegas SF, Patterson RM, Hokanson JA, Davis J (1993) Wrist anatomy: incidence, distribution, and correlation of anatomic variations, tears, and arthrosis. J Hand Surg 18:463–475

Wechsler RJ, Wehbe MA, Rifkin MD, Edeiken J, Branch HM (1987) Computed tomography diagnosis of distal radioulnar subluxation. Skeletal Radiol 16:1–5

Wijffels M, Stomp W, Krijnen P, Reijnierse M, Schipper I (2016) Computed tomography for the detection of distal radioulnar joint instability: normal variation and reliability of four CT scoring systems in 46 patients. Skeletal Radiol 45:1487–1493

Yang Z, Mann FA, Gilula LA, Haerr C, Larsen CF (1997) Scaphopisocapitate alignment: criterion to establish a neutral lateral view of the wrist. Radiology 205:865–869

Yoshioka H, Burns JE (2012) Magnetic resonance imaging of triangular fibrocartilage. J Magn Reson Imaging 35:764–778. https://doi.org/10.1002/jmri.22840

Yoshioka H, Tanaka T, Ueno T, Shindo M, Carrino JA, Lang P, Winalski CS (2006) High-resolution MR imaging of the proximal zone of the lunotriquetral ligament with a microscopy coil. Skeletal Radiol 35:288–294. https://doi.org/10.1007/s00256-005-0070-4

Yuen JC, Wright E, Johnson LA, Culp WC (2011) Hypothenar hammer syndrome: an update with algorithms for diagnosis and treatment. Ann Plast Surg 67:429–438

Zhan H, Bai R, Qian Z, Yang Y, Zhang H, Yin Y (2020) Traumatic injury of the triangular fibrocartilage complex (TFCC)—a refinement to the Palmer classification by using high-resolution 3-T MRI. Skeletal Radiol 49:1567–1579

Zhao X, Sun J, Duan F, Xin F, Shi LL, Yu T (2024a) Qualitative and quantitative anatomy of the deep radioulnar ligaments' insertion on ulna: cadaveric, histologic, and MRI study. J Hand Surg 49:377.e1–377.e9. https://doi.org/10.1016/j.jhsa.2022.06.003

Zhao X, Yu A, Zhao H, Qiu Y (2024b) Diagnostic value of MRI in traumatic triangular fibrocartilage complex injuries: a retrospective study. BMC Musculoskelet Disord 25:63. https://doi.org/10.1186/s12891-023-07140-z

Applications of Imaging for Nerve Entrapment at Wrist

Alex Zhu, Sadeem Lodhi, and Avneesh Chhabra

Contents

A. Zhu · S. Lodhi
Department of Radiology, UT Southwestern Medical Center, Dallas, TX, USA

A. Chhabra (✉)
Department of Radiology, UT Southwestern Medical Center, Dallas, TX, USA

Department of Orthopedic Surgery, UT Southwestern Medical Center, Dallas, TX, USA

Radiology & Orthopedic Surgery, UT Southwestern, Dallas, TX, USA

Johns Hopkins University, Maryland, MD, USA

University of Dallas, Richardson, TX, USA

Walton Centre for Neuroscience, Liverpool, UK
e-mail: avneesh.chhabra@utsouthwestern.edu

Med Radiol Diagn Imaging (2025)
https://doi.org/10.1007/174_2025_594,
Published Online: 24 August 2025

Abstract

Wrist mononeuropathies, primarily compression neuropathies, result from entrapment of the median, radial sensory, and less frequently, ulnar nerves within narrow anatomical passages, such as the carpal tunnel and Guyon's canal. Prolonged or severe compression leads to venous congestion and/or ischemia, inflammation, scarring, and demyelination, further impairing nerve function. Diagnostic imaging plays a critical role in the assessment of wrist entrapment neuropathies. Ultrasound (US) and Magnetic Resonance Imaging (MRI) provide superior soft tissue contrast for detailed evaluation of small nerves and their branches. US is particularly useful for assessing entrapment neuropathies, including carpal tunnel syndrome, by identifying changes in nerve size, signal alterations, and fascicular structure. MRI offers additional advantages, including less operator dependence, comprehensive visualization of carpal tunnel contents, and detailed evaluation of associated joint structures, cartilage, and tendons. MR neurography and functional diffusion tensor imaging further allows nerve selective imaging and lesion characterization. After learning from this chapter, the reader will be able to apply these imaging principles in their practices for the benefit of peripheral neuropathy patients.

1 Introduction

The understanding of wrist innervation is still evolving due to advancements in anatomical investigation techniques. Initially, the anatomic knowledge was based on dissecting nerves and their branches at 3.5x magnification. This was later improved by microdissection using a microscope. Histological examinations of the wrist capsule stained with the S-100 method revealed the paths of small nerve branches not visible during dissection, connections between nerves, and their entry points into the wrist joints.

Nerve branches to the wrist come from the ulnar, median, radial, lateral antebrachial cutaneous, and medial antebrachial cutaneous nerves. Most wrist mononeuropathies are compression neuropathies, caused by the entrapment of the median, radial sensory nerve, and less commonly the ulnar nerves in narrow passages—the carpal tunnel, radial tunnel, and the Guyon's canal. These can lead to pain and/or muscle and joint or limb dysfunction. This chapter discusses the anatomy and lesions causing nerve entrapments at the wrist with illustrative case examples. The reader will be able to apply the gained knowledge in their practices for the benefit of patients with upper extremity peripheral nerve entrapments.

2 Carpal Tunnel

The carpal tunnel is formed by the tubercles of the scaphoid and trapezium on the lateral side, bridged by the flexor retinaculum (or transverse carpal ligament), and the pisiform and hook of the hamate on the ulnar side. The dorsal roof is made of carpal bones. Nine tendons and the median nerve pass through the tunnel: four flexor digitorum superficialis, four flexor digitorum profundus, one flexor pollicis longus tendon, and the median nerve (Fig. 1). The palmar cutaneous branch of the median nerve branches off before entering the tunnel, coursing near the flexor carpi radialis tendon, superficially to the flexor retinaculum. After exiting the tunnel, the median nerve innervates (via recurrent branch) the three thenar muscles (abductor pollicis brevis, opponens pollicis, and superficial part of flexor pollicis brevis) and the first and second lumbricals. The terminal sensory branches of the median nerve provide sensation to the palmar surface of the lateral three and a half fingers. The palmar cutaneous branch pierces the superficial palmar fascia, providing sensation to the thenar eminence and the proximal radial aspect of the palm.

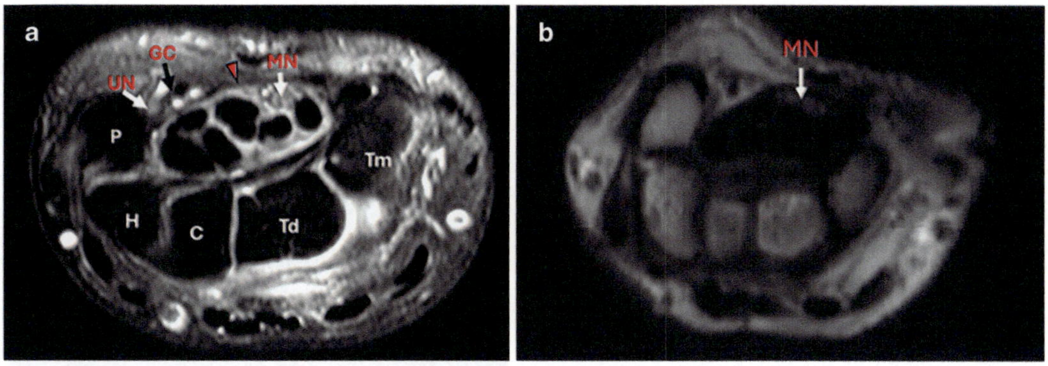

Fig. 1 Normal anatomy. The axial water (**a**) and in-phase (**b**) images of the wrist using T2W Dixon imaging show low signal flexor retinaculum (red arrow) in the carpal tunnel. MN, median nerve (MN); UN, ulnar nerve; GC, Guyon's canal; Tm, trapezium; Td, trapezoid; C, capitate; H, hamate; P, pisiform

3 Guyon's Canal

Guyon's canal, also known as the ulnar tunnel, is on the medial side of the hand. It runs from the pisiform bone to the hook of the hamate. The tunnel's roof is formed by the volar (superficial transverse) carpal ligament, and the floor is the flexor retinaculum (deep transverse carpal ligament). The radial border is formed by hook of the hamate and the medial border by the pisiform bone and pisohamate ligament.

Guyon's canal contains the ulnar nerve, ulnar artery, fat, and sometimes veins (Fig. 1). Before entering the canal, the ulnar nerve branches into a dorsal branch, which provides sensation to the dorsal ulnar hand, and a palmar branch, which supplies the skin over the hypothenar eminence.

Inside the canal, the ulnar nerve splits into superficial sensory and deep motor branches. The superficial branch supplies the palmaris brevis muscle and provides sensation to the fifth finger and the ulnar half of the fourth finger. The deep motor branch, along with the ulnar artery, makes a sharp turn at the hook of the hamate coursing under a fibrotendinous arch called the pisohamate hiatus, a known compression site. The deep motor branch innervates the hypothenar muscles (abductor digiti minimi, flexor digiti minimi brevis, and opponens digiti minimi), the adductor pollicis, the third and fourth lumbricals, and all the interossei muscles.

4 Radial Sensory Nerve

At the level of the elbow, the radial nerve splits into two branches: the superficial (sensory) branch and the deeper posterior interosseous nerve (PIN). The superficial radial sensory nerve (SRN) emerges between the brachioradialis and extensor carpi radialis longus, then travels distally toward the wrist. It provides sensory innervation to the lateral dorsum of the hand, the dorsal thumb, and the dorsal proximal portions of the second to fourth digits. Meanwhile, the PIN innervates the extensor compartment muscles of the forearm.

After piercing the deep fascia, the SRN lies superficially, immediately beneath the skin. As it crosses the wrist, it becomes vulnerable to mechanical compression, repetitive trauma, or penetrating injury (Fig. 2).

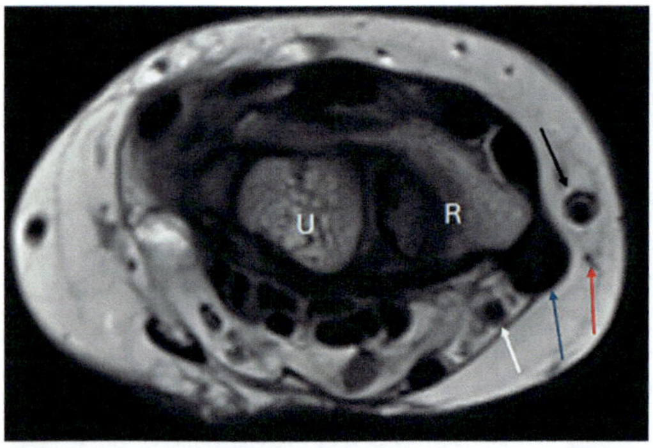

Fig. 2 Axial PDW Dixon in-phase image showing normal superficial branch of radial nerve (red arrow), cephalic vein (black arrow), radial artery (white arrow), radius (R), ulna (U), abductor pollicis longus APL tendon (blue arrow)

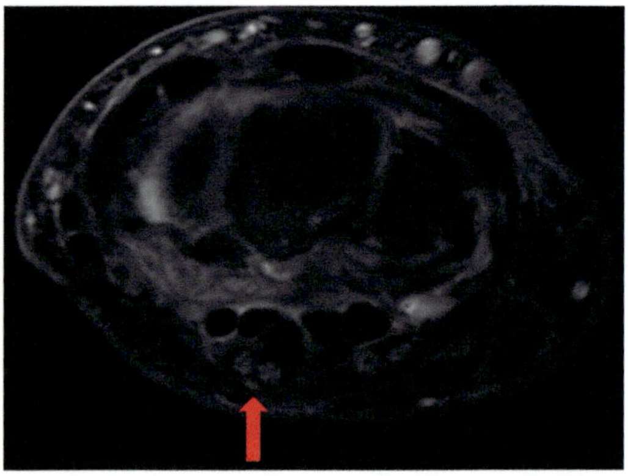

Fig. 3 Axial T2W Dixon water image showing otherwise normal median nerve. Arrow pointing towards bifid median nerve with persistent median vessel

5 Major Anatomical Variations of Nerves in the Carpal Tunnel and Ulnar Tunnel

5.1 Variations of the Motor Branch of the Median Nerve

Typically, the median nerve passes through the carpal tunnel as a single nerve, dividing into digital nerves distal to the flexor retinaculum. Bifurcation of the median nerve occurs when median nerve splits proximally to the flexor retinaculum, seen as a bifid nerve or early branching variation, and it may be associated with carpal tunnel syndrome (CTS). Other variations include persistent median artery or an accessory muscle belly of the long finger flexor superficialis (Figs. 3 and 4).

Variations of the median nerve motor branching include branches arising from the median nerve distal to the flexor retinaculum on the radial side or branches arising within the carpal tunnel or from an ulnar and anterior location and piercing the radial side on its course toward the thenar musculature. The median nerve motor branch may also have branches superficial to the flexor retinaculum.

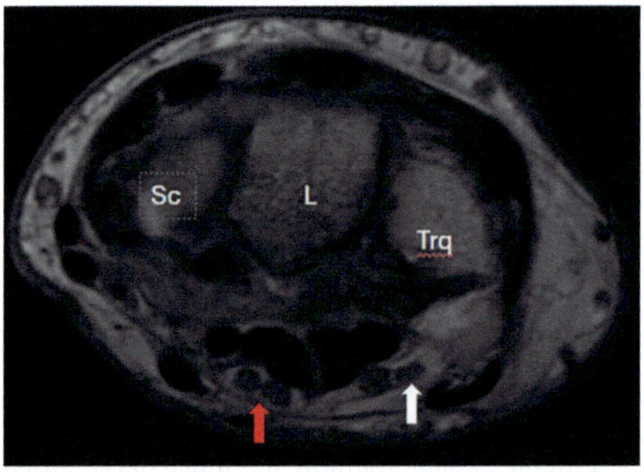

Fig. 4 Axial T2W Dixon water image showing otherwise normal, bifid median nerve (red arrow), ulnar nerve (white arrow), scaphoid (Sc), lunate (L), triquetrum (Trq)

5.2 Variations of the Palmar Cutaneous Branch of the Median Nerve

The palmar cutaneous branch of the median nerve arises from the main stem of the nerve prior to entering the carpal tunnel, superficial to the flexor retinaculum, and passing between the superficial and deep layers of forearm fascia. It then divides into three terminal branches supplying the dermis. The course of the palmar cutaneous branch varies where the nerve has a trans-ligamentous course piercing the flexor retinaculum or the nerve coursing ulnar to the median nerve.

5.3 Variations of the Ulnar Nerve

Aberrant position of the ulnar nerve within the carpal tunnel has been described in patients undergoing carpal tunnel release surgery. Such patients had presented with carpal tunnel syndrome associated with symptoms of ulnar nerve compression including intrinsic muscle wasting and paresthesia involving the little finger and the ulnar half of the ring finger.

6 Nerve Compression Conditions and Their Pathophysiology

Compressive forces affect the small blood vessels of the nerves and their myelin sheaths. Mild compression can block venous flow, causing nerve congestion and swelling, while more severe and persistent compression leads to arterial ischemia. Prolonged or repeated compression causes inflammation, scarring, and loss of myelin. Such scarring worsens the compression by affecting nerve pliability and mobility. Loss of myelin slows down the nerve conduction signals and, in severe cases, can completely block them. Persistent compression can further lead to nerve fiber (axonal and myelin sheath) degeneration.

6.1 Compression of Median Nerve in Carpal Tunnel: Carpal Tunnel Syndrome

Carpal tunnel syndrome (CTS) occurs when the median nerve is compressed in the carpal tunnel. Early clinical features include pain, numbness, and tingling in the first three fingers and the lateral half of the fourth finger. Symptoms can vary, from pain in the wrist to the entire hand, and sometimes radiating up the forearm or beyond the elbow. As CTS progresses, individuals may experience hand weakness, reduced fine motor skills, clumsiness, and eventually, atrophy of the thenar muscles.

Conditions that reduce the caliber of the carpal tunnel or increase the bulk of its contents can compress the median nerve. Factors that shrink the tunnel include overuse, osteoarthritis, trauma, and acromegaly. Factors that increase tunnel contents include tumor-like lesions like ganglion or flexor tenosynovitis, nerve sheath tumor, amyloid deposits, synovial thickening and tenosynovitis in rheumatoid arthritis, and hematoma from trauma, etc.

6.2 Ulnar Nerve Entrapment at the Wrist: Guyon's Canal Syndrome

Guyon canal syndrome involves entrapment and/or injury to the distal portion of the ulnar nerve as it travels through the Guyon canal.

Ulnar neuropathies at the wrist commonly result from bone (hook of hamate) fractures that impinge on the nerve, repetitive trauma from external compression, or internal compression such as ganglion cysts and thrombosed ulnar artery, e.g., in the setting of fibromuscular dysplasia or hypothenar hammer syndrome. Penetrating trauma limited to the ulnar artery may also secondarily cause nerve injury from compression by the formation of a space occupying lesion such as a pseudoaneurysm. Internal causes for chronic compression include vascular etiologies and other space occupying lesions as with CTS.

Guyon's canal is divided into 3 zones from its proximal to distal extent: zone 1 is proximal to the bifurcation of the ulnar nerve into the deep motor branch and the superficial sensory branch. Zone 2 is distal to zone 1, containing only the motor branch. Zone 3 is distal to zone 2 and surrounds only the superficial sensory branch of the ulnar nerve.

Compression in zone 1 at the proximal end of Guyon's canal is most likely caused by ganglion or hook of the hamate fractures. Injury in this area results in mixed motor and sensory symptoms. Compression in zone 2 is also most likely caused by ganglion, arterial pseudoaneurysm, or hook of the hamate fractures and causes weakness of interosseous muscles, fourth and fifth lumbricals, hypothenar muscles, and adductor pollicis muscle. Compression in zone 3 is caused by an ulnar artery thrombosis or aneurysm and produces sensory findings of numbness, tingling, and burning sensation.

6.3 Entrapment of the Radial Sensory Nerve: Wartenberg's Syndrome

Wartenberg's syndrome, also known as cheiralgia paresthetica, refers to repeated irritation of the superficial branch of the radial nerve as it courses along the dorsum and lateral side of the wrist. This condition can result from direct trauma to the area or from external compression, such as from a bracelet or watch, common in cyclists. Other causes include cephalic venipuncture and cannulation and radial arterial line removal complicated by thrombosis. Clinically, it presents with intense paresthesia or pain along the radial side of the hand, thumb, and index finger, accompanied by increased sensitivity of the affected nerve to tension and percussion. Specific motions, including flexion and ulnar deviation of the wrist, exacerbate the symptoms and can be magnified with pinching and gripping through this motion.

7 Imaging Modalities

Radiography, ultrasound (US), CT, and MRI are available for peripheral nerve assessment. While radiography and CT can show degenerative osteophytosis or fractures possibly affecting the nerves at wrist or hand, US and MRI exhibit superior soft tissue contrast and adequate spatial resolution to optimally assess these small nerves and their branches. The following discussion will be focused on US and MRI findings of wrist entrapment neuropathies.

8 Common Ultrasound Findings in Entrapment Neuropathies

US evaluation of wrist is ideally performed by a high frequency transducer (18 MHz linear or hockey-stick probe in our practice). It is prudent to obtain both long axis and short axis images of the nerve, adjacent soft tissues, and tendons. If a tumor like lesion is identified, color Doppler images should be obtained as well. The hallmark of nerve entrapment is fusiform enlargement immediately proximal to the entrapment site. Quantitatively assessing this enlargement by measuring the nerve's cross-sectional area serves as a diagnostic criterion. Comparison with other asymptomatic side can be obtained. Other findings include changes in nerve echotexture (more hypoechoic), shape (flattening and pinching at the entrapment site), fascicle size (enlargement of single or multiple fascicles and hypoechogenecity), and increased vascularity within the nerve on Doppler imaging. Sonopalpation or sonographic Tinel sign can be performed with US probe pressure on the nerve leading to tenderness if compressed nerve.

9 Evaluation of Carpal Tunnel Syndrome with Ultrasound

The hallmark of CTS on Ultrasound is the hypoechoic enlargement of median nerve at and proximal to the level of entrapment. A longitudinal view typically shows hypoechoic enlargement of the median nerve entering carpal tunnel with flattening of nerve (called Notch sign) under the transverse ligament (Fig. 5). On the transverse view, palmar bowing of the flexor retinaculum is more than 2 mm beyond a line connecting the pisiform and the scaphoid is suggestive of CTS in the appropriate setting of suspected CTS (Fig. 6).

Studies have also shown that enlargement of the nerve distal to the flexor retinaculum is a sensitive and specific criterion, but the reference value for the cross-sectional area of the median nerve

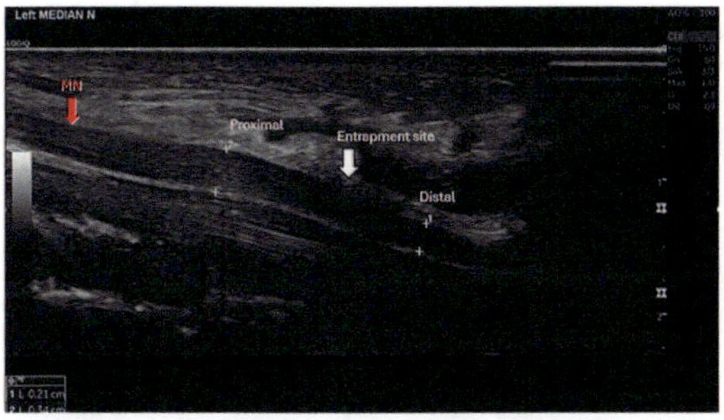

Fig. 5 Ultrasound grey scale long axis image at volar aspect of wrist showing median nerve (red arrow) with proximal enlargement at 34 mm above the entrapment site as compared to distal 21 mm at the wrist level

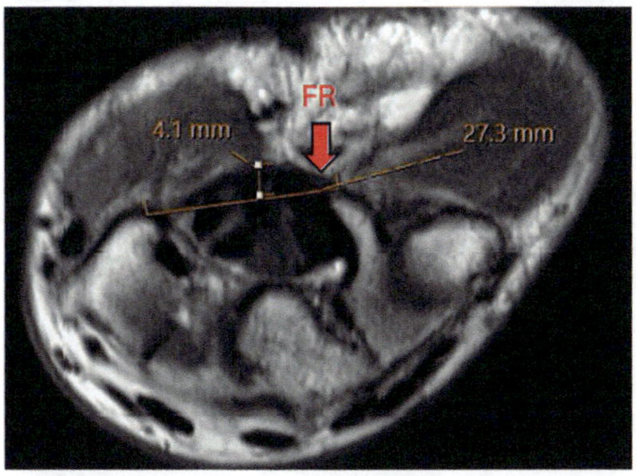

Fig. 6 Axial T2W Dixon in-phase image at wrist showing 4.1 mm palmar bowing of flexor retinaculum (FR) perpendicular to a line connecting the pisiform and the scaphoid. More than 2 mm is suggestive of carpal tunnel syndrome in appropriate clinical context

remains debated. Several studies, including a meta-analysis, suggest that a cutoff of greater than 9–10 mm^2 is sensitive for the diagnosis of CTS, whereas others use a more specific cutoff of greater than 11 mm^2. The more accurate way for CTS diagnosis is to compare the difference in median nerve area at the levels of proximal pronator quadratus muscle and the carpal tunnel. An increase of ≥2 mm^2 from the proximal to distal has 99% sensitivity and 100% specificity for CTS. The measurement should be made inside echogenic epineurium, outer connective tissue covering the nerve. An increase of 3 mm^2 or 30% change in size is consistent with CTS (Figs. 7 and 8). High division (proximal branching) of the median nerve is a

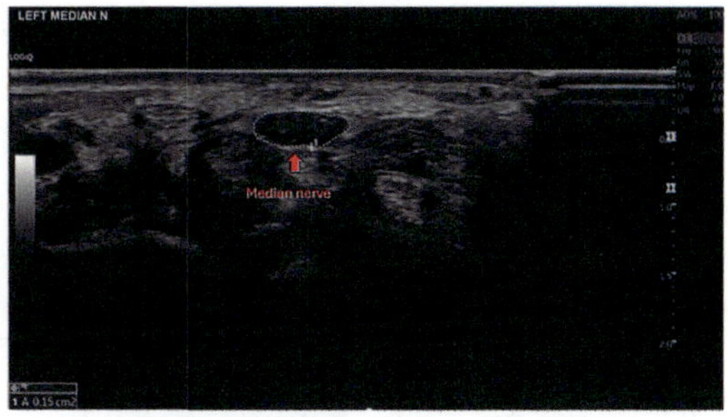

Fig. 7 Ultrasound axial image of median nerve at the level of wrist proximal to entrapment showing cross sectional area of 15 mm^2

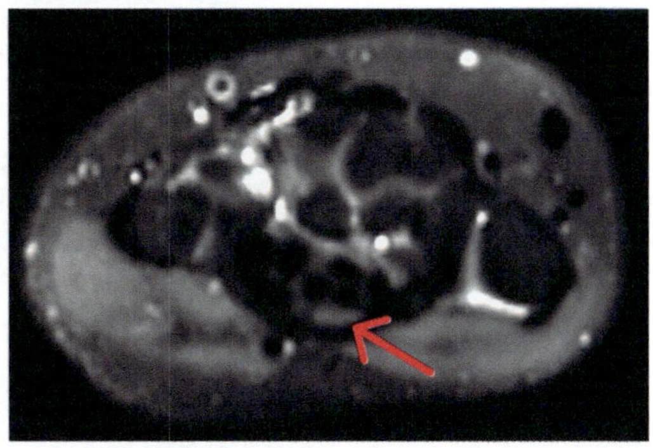

Fig. 8 3D PDW axial SPAIR image showing thickening of flexor retinaculum (red arrow) resulting in compression and consequently carpal tunnel syndrome

normal variant in 15% of population. One of the trunks may take an aberrant course through flexor digitorum superficialis muscle before reaching the carpal tunnel. The bifid nerves are often associated with persistent median vessel coursing between the two trunks. To diagnose CTS in these patients with bifid median nerve, the diameters of both branches should be measured, and an increase of ≥4 mm^2 from the proximal to distal suggests the diagnosis of CTS. Such enlargement can mimic a neuroma in continuity from injury, but fascicular continuity and homogeneity of signal are maintained (Fig. 9). Other anatomic abnormalities that ultrasound can identify as causes or mimics of CTS include traumatic neuroma, peripheral nerve sheath tumor, fibrolipoma of the nerve, ganglion, thrombosed persistent median artery, abscess, tenosynovitis, and compressive gouty tophi, etc.

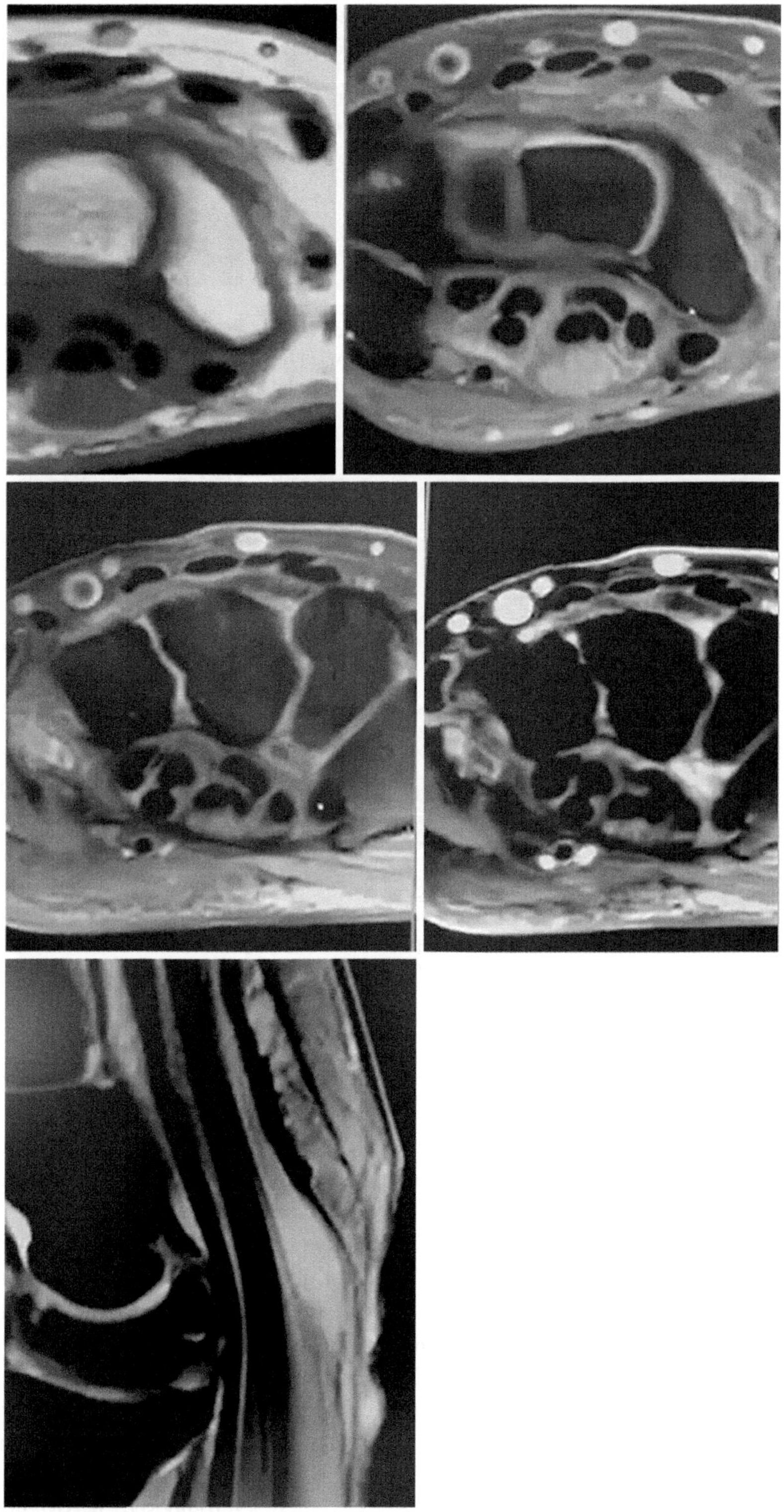

Fig. 9 Axial PDW and fsPDW images at the levels of pisiform and hamate show enlarged median nerve with distal flattening, pseudoneuroma formation due to entrapment. Notice fascicular continuity is maintained

CTS patients can be treated with conservative management with the use of splint, activity modification, ergonomic mouse for computers, and pain medications, etc. Persistent symptoms can be relieved with carpal tunnel injections of steroids, or US-guided percutaneous release of carpal tunnel ligament using thread technique or cutting device. Surgical resection of transverse carpal ligament and/or neurolysis is reserved for recalcitrant cases. On US, one may see divided ligament and the median nerve may return to normal diameter or remain mildly enlarged regardless of clinical outcome. Thickened or disrupted retinaculum or volar displacement of the nerve is normally seen after the surgery. Persistent moderate to severe enlargement and perineural scarring or iatrogenic injury of the nerve with or without neuroma formation confirm the clinical suspicion of incomplete release or persistent-worsening neuropathy.

10 MRI Imaging of Wrist

MRI offers advantages over ultrasound as it is less operator-dependent, provides clearer delineation of carpal tunnel contents, and allows for comprehensive measurement of the entire median nerve and regional joint structures, cartilage, and tendons.

10.1 MRI Protocol

Typical wrist MRI protocol uses a small field of view (10–12 cm) and a slice thickness of 2.0–3.0 mm using 2D (dimensional) MRI sequences. A thinner slice sequence (<1 mm) is possible on 3D turbo spin echo proton density fat saturation sequence, allowing for multiplanar reconstruction in isotropic voxel acquisitions. A 3T MRI with multichannel wrist or flex coil provides better signal-to-noise ratio, contrast, and image resolution. Dedicated MR imaging of the nerves is performed using MR neurography (MRN) protocol. This protocol outlines the nerve in its long axis like angiography does for vessels. A 3D, reverse steady state sequence in free precession (3D PSIF) or 3D DESS (dual echo steady state) sequence is ideal for vascular signal suppression and fat signal suppression to selectively visualize the nerve in multiple planes. Thick slab maximum intensity projection allows beautiful nerve depiction with improved background suppression. Diffusion tensor imaging (DTI) or DWI (diffusion weighted imaging) can be further used as part of MRN protocol to map out the nerve, detect signal abnormality in pathologic nerves, and measure quantitative information like apparent diffusion coefficient (ADC). DTI further allows tractography and calculation of fractional anisotropy (FA) values.

11 Diagnosis of CTS with MRI and MRN

Qualitative MRI features suggesting CTS include abnormally hyperintense median nerve on T2W images approaching the signal alteration of nearby vessels, effacement of deep fat pad in the proximal carpal tunnel at the level of pisiform, and flattening of the nerve in the carpal tunnel with proximal enlargement and increased signal of distal median nerve branches on T2W images. One or more features may be present apart from thenar muscle denervation changes and space occupying lesion adjacent to the nerve. Thenar muscle denervation changes though a key finding of median neuropathy is uncommon and only seen in more advanced cases of nerve entrapment or injury. The nerve also becomes abnormally hyperintense on DWI/DTI images. The flattening or caliber change of the nerve is best seen in long-axis on 3D MRN images. MRI-based neuropathy scoring reporting and data system (NS-RADS) is used for scoring the severity of qualitative nerve lesions. NS-RADS-mild entrapment E1 refers to abnormal increased T2W signal of the nerve at the carpal tunnel. NS-RADS moderate entrapment E2 refers to increased T2W signal and proximal enlargement of the nerve above the entrapment site. NS-RADS moderate entrapment E2 refers to increased T2W signal and proximal enlargement of the nerve above the entrapment site. Finally, NS-RADS severe entrapment E3 refers to increased T2W signal and proximal and distal enlargement of the nerve above and below the entrapment site. It may be associated with alternating bright-black-bright T2W signal alteration at the entrapment site with black signal at the site of constriction or hourglass appearance of the nerve across the entrapment site. In addition, thenar muscle denervation changes may be present in E2 and E3 classes.

Several quantitative parameters, including cross-sectional area (CSA), flattening ratio (FR), and signal intensity (SI) of the median nerve as well as palmar retinacular bowing ratio (BR), have been explored for CTS diagnosis. The most useful discriminatory parameters identified to date are the median CSA proximal to the carpal tunnel and palmar retinacular bowing. However, diagnostic criteria have not been firmly established. The median nerve is compared at three different locations:

1. Distal radioulnar joint proximal to the tunnel
2. Proximal tunnel at the level of pisiform
3. Distal tunnel at the level of the hook of hamate

Cross-sectional area (CSA) is measured by tracing the outer border of the median nerve on non-fat-suppressed images. The abrupt change in median nerve CSA from proximal to the tunnel to within the tunnel is diagnostic for CTS. The flattening ratio (FR) of the median nerve is the major axis divided by the minor axis. It is also used for assessing nerve compression. Median nerve edema/congestion, indicated by T2-hyperintensity, is measured by the signal intensity (SI) ratio, which is obtained by dividing the median nerve SI by the hypothenar muscle SI at the tunnel outlet. The maximum median nerve signal intensity is measured at the level proximal to the tunnel. Palmar retinacular bowing (BR) is measured at the inlet and outlet levels of the carpal tunnel. It is defined as the height from the deep margin of the retinaculum to a line drawn between the most volar points of the pisiform and scaphoid bones at the tunnel inlet or the trapezium and hook of hamate at the tunnel outlet. A positive value indicates the retinaculum is above the line, while a negative value indicates it is below the line. MRI after carpal tunnel release may be used to evaluate recurring symptoms. Normal postoperative findings include a complete surgical defect of the flexor retinaculum, volar extrusion of carpal tunnel contents, and improvement in neuro-muscular T2W signal changes. Persistent mild nerve thickness may still be observed (post-intervention class NS-RADS PI1). Moderate to severe nerve enlargement, moderate to severe increased T2W signal hyperintensity, reformation of the transverse carpal ligament with perineural scarring, alternating bright-black nerve signals along its course, and angulated nerve course are findings seen in isolation or combination, suggesting possible persistent neuropathy (PI2) or definitely worsening neuropathy (PI3), respectively. Post-injury neuroma in continuity and discontinuity of portion of the nerve are consistent with PI3 (Figs. 11 and 12). Thenar muscle denervation or worsening denervation changes are typically presented in PI2 and PI3 cases.

MRI is also useful for imaging characterization of neural or perineural mass lesions. For example, median nerve lipomatosis (fibrolipoma of the nerve) may be seen in the setting of macrodystrophia lipomatosa or in suspected carpal tunnel syndrome, where the nerve appears "spaghetti-like" or "multi-cable-like" with thickened fascicles and prominent intraneural fatty tissue. A common nerve sheath tumor is a schwannoma of the median nerve (Fig. 10). Other mass lesions include perineural cyst, ganglion, or post-traumatic hematoma.

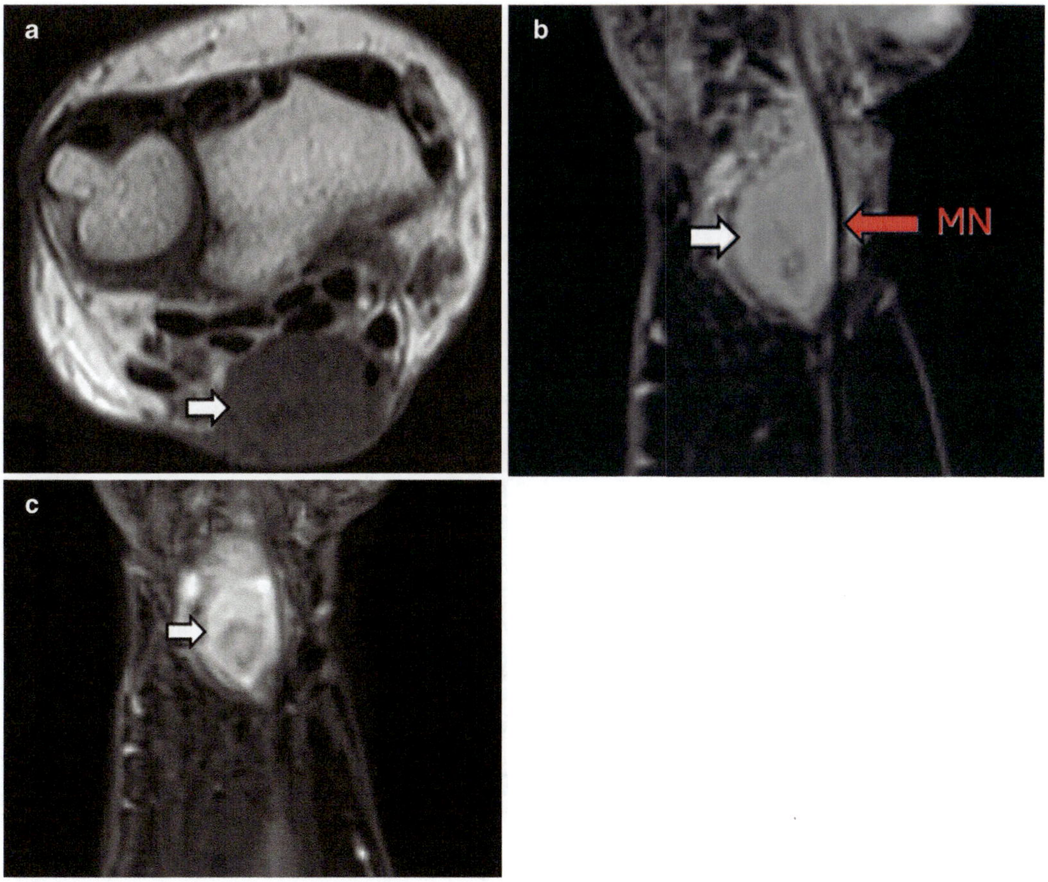

Fig. 10 (**a**) Axial T1W, (**b**) coronal 3D T1W pre- and (**c**) coronal 3D T1W post-contrast showing median nerve (red arrow) sheath tumor at carpal tunnel (white arrow). A biopsy proven schwannoma

12 Ultrasound Imaging of Guyon's Canal

Ultrasound can be used to assess the ulnar nerve and its branches, revealing trauma, ganglion cysts, and ulnar artery thrombosis and aneurysm, but it is not commonly used for diagnosing ulnar neuropathies at the wrist. Diagnosis based on measuring the cross-sectional area of the ulnar nerve at the wrist is hindered by the rarity of the condition, even though the upper limit of normal has been established as 8 mm^2.

13 MRI Imaging of Guyon's Canal

The ulnar nerve is visualized using a 3T MRI scanner. An optimal visualization is achieved when with T1W, fat-saturated T2W or fat-saturated PDW sequences are acquired with a 3 mm slice thickness and a 0.3 mm interslice gap. MRN uses T2W SPAIR imaging and 3D PSIF imaging with or without DWI/DTI. An MRI of the hand at the level of the hook of the hamate can be helpful for viewing the branching pattern

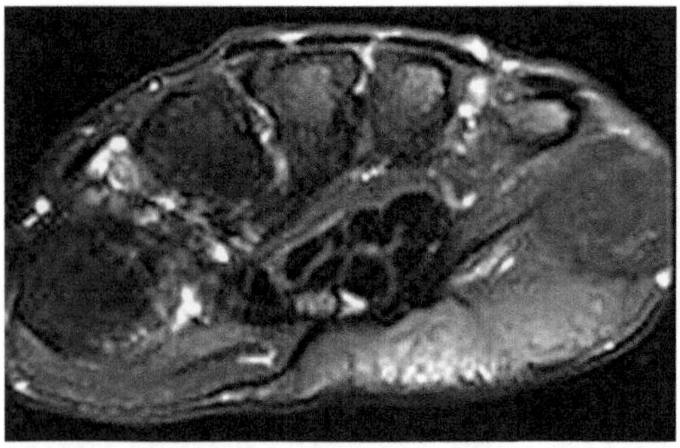

Fig. 11 Axial T2W SPAIR image showing discontinuity of ulnar bundle of the median nerve (red arrow) at carpal tunnel. Notice post-carpal tunnel release changes with subcutaneous scarring

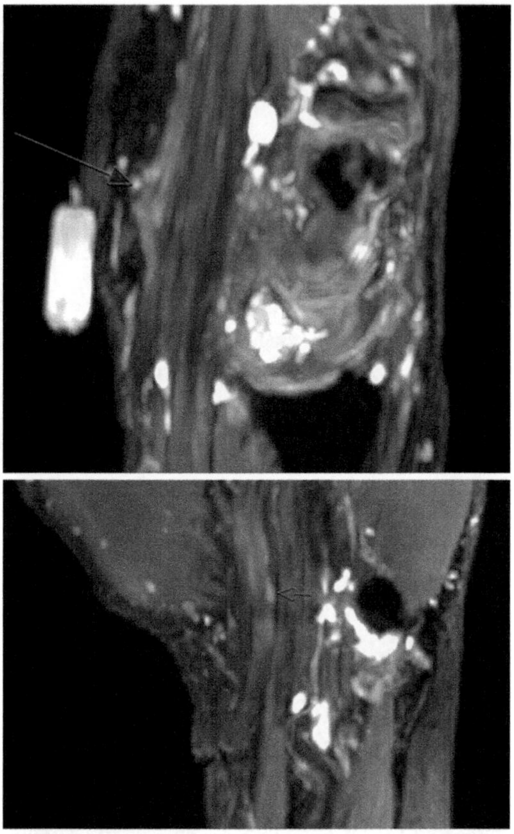

Fig. 12 3D PSIF MRN reconstruction images showing partial discontinuity of the epineurium with an enlarged fascicle along the volar ulnar aspect of the nerve, extending volar to the resected transverse carpal ligament consistent with neuroma in continuity, Sunderland Class IV injury

of the ulnar nerve in the Guyon canal and detecting anomalous musculature and ganglia, which are commonly reported causes of distal ulnar neuropathy. The entrapments are again recorded as NS-RADS E1–3 as described for the median nerve (Figs. 11 and 12). The superficial sensor branch of the ulnar nerve has a high risk of being injured in penetrating injuries to the wrist or main stem of the nerve by hook of hamate fracture (Figs. 13 and 14). Injury-related findings can be low grade (class I-III injuries, recorded as NS-RADS I1-3, with enlarged and hyperintense nerve) or high grade (class IV and V injuries, recorded as NS-RADS I4-5, with neuroma in continuity and complete nerve discontinuity, respectively).

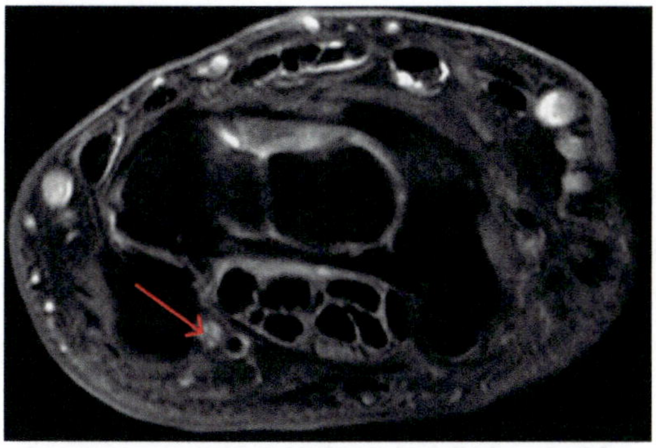

Fig. 13 Axial PD FS image showing increased signal of ulnar nerve (red arrow) in Guyon's canal adjacent to pisiform bone consistent with suspected neuropathy

14 Diagnosing Wartenberg's Syndrome with Ultrasound and MRI

Ultrasonography and MRI are valuable tools for identifying the precise location and extent of nerve injury in Wartenberg's syndrome. On ultrasound, the affected nerve exhibits a loss of its normal fibrillary pattern, swelling, and increased vascularity on color flow imaging. T2-weighted MRI or MRN reveals a characteristic increase in signal intensity, along with nerve swelling, providing a detailed view of the affected area with surrounding scarring, etc.

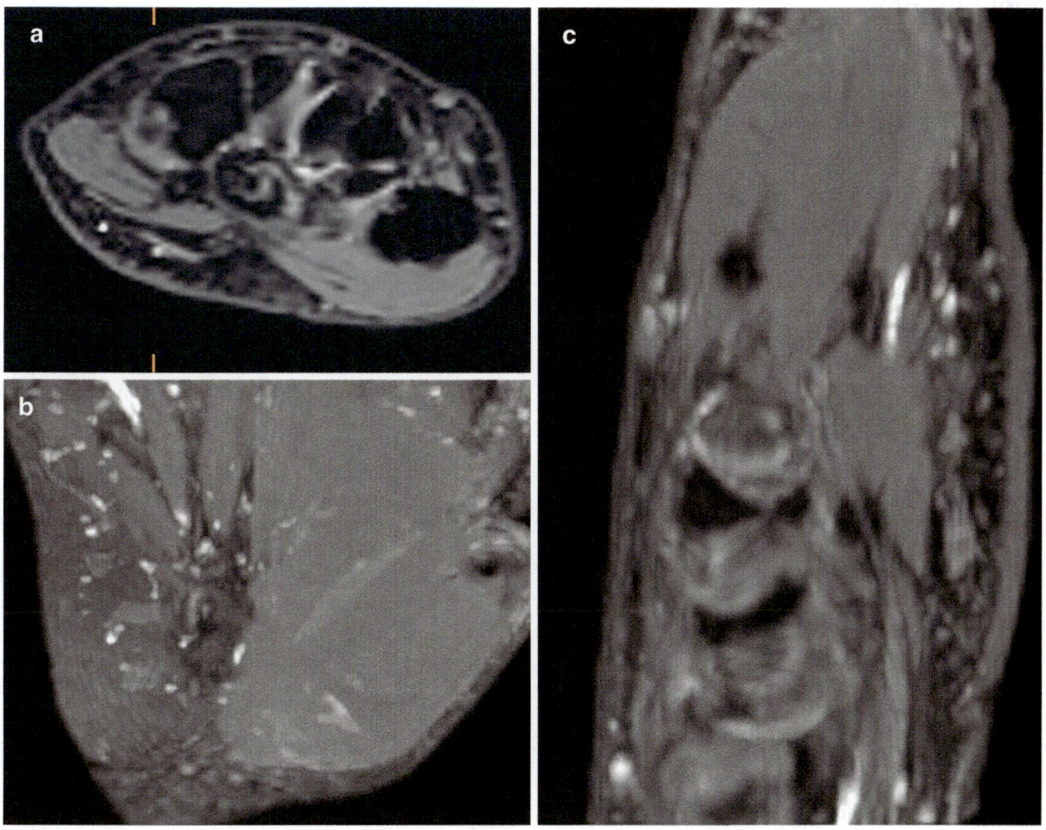

Fig. 14 (**a**) Axial reconstructed 3D PSIF image showing mildly displaced hook of hamate fracture (arrow). (**b**) MIP coronal reconstruction of the same sequence shows selective denervation edema of adductor pollicis (arrow). (**c**) Sagittal reconstruction of 3D PSIF image shows enlarged and hyperintense ulnar nerve at the site of fracture with distal normalization (arrows) consistent with suspected ulnar neuropathy

15 Conclusion

To conclude, wrist nerve entrapments are common with carpal tunnel syndrome being the dominant entrapment lesion. Knowledge of regional anatomy, US, and MRI findings of wrist entrapments can aid in their timely diagnosis and management.

Disclosures AC: Consultant: ICON Medical and TREACE Medical Concepts Inc., Book Royalties: Jaypee, Wolters, Medical advisor: Image biopsy Lab Inc., Research grant: Image biopsy Lab Inc., Qure-AI, Speaker: Telemedicine clinics.

The authors report no conflicts of interest.

Bibliography

Agarwal A, Chandra A, Jaipal U, Saini N (2019) Imaging in the diagnosis of ulnar nerve pathologies-a neoteric approach. Insights Imaging 10(1):37

Allmann KH, Horch R, Uhl M, Gufler H, Altehoefer C, Stark GB et al (1997) MR imaging of the carpal tunnel. Eur J Radiol 25(2):141–145

Andreisek G, Crook DW, Burg D, Marincek B, Weishaupt D (2006) Peripheral neuropathies of the median, radial, and ulnar nerves: MR imaging features. Radiographics 26(5):1267–1287

Bao H, Wang S, Wang G, Yang L, Hasan MU, Yao B, Wu C, Zhang X, Chen W, Chan Q, Wu L, Chhabra A (2017) Diffusion-weighted MR neurography of median and ulnar nerves in the wrist and palm. Eur Radiol 27(6):2359–2366. https://doi.org/10.1007/s00330-016-4591-0. Epub 2016 Sep 15. PMID: 27631109

Bayrak IK, Bayrak AO, Kale M, Turker H, Diren B (2008) Bifid median nerve in patients with carpal tunnel syndrome. J Ultrasound Med 27(8):1129–1136

Bordalo-Rodrigues M, Amin P, Rosenberg ZS (2004) MR imaging of common entrapment neuropathies at the wrist. Magn Reson Imaging Clin N Am 12(2):265–279, vi

Cartwright MS, Walker FO (2013) Neuromuscular ultrasound in common entrapment neuropathies. Muscle Nerve 48(5):696–704

Cartwright MS, Shin HW, Passmore LV, Walker FO (2007) Ultrasonographic findings of the normal ulnar nerve in adults. Arch Phys Med Rehabil 88(3):394–396

Cartwright MS, White DL, Demar S, Wiesler ER, Sarlikiotis T, Chloros GD et al (2011) Median nerve changes following steroid injection for carpal tunnel syndrome. Muscle Nerve 44(1):25–29

Cha JG, Han JK, Im SB, Kang SJ (2014) Median nerve T2 assessment in the wrist joints: preliminary study in patients with carpal tunnel syndrome and healthy volunteers. J Magn Reson Imaging 40(4):789–795

Chhabra A, Soldatos T, Subhawong TK, Machado AJ, Thawait SK, Wang KC et al (2011) The application of three-dimensional diffusion-weighted PSIF technique in peripheral nerve imaging of the distal extremities. J Magn Reson Imaging 34(4):962–967

Chhabra A, Madhuranthakam AJ, Andreisek G (2018) Magnetic resonance neurography: current perspectives and literature review. Eur Radiol 28(2):698–707

Chhabra A, Ratakonda R, Zaottini F, Picasso R, Martinoli C (2021) Hand and wrist neuropathies: high-resolution ultrasonography and MR neurography. Semin Musculoskelet Radiol 25(2):366–378

Chhabra A, Deshmukh SD, Lutz AM, Fritz J, Sneag DB, Mogharrabi B et al (2022) Neuropathy score reporting and data system (NS-RADS): MRI reporting guideline of peripheral neuropathy explained and reviewed. Skeletal Radiol 51(10):1909–1922

Coulier B, Goffin D, Malbecq S, Mairy Y (2003) Colour duplex sonographic and multislice spiral CT angiographic diagnosis of ulnar artery aneurysm in hypothenar hammer syndrome. JBR-BTR 86(4):211–214

Daniels SP, De Tolla JE, Azad A, Petchprapa CN (2022) Nerve imaging in the wrist. Semin Musculoskelet Radiol 26(2):140–152

Depukat P, Mizia E, Kuniewicz M, Bonczar T, Mazur M, Pelka P et al (2015) Syndrome of canal of Guyon – definition, diagnosis, treatment and complication. Folia Med Cracov 55(1):17–23

Doughty CT, Bowley MP (2019) Entrapment neuropathies of the upper extremity. Med Clin North Am 103(2):357–370

Elsaidi GA, Wiesler ER (2004) Lipofibromatous hamartoma of the median nerve: case presentation of MRI, ultrasound, electrodiagnostic, histologic, and surgical findings. Am J Orthop (Belle Mead NJ) 33(10):514–516

Feintisch AM, Ayyala HS, Datiashvili R (2017) An anatomic variant of persistent median artery in association with carpal tunnel syndrome: case report and review of the literature. J Hand Surg Asian Pac Vol 22(4):523–525

Genova A, Dix O, Saefan A, Thakur M, Hassan A (2020) Carpal tunnel syndrome: a review of literature. Cureus 12(3):e7333

Geoghegan JM, Clark DI, Bainbridge LC, Smith C, Hubbard R (2004) Risk factors in carpal tunnel syndrome. J Hand Surg Br 29(4):315–320

Ghasemi-Esfe AR, Khalilzadeh O, Vaziri-Bozorg SM, Jajroudi M, Shakiba M, Mazloumi M et al (2011) Color and power Doppler US for diagnosing carpal tunnel syndrome and determining its severity: a quantitative image processing method. Radiology 261(2):499–506

Guggenberger R, Markovic D, Eppenberger P, Chhabra A, Schiller A, Nanz D et al (2012) Assessment of median nerve with MR neurography by using diffusion-tensor imaging: normative and pathologic diffusion values. Radiology 265(1):194–203

Guirguis M, Sharan G, Wang J, Chhabra A (2022) Diffusion-weighted MR imaging of musculoskeletal tissues: incremental role over conventional MR imaging in bone, soft tissue, and nerve lesions. BJR Open 4(1):20210077

Guirguis M, Pezeshk P, Ashikyan O, Gowda P, Archer H, Hoang D et al (2023) Incremental value of diffusion weighted imaging over conventional MRI for the diagnosis of osteomyelitis of extremities. Skeletal Radiol 52(9):1669–1682

Hobson-Webb LD, Walker FO (2004) Traumatic neuroma diagnosed by ultrasonography. Arch Neurol 61(8):1322–1323

Inaparthy PK, Anwar F, Botchu R, Jahnich H, Katchburian MV (2008) Compression of the deep branch of the ulnar nerve in Guyon's canal by a ganglion: two cases. Arch Orthop Trauma Surg 128(7):641–643

Jarvik JG, Kliot M, Maravilla KR (2000) MR nerve imaging of the wrist and hand. Hand Clin 16(1):13–24, vii

Karvelas KR, Walker FO (2019) Clinical and ultrasonographic features of distal ulnar neuropathy: a review. Front Neurol 10:632

Kele H, Verheggen R, Reimers CD (2002) Carpal tunnel syndrome caused by thrombosis of the median artery: the importance of high-resolution ultrasonography for diagnosis. Case report. J Neurosurg 97(2):471–473

Klauser AS, Halpern EJ, De Zordo T, Feuchtner GM, Arora R, Gruber J et al (2009) Carpal tunnel syndrome assessment with US: value of additional cross-sectional area measurements of the median nerve in patients versus healthy volunteers. Radiology 250(1):171–177

Kostoris F, Bassini S, Longo E, Murena L (2019) Carpal tunnel syndrome associated with bifid median nerve and palmaris profundus – case report and literature review. J Hand Surg Asian Pac Vol 24(2):238–242

Mallouhi A, Pulzl P, Trieb T, Piza H, Bodner G (2006) Predictors of carpal tunnel syndrome: accuracy of gray-scale and color Doppler sonography. AJR Am J Roentgenol 186(5):1240–1245

Maroukis BL, Ogawa T, Rehim SA, Chung KC (2015) Guyon canal: the evolution of clinical anatomy. J Hand Surg Am 40(3):560–565

Mitchell R, Chesney A, Seal S, McKnight L, Thoma A (2009) Anatomical variations of the carpal tunnel structures. Can J Plast Surg 17(3):e3–e7

Naraghi AM, Awdeh H, Wadhwa V, Andreisek G, Chhabra A (2015) Diffusion tensor imaging of peripheral nerves. Semin Musculoskelet Radiol 19(2):191–200

Ng AWH, Griffith JF, Tong CSL, Law EKC, Tse WL, Wong CWY et al (2020) MRI criteria for diagnosis and predicting severity of carpal tunnel syndrome. Skeletal Radiol 49(3):397–405

Oge HK, Acu B, Gucer T, Yanik T, Savlarli S, Firat MM (2012) Quantitative MRI analysis of idiopathic carpal tunnel syndrome. Turk Neurosurg 22(6):763–768

Padua L, Liotta G, Di Pasquale A, Granata G, Pazzaglia C, Caliandro P et al (2012) Contribution of ultrasound in the assessment of nerve diseases. Eur J Neurol 19(1):47–54

Pasternack II, Malmivaara A, Tervahartiala P, Forsberg H, Vehmas T (2003) Magnetic resonance imaging findings in respect to carpal tunnel syndrome. Scand J Work Environ Health 29(3):189–196

Polatsch DB, Melone CP Jr, Beldner S, Incorvaia A (2007) Ulnar nerve anatomy. Hand Clin 23(3):283–289, v

Radack DM, Schweitzer ME, Taras J (1997) Carpal tunnel syndrome: are the MR findings a result of population selection bias? AJR Am J Roentgenol 169(6):1649–1653

Solomon DH, Katz JN, Bohn R, Mogun H, Avorn J (1999) Nonoccupational risk factors for carpal tunnel syndrome. J Gen Intern Med 14(5):310–314

Soubeyrand M, Melhem R, Protais M, Artuso M, Creze M (2020) Anatomy of the median nerve and its clinical applications. Hand Surg Rehabil 39(1):2–18

Tai TW, Wu CY, Su FC, Chern TC, Jou IM (2012) Ultrasonography for diagnosing carpal tunnel syndrome: a meta-analysis of diagnostic test accuracy. Ultrasound Med Biol 38(7):1121–1128

Thawait GK, Subhawong TK, Thawait SK, Andreisek G, Belzberg AJ, Eng J et al (2012) Magnetic resonance neurography of median neuropathies proximal to the carpal tunnel. Skeletal Radiol 41(6):623–632

Therimadasamy A, Peng YP, Putti TC, Wilder-Smith EP (2011) Carpal tunnel syndrome caused by gouty tophus of the flexor tendons of the fingers: sonographic features. J Clin Ultrasound 39(8):463–465

Wiesler ER, Chloros GD, Cartwright MS, Smith BP, Rushing J, Walker FO (2006) The use of diagnostic ultrasound in carpal tunnel syndrome. J Hand Surg Am 31(5):726–732

Yu JS, Habib PA (2004) Normal MR imaging anatomy of the wrist and hand. Magn Reson Imaging Clin N Am 12(2):207–219, v

Osteonecrosis and Osteochondrosis

Robert D. Henderson and Jonathan Erickson

Contents

The original version of the chapter has been revised. Dr. Robert D. Henderson's affiliations were corrected.

R. D. Henderson (✉)
Musculoskeletal Imaging Division, Joint Department of Medical Imaging, University Health Network, Toronto, ON, Canada

Department of Musculoskeletal Radiology, Royal Orthopaedic Hospital NHS Foundation Trust, Birmingham, UK

Department of Medical Imaging, Perth Children's Hospital, Perth, WA, Australia
e-mail: hendo.rd@gmail.com

J. Erickson
Radiology Department, National Orthopaedic Hospital at Cappagh, Dublin, Ireland

Department of Medical Imaging, Perth Children's Hospital, Perth, WA, Australia
e-mail: jon.erickson@health.wa.gov.au

Abstract

This concise chapter on osteonecrosis and osteochondrosis in the wrist and hand details the aetiology and typical bones involved in these conditions, and provides detailed descriptions of the available imaging modalities including plain radiograph, computed tomography, scintigraphy and magnetic resonance imaging, each with their strengths and weaknesses. Individual descriptions and classification of carpal bone osteonecrosis and osteochondrosis including Kienbock's disease of the lunate and the rarer Preiser's disease of the scaphoid are included.

1 Introduction

Osteonecrosis or avascular necrosis of the carpal bones is a common cause for chronic wrist pain, resulting in limited movement and weakened grip strength. Osteonecrosis is a complex and multifactorial disease process, most frequently occurring as a result of disruption to the arterial blood supply following trauma. The scaphoid is the most commonly affected bone in the wrist; however, the process can occur in any of the carpal

Med Radiol Diagn Imaging (2025)
https://doi.org/10.1007/174_2025_605,
Published Online: 17 September 2025

bones with involvement of multiple bones also having been described (Beckers et al. 2022; De Smet et al. 1993; Garcia and Vaca 2006; Humphrey et al. 2006; Pickrell and Harper 2022; Telfer et al. 1994; Zafra et al. 2004).

Osteochondroses refer to a heterogeneous group of conditions which tend to affect the skeletally immature with a variety of proposed mechanisms and risk factors. Those affecting the hand and wrist are characterised by features of osteonecrosis which is favoured to occur through a process of repetitive microtrauma, the most recognised being Kienböch's disease of the lunate.

Whilst there are many potential causes for both osteonecrosis and osteochondrosis, both processes typically cause insidious pain early in the disease process and which may progress to collapse of the subchondral bone plate leading to early advanced and progressive arthritis. The resulting chronic and often debilitating pain underlines the importance of early diagnosis with appropriate intervention and treatment (Wells and Dunn 2022).

Conventional radiographs remain the first-line imaging investigation noting that radiographic changes are typically seen relatively late in the disease process. MR imaging is both a sensitive and specific method enabling diagnosis of the early stages of osteonecrosis and avascular necrosis before carpal collapse occurs (Golimbu et al. 1995).

2 Aetiology

Osteonecrosis can be secondary to a variety of insults culminating in necrotic aseptic and avascular bone, implicating perfusional and vascular insufficiency as an underlying mechanism. The carpal bones are particularly vulnerable to insults given their relatively high frequency of traumatic injury and poor collateral circulation. Osteonecrosis within the wrist and hand most commonly involves the scaphoid, lunate and capitate bones, all of which have particularly tenuous vascularity (Botte et al. 2004; Gelberman and Gross 1986).

Various causes of osteonecrosis have been described including radiation, vascular, metabolic and systemic conditions. In the wrist, however, the most common cause is trauma, with the scaphoid and capitate most frequently affected. In some instances, a clear cause for osteonecrosis is not always established, and this is most clearly illustrated in the lunate, where it is termed 'Kienboch's disease'. Despite the absence of a definite or convincing traumatic event, repetitive microtrauma and subsequent vascular compromise is a favoured underlying mechanism (Resnick 2002). Regardless of the many potential causes, the final mechanism is always critical ischaemia with treatment goals aimed at pain improvement, reducing the risk of progressive degenerative disease and maximising functional outcomes (Wells and Dunn 2022). Other osteochondroses described in the hand and wrist are Prieser's disease (scaphoid), Thiemann's disease (phalanges) and Dietrich's disease (metacarpal head) (Botte et al. 2004; de Smet 2000; Ferlic and Morin 1989; Herbert and Lanzetta 1994; Tashjian et al. 2004).

Different cellular elements contained within bone vary in their susceptibility to anoxia and following the physical disruption to blood flow, the haematopoietic elements are generally accepted to be the first cell type to succumb followed by bone cells and subsequently bone marrow fat cells (Cruess 1986; Glimcher and Kenzora 1979a, b, c). As a result, temporary anoxia can produce variable degrees of cell death, potentially affecting the haematopoietic elements without involving the other cells. Once marrow fat cell death occurs, the involved segment of bone can be labelled as infarcted. The associated bone marrow changes during infarction make MRI a crucial tool in detecting early changes of osteonecrosis.

3 Imaging Techniques

3.1 Radiography

Typically, the X-ray findings of osteonecrosis lag behind the clinical manifestations with the initial radiographs often normal. The surrounding bone has maintained vascularity and perfusion whereby the influx of inflammatory cells evokes a response of increased osteoclastic activity

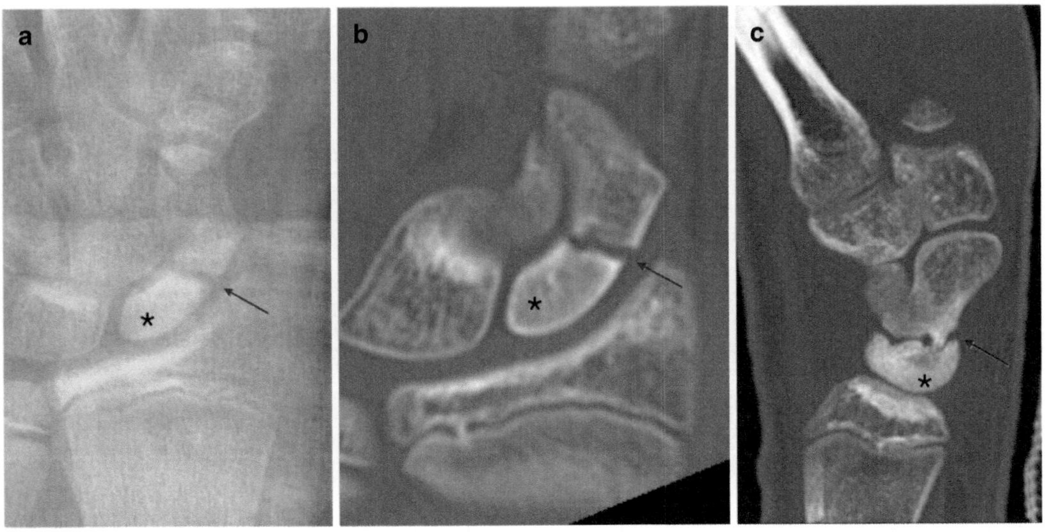

Fig. 1 (**a–c**) Early avascular necrosis at 6 weeks following transverse scaphoid waist fracture (→). (**a**) Even through the plaster cast the difference in bone density is appreciated on in-cast PA wrist radiograph, with the relative osteosclerosis (*) further accentuated on contemporary (**b**) coronal and (**c**) sagittal CT. (Images courtesy of Jennifer Stimec MD, Sick Kids Hospital, Toronto, Canada)

towards removal of the dead bone. As a result there is relative progressive osteopaenia in the surrounding viable bone, whereas the non-viable bone maintains its density becoming relatively sclerotic (Fig. 1a) with progressive sclerosis, and ultimately collapse and fragmentation (Fig. 2a) of the devitalised bone.

3.2 Computed Tomography

Computed tomography (CT) is rarely used in the primary assessment of carpal bone osteonecrosis; however, it can provide useful information from both an anatomical perspective and subtle bone detail not afforded by X-ray. Given the complexity of carpal bone anatomy, CT delivers superior quantitative evaluation of progressive volume reduction in the affected bone. It is capable of detecting favourable changes of early fracture healing, but more importantly deleterious features of sclerosis (Fig. 1b, c), subchondral osteolysis, collapse and fragmentation (Fig. 2a–c). Microcystic change is also a feature seen following subchondral collapse, plus also along the margins of a non-united fracture (Bush et al. 1987). Characterisation of secondary degenerative changes is also superior with CT.

The base of the hook of hamate is at relatively high risk for avascular necrosis following fracture (Telfer et al. 1994) and given the complex anatomy, avascular necrosis of this bone is often best detected with CT.

3.3 Magnetic Resonance Imaging

Magnetic resonance imaging remains the gold standard for the early detection of osteonecrosis with the ability to pre-emptively detect early marrow signal alteration before changes become apparent on CT or plain radiography (Imhof et al. 1997).

MRI changes characteristic of avascular necrosis include oedema-like marrow high signal on STIR (short tau inversion recovery) or T2 fat-saturated sequences, with corresponding loss of normal intrinsic marrow fat signal on T1-weighted sequences (Imhof et al. 1997; Mitchell et al. 1989) (Fig. 3a–c). As the process progresses, a pattern of reduced signal on T2-weighted sequences with surrounding increased T2 signal

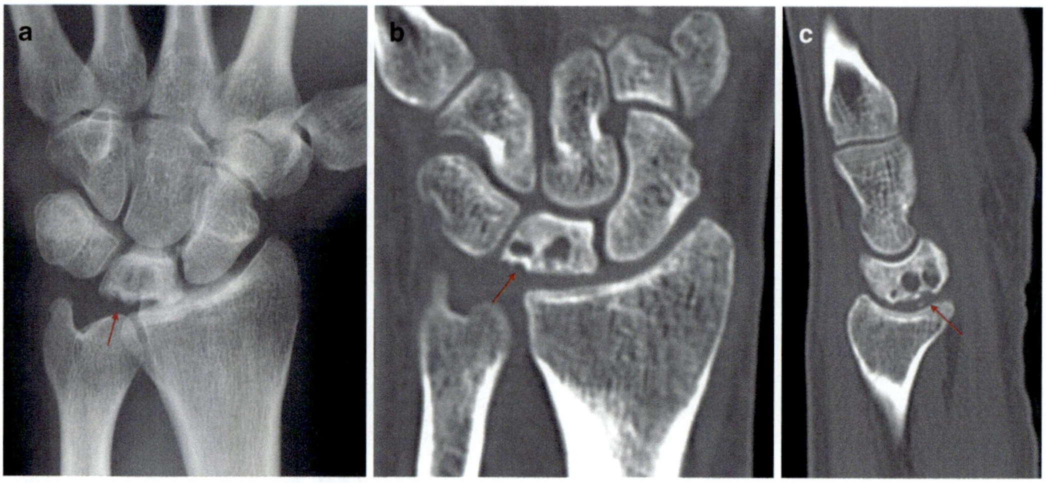

Fig. 2 (**a–c**) Features of progressive avascular necrosis of the lunate on PA wrist radiograph (**a**) with relative osteopaenia of the carpus and characteristic sclerosis, early subchondral bone plate collapse and corrugation, secondary cystic changes of the lunate (→). Coronal (**b**) and sagittal (**c**) CT images better delineate the above changes. (Images courtesy of Dr Bob Bleakney, University Health Network, Toronto, Canada)

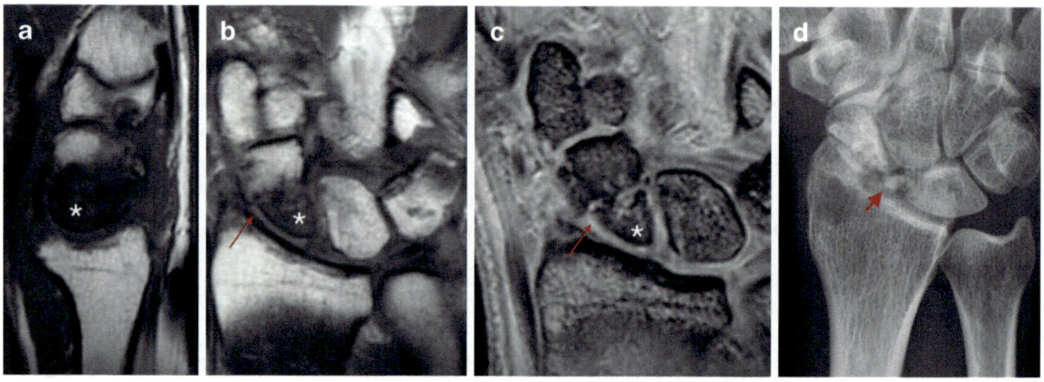

Fig. 3 (**a–d**) (**a**) Sagittal and (**b**) coronal PD sequences of a scaphoid waist fracture (→) demonstrating abnormal loss of intrinsic marrow fat signal of the proximal scaphoid pole (*), with corresponding appearances on coronal 3D SPACE. Follow-up PA wrist radiograph demonstrative sclerosis, collapse and fragmentation of the affected proximal scaphoid pole (→)

ensues and represents the interface between non-viable bone and surrounding reparative granulation tissue. MRI at this stage may show a characteristic serpiginous double line at this interface (Fig. 4a–c), representing granulation tissue adjacent to reactive bone formation (Imhof et al. 1997; Mitchell et al. 1989). Contrast-enhanced imaging is not typically required but may be a useful adjunct in helping distinguish viable from non-viable bone.

3.4 Bone Scintigraphy

The increased availability and accessibility of MRI has made the use of bone scintigraphy less common. Whilst this method remains very sensitive for the early detection of osteonecrosis, it is relatively non-specific and must be interpreted alongside conventional radiography. In the early stages of avascular necrosis, increased metabolic activity in the bone is characterised by higher

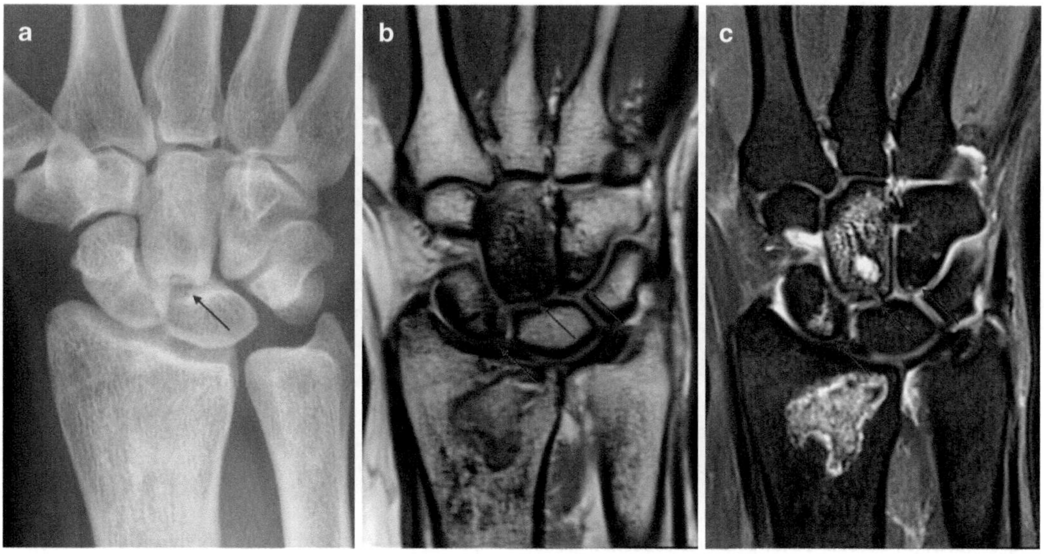

Fig. 4 (**a–c**) PA wrist radiograph (**a**) demonstrating multifocal avascular necrosis around the wrist of a patient with SLE. Characteristic subchondral collapse of the proximal capitate margin and proximal scaphoid pole, better delineated on MRI with pathognomonic marginal findings of an outer low signal band of sclerotic bone with inner lining of T2 high signal granulation tissue on coronal T1 (**b**) and STIR (**c**) sequences (→)

uptake in bone scintigraphy on both early and late phase scanning. Later bone scintigraphy uptake typically indicates an area of decreased tracer uptake represented by a focus of photopaenia or cold-spot. Whilst this may represent a focus of osteonecrosis, other conditions including myeloma, various skeletal metastasis, irradiation, haemangiomas and infection can also result in reduced tracer uptake, and this finding should be treated with caution.

4 Scaphoid

The scaphoid is the most common site for carpal bone osteonecrosis due to its high susceptibility to trauma and tenuous blood supply. Arterial supply to the proximal pole of the scaphoid is delivered in a retrograde fashion, arising from small dorsal ridge vessels entering the waist of the scaphoid from the radial artery. These vessels provide around 70–80% of the internal vascularity of the bone and in particular to the proximal pole. The remaining internal vascularity is supplied from the palmar aspect and provides blood to the distal pole (Botte et al. 2004). This unique blood supply makes the proximal pole vulnerable to osteonecrosis following fracture with a reported frequency of between 11% and 65% (Mazet Jr and Hohl 1963). Fractures of the proximal third have the highest incidence of osteonecrosis, with the frequency reducing with more distally located fractures. Whilst extremely rare, osteonecrosis of the distal scaphoid pole has been reported following fracture (Sherman et al. 1983).

In established cases, plain radiographs show an increase in bone density in the affected scaphoid at between 4 and 8 weeks and which is associated with non-union (Fig. 1a–c). Later, reduction in size, fragmentation and secondary degenerative changes can be seen (Fig. 3d).

MR imaging is the modality of choice for detecting early avascular necrosis. Typically, MR will show low signal intensity within the bone marrow of the proximal scaphoid pole on both the T1- and T2-weighted images. Contrast enhancement significantly increases the detection of non-viable bone; however, dynamic contrast enhancement has not been shown to increase

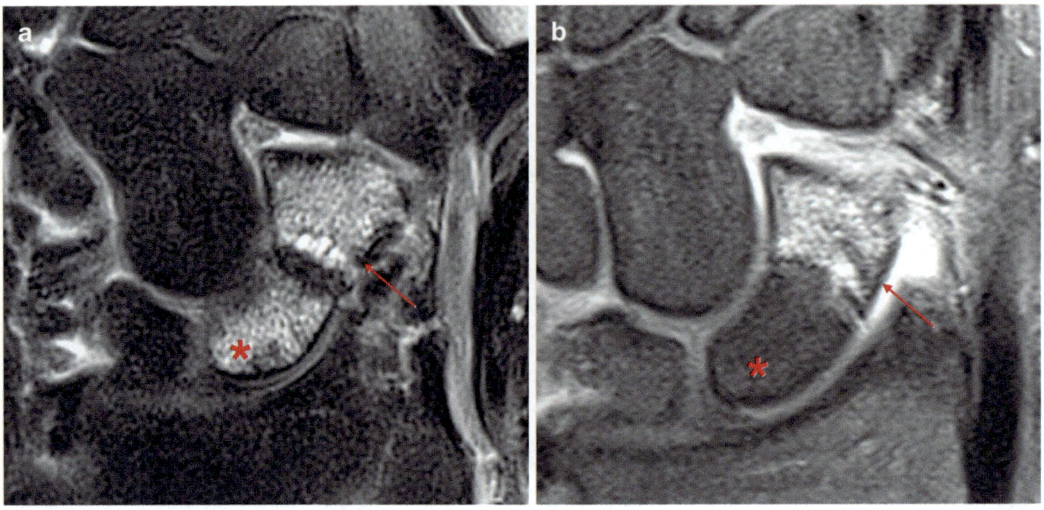

Fig. 5 (**a**, **b**) (**a**) Coronal T2 fat-saturated sequence shows scaphoid fracture non-union with persisting marrow oedema in both proximal (*) and distal (→) fracture segments. Following intravenous gadolinium contrast administration (**b**), the coronal T1 fat-saturated post-contrast sequence confirms devitalisation of the proximal scaphoid pole demonstrated by relative lack of contrast enhancement compared to the distal segment. (Courtesy of Dr Waqar Bhatti and Dr Andrew Grainger from first edition)

sensitivity (Cerezal et al. 2000; Megerle et al. 2011; Donati et al. 2011) (Fig. 5b). Whilst MR imaging has been shown to provide a good assessment of the vascularity of the bone as assessed with punctate bleeding at the time of surgery, it is not good at predicting outcomes of surgery in terms of union and revascularisation (Cerezal et al. 2000; Megerle et al. 2011; Schmitt et al. 2011; Singh et al. 2004; Dawson et al. 2001).

4.1 Preiser's Disease

Preiser's disease (idiopathic avascular necrosis of the scaphoid) is a rare condition first described in the early twentieth century (Preiser 1910). The condition results in ischaemia of the scaphoid bone without preceding trauma. Rarely, the condition can occur bilaterally and has also been described in association with Kienböch's disease (Lenoir et al. 2012; de Smet 2000; Ferlic and Morin 1989; Herbert and Lanzetta 1994) (Fig. 6a, b). Implicated risk factors include excessive alcohol intake, corticosteroid administration, chemotherapy and other disease processes. Histologically, there are empty bony lacunae, necrotic marrow and partly degenerated articular cartilage. Clinically, patients typically present with insidious pain along the dorsal and radial aspects of the wrist.

Radiographic and CT appearances show sclerosis, volume loss and cystic change which can progress to collapse and fragmentation (Fig. 3a–d). Two MRI patterns have been described, either a partial or focal form with ischaemic of the proximal scaphoid (Fig. 7a) which has a better prognosis, and a diffuse form with complete ischaemia and necrosis (Fig. 7b) (Kalainov et al. 2003). Isolated non-traumatic osteonecrosis of the distal pole of the scaphoid has also been described (Garg et al. 2011).

Conservative treatment for Preiser's disease includes wrist immobilisation and cortisone injections. Surgical options include partial excision with replacement by non-vascularised or vascularised bone graft, proximal row carpectomy, scaphoid excision with midcarpal fusion and total wrist fusion.

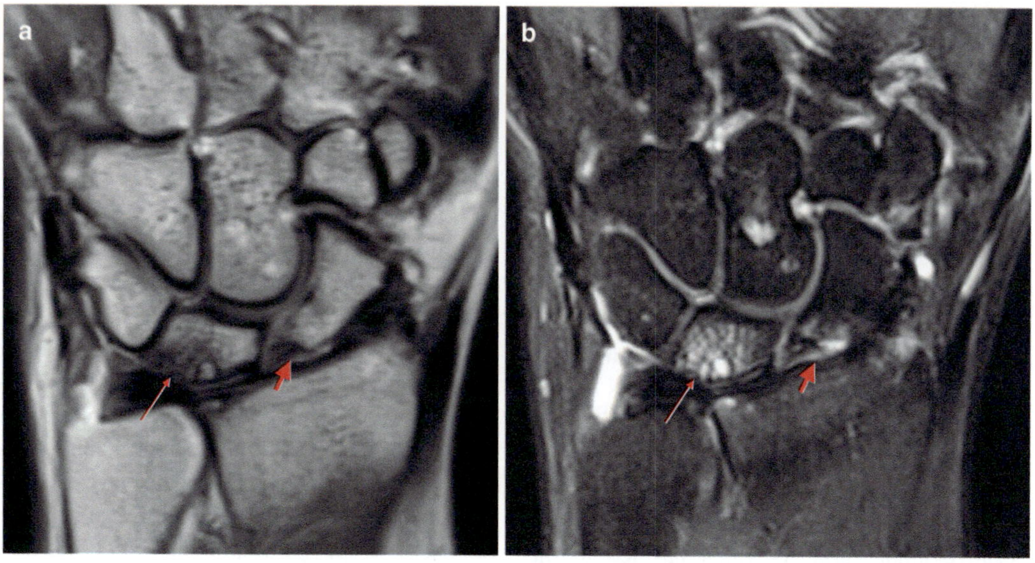

Fig. 6 (**a**, **b**) Corontal (**a**) PD and (**b**) STIR sequences demonstrating features of concurrent osteonecrosis of the lunate (Kienboch →) and scaphoid (Preiser →) characterised by subtle subchondral collapse and oedema of the proximal articular margins

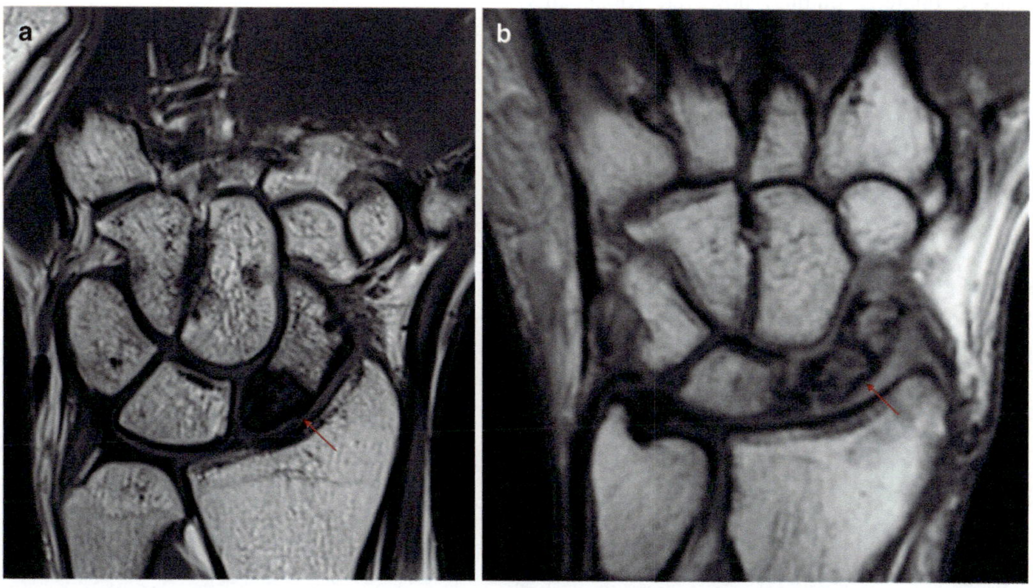

Fig. 7 (**a**, **b**) Coronal PD (**a**) MRI sequence demonstrating avascular necrosis of the proximal scaphoid pole (→), with comparison coronal PD (**b**) sequence demonstrating evolving patchy but diffuse avascular necrosis of the entire scaphoid with early volume loss and subtle contour irregularity

5 Lunate

5.1 Kienböch's Disease

Kienböch's disease is most commonly observed in patients between the ages of 20 and 40 years, having a predilection for the dominant (typically right) hand in persons engaged in manual labour. Whilst some patients have a history of preceding trauma, the majority of cases are idiopathic. The disease also occurs in the skeletally immature and the elderly, having a better prognosis in children following non-operative treatment, whereas better outcomes for the elderly require surgical intervention (Lichtman et al. 2017).

Kienböch's disease is strongly associated with negative ulnar variance which has led to the hypothesis that altered loading and biomechanics are implicated in the aetiology, although 40% of cases are seen in neutral ulnar variance (Fig. 8a–c). In addition, negative ulnar variance is typically a bilateral finding; however, Kienböch's disease is rarely bilateral. Other postulated theories include medialisation of the lunate, horizontalisation of the radial epiphysis or abnormal/variant lunate morphology. In some individuals, a variation in the blood supply to the lunate is seen with a single dominant branch (8%) rather than dual supply from the volar and dorsal branches with an intervening anastomosis, potentially increasing the risk of osteonecrosis (Gelberman and Gross 1986).

5.1.1 Imaging

On conventional radiographs, established lunate osteonecrosis demonstrates sclerosis (Fig. 9) followed by progressive collapse and fragmentation (Figs. 2, 6, 8, and 10). Associated findings such as negative ulnar variance and late stage secondary degenerative osteoarthritis may also be seen. Radiographs are an important initial imaging modality to differentiate lunate osteonecrosis from alternative causes of wrist pain such as ulna-lunate abutment, fracture, carpal malalignment, instability and arthritis.

CT is more sensitive than plain films for demonstrating sclerosis, compression and fractures of the lunate. Fractures are more common in

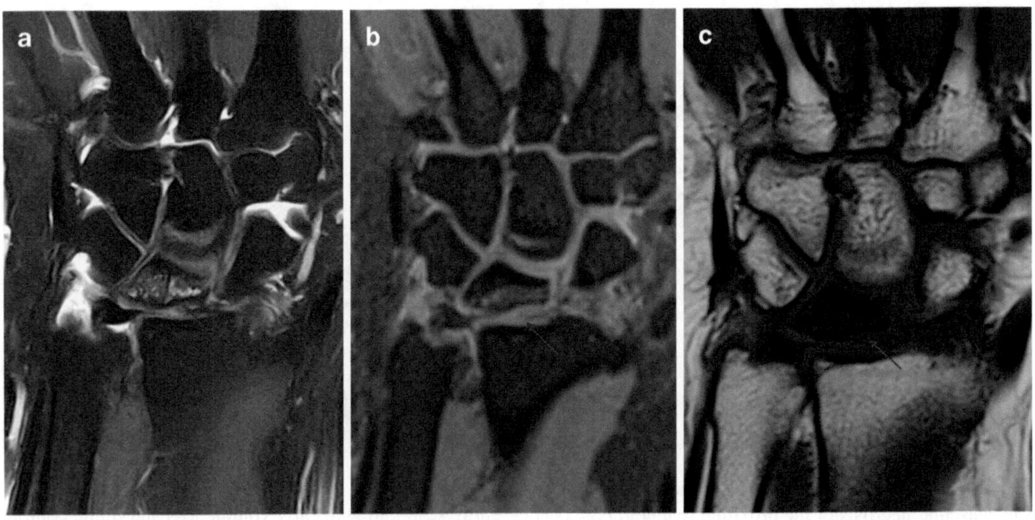

Fig. 8 (**a**–**c**) Coronal images of the wrist following injury, where arrows (→) indicate the marrow oedema throughout the lunate on STIR (**a**), subchondral collapse of the proximal lunate pole best seen on PD SPACE (**b**), whilst there is complete loss of normal fat signal on T1 (**c**). Additional injuries to the trifibrocartilage complex insertion at the styloid and contusion to the proximal capitate pole. (Images courtesy of Dr Bob Bleakney, University Health Network, Toronto, Canada)

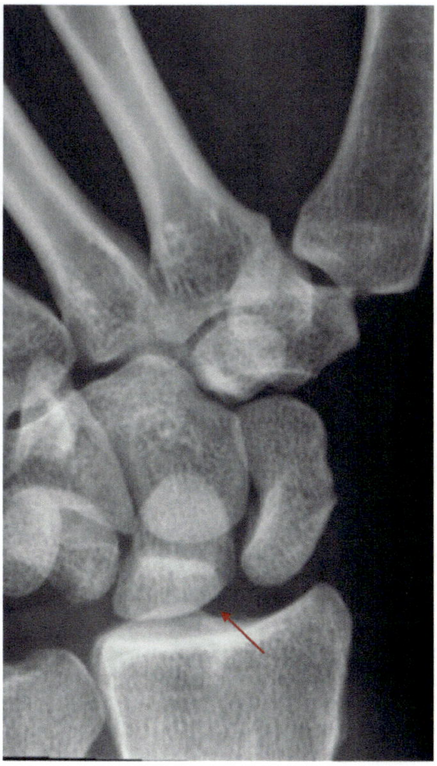

Fig. 9 Plain PA wrist radiograph showing early sclerosis of the lunate, typical features of Kienböch's disease (→). This is in the presence of mild negative ulnar variance

Kienböch's disease than previously reported and earlier detection with CT may allow preventative treatment and avoid lunate collapse (Friedman et al. 1991).

MRI and scintigraphy provide earlier evidence of Kienböch's disease and can help establish the diagnosis in the presence of normal radiographs. Two patterns of abnormality have been described on MRI, one with focal involvement of the radial half of the lunate and the other with diffuse lunate marrow signal changes (Sowa et al. 1989 Nov). As with osteonecrosis elsewhere, high T2-weighted imaging marrow signal may be seen in the initial stages of disease and which may be focal or patchy in distribution. Later in the disease process, T2 signal becomes low and accompanying cystic changes, collapse and fragmentation may be seen (Fig. 8a–c).

5.1.2 Staging of Kienböch's Disease

Several classification systems have been proposed for staging of Kienboch's disease, albeit with similar grading systems. The commonly used osseous Lichtman classification system uses four stages to diagnose and follow the progression of the disease (Lichtman et al. 1977, 2017).

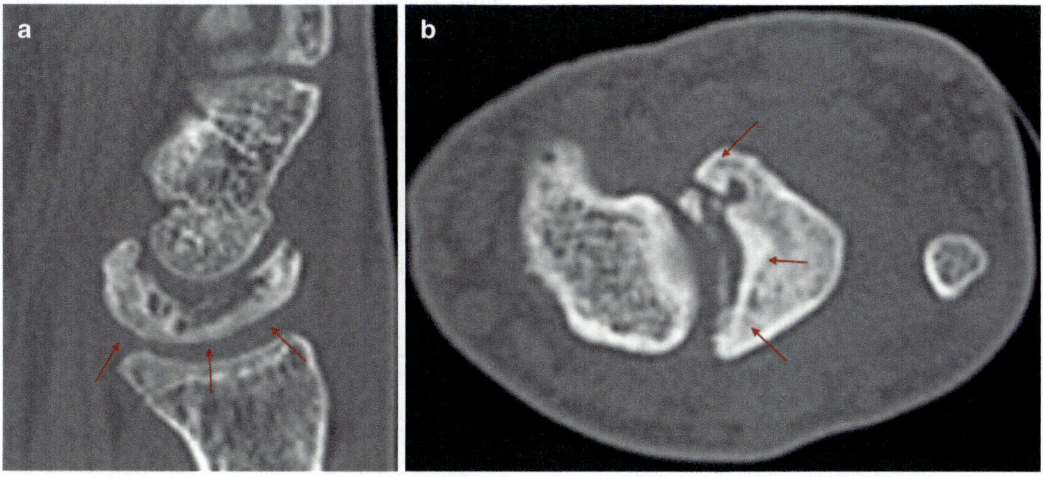

Fig. 10 (**a**, **b**) Sagittal (**a**) and axial (**b**) CT images demonstrating advanced Kienböch's disease (→) with sclerosis, collapse, subchondral cystic change and fragmentation

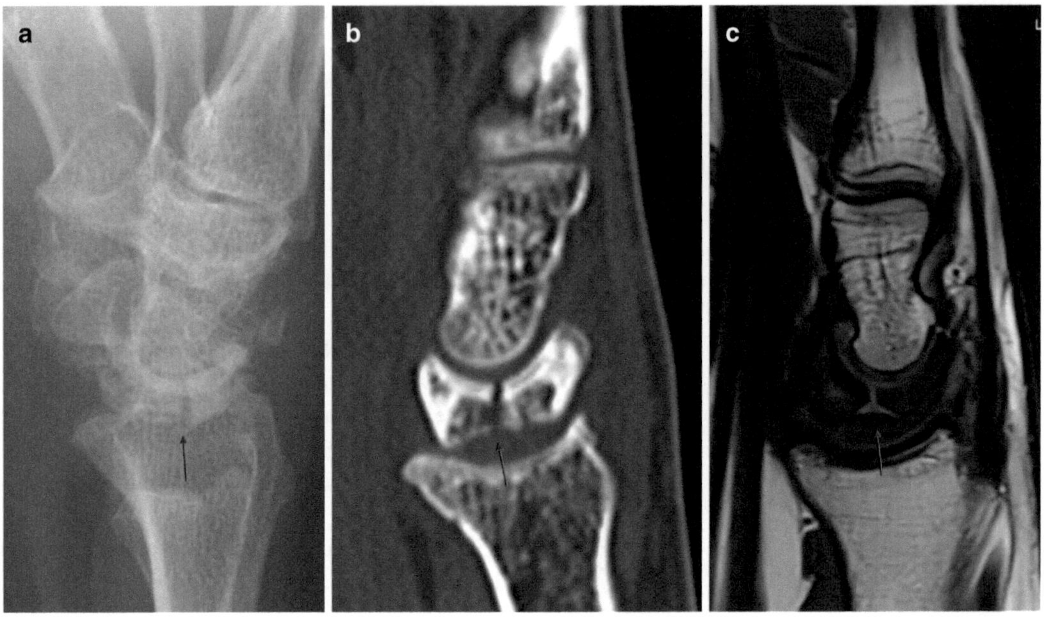

Fig. 11 (**a**–**c**) Multimodality correlation from lateral wrist radiograph (**a**), sagittal CT reformat (**b**) and sagittal PD sequence (**c**) demonstrating the subchondral collapse with flattened proximal lunate articular margin, and characteristic coronal-oriented fragmentation cleft (→). Additional early radiolunate degenerative changes. (Images courtesy of Dr Bob Bleakney, University Health Network, Toronto, Canada)

Stage 1:	Pre-radiological disease.
	The plain radiograph is normal except for possible predisposing factors such as negative ulnar variance. Detection of stage 1 disease is by MRI where there is typically internal bone marrow signal change with low T1 signal and low or patchy high T2 signal. Stage 1 disease can also be detected by bone scintigraphy.
Stage II:	Sclerosis of the lunate bone without collapse (Fig. 9).
Stage III:	Lunate fragmentation and collapse (Figs. 2, 6, 8, 10, and 11).
	As a consequence of collapse, there may be associated scapholunate dissociation and rotatory subluxation of the scaphoid. This has led to subdivision of stage III into stage IIIA: no rotatory subluxation and IIIB: associated scapholunate dissociation and rotatory subluxation with fixed scaphoid palmar flexion.
Stage IV:	Radiocarpal or midcarpal degenerative arthritis.

Whilst the diagnosis of Kienböch's disease with MRI is easily achieved, there are many therapeutic options available, typically beginning with non-operative management for at least 3 months in the early stages of disease. Multiple surgical options, including revascularisation of the lunate, lunate unloading by ulnar lengthening or radial shortening and pedicle or free vascularised bone grafting, are available; however, there is no strong consensus on the indications and results are variable (Kristensen et al. 1986; Weiss et al. 1991).

6 Capitate

Osteonecrosis of the capitate usually occurs following fracture and has been reported in the setting of rare midcarpal fracture dislocation (scaphocapitate syndrome) (Tashjian et al. 2004). Atraumatic associations include steroid use, SLE

(Fig. 4a–c), gout and haematological malignancy. Idiopathic osteonecrosis of the capitate without antecedent trauma has been described but is rare and is most commonly reported in women and younger patients (Kutty and Curtin 1995; Lapinsky and Mack 1992). Similar to the scaphoid, the capitate has a retrograde arterial supply from nutrient vessels entering the distal pole and potentially explaining the predominant proximal pole pattern of necrosis (Pickrell and Harper 2022).

Radiographic changes are of initial proximal pole osteopaenia with subsequent sclerosis and which may progress to fragmentation and collapse. MRI will show the typical features of osteonecrosis described previously. Treatment often involves excision of the capitate and carpal fusion with revascularisation also having been successfully achieved (Murakami et al. 2002).

7 Hamate

Hamate osteonecrosis is a relatively uncommon entity and follows trauma in the reported cases. Post-traumatic osteonecrosis involving both the hook of hamate and the body has been described (Telfer et al. 1994; Failla 1993). Like the scaphoid and capitate, the hamate is also vascularised via retrograde circulation with the proximal pole more vulnerable to osteonecrosis (Botte et al. 2004; Tashjian et al. 2004) (Fig. 12a–c).

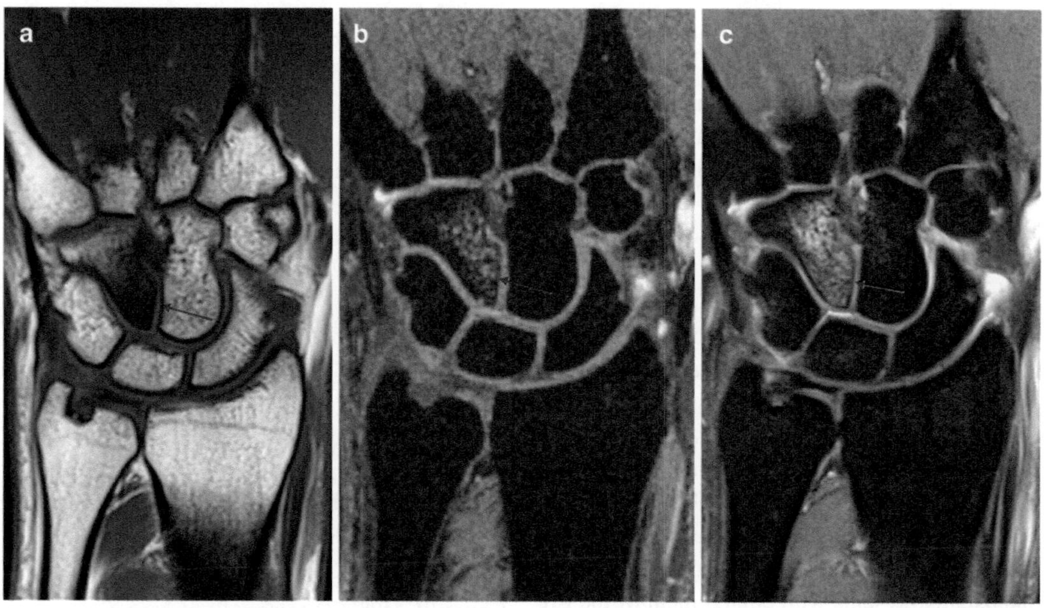

Fig. 12 (**a**–**c**) Coronal (**a**) T1-weighted, (**b**) 3D PD SPACE and (**c**) STIR sequences demonstrating the confluent T1 low signal marrow changes with corresponding oedema through the proximal to radial aspect of the capitate (→). (Images courtesy of Dr Lawrence White, University Health Network, Toronto, Canada)

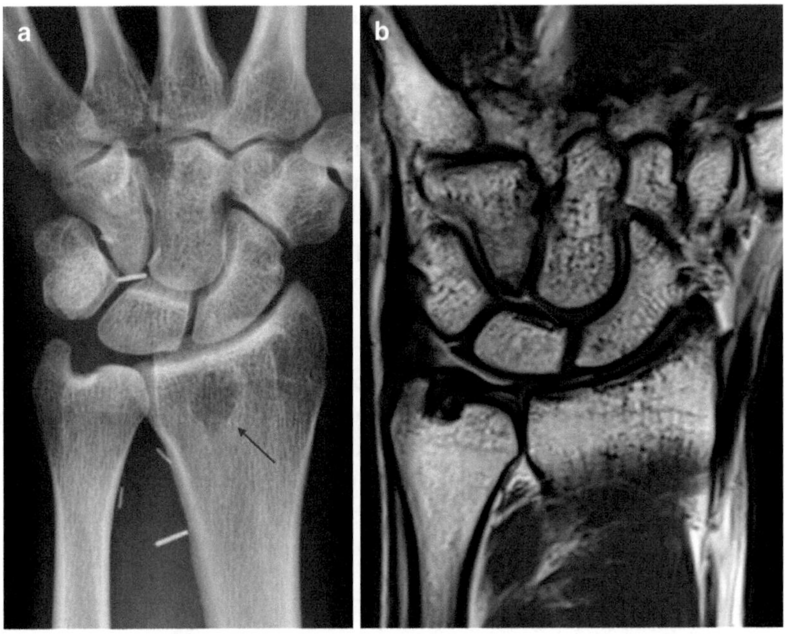

Fig. 13 (**a**, **b**) Post-operative scan following Fig. 6 whereby successful vascularised bone graft from the distal radius to the proximal hamate characterised on (**a**) PA wrist radiograph (blue→), with restoration of the normal T1 marrow signal characteristics on (**b**) coronal PD (red→). (Images courtesy of Dr Lawrence White, University Health Network, Toronto, Canada)

Subsequent restoration of normal MRI marrow signal alteration following vascularised bone graft transfer (Fig. 13a, b) to the hamate.

8 The Hand

The most common site for osteonecrosis in the hand is the metacarpal heads and about the proximal interphalangeal (PIP) joints of the fingers. Thiemann's disease is a rare autosomal-dominant form of avascular necrosis affecting the PIP joint (Tashjian et al. 2004). The condition has also been referred to as juvenile osteochondropathy of the fingers and multiple phalangeal epiphysitis and usually presents with enlargement of the PIP joints, frequently starting with the middle finger and progressing to involve the index and ring fingers, often sparing the little finger and thumb IP joints. Whilst the condition is usually painless, contractures, finger shortening and deformity can feature (Rubinstein 1975). Radiographic features include flattening, sclerosis and fragmentation of the epiphyses.

Osteonecrosis of the metacarpal heads (Dietrich's disease) has been described in association with trauma, systemic lupus erythematosus (SLE) and steroid use.

References

Beckers G, Mazy D, Cermak K, Van den Dungen S, Van Nieuwenhove O, Kinnen L (2022) Osteonecrosis of the trapezium: a case report and review of the literature. Acta Orthop Belg 88(1):186–189

Botte MJ, Pacelli LL, Gelberman RH (2004) Vascularity and osteonecrosis of the wrist. Orthop Clin North Am 35(3):405–421, xi

Bush C, Gillespy T III, Dell P (1987) High-resolution CT of the wrist: initial experience with scaphoid disorders and surgical fusions. Am J Roentgenol 149(4):757–760

Cerezal L, Abascal F, Canga A, Garcia-Valtuille R, Bustamante M, Pinal F (2000) Usefulness of gadolinium-enhanced MR imaging in the evaluation of the vascularity of scaphoid nonunions. Am J Roentgenol 174(1):14–19

Cruess RL (1986) Osteonecrosis of bone. Current concepts as to etiology and pathogenesis. Clin Orthop Relat Res 208:30–39

Dawson JS, Martel AL, Davis TRC (2001) Scaphoid blood flow and acute fracture healing: a dynamic MRI study with enhancement with gadolinium. J Bone Joint Surg Br 83-B(6):809–814

De Smet L (2000) Avascular nontraumatic necrosis of the scaphoid. Preiser's disease? Chir Main 19(2):82–85

De Smet L, Willemen D, Kimpe E, Fabry G (1993) Nontraumatic osteonecrosis of the capitate bone associated with gout. Ann Chir Main Memb Super 12(3):210–212

Donati OF, Zanetti M, Nagy L, Bode B, Schweizer A, Pfirrmann CWA (2011) Is dynamic gadolinium enhancement needed in MR imaging for the preoperative assessment of scaphoidal viability in patients with scaphoid nonunion? Radiology 28:808–816

Failla JM (1993) Hook of hamate vascularity: vulnerability to osteonecrosis and nonunion. J Hand Surg 18(6):1075–1079

Ferlic DC, Morin P (1989) Idiopathic avascular necrosis of the scaphoid: Preiser's disease? J Hand Surg Am 14(1):13–16

Friedman L, Yong-Hing K, Johnston GH (1991) The use of coronal computed tomography in the evaluation of Kienbock's disease. Clin Radiol 44(1):56–59

Garcia LA, Vaca JB (2006) Avascular necrosis of the pisiform. J Hand Surg Br 31(4):453–454

Garg B, Giupta H, Kotwal PP (2011) Nontraumatic osteonecrosis of the distal pole of the scaphoid. Indian J Orthop 45(2):185–187

Gelberman RH, Gross MS (1986) The vascularity of the wrist. Identification of arterial patterns at risk. Clin Orthop Relat Res 202:40–49

Glimcher MJ, Kenzora JE (1979a) The biology of osteonecrosis of the human femoral head and its clinical implications: I. Tissue biology. Clin Orthop Relat Res 138:284–309

Glimcher MJ, Kenzora JE (1979b) The biology of osteonecrosis of the human femoral head and its clinical implications: II. The pathological changes in the femoral head as an organ and in the hip joint. Clin Orthop Relat Res 139:283–312

Glimcher MJ, Kenzora JE (1979c) The biology of osteonecrosis of the human femoral head and its clinical implications. III. Discussion of the etiology and genesis of the pathological sequelae; comments on treatment. Clin Orthop Relat Res 140:273–312

Golimbu CN, Firooznia H, Rafii M (1995) Avascular necrosis of carpal bones. Magn Reson Imaging Clin N Am 3(2):281–303

Herbert TJ, Lanzetta M (1994) Idiopathic avascular necrosis of the scaphoid. J Hand Surg Br 19(2):174–182

Humphrey CS, Izadi KD, Esposito PW (2006) Case reports: osteonecrosis of the capitate: a pediatric case report. Clin Orthop Relat Res 447:256–259

Imhof H, Breitenseher M, Trattnig S, Kramer J, Hofmann S, Plenk H et al (1997) Imaging of avascular necrosis of bone. Eur Radiol 7(2):180–186

Kalainov DM, Cohen MS, Hendrix RW, Sweet S, Culp RW, Osterman AL (2003) Preiser's disease: identification of two patterns. J Hand Surg Am 28(5):767–778

Kristensen SS, Thomassen E, Christensen F (1986) Kienbock's disease–late results by non-surgical treatment. A follow-up study. J Hand Surg Br 11(3):422–425

Kutty S, Curtin J (1995) Idiopathic avascular necrosis of the capitate. J Hand Surg Br 20(3):402–404

Lapinsky AS, Mack GR (1992) Avascular necrosis of the capitate: a case report. J Hand Surg (Case Rep Rev) 17(6):1090–1092

Lenoir H, Coulet B, Lazerges C, Mares O, Croutzet P, Chammas M (2012) Idiopathic avascular necrosis of the scaphoid: 10 new cases and a review of the literature. Indications for Preiser's disease. Orthop Traumatol Surg Res 98(4):390–397

Lichtman DM, Mack GR, MacDonald RI, Gunther SF, Wilson JN (1977) Kienbock's disease: the role of silicone replacement arthroplasty. J Bone Joint Surg Am 59(7):899–908

Lichtman DM, Pientka WF II, Bain GI (2017) Kienböck disease: a new algorithm for the 21st century. J Wrist Surg 6(01):002–010

Mazet R Jr, Hohl M (1963) Fractures of the carpal navicular: analysis of ninety-one cases and review of the literature. J Bone Joint Surg Am 45-A:82–112

Megerle K, Worg H, Christopoulos G, Schmitt R, Krimmer H (2011) Gadolinium-enhanced preoperative MRI scans as a prognostic parameter in scaphoid nonunion. J Hand Surg Eur Vol 36(1):23–28

Mitchell DG, Steinberg ME, Dalinka MK, Rao VM, Fallon M, Kressel HY (1989) Magnetic resonance imaging of the ischemic hip. Alterations within the osteonecrotic, viable, and reactive zones. Clin Orthop Relat Res 244:60–77

Murakami H, Nishida J, Ehara S, Furumachi K, Shimamura T (2002) Revascularization of avascular necrosis of the capitate bone. Am J Roentgenol 179(3):664–666

Pickrell BB, Harper CM (2022) Avascular necrosis of capitate and other uncommon presentations of carpal avascular necrosis. Hand Clin 38(4):479–485

Preiser G (1910) Eine typische posttraumatische und zur spontanfraktur führende Ostitis des Naviculare carpi. Fortschr Geb Roentgenstr 15:189–197

Resnick D (2002) Osteochondroses. In: Resnick D (ed) Diagnosis of bone and joint disorders, 4th edn. Saunders, Philadelphia, pp 3686–3741

Rubinstein HM (1975) Thiemann's disease. A brief reminder. Arthritis Rheum 18(4):357–360

Schmitt R, Christopoulos G, Wagner M, Krimmer H, Fodor S, van Schoonhoven J et al (2011) Avascular necrosis (AVN) of the proximal fragment in scaphoid nonunion: is intravenous contrast agent necessary in MRI? Eur J Radiol 77(2):222–227

Sherman SB, Greenspan A, Norman A (1983) Osteonecrosis of the distal pole of the carpal scaphoid following fracture–a rare complication. Skeletal Radiol 9(3):189–191

Singh AK, Davis TR, Dawson JS, Oni JA, Downing ND (2004) Gadolinium enhanced MR assessment of proximal fragment vascularity in nonunions after scaphoid fracture: does it predict the outcome of reconstructive surgery? J Hand Surg Br 29(5):444–448

Sowa DT, Holder LE, Patt PG, Weiland AJ (1989) Application of magnetic resonance imaging to ischemic necrosis of the lunate. J Hand Surg 14(6):1008–1016

Tashjian RZ, Patel A, Akelman E, Weiss A-pC (2004) Avascular necrosis of the wrist and hand excluding the scaphoid and lunate. J Am Soc Surg Hand 4(2):109–116

Telfer JR, Evans DM, Bingham JB (1994) Avascular necrosis of the hamate. J Hand Surg Br 19(3):389–392

Weiss AP, Weiland AJ, Moore JR, Wilgis EF (1991) Radial shortening for Kienbock's disease. J Bone Joint Surg Am 73(3):384–391

Wells ME, Dunn JC (2022) Pathophysiology of avascular necrosis. Hand Clin 38(4):367–376

Zafra M, Carpintero P, Cansino D (2004) Osteonecrosis of the trapezium treated with a vascularized distal radius bone graft. J Hand Surg Am 29(6):1098–1101

Metabolic and Endocrine Disorders

Maria Pilar Aparisi Gómez,
Violeta Vasilevska Nikodinovska,
Miriana Rosaria Petrera,
Maria Alejandra Ferrando Fons, Catherine Phan,
Nuran Sabir, and Alberto Bazzocchi

Contents

M. P. Aparisi Gómez
Department of Radiology, Te Toka Tumai Auckland (Auckland District Health Board), Grafton, Auckland, New Zealand

Department of Anatomy and Medical Imaging, Faculty of Medical and Health Sciences, Waipapa Taumata Rau | University of Auckland, Auckland, New Zealand

Department of Radiology, IMSKE, Valencia, Spain

V. Vasilevska Nikodinovska
Medical Faculty, Ss. Cyril and Methodius University, Skopje, Macedonia

Department of Radiology, University Surgical Clinic "St. Naum Ohridski" Skopje, Skopje, Macedonia

M. R. Petrera · A. Bazzocchi (✉)
Diagnostic and Interventional Radiology, IRCCS Istituto Ortopedico Rizzoli, Bologna, Italy

M. A. Ferrando Fons
Sporthospine Praxis für Orthopäedie, Unfall- und Handchirurgie, Kaarst, Germany

C. Phan
Service de Radiologie Ostéo-Articulaire, APHP, Nord-Université de Paris, Hôpital Lariboisière, Paris, France

N. Sabir
Department of Radiology, Faculty of Medicine, Pamukkale University, Denizli, Turkey

Med Radiol Diagn Imaging (2025)

https://doi.org/10.1007/174_2025_617,
Published Online: 17 September 2025

Abstract

Metabolic diseases may cause alterations in mass, mineralization, turnover, and growth of bone. They may be caused by genetic, endocrine, nutritional, or biochemical disorders. The bone is affected as a tissue, but radiological features may not be always evident, or evident in every bone. A basic knowledge of the pathophysiology of metabolic bone diseases is essential to the understanding of the effects that metabolic bone disorders have on the skeleton, to help interpret the abnormal features which they cause on imaging of the wrist and hand.

Osteoporosis is the most common metabolic disease, characterized by low bone mass and microarchitecture degeneration with impaired bone quality, resulting in increased skeletal frailty and thus increased risk of fractures, which are particularly common around the wrist. Other metabolic conditions affect bone around the wrist and hand in diverse ways, and have distinctive features, in some cases, virtually diagnostic.

In this chapter we will review the manifestations of metabolic bone disease around the wrist and hand, reviewing the essentials for diagnosis. We will also focus on the possibilities the wrist and hand offer to the quantitative diagnosis of metabolic bone disease, through established and advanced techniques.

1 Introduction

Metabolic bone diseases are a heterogeneous group of disorders that cause alterations in mineralization, mass, turnover, and bone growth.

The causes can be genetic, nutritional deficiencies, or acquired conditions, and affect the skeleton as a whole, with specific manifestations depending on the different anatomical region, leading to different radiological presentations (Chang et al. 2016).

These unbalanced situations in bone metabolism may lead to bone deformities, fragility, and increased risk of fractures.

Osteoporosis is the most common metabolic disease. This is characterized by low bone mass and microarchitecture degeneration, leading to impaired bone quality, with in turn results in increased skeletal frailty and subsequent increase on the risk of fracture. Pathophysiologically, there is an imbalance in bone turnover, with bone reabsorption being greater than bone deposition.

Bone mass reaches its peak in puberal age, and then begins a gradual reduction. With aging, the overall amounts of resorbed and formed bone remodeling balance become negative, resulting in a decreased bone mass associated with reduced bone strength, which may result in osteoporosis. In this context, osteoporosis is aggravated when a suboptimal bone peak is reached in adolescence (Syed and Ng 2010; Gabet and Bab 2011; Siris et al. 2014).

There are two types of osteoporosis, based on the metabolic alteration.

Primary osteoporosis, due to endocrinological and physiological changes, is further divided into type I—menopausal form characterized by estrogen deficit (loss of their protective effect on bone mass) resulting in predominant loss of trabecular bone, and type II—senile osteoporosis in which stem cell reduction induces a predominant loss of cortical bone.

There are three major age-related processes that lead to bone loss. The most important is trabecular bone loss caused by thinning of the trabeculae, by disruption of the trabecular microstructure, and loss of trabecular elements that especially appears in early postmenopausal women. Trabecular bone loss over life is one-quarter at the radius. Decrease in cortical bone is the second process contributing to bone loss, which is mainly caused by increased porosity due to increased resorption cavities and due to accumulation of incompletely closed osteons with aging. The third process for bone loss is continued net resorption at the endocortical surface.

The peak of BMD in women is in their 30s. This declines with aging, greatly decreasing during the perimenopausal period (Sorenson and Cameron 1967).

Secondary osteoporosis is associated with several conditions, such as corticosteroid intake, endocrine disorders (e.g., Cushing syndrome, hypogonadism), gastrointestinal disorders (e.g., malabsorption, IBD), genetic and rheumatological disease (Sozen et al. 2017).

The prevalence of osteoporosis worldwide has been reported to be around 23.1% in women and 11.7% in men (Salari et al. 2021). It affects about 5000 million people, approximately ten million Americans over 50 years old (Clynes et al. 2020), and 32 million across Europe (25.5 million women and 6.5 million men) (Kanis et al. 2021), representing a public health problem, given it is responsible for the occurrence of fragility fractures.

2 Implications of Metabolic Bone Diseases

Fragility fractures due to osteoporosis are one of the most substantial challenges to public health. The World Health Organization considers osteoporosis to be second to cardiovascular risk as a critical health problem. The prompt diagnosis of osteoporosis, and its management, is therefore crucial, as a means to decrease the incidence of fractures and their consequences.

Osteoporotic fractures should be considered as the first sign of an evolving disease.

Bone loss over life is approximately 25%–40% at the femoral neck and distal radius (Chen et al. 2013), thus, fragility fractures typically caused by osteoporosis, occur in areas exhibiting a greater tendency for bone loss, such as the spine, hip, or wrist (Riggs et al. 2004; Khosla et al. 2006; Macdonald et al. 2011; Rozental et al. 2013).

However, the effect of osteoporosis is systemic, so there is increased risk for all types of fractures.

The combined lifetime risk for a hip, forearm, and vertebral fracture is approximately 40%, which is equivalent to the risk of developing cardiovascular disease (Kanis 2002). Approximately 1 in 3 women and 1 in 5 men over the age of 50 will have a fragility fracture in their remaining lifetime, as per data in Caucasian populations, from the International Osteoporosis Foundation (Link 2012). The global population aging increases the risk of fragility fractures related to osteoporosis in older adults (Samelson et al. 2019).

In patients with hip fractures, mortality is up to 20% within the following year due to associated morbidity, with mortality at 5 years 20% greater than expected. 20% will require ongoing care (Delmas et al. 2005). Mortality of hip fractures is similar to mortality from breast cancer, with a 5% rate of acute mortality and 15%–25% rate of death in the first year after the fracture (Keene et al. 1993).

The number of total hip fractures, according to trend projection, is expected to double until 2050 (Sing et al. 2023), increasing the burden on population and healthcare systems. Patients with vertebral fractures have less severe complications but are the most frequent. It is estimated that only 30% of these fractures come to clinical attention (Sambrook and Cooper 2006).

Wrist fractures increase almost twofold the risk of subsequent hip or vertebral fractures, but also the risk of new forearm fracture is increased by 3.3 times and other skeletal fractures by 2.4 times.

Humeral fractures, which are the third most common fracture in people over 65 years of age, are associated with a higher risk of subsequent hip fractures, to more than five times in the following year.

Even fractures at the foot or ribs have been found to double the risk of subsequent hip, vertebral, forearm, or other skeletal fractures (Klotzbuecher et al. 2000).

In 2006 it was estimated that osteoporosis caused more than 8.9 million fractures annually worldwide, resulting in an osteoporosis fracture every 3 s (Johnell and Kanis 2006).

2.1 Insufficiency Fractures Around the Wrist/Hand

Distal radius fractures are one of the most common types of fractures, accounting for up to 18% of all fractures in the elderly age group. They account for approximately 37% of overall osteoporotic fractures (Chung et al. 2009).

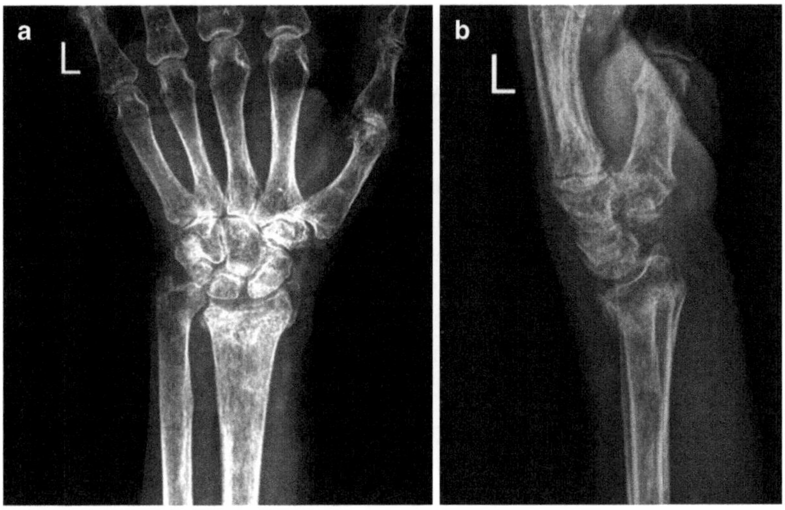

Fig. 1 Distal radius fragility fracture. (**a**) Anteroposterior projection showing an impacted fracture of the distal radius. Note the typical features of osteoporosis, with loss of bone mineralization. Radiographs have limited sensitivity, as a bone loss of 30%–50% should have occurred for this to be evident on radiographs. (**b**) lateral projection demonstrating the fracture has a Colles pattern, the most common configuration

The growth of the elderly population and a rise in the number of active elderly are directly responsible for the increase seen in this age group (Diamantopoulos et al. 2012; Nellans et al. 2012).

Fragility fractures of the distal forearm normally occur as a result low energy trauma, typically of a fall on an outstretched hand, from standing height.

They predominantly occur in the distal metaphysis, which is comprised of both rich cortical and trabecular bone, rather than the diaphysis which is predominantly comprised of cortical bone (Bala et al. 2015). The distal radial metaphysis seems to be more affected by age-related changes, reflected by the earlier loss of BMD at the ultradistal radius compared with other sites (Wilson et al. 2009; Chen et al. 2013). Premenopausal women with forearm fractures show deficit only in trabecular bone volume with the normal cortical area, while older postmenopausal women with forearm fractures show deficits in the trabecular bone volume and cortical porosity (Bala et al. 2015). Cortical porosity is reported as an important component of bone quality at the distal radius that deteriorates with aging (Chen et al. 2013). Distal radial fractures occur at younger ages in comparison to other osteoporotic fractures (Ahlborg et al. 2003; Barrett-Connor et al. 2008).

Fractures normally have the pattern of a Colles fracture (extra-articular) (Kanterewicz et al. 2002). They do not normally present a diagnostic challenge and are easily identified on plain radiographs (Fig. 1).

Fractures are slightly more frequent on the left, but that can be explained by the difference in bone mass in between the nondominant and dominant hand, considering that right-handed people are more prevalent (Nellans et al. 2012).

A study that aimed at investigating the association of patient characteristics, BMD, bone microarchitecture, and bone strength with the pattern complexity of distal radius fractures concluded that older age and male gender were independently associated with the pattern complexity of distal radius fractures. Other factors known to be associated with fracture risk, such as BMI, osteoporosis, number and severity of prevalent VFs, smoking, and alcohol use were not associated with pattern complexity (Daniels et al. 2019).

On the occasions in which the degree of complexity is greater, the fractures can associate distal radioulnar joint injuries, radial styloid fractures, and soft tissue injuries, such as injuries to the triangular fibrocartilage, scapholunate, or lunotriquetral ligaments. MRI has a very important role on the characterization of associated soft tissue injuries, and also on the assessment of post-treatment complications. In cases of complex fractures, with articular involvement, CT is especially useful for surgical planning.

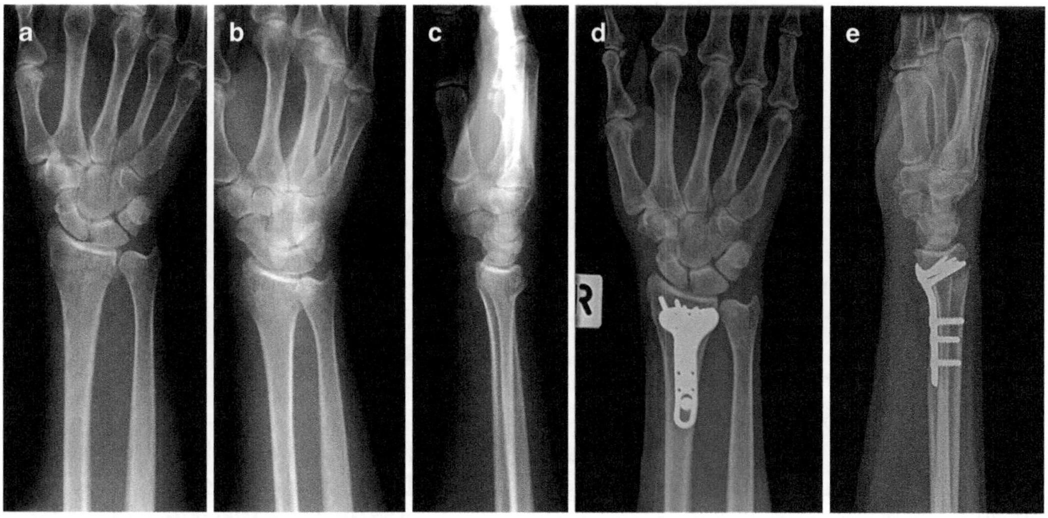

Fig. 2 Distal radius fragility fracture in a 62-year-old, after a fall. (**a**) Anteroposterior projection showing an impacted fracture of the distal radius. Osteoporosis may not be obvious until a significant amount of bone is lost. (**b**) oblique projection demonstrating a fracture line through the scaphoid fossa. (**c**) lateral projection demonstrating the fracture has a Colles pattern, and there is mild cortical comminution and dorsal displacement of fragments. (**d**) AP after fixation with plate and screws. (**e**) lateral projection demonstrates the screws are correctly placed, lodged within bone, and not proud from the dorsal cortex

Treatment can be nonoperative or operative depending on fracture stability and fracture displacement as well as patient age and activity demands.

Extra-articular fractures, with less than 5 mm of radial shortening and no significant dorsal angulation (less than 5° or within 20° of contralateral distal radius) are typically managed with closed reduction and immobilization, with a below arm cast or splint. In some extra-articular fractures with stable volar cortex, closed reduction with percutaneous pinning may be useful, but this is unusual in the elderly and context of fragility fractures. Open reduction with internal fixation is needed in cases of comminute or significantly displaced or angulated extra-articular fractures, severe osteoporosis, or in cases of displaced intra-articular fractures (>2 mm), when there are radiographic signs of instability or other fractures (Diaz-Garcia et al. 2011; Ju et al. 2015). The threshold for intervention appears to be becoming lower (Fig. 2).

Complications can be diverse, directly related to the mechanism of injury or post-surgical. Median nerve neuropathy is the most frequent neurologic complication, and may occur in cases in which there is immobilization in excessive wrist flexion and ulnar deviation. It is less common in low-energy trauma than in high-energy trauma (Niver and Ilyas 2012). Ulnar nerve neuropathy is more commonly seen in distal radio-ulnar joint involvement.

Extensor pollicis longus rupture is a known complication after distal radius fractures and is believed to occur more frequently after minimally displaced and nondisplaced distal radius fractures (Roth et al. 2012). The suggested mechanism is repetitive impingement of the extensor mechanism on the tendon after a non-displaced fracture, causing either a mechanical attrition or a local area of ischemia in the tendon. In a postsurgical context, volar plating with screw fixation that penetrates the dorsal cortex and is proud dorsally may be causative.

Other acute tendon injuries may also occur, but are much less frequent.

Osteoarthritis is also frequent after intra-articular fractures. Low BMD is a predisposing factor for poor functional outcomes (Diaz-Garcia et al. 2011; Ju et al. 2015). Additionally, ulnar impaction due to residual shortening of the radius and development of complex regional pain syndrome (CRPS), although less seen in older people, can also occur (Diaz-Garcia et al. 2011; Ju et al. 2015).

A key point in the context of a fragility fracture is to draw attention to underlying osteoporosis and raise clinical awareness to either trigger further investigation with DXA or indicate treatment. Distal radius fractures are considered to be a predictor of subsequent osteoporotic fractures.

The prevalence of osteoporosis in patients with distal radius fractures is high, diagnosed in 51.5% of the cases, with rates of newly diagnosed osteoporosis of 29.6% in patients aged 50–59 years, 54.8% in patients aged 60–69 years, and 92.8% in patients aged 70–79 years (Löfman et al. 2007; Gong et al. 2009; Oyen et al. 2011; Jung et al. 2016). Several studies reported occurrence of distal radius fractures approximately 15 years prior to hip fracture (Earnshaw et al. 1998; Barrett-Connor et al. 2008; Oyen et al. 2011; Schousboe 2016) with 1.4-fold and 5.2-fold increase of hip and vertebral fracture compared to women without prior distal radius fractures (Kanis et al. 2004; Siris et al. 2014). An osteoporotic hip fracture can occur after a distal radius fracture in younger postmenopausal women with distal radius fractures due to low BMD values (Jung et al. 2016). A 24-year follow-up study showed that osteoporotic fractures of the distal radius are highly associated with future risk of fracture (Mallmin et al. 1993). The risk of new forearm fracture is increased by 3.3 times and other skeletal fractures by 2.4 times (Klotzbuecher et al. 2000).

Orthopedic surgeons treating patients with a distal radius fracture with a low-energy mechanism of injury should recommend further evaluation of the patient's bone mineral density with DXA (Olschewski et al. 2001). Distal radius DXA performed in addition to a central DXA may be an effective tool for early detection of osteoporosis of the distal radius (Miyamura et al. 2020).

Distal radial fractures occur at younger ages in comparison to other osteoporotic fracture sites with incidence in the perimenopausal period approximately two-fold higher than that at other sites (Ahlborg et al. 2003; Barrett-Connor et al. 2008).

Therefore, in order to prevent osteoporotic fractures of the hip and spine, in postmenopausal women at 50–59 years of age with low-energy distal radius fractures should be evaluated for osteoporosis (Rozental et al. 2008; Jung et al. 2016).

3 Particular Metabolic Bone Disease Manifestations Around the Wrist/Hand

3.1 Hyperparathyroidism and Renal Osteodystrophy

Hyperparathyroidism is characterized by increased levels of parathyroid hormone that induces an increase in serum calcium, through increased intestinal absorption, mobilization of bone calcium, and reduced urinary excretion (Baig et al. 2018).

The condition may be primary, caused by parathyroid adenoma or secondary, more frequent than the primary form, in response to reduced serum calcium levels in the context of chronic renal failure.

Radiographic features described in hyperparathyroidism are mainly due to bone resorption, which could be subperiosteal, subchondral, subligamentous, cortical, and trabecular. The findings in bone overlap in these two scenarios (Bennett et al. 2020).

The main skeletal manifestations of hyperparathyroidism involve the hands, and in more advanced stages, the periosteal resorption typical of the pathology occurs also at other levels (Chang et al. 2016).

The occurrence of sub-periosteal erosions in the cortical bone is pathognomonic of hyperpara-

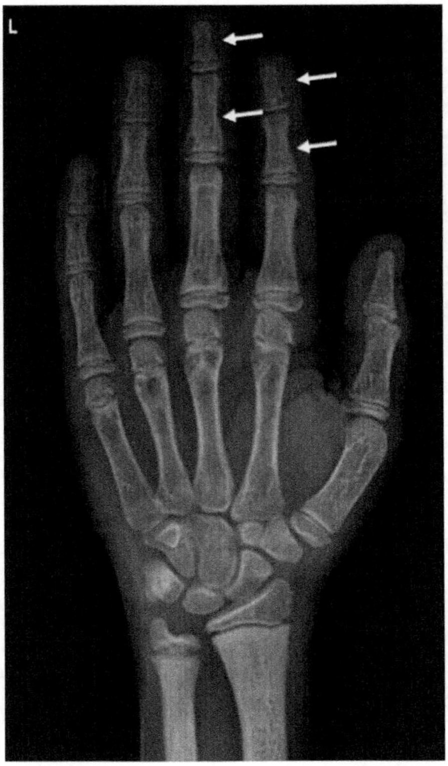

Fig. 3 14-year-old male. The occurrence of subperiosteal erosions in the cortical bone is pathognomonic of hyperparathyroidism. The typical and most sensitive site to identify these erosions is in the radial aspects of the middle phalanges of the index and middle fingers (white arrows)

thyroidism (Genant et al. 1973; Hayes and Conway 1990).

The typical and most sensitive site to identify these erosions is in the radial aspects of the middle phalanges of the index and middle fingers (Fig. 3). They also occur in the phalangeal tufts, neck of humerus and femur, and distal end of clavicle (Fig. 4). They appear as lace-like subperiosteal—intracortical irregular margins of the phalangeal bone.

If no subperiosteal erosions are identified on radiographs in the phalanges, they are unlikely to be evident in other locations in the skeleton. Involvement of in sites other than the phalanges indicates a more severe and long-standing hyperparathyroidism, probably secondary, the most frequent cause being chronic renal impairment (Figs. 5 and 6).

Subchondral bone resorption results in pseudo-widening of the joint space and can be seen commonly in small joints of the hand, sacroiliac joints, acromioclavicular joints, and pubic symphysis. Subligamentous bone resorption is seen at insertions of ligaments and tendons. Common sites of occurrence are in the pelvic bones, ribs, clavicles, and bones of extremities.

Intracortical bone resorption is another form of bone resorption that results from increased osteoclastic activity in haversian canals. This is not specific, and radiographically causes linear translucencies within the cortex (appearances of cortical "tunneling") (Hayes and Conway 1990). It can be seen as well in nutritional osteomalacia, renal osteodystrophy, thyrotoxicosis, and sometimes in acromegaly (Meema 1991).

The deposition of calcium pyrophosphate dihydrate (CPPD) in cartilage and fibrocartilage is more common in the hand and knee (also involving menisci). Chondrocalcinosis is typical of primary disease, rather than that secondary to chronic renal impairment (Dodds and Steinbach 1968).

CPPD in the wrist/hand may be seen in the triangular fibrocartilage complex, and the lunotriquetral ligament (Fig. 7).

Clinically, patients may present with acute pain resembling gout, because of the occurrence of arthritis and periarthritis. In these cases, joint effusions, synovitis, and crystal deposits may be seen on ultrasound, appearing as echogenic foci in the hyaline and fibrous cartilage, and in the tendons (parallel to the fiber orientation). The joints involved are usually the second and third MCPJ and the ulnocarpal joint. Normally there is concomitant osteoarthritis, which sometimes can have more aggressive appearances—with hook-like osteophytes in the metacarpal heads, large subchondral cysts, and a pattern of destruction, with subchondral collapse, loose bodies, and microfractures (Fig. 8). CPPD may be also asymptomatic (Aparisi Gómez et al. 2024).

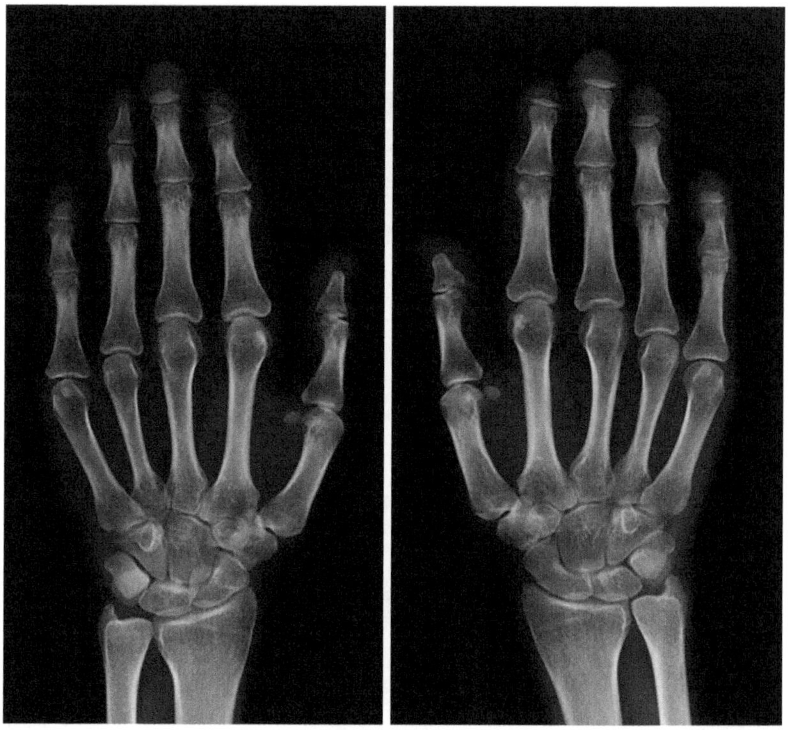

Fig. 4 Example of acroosteolysis in the context of hyperparathyroidism. Note the resorption of the distal phalanx tufts (every finger, different degrees)

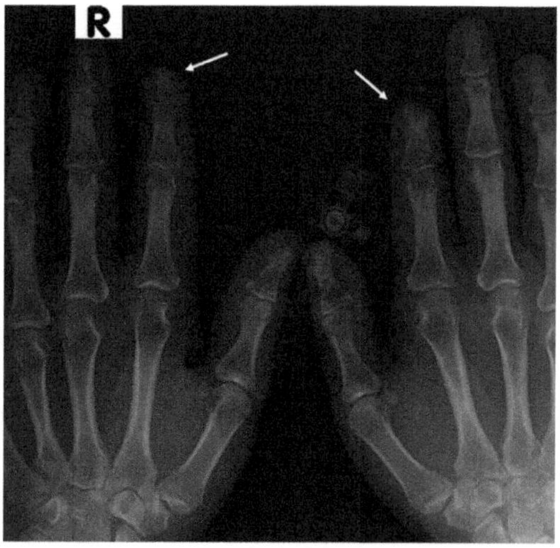

Fig. 5 Example of acroosteolysis in the context of hyperparathyroidism secondary to renal insufficiency

Brown tumors are cystic lesions (Osteitis fibrosa cystica) within bone due to excessive osteoclastic resorption, in the context of untreated severe primary or secondary hyperparathyroidism. Brown tumors are composed of numerous multinucleated osteoclasts (giant cells) admixed with stromal cells and matrix, which are found most often in trabecular portions of the jaw, long bones, and ribs. Radiographically, brown tumors appear as lucent lesions, sometimes expansile, which may be multi-loculated and can occur in any skeletal site. They are rare in the hands, but have been described (Franco et al. 2002; Browne et al. 2003; Nagaraj et al. 2012).

The differential diagnosis of brown tumors includes other lytic bone lesions, such as true giant cell tumors, multiple myeloma, fibrous dysplasia, and metastases.

Brown tumors can be clinically differentiated based off of serum calcium, serum electrophoresis, and correlated with an isotope bone scan or other radiographic findings suggestive of hyperparathyroidism (Bennett et al. 2020).

Osteosclerosis is a common feature of disease secondary to chronic renal impairment and not so

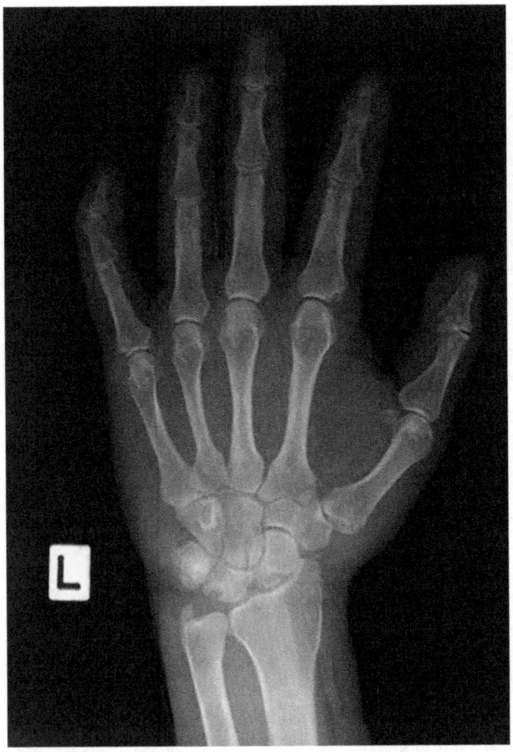

Fig. 6 Renal osteodystrophy, 44-year-old male. There are small regions of cortical bone resorption along the medial phalanges in the index and ring fingers, as well as poor definition of the cortices of the terminal tufts. There are small erosions in the ulnar styloid, and in the lunate. Small erosions are also present at the margins of the second and fifth metacarpophalangeal joint. They are less evident but also present in the interphalangeal joints. Findings are in keeping with renal osteodystrophy

common in primary hyperparathyroidism. It normally results from excessive accumulation of poorly mineralized osteoid, which appears denser radiographically than normal bone. In cases of primary disease, with normal renal function, it is the result of an exaggerated osteoblastic response subsequent to bone resorption. The increase in bone density affects particularly the axial skeleton ("rugger jersey" spine), which may be picked on pelvic radiographs (Sundaram 1989).

The bone resorption also affects the trabecular bone with spotty deossification and indistinct trabecular pattern in the skull, a typical granular "salt and pepper" appearance.

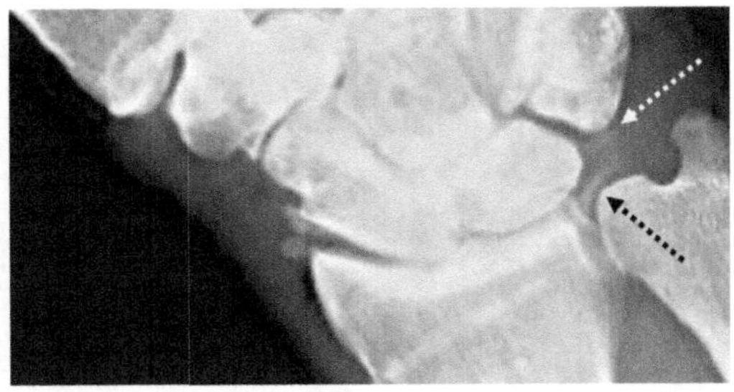

Fig. 7 Calcium pyrophosphate dihydrate (CPPD) deposit in the lunotriquetral (white dotted arrow) and triangular fibrocartilage (black dotted arrow)

The excessive bone resorption in the context of hyperparathyroidism at every level results in osteoporosis. In primary hyperparathyroidism there is a pattern of skeletal involvement that preferentially affects the cortical, as opposed to the trabecular, bone. BMD measurements made in sites in which cortical bone predominates, for example in the distal forearm, may be lower. In fact, hyperparathyroidism is an indication for the obtention of BMD measurement in the forearm to screen for osteoporosis (Aparisi Gómez et al. 2025).

In primary hyperparathyroidism, bone density improves after surgical removal. The demineralizing effect on cortical bone at the femoral neck and distal one-third radius has been found to be at least partially reversible by parathyroidectomy 10–15 years post-op (Rubin et al. 2008).

Soft tissue calcification, other than in articular cartilage and fibrocartilage, is not typical of primary hyperparathyroidism, however it may be seen with reduced glomerular function resulting in phosphate retention (secondary forms). The calcification may be vascular or around joints (in the pelvis, around the arteries, hips, and ischium) (Parfitt 1969) (Fig. 9).

3.2 Hypoparathyroidism

Hypoparathyroidism can result from reduced or absent parathyroid hormone production or from organ resistance (kidney, bone, or both). Idiopathic hypoparathyroidism usually presents

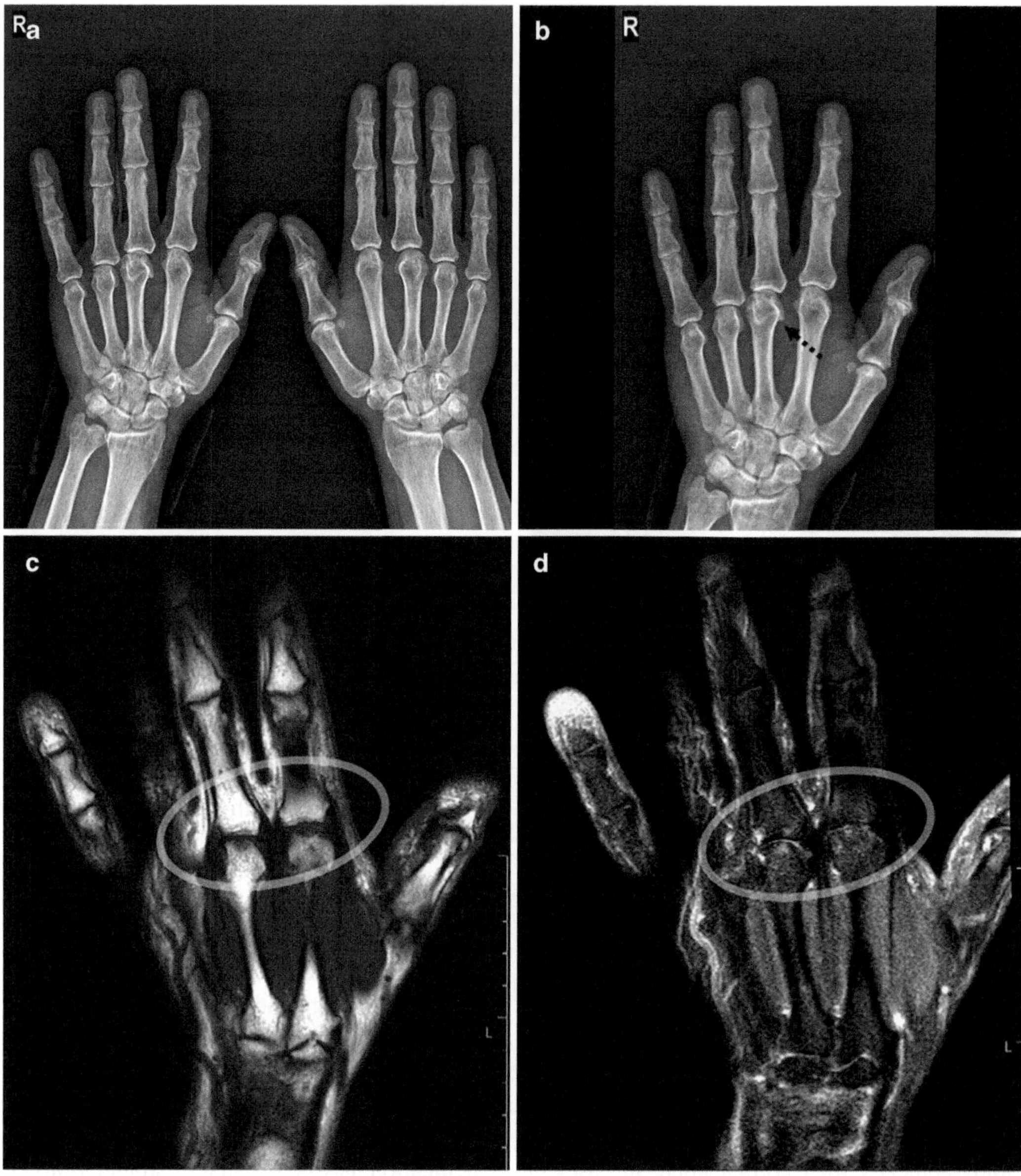

Fig. 8 61-year-old male, with pain and swelling in the second and third fingers of the right hand. (**a**) AP view of hands, demonstrating narrowing of the joint space in the second and third metacarpophalangeal joints of the right hand. (**b**) Right hand detail, note the hook-like osteophyte (black dotted arrow). On MRI, there is evidence of loss of articular cartilage, with narrowing of the joint space, and foci of subchondral bone marrow edema. (**c**) coronal T1 and (**d**) coronal STIR (second and third metacarpophalangeal joints circled)

during childhood, is more common in girls and rare in black races. It may be associated with pernicious anemia and Addison's disease, and may be part of a generalized autoimmune disorder. Acquired hypoparathyroidism can result from surgical removal of the parathyroid glands or from autoimmune disorders. Post-surgical hypoparathyroidism is more common. The biochemical alteration is hypocalcemia, which may manifest as tingling or burning sensation in the hands or around the mouth and muscle cramps. In severe cases, tetany occurs.

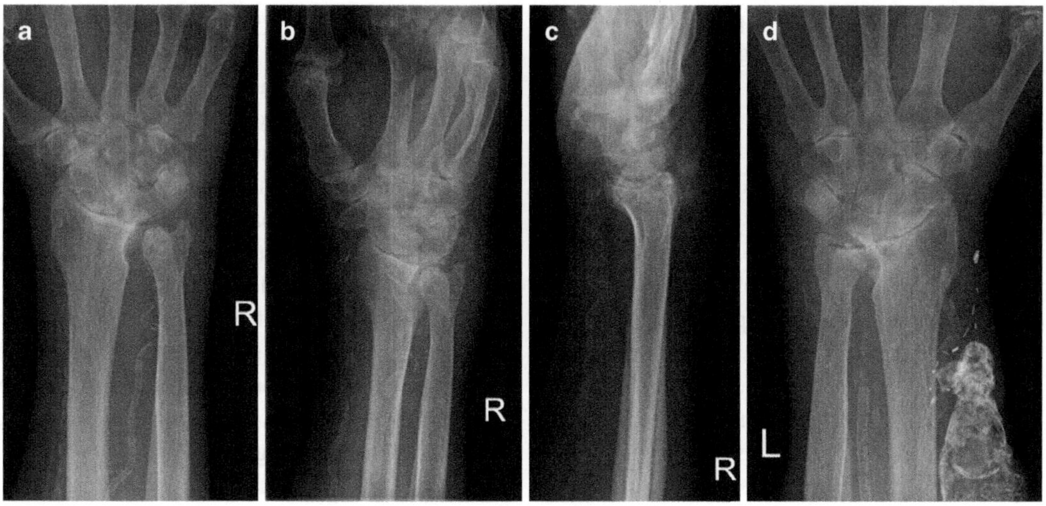

Fig. 9 (**a**) AP radiograph. Scalloping and remodeling of the sigmoid notch and spurring of the ulnar head. Severe radiocarpal arthrosis best seen in **b**, oblique view. (**c**) lateral view, showing soft tissue mineralization, reflecting CPPD. Note extensive arterial calcification. (**d**) AP left wrist, demonstrates even more evident vascular calcification, with a calcified pseudoaneurysm

Chronic deficiency of PTH in patients with hypoparathyroidism is associated with a profound reduction in bone remodeling, with consequent increases in bone density and abnormalities in microarchitecture and bone strength. It is still not clear whether there is an increase in fracture risk (Silva and Bilezikian 2021).

The typical radiological feature of hypoparathyroidism is osteosclerosis, which may be localized (23%) or generalized (9%). Metastatic calcification may be present in the basal ganglia and also in the subcutaneous tissue, and it is typical to find it around the hips and shoulders. A rare feature is enthesopathy with ossification in a paraspinal distribution, which also affects insertions around the pelvis and hips. It can be differentiated from ankylosing spondylitis in the fact that there is no erosive arthropathy in the sacroiliac joints (Adams and Davies 1977).

Pseudohypoparathyroidism (PHP) describes a group of genetic disorders characterized by hypocalcemia, hyperphosphatemia, raised PTH, and bone and kidney lack of response to PTH. The parathyroid glands are normal and produce PTH. It was first described by Albright et al. in 1942.

Patients are short in stature, have reduced intellect, rounded faces, and shortened metacarpals, particularly the fourth and fifth. Tetany, cataracts, and nail dystrophy are other features found. Metastatic calcification, which may be periarticular in hands and feet, bowing of long bones, and exostoses can occur. There is usually absence of the normal caudal widening of the lumbar inter-pedicular distances. Cord compression has been reported, from lumbar or cervical spinal stenosis or ossifications of the paravertebral ligaments (Okada et al. 1994).

Pseudo-pseudohypoparathyroidism (PPHP) is similar to PHP, but there is no resistance to PTH. Features are the same as PHP, but there are no associated parathyroid or other biochemical abnormalities. The abnormalities of metacarpal and metatarsal shortening, calvarial thickening, exostoses, soft tissue calcification, and ossification are seen. Bone density may be normal, reduced, or increased (Albright et al. 1952).

3.3 Hypothyroidism

The thyroid hormones mediate the growth, development, and maturation of the skeleton by regulating chondrocyte proliferation, promoting differentiation of bone progenitor cells, mineralization, and angiogenesis. It promotes GH secretion from the pituitary gland, as well as GH-dependent Insulin-Like Growth Factor 1 (IGF 1) production in the bone (Bassett and Williams 2016).

When the thyroid hormone is absent from birth, it leads to growth arrest, delayed bone age, and short stature. Ossification centers are defective, and they appear in an irregular and mottled pattern, with a fragmented appearance known as "stippled epiphyses", most frequently noted in the head of the femur, head of humerus, and the tarsal bone. When hypothyroidism is acquired during the growing age (juvenile hypothyroidism), manifestations are different. Skeletal maturation, defined as the appearance of secondary centers of ossification, is predominantly affected, with delayed fusion of epiphysis and delayed bone age. The epiphyseal centers are heterogeneous with irregular ossification, and the metaphyses of long bones usually have a thickened, sclerotic band (Cavallo et al. 2021).

Delayed bone age in the hand is a significant finding in children with hypothyroidism, as it can indicate the extent of the condition's impact on skeletal development. It's often used to help assess the severity of hypothyroidism and to monitor the effectiveness of treatment making adjustments to treatment as needed.

Early diagnosis and treatment of hypothyroidism, usually with thyroid hormone replacement therapy, can help to improve bone development and minimize long-term growth deficits.

Delayed bone age may also be seen in the context of growth hormone (GH) deficiency, hypophyseal alterations secondary to malformation, tumor, or infiltrative pathologies may also be associated with bone age delay consequently to a secondary GH deficiency or hypothyroidism. The presence of hypogonadism with the consequent lack of circulating estrogens, androgens, and other pubertal hormones may cause an important delay in bone maturation (Cavallo et al. 2021).

Thyroid acropachy is an unusual presentation of autoimmune thyroid disease (~1% of patients with Graves disease) (Fatourechi et al. 2002). It can occur in hyperthyroid, euthyroid, hypothyroid, or even post-treatment patients. It consists of digital clubbing, swelling of digits and toes, and periosteal reaction of extremity bones. It is almost always associated with ophthalmopathy and thyroid dermopathy.

The differential includes other conditions causing diffuse periostitis, such as hypertrophic pulmonary osteoarthropathy and pachydermoperiostosis (primary hypertrophic osteoarthropathy). The latter is a rare self-limiting osteoarthrodermopathic syndrome with familial and idiopathic forms, in which there is symmetrical subperiosteal bone formation in the long bones, especially of the forearm and leg bones, but also of the metacarpals, metatarsals, and phalanges.

Hypervitaminosis A and fluorosis are other causes for symmetric periostitis (Rana et al. 2009).

Thyroid acropachy always affects the ulnar side of the fifth metacarpal, a feature that can be used to differentiate thyroid acropachy from other conditions causing diffuse periostitis (Klein et al. 2018).

3.4 Acromegaly

Acromegaly is a rare metabolic disorder with an insidious evolution, distinguished by chronically elevated circulating levels of growth hormone and IGF 1. Diagnosis may be significantly delayed, increasing comorbidity. The recognition of radiographic changes is important for the early diagnosis and treatment of acromegaly, improving the prognosis and avoiding sequelae.

The effects of growth hormone on the skeleton depend on the degree of skeletal maturation. If the growth plates are still open, hormonal excess stimulates endochondral bone growth, in length and in width (gigantism). In the mature skeleton, in which growth plates are closed, hypersecretion of growth hormone may result in reactivation of endochondral bone formation at the junction sites between cartilage and bone, such as the costochondral junctions, as well as promoting periosteal reactions, with consequent bone enlargement (Resnick et al. 2025).

The high concentrations of growth hormone and IGF 1 promote hypertrophy and anabolism of the joint connective tissue, as well as of the periarticular ligaments (Anthony and Ioachimescu 2014).

In the hand, acromegaly causes thickening of the soft parts of the fingers due to a direct hormonal effect, together with enlargement of the sesamoid bones, phalanges, and metacarpals, mainly of the terminal tufts of the distal phalanges (classic spade-like appearance), resulting from excessive periosteal bone formation (Chang et al. 2016; Resnick et al. 2025). When accompanied by pronounced enlargement and hypertrophy of the phalangeal base, that can lead to the formation of a pseudoforamen in the lateral aspects of the phalanx. There can also be narrowing of the phalangeal diaphyses, caused by simultaneous formation and resorption of bone (Resnick et al. 2025).

4 Role of Radiography-Based Techniques and Radiogrammetry for Osteoporosis Assessment/Quantification

Radiographic absorptiometry (RA) and metacarpal radiogrammetry are the oldest radiographic methods devised to quantitatively evaluate osteoporosis. They are both applied to the hand (Adams 2010).

The development of the principles behind RA facilitated BMD estimation (Mack et al. 1939). RA consists of the obtention of a radiograph of a peripheral site (typically metacarpals and phalanges), placing a reference wedge of hydroxyapatite or aluminum close to the bone. BMD is then expressed relative to the density of this material (Cosman et al. 1991). RA was limited to peripheral skeletal sites, however, it showed a good correlation with the standard measurements of BMD derived by DXA ($r = 0.69$ and 0.68 respectively, at lumbar spine; $r = 0.63$ and 0.67 respectively, at the femoral neck) (Cosman et al. 1991). This makes it extrapolable to other sites.

However, RA is time-consuming and the results are influenced by multiple factors including operator experience, intensity of the X-ray beam, and soft tissue thickness (Adams 2010).

Radiogrammetry is a simple and inexpensive method to evaluate cortical bone changes in tubular bones using plain radiographs. It can be used in different bone segments, but the second metacarpal of the non-dominant hand is the most common site (Adams 2010).

The metacarpal index (MCI) (also called Barnett-Nordin index) is the ratio between the combined cortical thickness (radial and the ulnar cortex) of the mid second metacarpal and the diameter of the shaft at this level (Barnett and Nordin 1960; Hyldstrup and Nielsen 2001). As medullary width and bone width both increase with aging due to endosteal reabsorption and periosteal apposition, the MCI was used for a long time to obtain an objective evaluation of the degree of cortical bone loss in osteoporosis (Adams 2010). However, the manual measurement technique represented an important limitation, with a great inter-observer variation and a high precision error (Hyldstrup and Nielsen 2001).

Recently, technological advances have brought this technique back into focus: digital X-ray radiogrammetry (DXR) allows automatic identification of the average cortical thickness and bone width of the second, third, and fourth metacarpal midshafts. Measurements are averaged, enhancing accuracy and precision. From these measurements a compound measurement called "bone volume per projected area" (VPA) is determined and BMD is then derived through a geometrical operation (Rosholm et al. 2001; Adams 2010).

In 1999 DXR was approved by the Food and Drug Administration (FDA) as a reliable method for estimating BMD. A significant correlation was proved to exist between DXR-derived BMD at the three mid-metacarpals and DXA-derived BMD at the spine, total hip, and distal radius ($r = 0.52$, 0.55 and 0.76, respectively; $P < 0.0001$ for all) (Hyldstrup and Nielsen 2001). If five regions of interest (second, third, and fourth mid-metacarpals and the distal radius and ulna) were used to derive DXR-BMD the level of correlation with DXA-derived BMD was even higher

(r = 0.86 at the distal forearm; r = 0.79 at the ultradistal forearm; $r = 0.62$ at the spine; $r = 0.69$ at the total hip; r = 0.73 at femoral neck; $P < 0.0001$ for all) (Rosholm et al. 2001).

In the context of techniques based on radiographs to evaluate metabolic bone disease, microradioscopy, a relatively simple radiologic method that uses fine-detail hand radiographs magnified 6–8 times, can help recognize subtle abnormalities on the three surfaces of bone (Meema 1991).

5 Dual-Energy X-ray Absorptiometry

Dual-energy X-ray absorptiometry (DXA) is the technique of choice in the assessment of bone mineral density (BMD), with assessment of the average concentration of mineral in a defined section of bone (Wahner 1989; Lewiecki et al. 2004). DXA-based BMD values are cornerstone of diagnostic algorithms of osteoporosis. DXA is accurate (exact measurement of BMD), precise (reproducible), and flexible (different regions can be scanned) (Lentle and Prior 2003).

The World Health Organization (WHO) recommends using DXA as the standard measurement method and the global diagnostic criterion for osteoporosis, with spine or hip as the gold standard for osteoporosis screening. According to the diagnostic criteria of the WHO, osteoporosis is defined as any T-score lower than −2.5, osteopenia as any T-scores between −2.5 and −1.0, and normal bone density as any T-scores equal to or greater than −1.0 (Kanis et al. 2005). The T-score is defined as the number of standard deviations (SD) of a measured BMD value from the average BMD of the reference population (young adult females) (Kanis et al. 2005; Laster 2014).

The most commonly used sites for routine BMD measurements include the lumbar spine and proximal femur. As per International Society of Clinical Densitometry (ISCD) recommendations, the forearm is only targeted when the spine and hip are unmeasurable or spine and hip BMD data are unusable or uninterpretable (https://iscd.org/learn/official-positions/). Forearm BMD is reported as a superior predictor of forearm fracture risk compared to BMD at other skeletal sites (Miller et al. 2002; Baim et al. 2008). Additionally, BMD measured at the distal radius may represent the risk of osteoporotic humeral fracture better than that measured at the axial skeleton or lower limbs (Wilson et al. 2009). Peripheral BMD was found as highly predictive of fracture risk, since the decreased local BMD tends to correlate more closely with local fracture prevalence (Siris et al. 2014; Cosman et al. 2014). The significant association between lower distal forearm BMD and the occurrence of a forearm fracture was also reported in the pediatric population (Kalkwarf et al. 2011).

As such, DXA of the distal forearm is proposed as a better method for screening BMD and the risk assessment of a distal forearm fracture, compared with a central DXA, in the lumbar spine or hip (Wilson et al. 2009; Kalkwarf et al. 2011; Miyamura et al. 2020). Moreover, increased risk of osteoporotic fracture of distal radius related to lower BMD of the distal forearm can be underestimated when only central DXA scan is performed (Wilson et al. 2009; Miyamura et al. 2020).

In hyperparathyroidism, the forearm BMD is recommended (by the ISCD) because it best reflects cortical bone damage since in this condition mainly the cortical bone is affected (https://iscd.org/learn/official-positions/) (Shepherd et al. 2013). Not measuring the BMD at the forearm, may result in an underestimation of osteoporosis for patients with hyperparathyroidism (Wood et al. 2012; Silverberg et al. 2013) (Fig. 10).

In patients with distal radial fracture some studies found global decline in BMD (Kanterewicz et al. 2002), whereas other studies reported in addition to generalized reduction in BMD a regional decline in BMD at the distal part of the radius in men (Hanusch et al. 2017), as well as in postmenopausal women, who exhibit preferential bone loss at the distal part of the radius and are more vulnerable to fracture at this particular site (Miyamura et al.

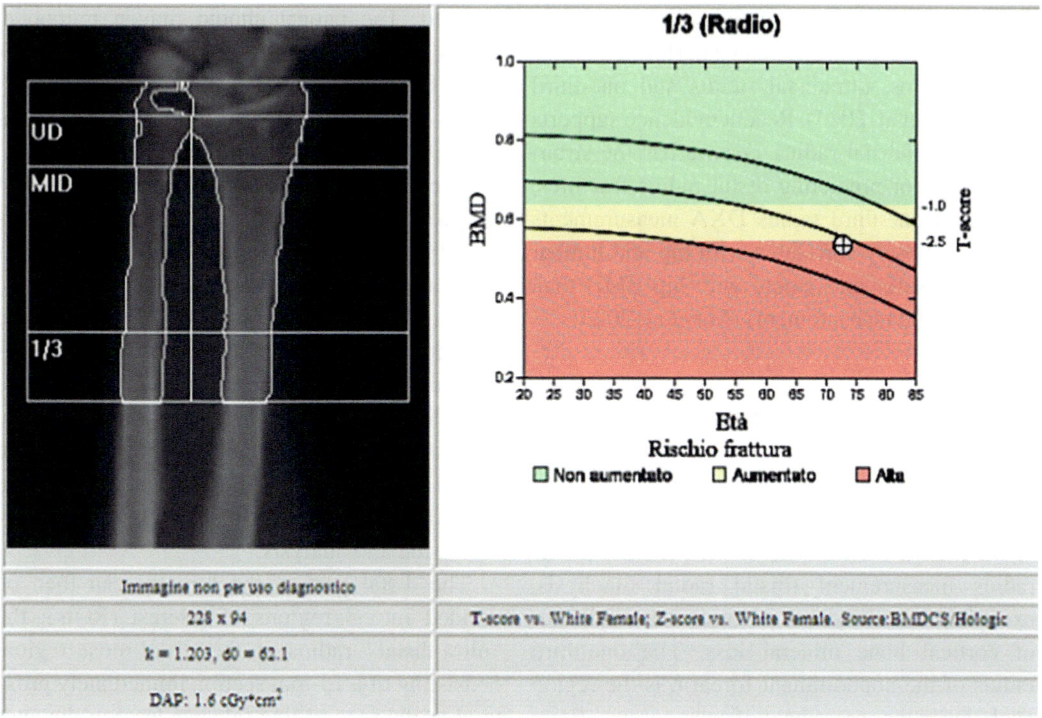

Fig. 10 In hyperparathyroidism, cotention of forearm BMD is recommended by the ISCD, because it best reflects cortical bone damage since in this condition mainly the cortical bone is affected. Not measuring the BMD at the forearm, may result in an underestimation of osteoporosis for patients with hyperparathyroidism

2020). There are cases showing preferential bone loss at the distal part of the radius without meeting osteoporosis criterion at the spine and hip. This suggests BMD measurements at the distal part of the forearm are a reliable and promising screening tool for early detection of osteoporosis and for early identification of patients who require intervention for osteoporosis (Kalkwarf et al. 2011; Miyamura et al. 2020).

There is a stronger correlation between wrist and hip BMD than correlation between wrist and lumbar BMD (Eftekhar-Sadat et al. 2016). Distal one-third radius BMD is closely related to the hip BMD (Ma et al. 2023), explained by a larger portion of cortical bone affecting the hip BMD, similar to the distal one-third of radial diaphysis (Wilson et al. 2009). Wrist BMD could therefore be used for predicting BMD of the hip, when hip BMD evaluation is not applicable due to some musculoskeletal burdens, such as hip prosthesis (Eftekhar-Sadat et al. 2016).

However, a study showed ultradistal radius BMD measurements showed significant differences and independence from the other sites, so authors suggested that distal forearm DXA scans would be valuable only when performed in addition to a central DXA (Ma et al. 2023).

The evaluation of osteoporosis includes BMD measurements and risk stratification in the hip and lumbar spine (Kanis et al. 2005; Siris et al. 2014), with measurement of T-score of hip and spine (central DXA). Currently, peripheral DXA scan of the distal radius is recommended in three conditions: when the hip and spine cannot be measured, than in patients with hyperparathyroidism and those whose weight exceeds the limit for the table (https://iscd.org/learn/official-positions/).

In patients with low energy-induced distal radius fractures, forearm DXA scan is indicated for identification of bone deficits. Forearm DXA scan on contralateral site can be performed at two different sites, ultradistal radius and one-third radius (Ma et al. 2023). Recent evidence supports that the ultradistal radius *T*-score has the strongest value for predicting distal radius fractures, and distal one-third radius DXA measurements are more closely correlated with hip and lumbar BMD measurements (more with hip BMD than lumbar BMD measurement) (Ma et al. 2023).

5.1 DXA Forearm Measurements

For assessment of trabecular bone loss the measurements are performed at the ultradistal portion of the radius, whereas the distal one-third of the radius measurement (distal radial diaphysis, excluding the ultradistal portion) is an indicator of cortical bone mineral loss. The one-third radius of the nondominant forearm is the region of choice in the assessment of osteoporosis (Baim et al. 2008).

Hand dominance would affect the measurements because forearm BMD is expected to differ between dominant and nondominant limbs (Miyamura et al. 2020). However, similarity in BMD between the dominant and non-dominant forearms of healthy patients has been reported (Min et al. 2016). Current recommendations are to use the one-third radius of the non-dominant arm to diagnose osteoporosis (https://iscd.org/learn/official-positions/). When the non-dominant wrist is fractured, then BMD can be measured on the dominant side.

The patient should be positioned sitting beside the scanning table in a chair. The forearm is scanned parallel to the long axis of the table. The examined limb should be bent at the elbow, wrist placed in pronation on the table, and the hand clenched into a fist (Sawicki et al. 2021). The scan should show the bones of the forearm centered, with the distal epiphysis of the ulna and radius visible.

The area of interest exceeding 1–2 cm and superior and inferior limits should be included to verify that the complete anatomic region is scanned. The patient should remain immobile, which is essential for optimizing BMD measurement (Lorente-Ramos et al. 2011). Important landmarks are the styloid process of the ulna, radial endplate, and bifurcation of the ulna and radius.

The scan should start at the distal contact point between the radius and ulna, placing the reference line at the styloid process of the ulna. This ensures the region of interest (ROI) includes the relevant bone tissue for analysis. The second line is placed at the radial endplate to define the proximal end of the ROI. Alternatively, it can be placed at the bifurcation of the radius and ulna. The radius endplate should be left outside the region for analysis. A vertical line placed between the radius and ulna can help with accurate segmentation and analysis.

The distal part of the forearm can then be divided into 3 regions of interest (ROIs): the "ultra-distal" radius is the distal-most region, consisting of a 15-mm section immediately proximal to the second line (always leaving the endplate of the radius outside); the "one-third distal" radius (one-third radius), consisting of a 20-mm section one-third of the distance between the ulnar styloid and the olecranon; and the "mid-distal" radius is the intermediate region, consisting of the remaining section between the 2 aforementioned sites (Sawicki et al. 2021) (Fig. 11).

BMD values are then calculated based upon each of the reference points. Areal BMD is expressed in absolute terms of grams of mineral per square centimeter (g/cm^2), and *T*-or *Z*-scores calculated.

BMD measures of the one-third radius remain stable regardless of the second line used to derive the ROI, with no statistical difference between measurements (Yu et al. 2019). The recommendation is the radial endplate and the bifurcation of the ulna and radius to be preferentially used as the reference point for routine forearm BMD measurement. The follow-up BMD measurements of the one-third radius should be performed using the same reference point as the initial measurement to ensure comparison of the same ROI (Yu et al. 2019).

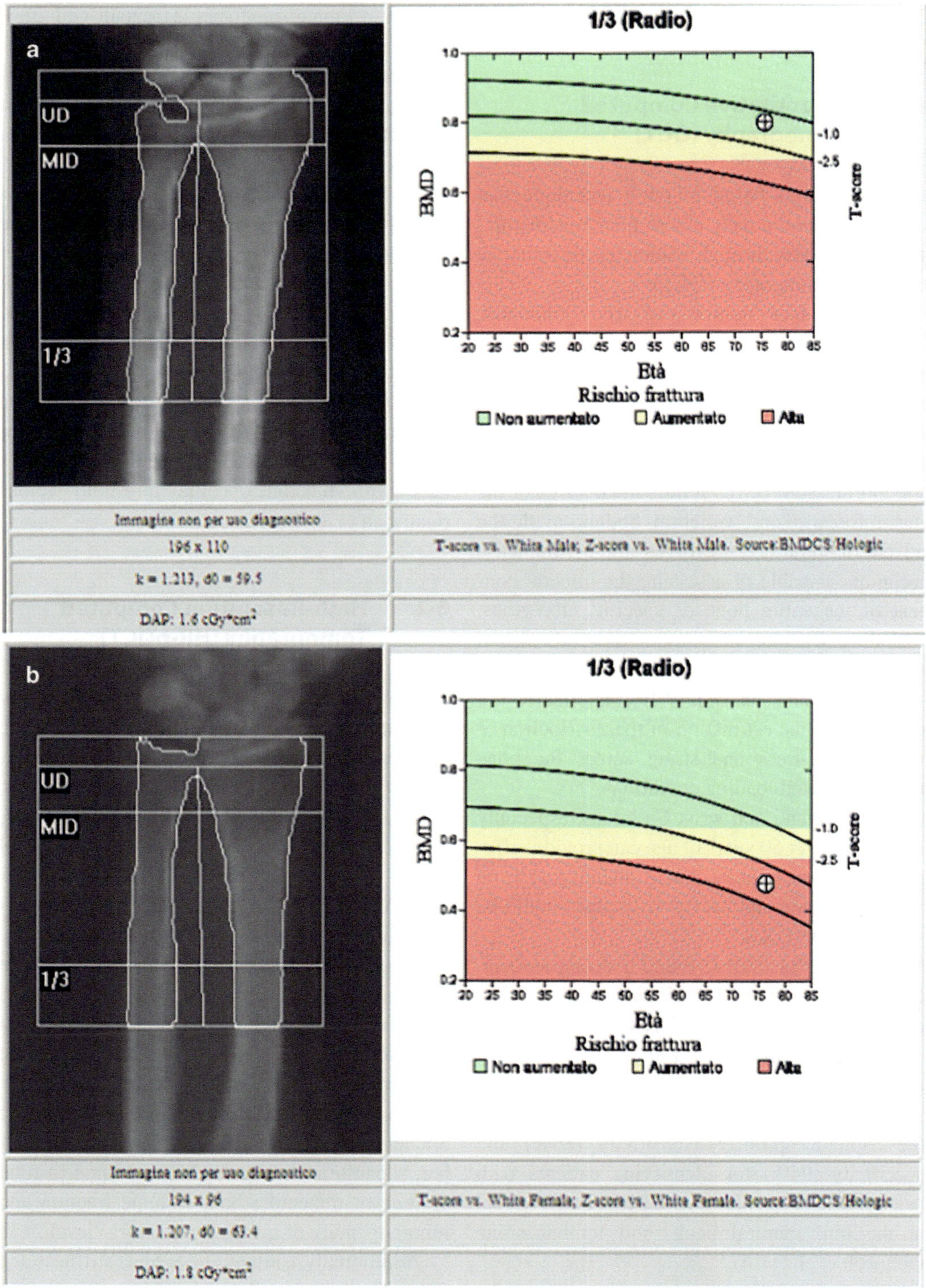

Fig. 11 The distal part of the forearm can then be divided into 3 regions of interest (ROIs): the "ultra-distal" radius is the distal-most region (UD), consisting of a 15-mm section immediately proximal to the second line (always leaving the endplate of the radius outside); the "one-third distal" radius (one-third radius) (1/3), consisting of a 20-mm section one-third of the distance between the ulnar styloid and the olecranon; and the "mid-distal" radius is the intermediate region, consisting of the remaining section between the 2 aforementioned sites (MID). (**a**) BMD within normal. (**b**) Osteoporotic patient

6 Computed Tomography -Based Techniques

6.1 Quantitative Computed Tomography (QCT)

CT is an X-ray-based imaging technique that allows to quantitatively assess bone macrostructure, particularly through volumetric quantitative computed tomography (QCT).

QCT enables noninvasive true volumetric bone mineral density assessment in mg/cm3. Phantoms with known concentrations of bone mineral equivalents are used to calibrate the attenuation coefficients (HU) of the CT dataset to bone mineral density (BMD). Initially, QCT was used to measure BMD in individual slices of the distal forearm and vertebral bodies. With the advent of spiral CT, it evolved into a volumetric technique capable of assessing the mineral content of the entire bone or specific subregions, including separate analyses of the cortical and trabecular components (Firoozabadi et al. 2008).

Final element analysis (FEA) applied to CT data enables the estimation of the distribution of mechanical stress and strain across the bone under simulated loading conditions.

Routine hand and wrist CT scans, especially in patients over 50 years of age can provide information on bone mineral density, identifying those with osteopenia and osteoporosis that should be screened with DXA.

Wagner et al. (2017) found a strong association between ulnar ≤146 Hounsfield Unit (HU) and low BMD assessed with DXA of forearm.

HU measurements from clinical CT scans at the capitate are also useful for the diagnosis of osteoporosis. A HU measurement below 307 at the capitate optimizes sensitivity (86%) and specificity (94%) for identifying patients with osteoporosis, correlating with BMD and T-scores at the hip, femoral neck, and lumbar spine (Johnson et al. 2016).

A recent study identified the strongest correlation between CT attenuation (HU) and total hip BMD T-score in the scaphoid, pisiform, and first metacarpal, while femoral neck BMD T-scores were most strongly correlated with ulnar HU, scaphoid, lunate, pisiform, trapezoid, and capitate. Furthermore, the highest sensitivity (69.2%) and specificity (77.1%) for identifying osteoporosis patients were found for a hamate CT attenuation threshold of 170.2 HU (Sebro and De La Garza-Ramos 2022).

While the measurement of HU from diagnostic CT scans holds promise for opportunistic osteoporosis screening, it is not yet ready for routine clinical implementation due to patient demographic differences, the lack of standardized thresholds, and variability between machines. According to the official positions of the ISCD (https://iscd.org/learn/official-positions/), the opportunistic use of diagnostic CT scans for assessing bone quality should be limited to scanners with machine-specific threshold values (Gausden et al. 2017).

6.2 High-Resolution Computed Tomography (HR-pQCT)

CT-based techniques for evaluating the microstructure of trabecular bone in a noninvasive manner include high-resolution computed tomography (HR-pQCT) (Genant and Jiang 2006).

HR-pQCT is a low-dose (3–5 μSv per scan), high-resolution (61–82 μm), three-dimensional imaging technique originally developed for in vivo assessment of bone density and microarchitecture. It allows differentiation between cortical and trabecular bone compartments at peripheral sites, such as the distal radius and tibia, through the assessment of density parameters (total, cortical and trabecular volumetric bone mineral density) and structural parameters at the cortical (area, thickness, porosity and pore diameter) and trabecular (area, thickness, number, separation, trabecular bone volume to total volume or trabecular bone volume fraction and inhomogeneity of trabecular network) level.

Additionally, estimations of bone stiffness and failure load can be calculated using finite element analysis (FEA) based on HR-pQCT data.

Although HR-pQCT is primarily used in research and not yet part of routine clinical practice, increasing evidence supports its value in evaluating osteoporosis and other metabolic bone diseases (Gazzotti et al. 2023).

For primary osteoporosis, recent studies (Mikolajewicz et al. 2020; Cheung et al. 2020) have confirmed that HR-pQCT parameters, particularly cortical volumetric BMD, trabecular thickness, and bone stiffness, can predict incident and major osteoporotic fractures, offering enhanced prediction beyond areal BMD measured by DXA. HR-pQCT of the forearm at the ultradistal radius has shown predictive value for hip fragility fractures, though evidence for predicting spine fractures remains insufficient in postmenopausal women. According to the ISCD's 2019 official positions, HR-pQCT is not yet recommended for osteoporosis diagnosis, as reference data for HR-pQCT is lacking. DXA remains the gold standard (https://iscd.org/learn/official-positions/).

HR-pQCT may be useful in monitoring bone structural changes during anti-osteoporotic therapy, as different drugs have varying effects on bone parameters. For instance, anabolic agents can increase cortical porosity and decrease cortical volumetric BMD without altering estimated bone strength, whereas anti-remodeling agents can cause slight increases in volumetric BMD without enhancing bone strength (Lespessailles et al. 2016).

Alongside osteoporosis, other metabolic conditions are associated with increased fracture risk, and the use of HR-pQCT may be useful in guiding treatment decisions (Van Den Bergh et al. 2021).

In secondary glucocorticoid-induced osteoporosis, HR-pQCT has revealed abnormal cortical and trabecular volumetric BMD and microarchitecture at the distal radius in postmenopausal women who have been treated with oral glucocorticoids for more than 3 months, despite showing similar areal BMD results by DXA (Sutter et al. 2014).

In addition to osteoporosis, other metabolic disorders are linked to a higher risk of fractures, and HR-pQCT could be valuable in helping to guide treatment decisions (Van Den Bergh et al. 2021).

In contrast to type 2 diabetes mellitus (T2DM), recent meta-analyses have shown that type 1 diabetes mellitus (T1DM) is specifically linked to detrimental trabecular characteristics (Walle et al. 2022). In adolescents with T1DM, estimated trabecular loading at both the distal radius was found to be significantly lower compared to healthy controls (Devaraja et al. 2020).

T2DM is associated with an increased fracture risk, despite areal BMD being normal or even elevated, which can lead to an underestimation of fracture risk. Several studies have shown that both cortical and trabecular microstructures are impaired in T2DM. HR-pQCT studies have yielded varying results depending on glycated hemoglobin (HbA1c) levels and the presence of microvascular disease. Poorly controlled T2DM (HbA1c > 7%) has been linked to lower cortical BMD (Ct.BMD) and cortical thickness (Ct.Th), as well as higher cortical porosity (Ct.Po) and reduced trabecular number (Tb.N) at the radius. Lower cortical BMD and thickness have been particularly reported in the presence of microvascular disease.

Chronic kidney disease (CKD) is a metabolic disorder linked to changes in bone microarchitecture and an increased fracture risk, which becomes clinically significant from CKD stage 3 onward (Kidney Int 2017). Bone microarchitectural alterations begin early in the disease, with a reduction in trabecular number (Tb.N) and a more irregular trabecular distribution in both men and women, along with a decrease in cortical thickness (Ct.Th) in men when compared to healthy controls (Bacchetta et al. 2010). As CKD progresses, especially in stage 4, there is a more notable decline in total bone mineral density (Tt.BMD), cortical bone mineral density (Ct.BMD), and trabecular bone mineral density (Tb.BMD). In addition, patients experience lower trabecular bone volume/total volume (Tb.BV/TV), trabecular thickness (Tb.Th), and cortical thickness (Ct.Th), with the trabecular network becoming increasingly heterogeneous (Paranhos-Neto et al. 2018). HR-pQCT of the distal radius has been shown to effectively distinguish between low and non-low bone turnover in CKD patients not yet on dialysis, particularly when combined with other biomarkers (Salam et al. 2018).

Female hemodialysis patients exhibited lower total bone mineral density (Tt.BMD), trabecular bone mineral density (Tb.BMD), trabecular number (Tb.N), cortical bone mineral density (Ct.BMD), cortical thickness (Ct.Th), and cortical area (Ct.Ar) in both the radius and tibia, when compared to age- and sex-matched controls (Negri et al. 2012).

The altered metabolism of parathyroid hormone (PTH) induces bone remodeling and affects bone density, as shown by HR-pQCT evaluation. In hyperparathyroidism, this is evidenced by lower cortical and trabecular vBMD, thinner cortices, and more widely spaced trabeculae (Wang et al. 2020). In contrast, in hypoparathyroidism, there is an increase in cortical vBMD at the radius in both females and males, as well as a decrease in cortical porosity (Ct.Po) in females (Cusano et al. 2016).

HR-pQCT shows significant differences in bone mass and architecture in patients with the first four types of osteogenesis imperfecta, against the low discriminative power of DXA (Gazzotti et al. 2023).

6.3 Dual-Energy CT (DECT)

Dual-energy CT (DECT) has become an invaluable tool in the diagnosis and management of crystal arthropathies, such as gout and calcium pyrophosphate deposition disease (CPPD), particularly in the hand and wrist. DECT is highly sensitive and specific for detecting monosodium urate (MSU) crystals and calcium pyrophosphate crystals, allowing for precise identification of both intra- and extra-articular deposits. This imaging modality provides detailed, color-coded images that enhance the visualization of crystal deposits within the joints and surrounding soft tissues of the hand and wrist, which is crucial for accurate diagnosis and differentiation from other joint conditions. DECT's ability to quantify crystal burden and monitor changes over time supports its use in assessing disease progression and treatment efficacy. Moreover, DECT can differentiate crystal deposits from other entities with similar radiographic appearances, such as erosions and calcifications, thus improving diagnostic confidence and patient outcomes (Fukuda et al. 2024).

The typical CT density of gouty tophi ranges between 160 and 170 Hounsfield Units (HU). It has been suggested that a threshold of 150 HU is optimal for diagnosing gout using DECT. However, DECT may yield false negatives in early-stage gout, where the MSU crystal volume is too small to be detected (Tiegs-Heiden et al. 2024).

On the other hand, CPPD deposition in tendon, synovial membrane, and fibrocartilage appear on DECT as well-defined, linear or punctate, thin calcifications, less dense than cortical bone (HU < 300) with a dual-energy index (DEI) between 0.016 and 0.036 (Tedeschi et al. 2023).

7 Ultrasound-Based Techniques

7.1 Quantitative Ultrasound (QUS)

QUS represents an effective alternative method for non-invasive evaluation of bone status. This technique is based on the interaction and the propagation of ultrasounds (mechanical waves) across cortical and trabecular bone; QUS parameters reflect the structural anisotropy of bone, allowing to deduce its mechanical proprieties (Glüer 1997). Major advantages are low cost, the portability, and the lack of ionizing radiation. However, reproducibility of the results is a major concern and comparing measurements is difficult and sometimes misleading (Glüer 1997).

The commercially available devices show great technological diversity (larger than with DXA) and employ different methods for calibration.

For these reasons, results from different devices cannot be directly compared (Krieg et al. 2008).

QUS-specific measures of bone status include speed of sound (SoS), a parameter closely related to bone mineralization, and broadband ultrasound attenuation (BUA), which is a reflection of the structural characteristics of trabecular bone (Guglielmi et al. 2010).

QUS is generally applied to peripheral skeletal sites, including the distal metaphysis of the phalanx, calcaneus (heel), radius, and tibia (locations with only a small amount of soft tissue over the bone);

In a study on postmenopausal women, promising results were seen in the application of phalangeal QUS (SoS) as a prescreening tool for DXA. Phalangeal QUS was able to identify groups of women with osteopenia and osteoporosis at both lumbar spine and total hip and distinguish women who used estrogen. Authors found that subjects identified by DXA as having osteopenia or osteoporosis had significantly lower SoS values in comparison with normals. Estrogen users had significantly higher spine and hip BMD and SoS values compared with non-estrogen users (Benitez et al. 2000).

However, the only validated measurement site in osteoporosis management is the heel.

A strong level of correlation has been found between heel trabecular transmission parameters (SoS and BUA) and BMD derived by DXA at lumbar spine and femoral neck (Krieg et al. 1996; Roux et al. 1996). Validated heel QUS devices have been proved to predict fragility fractures in postmenopausal women (hip, vertebral, and global fracture risk) and in men over 65 years of age (hip and all non-VFs), independently of central DXA BMD (Krieg et al. 2008).

Other more complex parameters can be derived from the combination of SoS and BUA, such as amplitude-dependent speed of sound (AD-SoS), stiffness, and quantitative ultrasound index (QUI) (Hans et al. 1996; Guglielmi et al. 2010).

QUS for the study of osteoporosis is completely validated and supported by scientific evidence. According to ISCD official positions, even though DXA remains the method of choice in clinical practice for therapeutic decisions, if a DXA scan cannot be performed, pharmacologic treatment can be initiated on the basis of a sufficient high fracture probability, assessed by heel QUS (using device-specific thresholds) in conjunction with clinical risk factors (Krieg et al. 2008). In particular, age over 75 years, BMI <20 kg/m^2, history of previous fractures after the age of fifty or falls within the last 12 months, maternal history of hip fracture, current smoking, DM, previous/current glucocorticoid treatment and use of arms to stand up from a chair are the clinical risk factors to take in account for decision making (Durosier et al. 2006; Kanis et al. 2007; Krieg et al. 2008).

8 Advanced MR Imaging

Clinical assessment of bone health and wrist fracture risk is based on bone mineral density (BMD) measurements obtained with Dual Energy X-ray Absorptiometry (DXA). Half of the women who sustain a fragility fracture in the wrist would not qualify for osteoporosis treatment on current DXA-estimated bone mineral density criteria. Therefore, a better approach is needed to determine individual risk of wrist fracture from a fall.

MRI of bone microarchitecture was first described approximately two decades ago in the distal radius and calcaneus (Majumdar et al. 1997; Wehrli et al. 1998; Link et al. 1998). MRI of trabecular microarchitecture refers to imaging of the marrow contents of the trabecular bone tissue compartment; hyperintense marrow signal provides contrast to trabecular plates and rods, which are hypointense on conventional MR images. The technical requirements to perform MRI of bone microarchitecture have been described in detail (Wehrli 2007). The main requirement to perform MRI of trabecular microarchitectures is the signal-to-noise ratio (SNR). A minimum SNR of 10 is recommended, which allows voxel sizes of 0.137–0.250 mm and slice thicknesses of 0.4–1.5 mm in scan times of approximately 10–15 min. Voxel size is directly proportional to SNR, so decreasing both in-plane dimensions by approximately 30% will result in a 50% reduction in SNR. Superficial anatomic sites, such as the distal radius (0–2 cm from the skin surface), provide higher SNR than deeper anatomic sites, such as the hip (6–10 cm from the skin surface), due to their close proximity to the radiofrequency coil (Wehrli 2007). As a result, for a given SNR, voxel sizes in the distal radius can be smaller than those that can be achieved in the hip. SNR gains can be facilitated by scanning at higher field strength, using multichannel coils (with smaller coil dimensions), and using SNR efficient pulse sequences (Techawiboonwong et al. 2005; Wehrli 2007; Chang et al. 2017). However, 7T units for clinical use are still extremely uncommon.

Peripheral extremity MRI scanners, capable of imaging only the knee, wrist, or ankle, could provide another means for widespread clinical use given their smaller physical footprint and lower cost, despite having lower field strength.

Approaches to assess trabecular bone microstructure in vivo have been performed at 1.5T and 3T. High-resolution imaging to depict the trabecular bone microarchitecture of the proximal femur has been challenging due to its deep location and high amounts of hematopoietic BM compared to fattier BM in the extremities such as in the wrist. Hematopoietic BM has longer T1 recovery times and therefore is darker in MRI.

Different quantitative MRI methods have been developed for imaging of osteoporosis. Initially based on high-resolution trabecular bone imaging and T2* mapping, quantitative susceptibility mapping (QSM) demonstrated its superiority over T2* mapping. Ultrashort echo time (UTE) imaging provides meaningful markers of cortical bone quality and quantity. Bone marrow (BM) which fills the cavities of trabecular bone and consists of adipocytes (yellow marrow regions) and hematopoietic red blood cells (red marrow regions) may play a key role in bone health and metabolism. Therefore, magnetic resonance spectroscopy (MRS) and chemical shift encoding-based water-fat MRI (CSE-MRI) have been developed for the evaluation of the nonmineralized bone compartment, represented by bone marrow, and for extraction of the BM fat fraction (BMFF). Novel postprocessing and analysis approaches, such as finite element analysis, and radiomics have shown a potential to further improve assessment of fracture risk in osteoporotic patients.

Image postprocessing plays an important role in trabecular bone microstructure assessment. After correcting for the coil inhomogeneity and segmentation, the trabecular bone microstructure data can be extracted: bone volume fraction (BVF) or bone volume to total volume fraction, trabecular thickness, trabecular spacing, and trabecular number. All these parameters are "apparent" as they correlate well with true values from Micro-CT (Majumdar et al. 1997). Several other methods can achieve postprocessing including digital topological analysis, geodesic topological analysis, and tensor scale analysis (Wehrli et al. 2001; Carballido-Gamio et al. 2009; Vasilić et al. 2009; Chen et al. 2016).

In vivo microstructural analysis of high-resolution MRI of the distal radius has been clinically applied to postmenopausal women with osteoporosis (Ladinsky et al. 2008; Kijowski et al. 2012), males on antiandrogen therapy (Greenspan et al. 2013), and diabetes (Pritchard et al. 2012).

While early MRI methods exploited the signal arising from BM to image trabecular microarchitecture of bone, more recent approaches like QSM and UTE imaging enable direct imaging of bone tissue.

T2* mapping was the first quantitative MRI technique for the assessment of bone (Majumdar et al. 1991; Wehrli et al. 2006). Bone is more diamagnetic than marrow. In the trabecular bone and BM interface, the two coexisting phases induce local magnetic field inhomogeneities. This can be measured as a shortening of the effective transverse relaxation time. It has been demonstrated that T2* correlates with the density and orientation of the trabecular bone (Wehrli et al. 2006). T2 mapping is affected by the anisotropic orientation of trabecular bone microstructure. A more direct measurement of the susceptibility difference between the trabecularized BM and surrounding tissues is based on QSM.

The method of quantitative susceptibility mapping (QSM) can overcome the limitation of T2* relaxometry that para- and diamagnetic susceptibility sources similarly result in an increased relaxation rate. In general, QSM has been proven to be capable of providing quantitative and reproducible data on magnetic susceptibility of different tissues of the body (Reichenbach et al. 2015). QSM needs moderate resolution but requires extensive postprocessing and is still in early stages of validation, and only for the spine.

Ultrashort echo time (UTE) MRI techniques of measuring cortical bone porosity and geometry have been extensively validated in preclinical studies (Seeman 2013; Rajapakse et al. 2015; Ma et al. 2020) and in vivo (Manhard et al. 2015). They have also been shown to detect impaired bone quality in vivo in patients with osteoporosis (Abbasi-Rad and Saligheh Rad 2017; Xiong et al. 2021; Jones et al. 2023).

The UTE technique provides valuable surrogate markers of cortical bone quantity and quality. Cortical bone comprises 80% of whole-body osseous mass and undergoes morphological and microstructural impairments during aging and in response to hormone depletion following menopause. The hallmark of morphological impairment is periosteal expansion outspaced by resorption and trabeculization of the endosteum, resulting in a reduction in cortical cross-sectional area. Microstructural impairment manifests as an expansion of intracortical pores while the total number of pores remains unchanged (Seeman 2013; Rajapakse et al. 2015). Imaging biomarkers of cortical geometry and porosity are meaningful complementary parameters for assessing bone quality and are associated with fracture independent of BMD, age, sex, height, and weight (Kral et al. 2017; Samelson et al. 2019). While cortical bone signal is anechoic in conventional MRI sequences due to its short T2* decay rate, UTE MRI captures the signal before it has decayed and enables assessment of the two cortical bone water pools: pore water (PW) and bound water (BW). Pore water and bound water have been demonstrated to correlate with porosity at Micro-CT and mechanical strength. Most of the studies using UTE MRI sequences were performed on the tibia or distal radius.

Magnetic resonance spectroscopy (MRS) and chemical shift encoding-based water-fat MRI (CSE-MRI) enable the quantitative assessment of the nonmineralized bone compartment through extraction of bone marrow fat fraction (BMFF).

In addition, parallel imaging and compressed sensing (PICS) techniques can reduce the scan duration of imaging protocol (6 min) without decreasing imaging quality (Vu et al. 2023). The challenge of accelerating scans by acquiring less data is to develop a method capable of reconstructing an image from fewer measurements. Parallel imaging methods learn spatial correlations between multiple receive channels to fill in unacquired data from accelerated scans.

One clinical application of the PICS is for monitoring the effects of treatment or disease on the proximal femur trabecular microarchitecture (Vu et al. 2023).

Further studies are needed to test the absolute agreement of advanced reconstruction methods with the fully-sampled scan and to investigate from larger cohorts the sensitivity of trabecular measurements in osteoporotic subjects and treatment effect on bone remodeling.

Currently, an increasing number of musculoskeletal research groups are investigating the potential benefits of utilizing magnetic resonance imaging (MRI) for bone evaluation, particularly for assessing bone quality by the mean of trabecular bone microarchitecture or by quantifying the nonmineralized component. Considerable efforts have been performed to improve MRI sequences and image processing with the perspective of developing clinical applications.

9 Quality Assurance

Quality assurance (QA) is necessary to assess and systematically monitor the various aspects of a service or structure to ensure that quality standards are respected.

For each technique used in the assessment of bone status and in particular in osteoporosis management (DXA, QCT, pQCT, HR-pQCT, MRI, and QUS) QA programs have been developed (Ihalainen et al. 2011; Guglielmi et al. 2012).

Upon the installation of a piece of equipment, the clinical application must be provided by the supplier as well as accuracy and precision as performance indicators. Furthermore, a reference database should be incorporated in DXA and QCT to compare patients' measured BMD with that of age- and sex-matched normal subjects and with normal young adults (Damilakis and Guglielmi 2010).

According to ISCD (https://iscd.org/official-positions-2023/) for women of all ethnic groups a uniform white (non-race/ethnicity) female normative database should be used and for men of all ethnic groups a uniform white (non-race/ethnicity) female reference.

The manufacturer should use NHANES III data as reference standard for total hip and femoral neck *T*-score, and their own database as the reference standard for lumbar *T*-scores; if local reference standards are available, they should be used to calculate only *Z*-scores, and not *T*-scores.

Accuracy is the ability of a measurement to match the actual value and is expressed in accuracy error, while precision is the degree of reproducibility of measures obtained under the same conditions and is expressed in precision error (PE); for DXA, the first one determines its ability to differentiate between healthy and unhealthy individuals and to estimate the fracture risk and the latter to monitor bone loss and therapy response (Damilakis and Guglielmi 2010).

The accuracy of DXA is determined by scanning a phantom of known density at least once a week, as system calibration (Guerri et al. 2018). Since the BMD value provided for the same anatomical area and accuracy differ among DXA scanners developed by different manufacturers, a standardized BMD obtained with cross-calibration techniques has been introduced to reduce to less than 6% the equipment differences. (Damilakis and Guglielmi 2010).

According to the ISCD official position each facility should calculate its DXA precision error, expressed in %CV (coefficient variation) and LSC (least significant change) which is the smallest statistically significant BMD change and the minimum time interval for follow-up measurements (Damilakis and Guglielmi 2010). For each technologist a precision error and LSC should be established, with the minimum acceptable values for total hip PE being 1.8%, 5% as LSC and for femoral neck 2.5% and LSC 6.9%. Each technologist should perform in vivo precision assessment after acquiring basic skills, after having performed 100 scans and after every skill level changes.

LSC as well as BMD obtained with different instruments not cross-calibrated cannot be compared (https://iscd.org/official-positions-2023/).

For QCT precision error depends on several factors as CT scanner model, technologist skills, the position of the ROIs. Patient movements with partial volume artifact represent the main cause of error in determining Ct.BMD and Tb. BMD. The presence of bone marrow at hip and spine leads to underestimation of bone density determining an accuracy error between 5% and 15%, a problem that could be overcome using an age-reference database and dual-energy CT (Guerri et al. 2018).

Movement artifacts and repositioning represent the main source of error in HR-pQCT, with reproducibility of density, morphological, and stiffness measurement found around 1%, 4.5%, and 3% (MacNeil and Boyd 2008).

Periodic checks and measurements of radiation dosimetry, patients, and occupational radiation exposure are compulsory to obtain optimal image quality maintaining the radiation exposure levels as low as achievable.

Patient positioning, coupling between the transducer and the skin, and soft tissue properties represent the main source of precision error for quantitative US (Damilakis and Guglielmi 2010).

Calibration check of the apparatus in the ultrasound signal emitted and determination of the propagation speed of the impulse emitted by the probes are required to guarantee the technique reliability along with a calibration of each device with its own phantom (Guglielmi et al. 2010).

Several technical problems may affect the image quality of MRI examinations, to guarantee high quality in clinical and radiological practice the American College of Radiologists (ACR) has proposed an accreditation program to provide a complete method to asses to MRI performance and QA procedures (Weinreb et al. 2005; Guerri et al. 2018).

Conflict of Interest The authors declare that they have no conflict of interest related to the present work.

References

Abbasi-Rad S, Saligheh Rad H (2017) Quantification of human cortical bone bound and free water in vivo with ultrashort echo time MR imaging: a model-based approach. Radiology 283:862–872. https://doi.org/10.1148/radiol.2016160780

Adams JE (2010) Radiogrammetry and radiographic absorptiometry. Radiol Clin North Am 48:531–540. https://doi.org/10.1016/j.rcl.2010.03.006

Adams JE, Davies M (1977) Paravertebral and peripheral ligamentous ossification: an unusual association of hypoparathyroidism. Postgrad Med J 53:167–172. https://doi.org/10.1136/pgmj.53.617.167

Ahlborg HG, Johnell O, Turner CH et al (2003) Bone loss and bone size after menopause. N Engl J Med 349:327–334. https://doi.org/10.1056/NEJMoa022464

Albright F, Forbes AP, Henneman PH (1952) Pseudo-pseudohypoparathyroidism. Trans Assoc Am Phys 65:337–350

Anthony JR, Ioachimescu AG (2014) Acromegaly and bone disease. Curr Opin Endocrinol Diabetes Obes 21:476–482. https://doi.org/10.1097/MED.0000000000000109

Aparisi Gómez MP, Boitsios G, Rosaria Petrera M et al (2024) How to approach the imaging differential diagnosis of rheumatic diseases by anatomic location. Radiol Clin North Am 62:755–782. https://doi.org/10.1016/j.rcl.2024.03.005

Aparisi Gómez MP, Wáng Y-XJ, Yu JS et al (2025) Dual-energy X-ray absorptiometry for osteoporosis screening: AJR expert panel narrative review. AJR Am J Roentgenol. https://doi.org/10.2214/AJR.25.32802

Bacchetta J, Boutroy S, Vilayphiou N et al (2010) Early impairment of trabecular microarchitecture assessed with HR-pQCT in patients with stage II–IV chronic kidney disease. J Bone Miner Res 25:849–857. https://doi.org/10.1359/jbmr.090831

Baig M, Mac Dhaibheid C, Shannon FJ (2018) Hip fracture in a patient with primary hyperparathyroidism: medical and surgical lessons. Cureus. https://doi.org/10.7759/cureus.2104

Baim S, Binkley N, Bilezikian JP et al (2008) Official positions of the International Society for Clinical Densitometry and executive summary of the 2007 ISCD Position Development Conference. J Clin Densitom 11:75–91. https://doi.org/10.1016/j.jocd.2007.12.007

Bala Y, Bui QM, Wang X-F et al (2015) Trabecular and cortical microstructure and fragility of the distal radius in women. J Bone Miner Res 30:621–629. https://doi.org/10.1002/jbmr.2388

Barnett E, Nordin BE (1960) The radiological diagnosis of osteoporosis: a new approach. Clin Radiol 11:166–174. https://doi.org/10.1016/s0009-9260(60)80012-8

Barrett-Connor E, Sajjan SG, Siris ES et al (2008) Wrist fracture as a predictor of future fractures in younger versus older postmenopausal women: results from the National Osteoporosis Risk Assessment (NORA). Osteoporos Int 19:607–613. https://doi.org/10.1007/s00198-007-0508-8

Bassett JHD, Williams GR (2016) Role of thyroid hormones in skeletal development and bone maintenance. Endocr Rev 37:135–187. https://doi.org/10.1210/er.2015-1106

Benitez CL, Schneider DL, Barrett-Connor E, Sartoris DJ (2000) Hand ultrasound for osteoporosis screening in postmenopausal women. Osteoporos Int 11:203–210. https://doi.org/10.1007/s001980050282

Bennett J, Suliburk JW, Morón FE (2020) Osseous manifestations of primary hyperparathyroidism: imaging findings. Int J Endocrinol 2020:3146535. https://doi.org/10.1155/2020/3146535

Browne RFJ, Murphy SM, Torreggiani WC et al (2003) Musculoskeletal case 27. Primary hyperparathyroidism-induced brown tumour of the third metacarpal. Can J Surg 46:122, 150–151

Carballido-Gamio J, Krug R, Huber MB et al (2009) Geodesic topological analysis of trabecular bone microarchitecture from high-spatial resolution magnetic resonance images. Magn Reson Med 61:448–456. https://doi.org/10.1002/mrm.21835

Cavallo F, Mohn A, Chiarelli F, Giannini C (2021) Evaluation of bone age in children: a mini-review. Front Pediatr 9:580314. https://doi.org/10.3389/fped.2021.580314

Chang CY, Rosenthal DI, Mitchell DM et al (2016) Imaging findings of metabolic bone disease. Radiographics 36:1871–1887. https://doi.org/10.1148/rg.2016160004

Chang G, Boone S, Martel D et al (2017) MRI assessment of bone structure and microarchitecture. Magn Reson Imaging 46:323–337. https://doi.org/10.1002/jmri.25647

Chen H, Zhou X, Fujita H et al (2013) Age-related changes in trabecular and cortical bone microstructure. Int J Endocrinol 2013:213234. https://doi.org/10.1155/2013/213234

Chen C, Jin D, Liu Y et al (2016) Trabecular bone characterization on the continuum of plates and rods using in vivo MR imaging and volumetric topological analysis. Phys Med Biol 61:N478–N496. https://doi.org/10.1088/0031-9155/61/18/N478

Cheung W-H, Hung VW-Y, Cheuk K-Y et al (2020) Best performance parameters of HR-pQCT to predict fragility fracture: systematic review and meta-analysis. J Bone Miner Res 36:2381–2398. https://doi.org/10.1002/jbmr.4449

Chung KC, Shauver MJ, Birkmeyer JD (2009) Trends in the United States in the treatment of distal radial fractures in the elderly. J Bone Joint Surg Am 91:1868–1873. https://doi.org/10.2106/JBJS.H.01297

Clynes MA, Harvey NC, Curtis EM et al (2020) The epidemiology of osteoporosis. Br Med Bull ldaa005. https://doi.org/10.1093/bmb/ldaa005

Cosman F, Herrington B, Himmelstein S, Lindsay R (1991) Radiographic absorptiometry: a simple method for determination of bone mass. Osteoporos Int 2:34–38. https://doi.org/10.1007/BF01627076

Cosman F, de Beur SJ, LeBoff MS et al (2014) Clinician's guide to prevention and treatment of osteoporosis. Osteoporos Int 25:2359–2381. https://doi.org/10.1007/s00198-014-2794-2

Cusano NE, Nishiyama KK, Zhang C et al (2016) Noninvasive assessment of skeletal microstructure and estimated bone strength in hypoparathyroidism. J Bone Miner Res 31:308–316. https://doi.org/10.1002/jbmr.2609

Damilakis J, Guglielmi G (2010) Quality assurance and dosimetry in bone densitometry. Radiol Clin North Am 48:629–640. https://doi.org/10.1016/j.rcl.2010.02.011

Daniels AM, Theelen LMA, Wyers CE et al (2019) Bone microarchitecture and distal radius fracture pattern complexity. J Orthop Res 37:1690–1697. https://doi.org/10.1002/jor.24306

Delmas PD, van de Langerijt L, Watts NB et al (2005) Underdiagnosis of vertebral fractures is a worldwide problem: the IMPACT study. J Bone Miner Res 20:557–563. https://doi.org/10.1359/JBMR.041214

Devaraja J, Jacques R, Paggiosi M et al (2020) Impact of type 1 diabetes mellitus on skeletal integrity and strength in adolescents as assessed by HRpQCT. JBMR Plus 4:e10422. https://doi.org/10.1002/jbm4.10422

Diamantopoulos AP, Rohde G, Johnsrud I et al (2012) The epidemiology of low- and high-energy distal radius fracture in middle-aged and elderly men and women in Southern Norway. PLoS One 7:e43367. https://doi.org/10.1371/journal.pone.0043367

Diaz-Garcia RJ, Oda T, Shauver MJ, Chung KC (2011) A systematic review of outcomes and complications of treating unstable distal radius fractures in the elderly. J Hand Surg Am 36:824–835.e2. https://doi.org/10.1016/j.jhsa.2011.02.005

Dodds WJ, Steinbach HL (1968) Primary hyperparathyroidism and articular cartilage calcification. Am J Roentgenol Radium Therapy, Nucl Med 104:884–892. https://doi.org/10.2214/ajr.104.4.884

Durosier C, Hans D, Krieg M-A, Schott A-M (2006) Prediction and discrimination of osteoporotic hip fracture in postmenopausal women. J Clin Densitom 9:475–495. https://doi.org/10.1016/j.jocd.2006.06.002

Earnshaw SA, Cawte SA, Worley A, Hosking DJ (1998) Colles' fracture of the wrist as an indicator of underlying osteoporosis in postmenopausal women: a prospective study of bone mineral density and bone turnover rate. Osteoporos Int 8:53–60. https://doi.org/10.1007/s001980050048

Eftekhar-Sadat B, Ghavami M, Toopchizadeh V, Ghahvechi Akbari M (2016) Wrist bone mineral density utility in diagnosing hip osteoporosis in postmenopausal women. Ther Adv Endocrinol Metab 7:207–211. https://doi.org/10.1177/2042018816658164

Fatourechi V, Ahmed DDF, Schwartz KM (2002) Thyroid acropachy: report of 40 patients treated at a single institution in a 26-year period. J Clin Endocrinol Metab 87:5435–5441. https://doi.org/10.1210/jc.2002-020746

Firoozabadi R, Morshed S, Engelke K et al (2008) Qualitative and quantitative assessment of bone fragility and fracture healing using conventional radiography and advanced imaging technologies-focus on wrist fracture. J Orthop Trauma 22:S83–S90. https://doi.org/10.1097/BOT.0b013e31815ea2a4

Franco M, Bendini JC, Albano L et al (2002) Radiographic follow-up of a phalangeal brown tumor. Joint Bone Spine 69:506–510. https://doi.org/10.1016/s1297-319x(02)00439-6

Fukuda T, Subramanian M, Noda K et al (2024) The comprehensive role of dual-energy CT in gout as an advanced diagnostic innovation. Skeletal Radiol. https://doi.org/10.1007/s00256-024-04856-4

Gabet Y, Bab I (2011) Microarchitectural changes in the aging skeleton. Curr Osteoporos Rep 9:177–183. https://doi.org/10.1007/s11914-011-0072-1

Gausden EB, Nwachukwu BU, Schreiber JJ et al (2017) Opportunistic use of CT imaging for osteoporosis screening and bone density assessment: a qualitative systematic review. J Bone Joint Surg 99:1580–1590. https://doi.org/10.2106/JBJS.16.00749

Gazzotti S, Aparisi Gómez MP, Schileo E et al (2023) High-resolution peripheral quantitative computed tomography: research or clinical practice? Br J Radiol 96:20221016. https://doi.org/10.1259/bjr.20221016

Genant HK, Jiang Y (2006) Advanced imaging assessment of bone quality. Ann N Y Acad Sci 1068:410–428. https://doi.org/10.1196/annals.1346.038

Genant HK, Heck LL, Lanzl LH et al (1973) Primary hyperparathyroidism. A comprehensive study of clinical, biochemical and radiographic manifestations. Radiology 109:513–524. https://doi.org/10.1148/109.3.513

Glüer CC (1997) Quantitative ultrasound techniques for the assessment of osteoporosis: expert agreement on current status. The International Quantitative Ultrasound Consensus Group. J Bone Miner Res 12:1280–1288. https://doi.org/10.1359/jbmr.1997.12.8.1280

Gong HS, Oh WS, Chung MS et al (2009) Patients with wrist fractures are less likely to be evaluated and managed for osteoporosis. J Bone Joint Surg Am 91:2376–2380. https://doi.org/10.2106/JBJS.H.01871

Greenspan SL, Wagner J, Nelson JB et al (2013) Vertebral fractures and trabecular microstructure in men with prostate cancer on androgen deprivation therapy. J Bone Miner Res 28:325–332. https://doi.org/10.1002/jbmr.1771

Guerri S, Mercatelli D, Aparisi Gómez MP et al (2018) Quantitative imaging techniques for the assessment of osteoporosis and sarcopenia. Quant Imaging Med Surg 8:60–85. https://doi.org/10.21037/qims.2018.01.05

Guglielmi G, Scalzo G, de Terlizzi F, Peh WCG (2010) Quantitative ultrasound in osteoporosis and bone metabolism pathologies. Radiol Clin North Am 48:577–588. https://doi.org/10.1016/j.rcl.2010.02.013

Guglielmi G, Damilakis J, Solomou G, Bazzocchi A (2012) Quality assurance of imaging techniques used in the clinical management of osteoporosis. Radiol Med 117:1347–1354. https://doi.org/10.1007/s11547-012-0881-z

Hans D, Dargent-Molina P, Schott AM et al (1996) Ultrasonographic heel measurements to predict hip fracture in elderly women: the EPIDOS prospective study. Lancet 348:511–514. https://doi.org/10.1016/s0140-6736(95)11456-4

Hanusch BC, Tuck SP, McNally RJQ et al (2017) Does regional loss of bone density explain low trauma distal forearm fractures in men (the Mr F study)? Osteoporos Int 28:2877–2886. https://doi.org/10.1007/s00198-017-4122-0

Hayes CW, Conway WF (1990) Calcium hydroxyapatite deposition disease. Radiographics 10:1031–1048. https://doi.org/10.1148/radiographics.10.6.2175444

https://iscd.org/official-positions-2023/

Hyldstrup L, Nielsen SP (2001) Metacarpal index by digital X-ray radiogrammetry: normative reference values and comparison with dual X-ray absorptiometry. J Clin Densitom 4:299–306. https://doi.org/10.1385/jcd:4:4:299

Ihalainen TM, Lönnroth NT, Peltonen JI et al (2011) MRI quality assurance using the ACR phantom in a multi-unit imaging center. Acta Oncol 50:966–972. https://doi.org/10.3109/0284186X.2011.582515

Johnell O, Kanis JA (2006) An estimate of the worldwide prevalence and disability associated with osteoporotic fractures. Osteoporos Int 17:1726–1733. https://doi.org/10.1007/s00198-006-0172-4

Johnson CC, Gausden EB, Weiland AJ et al (2016) Using Hounsfield Units to assess osteoporotic status on wrist computed tomography scans: comparison with dual energy X-ray absorptiometry. J Hand Surg Am 41:767–774. https://doi.org/10.1016/j.jhsa.2016.04.016

Jones BC, Lee H, Cheng C-C et al (2023) MRI quantification of cortical bone porosity, mineralization, and morphologic structure in postmenopausal osteoporosis. Radiology 307:e221810. https://doi.org/10.1148/radiol.221810

Ju J-H, Jin G-Z, Li G-X et al (2015) Comparison of treatment outcomes between nonsurgical and surgical treatment of distal radius fracture in elderly: a systematic review and meta-analysis. Langenbeck's Arch Surg 400:767–779. https://doi.org/10.1007/s00423-015-1324-9

Jung HJ, Park HY, Kim JS et al (2016) Bone mineral density and prevalence of osteoporosis in postmenopausal Korean women with low-energy distal radius fractures. J Korean Med Sci 31:972. https://doi.org/10.3346/jkms.2016.31.6.972

Kalkwarf HJ, Laor T, Bean JA (2011) Fracture risk in children with a forearm injury is associated with volumetric bone density and cortical area (by peripheral QCT) and areal bone density (by DXA). Osteoporos Int 22:607–616. https://doi.org/10.1007/s00198-010-1333-z

Kanis JA (2002) Diagnosis of osteoporosis and assessment of fracture risk. Lancet 359:1929–1936. https://doi.org/10.1016/S0140-6736(02)08761-5

Kanis JA, Johansson H, Oden A et al (2004) A meta-analysis of prior corticosteroid use and fracture risk. J Bone Miner Res 19:893–899. https://doi.org/10.1359/JBMR.040134

Kanis JA, Borgstrom F, De Laet C et al (2005) Assessment of fracture risk. Osteoporos Int 16:581–589. https://doi.org/10.1007/s00198-004-1780-5

Kanis JA, Oden A, Johnell O et al (2007) The use of clinical risk factors enhances the performance of BMD in the prediction of hip and osteoporotic fractures in men and women. Osteoporos Int 18:1033–1046. https://doi.org/10.1007/s00198-007-0343-y

Kanis JA et al (2021) SCOPE 2021: a new scorecard for osteoporosis in Europe. Arch Osteoporos 16(1):82

Kanterewicz E, Yañez A, Pérez-Pons A et al (2002) Association between Colles' fracture and low bone mass: age-based differences in postmenopausal women. Osteoporos Int 13:824–828. https://doi.org/10.1007/s001980200114

Keene GS, Parker MJ, Pryor GA (1993) Mortality and morbidity after hip fractures. BMJ 307:1248–1250. https://doi.org/10.1136/bmj.307.6914.1248

Khosla S, Riggs BL, Atkinson EJ et al (2006) Effects of sex and age on bone microstructure at the ultradistal radius: a population-based noninvasive in vivo assessment. J Bone Miner Res 21:124–131. https://doi.org/10.1359/JBMR.050916

Kidney Int 2017 Kidney Disease: Improving Global Outcomes (KDIGO) CKD-MBD Update Work Group (2017) Clinical practice guideline update for the diagnosis, evaluation, prevention, and treatment of chronic kidney disease-mineral and bone disorder (CKD- MBD). Kidney Int Suppl 7:1–59. https://doi.org/10.1016/j.kisu.2017.10.001

Kijowski R, Tuite M, Kruger D et al (2012) Evaluation of trabecular microarchitecture in nonosteoporotic postmenopausal women with and without fracture. J Bone Miner Res 27:1494–1500. https://doi.org/10.1002/jbmr.1595

Klein J, Brant WE, Vinson EN, Helms CA (2018) Brant and Helms' fundamentals of diagnostic radiology. Wolters Kluwer, Philadelphia

Klotzbuecher CM, Ross PD, Landsman PB et al (2000) Patients with prior fractures have an increased risk of future fractures: a summary of the literature and statistical synthesis. J Bone Miner Res 15:721–739. https://doi.org/10.1359/jbmr.2000.15.4.721

Kral R, Osima M, Borgen TT et al (2017) Increased cortical porosity and reduced cortical thickness of the proximal femur are associated with nonvertebral fracture independent of Fracture Risk Assessment Tool and Garvan estimates in postmenopausal women. PLoS One 12:e0185363. https://doi.org/10.1371/journal.pone.0185363

Krieg MA, Thiébaud D, Landry M, Burckhardt P (1996) Evaluation of bones using quantitative ultrasonography. Schweiz Med Wochenschr 126:159–163

Krieg M-A, Barkmann R, Gonnelli S et al (2008) Quantitative ultrasound in the management of osteoporosis: the 2007 ISCD official positions. J Clin Densitom 11:163–187. https://doi.org/10.1016/j.jocd.2007.12.011

Ladinsky GA, Vasilic B, Popescu AM et al (2008) Trabecular structure quantified with the MRI-based virtual bone biopsy in postmenopausal women contributes to vertebral deformity burden independent of areal vertebral BMD. J Bone Miner Res 23:64–74. https://doi.org/10.1359/jbmr.070815

Laster AJ (2014) Dual-energy x-ray absorptiometry: overused, neglected, or just misunderstood? N C Med J 75:132–136. https://doi.org/10.18043/ncm.75.2.132

Lentle BC, Prior JC (2003) Osteoporosis: what a clinician expects to learn from a patient's bone density examination. Radiology 228:620–628. https://doi.org/10.1148/radiol.2283020093

Lespessailles E, Hambli R, Ferrari S (2016) Osteoporosis drug effects on cortical and trabecular bone microstructure: a review of HR-pQCT analyses. Bonekey Rep 5. https://doi.org/10.1038/bonekey.2016.59

Lewiecki EM, Watts NB, McClung MR et al (2004) Official positions of the international society for clinical densitometry. J Clin Endocrinol Metab 89:3651–3655. https://doi.org/10.1210/jc.2004-0124

Link TM (2012) Osteoporosis imaging: state of the art and advanced imaging. Radiology 263:3–17. https://doi.org/10.1148/radiol.2631201201

Link TM, Majumdar S, Augat P et al (1998) In vivo high resolution MRI of the calcaneus: differences in trabecular structure in osteoporosis patients. J Bone Miner Res 13:1175–1182. https://doi.org/10.1359/jbmr.1998.13.7.1175

Löfman O, Hallberg I, Berglund K et al (2007) Women with low-energy fracture should be investigated for osteoporosis. Acta Orthop 78:813–821. https://doi.org/10.1080/17453670710014608

Lorente-Ramos R, Azpeitia-Armán J, Muñoz-Hernández A et al (2011) Dual-energy x-ray absorptiometry in the diagnosis of osteoporosis: a practical guide. AJR Am J Roentgenol 196:897–904. https://doi.org/10.2214/AJR.10.5416

Ma Y-J, Chen Y, Li L et al (2020) Trabecular bone imaging using a 3D adiabatic inversion recovery prepared ultrashort TE Cones sequence at 3T. Magn Reson Med 83:1640–1651. https://doi.org/10.1002/mrm.28027

Ma SB, Lee SK, An YS et al (2023) The clinical necessity of a distal forearm DEXA scan for predicting distal radius fracture in elderly females: a retrospective case-control study. BMC Musculoskelet Disord 24:177. https://doi.org/10.1186/s12891-023-06265-5

Macdonald HM, Nishiyama KK, Kang J et al (2011) Age-related patterns of trabecular and cortical bone loss differ between sexes and skeletal sites: a population-based HR-pQCT study. J Bone Miner Res 26:50–62. https://doi.org/10.1002/jbmr.171

Mack PB, O'Brien AT, Smith JM, Bauman AW (1939) A method for estimating the degree of mineralization of bones from tracings of roentgenograms. Science 89:467. https://doi.org/10.1126/science.89.2316.467

MacNeil JA, Boyd SK (2008) Improved reproducibility of high-resolution peripheral quantitative computed tomography for measurement of bone quality. Med Eng Phys 30:792–799. https://doi.org/10.1016/j.medengphy.2007.11.003

Majumdar S, Thomasson D, Shimakawa A, Genant HK (1991) Quantitation of the susceptibility difference between trabecular bone and bone marrow: experimental studies. Magn Reson Med 22:111–127. https://doi.org/10.1002/mrm.1910220112

Majumdar S, Genant HK, Grampp S et al (1997) Correlation of trabecular bone structure with age, bone mineral density, and osteoporotic status: in vivo studies in the distal radius using high resolution magnetic resonance imaging. J Bone Miner Res 12:111–118. https://doi.org/10.1359/jbmr.1997.12.1.111

Mallmin H, Ljunghall S, Persson I et al (1993) Fracture of the distal forearm as a forecaster of subsequent hip fracture: a population-based cohort study with 24 years of follow-up. Calcif Tissue Int 52:269–272. https://doi.org/10.1007/BF00296650

Manhard MK, Horch RA, Gochberg DF et al (2015) In vivo quantitative MR imaging of bound and pore water in cortical bone. Radiology 277:221–229. https://doi.org/10.1148/radiol.2015140336

Meema HE (1991) Radiologic study of endosteal, intracortical, and periosteal surfaces of hand bones in metabolic bone diseases. Hand Clin 7:37–51

Mikolajewicz N, Bishop N, Burghardt AJ et al (2020) HR-pQCT measures of bone microarchitecture predict fracture: systematic review and meta-analysis. J Bone Miner Res 35:446–459. https://doi.org/10.1002/jbmr.3901

Miller PD, Siris ES, Barrett-Connor E et al (2002) Prediction of fracture risk in postmenopausal white women with peripheral bone densitometry: evidence from the National Osteoporosis Risk Assessment. J Bone Miner Res 17:2222–2230. https://doi.org/10.1359/jbmr.2002.17.12.2222

Min DG, Lee JH, Choe HS et al (2016) Comparison of bone density on the dominant and nondominant sides between healthy elderly individuals and stroke patients. J Phys Ther Sci 28:2533–2536. https://doi.org/10.1589/jpts.28.2533

Miyamura S, Kuriyama K, Ebina K et al (2020) Utility of distal forearm DXA as a screening tool for primary osteoporotic fragility fractures of the distal radius: a case-control study. JB JS Open Access 5:e0036. https://doi.org/10.2106/JBJS.OA.19.00036

Nagaraj C, Oommen R, Jacob PM, Irodi A (2012) Solitary phalangeal brown tumour in primary hyperparathyroidism: report of a rare presentation. Indian J Nucl Med 27:107–110. https://doi.org/10.4103/0972-3919.110700

Negri AL, Del Valle EE, Zanchetta MB et al (2012) Evaluation of bone microarchitecture by high-resolution peripheral quantitative computed tomography (HR-pQCT) in hemodialysis patients. Osteoporos Int 23:2543–2550. https://doi.org/10.1007/s00198-011-1890-9

Nellans KW, Kowalski E, Chung KC (2012) The epidemiology of distal radius fractures. Hand Clin 28:113–125. https://doi.org/10.1016/j.hcl.2012.02.001

Niver GE, Ilyas AM (2012) Carpal tunnel syndrome after distal radius fracture. Orthop Clin North Am 43:521–527. https://doi.org/10.1016/j.ocl.2012.07.021

Okada K, Iida K, Sakusabe N et al (1994) Pseudohypoparathyroidism-associated spinal stenosis. Spine (Phila Pa 1976) 19:1186–1189. https://doi.org/10.1097/00007632-199405001-00019

Olschewski E, Murray P, Buckley R et al (2001) Assessment of osteoporosis using standard radiographs of the wrist. J Trauma 51:912–916. https://doi.org/10.1097/00005373-200111000-00014

Oyen J, Brudvik C, Gjesdal CG et al (2011) Osteoporosis as a risk factor for distal radial fractures: a case-control study. J Bone Joint Surg Am 93:348–356. https://doi.org/10.2106/JBJS.J.00303

Paranhos-Neto FP, Lima GAC, Silva LC et al (2018) HR-pQCT detects alterations in bone microstructure in men with CKD stages 3 and 4, which are influenced by hormonal changes and body composition. Clin Nephrol 89:10–17. https://doi.org/10.5414/CN109006

Parfitt AM (1969) Soft-tissue calcification in uremia. Arch Intern Med 124:544–556

Pritchard JM, Giangregorio LM, Atkinson SA et al (2012) Association of larger holes in the trabecular bone at the distal radius in postmenopausal women with type 2 diabetes mellitus compared to controls. Arthritis Care Res (Hoboken) 64:83–91. https://doi.org/10.1002/acr.20602

Rajapakse CS, Bashoor-Zadeh M, Li C et al (2015) Volumetric cortical bone porosity assessment with MR imaging: validation and clinical feasibility. Radiology 276:526–535. https://doi.org/10.1148/radiol.15141850

Rana RS, Wu JS, Eisenberg RL (2009) Periosteal reaction. AJR Am J Roentgenol 193:W259–W272. https://doi.org/10.2214/AJR.09.3300

Reichenbach JR, Schweser F, Serres B, Deistung A (2015) Quantitative susceptibility mapping: concepts and applications. Clin Neuroradiol 25(Suppl 2):225–230. https://doi.org/10.1007/s00062-015-0432-9

Resnick D, Jacobson JA, Chung CB et al (2025) Resnick's bone and joint imaging, 4th edn. Elsevier, St. Louis

Riggs BL, Melton Iii LJ, Robb RA et al (2004) Population-based study of age and sex differences in bone volumetric density, size, geometry, and structure at different skeletal sites. J Bone Miner Res 19:1945–1954. https://doi.org/10.1359/JBMR.040916

Rosholm A, Hyldstrup L, Backsgaard L et al (2001) Estimation of bone mineral density by digital X-ray radiogrammetry: theoretical background and clinical testing. Osteoporos Int 12:961–969. https://doi.org/10.1007/s001980170026

Roth KM, Blazar PE, Earp BE et al (2012) Incidence of extensor pollicis longus tendon rupture after nondisplaced distal radius fractures. J Hand Surg Am 37:942–947. https://doi.org/10.1016/j.jhsa.2012.02.006

Roux C, Fournier B, Laugier P et al (1996) Broadband ultrasound attenuation imaging: a new imaging method in osteoporosis. J Bone Miner Res 11:1112–1118. https://doi.org/10.1002/jbmr.5650110810

Rozental TD, Makhni EC, Day CS, Bouxsein ML (2008) Improving evaluation and treatment for osteoporosis following distal radial fractures: a prospective randomized intervention. J Bone Joint Surg-Am Vol 90:953–961. https://doi.org/10.2106/JBJS.G.01121

Rozental TD, Deschamps LN, Taylor A et al (2013) Premenopausal women with a distal radial fracture have deteriorated trabecular bone density and morphology compared with controls without a fracture. J Bone Joint Surg Am 95:633–642. https://doi.org/10.2106/JBJS.L.00588

Rubin MR, Bilezikian JP, McMahon DJ et al (2008) The natural history of primary hyperparathyroidism with or without parathyroid surgery after 15 years. J Clin Endocrinol Metab 93:3462–3470. https://doi.org/10.1210/jc.2007-1215

Salam S, Gallagher O, Gossiel F et al (2018) Diagnostic accuracy of biomarkers and imaging for bone turnover in renal osteodystrophy. J Am Soc Nephrol 29:1557–1565. https://doi.org/10.1681/ASN.2017050584

Salari N, Ghasemi H, Mohammadi L et al (2021) The global prevalence of osteoporosis in the world: a comprehensive systematic review and meta-analysis. J Orthop Surg Res 16:609. https://doi.org/10.1186/s13018-021-02772-0

Sambrook P, Cooper C (2006) Osteoporosis. Lancet 367:2010–2018. https://doi.org/10.1016/S0140-6736(06)68891-0

Samelson EJ, Broe KE, Xu H et al (2019) Cortical and trabecular bone microarchitecture as an independent predictor of incident fracture risk in older women and men in the Bone Microarchitecture International Consortium (BoMIC): a prospective study. Lancet Diabetes Endocrinol 7:34–43. https://doi.org/10.1016/S2213-8587(18)30308-5

Sawicki P, Tałałaj M, Życińska K et al (2021) Current applications and selected technical details of dual-energy X-ray absorptiometry. Med Sci Monit 27. https://doi.org/10.12659/MSM.930839

Schousboe JT (2016) Epidemiology of vertebral fractures. J Clin Densitom 19:8–22. https://doi.org/10.1016/j.jocd.2015.08.004

Sebro R, De La Garza-Ramos C (2022) Machine learning for opportunistic screening for osteoporosis from CT scans of the wrist and forearm. Diagnostics 12:691. https://doi.org/10.3390/diagnostics12030691

Seeman E (2013) Age- and menopause-related bone loss compromise cortical and trabecular microstructure. J Gerontol A Biol Sci Med Sci 68:1218–1225. https://doi.org/10.1093/gerona/glt071

Shepherd JA, Baim S, Bilezikian JP, Schousboe JT (2013) Executive summary of the 2013 international society for clinical densitometry position development conference on body composition. J Clin Densitom 16:489–495. https://doi.org/10.1016/j.jocd.2013.08.005

Silva BC, Bilezikian JP (2021) Skeletal abnormalities in hypoparathyroidism and in primary hyperparathyroidism. Rev Endocr Metab Disord 22:789–802. https://doi.org/10.1007/s11154-020-09614-0

Silverberg SJ, Walker MD, Bilezikian JP (2013) Asymptomatic primary hyperparathyroidism. J Clin Densitom 16:14–21. https://doi.org/10.1016/j.jocd.2012.11.005

Sing C, Lin T, Bartholomew S et al (2023) Global epidemiology of hip fractures: secular trends in incidence rate, post-fracture treatment, and all-cause mortality. J Bone Miner Res 38:1064–1075. https://doi.org/10.1002/jbmr.4821

Siris ES, Adler R, Bilezikian J et al (2014) The clinical diagnosis of osteoporosis: a position statement from the National Bone Health Alliance Working Group. Osteoporos Int 25:1439–1443. https://doi.org/10.1007/s00198-014-2655-z

Sorenson JA, Cameron JR (1967) A reliable in vivo measurement of bone-mineral content. J Bone Joint Surg Am 49:481–497

Sozen T, Ozisik L, Calik Basaran N (2017) An overview and management of osteoporosis. Eur J Rheumatol 4:46–56. https://doi.org/10.5152/eurjrheum.2016.048

Sundaram M (1989) Renal osteodystrophy. Skeletal Radiol 18:415–426. https://doi.org/10.1007/BF00368608

Sutter S, Nishiyama KK, Kepley A et al (2014) Abnormalities in cortical bone, trabecular plates, and stiffness in postmenopausal women treated with glucocorticoids. J Clin Endocrinol Metabol 99:4231–4240. https://doi.org/10.1210/jc.2014-2177

Syed FA, Ng AC (2010) The pathophysiology of the aging skeleton. Curr Osteoporos Rep 8:235–240. https://doi.org/10.1007/s11914-010-0035-y

Techawiboonwong A, Song HK, Magland JF et al (2005) Implications of pulse sequence in structural imaging of trabecular bone. J Magn Reson Imaging 22:647–655. https://doi.org/10.1002/jmri.20432

Tedeschi SK, Becce F, Pascart T et al (2023) Imaging features of calcium pyrophosphate deposition disease: consensus definitions from an International Multidisciplinary Working Group. Arthritis Care Res 75:825–834. https://doi.org/10.1002/acr.24898

Tiegs-Heiden CA, Baffour FI, Powell GM et al (2024) Dual energy CT for the diagnosis of gout: evaluating the optimal Hounsfield Unit setting for dual energy processing. RCR Open 2:100150. https://doi.org/10.1016/j.rcro.2024.100150

Van Den Bergh JP, Szulc P, Cheung AM et al (2021) The clinical application of high-resolution peripheral computed tomography (HR-pQCT) in adults: state of the art and future directions. Osteoporos Int 32:1465–1485. https://doi.org/10.1007/s00198-021-05999-z

Vasilić B, Rajapakse CS, Wehrli FW (2009) Classification of trabeculae into three-dimensional rodlike and platelike structures via local inertial anisotropy. Med Phys 36:3280–3291. https://doi.org/10.1118/1.3140582

Vu B-TD, Jones BC, Lee H et al (2023) Six-minute, in vivo MRI quantification of proximal femur trabecular bone 3D microstructure. Bone 177:116900. https://doi.org/10.1016/j.bone.2023.116900

Wagner SC, Dworak TC, Grimm PD et al (2017) Measurement of distal ulnar Hounsfield Units accurately predicts bone mineral density of the forearm. J Bone Joint Surg 99:e38. https://doi.org/10.2106/JBJS.15.01244

Wahner H (1989) Technical aspects and clinical interpretation of bone mineral measurements. Public Health Rep 104(Suppl):27–30

Walle M, Whittier DE, Frost M et al (2022) Meta-analysis of diabetes mellitus-associated differences in bone structure assessed by high-resolution peripheral quantitative computed tomography. Curr Osteoporos Rep 20:398–409. https://doi.org/10.1007/s11914-022-00755-6

Wang W, Nie M, Jiang Y et al (2020) Impaired geometry, volumetric density, and microstructure of cortical and trabecular bone assessed by HR-pQCT in both sporadic and MEN1-related primary hyperparathyroidism. Osteoporos Int 31:165–173. https://doi.org/10.1007/s00198-019-05186-1

Wehrli FW (2007) Structural and functional assessment of trabecular and cortical bone by micro magnetic resonance imaging. J Magn Reson Imaging 25:390–409. https://doi.org/10.1002/jmri.20807

Wehrli FW, Hwang SN, Ma J et al (1998) Cancellous bone volume and structure in the forearm: noninvasive assessment with MR microimaging and image processing. Radiology 206:347–357. https://doi.org/10.1148/radiology.206.2.9457185

Wehrli FW, Gomberg BR, Saha PK et al (2001) Digital topological analysis of in vivo magnetic resonance microimages of trabecular bone reveals structural implications of osteoporosis. J Bone Miner Res 16:1520–1531. https://doi.org/10.1359/jbmr.2001.16.8.1520

Wehrli FW, Song HK, Saha PK, Wright AC (2006) Quantitative MRI for the assessment of bone structure and function. NMR Biomed 19:731–764. https://doi.org/10.1002/nbm.1066

Weinreb J, Wilcox PA, Hayden J et al (2005) ACR MRI accreditation: yesterday, today, and tomorrow. J Am

Coll Radiol 2:494–503. https://doi.org/10.1016/j.jacr.2004.11.004

Wilson J, Bonner TJ, Head M et al (2009) Variation in bone mineral density by anatomical site in patients with proximal humeral fractures. J Bone Joint Surg Br 91:772–775. https://doi.org/10.1302/0301-620X.91B6.22346

Wood K, Dhital S, Chen H, Sippel RS (2012) What is the utility of distal forearm DXA in primary hyperparathyroidism? Oncologist 17:322–325. https://doi.org/10.1634/theoncologist.2011-0285

Xiong Y, He T, Wang Y et al (2021) CKD stages, bone metabolism markers, and cortical porosity index: associations and mediation effects analysis. Front Endocrinol (Lausanne) 12:775066. https://doi.org/10.3389/fendo.2021.775066

Yu W, Ying Q, Guan W et al (2019) Impact of reference point selection on DXA-based measurement of forearm bone mineral density. Arch Osteoporos 14:107. https://doi.org/10.1007/s11657-019-0658-2

Arthritis of the Hand and Wrist

Shweta Kataria and Girish Gandikota

Contents

S. Kataria · G. Gandikota (✉)
Department of Radiology, University of North Carolina at Chapel Hill, Chapel Hill, NC, USA
e-mail: Shweta_Kataria@med.unc.edu; Girish_Gandikota@med.unc.edu

Med Radiol Diagn Imaging (2025)
https://doi.org/10.1007/174_2025_623,

Published Online: 12 November 2025

Abstract

This chapter provides an in-depth look at how imaging plays a crucial role in diagnosing and managing hand and wrist arthritis. It starts with an introduction to arthritis, covering its clinical impact and how different types of arthritis affect the joints in unique ways. This chapter then explores the various imaging techniques used to evaluate arthritis in the hand and wrist, such as radiographs, ultrasound, MRI, and CT. It also highlights some of the exciting recent advancements in imaging, including dual-energy CT (DECT), high-resolution peripheral quantitative Ct (HR-pQCT), PET-MRI, and the role of Artificial Intelligence (AI), which are improving our ability to detect and understand arthritis. The focus then shifts to the specific radiographic features of different types of arthritis, including osteoarthritis, rheumatoid arthritis, psoriatic arthritis, calcium pyrophosphate dihydrate deposition disease (CPPD), and septic arthritis. By focusing mainly on radiographic features, this chapter provides valuable insights into how imaging can help clinicians better understand and manage these conditions.

1 Introduction

Arthritis is a common yet complex condition that affects millions worldwide. It manifests as more than 100 different types of joint disorders, characterized by joint pain, stiffness, swelling, and reduced range of motion. The ability to perform commonplace tasks, such as grasping objects, writing, or even buttoning a shirt, can be significantly disrupted when arthritis affects the hands, resulting in significant disability. Radiological imaging is essential for diagnosing, evaluating, and managing hand arthritis, providing critical information regarding the underlying pathology and disease progression.

In 2022, the age-adjusted prevalence of diagnosed arthritis among adults in the USA was 18.9% (Elgaddal et al. 2024). The incidence of arthritis increases with age, and women have a higher likelihood than males of having arthritis (Arthritis Foundation 2020). The hand's complex architecture, consisting of 27 bones along with many joints, tendons, and ligaments, renders it especially susceptible to arthritis-related damage. Arthritis may arise from various underlying factors, including degeneration, inflammatory or autoimmune disorders, infection, crystal deposition, and metabolic problems. Hand arthritis predominantly occurs in osteoarthritis (OA) and rheumatoid arthritis (RA), while other types, such as psoriatic arthritis, gout, and calcium pyrophosphate dihydrate deposition disease CPPD, account for a lesser proportion of cases. Each of these disorders exhibits unique clinical manifestations and radiological characteristics. Osteoarthritis is characterized by joint space narrowing, subchondral sclerosis, and osteophyte formation, especially in the distal interphalangeal (DIP) and first carpometacarpal (CMC) joints. In contrast, inflammatory arthritis typically presents as periarticular osteopenia, erosions, and joint deformities, commonly affecting the metacarpophalangeal (MCP) joints and wrists. The variations in joint involvement underscore the need for imaging in differentiating arthritis subgroups and tailoring treatment accordingly.

Radiological imaging offers insight into the structural alterations occurring within the joints. Radiography remains the first-line tool for imaging arthritis, owing to its accessibility and capacity to reveal alterations in bone structure. It provides critical insights into structural alterations, such as joint space narrowing, osteophytes, and erosions. Nonetheless, radiographs are limited in their ability to identify early disease alterations and soft tissue involvement. Advances in imaging techniques, including ultrasound, magnetic resonance imaging (MRI), and computed tomography (CT), have enhanced our capacity to identify early disease alterations, assess soft tissue involvement, and monitor treatment response. These techniques enable the visualization of subtle characteristics such as synovitis, tenosynovitis, and bone marrow edema, which are essential for the early diagnosis of inflammatory arthritis.

This chapter will explore the various imaging modalities utilized for assessing hand and wrist arthritis, emphasizing their applications, advantages, and limitations. Particular emphasis will be placed on the radiological characteristics that distinguish various types of arthritis, as well as briefly discuss the evolving role of novel technologies such as DECT and artificial intelligence in imaging interpretation. This chapter offers an in-depth review of imaging to enhance understanding and facilitate evidence-based decision-making in the diagnosis and management of hand and wrist arthritis.

2 Modalities for Radiological Investigation

2.1 Conventional Radiography

Radiographs are the first-line imaging modality to assess a patient for hand arthritis. It is a quick, cost-effective, widely available method. Radiography is particularly helpful in identifying structural changes such as joint space narrowing, subchondral sclerosis, osteophyte formation, and bone erosions. Serial radiographs can assess disease severity and track the progression of joint damage over time, aiding in evaluating the efficacy of therapeutic interventions. Radiography provides an excellent baseline for monitoring long-term structural changes in arthritis patients. Specific radiographic features can help distinguish between various forms of arthritis.

A comprehensive evaluation of hand radiographs should include assessment for joint space narrowing, which is an indirect indicator of cartilage loss, joint subluxation or dislocation, bone destruction, bone density, demineralization, presence and pattern of erosions, soft tissue swelling due to synovitis and inflammation, and soft tissue calcifications.

2.1.1 Limitations of Radiography

While radiography is an essential tool, it has certain limitations. Radiographs are less sensitive or limited in ability to detect early disease features such as synovitis, bone marrow edema, and soft tissue involvement, which are better visualized on modalities like MRI or ultrasound (Sudoł-Szopińska et al. 2017). Radiographs cannot directly visualize soft tissue abnormalities like tendons, ligaments, or synovial inflammation. Lack of three-dimensional imaging and overlapping structures can obscure subtle findings and fail to capture the full extent of joint damage. Radiation exposure may be a concern for certain patients.

2.1.2 Standard Views

A standard hand series includes posteroanterior (PA) view, oblique, and lateral views. Norgaard or posterior oblique view of both hands is obtained in suspected cases of inflammatory arthritis (Ezzati and Pezeshk 2022; Kluckman et al. 2021). PA view (Fig. 1a) provides a clear overall picture of the bone and joint anatomy of the hand. It is useful for assessing joint spaces, joint alignment, bone mineralization, and soft tissues. Norgaard view (Fig. 1b) is excellent for evaluating erosions at the MCP joints.

A standard wrist series includes PA, external oblique, and lateral views. A thumb series is sometimes obtained to evaluate for thumb base osteoarthritis, which includes an AP or PA, oblique, and lateral views of the thumb.

2.2 Ultrasound (US)

Ultrasound has become an essential tool in the assessment of hand arthritis due to its ability to provide real-time, high-resolution imaging of soft tissues, cartilage, and early bony erosive changes. Ultrasound can be performed in clinics, is low-cost, easily available, and radiation-free. It has the advantage of being able to detect early inflammatory changes, including synovitis, tenosynovitis, and erosions, before structural changes develop (Sahu et al. 2023). Power Doppler imaging further enhances the detection of active inflammation, which helps monitor disease activity and treatment response. It is ideal for dynamic assessment of tendon motion or joint mechanics. It also identifies characteristic findings in specific arthritis types. Ultrasound can be employed for

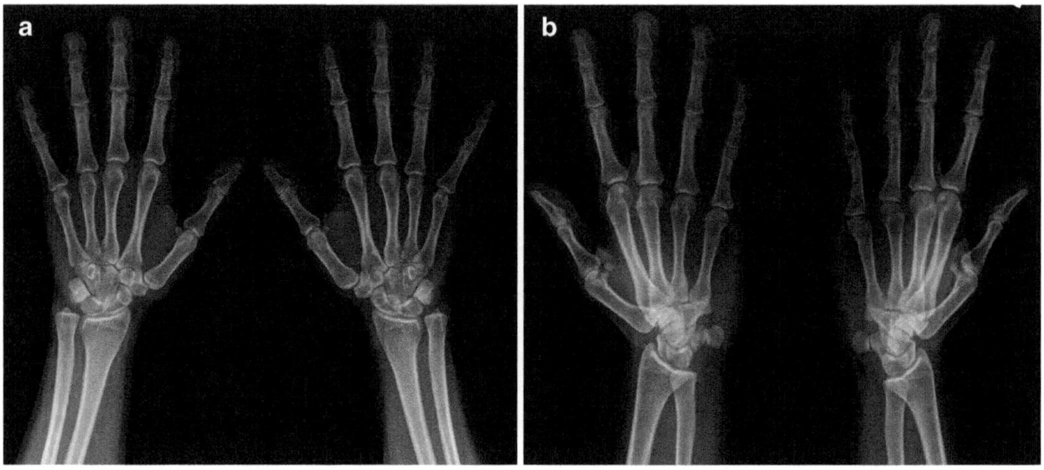

Fig. 1 Radiographic projections of the hand. (**a**) PA view; (**b**) Norgaard view

guided interventions, as it enables precise aspiration or injection of joints and soft tissues. It is useful for monitoring response to treatment.

Ultrasound can assess hand and wrist arthritis by demonstrating features such as synovitis, tenosynovitis, tendon abnormalities like thickening or disruption, joint effusion, erosions, and cartilage loss (Kaeley et al. 2020). Osteophytes can be seen as echogenic protruding bony excrescences. Synovial proliferation is hypoechoic and non-displaceable and poorly compressible thickening of the synovium, whereas joint effusion is displaceable. Synovial hyperemia in active inflammation demonstrates increased Doppler uptake. Erosions appear as disruption of the echogenic cortical line, sometimes with increased Doppler activity. Enthesitis is seen as loss of fibrillar echotexture and tendon thickening and peri-entheseal increased Doppler signal. Tenosynovitis is thickening of the tendon sheath and/or effusion. A typical ultrasound assessment for inflammatory arthritis includes investigating the second and third MCP joints, the dorsal aspect of the wrist for midcarpal, radiocarpal, and distal radioulnar joints, the most symptomatic joint, and the integrity of the flexor and extensor tendons.

2.2.1 Limitations of Ultrasound

Ultrasound is operator dependent and requires skilled interpretation for consistent results. While it is sensitive for detecting early inflammatory changes, it is less effective for assessment of deep-seated bony and joint structures compared to CT or MRI (McNally 2007). Its evaluation of bone is limited to cortical surface; hence, subchondral cysts, sclerosis, and osteitis cannot be detected on US. Comprehensive evaluation of multiple joints with ultrasound can be time-consuming.

2.3 Magnetic Resonance Imaging (MRI)

Magnetic resonance imaging (MRI) is an indispensable tool in the diagnosis and management of arthritis that provides detailed, high-resolution images of soft tissues. MRI excels in visualizing joint inflammation, synovitis, effusion, cartilage damage, tendons, tenosynovitis, and soft tissue abnormalities (Fig. 2). The ability to detect bone marrow edema, which is considered an early marker of inflammation and a precursor to erosions, makes it especially useful for the evaluation of early inflammatory arthritis (Sudoł-Szopińska

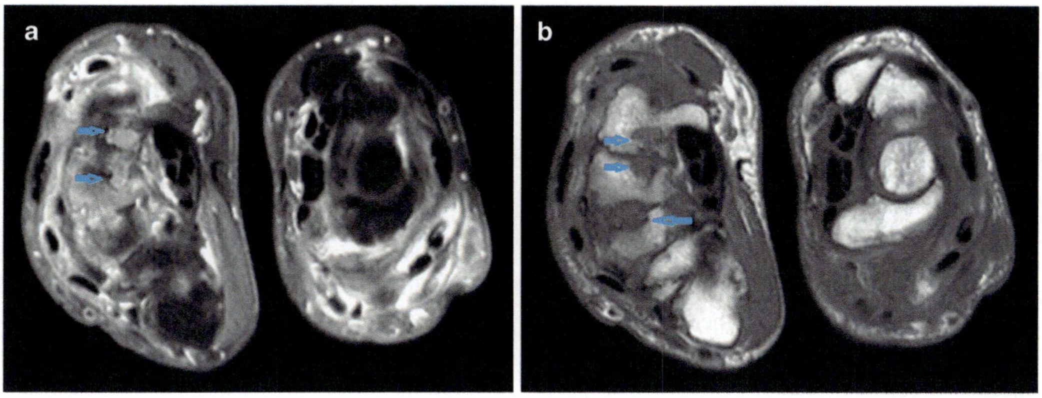

Fig. 2 (**a**) Postcontrast T1 FS and (**b**) T1 axial MR images of the wrist demonstrating erosions (arrows) and synovitis

et al. 2017). It correlates with disease activity and elevated inflammatory phase markers. This makes MRI an invaluable tool in the early diagnosis and management of arthritis even before the radiographic abnormalities appear. Its ability to detect subtle early changes, monitor disease progression, track disease activity, assess treatment response, and guide treatment decisions makes it invaluable for a wide range of arthritic conditions.

2.3.1 Limitations of MRI

MRI is more expensive and less widely available than radiographs or ultrasound, which may limit its accessibility in certain regions or healthcare settings. MRI takes longer compared to other modalities, which may be challenging for patients who cannot remain still for extended periods. Some patients may experience discomfort in the MRI scanner, especially those with claustrophobia, limiting its use in certain populations.

2.4 Computed Tomography (CT)

CT provides detailed cross-sectional, multiplanar, and 3D reconstructions of bone architecture. While its use is less common than radiography, CT plays a critical role in certain arthritic conditions, particularly in complex cases requiring high-resolution bone imaging. Although less commonly used for routine arthritis evaluation, CT excels in depicting bone details, particularly in cases where subtle erosions or structural abnormalities are suspected. It is useful for surgical planning in severe OA requiring joint replacement or fusion. CT is superior to radiography for detecting subtle calcifications, small erosions, and visualizing complex joint deformities. Dual-energy CT (DECT) is a powerful tool for diagnosing gout. DECT can visualize monosodium urate crystal deposits within joints and soft tissues with high specificity (Sotniczuk et al. 2022). It works on the principle of material decomposition, allowing for the differentiation of tissues based on their ability to attenuate X-rays at different energies. It helps in monitoring urate burden over time, assessing the effectiveness of urate-lowering therapy, and identifying subclinical deposition in asymptomatic joints.

2.4.1 Limitations of CT in Hand Arthritis

The use of CT is limited due to a higher radiation dose compared to radiography or ultrasound, limiting repeat use. Soft tissue changes are better evaluated with ultrasound or MRI. CT lacks sensitivity for detecting synovitis or tenosynovitis. CT is more expensive compared to radiography or ultrasound.

2.5 Fluoroscopy

Fluoroscopy is a dynamic imaging technique that uses continuous X-ray visualization to guide interventional procedures and assess joint function in real time. While not primarily a diagnostic tool, fluoroscopy plays a critical role in the management of hand arthritis, particularly for guidance for intra-articular injections, joint aspiration, and arthrography. Fluoroscopy ensures precise delivery of corticosteroids, anesthetics, or other therapeutic agents into affected joints. This is especially useful for small joints in the hand, where accurate placement is essential to maximize therapeutic efficacy and minimize complications. Arthrography is the injection of contrast media to visualize joint spaces and is followed by MRI. Arthrography is useful in the assessment of the integrity of the triangular fibrocartilage complex (TFCC) and intrinsic or extrinsic wrist ligaments. Continuous fluoroscopic imaging involves higher radiation exposure compared to static radiographs. Like conventional radiography, fluoroscopy does not provide imaging of soft tissues, which are better assessed with MRI or ultrasound.

2.6 Recent Advances and Other Imaging Modalities

- *Dual-Energy CT (DECT)*: It utilizes tissue-specific attenuation characteristics at different X-ray energy levels. Imaging is typically performed at 80 kV and 140 kV and analyzed using material decomposition algorithms. DECT is widely used for detecting monosodium urate (MSU) crystals, the hallmark of gout. It enables noninvasive identification and differentiation of MSU crystals from other substances, such as calcium pyrophosphate dihydrate (CPPD) crystals, which are found in pseudogout.

  DECT also helps differentiate urate deposition from osteoarthritis (OA) changes, making it particularly useful in cases where gout coexists with OA.

  In inflammatory arthritis, dual-energy CT with iodine mapping and virtual noncalcium (VNCa) techniques can detect inflammatory lesions in addition to CT's traditional role in assessing structural changes (Shiraishi et al. 2020). VNCa imaging helps visualize bone marrow edema by subtracting trabecular bone. However, its use has been mainly explored in larger bones, and assessing bone marrow edema in smaller bones, like the distal phalanges, remains technically challenging. Limitations of DECT include radiation exposure and limited availability.
- *Dynamic Contrast-Enhanced MRI*: It can quantify the inflammatory activity in inflamed synovial tissue. It involves the rapid acquisition of sequential images during and after administration of intravenous contrast and assesses the rate of enhancement of the synovial tissue (Burke et al. 2019). This correlates with disease activity and can be useful in treatment monitoring. Studies have shown that it can differentiate synovitis in RA from OA.
- *Positron Emission Tomography-Computed Tomography (PET-CT) and Positron Emission Tomography-Magnetic Resonance Imaging (PET-MRI)*: These imaging modalities provide both metabolic and structural data simultaneously, making them valuable for the early detection of inflammatory changes in arthritis. Both these imaging modalities enable functional assessment by quantifying metabolic activity in affected joints, potentially detecting inflammation before structural changes become visible. This capability aids in diagnosis, disease monitoring, and treatment response evaluation (Singh et al. 2024).

  Hybrid PET-MRI offers the advantage of combining high-resolution soft tissue contrast from MRI with the metabolic insights of PET imaging. The use of 18F-fluoride and 18F-FDG PET provides metabolic information related to subchondral bone remodeling, making it particularly useful for osteoarthritis (OA) imaging (Kogan et al. 2016). By integrating these imaging techniques, PET-MRI enhances the ability to assess both inflammation and structural integrity, offering a more comprehensive evaluation of joint diseases.
- *High-Resolution Peripheral Quantitative CT (HR-pQCT)*: It enhances visualization providing ultra-high resolution of bone microarchitecture. It is useful for detecting early subchondral changes or early erosions. HR-

pQCT scans possess superior spatial resolution compared to traditional CT scans while maintaining a comparable radiation dosage (Harnden et al. 2022). A drawback is the susceptibility to motion artifacts.

- *Photoacoustic Tomography (PAT)*: A novel handheld PAT scanner developed for small joint imaging has enabled real-time, high-resolution 3D visualization of vascular changes in inflamed joints.
- *Artificial Intelligence (AI) and Machine Learning*: Both aid in improving automated detection and classification of OA severity in radiographic images. AI-assisted analysis in MRI and US improves the accuracy of detecting erosions, synovitis, and joint damage. Automated quantification of inflammation and structural changes aids in disease monitoring.

3 Pattern of Joint Involvement

Most arthritic disorders have a predilection to involve certain joints (Kluckman et al. 2021). The pattern of joint involvement (Table 1) aids in the diagnosis of the type of articular disease (Fig. 3).

Table 1 Pattern of hand/wrist joint involvement in different types of arthritis

Disease	Distribution	Affected joints	Key features
Osteoarthritis	Bilateral, symmetric, or asymmetric	DIP, PIP, first CMC, triscaphe	Joint space narrowing, osteophytes, capsular ossicles, subchondral sclerosis, radial subluxation at first CMC
Erosive osteoarthritis	Bilateral, symmetric, or asymmetric	DIP, PIP > MCP, first CMC, triscaphe	Joint space narrowing, osteophytes, central erosions, soft tissue swelling, potential ankylosis
Rheumatoid arthritis	Bilateral, symmetric	MCP, PIP, IP (thumb), all wrist compartments	Periarticular osteopenia, joint space narrowing, marginal bone erosions and soft tissue swelling, early distal ulna involvement, pancompartmental wrist changes
Juvenile idiopathic arthritis	Symmetric or asymmetric	Any hand joint, midcarpal, common carpometacarpal. Relative sparing of the first carpometacarpal and radiocarpal joints	Bone proliferation, periostitis, and joint ankylosis. Osteopenia, joint space narrowing, and erosions are seen in variable degree
Psoriatic arthritis	Bilateral or unilateral. Asymmetric. Can have a ray-like distribution	DIP, PIP, MCP, any wrist compartment	Periarticular bone proliferation, enthesitis, erosions, and joint ankylosis. DIP joint involvement can be prominent. Pancompartmental involvement can be seen at the wrist
Reactive arthritis	Asymmetric	Any hand or wrist joint	Similar to psoriatic arthritis, but more common in lower extremities
Ankylosing spondylitis	Bilateral, asymmetric	Any hand or wrist joint	Hands are not a common site of involvement. Bone proliferation with whiskering. Osteopenia, erosions, joint space narrowing, and joint deformities are less prominent than in rheumatoid arthritis. Less extensive wrist disease
Systemic lupus erythematosus	Bilateral, symmetric	MCP, IP (all digits), first CMC	Joint deformities which are initially reversible and, later become fixed. No erosions in early disease
Scleroderma & polymyositis	Bilateral	DIP > PIP, first CMC	Soft tissue calcification, acro-osteolysis, thumb deformities (polymyositis), first CMC erosions

(continued)

Table 1 (continued)

Disease	Distribution	Affected joints	Key features
Gouty arthritis	Bilateral, asymmetric	DIP, PIP, MCP, common carpometacarpal	Soft tissue masses, eccentric erosions with sclerotic margins, overhanging edges, lack of osteopenia, preserved joint space
CPPD (calcium pyrophosphate dihydrate) disease	Bilateral, symmetric	MCP (second & third most common), radiocarpal, triscaphe, first CMC	Joint space loss, chondrocalcinosis, beak-like osteophytes (hemochromatosis)
Septic arthritis	Monoarticular	Any joint	Joint space narrowing, erosions, periarticular osteopenia, soft tissue swelling

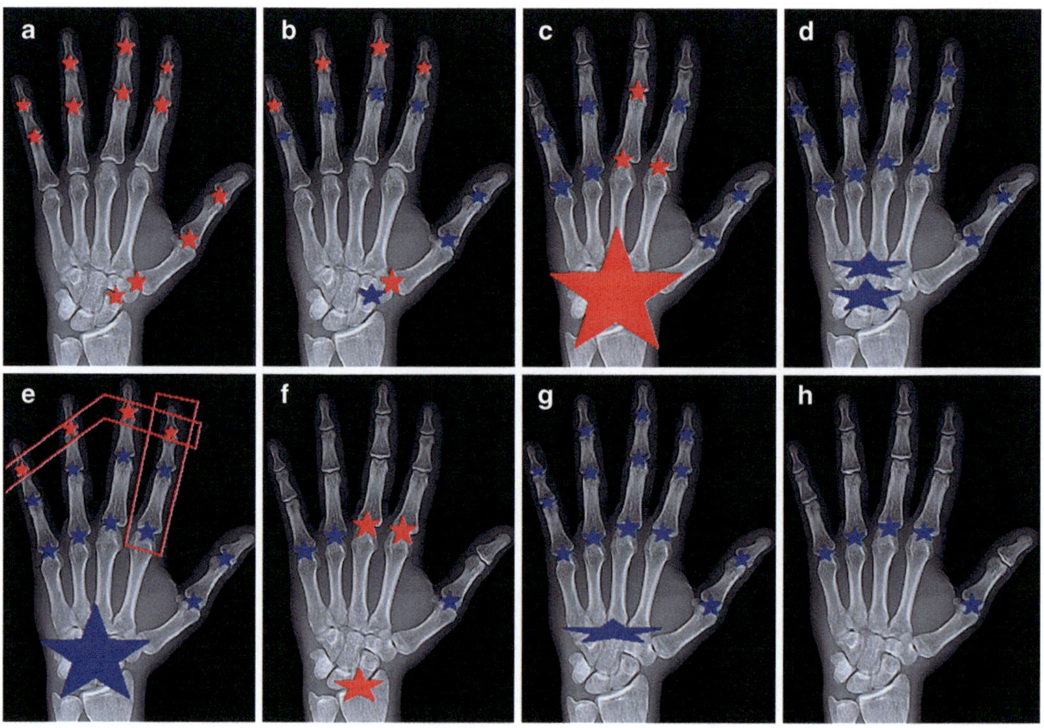

Fig. 3 Pattern of joint involvement. (**a**) Osteoarthritis. (**b**) Erosive osteoarthritis. (**c**) Rheumatoid arthritis. (**d**) Juvenile idiopathic arthritis; (**e**) Psoriatic arthritis; (**f**) Calcium pyrophosphate dihydrate deposition arthropathy. (**g**) Gout. (**h**) Systemic lupus erythematosus

4 Osteoarthritis (OA)

Osteoarthritis (OA), also known as degenerative joint disease, is a progressive disorder characterized by cartilage degradation, subchondral bone remodeling, osteophyte formation, and loss of joint function. It is the most prevalent form of arthritis, affecting over 528 million people globally. The hand is the second most commonly affected site after the knee, often leading to significant functional impairment (WHO 2023).

According to the Framingham Osteoarthritis Study, radiographic hand OA affects 44.2% of women and 37.7% of men, with erosive OA found more frequently in women (Haugen et al. 2011). Risk factors include advanced age, female sex, obesity, prior trauma, and metabolic comorbidities such as diabetes. While obesity has a weaker link with hand OA compared to knee or hip OA, systemic metabolic factors may accelerate disease progression.

Imaging plays a central role in OA diagnosis, staging, and monitoring. Conventional radiographs remain the cornerstone, demonstrating hallmark features such as joint space narrowing, subchondral sclerosis, osteophytes, and cysts. DIP, PIP, and first CMC joints are most frequently involved. Heberden's and Bouchard's nodes are common clinical manifestations related to DIP and PIP joint osteophytes, respectively.

Post-traumatic OA, particularly in the wrist, may develop after scaphoid fractures or ligament injuries, resulting in patterns like scapholunate advanced collapse (SLAC) or scaphoid nonunion advanced collapse (SNAC). These conditions involve progressive degeneration of the radiocarpal and midcarpal joints.

Advanced imaging provides further insight:

- MRI can detect early chondral changes, bone marrow edema, and synovitis, especially in atypical or early-stage disease (Feydy et al. 2009a, b). High-field MRI (3T and 7T) offers enhanced cartilage resolution.
- Ultrasound is sensitive to synovial inflammation, early osteophyte formation, and joint effusions.
- CT arthrography provides superior depiction of cartilage surfaces and subchondral bone, useful in surgical planning. Cone-beam CT arthrography has shown high accuracy in detecting cartilage lesions (Suojärvi et al. 2016).

Recent advances in quantitative imaging allow semi-automated grading of OA severity. AI models now support radiographic OA classification by detecting and quantifying structural changes.

Therapeutic approaches range from conservative management with NSAIDs, splinting, and physical therapy to image-guided corticosteroid injections and surgical interventions like arthrodesis or arthroplasty in advanced disease. In conclusion, OA of the hand and wrist is a common degenerative condition with a spectrum of clinical and imaging findings. Radiographs remain essential, but multimodality imaging enhances early detection, individualized management, and prognostication.

4.1 Imaging Features

Bilateral symmetric or asymmetric joint involvement. DIP, PIP, and thumb interphalangeal (IP) joints are commonly affected. Involvement of multiple fingers of both hands is characteristic. Joint space narrowing, subchondral sclerosis, osteophytes, and small capsular ossicles can be seen (Fig. 4). Heberden's nodes are palpable osteophytes about the DIP joints, and analogous changes at the PIP joints are referred to as Bouchard's nodes. Sometimes, small gelatinous mucoid cysts of the soft tissues appear on the dorsal aspects of involved interphalangeal joints. Joint deformities in osteoarthritis are characterized by horizontal instability.

Though less frequently involved than the interphalangeal joints, metacarpophalangeal OA presents with joint space narrowing and small osteophytes. The absence of marginal erosions helps differentiate it from rheumatoid

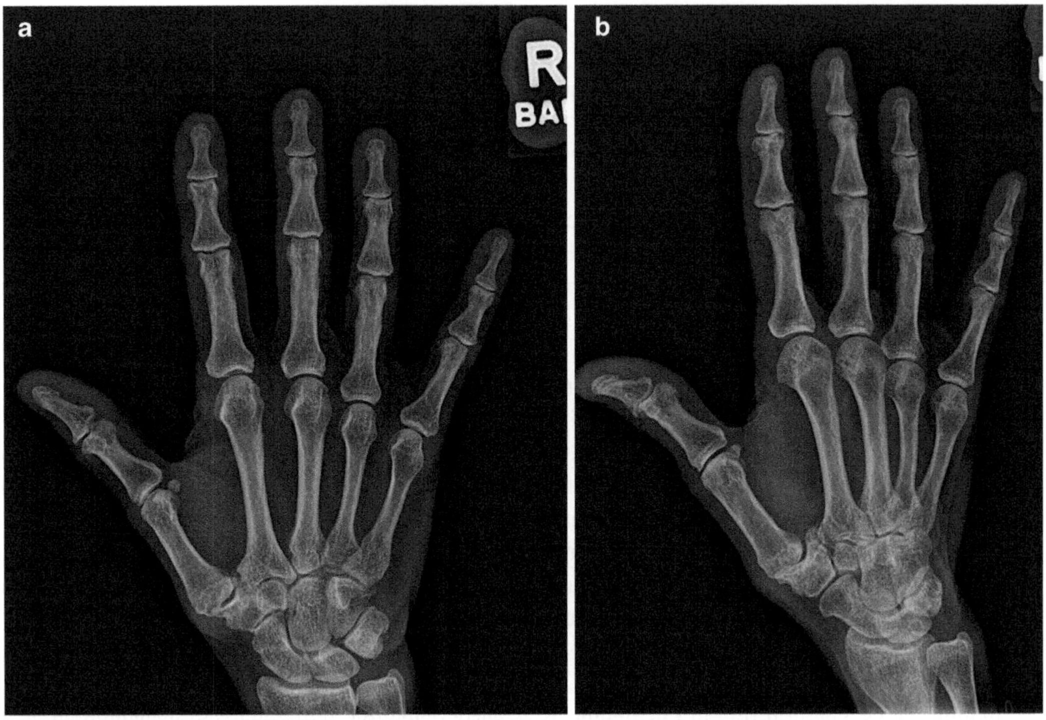

Fig. 4 Osteoarthritis. (**a**) PA and (**b**) Oblique radiographs of the right hand demonstrate joint space narrowing, subchondral sclerosis, and osteophytes at the thumb interphalangeal joint, index finger distal interphalangeal joint, and first carpometacarpal joint

arthritis. Distinguishing features of CPPD crystal deposition disease or hemochromatosis include the absence of large cystic lesions and periarticular calcifications.

At the wrist, the first carpometacarpal (trapeziometacarpal) and trapezio-trapezoid-scaphoid (triscaphe) joints are affected. Joint space loss, subchondral sclerosis, osteophytes, and radial subluxation can be evident at the first CMC joint (Fig. 5). At the triscaphe joint, joint space narrowing and subchondral sclerosis are the common features. Post-traumatic OA may involve any joint at the wrist. Scaphoid nonunion advanced collapse (SNAC) is a type of degenerative arthropathy involving the radiocarpal articulation occurring as a sequela of non-united scaphoid fractures. Scapholunate advanced collapse (SLAC) can occur with scapholunate separation, or dissociation, and subsequent degenerative changes at the lunate-capitate and radiocarpal joints.

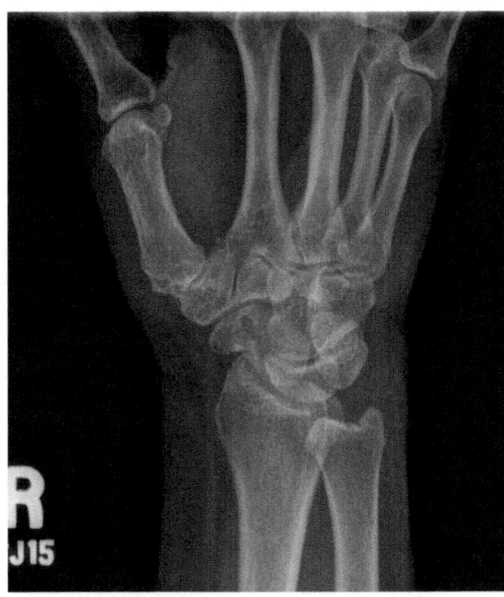

Fig. 5 Osteoarthritis. Oblique radiographs of the right wrist demonstrate joint space narrowing, subchondral sclerosis, subchondral cysts, and osteophytes at the first carpometacarpal joint

4.2 Conventional Radiography (Table 2)

Conventional radiographs remain the gold standard for diagnosing hand and wrist OA.

Table 2 Radiographic features of OA

Nonuniform joint space narrowing
Marginal osteophytes
Subchondral sclerosis
Subchondral cysts
Deformity & malalignment

4.3 Ultrasound (US)

- Detects early osteophyte formation and synovial inflammation
- Assesses joint effusion and synovial hypertrophy
- Can visualize cartilage thickness and vascularity via Doppler imaging

4.4 Computed Tomography (CT)

- Superior in evaluating bony anatomy and subtle cortical changes.
- Useful for preoperative planning in advanced cases.
- Cone-beam CT arthrography (CBCT-A) has emerged as a superior modality for articular cartilage evaluation. A study demonstrated high sensitivity and specificity comparable to MR arthrography for cartilage lesions and ligament tears (Suojärvi et al. 2016). The technique's ability to create isotropic 0.2 mm voxels allows three-dimensional assessment of cartilage thickness, surface congruity, and subchondral cyst communication.

4.5 Magnetic Resonance Imaging (MRI)

- Clinical and radiographic features are usually straightforward, and MRI is not used for primary diagnosis.
- MRI is highly sensitive for detecting early cartilage loss and bone marrow edema. It can identify soft tissue involvement and synovitis. Early osteoarthritic changes appear as areas of surface irregularity, fibrillation, and small focal defects in the articular cartilage with increased signal intensity on proton density or T2-weighted fast spin-echo images. Advanced disease is characterized by extensive chondral thinning, multiple focal defects with obtuse margins, and signal abnormalities within the subchondral bone marrow, subchondral cyst formation, edema-like changes, or fibrosis. Additional degenerative features, including osteophytes and synovitis, are frequently observed. While MRI is not typically used for primary diagnosis, it can be useful in atypical or early-stage cases. Some MRI findings, such as extensive subchondral bone marrow edema, gadolinium-enhanced cysts, and heterogeneous joint fluid signal, may be misleading.
- Recent advancements, such as 3T MRI and dedicated wrist coils, have improved spatial resolution to 0.3 mm in-plane, enhancing the detection of subtle synovitis and osteochondral defects. However, MRI's utility in hand and wrist OA remains limited due to small joint spaces, partial volume effects, and poor correlation between imaging findings and clinical symptoms.

4.6 Other Joints Involved

- Knee
- Hip joint
- Shoulder: Acromioclavicular and glenohumeral joints
- Spine OA: Degenerative changes in cervical and lumbar regions
- Foot OA: Particularly at the first metatarsophalangeal (MTP) joint

5 Erosive Osteoarthritis (EOA)

Erosive osteoarthritis (EOA) is a distinct and aggressive form of osteoarthritis that primarily affects the interphalangeal joints of the hands. It is characterized by predominant involvement of distal interphalangeal joints, an abrupt onset with inflammation, characteristic central erosions on radiographs, and "gull-wing" deformities. Clinically, it presents with pain, swelling, stiffness, and reduced function. EOA is considered an inflammatory subset of osteoarthritis, with a complex interplay of mechanical stress, metabolic factors, and local inflammation. Unlike non-inflammatory osteoarthritis, EOA exhibits simultaneous bone resorption and formation, leading to its characteristic radiographic features. Hormonal changes, particularly estrogen deficiency in postmenopausal women, may also play a role in disease progression. Genetic predisposition, metabolic factors like obesity and insulin resistance, and hormonal factors contribute to disease susceptibility. EOA progresses through stages of acute inflammation, joint destruction, and eventual stabilization. Some patients experience spontaneous remission, while others develop significant deformities, functional impairment, and joint ankylosis. Unlike rheumatoid arthritis (RA), EOA is not associated with systemic complications or extra-articular manifestations.

The estimated prevalence of EOA in the general population is 2.8%, rising to 10.2% in those with symptomatic osteoarthritis (Marshall et al. 2013). EOA predominantly affects postmenopausal women and primarily develops in individuals with baseline non-erosive osteoarthritis. It is more common in women (17.3%) than in men (9.6%) (Haugen et al. 2011). Among individuals over 60 years of age with radiographic hand osteoarthritis, 24.3% of women and 9.5% of men exhibit erosive disease.

5.1 Imaging Features (Table 3)

EOA primarily affects the interphalangeal joints of the hands, with a predilection for the distal interphalangeal (DIP) joints, followed by the proximal interphalangeal (PIP) joints (Marshall et al. 2013). The first carpometacarpal joint may also be involved, but the metacarpophalangeal joints and wrists are typically spared. On radiographs, erosions and soft tissue swelling are observed in addition to the typical features of non-inflammatory OA (Fig. 6).

Table 3 Radiographic features of EOA

Central erosions
Gull-wing deformities
Uniform joint space narrowing
Marginal osteophytes
Subchondral sclerosis
Symmetrical distribution
Soft tissue swelling

In the initial stages, joint space narrowing and subtle erosions may be seen. As the disease progresses, the destructive stage is characterized by prominent central erosions in the subchondral plate. Central erosions, combined with marginal osteophytes, create characteristic "gull-wing" or "saw-tooth" deformities. Some joints may show signs of repair, including the disappearance of osteolytic areas and reconstruction of the subchondral bone plate. In more advanced disease, severe joint deformity, ankylosis, and extensive osteophyte formation may be present.

5.2 Other Imaging Modalities

While conventional radiography remains the primary imaging method for diagnosing and monitoring EOA, other modalities can provide additional information:

- Ultrasound: It detects early inflammatory changes and erosions. It offers real-time imaging and is useful for monitoring disease progression and treatment response.
- Magnetic Resonance Imaging (MRI): It provides a detailed assessment of soft tissue involvement and early bone changes. It can detect synovitis, bone marrow edema, and subtle erosions not visible on radiographs.
- Computed Tomography (CT): It offers high-resolution images of bony changes and ero-

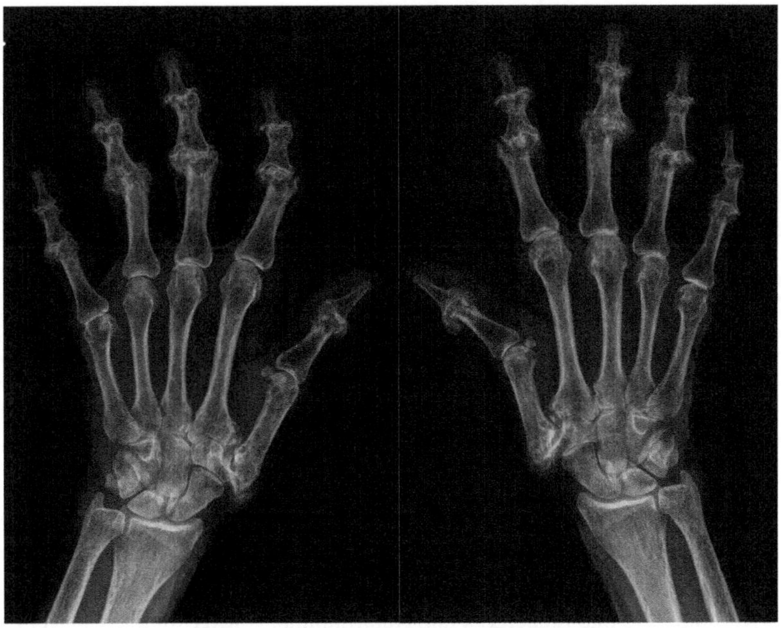

Fig. 6 Erosive osteoarthritis. PA radiographs of bilateral hands demonstrate symmetric joint space loss, subchondral sclerosis, central erosions, and osteophytes with gull-wing deformities at all the distal and proximal interphalangeal joints, and at the thumb interphalangeal joint. Joint space loss, subchondral sclerosis, and osteophytes are also present at the first carpometacarpal joint

sions. It is particularly useful for evaluating complex joint anatomy and subtle erosive changes.

6 Rheumatoid Arthritis

Rheumatoid arthritis (RA) is a chronic systemic autoimmune disease that primarily affects synovial joints, leading to inflammation, joint destruction, and deformities. The "bare area" of a synovial joint near the attachment of capsule which lacks cartilage is susceptible to synovitis-mediated bone destruction. RA has a predilection for small joints of the hands and feet and is characterized by a proximal distribution of joint involvement. The hand and wrist are among the earliest and most affected sites, often exhibiting symmetrical joint involvement that progressively leads to structural damage and functional impairment.

RA frequently affects individuals aged 25–55 years and is more common in women over 65 years. Women are affected 2–3 times more frequently than men. The global prevalence of RA increased by 14.1% from 1990 to 2020, with an estimated 17.6 million cases in 2020 (GBD 2021 Rheumatoid Arthritis Collaborators and Cross 2023). Mortality rates due to RA decreased by 23.8% globally from 1990 to 2020. The global burden of RA is projected to reach 31.7 million cases by 2050. Risk factors include genetic predisposition (HLA-DR4, HLA-DR1), environmental factors (smoking), autoimmune dysfunction, and hormonal influences.

RA can also present with extra-articular manifestations, including rheumatoid nodules, Raynaud's phenomenon, Sicca syndrome, episcleritis and keratoconjunctivitis, interstitial lung disease, pulmonary hypertension, pleurisy, pericarditis, peripheral neuropathy, mononeuropathy, anemia, neutropenia, thrombocytopenia, Felty's syndrome, weight loss, cachexia, malaise, fatigue, and fever.

Imaging plays a crucial role in the early detection, monitoring, and treatment response assessment of RA-related changes in the hand and wrist. While conventional radiography remains the standard tool for evaluating joint damage, ultrasound and magnetic resonance imaging (MRI) have emerged as more sensitive modalities for detecting early inflammatory changes such as synovitis, tenosynovitis, erosions, and bone marrow edema (Boutry et al. 2007). Early and precise imaging is critical in RA management, allowing for timely intervention to prevent irreversible joint damage. The *2010 ACR/EULAR classification criteria* for RA (Kay and Upchurch 2012), which include joint involvement, serology (Rheumatoid Factor or Anti-Cyclic Citrullinated Peptide Antibodies), acute phase reactants (ESR or CRP), and symptom duration, can help distinguish RA from other conditions.

The primary goal of RA treatment is to reduce inflammation, prevent joint damage, and preserve function (Johns Hopkins Arthritis Center 2020). Disease-modifying antirheumatic drugs (DMARDs), such as Methotrexate, Hydroxychloroquine, Sulfasalazine, and Leflunomide, form the cornerstone of therapy by slowing disease progression. Biologic therapies target specific immune pathways, including TNF inhibitors like Etanercept and Adalimumab, T-cell blockers such as Abatacept, and B-cell depleting agents like Rituximab. Supportive therapies such as nonsteroidal anti-inflammatory drugs (NSAIDs), corticosteroids, and physical and occupational therapy help manage symptoms and improve mobility. In cases where medical management is insufficient, surgical interventions like synovectomy, tendon repair, joint fusion, or arthroplasty may be considered to restore function and alleviate pain.

6.1 Imaging Features

Imaging is critical for early diagnosis, assessment of disease activity and progression, monitoring treatment response and guiding therapeutic decisions.

RA typically affects synovial joints with symmetric polyarticular involvement, particularly the proximal interphalangeal (PIP) and metacarpophalangeal (MCP) joints (Saltzherr et al. 2019).

The earliest changes in RA are observed in the second and third MCP joints and the third PIP joint, while distal interphalangeal (DIP) joint involvement is rare and tends to be mild. A characteristic early feature is the involvement of the distal ulna, and pancompartmental wrist involvement is often present. Rapid inflammatory progression may occur, leading to cartilage and bone destruction. Early signs of RA include soft tissue swelling, periarticular osteopenia, and synovitis. MRI findings in very early RA can reveal bone marrow edema, erosions, and synovitis (Kosta et al. 2011). Joint space narrowing and marginal erosions are particularly seen in the MCP joints, ulnar styloid, and carpal bones. Additionally, tendon involvement, leading to tenosynovitis and potential tendon rupture can be seen. Tenosynovitis is an important imaging finding in early RA that could improve the diagnostic performance of the 2010 ACR/EULAR classification criteria. Tenosynovitis of the extensor carpi ulnaris and flexor tendons of the second finger are prognostic and associated with RA progression (Navalho et al. 2012). The extensor carpi ulnaris is a common and early site involvement in RA of the wrist (Sommer et al. 2005). The inflammatory process may result in erosions of the adjacent ulnar styloid process. Over time, progressive deformities such as ulnar deviation, swan-neck deformity, boutonnière deformity, and radial deviation of the wrist can develop. In the late stages, complications such as joint ankylosis, ligamentous instability, and carpal collapse are observed.

Table 4 Radiographic features of RA (Figs. 7 and 8)

Early findings	Soft tissue swelling due to a combination of joint effusion, edema, or tenosynovitis Periarticular osteopenia
Late findings	Joint space narrowing (concentric and uniform) Marginal erosions—often seen in the "bare areas" of joints, frequently on the radial side of the metacarpophalangeal (MCP) joints
Joint deformities	Mallet finger, boutonnière deformity, swan-neck deformity, ulnar drift, thumb malalignment, zigzag deformity, ulnar deviation at MCP joints, radial deviation at the wrist

Conventional radiography (Table 4) is the first-line imaging modality due to its low cost and wide availability. However, it has low sensitivity for detecting soft tissue edema and synovial thickening, and erosions may take 6–12 months to appear on radiographs.

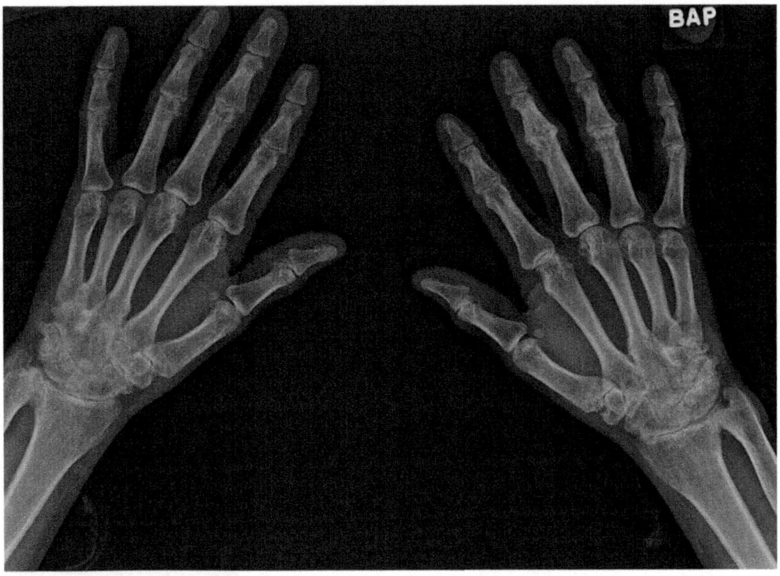

Fig. 7 Rheumatoid arthritis. PA radiographs of bilateral hands demonstrate symmetric joint space narrowing and marginal erosions at bilateral second and third metacarpophalangeal joints, and at third and fourth proximal interphalangeal joints. Severe intercarpal and radiocarpal joint space loss and multifocal carpal erosions are also present at the wrist

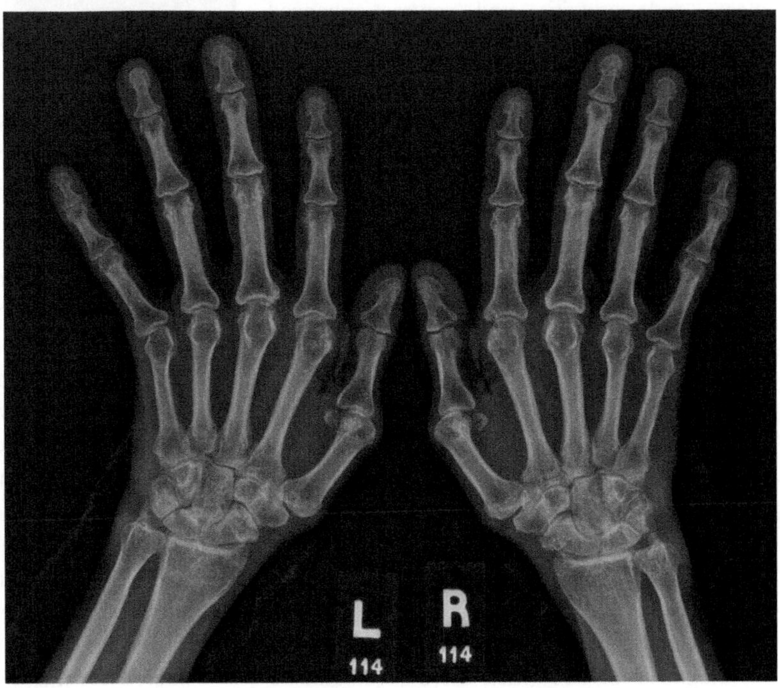

Fig. 8 Rheumatoid arthritis. PA radiographs of bilateral hands demonstrate periarticular osteopenia. Joint space narrowing and marginal erosions at bilateral second and third metacarpophalangeal joints, bilateral radiocarpal joint space narrowing, erosion at the right ulna styloid process with adjacent soft tissue swelling, and soft tissue swelling adjacent to the left ulna styloid process are also present

Ultrasound (Table 5) is more sensitive than radiography in detecting early inflammatory changes (Rubin 2019). It offers several advantages, including being non-ionizing, providing real-time dynamic assessment, and being useful for guiding interventions such as joint aspirations and injections.

MRI (Table 6) is the most sensitive imaging modality for detecting early inflammatory changes (Rubin 2019). MRI sequences used to

Table 5 Ultrasound features of RA (Figs. 9 and 10)

Synovial hypertrophy and effusion	Soft tissue swelling, periarticular osteopenia
Power Doppler signal	Assesses synovial vascularity which indicates active inflammation before structural changes occur. It can be utilized for quantification of synovial inflammation (Rowbotham and Grainger 2011)
Tenosynovitis	Tendon sheath thickening and/or effusion
Early bone erosions	Discontinuity of bony surface visible in two perpendicular planes especially in MCP, PIP, and wrist joints

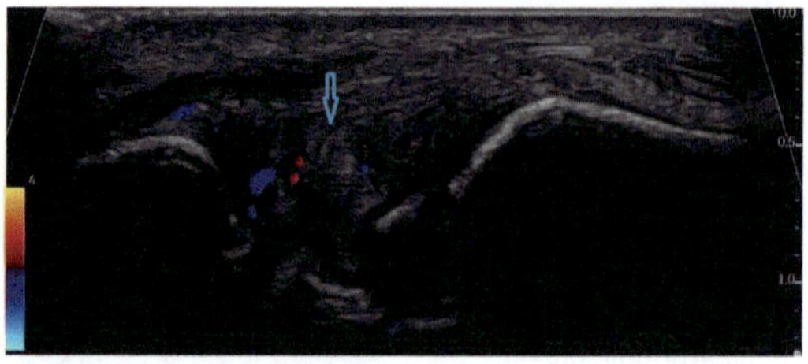

Fig. 9 Synovitis in rheumatoid arthritis. Ultrasound of the second metacarpophalangeal joint demonstrates synovial thickening and synovial hyperemia with increased Doppler signal

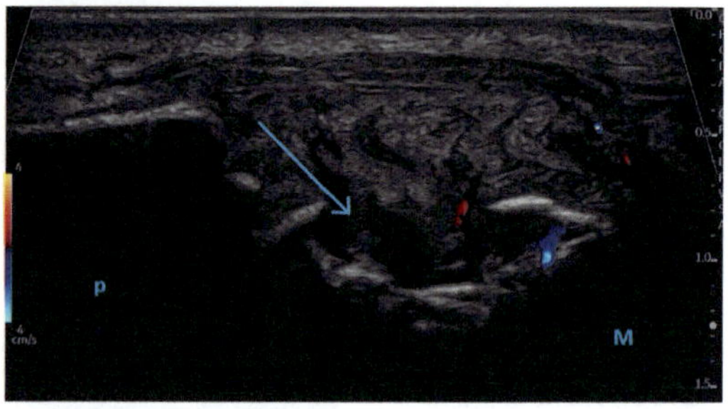

Fig. 10 Erosion in rheumatoid arthritis. Ultrasound of the third metacarpophalangeal joint demonstrates an erosion (arrow) at the metacarpal head (M) with adjacent synovial thickening and increased Doppler signal

evaluate rheumatoid arthritis (RA) include T1-weighted for anatomical detail and erosion detection, T2-weighted/STIR for bone marrow edema and synovitis, and contrast-enhanced T1-weighted for assessing active synovitis. However, MRI has limitations, including being costly, time-consuming, and having contraindications such as metallic implants and claustrophobia. While not routinely used in RA imaging, CT can provide detailed information about bony changes and is particularly useful for assessing complex joints. It is valuable for detecting bony erosions, joint alignment abnormalities, and joint ankylosis, especially in advanced cases involving the wrist.

The EULAR recommendations (Colebatch et al. 2013) highlight the role of imaging in improving the diagnosis and management of rheumatoid arthritis (RA). The following is a summary of EULAR Recommendations for Imaging in RA:

1. CR, ultrasound, or MRI can help confirm a diagnosis of RA when there is diagnostic uncertainty, improving upon clinical criteria alone.
2. Inflammation detected by ultrasound or MRI can predict the progression to clinical RA in cases of undifferentiated inflammatory arthritis.
3. Ultrasound and MRI are more effective than clinical examination in detecting joint inflammation and should be used for more accurate assessments.
4. Conventional radiographs (CR) of the hands and feet should be used initially to detect joint damage. If no damage is seen, ultrasound or MRI may be used for earlier detection, especially in early RA.
5. Bone marrow edema on MRI is a strong predictor of future radiographic progression in early RA and should be considered for prognosis. Synovitis on MRI or US, as well as joint damage detected by conventional radiographs, MRI, or ultrasound, can also be considered for the prediction of further joint damage.
6. Imaging may be more predictive of treatment response than clinical disease activity and may be used to predict response to treatment.
7. MRI and ultrasound, with better detection of inflammation than clinical examination, are useful for monitoring disease activity.

8. Periodic radiographs of the hands and feet should be considered to assess joint damage, while MRI (and possibly ultrasound) is more sensitive to changes and can be used to monitor progression.
9. Lateral radiographs in flexion and neutral position should be done if cervical spine involvement is suspected. MRI should be performed if abnormalities or neurological symptoms are present.
10. MRI and ultrasound can detect inflammation that might lead to future joint damage, even during clinical remission, and can be used to assess persistent inflammation.

6.2 Other Joints Involved

- Feet: MTP joint erosions, hallux valgus, hammer toe deformity
- Cervical spine: Atlantoaxial subluxation, odontoid erosion
- Knees: Synovial hypertrophy, Baker's cysts, joint effusion, cartilage loss
- Hips: Protrusio acetabuli
- Temporomandibular joint: Erosions, ankylosis
- Shoulders: Glenohumeral and acromioclavicular joint erosions

Table 6 MRI features of RA (Fig. 11)

Synovitis	Contrast-enhancing thickened synovium
Bone marrow edema	Precursor to erosions
Erosions	Sharply defined regions of bone loss with a cortical defect. Are detectable earlier than radiography or CT
Tenosynovitis	MRI detected tenosynovitis has been reported as the strongest predictor of progression to inflammatory arthritis in patients with clinically suspect arthralgia (Harnden et al. 2022)
Cartilage damage	Decreased thickness of articular cartilage

7 Juvenile Idiopathic Arthritis

Juvenile idiopathic arthritis (JIA) is the most common chronic rheumatic disease in children and encompasses a heterogeneous group of autoimmune arthritides with onset before age 16 and symptoms lasting more than 6 weeks (Tsujioka et al. 2023; Muller et al. 2015). JIA may affect one or multiple joints and varies widely in clinical presentation, disease course, and imaging findings. The global prevalence ranges from 16 to 150 per 100,000 children (Sheybani et al. 2013), with higher incidence in girls and peak onset between ages 11 and

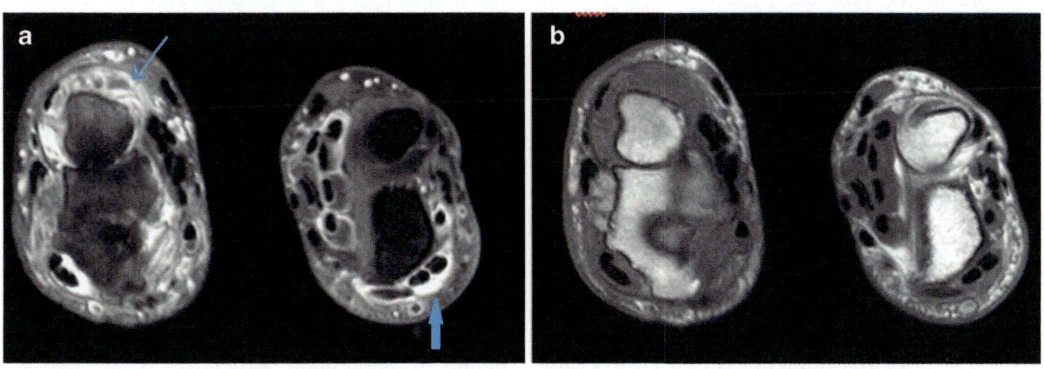

Fig. 11 Synovitis and tenosynovitis in rheumatoid arthritis. (**a**) Postcontrast T1 FS and (**b**) T1 axial MR images of the wrist demonstrate synovial proliferation about the distal ulna (thin arrow) and extensor tendons (solid arrow)

15 (Harrold et al. 2013). Risk factors include genetic predisposition, immune dysregulation, and environmental triggers.

JIA often affects the hand and wrist, which can have serious long-term consequences. At diagnosis, about 25% of JIA patients have wrist involvement, and this increases to 40% after 5 years. Early wrist involvement, along with distal small joint arthritis and symmetric arthritis, is considered a poor prognostic factor. A study (Selvaag et al. 2017) of 60 patients with long-term JIA and wrist arthritis found that over half had radiographic damage in their hands and wrists after 29 years. While most had modest damage, 25% experienced severe damage, particularly those with RF-positive or anti-CCP-positive JIA. The damage primarily involved the carpal bones and included erosions and joint space narrowing (JSN).

The International League of Associations for Rheumatology (ILAR) classifies JIA into subtypes based on joint involvement, symptoms, family history, and serologic findings (Tsujioka et al. 2023):

- Oligoarticular JIA (most common, ~40% of cases): Peak onset at 2–4 years; female-to-male ratio of 3:1.
- RF-positive polyarthritis: Primarily affects adolescent females (9:1 female-to-male ratio).
- RF-negative polyarticular JIA: Affects five or more joints; bimodal peak onset (2–4 years and 10–14 years). Female-to-male ratio is 3:1 in early onset and 10:1 in late onset.
- Enthesitis-related arthritis: More common in males (1:7 female-to-male ratio), with peak onset at 9–12 years.

7.1 Imaging Features

Imaging plays a crucial role in the diagnosis and management of JIA. Imaging is utilized to evaluate for the presence and activity of synovial inflammation, monitor disease progression, and exclude other joint diseases. Optimal imaging studies should be individualized. Common features include active synovitis, increased joint fluid, periarticular soft tissue edema, and periarticular osteopenia. Tenosynovial inflammation is often present in the tendon sheaths of the hands. Tenosynovitis and multicompartmental arthritis are common findings in the ankle and wrist in patients with juvenile idiopathic arthritis. In a study it was found that in patients referred for MRI, the extensor digitorum was the most commonly involved tendon, and the intercarpal joint was the most frequently affected joint (Javadi et al. 2014). Synovitis, bone marrow edema, and tenosynovitis are early signs of JIA that can be detected by MRI and ultrasound. Erosions, joint space narrowing, and growth disturbances are late findings that can be visualized on radiographs.

Imaging findings can be symmetric or asymmetric in distribution. Radiographic findings include bone proliferation, periostitis, and joint ankylosis (Fig. 12). Osteopenia, joint space narrowing, and erosions are seen in variable degree. Any joint of the hand and wrist may be involved. There may be osseous ankylosis at the midcarpal and common carpometacarpal joints, with relative sparing of the first carpometacarpal and radiocarpal joints (Resnick et al. 2024).

Imaging plays a vital role in diagnosing and managing JIA by detecting inflammation, tracking disease progression, and ruling out other joint conditions.

Conventional radiography (Table 7) is often the first imaging tool used for JIA. It aids in initial diagnosis by excluding fractures, infections, or tumors. Initial radiographs are good as baseline assessment tool and provide a reference for follow-up. Radiographs are helpful in detecting complications like bone overgrowth, premature physeal fusion, and limb length discrepancies.

Ultrasonography (Table 8) is a safe, cost-effective alternative to MRI for detecting synovitis, joint effusions, and tenosynovitis. High-frequency ultrasound provides excellent detail of superficial structures (e.g., tendons, ligaments, joint capsules). Power Doppler ultrasound detects increased blood flow in inflamed synovium, indicating active disease. US is also useful for guiding joint aspirations and injections.

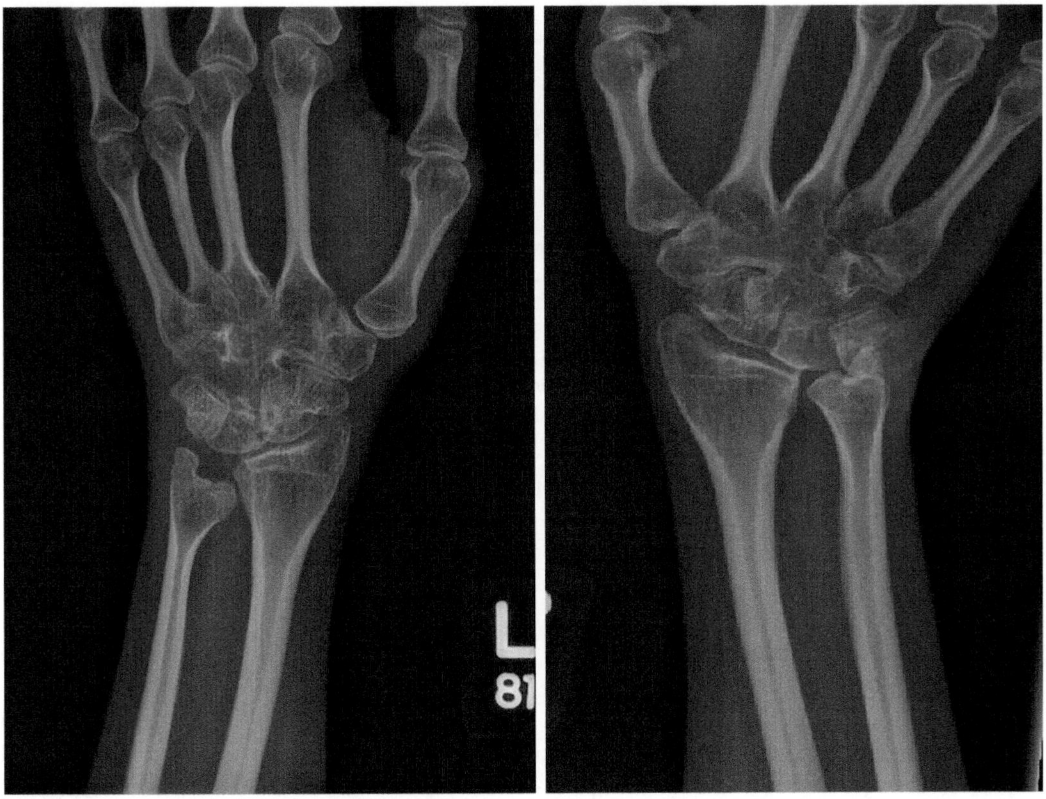

Fig. 12 Juvenile idiopathic arthritis. PA radiographs of bilateral wrists demonstrate periarticular osteopenia, ankylosis of the second and third carpometacarpal joints, and intercarpal ankylosis of the distal carpal row. Osseous erosions are present at the scapholunate joint

Table 7 Radiographic features of JIA

Soft tissue swelling
Joint effusion
Periarticular osteopenia
Erosions (less common in children due to thicker epiphyseal cartilage)
Periostitis
Joint space narrowing (an irreversible indicator of joint damage)
Premature ossification
Joint malalignment
Carpal ankylosis

Table 8 Ultrasound features of JIA

Synovitis
Joint effusion
Tenosynovitis
Enthesitis
Power Doppler signal indicating active inflammation

MRI (Table 9) is the gold standard for detecting early inflammatory changes in JIA. It has the highest sensitivity for detecting synovitis and bone marrow edema. MRI can visualize cartilage damage and early erosions before they appear on radiographs. It provides a comprehensive view of synovium, cartilage, growth plates, bone marrow, and soft tissues. Typical MRI protocol includes (Nusman et al. 2016) T1-weighted images to assess bone marrow and erosions, fat-suppressed T2-weighted or STIR images to evaluate joint fluid, cartilage, marrow edema, and tendons. Contrast-enhanced T1-weighted images can differentiate active synovitis from effusions or fibrotic pannus. Rheumatoid Arthritis MRI Score (RAMRIS), developed by the OMERACT study group, has been adapted for use in children

Table 9 MRI features of JIA

Bone marrow edema
Synovitis
Tenosynovitis
Joint effusion
Erosions
Periostitis
Enthesitis
Cartilage thinning, fissuring, and volume loss

despite skeletal differences. Some MRI findings, like bony depressions and minor bone marrow changes, can mimic pathology. Growth disturbances and periarticular osteopenia in long-standing JIA are more reliable markers of joint damage.

Table 10 Radiographic features of PsA (Fig. 13)

Asymmetrical joint involvement
Joint space widening or narrowing. Joint space widening is due to bone destruction and erosions
Predilection for DIP joints. PIP joints are also frequently involved, while the metacarpophalangeal (MCP) joints are often spared
Periarticular erosions with adjacent bone proliferation
Irregular bone growth around joints, sometimes described as "whiskering" or "fuzzy bone margins"
Enthesitis and periostitis
"Opera glass" and "pencil-in-cup" deformities from chronic joint damage, especially in the interphalangeal joints
"Sausage digit"—soft tissue swelling affecting an entire finger
Progressive joint ankylosis in chronic cases
"Ivory phalanx"—sclerosis of the distal phalanx, more common in the toes

8 Psoriatic Arthritis (PsA) and Other Seronegative Spondyloarthropathies

Seronegative spondyloarthropathies are a group of inflammatory joint diseases that include psoriatic arthritis, ankylosing spondylitis, reactive arthritis, and enteropathic arthritis. They are called "seronegative" because they lack rheumatoid factor. These conditions mainly affect the spine, peripheral joints, and areas where tendons and ligaments attach to bones (entheses) (Luong and Salonen 2000). While they can involve the hands and wrists, axial involvement is more common.

Psoriatic arthritis is a chronic inflammatory condition linked to psoriasis, influenced by both genetic and environmental factors. It affects both cartilage and synovial joints, as well as entheses in the axial and appendicular skeleton. Around 20–35% of affected individuals carry the HLA-B27 genetic marker (Menis et al. 2023). PsA occurs in about 30% of people with psoriasis (Crespo-Rodríguez et al. 2021) and can significantly impact daily function and quality of life. Symptoms include joint pain, swelling, functional impairment, and structural damage. The disease is characterized by inflammatory arthritis, enthesopathy, and bone proliferation, with a tendency to affect the distal interphalangeal (DIP) joints of the hands and feet (Table 10) (Spira et al. 2010). Nail involvement is often linked to DIP joint inflammation. MRI can detect soft tissue swelling and inflammatory changes.

Although wrist involvement is less common in PsA, it can affect the radiocarpal and intercarpal joints, leading to characteristic erosions and periostitis. Pancompartmental involvement of the wrist can occur. However, wrist involvement is rare without more typical distal joint changes. Axial involvement occurs in 20%–40% of people with peripheral PsA, often presenting as sacroiliitis, which can be asymmetric or symmetric, with subchondral erosions, joint space irregularity, and ankylosis.

Ultrasound (Table 11) helps detect early inflammatory changes and soft tissue involvement (Fig. 14). MRI (Table 12) is essential for early diagnosis and tracking disease progression. MRI protocols for PsA typically include T1-weighted images in multiple planes, T2-weighted, and

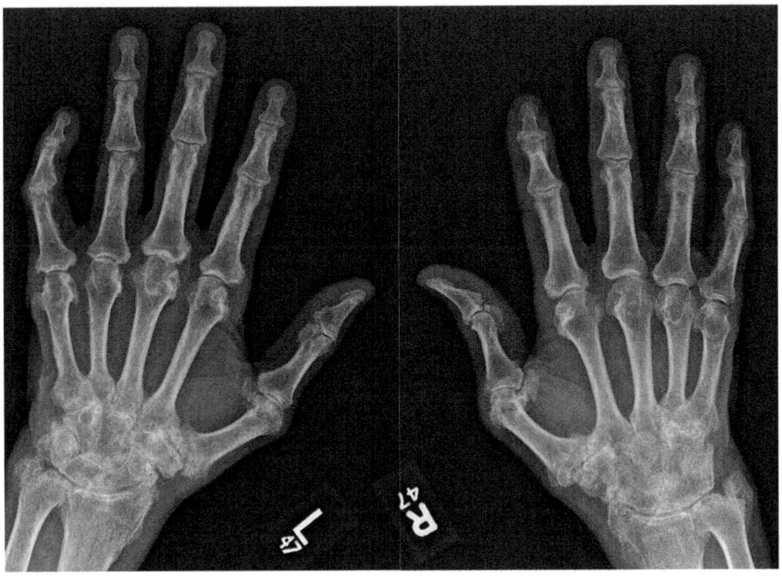

Fig. 13 Psoriatic arthritis. PA radiographs of bilateral hands demonstrate joint space narrowing, erosions, and bony proliferative changes at bilateral interphalangeal, metacarpophalangeal, and wrist joints

Table 11 Ultrasound features of PsA

Synovitis
Joint effusion
Tenosynovitis
Enthesitis
Power Doppler signal indicating active inflammation

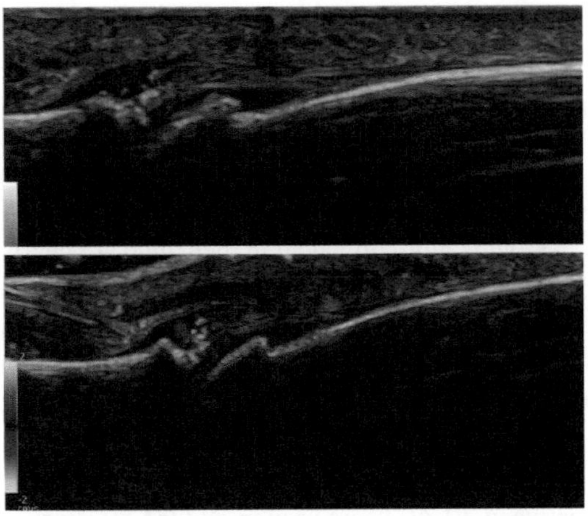

Fig. 14 Enthesitis in psoriatic arthritis. Ultrasound of the third proximal interphalangeal joint demonstrates cortical irregularity at the proximal base of the middle phalanx at the attachment site of the central slip of the extensor tendon. There is thickening of the distal tendinous attachment with adjacent increased Doppler signal

Table 12 MRI features of PsA

Enthesitis
Osteitis/bone marrow edema
Periostitis
Synovitis
Tenosynovitis
Dactylitis, presenting as widespread soft tissue swelling ("sausage digits"). This is due to the flexor tendon sheath tenosynovitis along with synovitis and soft tissue edema (Spira et al. 2010)

contrast-enhanced T1-weighted sequences. STIR sequences to highlight bone marrow edema. CT is less commonly used but can help assess bone erosions and ankylosis in advanced cases.

PsA presents in five clinical subtypes (Sudoł-Szopińska et al. 2016):

- Polyarthritis involving the DIP joints
- Deforming arthritis, which can lead to ankylosis or severe joint destruction (arthritis mutilans)
- Symmetric seronegative polyarthritis, resembling rheumatoid arthritis but without its typical lab markers
- Monoarthritis or asymmetric oligoarthritis
- Sacroiliitis and spondylitis

8.1 Other Seronegative Spondyloarthropathies Affecting the Hand and Wrist (Tables 13, 14, and 15)

Ankylosing spondylitis (AS) has a strong genetic link, with 96% of patients being HLA-B27 positive. AS primarily affects the spine but can involve peripheral joints. Bilateral, symmetric sacroiliitis is a key feature. Radiographs may show spinal syndesmophytes, facet joint inflammation, and eventual fusion. MRI is highly effective for detecting early sacroiliac joint inflammation (Canella et al. 2012).

Reactive arthritis often follows a GI or genitourinary infection. It typically affects young men (ages 25–35). It is more common in the lower limbs, but imaging features mimic PsA. It may present with sausage digits and pencil-in-cup deformities. Sacroiliitis can be asymmetric.

Enteropathic arthritis (EA) is associated with inflammatory bowel diseases (IBD) like Crohn's disease and ulcerative colitis. Peripheral arthritis is often mild and non-erosive. Imaging may show mild periostitis and synovial thickening.

8.2 Other Affected Joints

- Sacroiliitis in PsA is often bilateral and can be symmetric or asymmetric. In AS and enteropathic arthritis, sacroiliitis is often bilateral and symmetric.
- Other affected joints include the knees, elbows, ankles, and shoulders.
- Enthesophytes may develop at sites such as the calcaneus, greater trochanter, ischial tuberosities, medial and lateral malleoli, olecranon, and patella.

Table 13 Radiographic features of seronegative spondyloarthropathies

Bone erosions
Enthesitis
Periostitis
Joint space narrowing
Ankylosis

Table 14 Ultrasound features of seronegative spondyloarthropathies

Synovitis
Tenosynovitis
Enthesitis
Power Doppler signal indicating active inflammation

Table 15 MRI features of seronegative spondyloarthropathies

Enthesitis
Osteitis/bone marrow edema especially in periarticular or subchondral regions
Synovitis
Tenosynovitis

9 Gout

Gout is a common metabolic disorder caused by the deposition of monosodium urate (MSU) crystals in joints and soft tissues due to hyperuricemia. While the first metatarsophalangeal (MTP) joint is most commonly affected, gout can also involve the hand and wrist, presenting as a sudden and painful inflammatory arthritis. Symptoms include intense pain, redness, and swelling, which, if untreated, may lead to tophi formation, joint destruction, and functional impairment. Though less frequent in the upper extremities, gout in the hand and wrist can be significantly debilitating. The most commonly affected joints include the wrist, metacarpophalangeal (MCP) joints, and interphalangeal (IP) joints.

Gout is more prevalent in men, who are nearly three times more likely to develop the condition than women. Black males are the most common affected demographic (Arthritis Foundation 2020). While rare in premenopausal women, postmenopausal women have an increased risk. The incidence of gout rises with age, peaking between 30–60 years in men and 60–80 years in women. Prevalence exceeds 12% in individuals over 80 years old, and gout is strongly associated with metabolic syndrome.

Radiographic changes (Table 16) in gout typically appear 6–8 years after initial presentation. Tophaceous deposits can be found in periarticular soft tissues, synovium, and subchondral bone.

Table 16 Radiographic features of gout

Bilateral and asymmetric joint involvement
Lobulated soft tissue masses (tophi) may show calcification
Soft tissue swelling
Effusion
Well-defined, "punched-out" erosions with overhanging edges and sclerotic margins. Erosions are typically extra-articular but may also be intra-articular or juxta-articular
Preservation of joint space until very late stages
Normal bone mineralization
Widespread articular abnormalities involving the distal interphalangeal (DIP), proximal interphalangeal (PIP), and MCP joints
Prominent involvement of the carpometacarpal (CMC) compartment, often exhibiting large erosions

Erosions may occur intra-articularly or at a distance from the joint (Figs. 15 and 16). US (Table 17) has a sensitivity of 70.1% for diagnosing gout in the hand and wrist, with higher sensitivity for intra-articular (80.3%) compared to extra-articular (42.5%) findings (Klauser et al. 2018). US is helpful modality for guidance for joint aspiration.

CT is particularly useful for confirming tophi, which appear as high-density soft tissue masses (~160 Hounsfield units). This is lower than the density of calcium hydroxyapatite crystals seen in calcific tendinitis. DECT has transformed gout imaging by allowing specific identification and quantification of MSU crystal deposits. DECT

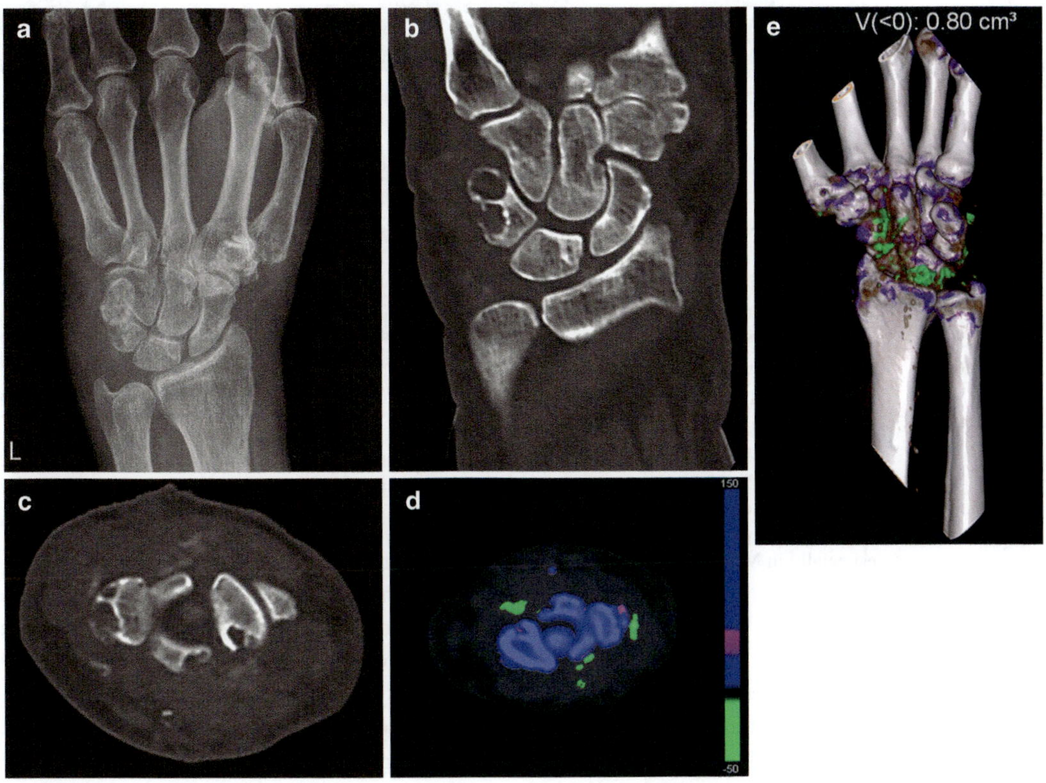

Fig. 15 Gout. (**a**) PA radiograph of the left wrist demonstrates soft tissue swelling at the ulnar aspect and lucent erosions of the triquetrum. (**b, c**) Coronal and axial CT sections of the left wrist show erosions of the triquetrum and diffuse soft tissue thickening with specks of calcification at the wrist. (**d**) Axial spectral dual-energy CT (DECT) image depicts monosodium urate (MSU) crystal deposition in green. (**e**) 3D-rendered DECT image depicts MSU crystal deposition about the wrist in green and volume of crystal burden

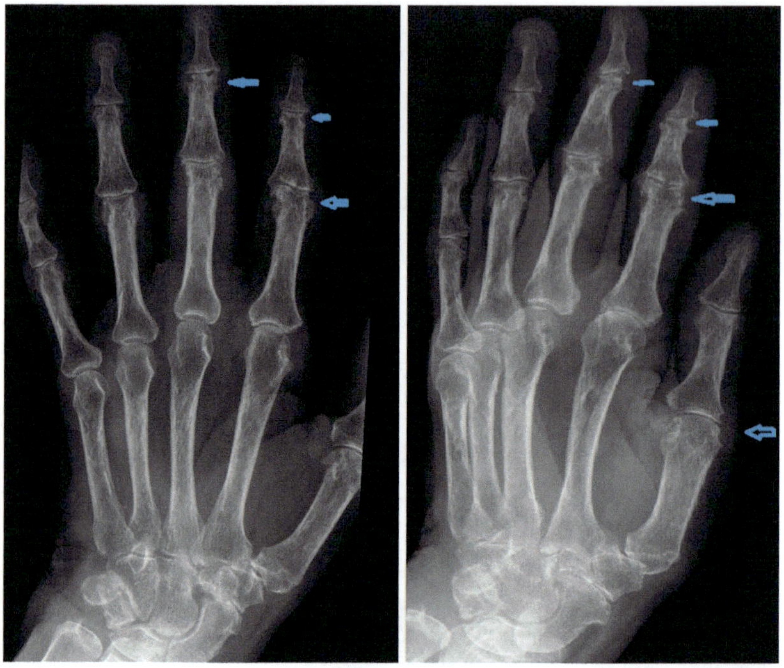

Fig. 16 Gout. PA and oblique radiographs of fingers demonstrate multifocal juxta-articular punched-out osseous erosions with overhanging edges and adjacent soft tissue swelling

Table 17 Ultrasound features of gout (Figs. 17, 18, and 19)

Double contour (DC) sign	Most sensitive indicator of intra-articular gout (Klauser et al. 2018), appearing as a hyperechoic band over the articular cartilage
Hyperechoic aggregates	Representing MSU crystal deposits, these are highly specific for gout
Tophi	Appearing as heterogeneous hyperechoic soft tissue masses, sometimes causing posterior acoustic shadowing
Early bone erosions	Discontinuity of bony surface visible in two perpendicular planes especially in MCP, PIP, and wrist joints

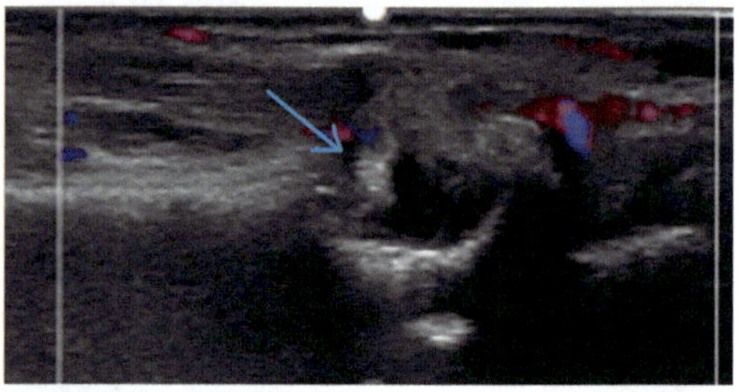

Fig. 17 Gout. Ultrasound of wrist shows erosion at the distal radius (arrow)

has high sensitivity and specificity for detecting MSU crystals in joints, tendons, and periarticular soft tissues. It can visualize both intra- and extra-articular urate deposits (Fig. 15). The ability of DECT to quantify crystal burden is useful for monitoring treatment response.

While not as specific as DECT, MRI provides a detailed assessment of soft tissue and osseous abnormalities (Fig. 20). It is particularly valuable for evaluating tophi size and location, extent of synovitis, erosions, bone marrow edema, and tendon or ligament involvement.

The gold standard for gout diagnosis is the identification of negatively birefringent MSU crystals in synovial fluid or tophus aspirates using polarized light microscopy.

Gout treatment includes medications, lifestyle modifications, and, in severe cases, surgery. NSAIDs, colchicine, and corticosteroids help manage acute attacks, while urate-lowering therapy (e.g., allopurinol, febuxostat) prevents recurrence by reducing uric acid levels. Lifestyle changes such as weight loss, reducing purine-rich foods, and limiting alcohol intake can further

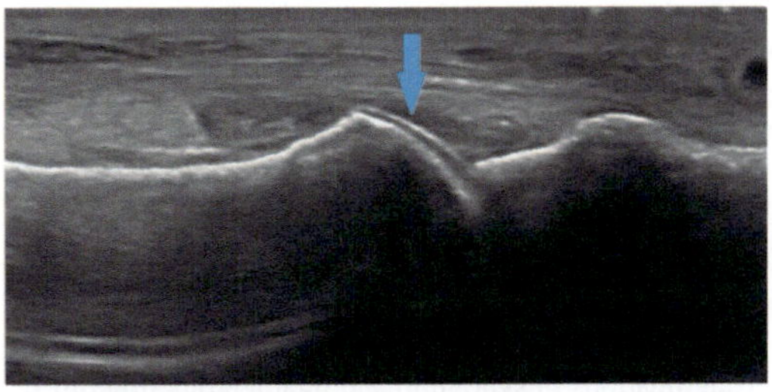

Fig. 18 Gout. Double contour sign on ultrasound (arrow)

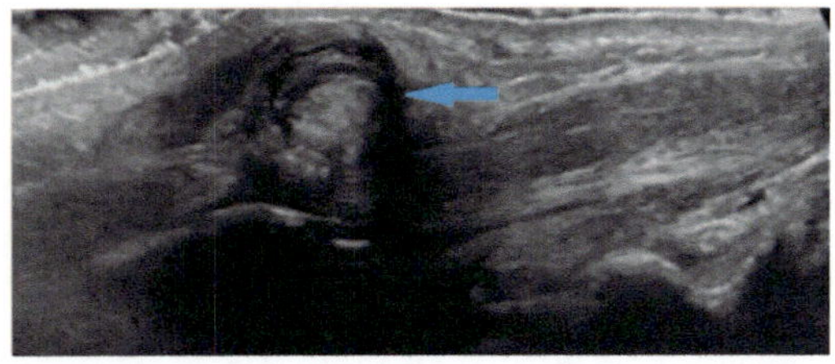

Fig. 19 Gout. Ultrasound of wrist shows gouty tophus adjacent to the extensor digitorum tendon (arrow)

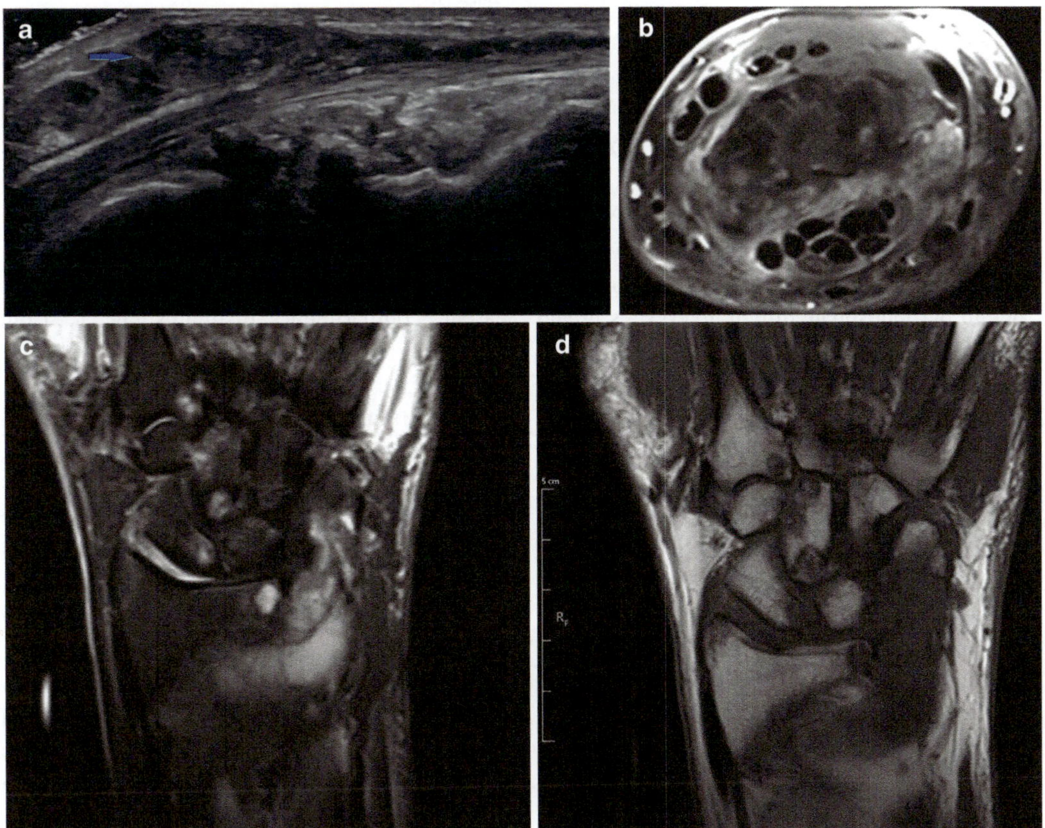

Fig. 20 Gout. (**a**) Ultrasound of wrist—extensive synovial proliferation about the extensor digitorum tendon (arrow). (**b**) Axial post contrast T1FS. (**c**) Coronal STIR. (**d**) Coronal T1 MR images of the wrist show extensive synovial proliferation about the extensor tendons and multifocal erosions

help control the disease. In severe or chronic cases, surgical options like wrist arthroscopy for synovectomy, joint fusion or replacement, and tophi removal may be necessary to restore joint function and alleviate pain.

Other Joints Affected by Gout

- Big toe (most common)
- Ankles
- Knees
- Elbows
- Fingers

Table 18 Radiographic features of CPPD (Fig. 21)

Bilateral distribution in MCP joints
Joint space narrowing, subchondral cysts, sclerosis, small osteophytes
Chondrocalcinosis: Linear or punctate calcifications in articular cartilage and fibrocartilage
Involvement of radiocarpal, midcarpal, and common carpometacarpal joints
Calcifications in synovium and ligamentous structures, particularly the triangular fibrocartilage complex (TFCC), scapholunate, and lunotriquetral ligaments
Carpal malalignment with potential scapholunate diastasis

10 Calcium Pyrophosphate Deposition Disease (CPPD)

Calcium pyrophosphate deposition (CPPD) disease, as the name suggests, is a metabolic arthropathy characterized by the deposition of calcium pyrophosphate dihydrate crystals in and around joints, particularly in articular cartilage and fibrocartilage. Less commonly, calcifications may occur in capsular, synovial, ligamentous, and tendinous structures. CPPD primarily affects middle-aged and elderly individuals, with prevalence increasing with age, with most patients affected being over the age of 65. It rarely occurs under the age of 60 (Zamora and Naik 2025).

Most individuals remain asymptomatic; some may experience intermittent acute attacks of arthritis resembling gout, hence the term "pseudogout."

CPPD arthropathy commonly affects the knee, wrist (radiocarpal and midcarpal joints), metacarpophalangeal (MCP) joints of the hand, shoulder, and hip. The joint changes resemble osteoarthritis and include joint space narrowing, bone sclerosis, and subchondral cyst formation (Table 18). However, CPPD arthropathy can be distinguished by its unusual distribution, relatively small osteophytes contrasting with the presence of severe arthropathy, multiple subchondral cysts, and the presence of chondrocalcinosis. CPPD arthropathy can mimic various conditions, including osteoarthritis, rheumatoid arthritis, and gout (Iqbal et al. 2019). Unlike RA, bone erosions are absent.

CPPD predominantly affects the second and third MCP joints (Miksanek and Rosenthal 2015), characterized by joint space narrowing, sclerosis, subchondral cyst formation, and bony collapse.

In the wrist, CPPD typically affects the radiocarpal compartment, distinguishing it from primary osteoarthritis. Calcification is most commonly observed in the triangular fibrocartilage, hyaline articular cartilage, synovium, and ligamentous structures, particularly the scapholunate and lunotriquetral ligaments. Carpal malalignment with scapholunate separation may occur due to scapholunate ligament disruption, resembling scapholunate advanced collapse (SLAC). However, CPPD-related changes are typically bilateral and occur in older individuals.

US can detect hyperechoic deposits in the hyaline cartilage and fibrocartilage. It has increased sensitivity compared to conventional radiography (Iqbal et al. 2019). US can detect crystal deposits in tendons and soft tissues. Computed tomography (CT) has higher sensitivity for detecting small calcifications (Miksanek and Rosenthal 2015). CT is useful for assessing the extent of joint damage and crystal distribution.

MRI has limited use in evaluation of CPPD arthropathy. MRI can identify presence of synovitis, joint effusion, associated soft tissue changes, and ligamentous involvement.

The definitive diagnosis of CPPD disease requires synovial fluid analysis: identification of characteristic rhomboid-shaped positively birefringent calcium pyrophosphate crystals under

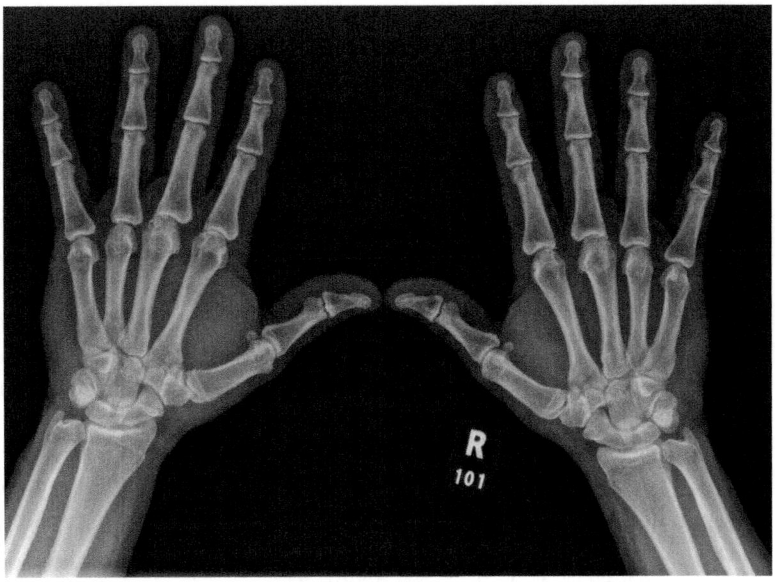

Fig. 21 CPPD. PA radiographs of bilateral hands demonstrate joint space narrowing, subchondral cysts, and small osteophytes in the bilateral second and third metacarpophalangeal joints

polarized light microscopy (Cowley and McCarthy 2023).

10.1 CPPD in Other Joints

CPPD disease can affect various other joints, including the following:

- Knee: Most commonly affected joint in CPPD disease (Krekeler et al. 2022); chondrocalcinosis of the menisci and articular cartilage
- Hip: Often presents with osteoarthritis-like symptoms
- Shoulder: Can mimic rotator cuff pathology
- Spine: May cause crowned dens syndrome or spinal stenosis

10.2 Hemochromatosis

Hemochromatosis is a disorder characterized by excessive iron accumulation in the body, which can lead to various complications, including arthropathy. The condition can be primary (genetic) or secondary (related to chronic diseases or multiple transfusions).

Hemochromatosis arthropathy in the hand and wrist presents with distinct radiographic features that can help differentiate it from other arthritic conditions. The arthropathy of hemochromatosis shares similarities with osteoarthritis but has unique features. Hemochromatosis involves all MCP joints. There is a predilection for the second and third MCP joints. This condition is characterized by uniform loss of joint space, more extensive than typical osteoarthritis. Large subchondral cysts are a common feature. Distinctive hook-like osteophytes projecting from the radial aspect of the second and third metacarpal heads are considered characteristic, though not specific (Table 19). Hemochromatosis arthropathy can involve joints not typically affected by osteoarthritis, such as MCP joints, wrists, elbows, and glenohumeral joints. Unlike CPPD disease, hemochromatosis is less likely to cause scapholunate dissociation. Chondrocalcinosis is similar to that seen in CPPD crystal deposition disease, affecting both hyaline and fibrocartilage. Common sites include knee menisci, triangular fibrocartilage, pubic symphysis, and spine. Hemochromatosis is generally symmetrical and polyarticular, affecting not only the hand and wrist but also other joints such as knees, hips, and shoulders.

Table 19 Radiographic features of hemochromatosis

Radiographic features of hemochromatosis
Symmetric and polyarticular
Diffuse osteopenia
Chondrocalcinosis
Uniform joint space narrowing, large subchondral cysts, sclerosis, osteophytes
Predilection for the second and third MCP joints. The fourth and fifth MCP joints are also frequently affected (Adamson III et al. 1983)
Distinctive hook-like (or beak-like) osteophytes projecting from the radial aspect of the second and third metacarpal heads

MRI is considered the most sensitive and specific imaging modality for diagnosing hemochromatosis. The accumulation of iron leads to a susceptibility effect, causing signal loss in affected tissues, particularly on T2*-weighted sequences (Queiroz-Andrade et al. 2009). This characteristic allows for *detection of iron overload* noninvasively. MRI techniques can estimate hepatic iron concentration, potentially avoiding the need for repeated biopsies.

While less specific than MRI, CT can provide valuable information. Nonenhanced CT may show a homogeneous increase in liver attenuation due to iron deposition. Routine abdominal CT scans can be used for opportunistic screening of liver attenuation, potentially revealing unsuspected iron overload (Lawrence et al. 2018).

Radiographic findings can help differentiate hemochromatosis arthropathy from other conditions. Hemochromatosis can mimic rheumatoid arthritis clinically, but radiographic features differ (Akgöl 2014). While there is overlap of imaging features with CPPD, the more frequent involvement of the fourth and fifth MCP joints and the hook-like osteophytes favor hemochromatosis.

11 Septic Arthritis

Septic arthritis is a medical emergency that necessitates prompt diagnosis and treatment. It should always be considered in cases of monoarticular joint involvement presenting with signs of inflammation. The most common route of infection is hematogenous spread. Other routes include direct extension from adjacent osteomyelitis or soft tissue infection, as well as direct inoculation following trauma or surgical intervention. Infections in the hand and wrist can progress rapidly if neglected, leading to joint destruction and diffuse spread. The definitive diagnosis is typically confirmed through joint aspiration and synovial fluid analysis.

Conventional radiography (Fig. 22; Table 20) is the initial imaging modality for suspected septic arthritis of the hand and wrist. Even if initial radiographic findings are unremarkable, baseline radiographs are valuable for follow-up imaging. Early findings include periarticular osteopenia, joint effusion, and blurring of periarticular fat planes. As the infection progresses, joint space narrowing due to cartilage destruction by pyogenic infection, bone erosions, and periosteal thickening develop. In tuberculous arthritis, periarticular osteopenia is the predominant early feature, while joint space narrowing and erosions occur much later in the disease course.

MRI (Table 21) is the modality of choice for detecting septic arthritis due to its superior soft tissue contrast and ability to visualize intra-articular structures. It is particularly useful for detecting early cartilage and bone involvement before radiographic changes appear. While less sensitive than MRI, ultrasonography is a useful modality, particularly in guiding interventional procedures such as joint aspiration. It is also an alternative imaging option for patients unable to undergo MRI. US findings suggestive of septic arthritis include joint effusion, soft tissue edema, synovial thickening, with power Doppler imaging aiding in the assessment of synovial hypervascularity.

Nuclear medicine techniques, such as three-phase bone scans and white blood cell (WBC) scans, are useful in specific cases, particularly when there is suspicion of concomitant osteomy-

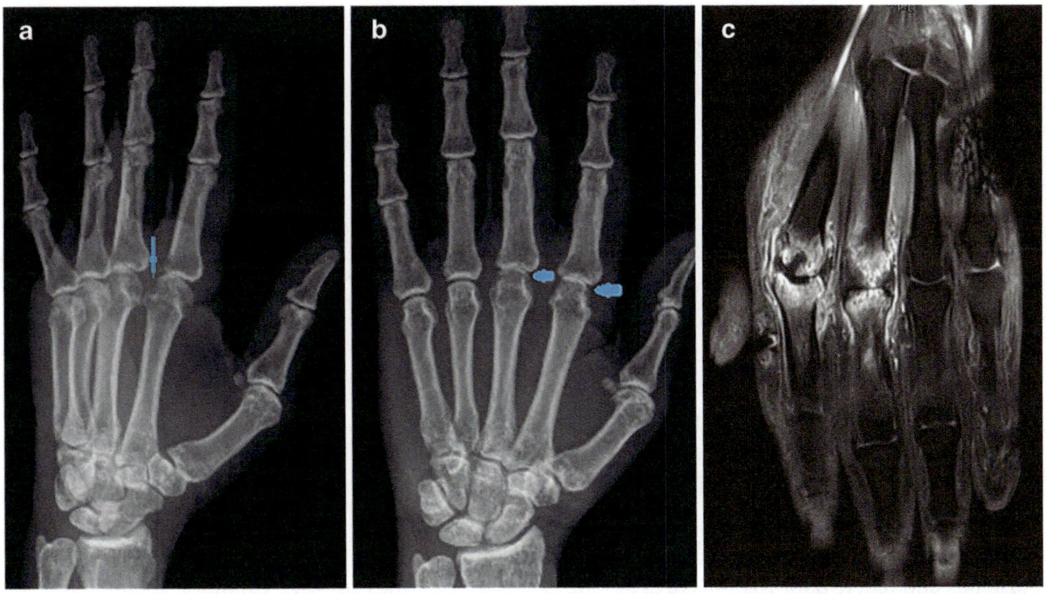

Fig. 22 Septic arthritis. (**a**, **b**) Oblique and PA hand radiographs demonstrate joint space narrowing and erosions at second and third metacarpophalangeal joints. (**c**) Coronal STIR MRI shows marrow edema, joint space loss, erosions, and surrounding soft tissue edema at second and third metacarpophalangeal joints

Table 20 Radiographic features of septic arthritis

Periarticular soft tissue swelling
Joint effusion
Blurring of periarticular fat planes
Joint space narrowing, indicative of cartilage degradation due to pyogenic infection
Osseous erosions
Juxta-articular osteopenia
Periosteal thickening

Table 21 MRI features of septic arthritis (Karchevsky et al. 2004)

Joint effusion
Synovial enhancement and thickening
Pericapsular edema
Bone marrow edema and enhancement, which may be reactive or indicative of osteomyelitis
Bone erosions and periosteal reaction

elitis or in patients with arthroplasty or other implanted intra-articular hardware, where conventional imaging may be limited. The Society of Nuclear Medicine and Molecular Imaging (SNMMI) provides guidelines on the appropriate use of nuclear medicine imaging in musculoskeletal infections (Palestro et al. 2021). Due to their high sensitivity, bone scintigraphy and 18F-FDG PET/PET-CT serve as effective rule-out tests for septic arthritis. When these are inconclusive and osteomyelitis is a diagnostic consideration, labeled leukocyte scintigraphy, either independently or combined with bone or bone marrow scintigraphy, can provide additional diagnostic value. However, Gallium-67 scintigraphy, whether used alone or in combination with bone scintigraphy, is not recommended for diagnosing septic arthritis.

12 Systemic Lupus Erythematosus (SLE) and Other Connective Tissue Diseases

12.1 Introduction

Connective tissue diseases frequently affect the musculoskeletal system, with the hands and wrists being common sites of involvement. Radiological imaging plays a crucial role in identifying characteristic features of these conditions, aiding in early diagnosis, disease monitoring, and treatment planning (Table 22).

In long-standing disease, a subset of patients develop Jaccoud's arthropathy (Fig. 23), a deforming but non-erosive arthropathy affecting the hands and feet (Sudoł-Szopińska et al. 2022). Musculoskeletal ultrasound (Table 23) is increasingly used to detect subclinical synovitis in SLE. Research suggests that a high proportion of patients show some form of joint abnormality on US, even in the absence of significant clinical symptoms (Tani et al. 2018). In one study, 95.1% of SLE patients had at least one joint abnormality, with synovitis being the most common finding, followed by tenosynovitis, joint effusion, and, less frequently, bone erosions (Tang et al. 2020). The third metacarpophalangeal (MCP) joint was identified as the most frequently affected site.

Table 22 Radiographic features of SLE

Non-erosive arthritis in the early stages
Bilateral and symmetric involvement of the small joints
Juxta-articular osteopenia
Subluxations and dislocations, which are initially reversible but may become irreversible with disease progression
Absence of erosions or joint space narrowing in early stages

Table 23 Ultrasound features of SLE

Synovitis
Tenosynovitis
Joint effusion
Bone erosions, though less common

Table 24 MRI features of SLE

Bone marrow edema
Periarticular edema
Joint effusion
Tenosynovitis
Erosions

MRI (Table 24) provides superior soft tissue contrast and is particularly useful for detecting bone marrow edema (BME) and other subtle abnormalities in SLE. Common findings include periarticular capsular edema, joint effusion, and mild synovial hypertrophy, which are often observed in patients with active disease (Sudoł-Szopińska et al. 2022). Bone marrow edema at the wrist has been reported in some studies to occur in 13%–35% of cases (Sudoł-Szopińska et al. 2022). Erosions at the MCP joints and wrists have been detected in a substantial number of patients (Ball et al. 2013). Extensor tenosynovitis at the wrist appears to be more common in SLE than in rheumatoid arthritis (RA) in comparative studies (Ball et al. 2013). MRI findings have been shown to correlate well with ultrasound assessments, particularly for synovitis at the MCP joints and wrist extensor tenosynovitis.

12.2 Mixed Connective Tissue Disease (MCTD) (Table 25)

MCTD shares overlapping features with SLE, scleroderma, and polymyositis/dermatomyositis. Imaging studies have identified common radiographic patterns, including involvement of MCP, PIP, midcarpal, and radiocarpal joints.

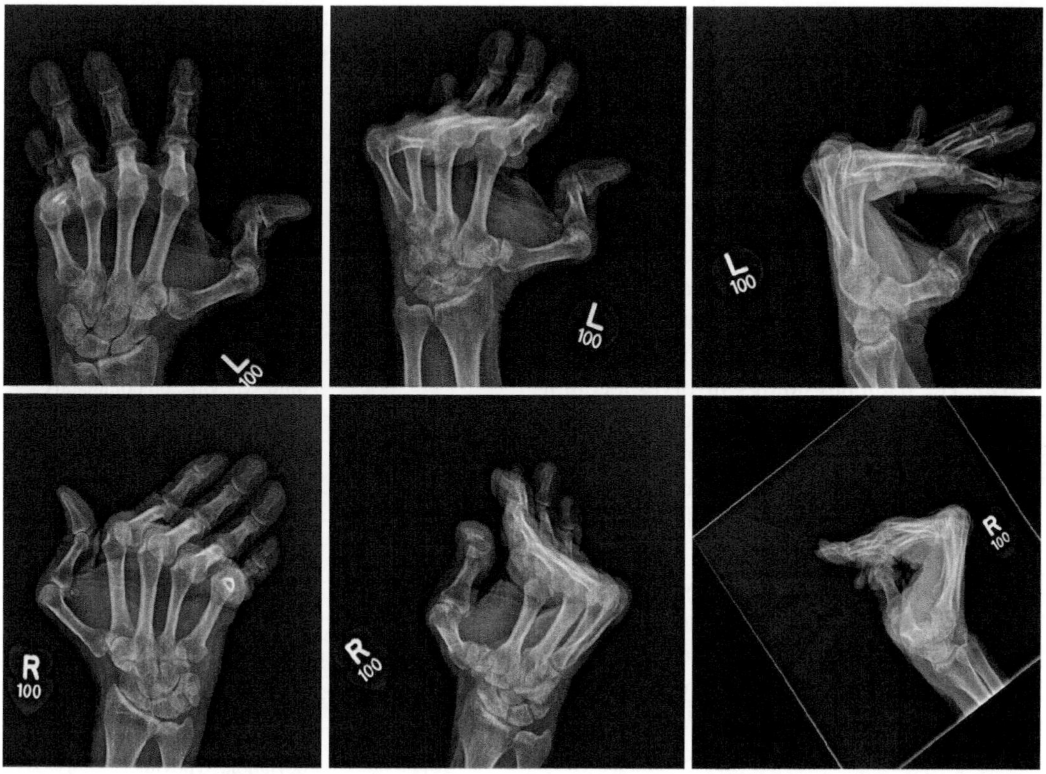

Fig. 23 Jaccoud arthropathy in SLE. PA, lateral, and oblique radiographs of bilateral hands demonstrate volar and ulnar subluxation at bilateral metacarpophalangeal joints. No osseous erosions

Table 25 Radiographic features of MCTD

Periarticular osteopenia
Diffuse joint space narrowing
Osseous erosions, which resemble those seen in rheumatoid arthritis (RA), including distal interphalangeal (DIP) joint involvement
Intra-articular bony ankylosis, which may develop in chronic disease

12.3 Systemic Sclerosis (Scleroderma) (Tables 26 and 27)

Table 26 Radiographic features of systemic sclerosis

Bilateral involvement, can affect first CMC joint, first MCP, distal radioulnar and intercarpal joints, and DIP joints
Osseous erosions—Erosions are common in distal phalanges (Vadher et al. 2023)
Periarticular soft tissue calcifications
Acro-osteolysis (resorption of distal phalanges)

Table 27 MRI features of systemic sclerosis

Synovitis
Bone marrow edema
Erosions
Tenosynovitis
Carpal bone necrosis (Hashimoto et al. 2014)

Ultrasound has proven useful in detecting early soft tissue and vascular changes in systemic sclerosis. Studies report a high prevalence of synovitis and tenosynovitis, often with characteristic imaging patterns. Ultrasound can detect synovitis, tenosynovitis, calcinosis, acro-osteolysis, and distal vascularization (Freire et al. 2013). In a study, the prevalence of synovitis as identified by ultrasound was substantially greater than that detected by clinical examination (Cuomo et al. 2009).

13 Neuropathic Arthropathy (Table 28)

Neuropathic arthropathy, also known as Charcot joint, is a progressive degenerative joint disorder characterized by joint destruction, dislocation, and deformity. While commonly associated with the foot in diabetic patients, it can also affect the hand and wrist, particularly in cases of syringomyelia or cervical spondylotic myelopathy (Jackson et al. 2012). The pathophysiology involves a combination of mechanical and neurovascular factors. Loss of protective sensation leads to repetitive microtrauma, while autonomic dysfunction results in increased blood flow and bone resorption (Dardari 2020).

MRI exhibits high sensitivity in detecting early-stage neuropathic arthropathy by revealing bone marrow edema, subchondral cyst formation, and cartilage damage before radiographic manifestations become apparent. Unlike conventional radiography, a crucial role of MRI in neuropathic arthropathy is distinguishing it from septic arthritis or osteomyelitis. While both conditions may present with bone marrow signal alterations, neuropathic arthropathy typically exhibits joint destruction with relatively mild periarticular inflammatory changes, absence of soft tissue abscess formation, and lack of sinus tracts—features that favor a non-infectious etiology (Noguerol et al. 2017).

Table 28 Radiographic features of neuropathic arthropathy

Joint space narrowing
Subchondral sclerosis
Osteophytes
Joint debris ("bag of bones" appearance)
Subluxation or dislocation
Fragmentation and bone destruction
Joint disorganization

14 Summary of Key Features of Various Arthritis (Table 29)

Table 29 Summary of key features of various arthritis

	Key features
Osteoarthritis (OA)	Nonuniform joint space narrowing, osteophytes, subchondral sclerosis, cysts, Heberden's/Bouchard's nodes, subchondral bone marrow edema and cartilage thinning or loss, mild synovitis, predominantly affects DIP and first CMC joints
Erosive osteoarthritis (EOA)	Uniform joint space narrowing, osteophytes, subchondral sclerosis, central erosions, gull-wing deformities, ankylosis in advanced cases, DIP joint involvement common, typically spares the MCP joints
Rheumatoid arthritis (RA)	Symmetrical, concentric joint space narrowing, wrist, second and third MCP, third PIP, periarticular osteopenia, marginal erosions, ulnar deviation, synovitis, tenosynovitis, bone marrow edema, increased signal on power Doppler US in active inflammation
Psoriatic arthritis (PsA)	Pencil-in-cup deformity, joint erosions, periostitis, enthesitis, dactylitis, synovitis, asymmetric DIP involvement, onycholysis or pitting of nails
Gout	Punched-out erosions with overhanging edges, soft tissue tophi, preserved joint space, MSU crystal deposition on DECT, double contour sign on US, any joint
CPPD (Pseudogout)	Prominent subchondral cysts, chondrocalcinosis, small osteophytes, scapholunate advanced collapse (SLAC), second and third MCP joints, radiocarpal joint, isolated triscaphe joint involvement at the wrist

(continued)

Table 29 (continued)

	Key features
Hemochromatosis	Joint space narrowing, prominent hook-like osteophytes at radial aspect of metacarpal heads, predominant MCP joint involvement
Systemic lupus erythematosus	Non-erosive arthritis, Jaccoud arthropathy, avascular necrosis, synovitis, extensor tenosynovitis
Septic arthritis	Monoarticular, soft tissue swelling, juxta-articular osteopenia, joint effusion, erosions, joint space narrowing when infection progresses, rapid joint destruction, systemic symptoms

15 Conclusion

Radiological imaging remains fundamental in diagnosing and managing various arthritic conditions affecting the hand and wrist. Patterns of joint involvement and characteristic imaging features help distinguish different types of arthritis. While conventional radiography is the cornerstone for initial assessment and chronic disease evaluation, advanced imaging modalities such as MRI, ultrasound, CT, and DECT significantly enhance early detection and disease monitoring. Ultrasound, in particular, plays a crucial role in detecting early inflammatory changes, guiding interventions, and assessing soft tissue involvement with high sensitivity. MRI is particularly valuable for detecting bone marrow edema, synovitis, and cartilage damage—often before these changes become visible on radiographs making it essential for early diagnosis and monitoring disease progression. Each arthropathy exhibits distinct imaging patterns:

- Osteoarthritis and erosive OA reveal joint space narrowing, osteophyte formation, and characteristic deformities.
- Inflammatory conditions like rheumatoid arthritis, psoriatic arthritis, and juvenile idiopathic arthritis display soft tissue swelling, erosions, and joint deformity, often detectable earlier on MRI or ultrasound.
- Crystal deposition diseases such as gout and CPPD show unique calcific or erosive patterns, with DECT and ultrasound providing high specificity.
- Metabolic and infectious arthropathies exhibit overlapping but distinguishable imaging characteristics that, in the appropriate clinical context, facilitate accurate diagnosis.

Emerging technologies, including PET-MRI and AI-driven analysis, are further refining diagnostic accuracy and patient management. In conclusion, a multimodal and tailored imaging approach—guided by clinical suspicion, patient history, and disease progression—is essential in the evaluation of hand and wrist arthritis. Radiologists must be familiar with the evolving imaging spectrum of arthritic diseases to contribute meaningfully to multidisciplinary care and improve patient outcomes.

References

Adamson TC III et al (1983) Hand and wrist arthropathies of hemochromatosis and calcium pyrophosphate deposition disease: distinct radiographic features. Radiology 147(2):377–381

Akgöl G (2014) Hemochromatosis mistakenly treated as rheumatoid arthritis. Arch Rheumatol 29(1):57–60. https://doi.org/10.5606/tjr.2014.3102

Arthritis Foundation (2020) Arthritis by the numbers. https://www.arthritis.org/getmedia/73a9f02d-7f91-4084-91c3-0ed0b11c5814/abtn-2020-final.pdf

Ball (2013) Defining hand arthritis in systemic lupus erythematosus, from an ultrasound, magnetic resonance imaging and antibody status perspective – ACR Meeting Abstracts. https://acrabstracts.org/abstract/defining-hand-arthritis-in-systemic-lupus-erythematosus-from-an-ultrasound-magnetic-resonance-imaging-and-antibody-status-perspective/

Boutry N et al (2007) Early rheumatoid arthritis: a review of MRI and sonographic findings. Am J Roentgenol 189(6):1502–1509. https://doi.org/10.2214/ajr.07.2548

Burke CJ et al (2019) MRI of synovitis and joint fluid. J Magn Reson Imaging 49(6):1512–1527. https://doi.org/10.1002/jmri.26618

Canella C et al (2012) MRI in seronegative spondyloarthritis: imaging features and differential diagnosis in the spine and sacroiliac joints. Am J Roentgenol 200(1):149–157. https://doi.org/10.2214/ajr.12.8858

Colebatch AN et al (2013) EULAR recommendations for the use of imaging of the joints in the clinical management of rheumatoid arthritis. Ann Rheum Dis. https://ard.bmj.com/content/annrheumdis/72/6/804.full.pdf?with-ds=yes

Cowley S, McCarthy G (2023) Diagnosis and treatment of calcium pyrophosphate deposition (CPPD) disease: a review. Open Access Rheumatol Res Rev 15:33–41. https://doi.org/10.2147/oarrr.s389664

Crespo-Rodríguez AM et al (2021) Role of diagnostic imaging in psoriatic arthritis: how, when, and why. Insights Imaging 12:121. https://doi.org/10.1186/s13244-021-01035-0

Cuomo G et al (2009) Ultrasonographic features of the hand and wrist in systemic sclerosis. Lara D Veeken 48(11):1414–1417. https://doi.org/10.1093/rheumatology/kep250

Dardari D (2020) An overview of Charcot's neuroarthropathy. J Clin Transl Endocrinol 22:100239. https://doi.org/10.1016/j.jcte.2020.100239. PMID: 33251117; PMCID: PMC7677697

Elgaddal N, Kramarow E et al (2024) Arthritis in adults age 18 and older: United States, 2022. https://doi.org/10.15620/cdc:145594

Ezzati F, Pezeshk P (2022) Radiographic findings of inflammatory arthritis and mimics in the hands. Diagnostics 12(9):2134. https://doi.org/10.3390/diagnostics12092134

Feydy A et al (2009a) Osteoarthritis of the wrist and hand, and spine. Radiol Clin North Am 47(4):723–759. https://doi.org/10.1016/j.rcl.2009.06.004

Feydy A et al (2009b) Role of imaging in spine, hand, and wrist osteoarthritis. Rheum Dis Clin N Am:605–649. https://doi.org/10.1016/j.rdc.2009.08.007

Freire V et al (2013) Hand and wrist involvement in systemic sclerosis: US features. Radiology 269(3):824–830. https://doi.org/10.1148/radiol.13121994

GBD 2021 Rheumatoid Arthritis Collaborators, Cross M (2023) Global, regional, and national burden of rheumatoid arthritis, 1990–2020, and projections to 2050: a systematic analysis of the Global Burden Of Disease Study 2021. Lancet Rheumatology:e594–e610. https://www.thelancet.com/pdfs/journals/lanrhe/PIIS2665-9913%2823%2900211-4.pdf

Harnden K, Di Matteo A, Mankia K (2022) When and how should we use imaging in individuals at risk of rheumatoid arthritis? Front Med 9. https://doi.org/10.3389/fmed.2022.1058510

Harrold LR et al (2013) Incidence and prevalence of juvenile idiopathic arthritis among children in a managed care population, 1996–2009. J Rheumatol 40(7):1218–1225. https://doi.org/10.3899/jrheum.120661

Hashimoto N et al (2014) FRI0486 analysis of wrist joints in patients with systemic sclerosis using magnetic resonance imaging. Ann Rheum Dis 73(Suppl 2):563.2–563. https://doi.org/10.1136/annrheumdis-2014-eular.1804

Haugen IK et al (2011) Prevalence, incidence and progression of hand osteoarthritis in the general population: the Framingham Osteoarthritis Study. Ann Rheum Dis 70(9):1581–1586. https://doi.org/10.1136/ard.2011.150078

Iqbal SM et al (2019) Updated treatment for calcium pyrophosphate deposition disease: an insight. Cureus [Preprint]. https://doi.org/10.7759/cureus.3840

Jackson K et al (2012) Charcot arthropathy of the wrist associated with cervical spondylotic myelopathy. Glob Spine J 2(4):227–230. https://doi.org/10.1055/s-0032-1315457

Javadi S et al (2014) Wrist and ankle MRI of patients with juvenile idiopathic arthritis: identification of unsuspected multicompartmental tenosynovitis and arthritis. Am J Roentgenol 202(2):413–417. https://doi.org/10.2214/ajr.13.10671

Johns Hopkins Arthritis Center (2020) Rheumatoid arthritis treatment options. Johns Hopkins Arthritis Center. https://www.hopkinsarthritis.org/arthritis-info/rheumatoid-arthritis/ra-treatment/

Kaeley GS, Bakewell C, Deodhar A (2020) The importance of ultrasound in identifying and differentiating patients with early inflammatory arthritis: a narrative review. Arthritis Res Ther 22(1). https://doi.org/10.1186/s13075-019-2050-4

Karchevsky M et al (2004) MRI findings of septic arthritis and associated osteomyelitis in adults. Am J Roentgenol 182(1):119–122. https://doi.org/10.2214/ajr.182.1.1820119

Kay J, Upchurch KS (2012) ACR/EULAR 2010 rheumatoid arthritis classification criteria. Lara D. Veeken 51(suppl 6):vi5–vi9. https://doi.org/10.1093/rheumatology/kes279

Klauser AS et al (2018) Gout of hand and wrist: the value of US as compared with DECT. Eur Radiol 28(10):4174–4181. https://doi.org/10.1007/s00330-018-5363-9

Kluckman ML, Bernard S, Bui-Mansfield LT (2021) A systematic approach to radiographic evaluation of arthritis of the hand and wrist. 44(11). https://cme.lww.com/ovidfiles/00219246-202105310-00001.pdf

Kogan F, Fan AP, Gold GE (2016) Potential of PET-MRI for imaging of non-oncologic musculoskeletal disease. Quant Imaging Med Surg 6(6):756–771. https://doi.org/10.21037/qims.2016.12.16

Kosta PE et al (2011) The usefulness of magnetic resonance imaging of the hand and wrist in very early rheumatoid arthritis. Arthritis Res Ther 13(3). https://doi.org/10.1186/ar3355

Krekeler M et al (2022) High prevalence of chondrocalcinosis and frequent comorbidity with calcium pyrophosphate deposition disease in patients with seronegative rheumatoid arthritis. RMD Open 8(2):e002383. https://doi.org/10.1136/rmdopen-2022-002383

Lawrence EM, Pooler BD, Pickhardt PJ (2018) Opportunistic screening for hereditary hemochromatosis with unenhanced CT: determination of an optimal liver attenuation threshold. Am J Roentgenol 211(6):1206–1211. https://doi.org/10.2214/ajr.18.19690

Luong AA, Salonen DC (2000) Imaging of the seronegative spondyloarthropathies. Curr Rheumatol Rep 2:288–296

Marshall M et al (2013) Erosive osteoarthritis: a more severe form of radiographic hand osteoarthritis rather than a distinct entity? Ann Rheum Dis 74(1):136–141. https://doi.org/10.1136/annrheumdis-2013-203948

McNally EG (2007) Ultrasound of the small joints of the hands and feet: current status. Skeletal Radiol 37(2):99–113. https://doi.org/10.1007/s00256-007-0356-9
Menis J et al (2023) Current characteristics of a population of psoriatic arthritis and gender disparities. J Clin Transl Res [Preprint]. https://doi.org/10.18053/jctres.09.202302.001
Miksanek J, Rosenthal AK (2015) Imaging of calcium pyrophosphate deposition disease. Curr Rheumatol Rep 17(3). https://doi.org/10.1007/s11926-015-0496-1
Muller L-SO, Humphries P, Rosendahl K (2015) The joints in juvenile idiopathic arthritis. Insights Imaging 6(3):275–284. https://doi.org/10.1007/s13244-015-0406-0
Navalho M et al (2012) Bilateral MR imaging of the hand and wrist in early and very early inflammatory arthritis: tenosynovitis is associated with progression to rheumatoid arthritis. Radiology 264(3):823–833. https://doi.org/10.1148/radiol.12112513
Noguerol TM et al (2017) Advanced MR imaging techniques for differentiation of neuropathic arthropathy and osteomyelitis in the diabetic foot. Radiographics 37(4):1161–1180. https://doi.org/10.1148/rg.2017160101
Nusman CM, Rosendahl K, Maas M (2016) MRI protocol for the assessment of juvenile idiopathic arthritis of the wrist: recommendations from the OMERACT MRI in JIA Working Group And Health-e-Child. J Rheumatol 43(6):1257–1258. https://doi.org/10.3899/jrheum.160094
Palestro CJ et al (2021) Appropriate use criteria for the use of nuclear medicine in musculoskeletal infection imaging. J Nucl Med 62(12):1815–1831. https://doi.org/10.2967/jnumed.121.262579
Queiroz-Andrade M et al (2009) MR imaging findings of iron overload. Radiographics 29(6):1575–1589. https://doi.org/10.1148/rg.296095511
Resnick DL et al (2024) Resnick's bone and joint imaging. Elsevier, St. Louis
Rowbotham EL, Grainger AJ (2011) Rheumatoid arthritis: ultrasound versus MRI. Am J Roentgenol 197(3):541–546. https://doi.org/10.2214/ajr.11.6798
Rubin DA (2019) MRI and ultrasound of the hands and wrists in rheumatoid arthritis. I. Imaging findings. Skeletal Radiol:677–695. https://doi.org/10.1007/s00256-019-03179-z
Sahu AK, Kataria S, Gandikota G (2023) Added value of high-resolution ultrasound and MRI in the evaluation of rheumatologic diseases. J Ultrason 23(95):283–296. https://doi.org/10.15557/jou.2023.0035
Saltzherr S et al (2019) Imaging of osteoarthritis and rheumatoid arthritis in hand joints. Erasmus Universiteit, Rotterdam
Selvaag AM et al (2017) Radiographic damage in hands and wrists of patients with juvenile idiopathic arthritis after 29 years of disease duration. Pediatr Rheumatol 15(1). https://doi.org/10.1186/s12969-017-0151-7
Sheybani EF et al (2013) Imaging of juvenile idiopathic arthritis: a multimodality approach. Radiographics 33(5):1253–1273. https://doi.org/10.1148/rg.335125178
Shiraishi M et al (2020) Differentiating rheumatoid and psoriatic arthritis of the hand: multimodality imaging characteristics. Radiographics 40(5):1339–1354. https://doi.org/10.1148/rg.2020200029
Singh SB et al (2024) Role of PET/CT in diagnosing and monitoring disease activity in rheumatoid arthritis: a review. Ann Nucl Med 38(3):165–175. https://doi.org/10.1007/s12149-023-01896-z
Sommer OJ et al (2005) Rheumatoid arthritis: a practical guide to state-of-the-art imaging, image interpretation, and clinical implications. Radiographics 25(2):381–398. https://doi.org/10.1148/rg.252045111
Sotniczuk M et al (2022) The clinical utility of dual-energy computed tomography in the diagnosis of GOUT—a cross-sectional study. J Clin Med 11(17):5249. https://doi.org/10.3390/jcm11175249
Spira D et al (2010) MRI findings in psoriatic arthritis of the hands. Am J Roentgenol 195(5):1187–1193. https://doi.org/10.2214/ajr.10.4281
Sudoł-Szopińska I et al (2016) Diagnostyka obrazowa łuszczycowego zapalenia stawów. Część I: etiopatogeneza, klasyfikacje i rentgenodiagnostyka. J Ultrason 16(64):65–77. https://doi.org/10.15557/jou.2016.0007
Sudoł-Szopińska I et al (2017) Rheumatoid arthritis: what do MRI and ultrasound show. https://doi.org/10.15557/JoU.2017.0001
Sudoł-Szopińska I et al (2022) Update on current imaging of systemic lupus erythematous in adults and juveniles. J Clin Med 11(17):5212. https://doi.org/10.3390/jcm11175212
Suojärvi N et al (2016) Radiocarpal injuries: cone beam computed tomography arthrography, magnetic resonance arthrography, and arthroscopic correlation among 21 patients. Scand J Surg 106(2):173–179. https://doi.org/10.1177/1457496916659226
Tang H et al (2020) Comparison of role of hand and wrist ultrasound in diagnosis of subclinical synovitis in patients with systemic lupus erythematosus and rheumatoid arthritis: a retrospective, single-center study. Med Sci Monit 26. https://doi.org/10.12659/msm.926436
Tani C et al (2018) Imaging of joints in systemic lupus erythematosus. Clin Exp Rheumatol 36:S68–S73
Tsujioka Y et al (2023) Imaging findings of juvenile idiopathic arthritis and autoinflammatory diseases in children. Jpn J Radiol 41(11):1186–1207. https://doi.org/10.1007/s11604-023-01447-6
Vadher AB et al (2023) Ultrasound and magnetic resonance imaging of hands in systemic sclerosis: a cross-sectional analytical study of prevalence of inflammatory changes in patients with subclinical arthropathy. J Scleroderma Relat Disord 8(1):72–78. https://doi.org/10.1177/23971983221140673
World Health Organization (2023) Osteoarthritis. Report
Zamora EA, Naik R (2025) Calcium pyrophosphate deposition disease. [Updated 2023 Jun 20]. In: StatPearls [Internet]. StatPearls Publishing, Treasure Island (FL). Available from: https://www.ncbi.nlm.nih.gov/books/NBK540151/

Imaging of Soft Tissue and Bone Infections of the Hand and Wrist

Thanat Kanthawang, Nuttaya Pattamapaspong, and Wilfred C. G. Peh

Contents

T. Kanthawang · N. Pattamapaspong
Department of Radiology, Faculty of Medicine, Chiang Mai University, Chiang Mai, Thailand
e-mail: thanatkanthawang@gmail.com; nuttaya.p@cmu.ac.th

W. C. G. Peh (✉)
Department of Diagnostic Radiology, Khoo Teck Puat Hospital, Singapore, Republic of Singapore
e-mail: Wilfred.peh@gmail.com

Abstract

Hand infections, whether acute or chronic, require prompt diagnosis and management to prevent complications like stiffness, contractures, or amputation. While most infections of the hand and wrist are confined to superficial soft tissues, deep infections such as necrotizing fasciitis, osteomyelitis, and septic arthritis often require surgical intervention. Imaging is crucial for assessing the infection extent, particularly in cases with suspected bone or joint involvement or deep abscesses, guiding treatment, and distinguishing infections from inflammatory arthritis or tumors. Radiographs are the first-line imaging tool and can be used for monitoring osteomyelitis, with changes appearing 8–10 days post-infection. Magnetic resonance imaging (MRI) is the gold standard for detecting and staging infections, with gadolinium-enhanced imaging aiding in detecting abscesses. Computed tomography (CT) is particularly useful in chronic osteomyelitis for detecting sequestra requiring surgical removal, while ultrasound (US) imaging effectively detects fluid collections, abscesses, and foreign bodies. Chronic infections should be considered in patients presenting with painless swelling or draining sinuses. Comprehensive clinical evaluation, along with pathogen identification through imaging-guided aspiration, is crucial for targeted antibiotic therapy. A multidisciplinary approach, involving radiolo-

Med Radiol Diagn Imaging (2025)
https://doi.org/10.1007/174_2025_595,
Published Online: 26 October 2025

gists, infectious disease specialists, and hand surgeons, is essential for optimizing treatment and minimizing morbidity.

Abbreviations

CRP	C-reactive protein
CT	Computed tomography
DECT	Dual-energy computed tomography
DWI	Diffusion-weighted imaging
ESR	Erythrocyte sedimentation rate
FBs	Foreign bodies
HIV	Human immunodeficiency virus
NF	Necrotizing fasciitis
MRI	Magnetic resonance imaging
MRSA	Methicillin-resistant *Staphylococcus aureus*
TB	Tuberculosis
US	Ultrasound
WBC	White blood cell

1 Introduction

Hand infections, commonly encountered by hand surgeons and primary care physicians, vary in anatomical extension, severity, and causative organisms (Flevas et al. 2019). Neglected wounds are the leading cause of hand infections, and patients with comorbidities such as diabetes mellitus and immunocompromised conditions significantly increase the risk of serious outcomes (Houshian et al. 2006). Superficial infections, which affect the skin, nail folds, or subcutaneous tissues, often resolve with antibiotic treatment. In contrast, deep infections involving tendons, bones, or joints typically require surgical intervention to prevent serious complications such as stiffness, contractures, or tissue necrosis. Differentiating between superficial and deep infections is essential for determining the appropriate treatment and promoting recovery (Houshian et al. 2006; Flevas et al. 2019). The hand's complex anatomy necessitates precise identification of affected structures for adequate removal of the infectious tissue, while maintaining the hand functions. Imaging studies play a vital role in diagnosing hand infections, particularly deep ones, by identifying affected compartments and distinguishing them from mimicking conditions such as non-infectious limb swelling, inflammatory arthritis, or crystal arthropathies (Louis and Jebson 1998). This chapter examines hand and wrist infections in terms of anatomy, patterns of spread, causative organisms, imaging findings, and treatment response evaluation.

2 Pathophysiology

2.1 Type of Infection

Hand and wrist infections are classified as either superficial or deep infections, depending on their location relative to tendons (Ahlawat et al. 2017). Superficial infections constitute 70–85% of cases (Brown and Young 1993), including cellulitis, lymphangitis, subcutaneous abscesses, and infection of the nail and fingertip such as paronychia, herpetic whitlow, and pulp space infection. These infections are typically managed in outpatient settings without the need for imaging studies. In contrast, deep infections, such as tenosynovitis, deep fascial space infections, septic arthritis, and osteomyelitis, often require hospitalization, intravenous antibiotics, and surgical intervention. Major hospital centers report 25–100 annual admissions for hand infections, with tenosynovitis being the most common (Brown and Young 1993; Turker et al. 2014). A review of 159 patients who required surgery for hand infections found that tenosynovitis was the most common diagnosis (67.3%), followed by soft tissue abscess (17.0%) and septic arthritis (11.9%), with these three entities collectively accounting for up to 95% of cases (Imahara and Friedrich 2010).

Penetrating injuries, including lacerations and animal or human bites, are the leading causes of infection (Imahara and Friedrich 2010; Fowler and Ilyas 2013; Turker et al. 2014). Retained foreign bodies (FBs) occur in as high as 7–15% of traumatic wounds, which can be unrecognized by clinical examination alone in up to 38% of cases (Anderson et al. 1982). The hand is easily injured during daily activities or minor trauma, and small wounds are often overlooked. Infections commonly affect the palm, dorsal hand (21%), middle finger or third web space (17%), and index finger or second web space (16%) (Turker et al. 2014).

2.2 Review of Anatomy

The soft tissue anatomy of the hand influences the patterns of infection spread and complications. To help gain an understanding of the relevant anatomy, the hand structures can be divided into three groups, comprising: (a) the nail complex and pulp space; (b) the synovial spaces, including the flexor and extensor tendon sheaths and the radial and ulnar bursae; and (c) the volar and dorsal spaces.

2.2.1 Nail Complex and Pulp Space

The nail complex (Fig. 1) consists of the nail plate and perionychium. The nail plate is the hard translucent part, while the perionychium includes the nail bed and soft tissue bordering the sides (paronychium). The nail bed, located beneath the plate, contains the germinal matrix proximally and the sterile matrix distally. The nail plate lies beneath the nail fold, with the eponychium being the portion where the fold attaches to the nail surface. The hyponychium, at the junction of the nail bed and fingertip skin, is composed of keratin and serves as a barrier against bacterial and fungal invasion (Zook 1990).

The distal pulp space is a "close sac" of connective tissue separated from the rest of the finger. Vertical trabeculations extend from the periosteum to the epidermis (Fig. 1), forming a latticework of septal compartments in the distal phalanx. The digital artery supplies the epiphysis of distal phalanges, then enters the pulp and supplies the diaphysis. Severe infection of the distal pulp can cause compression or thrombosis, leading to diaphyseal necrosis.

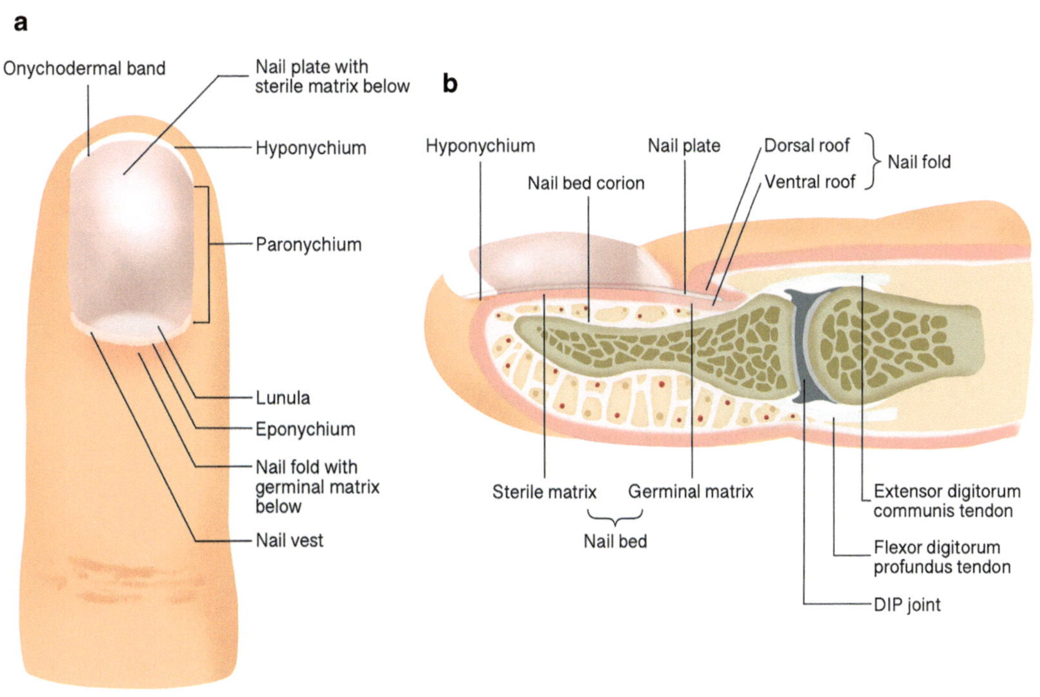

Fig. 1 (**a**, **b**) Line drawings illustrate the anatomy of the nail complex, including the nail plate, perionychium (nail bed and paronychium), eponychium, and hyponychium. The nail bed consists of the germinal matrix and sterile matrix (**b**). The pulp space contains vertical trabeculations and septal interstices. The extensor digitorum communis and flexor digitorum profundus tendons are also depicted (**b**)

2.2.2 Synovial Spaces

The tendon sheaths (Fig. 2) consist of two layers: the visceral layer, which adheres to the tendon as the epitenon, and the parietal layer. These two layers form a closed system, connecting proximally and distally. The flexor tendon sheath extends from the metacarpal neck (at the level of A1 pulley) to the distal interphalangeal joint (Doyle 1989). Typically, the flexor tendon sheaths of the thumb and little finger communicate with the radial and ulnar bursae, respectively. In about 15% of cases, variations connect the sheaths of the index, middle, or ring fingers to the radial or ulnar bursae (Scheldrup 1951; Fussey et al. 2009). Flexor tendons receive nutrients through the vascular system and diffusion from synovial fluid. Infection within this closed system increases pressure, obstructing the blood supply, leading to tendon necrosis and rupture (Schnall et al. 1996). The synovial sheaths for the six extensor compartments are located below the dorsal carpal ligament, extending slightly above and below it (Resnick 1975).

Radial and ulnar bursae (Fig. 2) are synovial spaces of the palm and wrist. The radial bursa, originating from the flexor pollicis longus tendon sheath at the metacarpophalangeal joint, extends 1–2 cm proximal to the transverse carpal liga-

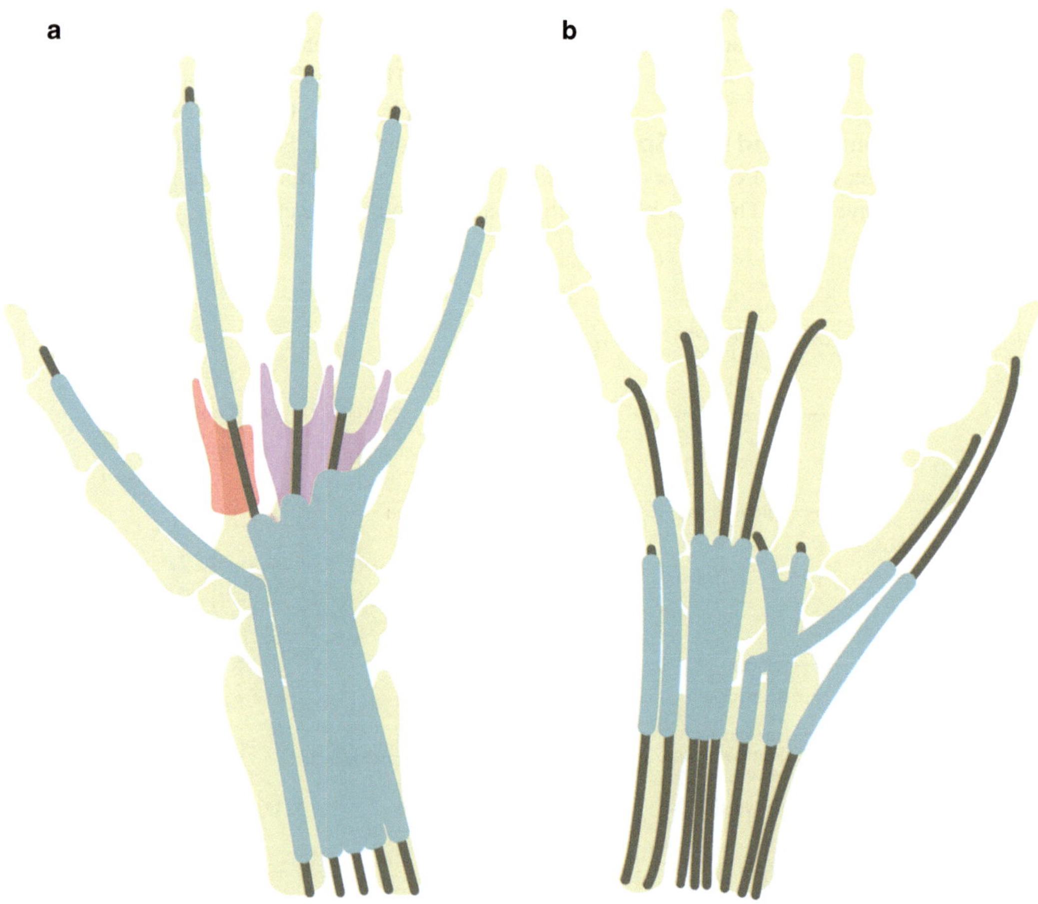

Fig. 2 Line drawings of the hand and finger tendons and tendon sheaths. (**a**) The volar view of the hand shows the flexor tendons (dark green), flexor tendon sheaths, and radial and ulnar bursae (light green), and deep spaces, including the thenar (orange) and midpalmar (purple) spaces. (**b**) The dorsal view of the hand shows the extensor tendons (dark green) and their associated tendon sheaths (light green). Typically, infection of the flexor tendon sheaths of the thumb and little finger spreads to the radial and ulnar bursae, respectively, whereas infection of the tendon sheaths of the second, third, and fourth digits does not spread to the bursae unless there is direct communication

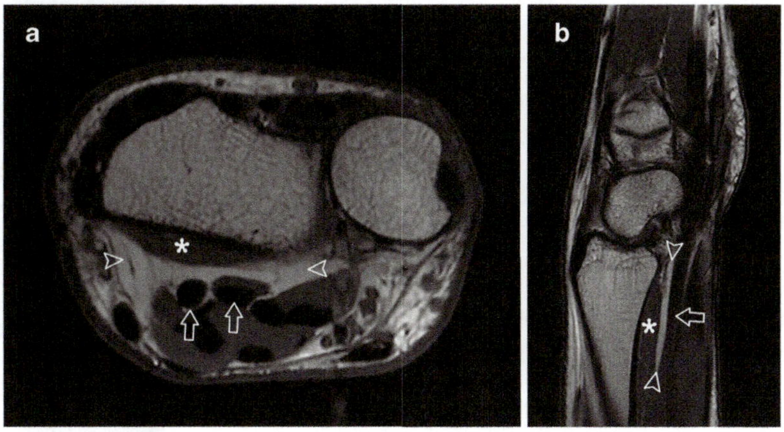

Fig. 3 (**a**) Axial and (**b**) sagittal T1-weighted MR images of the wrist show the space of Parona (open arrowheads), which is a potential space in the distal forearm between the fascia of the pronator quadratus muscle (asterisk) and the flexor digitorum profundus tendon sheath (open arrows)

ment. Similarly, the ulnar bursa continues from the flexor tendon sheath of the little finger, extending proximally past the transverse carpal ligament (Kanavel 1921; Scheldrup 1951; Doyle 1989). The ulnar bursa, wider at its proximal end, overlaps the bases of the third and fourth metacarpals and partially invaginates the flexor tendons without fully enclosing them. In up to 80% of individuals, these bursae extend to the carpal tunnel (Resnick 1975; Aguiar et al. 2006; Fussey et al. 2009). The radial and ulnar bursae can be directly connected (33–100% of cases) or may connect through the subfascial space of Parona in the forearm (Resnick 1975; Aguiar et al. 2006; Fussey et al. 2009) (Fig. 3).

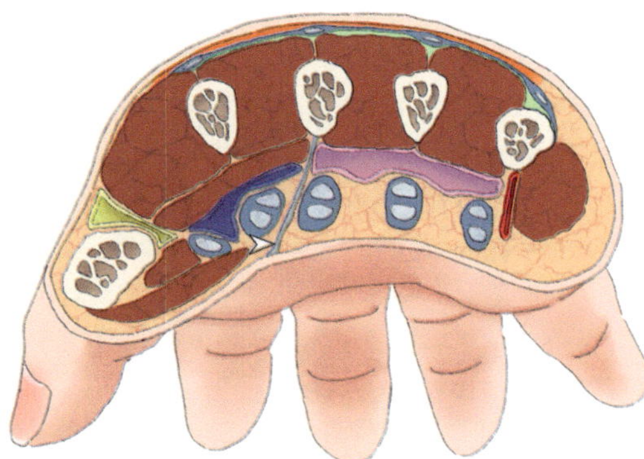

Fig. 4 Cross-sectional line drawing through the metacarpal bones outlines the two volar deep spaces—the midpalmar (pink) and thenar (purple) spaces—separated by a septum (arrowhead) and positioned deep to the digital flexor tendon sheaths. Notably, the sheath of the index finger is closely related to the thenar space (purple), while the sheaths of the third, fourth, and fifth fingers are associated with the midpalmar space (pink). A small hypothenar space (red) is also observed. The dorsal spaces include the superficial dorsal subcutaneous space (orange), the deeper dorsal subaponeurotic space (green), and the interdigital web spaces (yellow, representing the first interdigital web space)

2.2.3 Subfascial Deep Spaces

The volar deep subfascial spaces (Fig. 4) include the thenar, midpalmar, and hypothenar spaces in the hand and the space of Parona in the forearm. The thenar and midpalmar spaces are separated by the midpalmar septum, while the midpalmar and hypothenar spaces are divided by the hypothenar septum. The thenar space, which lies between the thenar eminence and the third metacarpal, is bordered dorsally by the adductor pollicis muscle, volarly by the index finger flexor tendon, radially by the adductor pollicis insertion, and ulnarly by the midpalmar septum (Jebson 1998). The midpalmar space lies in the center of the palm, bordered dorsally by the periosteum of metacarpals and interosseous muscles and ventrally by the flexor tendons and lumbrical muscles, with the midpalmar septum radially and the hypothenar muscles ulnarly (Jebson 1998).

The hypothenar space, located between the hypothenar septum and muscles, has its dorsal boundary formed by the fifth metacarpal periosteum and deep hypothenar fascia. The space of Parona is a potential space in the distal volar forearm, located between the fascia of the pronator quadratus muscle and the flexor digitorum profundus tendon sheath (Fig. 3). The space directly

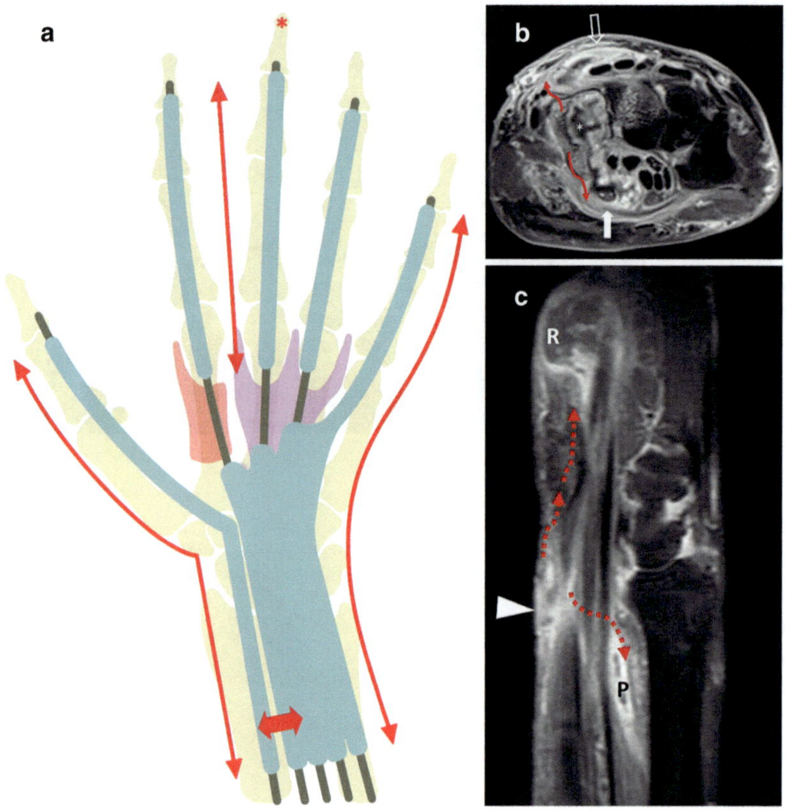

Fig. 5 (**a**) Line drawing (volar view) illustrates the spread of infection in the hand and fingers. Infection spreads from the flexor tendon sheaths of the thumb and little finger to the radial and ulnar bursae, respectively (curved double-headed red arrows). Infection may spread between the radial and ulnar bursae through a direct communication (short straight double-headed red arrow). In contrast, infections of the tendon sheaths of second, third, and fourth digits typically are limited in the finger (long straight double-headed red arrow) and do not typically spread to the bursae unless direct communication is present. The tips of digits are the common site of primary infection (*). (**b**) Axial fat-suppressed contrast-enhanced T1-weighted MR image of a 78-year-old-man shows the spread of infection from osteomyelitis in the hamate (*) to the extensor (open arrow) and flexor (solid arrow) tendon sheaths. The curved red arrows indicate the pathway of spread. (**c**) Sagittal fat-suppressed contrast-enhanced T1-weighted MR image of a 39-year-old man with a penetrating wound in the wrist (solid arrowhead). The infection spreads from the wound to the radial bursa in the forearm and hand (R) then to the space of Parona (P). The dotted red arrows indicate the pathway of spread

communicates with the midpalmar space but does not connect to the radial or ulnar bursae unless the bursae are ruptured (Fig. 5). Infection of the space connecting to either radial or ulnar bursae can form a large horseshoe-shaped abscess (Sharma et al. 2013).

The dorsal spaces include the dorsal subcutaneous space, dorsal subaponeurotic space, and interdigital web spaces (Fig. 4). The dorsal subcutaneous space is the superficial layer between the skin and the extensor tendon aponeurosis, containing loose connective tissue without distinct boundaries. The deeper dorsal subaponeurotic space lies between the extensor tendon aponeurosis and the periosteum of the metacarpals and dorsal interosseous muscle fascia (Jebson 1998). It forms a truncated cone, narrower proximally and wider distally (Kanavel 1921). The interdigital web spaces, located between the fingers, consist of loose connective tissue and extend around the deep intermetacarpal ligaments. The second through fourth web spaces are beneath the palmar fascia, with their dorsal boundary formed by the distal hand fascia and skin. The radial and ulnar borders are defined by the extensor mechanisms and metacarpophalangeal joint capsuloligamentous structures (Jebson 1998).

2.3 Routes and the Spread of Infection

The hand can be infected by three routes (Resnick 1976):

- *Direct implantation*. This occurs after penetrating injuries that disrupt the skin, which is the most common route. Infections can also be introduced during procedures such as arthrography, arthroscopy, open surgery, or pin insertion.
- *Hematogenous spread*. Pathogens enter via the bloodstream, often originating from the respiratory, genitourinary, or gastrointestinal systems. This route is unusual and occurs more commonly in children, elderly, immunocompromised individuals, and intravenous drug users (Koshy and Bell 2019).
- *Spread from a neighboring infection*. An infection can extend from one tissue layer to another, such as from the subcutis to bone or joint, or from bone marrow to an adjacent joint or soft tissue, or communication between bursae and tendon sheaths (Fig. 5).

Osteomyelitis of the hand is relatively rare due to its extensive blood supply (Ong and Levin 2009; Turker et al. 2014). It most often arises from direct inoculation following a penetrating injury or contiguous spread from adjacent soft tissue infections such as suppurative flexor tenosynovitis or felon. As a result, approximately 70% of cases involve a single bone, with the distal phalanx being the most commonly affected (38%), followed by the proximal phalanx and the metacarpals, often resulting from a clenched-fist injury (fight bite) (Reilly et al. 1997). The soft tissue infection initially leads to periostitis, followed by the invasion of the cortical bone, and eventually progresses to osteomyelitis as the infection spreads into the medullary bone through the cortical Haversian and Volkmann's canals (Resnick 1976). On rare occasions, osteomyelitis that occurs in the bone via hematogenous spread can extend to the soft tissues (Fig. 5c).

In septic arthritis of the hand, the location of the affected joint is related to the route of spread (Resnick 1976). Joints of the fingers are commonly infected by the spread of osteomyelitis from the phalanges. Penetrating injuries such as cuts, stabs, bites, or during diagnostic or surgical procedures lead to infection of metacarpophalangeal and proximal interphalangeal joints (Resnick 1976) (Fig. 6). Hematogenous seeding of pathogens, particularly in patients with severe sepsis or significant immunological deficiencies, affects carpal joints (Resnick 1976).

2.4 Causative Organisms

Hand infections are commonly caused by a range of pathogens, with *Staphylococcus aureus* being the most prevalent, accounting for 30% to 80% of positive cultures, followed by *Streptococcus* species (Fowler and Ilyas 2013; Turker et al. 2014; Kistler et al. 2019). *Staphylococcus aureus* is the primary pathogen responsible for clean surgical infections, whereas *Staphylococcus epidermidis* is more frequently associated with infections related to implants (Gastrin and Lovestad 1989). Methicillin-resistant *Staphylococcus aureus* (MRSA) is increasingly prevalent, particularly in urban areas, accounting for up to 65% of *Staphylococcus aureus* cases (Fowler and Ilyas 2013; Turker et al. 2014; Kistler et al. 2019). Table 1 outlines the types of infections and their common causative organisms.

Certain microorganisms are strongly associated with specific types of injuries. *Eikenella corrodens* is commonly linked to human bites, while *Pasteurella multocida* is frequently isolated in animal bites (Houshian et al. 2006). Group A β-hemolytic *Streptococcus* is the most commonly identified single organism in necrotizing soft tissue infections (DeLullo et al. 2013). Although *Staphylococcus aureus* is the most common pathogen in septic arthritis, *Neisseria gonorrhoeae* should also be considered a potential causative agent (Flevas

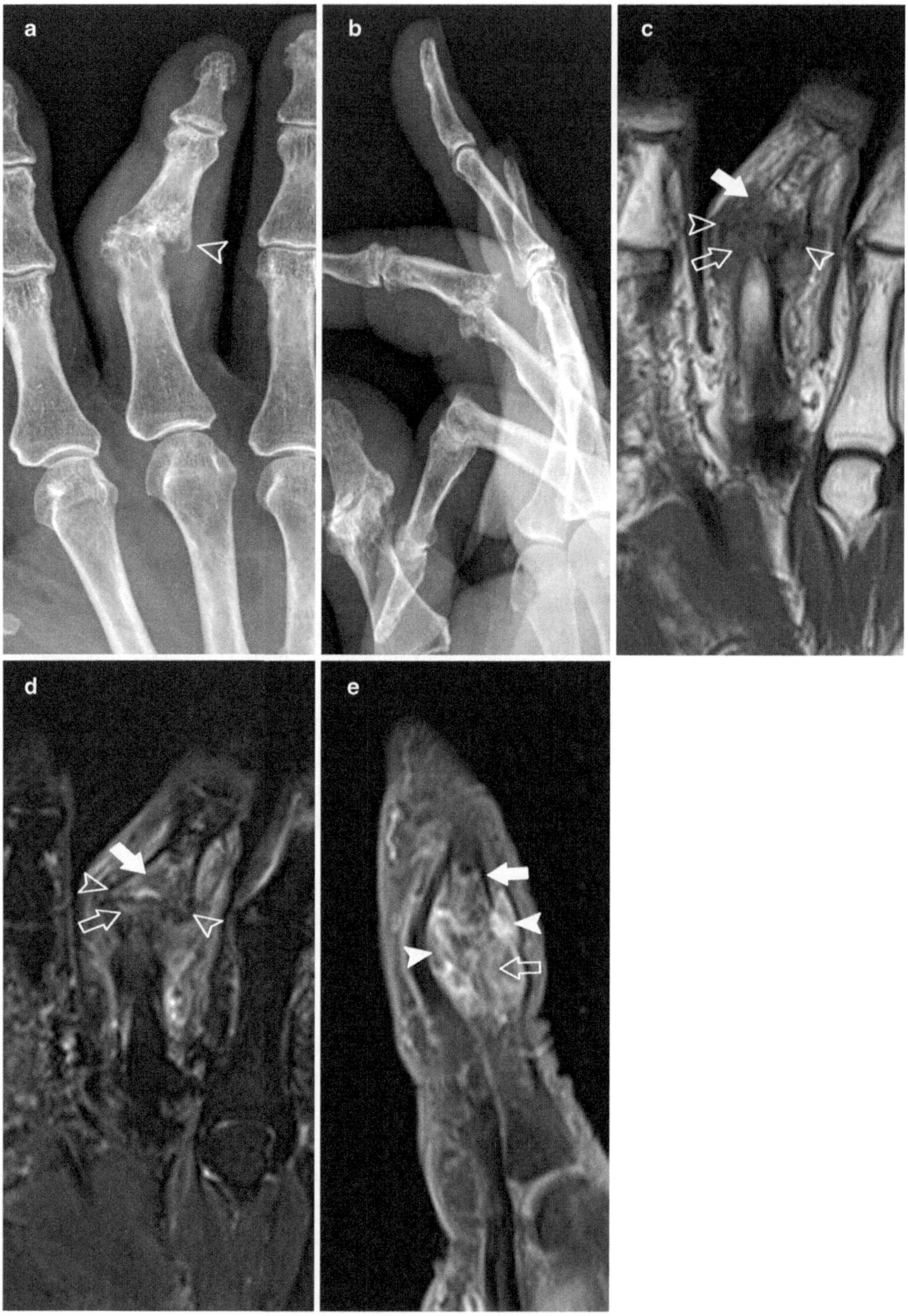

Fig. 6 Septic arthritis of the third proximal interphalangeal (PIP) joint in a patient who presented with joint swelling for 3 weeks. The patient had a history of a cut wound that had healed by the time of the MRI. (**a**) Posteroanterior and (**b**) lateral radiographs of the third finger show soft tissue swelling around the PIP joint, accompanied by ulnar and dorsal subluxation and bone erosions (open arrowhead). Coronal (**c**) T1-weighted and (**d**) short tau inversion recovery (STIR), and (**e**) sagittal fat-suppressed contrast-enhanced T1-weighted MR images show synovitis (solid arrowheads), a small joint effusion, and multiple bone erosions (open arrowheads). Subchondral bone changes (arrows) exhibit signal hyperintensity on STIR (**d**) and enhancement on contrast-enhanced (**e**) images. Marked T1 hypointensity in the middle phalanx (solid arrow in **c**) is suggestive of osteomyelitis, while preserved fatty marrow signal in the proximal phalanx (open arrows in **c**) indicates reactive bone marrow edema

Table 1 Types of infection and common causative organisms

Type of infection	Common causative organisms
Cellulitis	*S. aureus, Streptococcus* species
Necrotizing fasciitis	*Streptococcus* species, polymicrobes
Abscess (paronychia, felon, deep space infection)	*S. aureus*
Flexor tenosynovitis	*S. aureus, anaerobes*
Septic arthritis	*S. aureus*
Human bite	*S. aureus, Streptococcus* species, *Eikenella corrodens*, anaerobes
Animal bite	*Pasteurella multocida, S. aureus, Streptococcus* species

et al. 2019). Farm injuries, bite wounds, and infections in immunocompromised individuals, such as those with diabetes mellitus or human immunodeficiency virus (HIV) infection, are often polymicrobial (Ong and Levin 2009; Flevas et al. 2019). Anaerobic organisms are particularly prevalent in infections related to diabetes mellitus and intravenous drug use (Jalil et al. 2011; Flevas et al. 2019).

Atypical infections can also occur in the hand and wrist. *Candida albicans* frequently causes chronic paronychia in individuals exposed to wet environments (Shafritz and Coppage 2014). *Mycobacterium marinum* and *Vibrio* species are commonly associated with soft tissue infections following aquatic injuries (Diaz and Lopez 2015). Other atypical mycobacteria, such as *Mycobacterium avium*, can affect both immunocompromised and healthy individuals (Al-Qattan and Helmi 2014). In endemic areas, *Mycobacterium tuberculosis* and *Mycobacterium leprae* should also be considered in the setting of a chronic slowly progressing infection that is resistant to broad-spectrum antibacterial treatment. Recognizing these associations is essential for guiding appropriate antimicrobial therapy.

3 Clinical Features and Complications

A thorough history and physical examination are critical for diagnosing and treating hand infections. Key factors include the patient's age, occupation, handedness, comorbidities, and immune status. Detailed history-taking should identify the time of onset, nature of injury, previous treatments, and any signs of systemic febrile illness or hematogenous spread. Understanding the setting of inoculation and chronicity helps guide empiric antibiotic coverage.

Certain populations are at higher risk, including manual laborers, patients with diabetes mellitus, intravenous drug users, transplant recipients, and immunocompromised individuals (Clark 2003; Rerucha et al. 2019). Patients with diabetes mellitus are prone to deep infections caused by atypical organisms and often require multiple surgeries (Sharma et al. 2018; Schmidt et al. 2019), while transplant recipients and patients on immunosuppressive drugs, including biological disease-modifying antirheumatic drugs (DMARDs), face a higher risk of extensive infection, multiple debridement, and amputation (Schmidt et al. 2019). Elderly individuals, due to poor vascular perfusion and weakened skin barriers, and newborns with immature immune systems are also particularly vulnerable (Flevas et al. 2019).

Chronic hand infections, though uncommon, should be a concern in the setting of persistent hand ulcers, abscesses, or masses, particularly in immunocompromised individuals. While *Mycobacterium tuberculosis* was historically the leading cause of chronic hand infections, nontuberculous mycobacteria are now more prevalent (Patel et al. 2014). Musculoskeletal tuberculosis (TB) begins from a primary pulmonary infection developing in the post-primary stage, with hand involvement in about 5% of cases, but there is increased incidence in endemic areas (Pattamapaspong et al. 2024). Mycobacteria often target the synovium, with a tendency to involve tendon sheaths more frequently than bones or joints (Jaovisidha et al. 1996).

Clinical manifestations of hand infections are the result of inflammatory response and complications. Early infections are often localized due to the hand's compartmentalized anatomy, with symptoms like redness, warmth, swelling, pain, and functional impairment. Localized symptoms help identify infections such as paronychia, felon, or herpetic whitlow (Clark 2003; Shafritz and Coppage 2014). Fluctuance or unresolved cellulitis may indicate abscesses, while crepitus suggests gas gangrene or necrotizing infection (Koshy and Bell 2019).

Kanavel's signs (flexed position and fusiform swelling of the digit, tenderness to palpation along the flexor tendon sheath, and pain upon passive digit extension) are key for diagnosing flexor tenosynovitis, while pain with joint movement may signify septic arthritis (Kennedy et al. 2016; Koshy and Bell 2019). Tendon rupture associated with tenosynovitis should be carefully evaluated (Schnall et al. 1996). Osteomyelitis may present with bony pain, erythema, or occasionally draining sinuses, especially in the chronic stage (Koshy and Bell 2019). Neurovascular compression is crucial, especially for infections in enclosed spaces such as the carpal tunnel. Inappropriate or delayed treatment causes fibrous ankylosis, joint subluxation, pathological fractures, and limb deformities, especially in pediatric patients.

Patients should be evaluated for febrile illness and systemic infection. Laboratory tests, including white blood cell (WBC) count, erythrocyte sedimentation rate (ESR), and C-reactive protein (CRP), help in assessment of systemic inflammation and monitoring the treatment response. Nevertheless, the body temperature, ESR, and CRP levels may not always be abnormal and may therefore have limited diagnostic value (Houshian et al. 2006).

Necrotizing fasciitis (NF) is a medical emergency and should be suspected in patients with hemodynamic instability, even if the soft tissue infection appears mild or unimpressive (Chan et al. 2008). Early in the disease, the infection may seem benign, with delayed onset of clinical signs (Flevas et al. 2019). Strong indicators, such as skin necrosis, bullae, crepitus, detecting gas on imaging and hemodynamic instability, are not always present (Ong and Levin 2009). In cases of high clinical suspicion, particularly in hemodynamically unstable patients, imaging is not necessary prior to proceeding with surgery.

4 Imaging Features

Imaging is typically unnecessary for superficial infections such as paronychia and felon but essential for deep or complex cases, aiding diagnosis and surgical planning, as well as avoiding potential complications. Advanced imaging modalities play a crucial role in evaluating complex infections. Each modality has its own advantages, and occasionally, several modalities are used in combination.

4.1 Radiography

Radiographs serve as the initial modality and are complimented by spot views in equivocal cases. They help confirm inflammatory involvement of the hand. Radiographs are able to detect FBs, soft tissue gas, fractures, and osteoarticular conditions such as osteomyelitis and septic arthritis (Koshy and Bell 2019). Gas collections are derived either from skin disruption or from gas-forming pathogens. They also effectively identify radiodense FBs, e.g., metal and glass, which can act as infection niduses. On oblique views, subtle cortical lesions may sometimes be detected at the injury site after a deep bite down to the bone surface (Capitanio and Kirkpatrick 1970; Resnick 1976) (Fig. 6). Although limited in assessing soft tissue, radiographs can reveal para-articular swelling indicative of inflammatory change in septic arthritis, abscesses, tenosynovitis, or bursitis.

Early-stage osteomyelitis may not show radiographical changes until 2 weeks after onset, with osteolysis, osteopenia, and periostitis becoming visible (Reilly et al. 1997) (Fig. 7). Early signs of

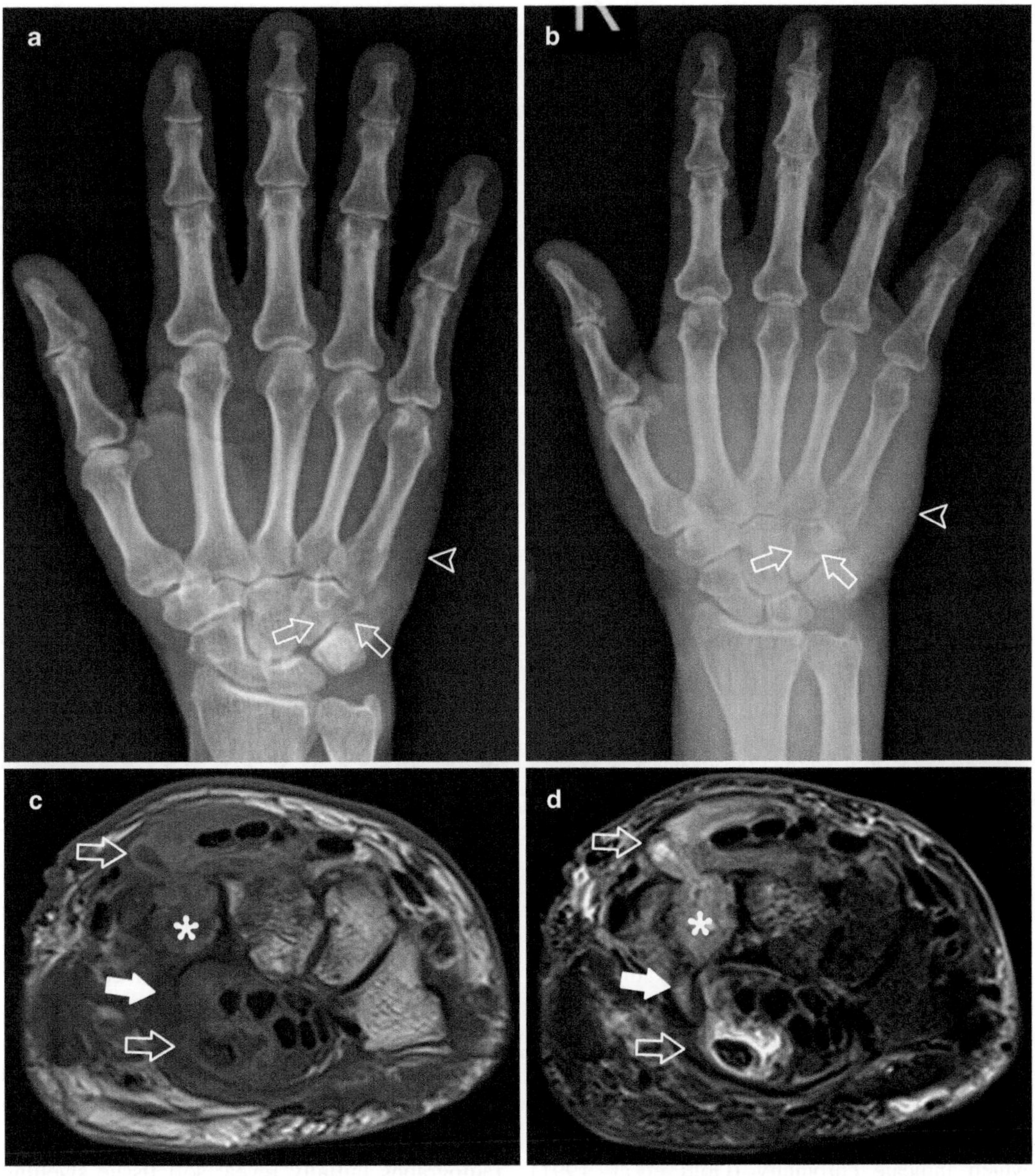

Fig. 7 Osteomyelitis and tenosynovitis in a 78-year-old man. Posteroanterior radiograph of the right hand taken (**a**) 1 week after the onset of wrist pain and (**b**) at 2-week follow-up shows a progressive osteolytic lesion in the hamate bone (open arrows), consistent with acute osteomyelitis. Increasing soft tissue swelling is noted around the wrist, particularly on the ulnar side, corresponding to progressive tenosynovitis (open arrowheads). Axial (**c**) T1-weighted, (**d**) fat-suppressed T2-weighted, (**e**) fat-suppressed-contrast-enhanced T1-weighted and (**f**) apparent diffusion coefficient (ADC) MR images (B-value = 800) obtained at 5 weeks after the onset of symptom show osteomyelitis with an intraosseous abscess in the hamate (asterisk), extensor and flexor tenosynovitis, and ulnar bursitis (open arrows). The restricted diffusion area on the ADC image (**f**) corresponds to the rim enhancement at the wall of abscesses (**e**). (**g**) Coronal fat-suppressed T2-weighted MR image of the hand and wrist shows flexor tenosynovitis, ulnar bursitis, and extension of the infection to the space of Parona, forming a characteristic horseshoe-shaped abscess (open arrows)

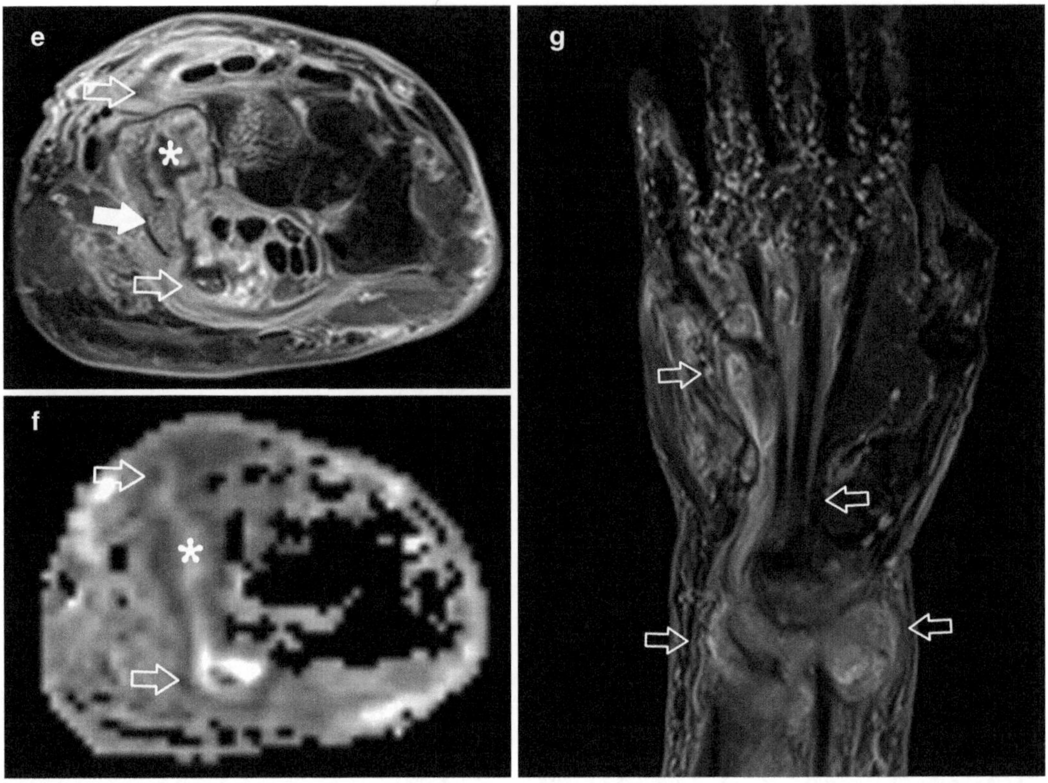

Fig. 7 (continued)

acute osteomyelitis include subtle periosteal reaction and focal subperiosteal osteopenia (Capitanio and Kirkpatrick 1970). In the subacute stage, a round or elongated radiolucency with surrounding osteosclerosis, tortuous shape, and a connection to the growth plate is characteristic of a Brodie's abscess (Pineda et al. 2009) (Fig. 8). Advanced osteomyelitis is characterized by osteosclerosis, sequestra, and involucrum which indicate chronicity (Gold et al. 1991) (Fig. 8). Presence of sequestra, and progression of bone destruction or periosteal reaction around the cortical bone defects, indicates active disease.

In septicemia, although rare, pathogens can spread hematogenously, leading to acute osteomyelitis or pyogenic arthritis around the wrist, with the infectious source remaining unknown in up to 50% of cases (Pineda et al. 2009). Hematogenous osteomyelitis typically originates in the metaphysis, where slow blood flow in venous sinusoids facilitates bacterial implantation. The pattern of spread is age-dependent. In infants, limited metaphyseal vessels penetrate the bone plate, causing simultaneous osteomyelitis and purulent arthritis. In children and adolescents, the sharp turn of vessels at the growth plate restricts infection to the diametaphysis. In adults, free vascular communication through the closed bone plate allows the infection to spread to the epiphysis (Resnick 1976). In septic arthritis, radiographs initially reveal soft tissue swelling and periarticular osteopenia, progressing to erosions, joint space narrowing, and eventual joint collapse with usually monoarticular distribution.

TB serves as an example for imaging findings in chronic hand infections. Radiographic changes, which are usually noticeable 2–4 months after the symptom onset, are named the Phemister triad comprising periarticular osteopenia and marginal erosions with preserved joint space (Phemister and Hatcher 1933) (Fig. 9). Advanced cases may show para-articular abscesses, calcification, and significant destruction of intercon-

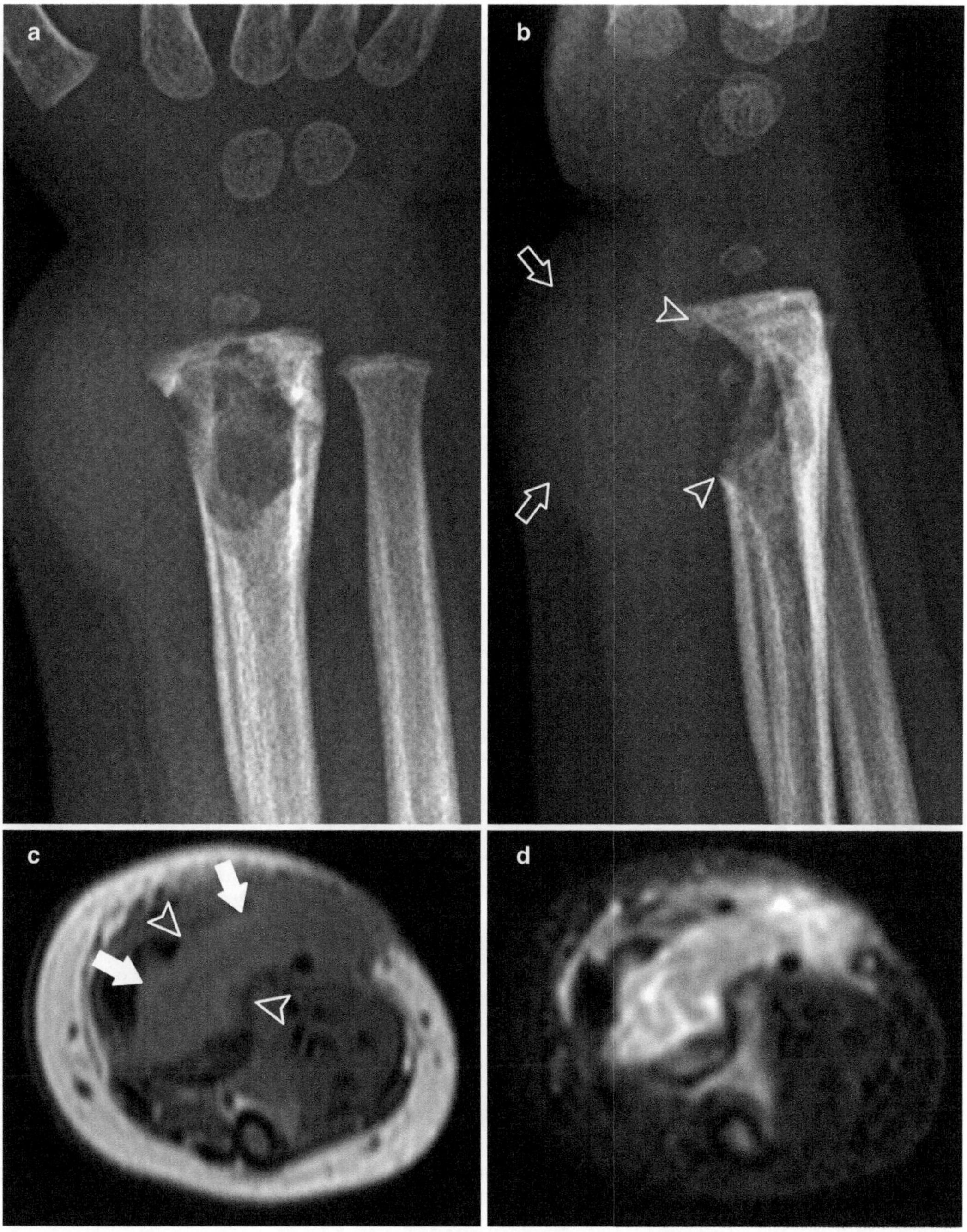

Fig. 8 Tuberculous osteomyelitis with transphyseal spread in an 11-month-old infant who presented with wrist pain and swelling for 1 month. (**a**) Posteroanterior and (**b**) lateral radiographs of the wrist show a geographical osteolytic lesion in the distal radial metaphysis with an associated soft tissue mass (open arrows), continuous periosteal reaction, and cortical destruction or cloaca (open arrowheads). Axial (**c**) T1-weighted, (**d**) STIR, and (**e**) fat-suppressed contrast-enhanced T1-weighted MR images show a penumbra sign with a T1-hyperintense wall in the intraosseous and soft tissue abscesses (solid arrows in **c**). Note the cloaca (open arrowheads in **c**). (**f**) Coronal spoiled gradient echo image of the wrist shows osteomyelitis in the distal radial metaphysis with transphyseal spread into the unossified epiphysis (solid arrowhead). The T2-hyperintense signal in the subperiosteal region indicates periosteal infectious materials (open arrows). Follow-up radiographs taken at (**g**) 4 months and (**h**) 1 year after drainage of the abscess and antibiotic treatment show healing of the cortical bone defect, and gradually reduced size of intramedullary bone destruction and periosteal reaction, with a persistent small osteolytic lesion in the metaphysis of distal radius at 1 year

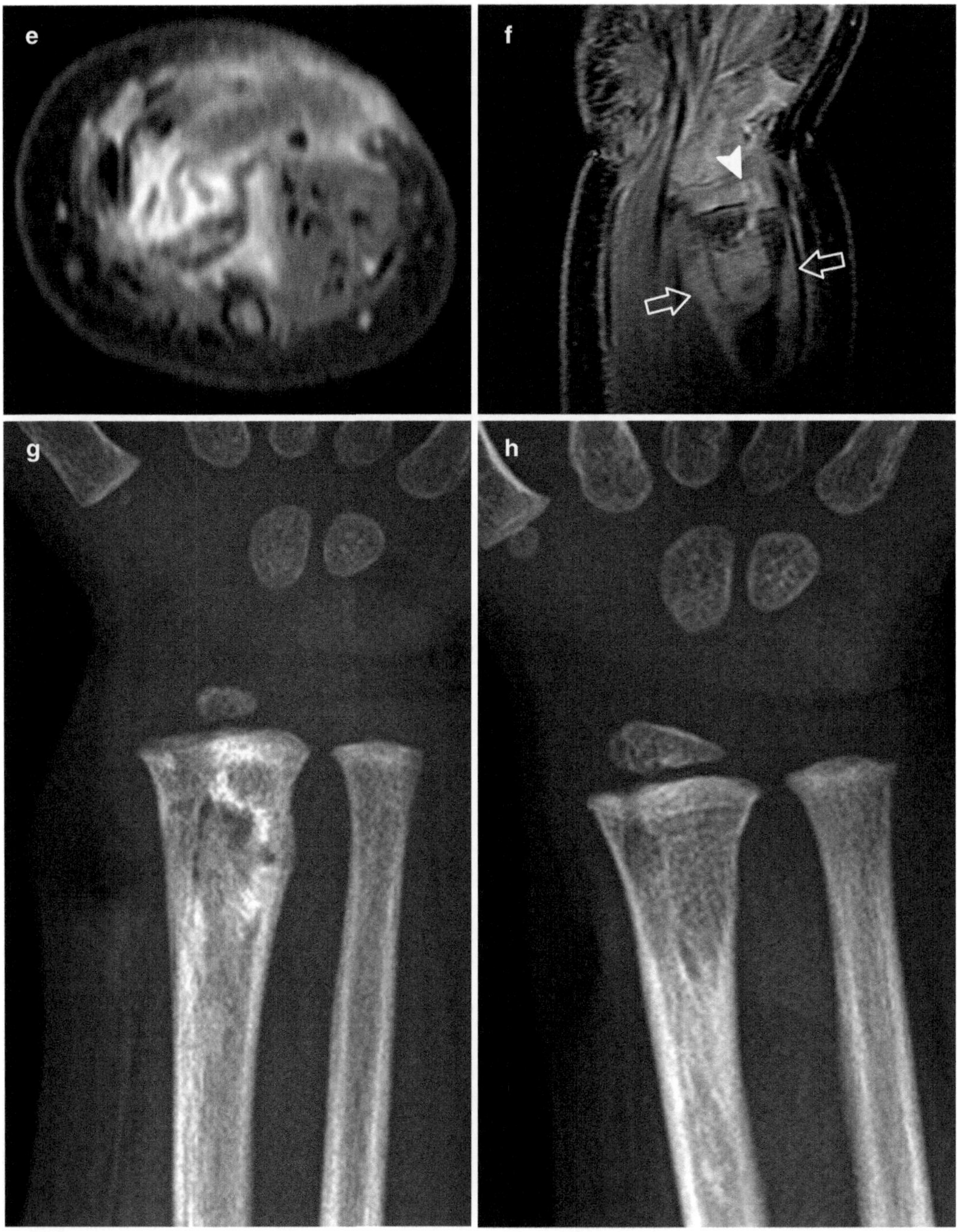

Fig. 8 (continued)

necting wrist joints (Singh et al. 2023). Calcifications are usually observed in soft tissue abscesses and tendon sheath involvement during the healing process. TB osteomyelitis is common in children and exhibits distinctive patterns, including transphyseal spread (Fig. 8), spina ventosa (or TB dactylitis, characterized by short tubular bone enlargement with subperiosteal proliferation), and cystic osteomyelitis resulting from hematogenous spread (Ranjan et al. 2019;

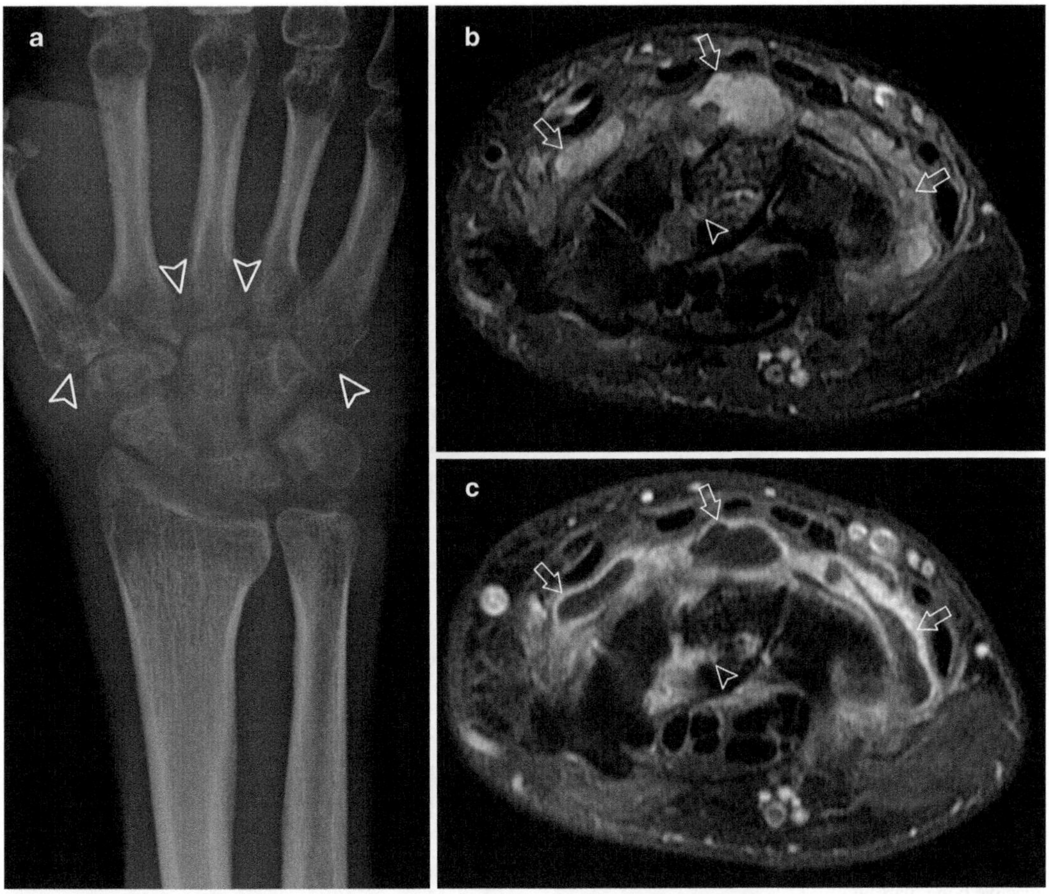

Fig. 9 Tuberculous (TB) arthritis in a 32-year-old man with a history of treated TB spondylodiscitis who presented with wrist pain for 2 months. (**a**) Posteroanterior radiograph of the wrist shows juxta-articular osteopenia and multiple bone erosions (open arrowheads) affecting the radiocarpal, distal radioulnar, intercarpal, and carpometacarpal joints. Despite these erosive changes, the joint spaces remain preserved, consistent with Phemister's triad, a classic radiographic feature of TB arthritis. Axial (**b**) fat-suppressed T2-weighted and (**c**) fat-suppressed contrast-enhanced T1-weighted MR images show thickened synovitis, bone erosions (open arrowheads), and periarticular abscesses (open arrows)

Pattamapaspong et al. 2024). Multiple cystic osteomyelitis, or osteitis cystica tuberculosa multiplex, is a rare pediatric condition in children under 5 years of age, characterized by multiple osteolytic lesions that heal with focal sclerosis (Agarwal et al. 2011).

Untreated or delayed treatment can cause complications such as fibrous ankylosis, joint subluxation or dislocation, early osteoarthritis, pathological fractures, and premature physeal closure, which are detectable on radiographs. In children, reactive hyperemia in growing ossification centers may lead to enlarged epiphyses.

4.2 Magnetic Resonance Imaging

Magnetic resonance imaging (MRI) is highly effective for assessing hand and wrist infections, including soft tissue involvement, early bone marrow changes, and abscesses. It delineates disease extension from bones (Figs. 7 and 8) and joints (Figs. 6 and 10) to surrounding soft tissues, tendon sheaths (Figs. 7 and 11), and bursae (Figs. 5 and 7), while detecting early structural damage such as erosions, tissue necrosis, and cartilage defects. It is also valuable for visualizing transphyseal extension in unossified epiphyses (Teo and Peh 2004) (Fig. 8).

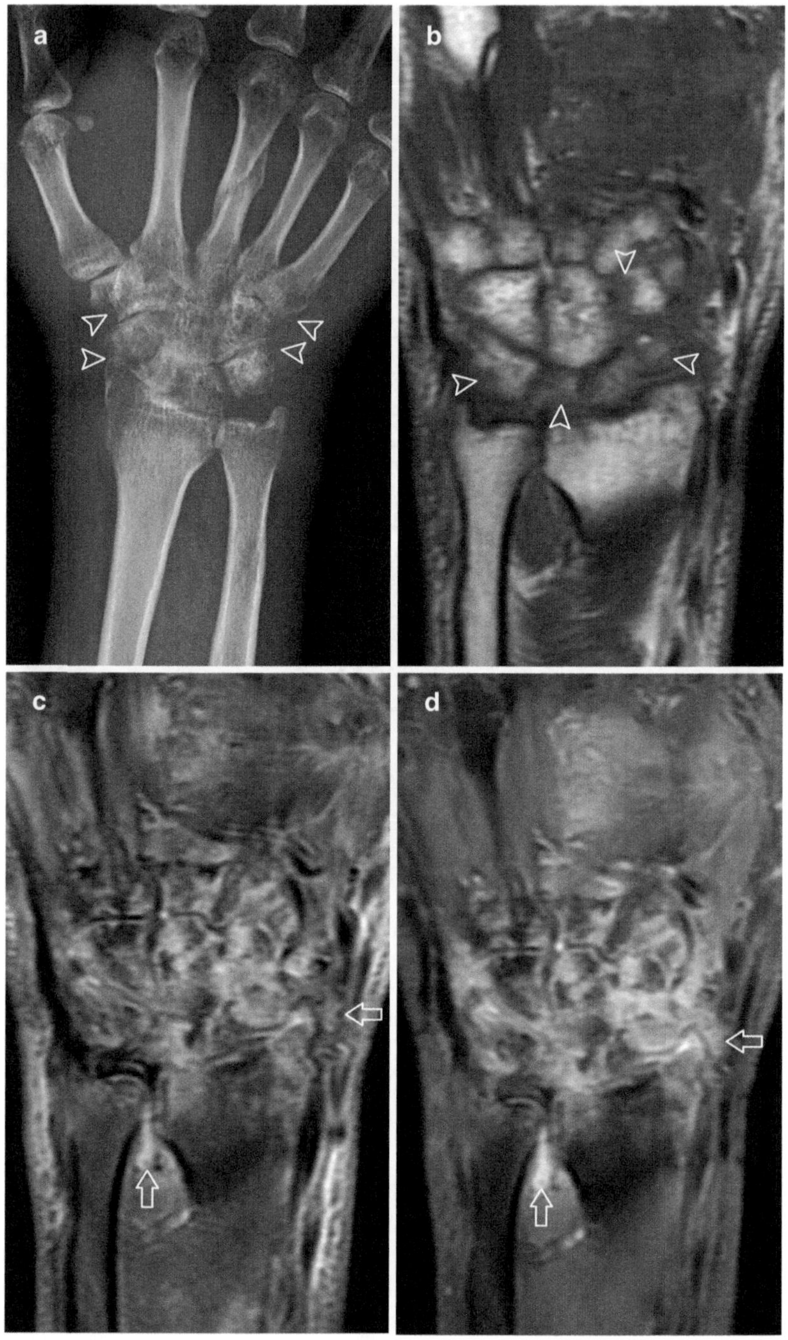

Fig. 10 Septic arthritis in a 40-year-old man who presented with wrist pain for 1 week. (**a**) Posteroanterior radiograph of the wrist shows juxta-articular osteopenia involving the radiocarpal, distal radioulnar, intercarpal, and carpometacarpal joints, with several bone erosions (open arrowheads). An old fracture in the third metacarpal shaft is also noted. Coronal (**b**) T1-weighted, (**c**) fat-suppressed T2-weighted, and (**d**) fat-suppressed contrast-enhanced T1-weighted MR images show several bone erosions (open arrowheads) with subchondral bone marrow edema and diffuse synovitis (open arrows). The absence of a T1-hypointense signal compared to the muscle around the bone erosions in (**b**) distinguishes reactive bone marrow edema from osteomyelitis

The use of dedicated surface or phased-array multi-channel coils enables high-resolution imaging, which is essential for evaluating small structures like the hand. T2-hyperintense and T1-hypointense signals in bone and soft tissue on MRI cannot reliably distinguish between infectious and non-infectious inflammation (Pineda et al. 2009). MRI may sometimes overestimate or underestimate the extent of infection. Contrast-enhanced MRI is highly sensitive for diagnosing musculoskeletal infections, with 100% sensitivity and 77% specificity (Hopkins et al. 1995). It is

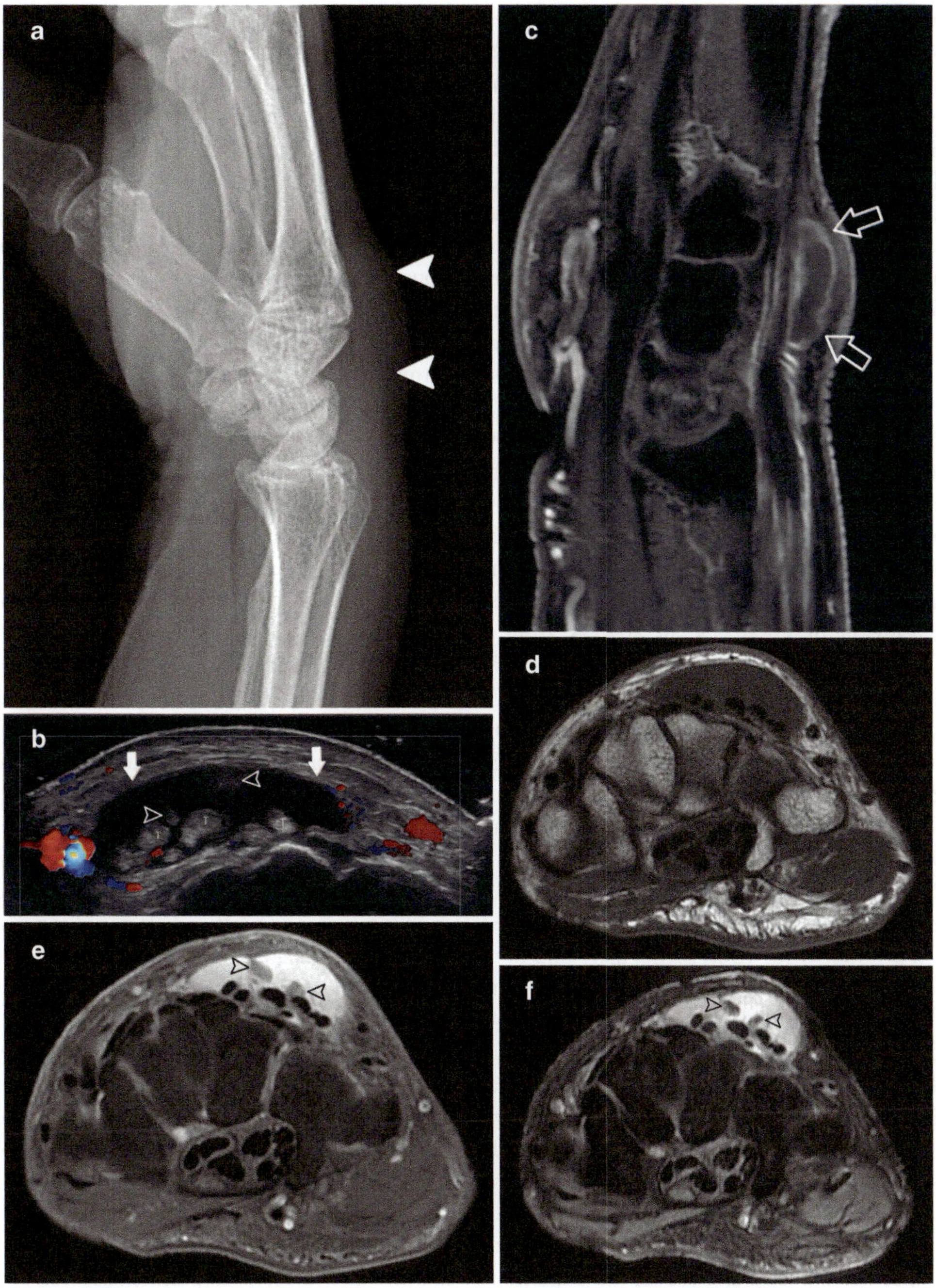

Fig. 11 Tuberculous (TB) tenosynovitis in a 69-year-old woman who had a palpable mass at dorsum of wrist for 4 months. (**a**) Lateral radiograph shows soft tissue swelling at the dorsal aspect of the wrist (solid arrowheads). (**b**) Transverse US image shows distension of extensor tendon sheath (solid arrows) filled with the echogenic debris (white open arrowheads) (T: tendon). The synovitis of the distended tendon sheath (open arrows) is well delineated on the (**c**) sagittal fat-suppressed contrast-enhanced T1-weighted MR image. The debris is imperceptible on the (**d**) axial T1-weighted MR image, but it is demonstrated as hypointense signal rice bodies (black open arrowheads) on (**e**) axial fat-suppressed proton density-weighted MR image without blooming on (**f**) axial gradient recalled echo MR image. Tissue obtained from debridement revealed granulomatous inflammation. The patient was treated by anti-TB drug with a good response

particularly useful for distinguishing liquefied abscesses from vascularized inflammatory tissue, identifying a sinus tract, and for differentiating synovitis from effusions and debris (Pattamapaspong et al. 2024) (Figs. 6c–e, 7c–h, and 8c–f). Lack of contrast enhancement effectively rules out infection, but intravenous contrast agent administration alone cannot reliably differentiate infectious from non-infectious inflammation (Hopkins et al. 1995). For patients with contraindications to gadolinium, diffusion-weighted imaging (DWI) can help detect abscess formation (Wudhikulprapan et al. 2024) (Fig. 7f).

MRI signal intensities in infections vary, based on inflammatory patterns ranging from reactive edema and abscess formation to non-caseating and caseating granulomas, with liquefaction being commonly observed in chronic infections. This peripheral rim of contrast enhancement differentiates an abscess from a phlegmon (Fig. 12) as well as from a serous fluid collection. T1-hyperintense signal indicates vascularized tissue or abscess walls, referred to as the "penumbra sign" (Grey et al. 1998) (Fig. 8), while T2-hypointense areas reflect fibrosis or paramagnetic free radicals (Sawlani et al. 2003).

MRI is the most reliable imaging modality for diagnosing NF, characterized by thickened deep fascia (>3 mm) with T2 hyperintensity and non-enhancing or mixed enhancement patterns in the necrotic fascia (Kim et al. 2011; Ali et al. 2014) (Fig. 13). Additional findings include fascial fluid, edema extending into intermuscular septa, peripheral band-like hyperintensity, muscle contrast enhancement, and involvement of multiple musculofascial compartments, which increase diagnostic confidence (Ali et al. 2014). However, T2-hyperintense signal in the deep fascia is again non-specific and can also occur in conditions such as non-infectious fasciitis, muscle tears, and radiation-induced changes. Subcutaneous and fascial emphysema, though more specific, have lower sensitivity and are better detected by computed tomography (CT) than MRI (Kothari et al. 2001). Gas pockets, appearing as signal voids on all sequences, are best visualized using gradient-echo sequences.

The high sensitivity of MRI makes it invaluable for early detection and for distinguishing NF from other clinically mimicking infections. In cellulitis, a superficial infection involving the dermis and superficial fascia, MRI reveals reticulated T1-hypointensity and T2-hyperintensity (Ali et al. 2014). Gadolinium-enhanced imaging aids in differentiating cellulitis from noninfectious causes of subcutaneous tissue edema, such as congestive heart failure (Figs. 12 and 13). Complicated cellulitis may progress to abscess formation, appearing as rim-enhanced fluid collections, but it does not involve the deep intermuscular fascia, distinguishing it from NF. Pyomyositis, a bacterial infection of skeletal muscles, is characterized by diffuse hyperintense signals and enhancement of affected muscles. Advanced stages are often characterized by intramuscular abscesses, while early pyomyositis may present with reactive muscle changes that can mimic NF (Ali et al. 2014). While both conditions may exhibit T2-hyperintense signal in superficial fascia and muscles, the patterns of involvement and associated features aid in differentiation (Seok et al. 2009). Diffuse hyperintense signal areas in muscles on fat-suppressed T2-weighted MR images, combined with thickened, irregular enhancement of the surrounding deep fascia, are suggestive features of pyomyositis (Seok et al. 2009) (Fig. 12).

MRI is the gold standard for diagnosing, planning treatment, and monitoring osteomyelitis due to its high sensitivity in detecting bone marrow edema, soft tissue involvement, abscesses, and osteonecrosis (Hopkins et al. 1995). It can identify osteomyelitis within 1–3 days of onset (Tehranzadeh et al. 1992), distinguishing it from reactive marrow edema with the presence of confluent T1-hypointense signals (Collins et al. 2005). Conversely, hyperintensity on fluid-sensitive images or contrast enhancement without corresponding T1-hypointensity usually suggests reactive marrow edema rather than osteomyelitis (Figs. 6 and 10).

The "penumbra sign," indicative of Brodie's abscess in subacute osteomyelitis (Grey et al. 1998), appears as a hypersignal rim on unenhanced T1-weighted MR images. This rim usu-

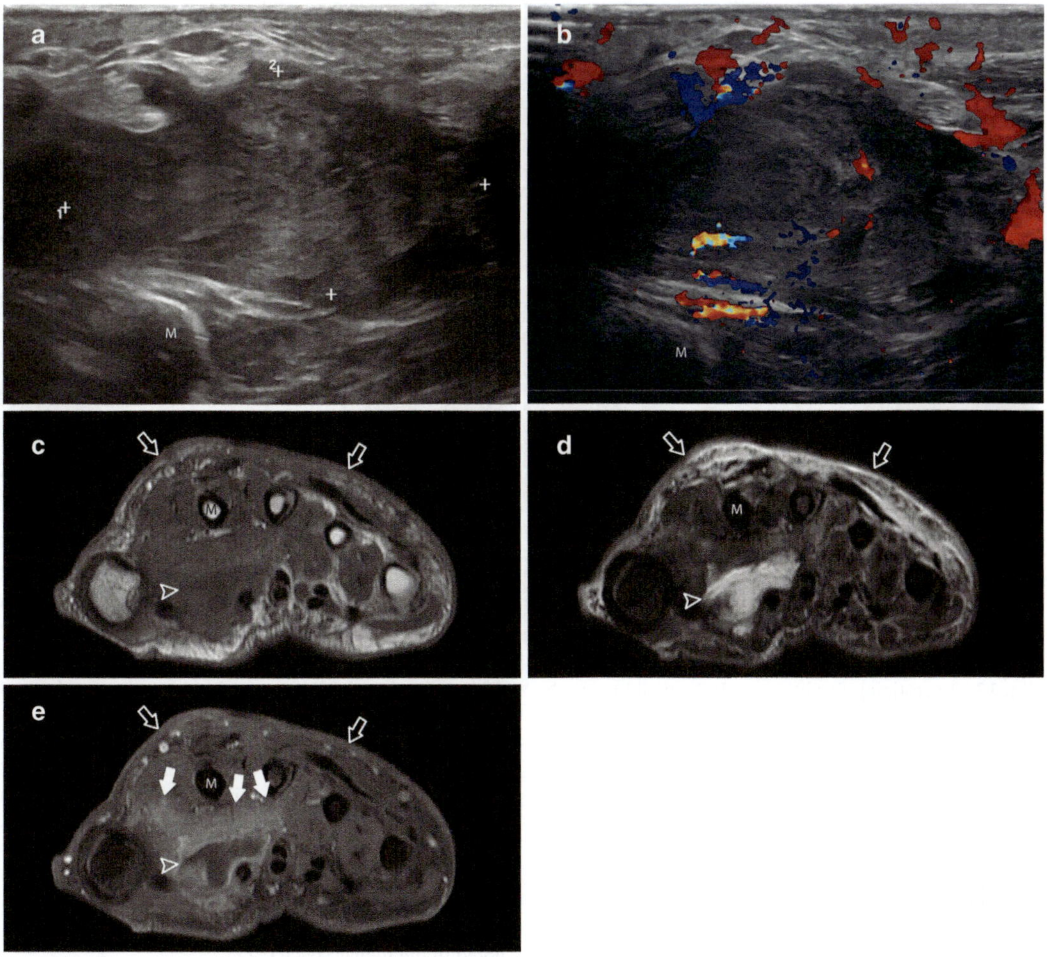

Fig. 12 Pyomyositis with an intramuscular abscess in a 40-year-old man who presented with septic arthritis of the wrist joint after a penetrating injury. Transverse (**a**) grayscale and (**b**) color Doppler US images of the palm show an irregular echogenic lesion in the thenar muscle which is noncompressible and contains internal vascularity suggestive of a phlegmon. Axial (**c**) T1-weighted, (**d**) fat-suppressed T2-weighted, and (**e**) fat-suppressed contrast-enhanced T1-weighted MR images performed 1 week later show a rim-enhancing abscess in the adductor pollicis muscle with a T1-penumbra sign at the wall and internal T2-hyperintense signal (open arrowheads). Surrounding thenar muscle shows diffuse T2-hyperintense signal and enhancement with irregular thickened fascia (solid arrows). The subcutaneous tissue edema (open arrows) on the dorsum of the hand shows no enhancement on the contrast-enhanced image (**e**), suggesting noninfectious edema. (M: second metacarpal bone)

ally shows contrast enhancement and surrounding bone marrow edema (Fig. 8c, d). In chronic osteomyelitis, MRI highlights sequestra surrounded by granulation tissue, along with involucrum, cloaca, and sinus tracts. Granulation tissue appears hyperintense on T2-weighted MR images and enhances, while sequestra remain hypointense across all sequences. The involucrum exhibits signal hypointensity and is separated from cortical bone by a zone of periosteal reaction (Fig. 8f), often appearing as a hyperintense mass on T2-weighted images, suggesting infectious material. Cortical bone breaks forming cloacae (Fig. 8c), often found with sinus tracts extending to the skin. CT complements MRI by detecting sequestra, essential for surgical planning and excision, and providing additional bony detail in complex cases (Gold et al. 1991; Santiago Restrepo et al. 2003; Pineda et al. 2009).

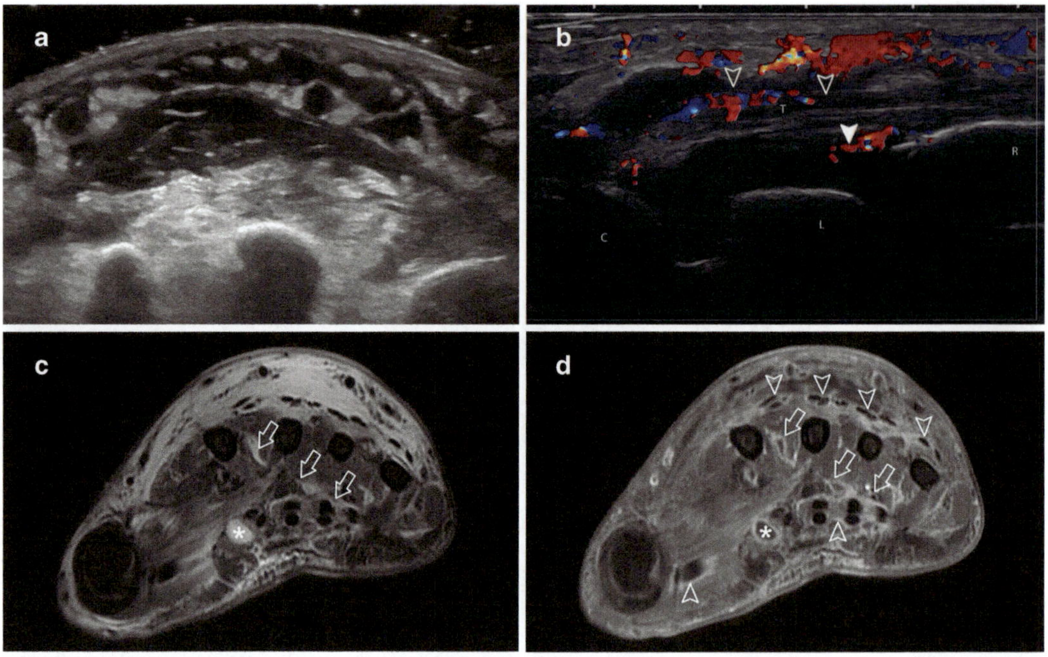

Fig. 13 Necrotizing fasciitis in a 59-year-old man who presented with a hemorrhagic bleb on the wrist. (**a**) Transverse gray-scale and (**b**) Longitudinal color Doppler US images of the dorsum of the hand shows diffuse subcutaneous tissue swelling with a cobblestone pattern, characterized by hypoechoic strands between hyperechoic fatty lobules (**a**) and increased vascularity (**b**), indicative of cellulitis. Tenosynovitis of the extensor tendon (open arrowheads) and synovitis in the radiocarpal joint (solid arrowheads) are also observed. (R: radius, L: lunate, C: capitate). Axial (**c**) fat-suppressed T2-weighted and (**d**) fat-suppressed contrast-enhanced T1-weighted MR images obtained 2 days later show diffuse muscle edema and enhancement, along with T2-hyperintense thickened fascia in the mid-palmar and interdigital spaces with mixed enhancement (open arrows), suggestive of necrotizing fasciitis. Tenosynovitis is evident in both the flexor and extensor tendon sheaths (open arrowheads). The diagnosis was confirmed by pathological examination following surgical debridement. Additionally, a small rim-enhancing abscess is noted in the thenar space (*)

Synovitis, periarticular soft tissue edema, subchondral bone marrow edema, and bone erosions can be seen in both septic and nonseptic inflammatory arthritis (Graif et al. 1999) (Fig. 10). Moreover, no single finding or combination of findings is pathognomonic or sufficient to definitively rule out joint infection (Graif et al. 1999). A thorough evaluation, including clinical history, laboratory tests, and joint aspiration, with or without ultrasound (US) imaging guidance, is crucial for an accurate diagnosis of septic arthritis. Chronic infectious arthritis causes cartilage damage via granulation tissue invasion, often leaving areas of intact cartilage and bone, unlike bacterial septic arthritis, which rapidly destroys it (Pattamapaspong et al. 2024). Chronic infections often cause joint, bursa, and tendon sheath effusions containing T2-hypointense particles due to caseating material and rice bodies (Pattamapaspong et al. 2024) (Fig. 11). Moreover, paraarticular abscess, thinner and smooth abscess wall, and less surrounding soft tissue swelling indicate chronic infection rather than bacterial septic arthritis (Hong et al. 2001). Patterns of disease in tendon sheaths may present as (a) synovial fluid distension with a normal-appearing tendon; (b) synovial thickening accompanied by hypointense material in the synovial fluid on T2-weighted MR images, often involving the tendon; and (c) peritendinous soft-tissue masses (Jaovisidha et al. 1996) (Fig. 11).

4.3 Computed Tomography

Multidetector computed tomography (MDCT), with a capability to display multiple levels of tissue density, is highly effective for the detection of cortical bone lesions and gas, making it invaluable for diagnosing NF and advanced osteomyelitis. It excels at identifying sequestra through their dense eburnation and location within granulation tissue (Gold et al. 1991). CT is faster, more accessible, and cost-effective compared to MRI but lacks the sensitivity for early bone marrow changes and soft tissue detail that MRI offers. It is frequently used in clinical practice to evaluate complex infections in the hand and wrist in severely ill patients, especially when MRI is unavailable (Fig. 14). Contrast-enhanced CT with iodinated contrast agents improves the assessment of soft tissue lesions, including abscesses and tenosynovitis (Kothari et al. 2001). In CT, abscesses have a semi-liquid density of about 30–50 Hounsfield Units with the peripheral enhancing wall (Jaovisidha et al. 1996). In summary, MRI provides unmatched sensitivity for early infection detection and detailed soft tissue evaluation, while CT is more effective for identifying gas, sequestra, calcifications, and cortical bone involvement. Both modalities complement each other in managing complex infections.

MDCT is superior to MRI for detecting radiodense FBs. FBs often trigger immune responses, forming granulomas characterized by inflammation, fibrosis, and encapsulation. MDCT is 5–15 times more sensitive than radiography for detecting FBs and is the preferred modality for materials such as plastic, glass, and stone, particularly in gas-filled cavities (Aras et al. 2010; Pattamapaspong et al. 2013). However, CT is less sensitive than US imaging for small, superficial FBs and may miss small objects if thick imaging slices are used. Common complications of FBs include cellulitis, granuloma formation, abscesses, osteomyelitis, and septic arthritis. While CT is effective for characterizing complications, it is less accurate than MRI. Given its higher cost, ionizing radiation exposure, and limitations in detecting inflammation, CT should be reserved for cases where radiography and US imaging fail to provide conclusive results for FBs.

Retrograde contrast agent filling (sinography) combined with CT can trace sinus tracts from the skin to their medullary bone origins (Santiago Restrepo et al. 2003). Additionally, CT and US imaging are invaluable for guiding percutaneous punctures to obtain fluid for bacteriological analysis.

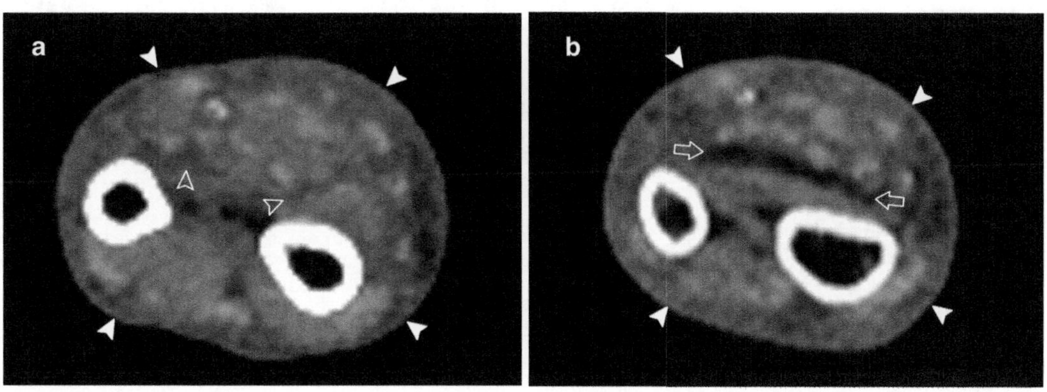

Fig. 14 Necrotizing fasciitis in an 87-year-old woman who presented with clinical sepsis and swelling of forearm and wrist. Axial unenhanced CT images obtained at the (**a**) distal forearm and (**b**) wrist show diffuse subcutaneous tissue edema (solid arrowheads). Fluid density along the deep intermuscular fascia (open arrowheads) is different from the unaffected inter-fascial fat in the space of Parona (open arrows). Surgical drainage revealed necrotizing fasciitis

4.4 Ultrasound Imaging

US imaging is the first-line imaging modality for evaluating soft tissue infections, detecting fluid collections, abscesses, and radiolucent FBs, particularly in soft tissues and joint spaces (Kothari et al. 2001) (Fig. 15). High-resolution probes (≥10 MHz) are essential for imaging small structures like the hand and wrist. US is also valuable for assessing soft tissue abscesses and joint effusion and guiding needle aspiration (Fig. 16).

Cellulitis appears as diffuse swelling or a cobblestone pattern with hypoechoic strands between hyperechoic fatty lobules in subcutaneous tissue, often accompanied by hyperemia on Doppler US images (Fig. 13). This appearance is nonspecific and may be present in noninfective subcutaneous edema. However, concurrent hyperemia is seen with cellulitis, which is not a feature of noninfective forms of edema. Abscesses are visualized as hypoechoic or heterogeneous fluid collections with hyperemic walls (Jeffrey Jr. et al. 1987) (Figs. 12 and 16). Gentle transducer compression can compress the fluid, aiding diagnosis, and confirm drainability. Tenosynovitis is characterized by variably thickened tendon sheaths, hypoechoic synovial fluid, and hyperemia on Doppler US imaging. Tendon function and gliding can be evaluated during a dynamic US study.

In cases of radiolucent FBs, US imaging is highly effective in detecting materials such as wood or plastic, which may be missed on radiographs (Aras et al. 2010; Pattamapaspong et al. 2013). On US images, all FBs appear as hyperechoic structures, often accompanied by posterior acoustic shadowing or reverberation artifacts, particularly in materials such as wood, glass, and metal (Fig. 15). Plastic and organic substances

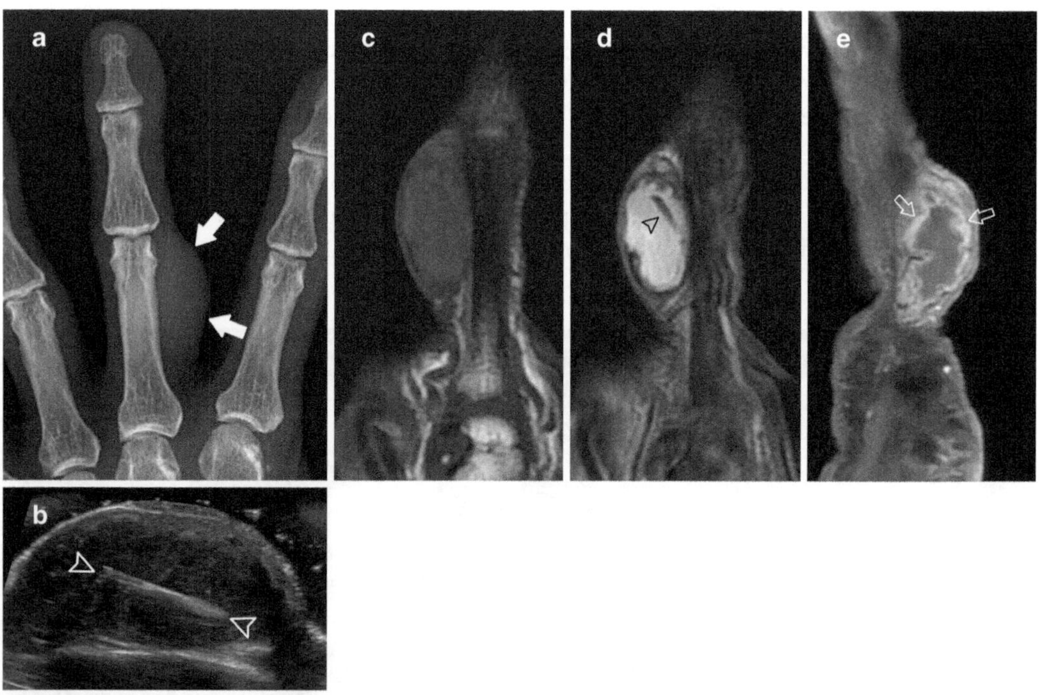

Fig. 15 Wooden foreign body with surrounding abscess in a 70-year-old man who presented with a slowly growing mass in the left middle finger. (**a**) Posteroanterior radiograph shows a soft tissue mass (solid arrows) without a visible radiopaque foreign body. (**b**) Longitudinal grayscale US image of the lesion, performed before MRI, shows a hyperechoic foreign body (white open arrowheads) with posterior reverberation artifacts, surrounded by a heterogeneous hypoechoic area consistent with a foreign body abscess. (**c**) Coronal T1-weighted, (**d**) coronal fat-suppressed T2-weighted, and (**e**) sagittal fat-suppressed contrast-enhanced T1-weighted MR images show the foreign body (black open arrowheads) surrounded by a thickened-wall, rim-enhancing foreign body abscess (white open arrows). The diagnosis was confirmed by surgery

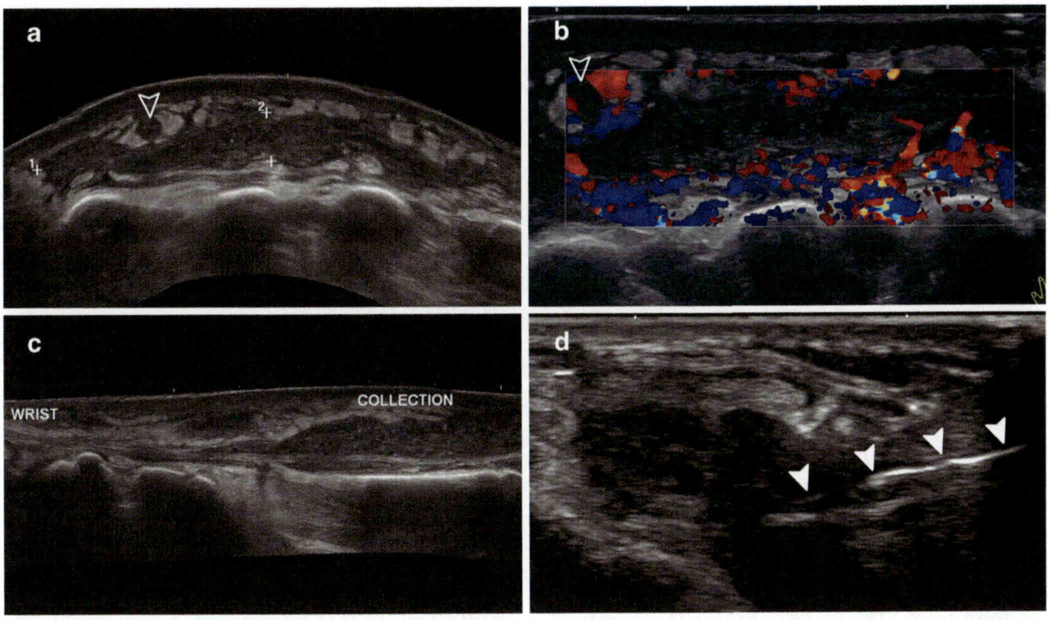

Fig. 16 Soft tissue abscess in a 56-year-old woman who presented with dorsal hand swelling and fluctuation on physical examination. (**a**) Transverse gray-scale US image of the dorsal hand shows an echogenic fluid collection (between cursors) in the deeper dorsal subaponeurotic space. (**b**) Transverse color Doppler US image shows peripheral hyperemia, and the collection appears compressible, further supporting the diagnosis. Additionally, thrombophlebitis is noted in the adjacent superficial vein (open arrowhead in **a**, **b**). (**c**) Longitudinal extended-field-of-view US image shows extent of the abscess. (**d**) US-guided needle aspiration (solid arrowheads) confirmed the diagnosis

tend to produce softer acoustic shadows. The inflammatory response or granuloma formation surrounding the FBs varies, depending on the material type and duration of retention, typically presenting as a hypoechoic rim or an area of mixed echogenicity (Fig. 15). Hyperemia on color Doppler imaging indicates active inflammation, while chronic cases may show encapsulated FBs surrounded by fibrous tissue, making detection more challenging. US imaging is also valuable for guiding FB removal, minimizing tissue damage, and ensuring complete extraction. Although highly effective for superficial FBs, deeper or more complex cases may require CT or MRI for further evaluation (Fig. 15c–e).

Doppler US imaging can differentiate synovial effusion from synovial thickening in conditions such as tenosynovitis or septic arthritis (Fig. 13). Joint effusions appear hypoechoic or hyperechoic without vascularity, distinguishable from the synovium and capsule. US imaging can occasionally detect superficial bone erosions in arthritis. It is also effective for diagnosing early suppurative flexor tenosynovitis or TB tenosynovitis, showing fluid, granulomatous tissue, and debris or rice bodies with variable echogenicity.

While limited for the diagnosis of NF, US imaging can show thickened fascial planes, hypoechoic fluid, and subcutaneous edema. Gas may be detected as echogenic foci with "dirty" posterior shadowing. Although less sensitive than MRI for osteomyelitis, US imaging can detect juxtacortical swelling, periosteal thickening, subperiosteal abscesses, and occasionally cloaca. US imaging may struggle to visualize small, deep abscesses, such as those in the carpal tunnel, and cannot reliably assess bony structures. While large abscesses are easily detected, multi-compartmental abscesses are challenging to differentiate from reactive fluid collection. For deep infections, MRI provides superior visualization of abscesses and multi-compartmental involvement (Fig. 13).

5 Imaging Differential Diagnoses

5.1 Osteomyelitis

Osteomyelitis is typically diagnosed through a combination of clinical and imaging findings. However, aggressive bone destruction with periostitis and soft tissue swelling may mimic malignant neoplasms (Fig. 17) such as Ewing sarcoma or osteosarcoma in children, lymphoma in young adults, and skeletal metastases in older individuals. Imaging features can also resemble bone infarction, particularly in the diaphysis. Diagnostic complexity increases in patients with predisposing conditions to osteomyelitis and osteonecrosis, such as sickle cell anemia, Gaucher disease, lymphoproliferative disorders, or long-term steroid use. Presence of extraosseous soft tissue masses supports the diagnosis (Fig. 17). The sharp and well-defined margin of the lesion helps distinguish between tumor (Fig. 17c) and the poorly marginated osteomyelitis (Fig. 6c) (Henninger et al. 2013).

Subacute to chronic osteomyelitis, including Brodie's abscess, can mimic bone cysts, aneurysmal bone cysts, or fibrous dysplasia. TB osteomyelitis in metaphyseal lesions with subarticular bone involvement may resemble aneurysmal bone cysts or giant cell tumors (Fig. 18), while epiphyseal abscesses mimic chondroblastoma or Langerhans cell histiocytosis. The "penumbra sign" on T1-weighted MR imaging is a key diagnostic feature for distinguishing osteomyelitis and abscesses from tumors (Grey et al. 1998; McGuinness et al. 2007) (Fig. 8). CT aids in identifying a nidus and vascular groove sign, particularly for osteoid osteoma resembling subacute to chronic osteomyelitis in the diaphysis with thick periositis (Liu et al. 2011).

Chronic nonbacterial osteomyelitis (CNO), formerly called as chronic recurrent multifocal osteomyelitis (CRMO), is an aseptic chronic condition primarily affecting children and adolescents, often linked to the SAPHO (synovitis, acne, pustulosis, hyperostosis, osteitis) syndrome (Greenwood et al. 2017). It also has been referred to as Garré's sclerosing osteomyelitis. It presents as multifocal osteomyelitic lesions with a mix of osteosclerotic and osteolytic features, typically in the metaphyses of lower extremity bones and medial ends of the clavicles. Radiographs reveal sclerosis, osteolysis, and, in some cases, massive clavicular enlargement. CRMO may be associated with conditions such as inflammatory bowel disease and Wegener's granulomatosis (Greenwood et al. 2017). Skin conditions, e.g., pustulosis and psoriasis, are common comorbidities. The diagnosis is challenging due to nonspecific laboratory findings and negative cultures. The metaphyses of the bones of the lower extremity and the medial ends of the clavicles are particularly vulnerable, and imaging screening for multifocal disease is essential. Scintigraphy and MRI are useful for detecting multifocal lesions and monitoring progression (Kothari et al. 2001) (Fig. 19). Diagnosis should be confined to cases of sclerosing osteomyelitis without evidence of sequestra or granulation tissue, especially in cases involving the clavicle and sternoclavicular region.

Spina ventosa presenting in TB dactylitis is not specific for TB and can occur in other infectious diseases such as fungal infection and melioidosis (Abid et al. 2024). The differential diagnoses of TB dactylitis also include non-infectious lesions such as fibrous dysplasia, sarcoidosis, hyperparathyroidism, and sickle cell anemia. In the early stage of TB dactylitis, expanded digits with bone marrow signal abnormality on MR images, together with periostitis, may clinically and radiologically mimic bone marrow ischemia and vascular occlusion of sickle cell disease (Kosaraju et al. 2017). On contrast-enhanced MRI, intense, ring-shaped enhancement is observed at the small tubular bone(s) affected in TB osteomyelitis (Hsu et al. 2004). Differential diagnoses of multifocal tuberculous osteomyelitis include Langerhans cell histiocytosis, sarcoidosis, multiple myeloma, and metastasis.

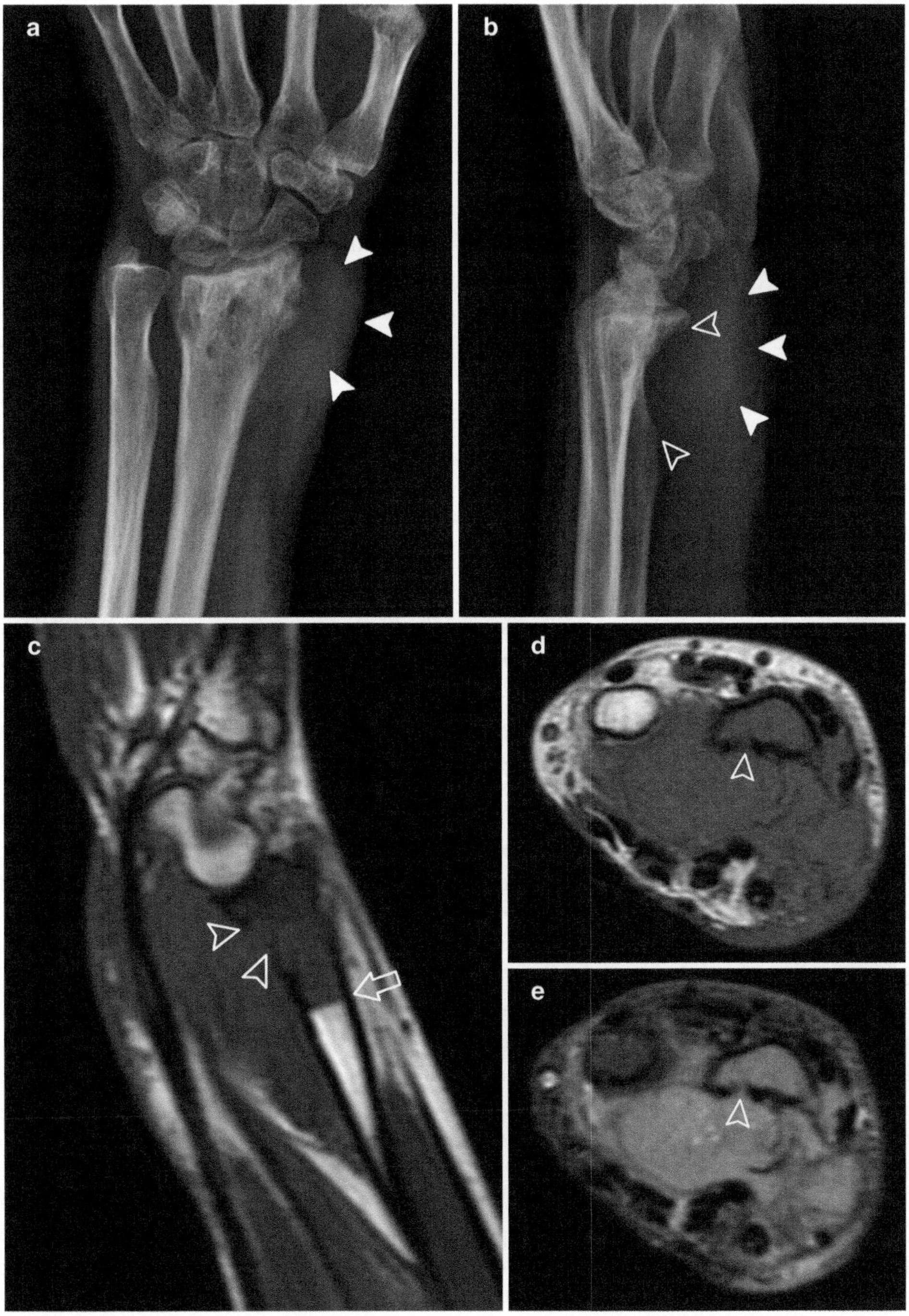

Fig. 17 Ewing sarcoma in a 25-year-old woman who presented with a palpable wrist mass. (**a**) Posteroanterior and (**b**) lateral radiographs of the wrist show a mixed osteosclerotic and osteolytic lesion in the metaphysis and epiphysis of the left distal radius, with cortical destruction (open arrowheads) and soft tissue mass on the volar side (solid arrowheads). (**c**) Sagittal T1-weighted MR image shows a well-defined margin of the intramedullary lesion (open arrow), aiding in differentiation from osteomyelitis. Note the cortical destruction (open arrowheads). Axial (**d**) T1-weighted, (**e**) fat-suppressed T2-weighted, and (**f**) fat-suppressed contrast-enhanced T1-weighted MR images show an enhancing tumor with a large extraosseous soft tissue mass (solid arrows), along with cortical remodeling and small areas of cortical destruction (open arrowhead), supporting the diagnosis of small round cell tumor like Ewing sarcoma

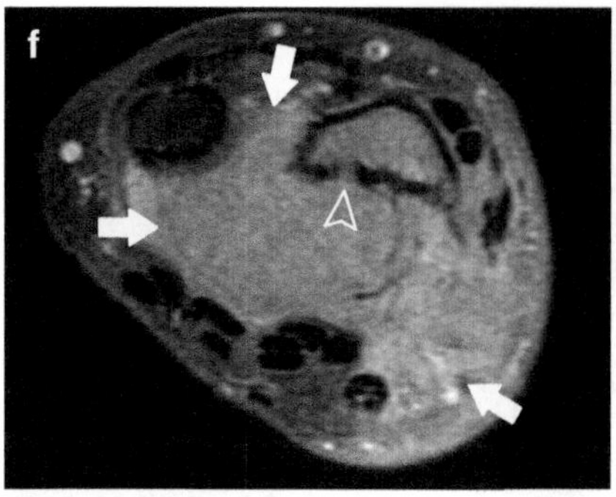

Fig. 17 (continued)

5.2 Septic Arthritis

Shared radiographical features, including marginal erosions and periarticular osteoporosis, are seen in infective arthritis, rheumatoid arthritis, and spondyloarthropathies. Advanced cases of any arthritis may result in intraarticular bony ankylosis. When clinical signs of hand and wrist arthritis are present, challenge arises in distinguishing infective arthritis from other arthropathies such as rheumatoid arthritis, gout, or calcium pyrophosphate deposition (CPPD) disease, especially when these conditions coexist. Clues to diagnosis include a poor response to treatment of the pre-existing joint disease or rapid deterioration of a joint compared to other affected joints (Fig. 20).

Unilateral hand and wrist arthritis with poorly defined margins of bone erosions accompanied by a large joint effusion and para-articular abscesses strongly suggest infective arthritis. However, unilateral disease may also occur in rheumatoid arthritis or gout, particularly in patients with hemiparalysis (Needs et al. 1985) (Fig. 21). While other joint diseases such as pigmented villonodular synovitis, synovial chondromatosis, gout, and osteoarthrosis may show bone erosions or cysts, these bone lesions are usually sharply marginated, unlike the poorly defined bone destruction seen in infective arthritis.

TB arthritis, slower in progression than bacterial arthritis, may mimic rheumatoid arthritis and other chronic arthropathies (Graif et al. 1999). TB arthritis is characterized by large bone erosions, para-articular abscesses, and homogeneous synovitis compared to the irregular synovial thickening of rheumatoid arthritis (Choi et al. 2009) (Fig. 9). Diffuse tenosynovial giant cell tumors, also known as pigmented nodular synovitis, present with T2-hypointense synovial thickening and hemosiderin deposition, detectable as signal blooming on T2*-weighted MR images. Similarly, intra-articular amyloid deposition shows T2-hypointense synovial thickening on MRI and hypoechoic synovium on US imaging, often mimicking TB synovitis. A definitive diagnosis of amyloidosis requires Congo red staining on histopathology.

US imaging and dual-energy CT (DECT) are valuable tools for confirming the diagnosis of crystal deposition diseases such as gout and CPPD. US imaging detects features like the double-contour sign, gouty tophi, intraarticular aggregate, and hyperechoic CPPD deposits in the cartilage, offering real-time, non-invasive assessment (Girish et al. 2013; Pattamapaspong et al. 2017) (Figs. 22 and 23). DECT maps monosodium urate (MSU) crystals with color-coded overlays, excelling in deep or asymptomatic deposits (Dalbeth et al. 2015) (Fig. 22). Despite the operator dependence of US imaging and limited ability for deep structures, and DECT's radiation exposure, these complementary techniques ensure an early and accurate diagnosis.

5.3 Soft Tissue Infections

On MRI, areas of T2-hyperintense signal in the fascia, muscles, and subcutaneous tissue are nonspecific and may occur in non-infectious conditions such as inflammatory fasciitis or myositis, traumatic injury, or radiation-induced changes (Fig. 24). Clinical correlation is essential for accurate diagnosis. Contrast-enhanced MRI can aid in distinguishing inflammatory from non-inflammatory causes.

TB myositis, tenosynovitis, and bursitis typically present as slow-growing masses with minimal inflammatory response, often resembling soft tissue tumors (Pattamapaspong et al. 2024).

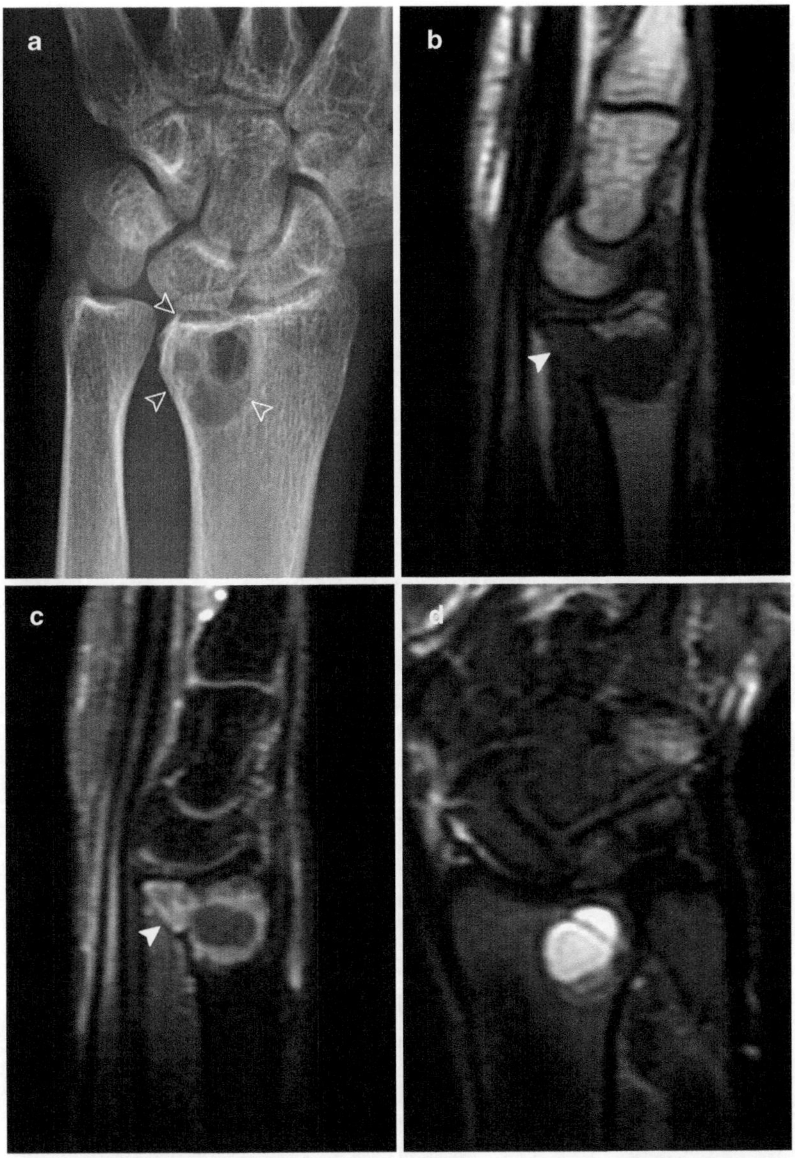

Fig. 18 Giant cell tumor in a 34-year-old man. (**a**) Posteroanterior radiograph of the wrist shows a well-defined geographical osteolytic lesion eccentrically located in the metaphysis of the distal radius (open arrowheads), extending subarticularly. The lesion exhibits cortical remodeling and thin internal trabeculation, creating a characteristic "soap bubble" appearance. No cortical destruction is observed. (**b**) Sagittal T1-weighted, (**c**) sagittal fat-suppressed contrast-enhanced T1-weighted, and (**d**) coronal fat-suppressed T2-weighted MR images show a thick-walled cystic lesion with an associated enhancing soft tissue mass (solid arrowheads)

Imaging techniques such as CT, MRI, and US imaging are crucial for detecting abscesses, evaluating the extent of disease, and identifying characteristic features like rim calcifications, which are common in TB granulomas and other chronic infections (Pattamapaspong et al. 2024). Rice bodies, often associated with TB, may also be found in other forms of chronic synovitis, including rheumatoid arthritis and fungal infections.

Differentiating TB from conditions such as synovial osteochondromatosis (Fig. 25), which presents with intra-articular loose bodies showing

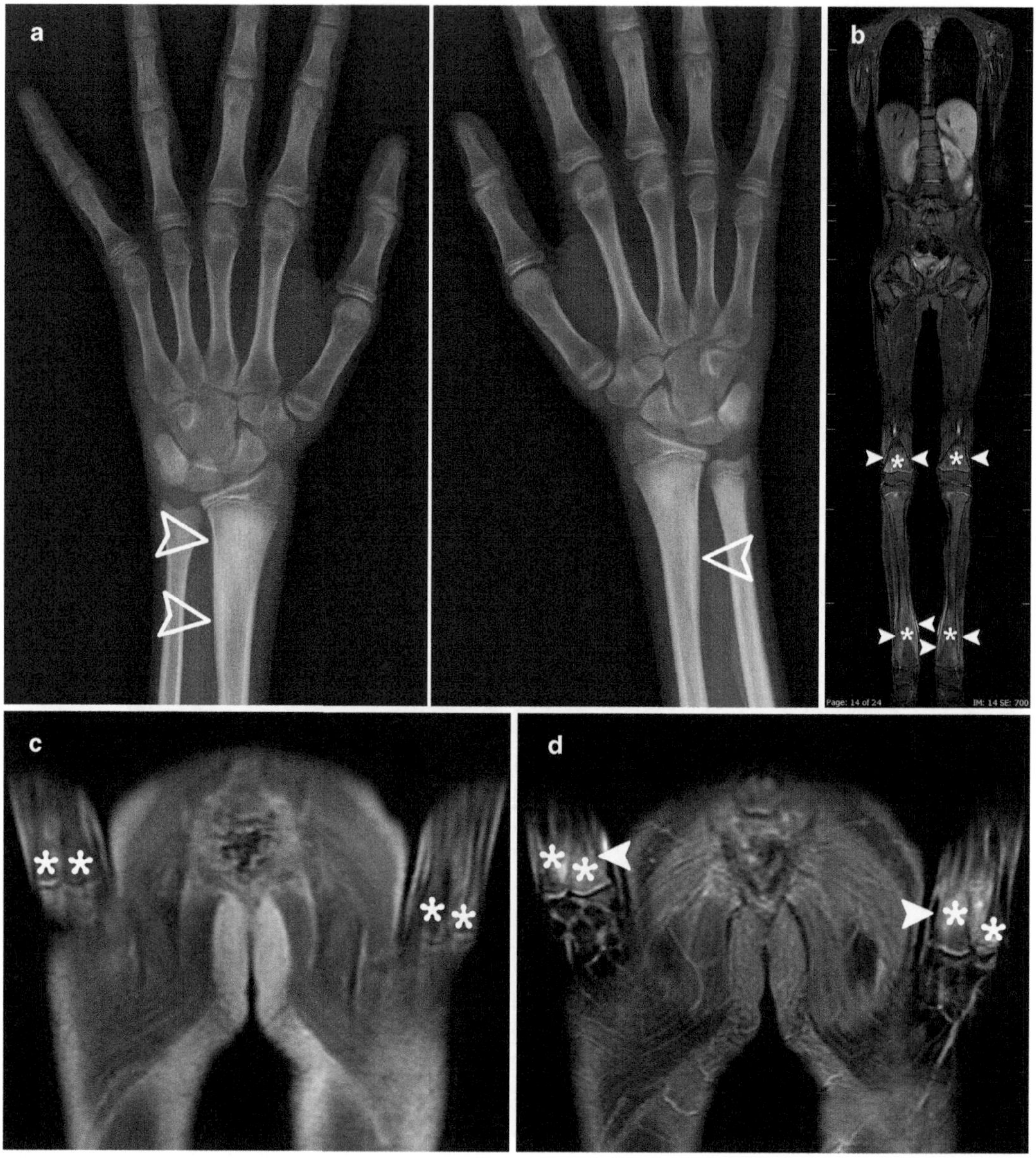

Fig. 19 Chronic recurrent multifocal osteomyelitis (CRMO) in a 13-year-old boy who presented with chronic limb pain and swelling predominantly in bilateral ankles. (**a**) Anteroposterior radiograph shows osteosclerotic lesions in the metaphyses of bilateral distal radii and ulnae, with a continuous periosteal reaction on the ulnar side of the bilateral distal radii (open arrowheads). (**b**) Coronal STIR whole-body MR image shows T2-hyperintense intramedullary lesions (*) in bilateral distal femurs and tibias with periostitis (solid arrowheads). Coronal (**c**) T1-weighted and (**d**) STIR MR images of both wrists show T2-hyperintense intramedullary lesions with periostitis in bilateral distal radii and ulnae. A biopsy of the distal tibia revealed inflammatory infiltration in the periosteum. The further investigation found chronic inflammatory bowel disease and the final diagnosis was enteropathic CRMO

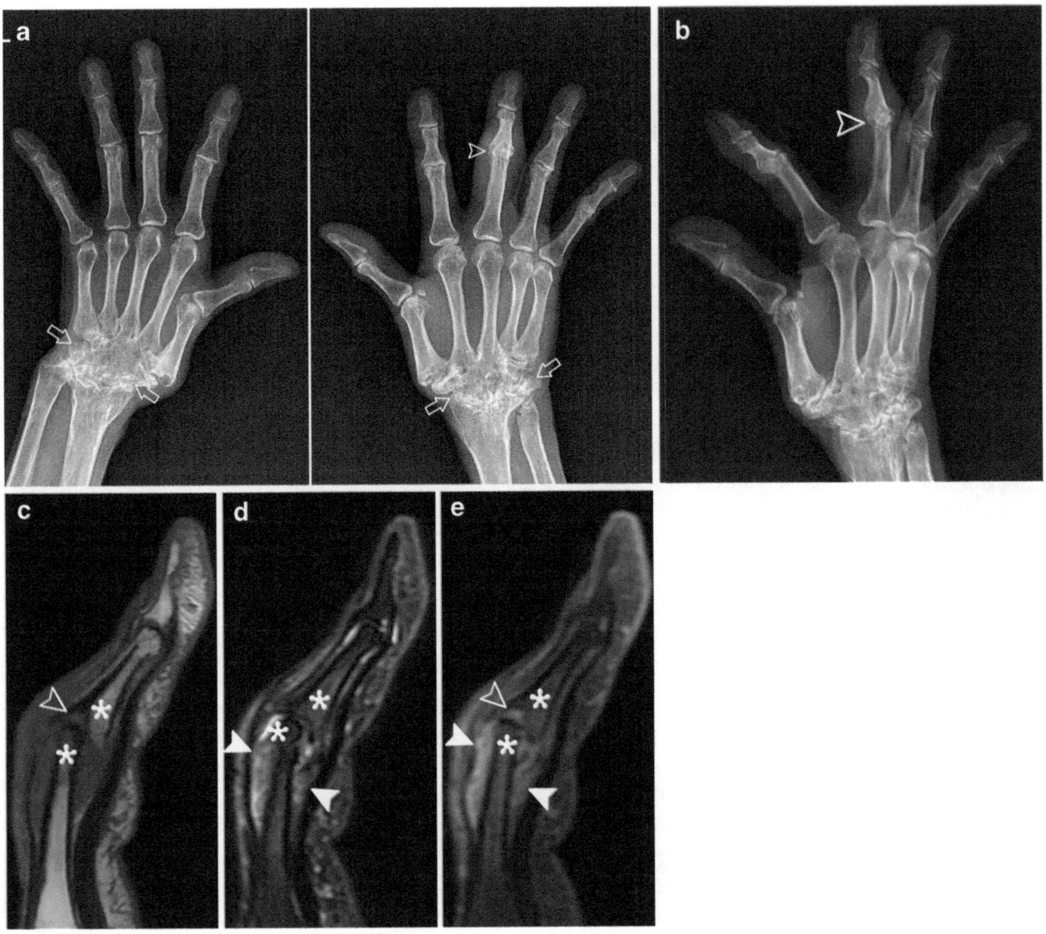

Fig. 20 Septic arthritis of the right third PIP joint in a 72-year-old woman with underlying rheumatoid arthritis. She presented with severe pain in the third PIP joint. (**a**) Posteroanterior radiograph of both hands and (**b**) oblique radiograph of the right hand show soft tissue swelling with joint space narrowing and bone erosions (open arrowheads) at the third PIP joint. Severe joint space narrowing and bone ankylosis are noted in both wrist joints (open arrows), consistent with underlying rheumatoid arthritis. Because of the rapid deterioration of the third PIP joint compared to other affected joints, septic arthritis was suspected. Sagittal (**c**) T1-weighted, (**d**) fat-suppressed T2-weighted, and (**e**) fat-suppressed contrast-enhanced T1-weighted MR images show synovitis (solid arrowheads), bone erosions (open arrowheads), subchondral bone marrow edema (*), and periarticular soft tissue edema. Preserved fatty marrow signal within the area of subchondral bone marrow edema on (**c**) suggests reactive changes rather than associated osteomyelitis. Joint aspiration and synovial fluid analysis confirmed septic arthritis

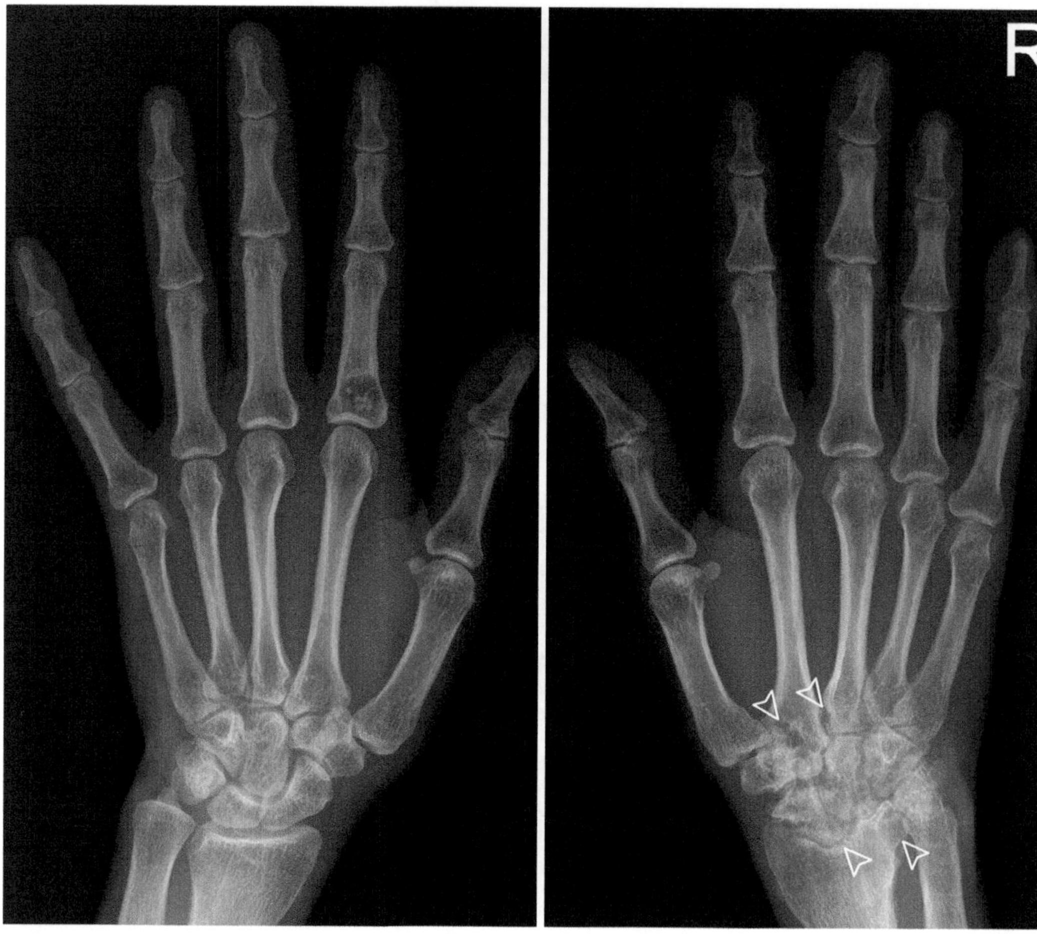

Fig. 21 Rheumatoid arthritis in a 46-year-old woman with left hemiparesis due to stroke. Posteroanterior radiograph of both hands shows unilateral joint destruction in the right wrist joint, while the left wrist is unaffected, suggesting a protective effect from left-sided hemiparesis. An enchondroma is noted at the base of the left second proximal phalanx, containing an internal chondroid matrix

"ring-and-arc" calcifications on radiographs, is essential. MRI helps distinguish calcified nodules (which are T2-hypointense) from non-mineralized ones (which are T2-hyperintense). On T1-weighted MRI images, synovial osteochondromatosis are typically visualized due to the presence of calcification or ossification, while rice bodies are almost imperceptible on imaging (Chen et al. 2002). On US imaging, TB tenosynovitis is characterized by synovial fluid and thickened tendon sheaths, appearing hyperechoic compared to non-tuberculous tenosynovitis (Jaovisidha et al. 1996). Foggy calcifications in a peritendinous location are highly suggestive of TB.

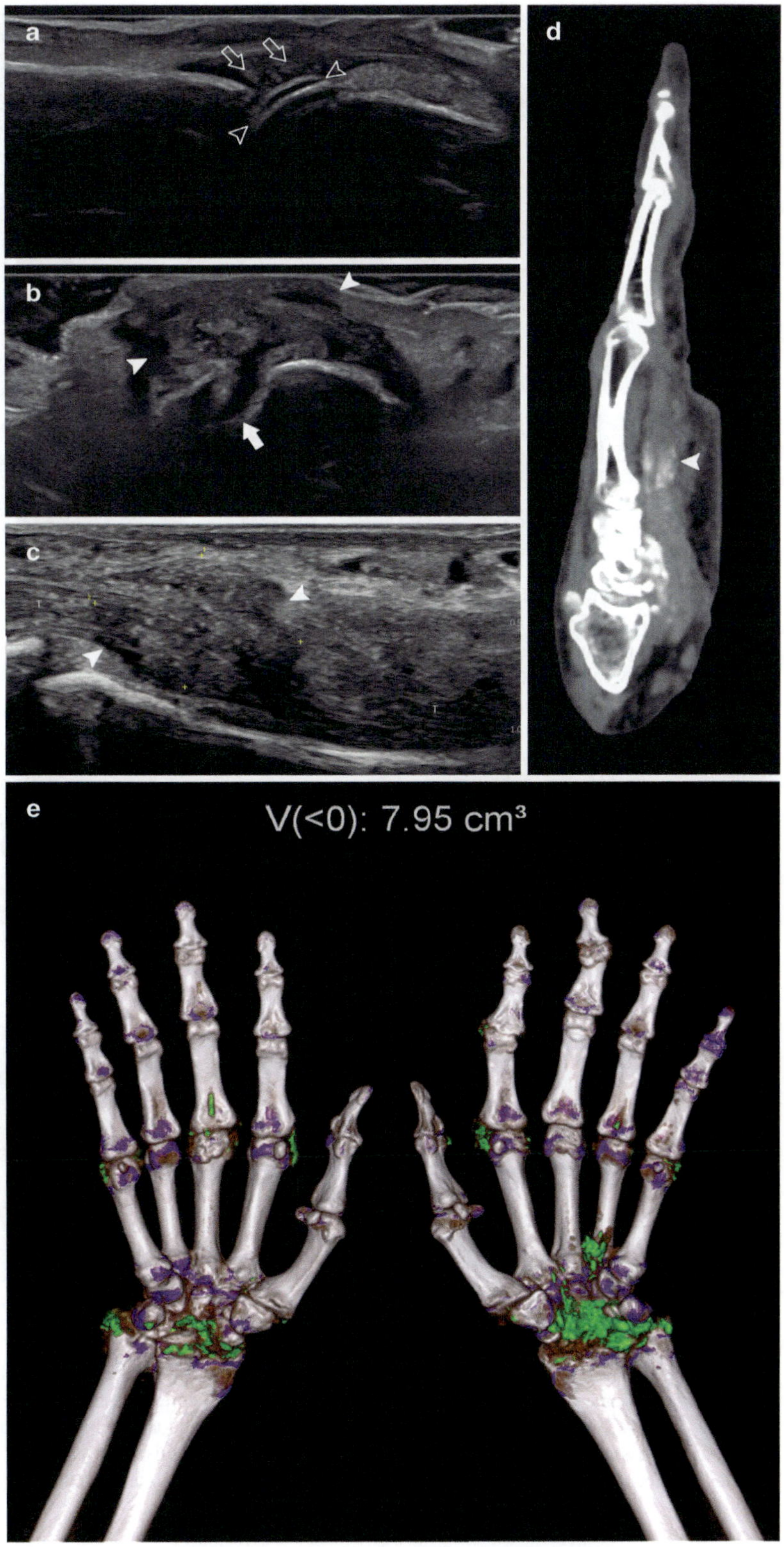

Fig. 22 Gouty deposition in a 70-year-old man with limited range of motion in the left little finger. (**a**) Longitudinal US image of the fifth metacarpophalangeal joint shows a thick echogenic line overlying the cartilage surface or a double contour sign (open arrowheads) and hyperechoic spots of gouty deposition (open arrows) within the thickened synovium. (**b**) Transverse US image of the same joint shows a heterogeneous hyperechoic tophus (solid arrowheads) and bone erosion in the metacarpal head (solid arrow). (**c**) Longitudinal US image of the little finger shows heterogeneous hyperechoic intratendinous tophus (solid arrowheads) in the flexor digitorum tendons (T), which is confirmed by the corresponding (**d**) sagittal unenhanced dual-energy CT (DECT) image (solid arrowhead). (**e**) Reformatted 3D DECT image shows areas of gouty depositions (green color coding) with a volume of 7.95 cm^3

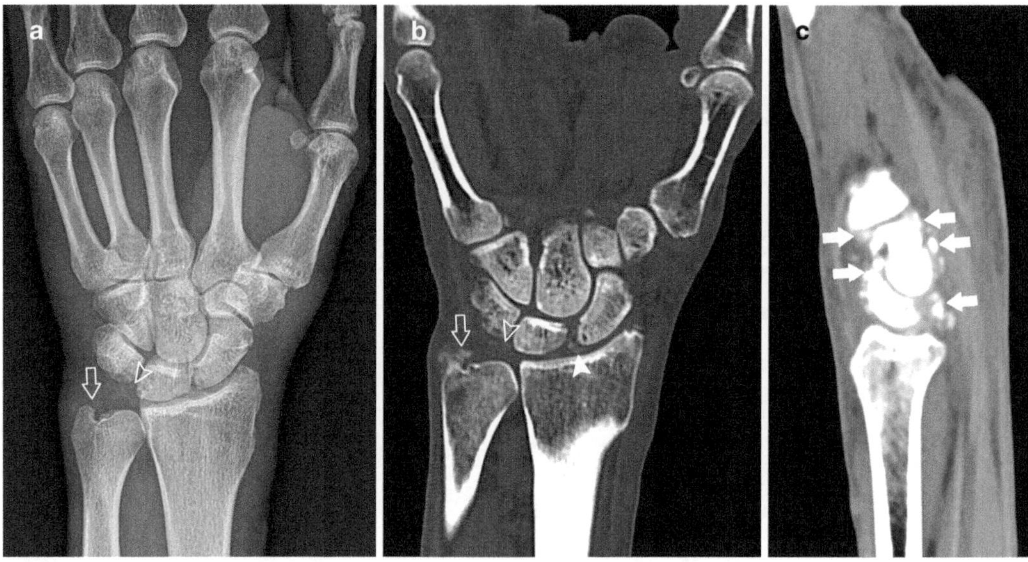

Fig. 23 Calcium pyrophosphate dihydrate (CPPD) deposition disease in a 77-year-old man. (**a**) Posteroanterior radiograph, and (**b**) coronal and (**c**) sagittal CT images of the left wrist show calcifications in the articular structures including the scapholunate ligament (solid arrowhead), lunotriquetral ligament (open arrowheads), triangular fibrocartilage complex (open arrows), and joint capsule (solid arrows)

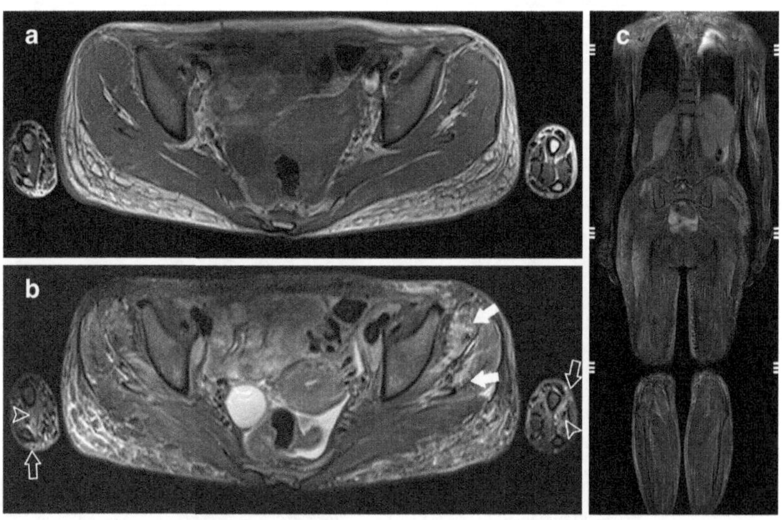

Fig. 24 Systemic sclerosis with inflammatory myopathy in a 47-year-old woman. (**a**) Axial T1-weighted, (**b**) axial STIR, and (**c**) coronal STIR whole-body MR images show patchy muscle edema in the pronator quadratus and left extensor muscles (open arrowheads), accompanied by subcutaneous tissue edema (open arrow). Additionally, muscle and subcutaneous tissue edema is noted bilaterally in the gluteal regions, more pronounced in the left gluteus minimus and medius muscles (solid arrows). No muscle atrophy is observed on the T1-weighted image (**a**), and no fluid collection is detected. While the imaging findings in the hand are non-specific and may resemble pyomyositis or cellulitis, the presence of multifocal lesions and clinical correlation are essential for an accurate diagnosis

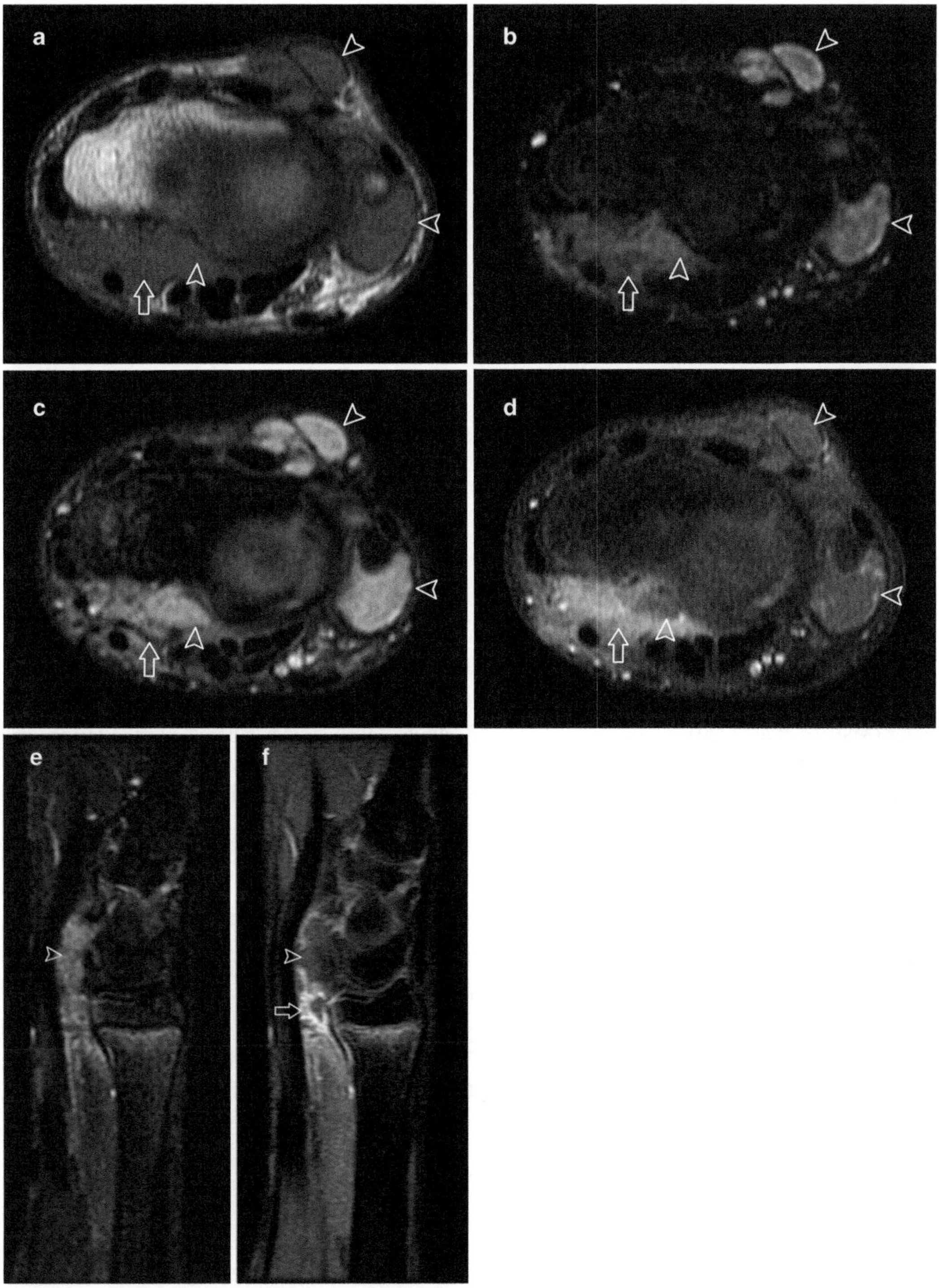

Fig. 25 Synovial chondromatosis in a 15-year-old boy. Axial (**a**) T1-weighted, (**b**) STIR, (**c**) gradient T2*-weighted and (**d**) fat-suppressed contrast-enhanced T1-weighted MR images along with sagittal (**e**) STIR and (**f**) fat-suppressed contrast-enhanced T1-weighted MR images show multiple non-enhancing T1-isointense and heterogeneous T2-hyperintense lesions around the radiocarpal joint (open arrowheads) with evidence of synovitis in volar aspect (open arrows). No blooming on the gradient image (**c**) is observed. These findings are in keeping with synovial chondromatosis

6 Diagnosis Confirmation

Clinical symptoms such as erythema, swelling, stiffness, and severe pain are critical indicators for the early diagnosis of infections. Imaging modalities like MRI and US imaging play an essential role in distinguishing infections from other conditions, such as inflammatory arthritis and tumors, while also aiding in the detection of abscess formation and potential complications.

Joint aspiration and fluid analysis, including Gram staining, cell count, and aerobic/anaerobic cultures, are vital diagnostic tools. For high-risk patients, additional testing for mycobacterial and fungal cultures may be necessary. Aspiration should also be performed when fluctuance is clinically evident (Malizos et al. 2020). Molecular methods, such as nucleic acid amplification tests (e.g., Xpert MTB/RIF for *M. tuberculosis*), further enhance pathogen identification. Cultures from multiple tissue samples are particularly crucial in cases of extrapulmonary TB or deep infections, while histological examination is invaluable for diagnosing granulomatous diseases (Malizos et al. 2020).

Careful selection of biopsy sites improves organism detection, with imaging guidance playing a pivotal role. Tissue sampling from at least three different areas is recommended for microbiological examination (Glaudemans et al. 2019). It has been suggested that culture is more effective at detecting organisms in tissue specimens compared to joint effusion, with similar diagnostic value to molecular testing (Smits et al. 2019). Aspiration or biopsy should always be conducted prior to starting antibiotics and must avoid traversing areas of overlying cellulitis to prevent the risk of inoculating organisms.

7 Treatment

NF requires immediate surgical debridement combined with intravenous broad-spectrum antibiotics. Early intervention, ideally within 6–12 h, significantly reduces mortality and morbidity (Malizos et al. 2020). Empirical antibiotics are started for most hand and wrist infections, targeting likely pathogens such as MRSA or gram-negative bacteria. Timely tetanus prophylaxis is crucial for contaminated wounds. Antibiotic regimens are tailored based on culture results and severity: 4–6 weeks for osteomyelitis and septic arthritis and 1–2 weeks for superficial soft tissue infections (Malizos et al. 2020). Chronic infections like tuberculous arthritis may necessitate prolonged treatment with anti-TB drugs guided by histological and molecular confirmation.

The high vascularity and reduced load-bearing activities of the hand support effective treatment outcomes. While mild early infections without abscess formation may respond to antibiotics, advanced infections with severe symptoms necessitate prompt debridement and drainage. Abscesses, septic arthritis, and osteomyelitis often require surgical intervention. Sequestra, i.e., dense fragments of necrotic bone, must be surgically removed for adequate treatment. Delayed drainage can lead to tissue necrosis, tendon rupture, systemic sepsis, and permanent disability. Severe infections may require multiple debridements.

Follow-up for hand and wrist infections entails clinical evaluations, laboratory monitoring, and imaging studies, depending on treatment strategies. Frequent assessments, especially post-surgery or in severe cases, are crucial for monitoring redness, swelling, pain, and systemic symptoms. Laboratory tests, including CRP, ESR, and WBC counts, help track resolution of the infection. Monitoring of wound healing and hand functions helps early detection of reinfections or complications.

Imaging plays a pivotal role in the follow-up of hand and wrist infections, especially in cases with persistent symptoms. US imaging or MRI is instrumental in identifying residual abscesses, fluid collections, or unresolved infections. Radiographs are valuable for monitoring bone healing in osteomyelitis (Fig. 8). During osteomyelitis healing, clinical and imaging findings must be evaluated together, as ongoing bone resorption may mimic progressive disease on radiographs despite clinical improvement (Erdman et al. 1991). For follow-up imaging of septic arthritis, MRI is considered the preferred modality. Repeat MRI scans are typically done to monitor treatment response, looking for reduction in joint effusion, synovial inflammation, and bone marrow changes (Abbod et al. 2018).

8 Conclusion

Hand infections, whether acute or chronic, require prompt diagnosis and management to prevent complications such as stiffness, contractures, or amputation. While most infections of the hand and wrist are confined to soft tissues, deep infections such as NF, osteomyelitis, and septic arthritis often require surgical intervention. Imaging is crucial for assessing the infection extent, particularly in cases with suspected bone or joint involvement or deep abscesses, guiding treatment, and distinguishing infections from inflammatory arthritis or tumors. Radiographs are the first-line imaging tool and can be used for monitoring osteomyelitis, with changes appearing 8–10 days post-infection. MRI is the gold standard for detecting and staging infections, with gadolinium-enhanced imaging aiding in detecting abscesses. CT is particularly useful in chronic osteomyelitis for detecting sequestra requiring surgical removal, while US imaging effectively detects fluid collections, abscesses, and FBs. Chronic infections should be considered in patients presenting with painless swelling or draining sinuses. Comprehensive clinical evaluation, along with pathogen identification through imaging-guided aspiration, is crucial for targeted antibiotic therapy. A multidisciplinary approach, involving radiologists, infectious disease specialists, and hand surgeons, is essential for optimizing treatment and minimizing morbidity.

Acknowledgment We thank Dr. Wattanapong Narueban and Dr. Krittinai Naiwatanakul for their contributions to illustrations (Figs. 1a, b, 2a, b, 4 and 5a).

References

Abbod H, Al-Otaibi L, Alshamiri K (2018) Septic arthritis. Int J Pediatr Adolesc Med 5:152–154. https://doi.org/10.1016/j.ijpam.2018.12.005

Abid W, Ladeb MF, Chidambaranathan N, Peh WCG, Vanhoenacker FM (2024) Imaging of musculoskeletal tuberculosis. Skeletal Radiol 53:2081–2097. https://doi.org/10.1007/s00256-023-04556-5

Agarwal A, Khan SA, Qureshi NA (2011) Multifocal osteoarticular tuberculosis in children. J Orthop Surg (Hong Kong) 19:336–340. https://doi.org/10.1177/230949901101900315

Aguiar RO, Gasparetto EL, Escuissato DL, Marchiori E, Trudell DJ, Haghighi P, Resnick D (2006) Radial and ulnar bursae of the wrist: cadaveric investigation of regional anatomy with ultrasonographic-guided tenography and MR imaging. Skeletal Radiol 35:828–832. https://doi.org/10.1007/s00256-006-0143-z

Ahlawat S, Corl FM, LaPorte DM, Fishman EK, Fayad LM (2017) MDCT of hand and wrist infections: emphasis on compartmental anatomy. Clin Radiol 72:338.e331–33338.e9. https://doi.org/10.1016/j.crad.2016.11.020

Ali SZ, Srinivasan S, Peh WCG (2014) MRI in necrotizing fasciitis of the extremities. Br J Radiol 87:20130560. https://doi.org/10.1259/bjr.20130560

Al-Qattan MM, Helmi AA (2014) Chronic hand infections. J Hand Surg Am 39:1636–1645. https://doi.org/10.1016/j.jhsa.2014.04.003

Anderson MA, Newmeyer WL 3rd, Kilgore ES Jr (1982) Diagnosis and treatment of retained foreign bodies in the hand. Am J Surg 144:63–67. https://doi.org/10.1016/0002-9610(82)90603-1

Aras MH, Miloglu O, Barutcugil C, Kantarci M, Ozcan E, Harorli A (2010) Comparison of the sensitivity for detecting foreign bodies among conventional plain radiography, computed tomography and ultrasonography. Dentomaxillofac Radiol 39:72–78. https://doi.org/10.1259/dmfr/68589458

Brown DM, Young VL (1993) Hand infections. South Med J 86:56–66. https://doi.org/10.1097/00007611-199301000-00013

Capitanio MA, Kirkpatrick JA (1970) Early roentgen observations in acute osteomyelitis. Am J Roentgenol Radium Therapy, Nucl Med 108:488–496. https://doi.org/10.2214/ajr.108.3.488

Chan T, Yaghoubian A, Rosing D, Kaji A, de Virgilio C (2008) Low sensitivity of physical examination findings in necrotizing soft tissue infection is improved with laboratory values: a prospective study. Am J Surg 196:926–930; discussion 930. https://doi.org/10.1016/j.amjsurg.2008.07.025

Chen A, Wong LY, Sheu CY, Chen BF (2002) Distinguishing multiple rice body formation in chronic subacromial-subdeltoid bursitis from synovial chondromatosis. Skeletal Radiol 31:119–121. https://doi.org/10.1007/s002560100412

Choi JA, Koh SH, Hong SH, Koh YH, Choi JY, Kang HS (2009) Rheumatoid arthritis and tuberculous arthritis: differentiating MRI features. AJR Am J Roentgenol 193:1347–1353. https://doi.org/10.2214/AJR.08.2164

Clark DC (2003) Common acute hand infections. Am Fam Physician 68:2167–2176

Collins MS, Schaar MM, Wenger DE, Mandrekar JN (2005) T1-weighted MRI characteristics of pedal osteomyelitis. AJR Am J Roentgenol 185:386–393. https://doi.org/10.2214/ajr.185.2.01850386

Dalbeth N, House ME, Aati O, Tan P, Franklin C, Horne A, Gamble GD, Stamp LK, Doyle AJ, McQueen FM (2015) Urate crystal deposition in asymptomatic hyperuricaemia and symptomatic gout: a dual energy CT study. Ann Rheum Dis 74:908–911. https://doi.org/10.1136/annrheumdis-2014-206397

DeLullo JA, Lubahn JD, Loeffler OP, Dominy DD (2013) Necrotizing soft tissue infections of the upper extremity: a case series. J Surg Orthop Adv 22:198–203. https://doi.org/10.3113/jsoa.2013.0198

Diaz JH, Lopez FA (2015) Skin, soft tissue and systemic bacterial infections following aquatic injuries and exposures. Am J Med Sci 349:269–275. https://doi.org/10.1097/MAJ.0000000000000366

Doyle JR (1989) Anatomy of the flexor tendon sheath and pulley system: a current review. J Hand Surg Am 14:349–351. https://doi.org/10.1016/0363-5023(89)90110-x

Erdman WA, Tamburro F, Jayson HT, Weatherall PT, Ferry KB, Peshock RM (1991) Osteomyelitis: characteristics and pitfalls of diagnosis with MR imaging. Radiology 180:533–539. https://doi.org/10.1148/radiology.180.2.2068324

Flevas DA, Syngouna S, Fandridis E, Tsiodras S, Mavrogenis AF (2019) Infections of the hand: an overview. EFORT Open Rev 4:183–193. https://doi.org/10.1302/2058-5241.4.180082

Fowler JR, Ilyas AM (2013) Epidemiology of adult acute hand infections at an urban medical center. J Hand Surg Am 38:1189–1193. https://doi.org/10.1016/j.jhsa.2013.03.013

Fussey JM, Chin KF, Gogi N, Gella S, Deshmukh SC (2009) An anatomic study of flexor tendon sheaths: a cadaveric study. J Hand Surg Eur Vol 34:762–765. https://doi.org/10.1177/1753193409344529

Gastrin B, Lovestad A (1989) Postoperative wound infection: relation to different types of operation and wound contamination categories in orthopaedic surgery. J Hosp Infect 13:387–393. https://doi.org/10.1016/0195-6701(89)90058-3

Girish G, Glazebrook KN, Jacobson JA (2013) Advanced imaging in gout. AJR Am J Roentgenol 201:515–525. https://doi.org/10.2214/ajr.13.10776

Glaudemans A, Jutte PC, Cataldo MA, Cassar-Pullicino V, Gheysens O, Borens O, Trampuz A, Wortler K, Petrosillo N, Winkler H, Signore A, Sconfienza LM (2019) Consensus document for the diagnosis of peripheral bone infection in adults: a joint paper by the EANM, EBJIS, and ESR (with ESCMID endorsement). Eur J Nucl Med Mol Imaging 46:957–970. https://doi.org/10.1007/s00259-019-4262-x

Gold RH, Hawkins RA, Katz RD (1991) Bacterial osteomyelitis: findings on plain radiography, CT, MR, and scintigraphy. AJR Am J Roentgenol 157:365–370. https://doi.org/10.2214/ajr.157.2.1853823

Graif M, Schweitzer ME, Deely D, Matteucci T (1999) The septic versus nonseptic inflamed joint: MRI characteristics. Skeletal Radiol 28:616–620. https://doi.org/10.1007/s002560050562

Greenwood S, Leone A, Cassar-Pullicino VN (2017) SAPHO and recurrent multifocal osteomyelitis. Radiol Clin North Am 55:1035–1053. https://doi.org/10.1016/j.rcl.2017.04.009

Grey AC, Davies AM, Mangham DC, Grimer RJ, Ritchie DA (1998) The ‘penumbra sign’ on T1-weighted MR imaging in subacute osteomyelitis: frequency, cause and significance. Clin Radiol 53:587–592. https://doi.org/10.1016/s0009-9260(98)80150-5

Henninger B, Glodny B, Rudisch A, Trieb T, Loizides A, Putzer D, Judmaier W, Schocke MF (2013) Ewing sarcoma versus osteomyelitis: differential diagnosis with magnetic resonance imaging. Skeletal Radiol 42:1097–1104. https://doi.org/10.1007/s00256-013-1632-5

Hong SH, Kim SM, Ahn JM, Chung HW, Shin MJ, Kang HS (2001) Tuberculous versus pyogenic arthritis: MR imaging evaluation. Radiology 218:848–853. https://doi.org/10.1148/radiology.218.3.r01fe27848

Hopkins KL, Li KCP, Bergman G (1995) Gadolinium-DTPA-enhanced magnetic resonance imaging of musculoskeletal infectious processes. Skeletal Radiol 24:325–330. https://doi.org/10.1007/BF00197059

Houshian S, Seyedipour S, Wedderkopp N (2006) Epidemiology of bacterial hand infections. Int J Infect Dis 10:315–319. https://doi.org/10.1016/j.ijid.2005.06.009

Hsu CY, Lu HC, Shih TT (2004) Tuberculous infection of the wrist: MRI features. AJR Am J Roentgenol 183:623–628. https://doi.org/10.2214/ajr.183.3.1830623

Imahara SD, Friedrich JB (2010) Community-acquired methicillin-resistant Staphylococcus aureus in surgically treated hand infections. J Hand Surg Am 35:97–103. https://doi.org/10.1016/j.jhsa.2009.09.004

Jalil A, Barlaan PI, Fung BK, Ip JW (2011) Hand infection in diabetic patients. Hand Surg 16:307–312. https://doi.org/10.1142/S021881041100559X

Jaovisidha S, Chen C, Ryu KN, Siriwongpairat P, Pekanan P, Sartoris DJ, Resnick D (1996) Tuberculous tenosynovitis and bursitis: imaging findings in 21 cases. Radiology 201:507–513. https://doi.org/10.1148/radiology.201.2.8888250

Jebson PJ (1998) Deep subfascial space infections. Hand Clin 14:557–566, viii

Jeffrey RB Jr, Laing FC, Schechter WP, Markison RE, Barton RM (1987) Acute suppurative tenosynovitis of the hand: diagnosis with US. Radiology 162:741–742. https://doi.org/10.1148/radiology.162.3.3544036

Kanavel AB (1921) Infections of the hand, 4th edn. Lea & Febiger, United States

Kennedy CD, Huang JI, Hanel DP (2016) In brief: Kanavel’s signs and pyogenic flexor tenosynovitis. Clin Orthop Relat Res 474:280–284. https://doi.org/10.1007/s11999-015-4367-x

Kim KT, Kim YJ, Won Lee J, Kim YJ, Park SW, Lim MK, Suh CH (2011) Can necrotizing infectious fasciitis be differentiated from nonnecrotizing infectious fasciitis with MR imaging? Radiology 259:816–824. https://doi.org/10.1148/radiol.11101164

Kistler JM, Thoder JJ, Ilyas AM (2019) MRSA incidence and antibiotic trends in urban hand infections: a 10-year longitudinal study. Hand (N Y) 14:449–454. https://doi.org/10.1177/1558944717750921

Kosaraju V, Harwani A, Partovi S, Bhojwani N, Garg V, Ayyappan S, Kosmas C, Robbin M (2017) Imaging of musculoskeletal manifestations in sickle cell disease patients. Br J Radiol 90:20160130. https://doi.org/10.1259/bjr.20160130

Koshy JC, Bell B (2019) Hand infections. J Hand Surg Am 44:46–54. https://doi.org/10.1016/j.jhsa.2018.05.027

Kothari NA, Pelchovitz DJ, Meyer JS (2001) Imaging of musculoskeletal infections. Radiol Clin North Am 39:653–671. https://doi.org/10.1016/s0033-8389(05)70304-3

Liu PT, Kujak JL, Roberts CC, de Chadarevian JP (2011) The vascular groove sign: a new CT finding associated with osteoid osteomas. AJR Am J Roentgenol 196:168–173. https://doi.org/10.2214/AJR.10.4534

Louis DS, Jebson PJ (1998) Mimickers of hand infections. Hand Clin 14:519–529, vii

Malizos KN, Papadopoulou ZK, Ziogkou AN, Rigopoulos N, Athanaselis ED, Varitimidis SE, Dailiana ZC (2020) Infections of deep hand and wrist compartments. Microorganisms 8. https://doi.org/10.3390/microorganisms8060838

McGuinness B, Wilson N, Doyle AJ (2007) The "penumbra sign" on T1-weighted MRI for differentiating musculoskeletal infection from tumour. Skeletal Radiol 36:417–421. https://doi.org/10.1007/s00256-006-0267-1

Needs CJ, Webb J, Tyndall A (1985) Paralysis and unilateral arthritis: is the association established? Clin Rheumatol 4:176–180. https://doi.org/10.1007/BF02032289

Ong YS, Levin LS (2009) Hand infections. Plast Reconstr Surg 124:225e–233e. https://doi.org/10.1097/PRS.0b013e3181b458c9

Patel DB, Emmanuel NB, Stevanovic MV, Matcuk GR Jr, Gottsegen CJ, Forrester DM, White EA (2014) Hand infections: anatomy, types and spread of infection, imaging findings, and treatment options. Radiographics 34:1968–1986. https://doi.org/10.1148/rg.347130101

Pattamapaspong N, Srisuwan T, Sivasomboon C, Nasuto M, Suwannahoy P, Settakorn J, Kraisarin J, Guglielmi G (2013) Accuracy of radiography, computed tomography and magnetic resonance imaging in diagnosing foreign bodies in the foot. Radiol Med 118:303–310. https://doi.org/10.1007/s11547-012-0844-4

Pattamapaspong N, Vuthiwong W, Kanthawang T, Louthrenoo W (2017) Value of ultrasonography in the diagnosis of gout in patients presenting with acute arthritis. Skeletal Radiol 46:759–767. https://doi.org/10.1007/s00256-017-2611-z

Pattamapaspong N, Kanthawang T, Bouaziz MC, Ladeb MF, Hammami N, Peh WCG (2024) Imaging of musculoskeletal tuberculosis. Br J Radiol 97:1–12. https://doi.org/10.1093/bjr/tqad019

Phemister D, Hatcher C (1933) Correlation of pathological and roentgenological findings in the diagnosis of tuberculous arthritis. AJR Am J Roentgenol 29:736–752

Pineda C, Espinosa R, Pena A (2009) Radiographic imaging in osteomyelitis: the role of plain radiography, computed tomography, ultrasonography, magnetic resonance imaging, and scintigraphy. Semin Plast Surg 23:80–89. https://doi.org/10.1055/s-0029-1214160

Ranjan R, Goel L, Sud A, Sinha A, Tulika KR (2019) Bilateral tubercular dactylitis: unusual presentation of an usual disease. Indian J Tuberc 66:346–352. https://doi.org/10.1016/j.ijtb.2017.05.002

Reilly KE, Linz JC, Stern PJ, Giza E, Wyrick JD (1997) Osteomyelitis of the tubular bones of the hand. J Hand Surg Am 22:644–649. https://doi.org/10.1016/S0363-5023(97)80122-0

Rerucha CM, Ewing JT, Oppenlander KE, Cowan WC (2019) Acute hand infections. Am Fam Physician 99:228–236

Resnick D (1975) Roentgenographic anatomy of the tendon sheaths of the hand and wrist: tenography. Am J Roentgenol Radium Therapy, Nucl Med 124:44–51. https://doi.org/10.2214/ajr.124.1.44

Resnick D (1976) Osteomyelitis and septic arthritis complicating hand injuries and infections: pathogenesis of roentgenographic abnormalities. J Can Assoc Radiol 27:21–28

Santiago Restrepo C, Gimenez CR, McCarthy K (2003) Imaging of osteomyelitis and musculoskeletal soft tissue infections: current concepts. Rheum Dis Clin N Am 29:89–109. https://doi.org/10.1016/s0889-857x(02)00078-9

Sawlani V, Chandra T, Mishra RN, Aggarwal A, Jain UK, Gujral RB (2003) MRI features of tuberculosis of peripheral joints. Clin Radiol 58:755–762. https://doi.org/10.1016/s0009-9260(03)00271-x

Scheldrup EW (1951) Tendon sheath patterns in the hand; an anatomical study based on 367 hand dissections. Surg Gynecol Obstet 93:16–22

Schmidt G, Piponov H, Chuang D, Gonzalez M (2019) Hand infections in the immunocompromised patient: an update. J Hand Surg Am 44:144–149. https://doi.org/10.1016/j.jhsa.2018.07.001

Schnall SB, Vu-Rose T, Holtom PD, Doyle B, Stevanovic M (1996) Tissue pressures in pyogenic flexor tenosynovitis of the finger. Compartment syndrome and its management. J Bone Joint Surg Br 78:793–795

Seok JH, Jee W-H, Chun K-A, Kim J-Y, Jung C-K, Kim YR, Eo W-K, Kim Y-S, Chung YG (2009) Necrotizing fasciitis versus pyomyositis: discrimination with using MR imaging. Korean J Radiol 10:121–128

Shafritz AB, Coppage JM (2014) Acute and chronic paronychia of the hand. J Am Acad Orthop Surg 22:165–174. https://doi.org/10.5435/JAAOS-22-03-165

Sharma KS, Rao K, Hobson MI (2013) Space of parona infections: experience in management and outcomes in a regional hand centre. J Plast Reconstr

Aesthet Surg 66:968–972. https://doi.org/10.1016/j.bjps.2013.03.020

Sharma K, Pan D, Friedman J, Yu JL, Mull A, Moore AM (2018) Quantifying the effect of diabetes on surgical hand and forearm infections. J Hand Surg Am 43:105–114. https://doi.org/10.1016/j.jhsa.2017.11.003

Singh M, Jeyaraman M, Jeyaraman N, Jayakumar T, Iyengar KP, Jain VK (2023) Mycobacterium tuberculosis infection of the wrist joint: a current concepts review. J Clin Orthop Trauma 44:102257. https://doi.org/10.1016/j.jcot.2023.102257

Smits M, van de Groes S, Thurlings RM (2019) Synovial tissue biopsy collection by rheumatologists: ready for clinical implementation? Front Med (Lausanne) 6:138. https://doi.org/10.3389/fmed.2019.00138

Tehranzadeh J, Wang F, Mesgarzadeh M (1992) Magnetic resonance imaging of osteomyelitis. Crit Rev Diagn Imaging 33:495–534

Teo HE, Peh WCG (2004) Skeletal tuberculosis in children. Pediatr Radiol 34:853–860. https://doi.org/10.1007/s00247-004-1223-7

Turker T, Capdarest-Arest N, Bertoch ST, Bakken EC, Hoover SE, Zou J (2014) Hand infections: a retrospective analysis. PeerJ 2:e513. https://doi.org/10.7717/peerj.513

Wudhikulprapan W, Phinyo P, Hadi A, Kanthawang T, Choudur HN (2024) Diagnosing osteomyelitis in diabetic foot by diffusion-weighted imaging and dynamic contrast material-enhanced magnetic resonance imaging: a systematic review and meta-analysis. Clin Radiol 79:805–817. https://doi.org/10.1016/j.crad.2024.07.015

Zook EG (1990) Anatomy and physiology of the perionychium. Hand Clin 6:1–7

Sports Injuries of Hand and Wrist

Malini Lawande, Aditya Daftary, and Ankita Ahuja

Contents

Abstract

Sports injuries are common in the wrist and hand. These may occur due to acute trauma or chronic overuse. Imaging modalities like radiograph, ultrasound, CT and MRI play an important role in early diagnosis and planning appropriate management ensuring early return to play. Understanding the mechanism of injury is useful to understand the structures injured and to select the appropriate imaging modality.

Acute as well as chronic overuse sports injuries are common in the wrist and hand. Early and accurate diagnosis by imaging plays an important role in management and early return to play.

These injuries may be osseous, tendon, or ligament injuries. Less commonly neural and vascular injuries may occur. Certain injuries are more common in certain sports due to the mechanism of play and overuse.

The imaging of these injuries has been discussed in greater detail in the individual chapters. Here we look at the mechanism of common sports injuries of the wrist and hand with a brief description of their typical imaging appearance.

M. Lawande (✉) · A. Daftary · A. Ahuja
Innovision Imaging, Mumbai, India
e-mail: malini.lawande@innovisionimaging.com

Med Radiol Diagn Imaging (2025)
https://doi.org/10.1007/174_2025_593,

Published Online: 09 September 2025

1 Wrist and Hand Injuries in Sports

1.1 Acute Fractures

Scaphoid is the most commonly fractured carpal bone and occurs due to fall on an outstretched hand with extended wrist. This is commonly seen in roller skating and contact sports (Chen et al. 2009). Plain radiographs are useful to detect the scaphoid fracture (Fig. 1). However, in some cases, the fracture may be occult. MRI is useful in these cases with STIR images showing marrow edema and the T1/Proton density images demonstrating the fracture line. The blood supply to the scaphoid enters through the distal pole. Fractures through the waist and proximal pole lead to disruption of the vascular supply and can further lead to avascular necrosis of the proximal pole (Fig. 2). Undiagnosed scaphoid fractures may lead to non-union and carpal instability, further leading to osteoarthritis (scaphoid non-union advanced collapse (SNAC)) (Howse 1994).

Fracture of the distal radius may occur due to fall on an outstretched hand and is common in sports like hockey and ice skating (Tedesco et al. 2020). Displacement, articular surface extension, and depression are assessed to decide the management.

Fractures of the hook of hamate occur due to transmission of the force from golf club, bat, or racquet to the palm. These occur in the dominant hand in tennis and other racquet sports (Gil and Kakar 2019). In cricket, hook of hamate fractures is seen in the non-dominant hand due to the double grip nature of holding the bat where the non-dominant hand holds the bat superiorly with the bat handle resting on the hamate hook (Batta et al. 2023). In golf, these fractures occur in the leading non-dominant hand due to blow from the butt of the handle of the golf club (Murray and Cooney 1996). These fractures may also be occult on radiographs and MRI or CT can be used for further evaluation (Fig. 3). Fracture of the hook of hamate needs to be differentiated from accessory ossicle (os hamuli proprium) in which the ossification center of the hook fails to fuse with the rest of the body. The accessory ossicle is smooth and well corticated with absence of marrow edema.

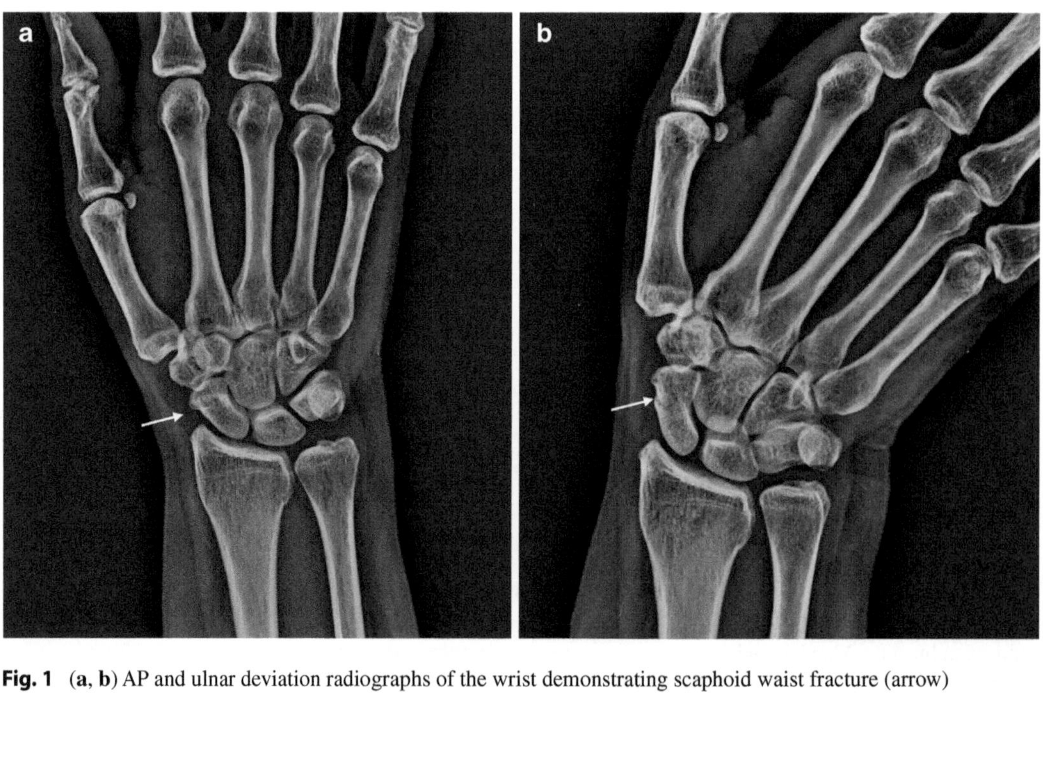

Fig. 1 (**a**, **b**) AP and ulnar deviation radiographs of the wrist demonstrating scaphoid waist fracture (arrow)

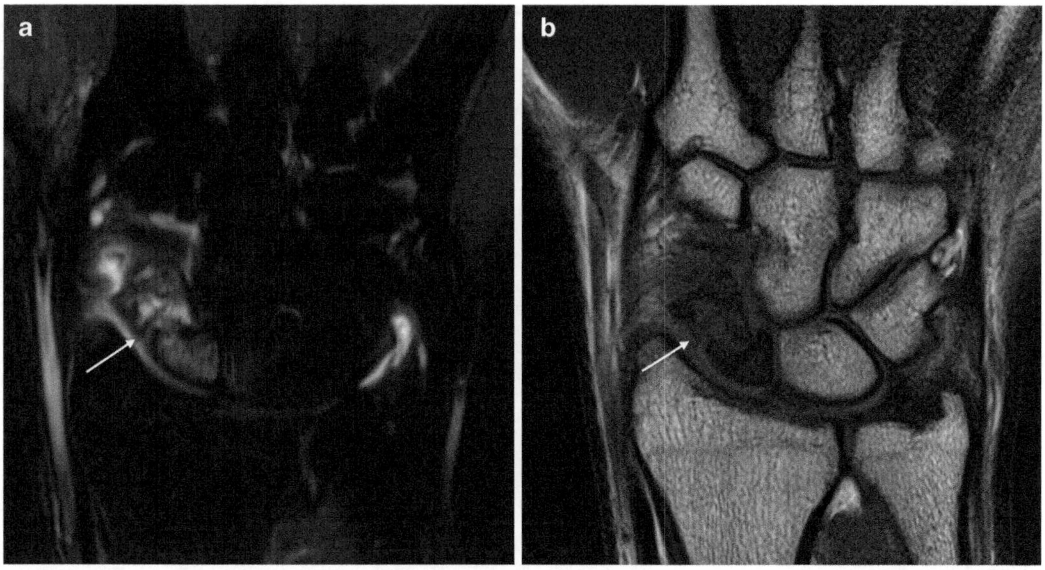

Fig. 2 (**a**, **b**) Coronal STIR and T1 weighted images reveal ununited scaphoid waist fracture (arrow) with avascular necrosis in the proximal pole

Ulnar styloid process fractures may occur associated with other fractures during fall or due to direct impact in contact sports (Cockenpot et al. 2016).

1.2 Stress Fractures

Stress injuries occur due to chronic microtrauma and repetitive impact on a normal bone.

Stress fractures of hamate hook are common due to repetitive impaction of the racquet, cricket bat, or golf club against it. Stress fractures of scaphoid are seen in gymnastics and shot put due to repeated dorsiflexion (Gabel 1998).

Metacarpal (second) stress fractures are seen in tennis players due to repetitive impact of the racquet handle and altered biomechanics of the grip (Waninger and Lombardo 1995). Other bones like pisiform (volleyball), triquetrum (break dancing), and fifth metacarpal (soft ball) are also prone to stress injuries (Lohman et al. 2003; Bhairo et al. 1992). These stress injuries are initially seen as marrow edema on STIR/fat-saturated T2-weighted images with subsequent development of T1 hypointense marrow signal. Later stages show discrete fracture line. Hence, MRI is a very useful modality in detecting early stress injuries before fracture develops.

Repetitive impact to the distal radial physes in pediatric gymnasts due to high axial load transmission while weight bearing during high impact maneuvers leads to growth plate injury and is called Gymnast's wrist (Albanese et al. 1989). This is seen on radiographs as widened and ill-defined distal radial physes. On MRI, it shows periphyseal edema and may lead to physeal arrest (Shih et al. 1995).

1.3 Osteonecrosis

Keinbock's disease is due to osteonecrosis of the lunate and may be seen in the dominant hand of athletes with repetitive wrist loading like gymnastics and handball. MRI is useful in diagnosing as well as staging of the disease. There is T1 hypointense and STIR hyperintense marrow signal in the lunate initially with further progress to sclerosis with fragmentation and collapse and finally osteoarthritis (Trumble and Katolik 2006).

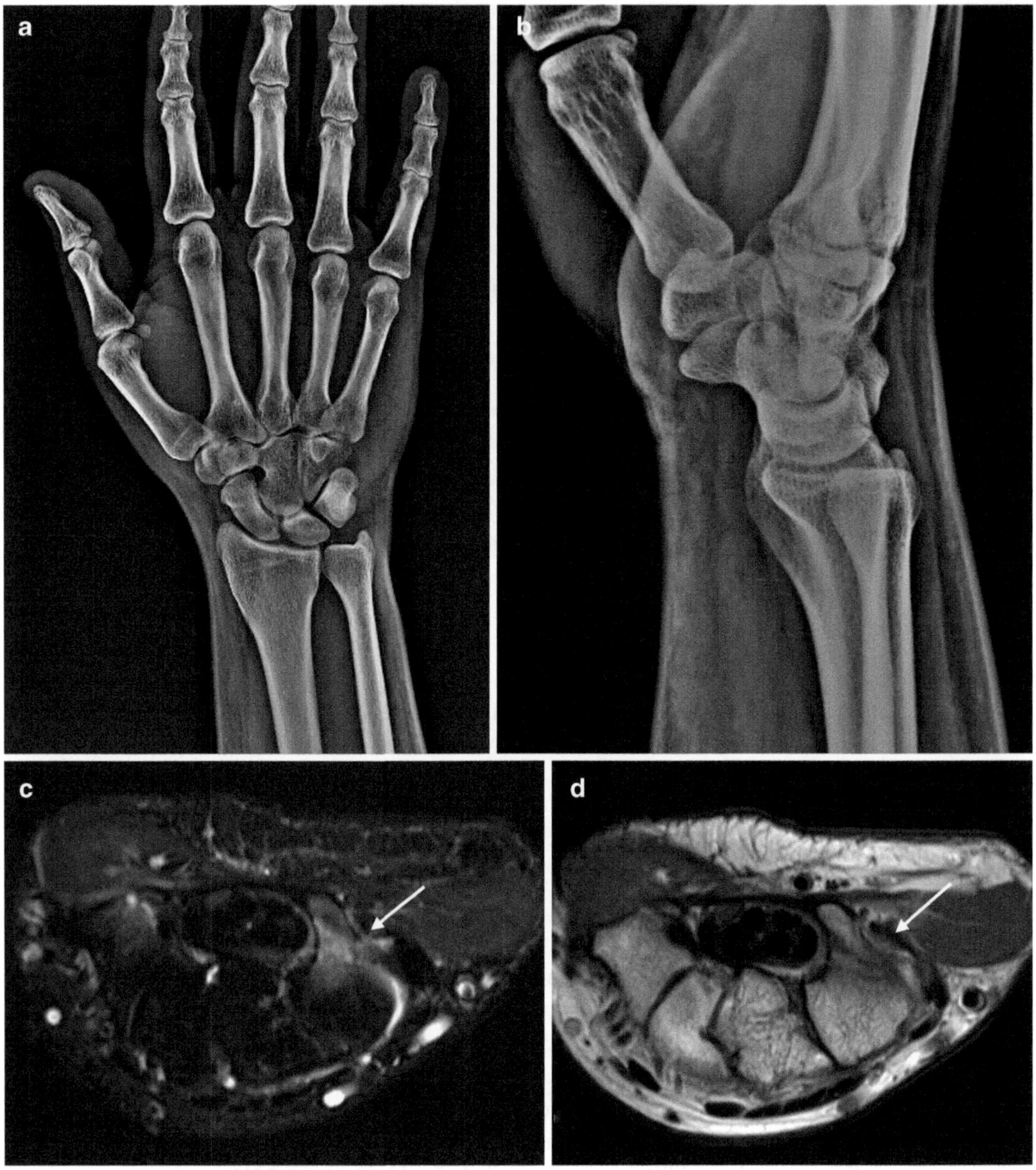

Fig. 3 (**a**, **b**) AP and lateral radiographs in a golf player with ulnar sided pain do not reveal any abnormality. (**c**, **d**) Axial fat saturated T2 and Proton density images show non-displaced fracture of the hook of hamate with moderate marrow edema (arrow)

1.4 Ligament Injuries

Scapholunate ligament injuries may occur in any sport due to impact against another player or the ground with wrist in hyperextended position. The dorsal component of the scapholunate ligament is the most important component in maintaining stability. On radiographs, there is widening of the scapholunate interval more than 2 mm (Terry Thomas sign) with foreshortened scaphoid. Clenched fist radiographs are useful as they stress the scapholunate ligament and accentuate the scapholunate interval widening in cases with ligament injuries. Dorsal intercalated segmental instability (DISI) may be seen as dorsal tilting of the lunate in the sagittal plane with increase in scapholunate and capitatolunate angles. The instability may further lead to osteo-

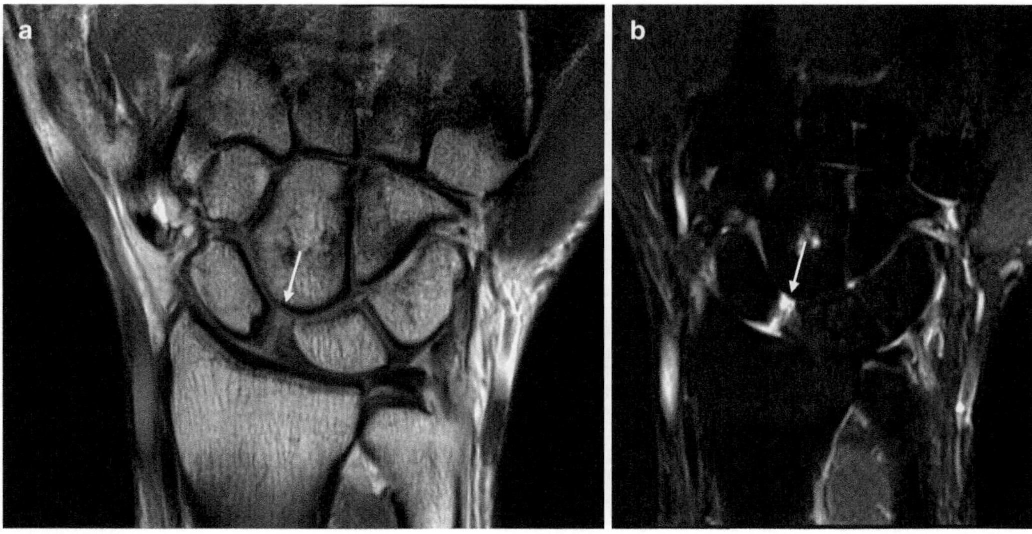

Fig. 4 (**a**, **b**) Coronal proton density and STIR images in a hockey player show full thickness scaphoid attachment scapholunate ligament tear with widening of the scapholunate interval (arrow)

arthritis and is called scapholunate advanced collapse (SLAC) (Connell et al. 2001). The dorsal, volar, and membranous components of the scapholunate ligament can be well evaluated on MRI (Fig. 4).

Lunotriquetral ligament injuries are less common and may occur due to fall on an outstretched hand. Radiographs may show widening of the lunotriquetral interval.

Hockey wrist is due to dorsal ulnotriquetral ligament injury and is common in ice hockey players. It occurs in the proximal hand which holds the stick and is in flexion pronation position. Superadded torque forces with radial deviation lead to dorsal ulnotriquetral ligament injury and ulnar sided pain (Tedesco et al. 2020).

MRI is useful to demonstrate the ligaments and their tears as full thickness or partial thickness disruption.

1.5 Triangular Fibrocartilage Injuries

Triangular fibrocartilage (TFCC) is the main stabilizer of the distal radioulnar joint. It may be injured due to fall on an outstretched hand or distraction force along the volar aspect in racquet sports. It is prone to degeneration and tears, which may occur due to rotational motion during grip of the cricket bat during bat swing (Batta et al. 2023).

TFCC injury may also be seen in cricket due to over swinging during batting or due to hitting the bat on the ground.

TFCC tears are classified as Palmer class 1 traumatic tears which is further subclassified based on the location of the tear. Palmer class 2 tears are degenerative and are further divided based on adjoining chondral loss and lunotriquetral ligament integrity (Oneson et al. 1996).

Triangular fibrocartilage complex consists of the triangular fibrocartilage proper (articular disc), dorsal and volar radioulnar ligaments, meniscal homologue, and the ulnocarpal ligaments. The triangular fibrocartilage proper and radioulnar ligaments (which are thickenings along the volar and dorsal aspects of the fibrocartilage proper) are the important structures to be evaluated on MRI.

The triangular fibrocartilage near its ulnar attachment reveals striated appearance with hyperintense signal due to the presence of loose connective tissue. Also, there is intermediate signal intensity at its radial attachment at the interface with the articular cartilage that should not be mistaken for a tear. The tear should be a defect of fluid signal intensity (Fig. 5). Traumatic ulnar attachment injuries are amenable to repair as this region is vascular (Yamabe et al. 2012).

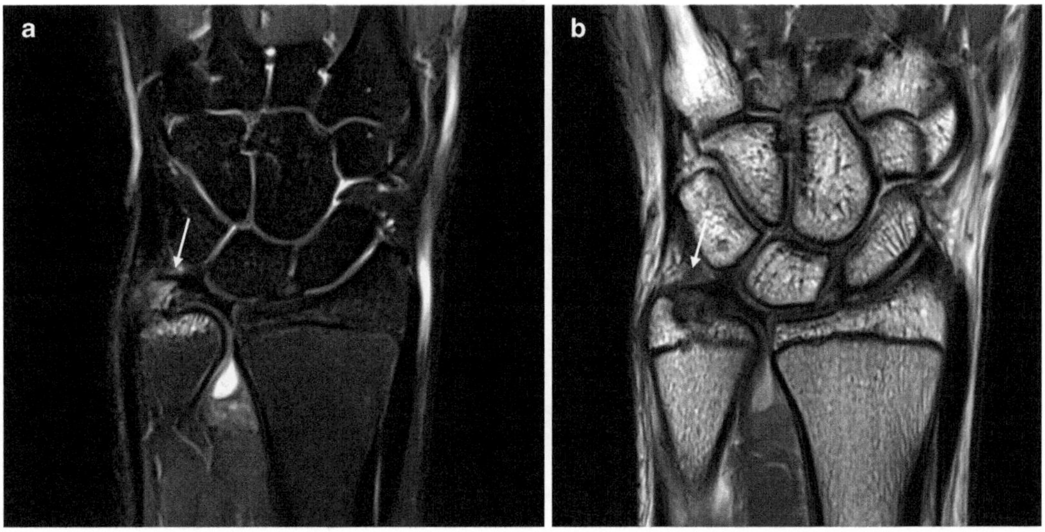

Fig. 5 (**a**, **b**) Coronal fat saturated T2 and proton density images of the wrist in a tennis player reveal high grade ulnar attachment triangular fibrocartilage injury (arrow) with mild adjoining distal ulnar marrow edema and mild distal radioulnar joint effusion

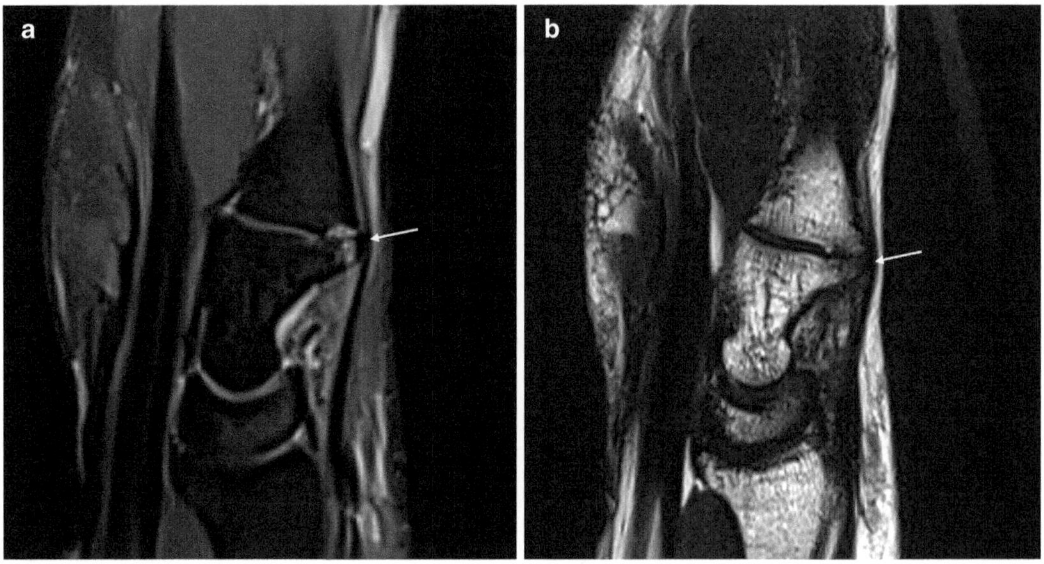

Fig. 6 (**a**, **b**) Sagittal STIR and proton density images in a boxer reveal carpal boss at third metacarpal base with mild marrow edema (arrow)

1.6 Carpal Boss

Carpal boss is an osseous prominence along the dorsal aspect of the bases of second or third metacarpals adjoining their articulation with trapezoid and capitate. It may be due to an osteophyte or accessory ossicle and common in boxers due to repeated impaction injuries (Melone et al. 2009). It may be symptomatic and show marrow edema as well as surrounding soft tissue edema on MRI with friction related changes in the overlying tendons (Figs. 6 and 7).

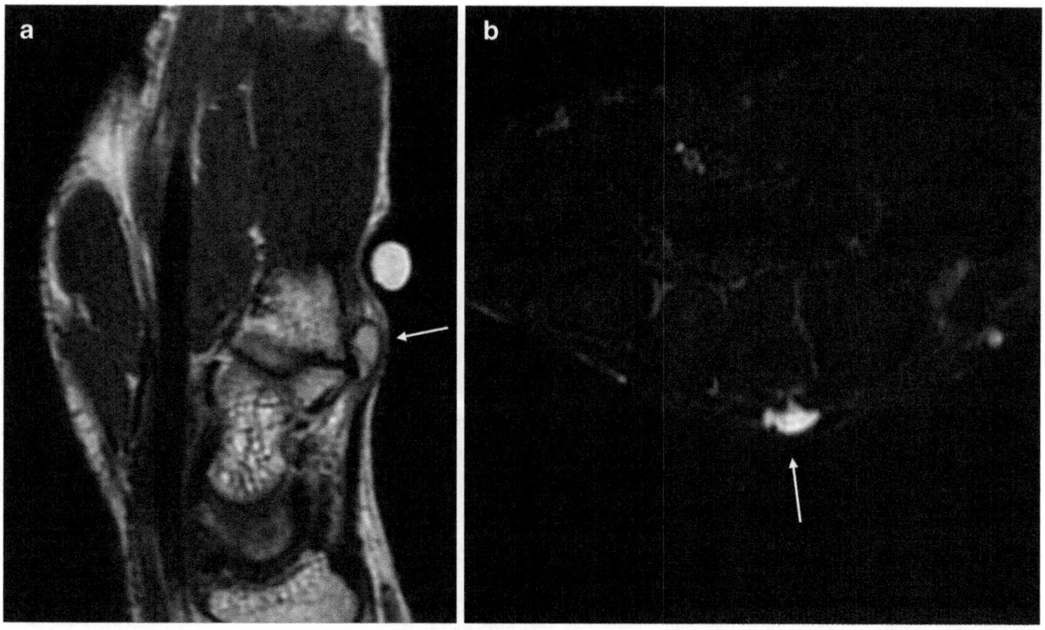

Fig. 7 (**a**, **b**) Sagittal proton density and axial STIR images reveal carpal boss at third metacarpal base with small overlying adventitious bursa/ganglion (arrow)

1.7 Bone Abutment Syndromes

Ulnocarpal abutment is a common cause of ulnar sided pain and occurs due to repeated impaction between the distal ulna and lunate. It is common in racquet sports, gymnastics, and baseball. The triad of imaging findings include positive ulnar variance, tear of the central portion of triangular fibrocartilage proper, and chondral loss with subchondral cystic changes in the adjoining lunate and/or triquetrum (Cerezal et al. 2002) (Fig. 8).

Ulnar styloid abutment is less common and is diagnosed when the ulnar styloid process is longer than 6 mm and impacts the triquetrum. MRI may show cystic changes and marrow edema with chondral loss along proximal triquetrum.

Hamatolunate abutment occurs when there is type II lunate which has a facet articulating with the adjoining hamate and resultant impaction-related changes along the contiguous surfaces.

1.8 Tendon Overuse Injuries

Chronic overuse injury of the tendons is common in the wrist and hand. These occur due to repeated stress and loading in sports like gymnastics and rowing. These are also seen commonly in sports which involve use of racquets, bats, or clubs (Werner and Plancher 1998).

Tendinosis or tendinopathy is seen as tendon enlargement with intrasubstance signal and tendon sheath fluid (tenosynovitis). If untreated, these may lead to tendon tear.

Ultrasound is an excellent modality in diagnosing these overuse tendon injuries. MRI can also demonstrate these tendon pathologies.

De Quervain's tenosynovitis occurs due to repetitive microtrauma due to the first compartment extensor tendons (abductor pollicis longus and extensor pollicis brevis) gliding over the radial styloid (Fig. 9). It is common in rowers, racquet sports, golf, and weight trainers. It is also common in professional gamers due to repeated movements of the thumb and wrist while playing video games and hence is also called "Gamer's thumb" (Reinstein 1983; Rossoni et al. 2023). It presents with dorsoradial pain and restricted thumb movements. These two tendons may be present in two separate sheaths or a common sheath. Identifying this is important in planning ultrasound guided pain relief injections.

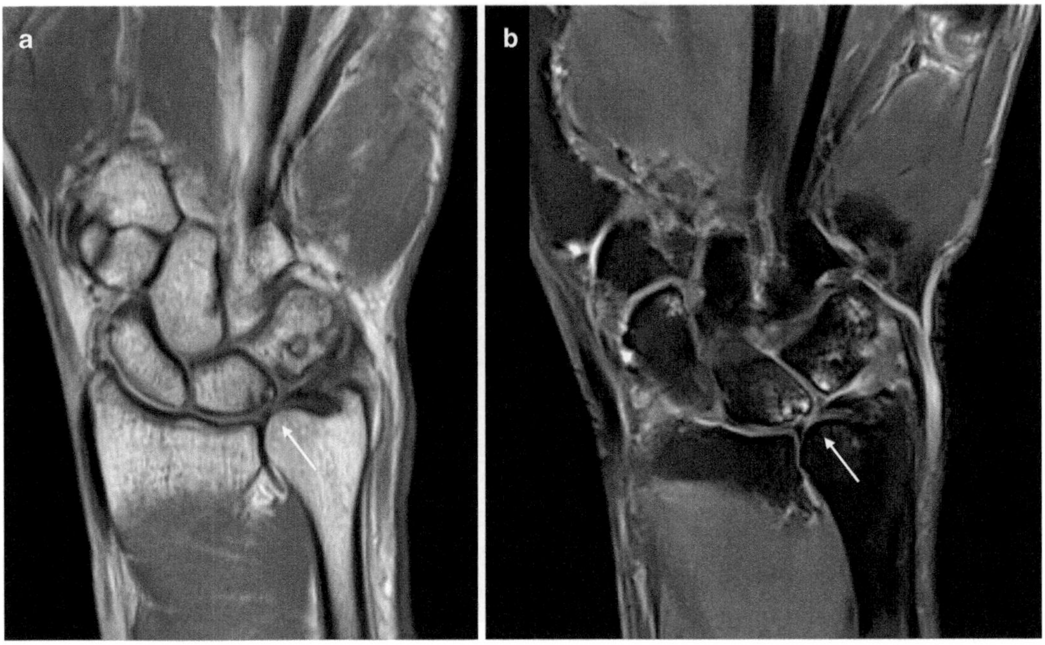

Fig. 8 (**a**, **b**) Coronal proton density and STIR images in a tennis player reveal ulnocarpal abutment with triad of central portion triangular fibrocartilage tear, chondral loss, and cystic changes in the adjoining lunate and triquetrum and positive ulnar variance (arrow)

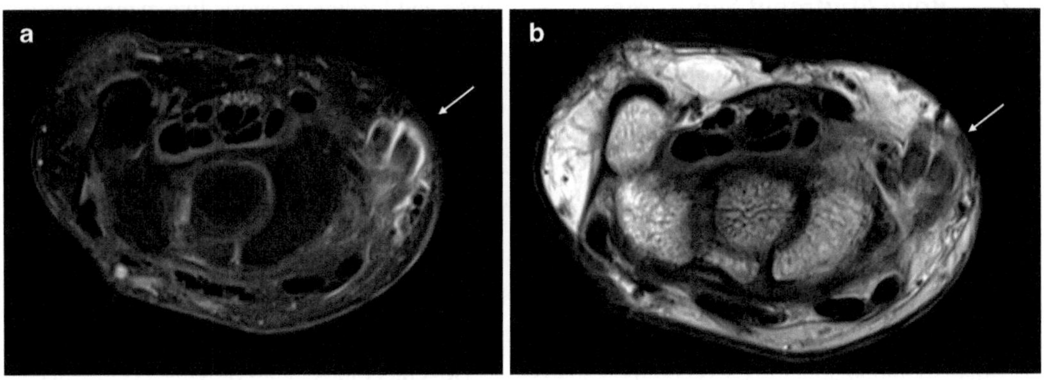

Fig. 9 (**a**, **b**) Axial fat saturated T2 weighted and proton density images in a patient with de Quervain's tenosynovitis demonstrating first extensor compartment tendinosis and tendon sheath fluid (arrow)

Extensor Carpi ulnaris tendinopathy occurs due to overuse in rowing and racquet sports. It is seen in the non-dominant hand of a tennis player due to the double-handed back hand. It is also seen in the non-dominant hand in cricket due to sudden ulnar deviation at the terminal end of the swing (Batta et al. 2023). This leads to tendinosis, tenosynovitis, or longitudinal split tears, commonly at the level of the ulnar styloid process.

The extensor carpi ulnaris tendon and its fibrous sheath are also prone to overuse injury in tennis players during forehand ground stroke due to repeated transmission of impact forces between the ball and racquet to the wrist (Gil and Kakar 2019) (Figs. 10 and 11).

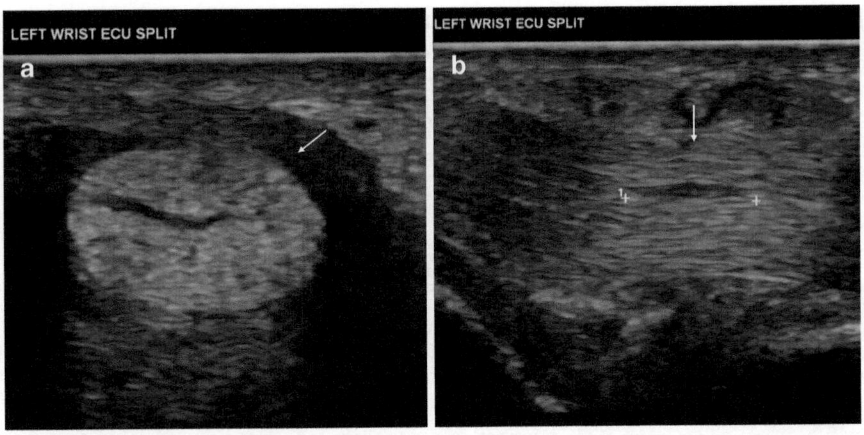

Fig. 10 (**a**, **b**) Ultrasound in axial and sagittal plane in a tennis player reveals extensor carpi ulnar tendon split tear (+) (arrow) at level of ulnar styloid process

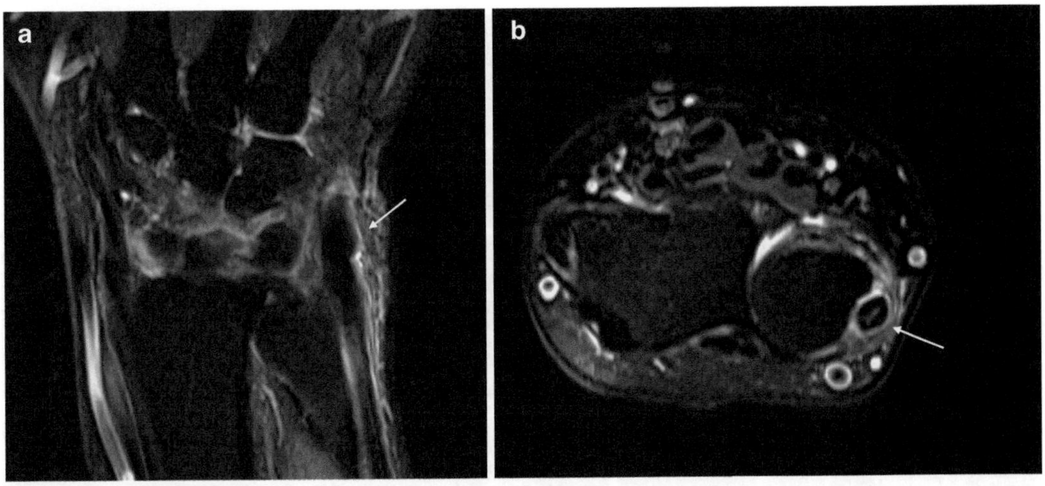

Fig. 11 (**a**, **b**) Coronal and axial STIR images in a cricketer reveal mild to moderate extensor carpi ulnaris tendinosis with tendon sheath fluid

The extensor carpi ulnaris tendon courses in a fibro osseous tunnel overlying the distal medial ulna and is held in place by a fibrous subsheath and an overlying extensor retinaculum. Acute injury or rupture of the fibrous subsheath may occur in tennis players during low forehand stroke due to sudden supination of the forearm with wrist in flexion and ulnar deviation (Burkhart et al. 1982). It may also be seen in golfers and weightlifters. This leads to subluxation of the extensor carpi ulnaris tendon especially during forced supination (Fig. 12). Dynamic ultrasound is very useful in demonstrating the tendon subluxation as well as defect in the subsheath.

Intersection syndromes occur due to friction between the tendons as they cross over each other. This may be seen as tendon sheath fluid and peritendinous edema at the site of crossing. Proximal intersection occurs at the site of crossing of first extensor compartment tendons over the second extensor compartment tendons in the distal forearm. This is commonly seen in rowing, racquet sports, skiing, and horse riding as well as

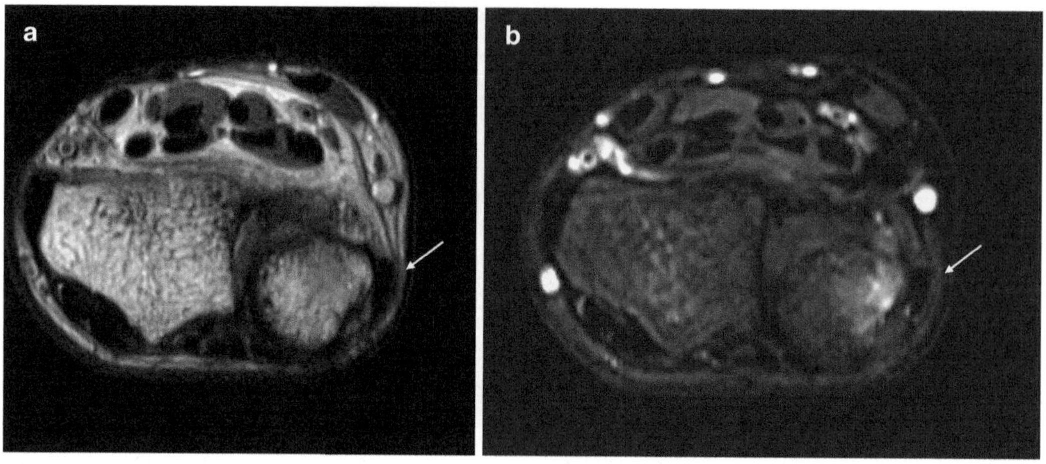

Fig. 12 (**a**, **b**) Axial Proton density and fat saturated T2 weighted images in a weight lifter show extensor carpi ulnaris tendons subsheath injury with palmar tendon subluxation and mild underlying ulnar styloid marrow edema (arrow)

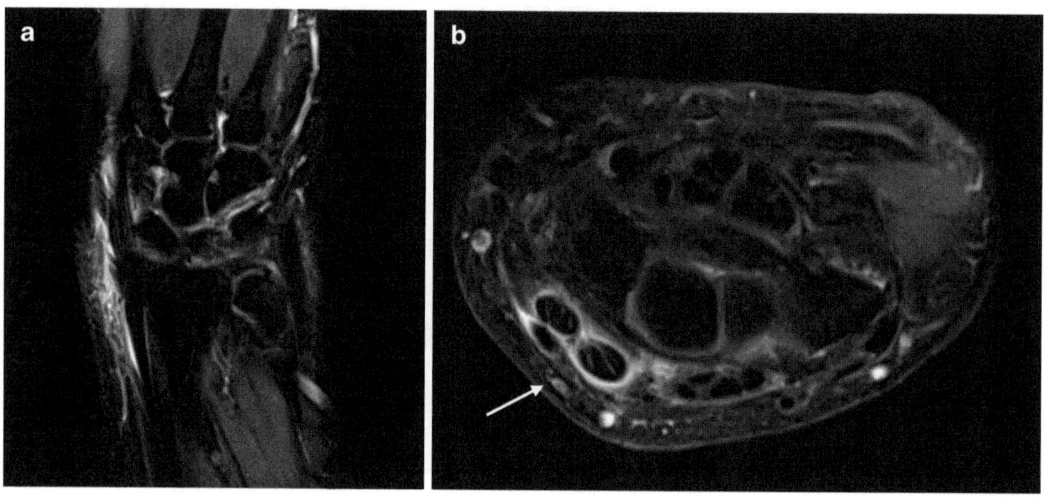

Fig. 13 (**a**, **b**) Coronal STIR and axial fat saturated T2 weighted images in a tennis player reveal distal intersection syndrome with tendon sheath fluid at site of crossing of second and third extensor compartment tendons (arrow)

in weight training due to repeated wrist extension (Costa et al. 2003; Lisle et al. 2009). Distal intersection is seen at the crossing of second and third extensor compartment. It is common in tennis players and video game players (Alter et al. 2023) (Figs. 13 and 14).

1.9 Hand and Finger Injuries

1.9.1 Joint Injuries

The metacarpophalangeal and interphalangeal joint stability is maintained by the collateral ligaments, volar plate, flexor, and extensor tendons. Common joint injuries are dislocations, subluxations, collateral ligament tears, volar plate injuries, and intra-articular fractures.

Most of these joint injuries are evaluated and managed based on radiograph findings. Additional investigations like MRI or ultrasound are required when the dislocation is irreducible, the injuries do not settle as expected, or collateral ligament injuries are suspected.

Acute ulnar collateral ligament injury at the first metacarpophalangeal joint is termed as Skier's thumb. It occurs due to sudden forceful radial deviation in an abducted thumb, which happens due to fall during skiing while holding the ski pole. It is commonly seen in contact and collision sports like football and basketball. Chronic ulnar collateral ligament injuries due to repetitive valgus stress are termed the Gamekeeper's thumb as it was initially described in Scottish gamekeepers who used the thumb to break the necks of the animals. Radiographs are useful to detect avulsion fractures at the site of attachments of the collateral ligament (Fig. 15). MRI is useful to demonstrate the degree of the collateral ligament tear and retraction (Abrahamsson et al. 1990).

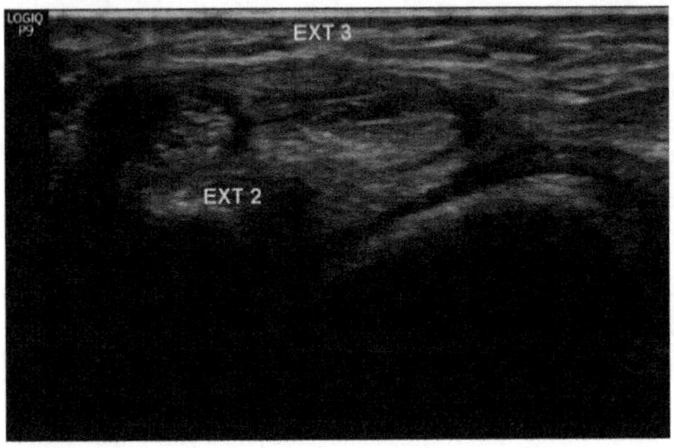

Fig. 14 Ultrasound in axial plane in a tennis player shows distal intersection syndrome with tendon sheath fluid at site of crossing of second and third extensor compartment tendons. EXT 2- Second compartment extensor tendon, EXT 3- third compartment extensor tendon

It is important to acquire coronal images parallel to the dorsal cortex of the first metacarpal head to allow adequate evaluation of the collateral ligaments. These tears are more common at the proximal phalangeal attachment. Non-Stener lesion is when the torn ulnar collateral ligament lies deep to the adductor aponeurosis and may heal with conservative management (Fig. 16). The torn ligament may be retracted and lie superficial to the adductor aponeurosis (Stener lesion), which will not heal on its own and require surgical intervention. On MRI, this is seen as "yo-yo on a string" appearance with the adductor aponeurosis representing the string and the retracted buckled and balled up ulnar collateral ligament as the yo-yo. (Lisle et al. 2009) (Fig. 17).

Radial collateral ligament injuries of the thumb metacarpophalangeal joint are common in sports like football and soccer.

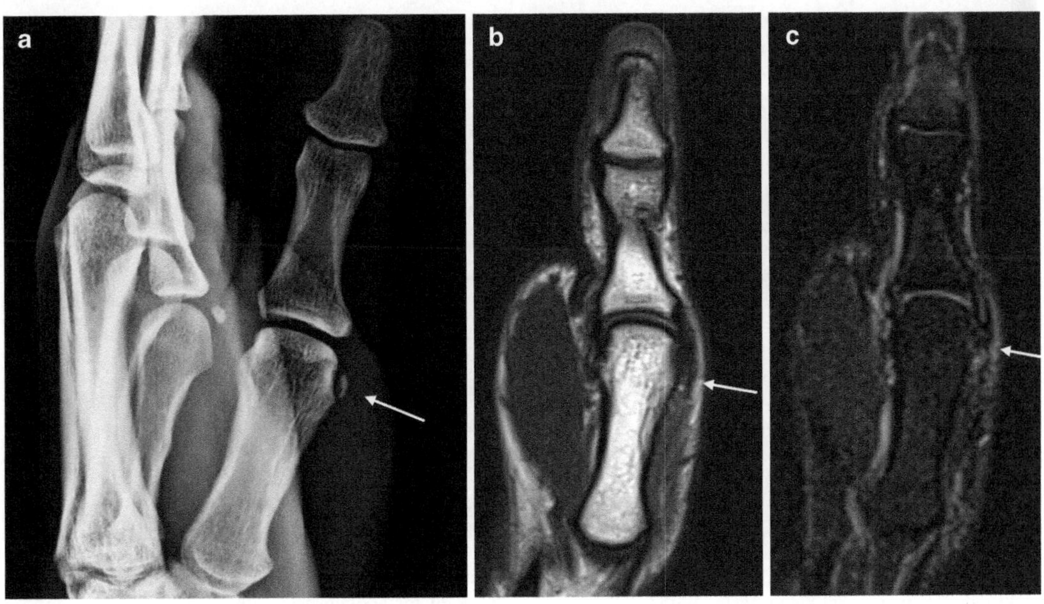

Fig. 15 (a–c) Frontal radiograph, coronal proton density, and STIR images of the thumb in a cricket player demonstrate avulsion fracture (arrow) at the proximal attachment of the first metacarpophalangeal joint radial collateral ligament

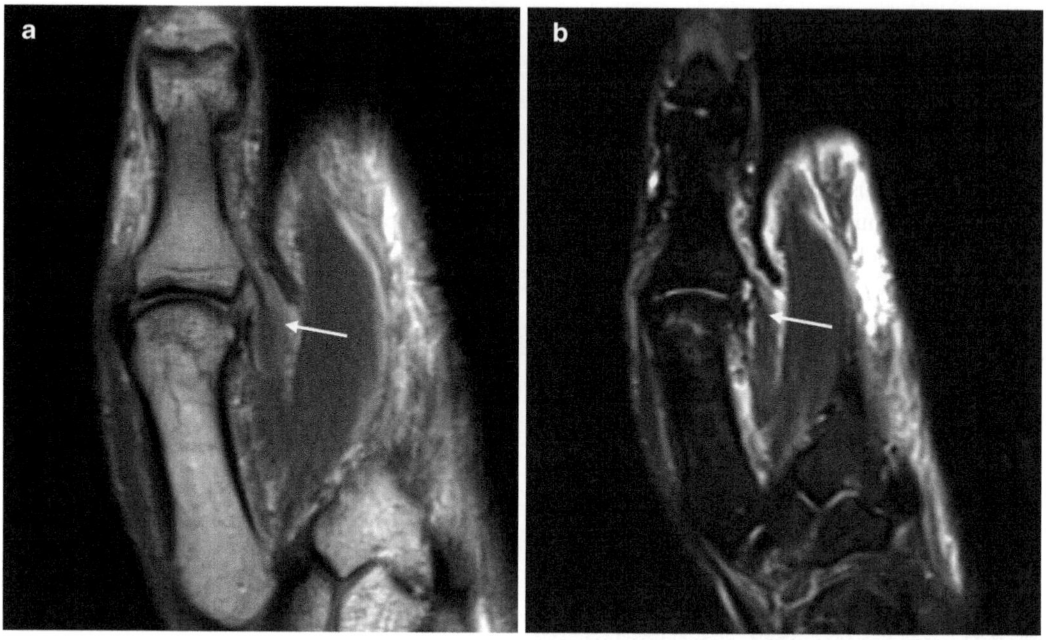

Fig. 16 (**a**, **b**) Coronal proton density and STIR images of thumb in a basketball player show full thickness tear (arrow) at the distal attachment of the ulnar collateral ligament of first metacarpophalangeal joint with intact adductor aponeurosis superficial to it suggestive of non Stener lesion

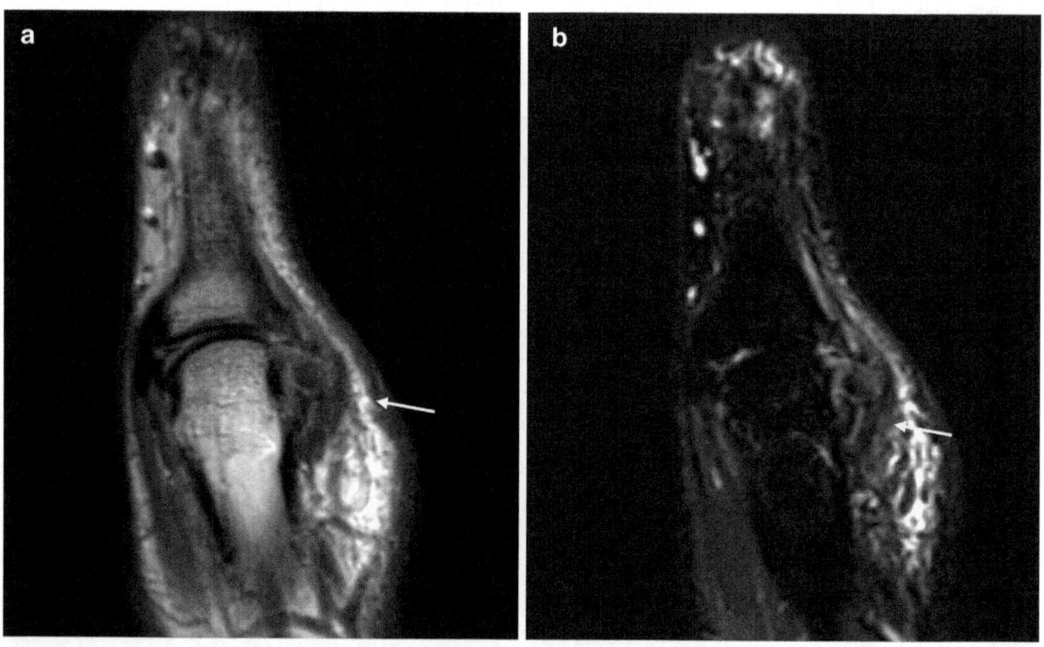

Fig. 17 (**a**, **b**) Coronal proton density and STIR images in a football player reveal Stener lesion with full thickness distal attachment first metacarpophalangeal joint ulnar collateral ligament tear with retraction, lying superficial to the adductor aponeurosis with 'yo-yo on string' appearance (arrow)

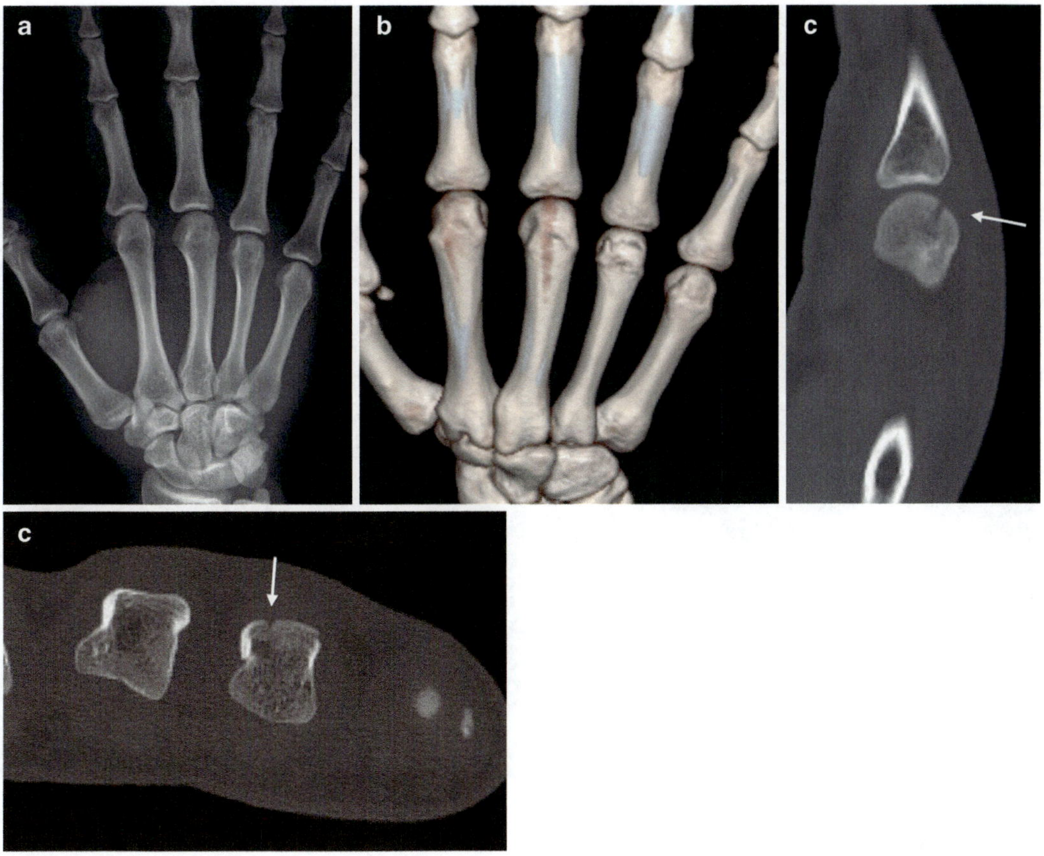

Fig. 18 (**a–d**) AP radiograph, CT 3D, sagittal, and axial images reveal subtle impacted dorsal radial aspect fourth metacarpal head fracture (arrow) in a cricket player due to direct impact by the ball during fielding

Bennett's fracture is a two-part intra-articular fracture of the first metacarpal base due to forced abduction. It is seen commonly in a quarterback's throwing hand when it impacts against the opponent's helmet during follow through. It is common in football, rugby, and boxing (Carpo and Hasting 1998). It yields a smaller fragment attached to the anterior oblique ligament that articulates with the trapezium. The remaining metacarpal is retracted laterally by the abductor pollicis longus. True lateral radiographs and CT are useful to assess size of the osseous fragment and displacement, which help in planning further management.

Dorsal dislocation of the thumb metacarpophalangeal joint is common in almost all the sports and is associated with volar plate rupture, usually at the distal attachment.

Mid phalanx fractures are common in fingers due to direct impact, while distal phalangeal fractures are seen due to crush injuries.

Boxer's fracture is usually a transverse fracture through the fifth metacarpal neck due to direct impact on hitting a solid surface with closed fist (Loosemore et al. 2017). Other metacarpal fractures may be seen due to direct impact (Fig. 18).

The proximal interphalangeal joint is the most commonly injured joint in the hand. Proximal and distal interphalangeal joint dislocations are common in sports with ball handling like basketball, baseball, and football (Lin et al. 2023; Deckey et al. 2020). These may be volar, dorsal, or lateral, the most common being dorsal due to axial loading in hyperextension. This leads to rupture or osseous avulsion at the distal attachment of the volar plate (Figs. 19 and 20).

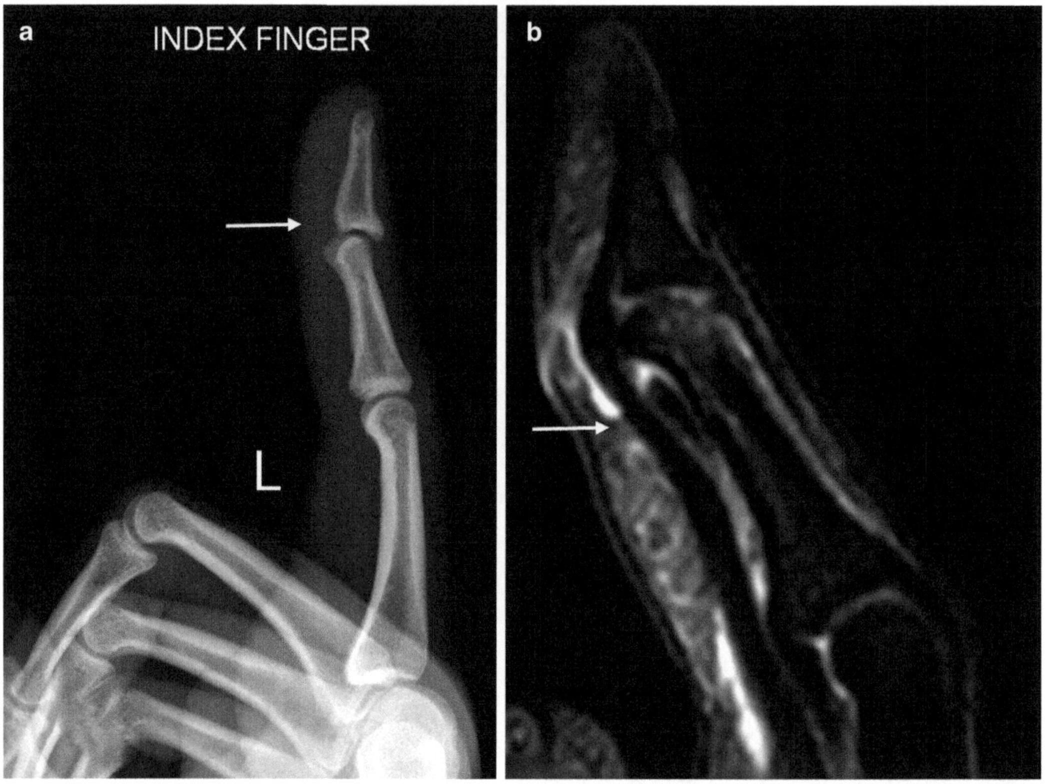

Fig. 19 (**a**, **b**) Lateral radiograph and sagittal STIR images reveal dorsal subluxation (arrow) at the distal interphalangeal joint of the index finger in a cricket player due to direct impact by the ball during fielding with full thickness disruption of distal attachment volar plate and mild middle phalanx head marrow edema (arrow)

Coach finger is the term used for dorsal dislocation at the proximal interphalangeal joint and is common in baseball coaches due to hyperextension while catching a ball (McCue et al. 1974). In these patients, MRI is useful to assess volar plate injuries. The volar plate is well seen on the sagittal images as a triangular hypointense structure. Untreated distal attachment volar plate injury leads to swan neck deformity, while proximal attachment injury leads to pseudo boutonniere deformity.

Collateral ligament injuries are common with axial loading in dorsiflexion. These injuries are common in football, rugby and other tackling sport, volleyball during blocking, as well as climbers (Isani and Melone 1986; Holtzhausen and Noakes 1996). Radial collateral ligament is most commonly injured at the proximal attachment (Rettig 2004). Collateral ligaments are seen as linear hypointense structures on the coronal images on MRI. Their injuries are seen as thickening and hyperintensity, partial thickness tears, or full thickness disruption (Fig. 21).

1.9.2 Closed Tendon Injuries

Mallet finger is the most common closed tendon injury of the fingers. It is seen due to impact of the ball at the distal interphalangeal joint, leading to its forced flexion and resultant avulsion at the terminal phalanx attachment of the extensor tendon. This injury leads to inability to extend the finger with flexion deformity at the distal interphalangeal joint which resembles a mallet and hence the name mallet finger. It is most commonly seen in sports which involves softball, basketball, volleyball, and baseball as well as receivers in football (Aronowitz and Leddy 1998; Lin and Strauch 2014). The avulsion may be osseous which is well depicted on the lateral radiograph (Fig. 22). More than one-third articular surface involvement by the fracture may

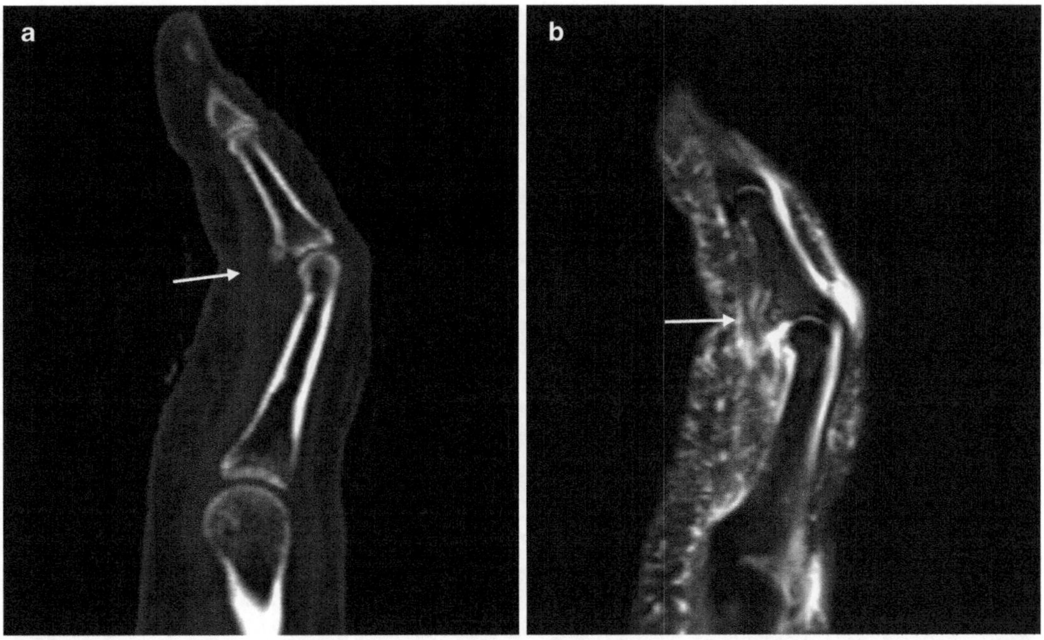

Fig. 20 (**a**, **b**) Sagittal CT and STIR images in a volleyball player reveal fracture at the volar base of middle phalanx with full thickness tear at the distal attachment of the volar plate (arrow). Mild proximal interphalangeal joint effusion and periarticular soft tissue edema

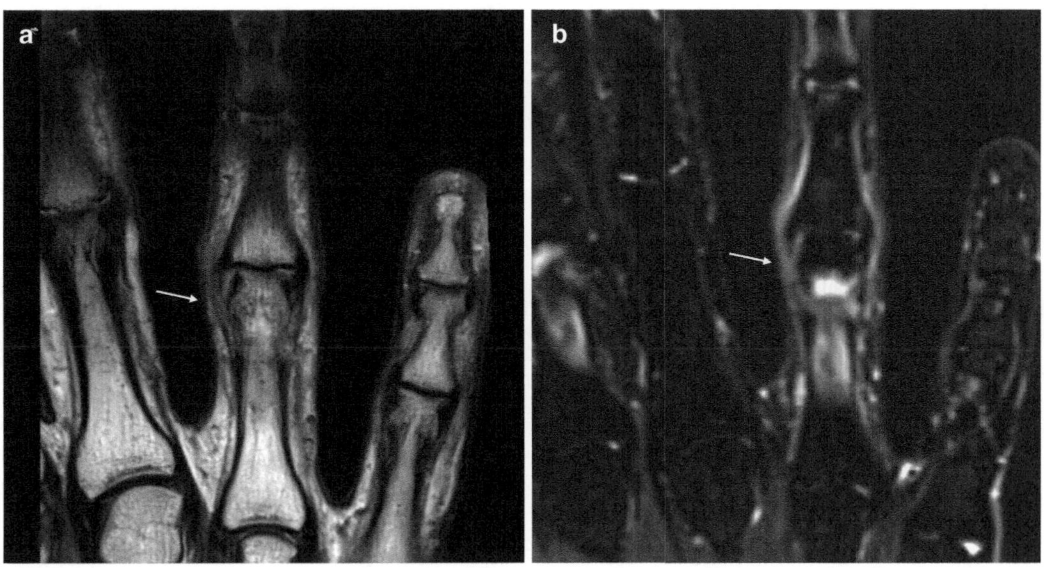

Fig. 21 (**a**, **b**) Coronal proton density and STIR images of the ring finger in a volleyball player reveal high grade tear of the radial collateral ligament at its proximal attachment (arrow)

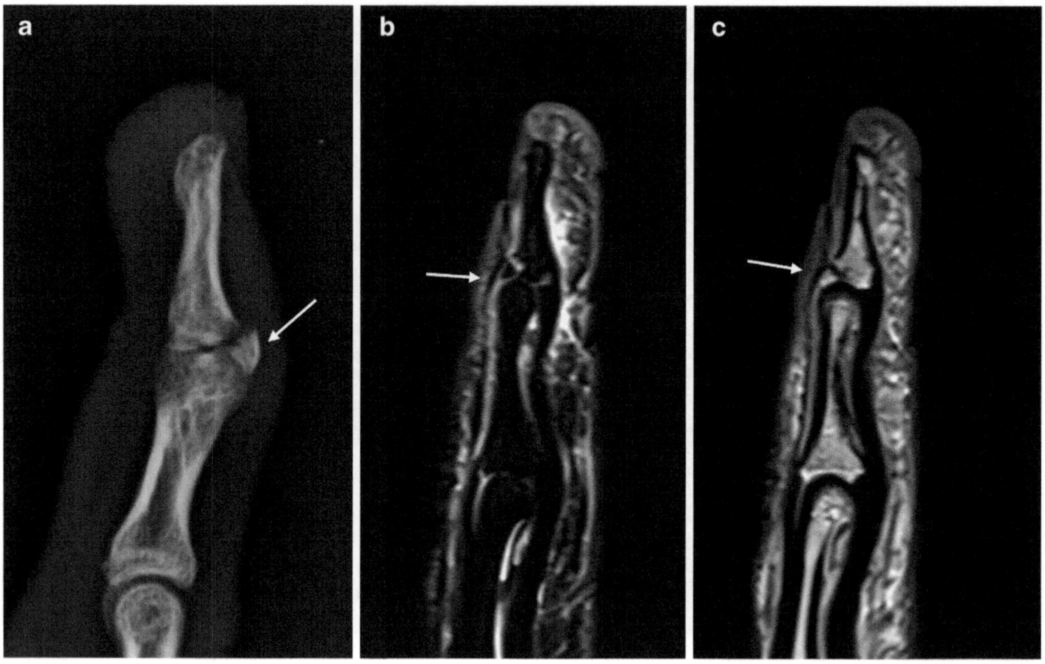

Fig. 22 (**a–c**) Lateral radiograph, sagittal STIR, and T2 weighted images of finger reveal mallet fracture of the dorsal distal phalanx base at site of attachment of the common extensor tendon (arrow)

require surgical fixation. Larger fracture fragment also leads to volar subluxation at the distal interphalangeal joint. Instead of osseous avulsion, there may be a tendinous avulsion at the distal phalangeal attachment of the extensor tendon (Fig. 23). MRI and ultrasound are useful to demonstrate the tear and the degree of retraction.

Boutonniere injury occurs due to disruption at the middle phalangeal base attachment of the central slip of extensor digitorum tendon. This leads to flexion deformity at proximal and hyperextension at the distal interphalangeal joint. This is common in volleyball and basketball players but may be difficult to diagnose in the acute phase as the extension may be maintained by the intact lateral bands. Later the lateral bands show lateral and volar displacement and may get attenuated leading to Boutonniere deformity (Elliott 1970; Lin and Strauch 2014). Radiographs may show osseous avulsion, while MRI and ultrasound are useful to diagnose the tendon disruption especially in acute injuries when clinical assessment is limited (Fig. 24).

Boxer's knuckle is caused by repetitive trauma leading to extensor hood injury (Loosemore et al. 2017). The extensor hood is an important stabilizer of the extensor digitorum tendon with sagittal bands forming its main component. This injury is common in boxers due to repeated landing of punches. It is most common in the ring finger metacarpophalangeal joint and involves the radial sagittal band with resultant medial subluxation of the extensor tendon. It can also lead to capsular tear and metacarpophalangeal joint cartilage loss. Ultrasound and MRI are useful delineating the extensor hood sagittal bands and their injuries which may be seen as thickening and hyperintense signal, partial tears, or full thickness disruption appreciated in the axial images. Dynamic ultrasound is very useful to detect dynamic subluxation or dislocation of the extensor tendon (Fig. 25).

Jersey finger is due to avulsion at the distal phalangeal attachment of the flexor digitorum profundus tendon. It is commonly seen in football and rugby players due to sudden hyperextension of the flexed distal interphalangeal joint due to the finger getting caught in the opponent's jersey while tackling or grabbing the player. It is most common in the ring finger. Osseous avulsion is

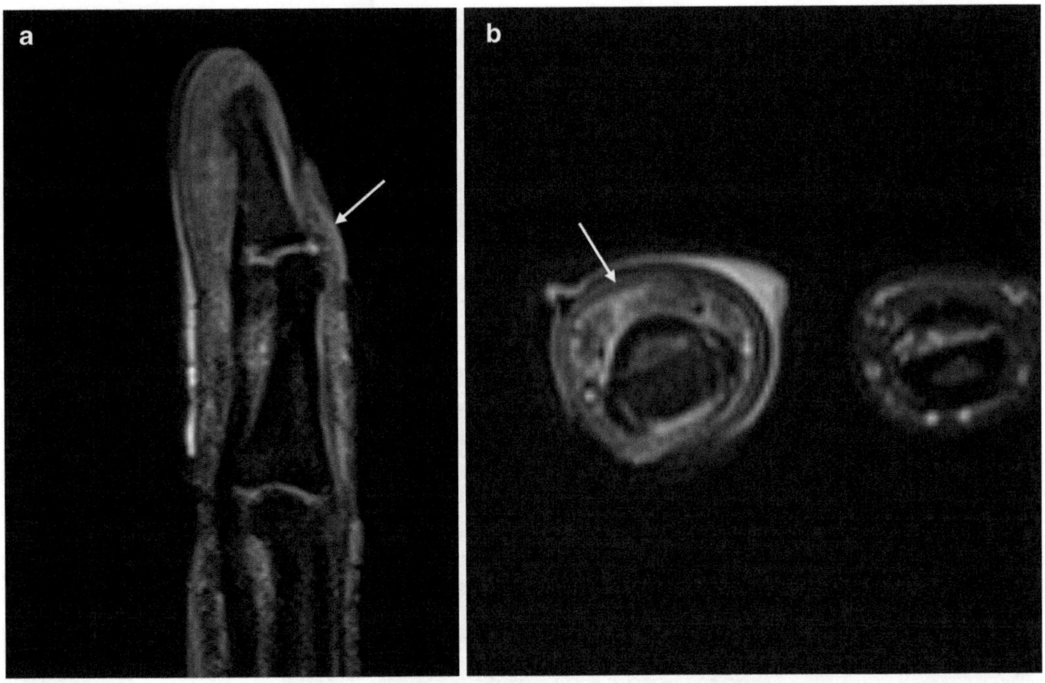

Fig. 23 (**a**, **b**) Sagittal and axial fat saturated T2 weighted images in a basketball player reveal full thickness tear at the distal phalanx attachment of extensor tendon (mallet finger) (arrow)

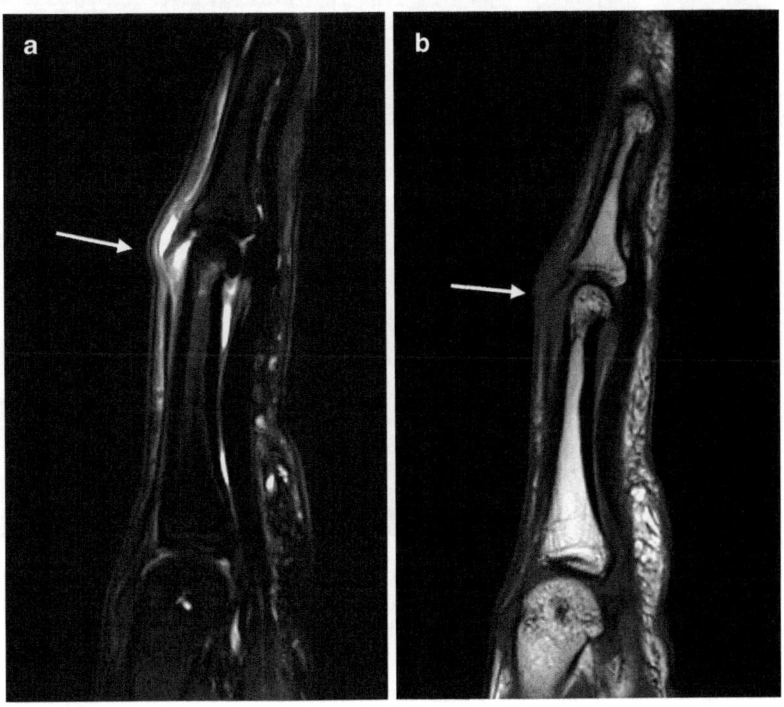

Fig. 24 (**a**, **b**) Sagittal fat saturated T2 and proton density images of the finger in a cricket player show full thickness tear of the extensor tendon central slip at the level of the proximal phalanx neck (arrow). Mild proximal phalanx neck marrow edema and mild proximal interphalangeal joint effusion. This can lead to boutonniere deformity

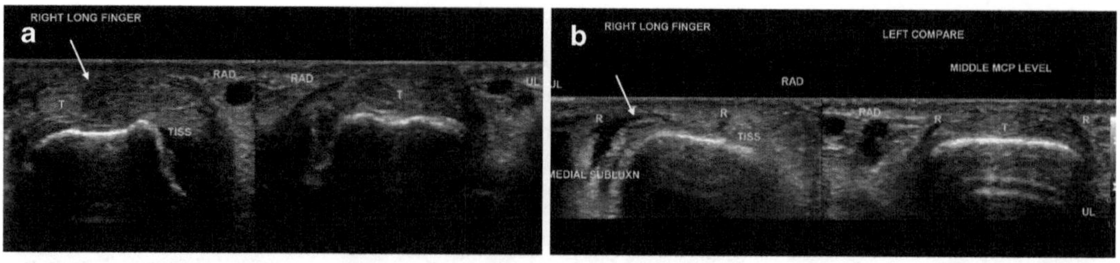

Fig. 25 (**a**, **b**) Ultrasound in axial plane reveals metacarpophalangeal joint radial collateral ligament and radial sagittal band high grade injury with resultant medial subluxation of the extensor tendon in a boxer (arrow)

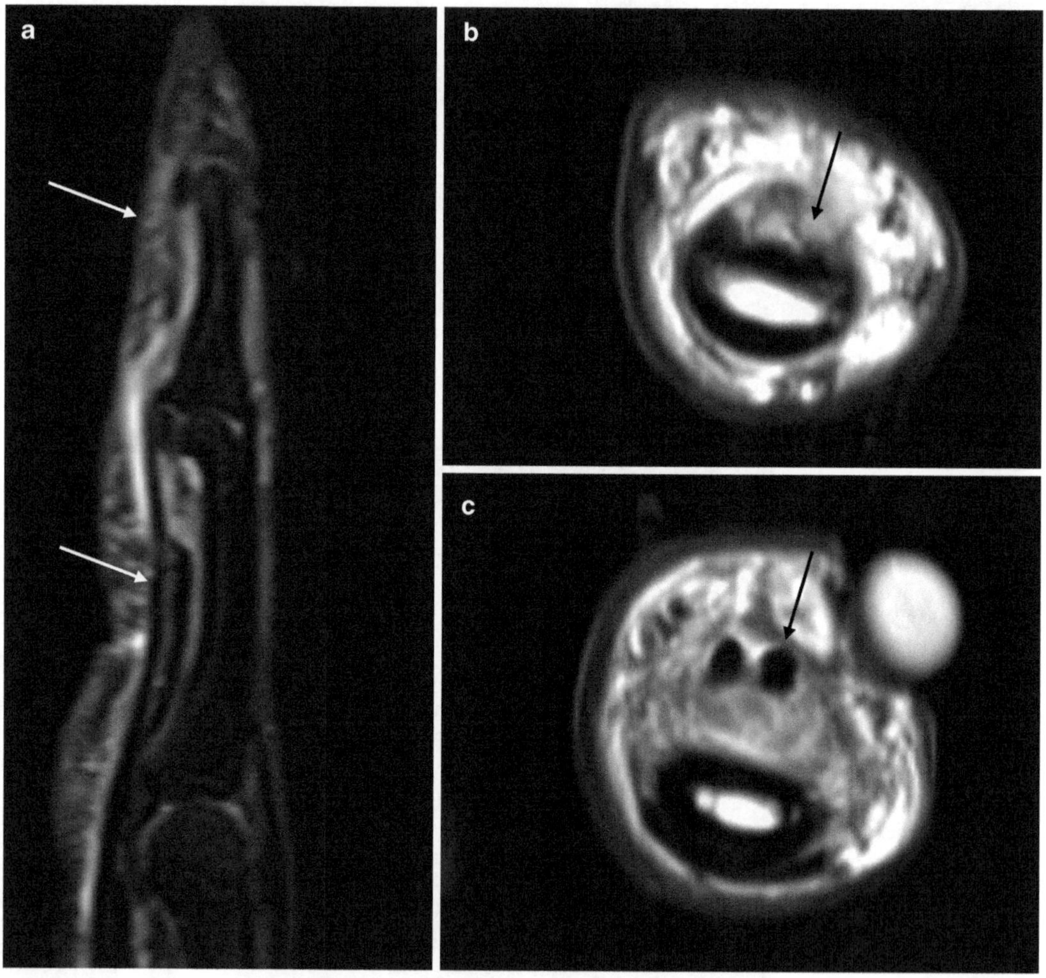

Fig. 26 Sagittal STIR and axial proton density images of the index finger in a footballer show full thickness tear of the flexor digitorum profundus tendon at distal phalanx insertion (**a**, **b**) (arrow). Axial images (**c**) at the level of the proximal phalanx reveal intact flexor digitorum superficialis (Jersey finger) (arrow)

seen on the radiograph. MRI and ultrasound are useful to delineate the tear in its retracted end helping in classification and planning the surgical management (Fig. 26). Flexor digitorum superficialis tendon tears are less common but may occur due to forced hyperflexion at proximal interphalangeal joint during active flexion (Fig. 27). Dynamic ultrasound scores over MRI in detecting small tears as well as its exact extent during active/passive movement of the finger.

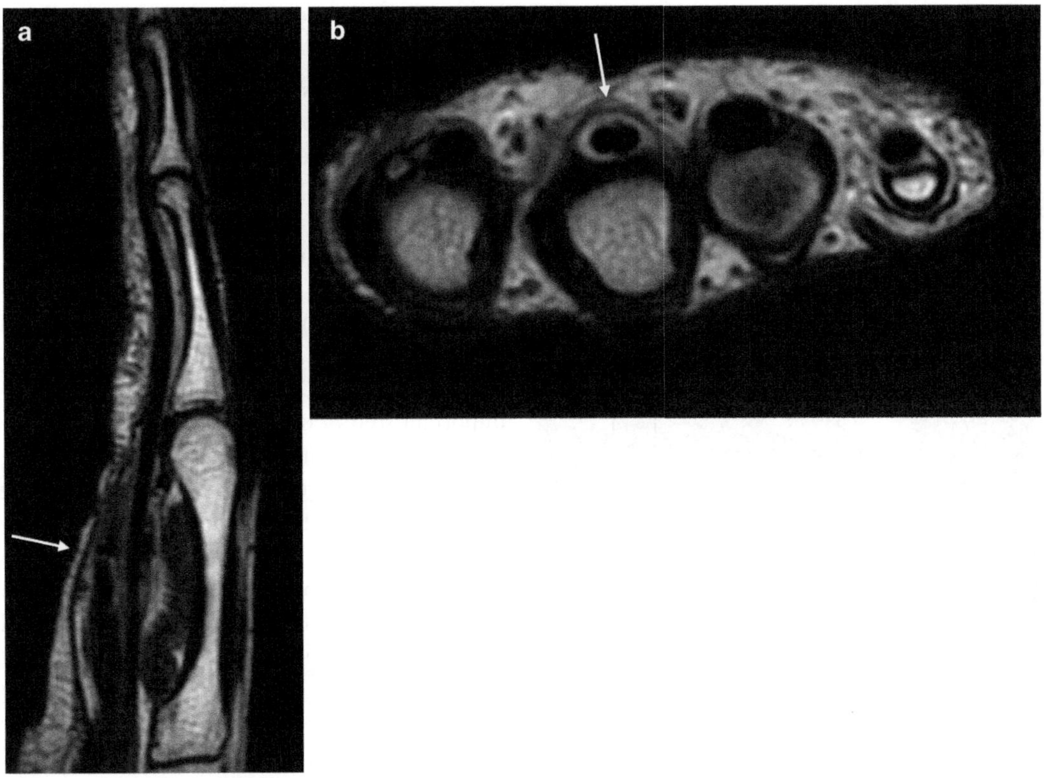

Fig. 27 (**a**, **b**) Sagittal and axial proton density images of the middle finger in a weightlifter show full thickness tear of the flexor superficialis tendon from its insertion with retraction into hand (arrow). Intact flexor digitorum profundus

Flexor pulley injuries are common in rock climbers due to forceful extension of the flexed fingers, hence the term "Climber's finger." These most commonly involve the middle and ring fingers. Five annular and three cruciate pulleys keep the flexor tendon in place and allow smooth gliding movements. During rock climbing, A2 pulley injuries are most common and may also be associated with A3 pulley injuries. Isolated A4 pulley injuries are seen in baseball pitchers (Schöffl et al. 2023).

Normally the flexor tendons course in close relation to the phalanges. With pulley injuries, the flexor tendons are displaced anteriorly leading to a bow stringing appearance (Fig. 28). Ultrasound and MRI are useful to assess continuity of the pulley on axial images.

1.10 Nerve Compression Syndromes

Carpal tunnel syndrome may be transient and is seen in sports which involve repeated flexion and extension of the wrist like swimming, body building, as well as para athletes like wheelchair athletics. It is also common in long distance cycling due to vibrations and repetitive direct force. It is also seen in electronic sports like video gaming due to repetitive pressing of buttons and gripping the controllers (Rossoni et al. 2023). It occurs due to compression of the median nerve in the carpal tunnel with resultant paresthesias in the median nerve distribution. Ultrasound and MRI demonstrate flattening of the median nerve at the level of hamate with swelling and edema at the level of pisiform. They may also demonstrate tenosynovitis in the flexor tendon sheaths. Severe cases show denervation changes in the thenar muscles.

Ulnar nerve injury may be seen following fracture of hook of hamate due to close relation of the nerve in the Guyon's canal. Repetitive ulnar sided wrist compression in sports like cycling and racquet sports may lead to ulnar neuropathy. Handle bar palsy is common in

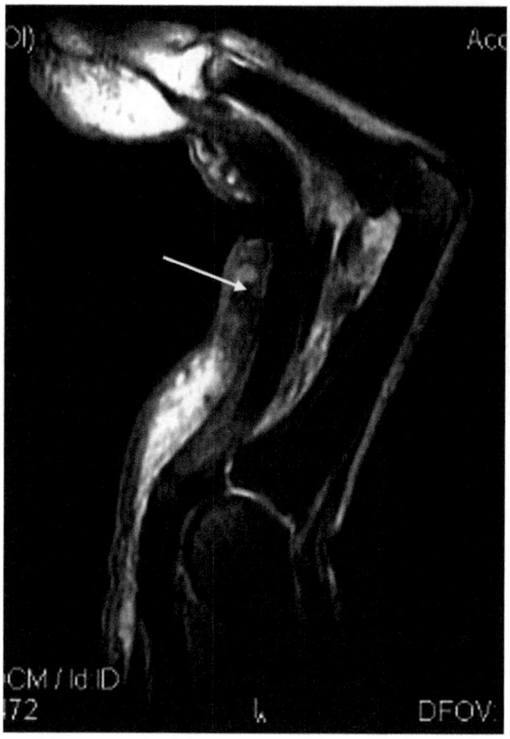

Fig. 28 Sagittal STIR images of the middle finger in a rock climber reveal rupture of A2 pulley with anterior displacement of the flexor tendons in relation to proximal phalanx (bowstringing) (arrow)

downhill mountain biking due to compression of the deep branch of ulnar nerve (Capitani and Beer 2002). Ultrasound and MRI are useful to assess the size, continuity, and internal architecture of the nerves.

1.11 Conclusion

Hand and wrist injuries are common in most sports and may be acute or due to chronic overuse (Tables 1 and 2). Imaging plays a very important role in diagnosing and assessing the extent of these injuries. This helps in deciding the further management as well as predicting the return to play. Radiographs and CT are useful in imaging osseous injuries, while ultrasound and MRI provide excellent soft tissue resolution to assess the tendons, muscles, and nerves. MRI enables detection of marrow edema and articular cartilage. The dynamic capability of ultrasound makes it the modality of choice in evaluating tendons. Ultrasound also allows guided injections for treatment of some of these injuries.

Table 1 Sports-related wrist and hand injuries

Sport	Common injuries
Cricket	Hook of hamate fractures (non-dominant hand due to double grip) Extensor carpi ulnaris tendinopathy (non-dominant hand, sudden ulnar deviation at end of swing) TFCC injuries (rotational motion during grip, over-swinging, hitting back on ground)
Tennis/racquet sports	Hook of hamate fractures (dominant hand) De Quervain's tenosynovitis Extensor carpi ulnaris tendinopathy (non-dominant hand in double-handed backhand) Extensor carpi ulnaris subsheath injury (during low forehand stroke) Proximal intersection syndrome Second metacarpal stress fractures (repetitive impact of racquet handle) Ulnocarpal abutment TFCC injuries from repetitive supination/pronation motions
Golf	Hook of hamate fractures (leading non-dominant hand from club handle) De Quervain's tenosynovitis Extensor carpi ulnaris subsheath injury

Table 1 (continued)

Sport	Common injuries
Gymnastics	Scaphoid stress fractures (repeated dorsiflexion) "Gymnast's wrist" (distal radial physeal injuries in pediatric athletes) Keinbock's disease (osteonecrosis of lunate) Ulnocarpal abutment Tendon overuse injuries
Boxing/martial arts	Carpal boss (repeated impaction injuries) Bennett's fractures Boxer's knuckle (extensor hood/sagittal band injury, especially ring finger) Boxer's fracture (5th metacarpal neck fracture from improper punching) Scaphoid fractures in martial arts from incorrect strikes
Basketball/volleyball	Proximal interphalangeal joint dislocations Mallet finger Boutonniere injury Pisiform stress fractures (volleyball) Ulnar collateral ligament injuries (thumb)
Football/rugby	Proximal interphalangeal joint dislocations Collateral ligament injuries Ulnar collateral ligament injuries (thumb) Radial collateral ligament injuries (thumb) Bennett's fractures (quarterback's throwing hand) Jersey finger (ring finger, flexor digitorum profundus avulsion)
Baseball/softball	Coach finger (dorsal dislocation at PIP joint) Mallet finger Fifth metacarpal stress injuries (softball) A4 pulley injuries (pitchers), Ulnocarpal abutment UCL injuries at the wrist level (pitchers) Hook of hamate fractures during batting
Hockey/lacrosse	Distal radius fractures (fall on outstretched hand) Specific patterns of finger fractures from stick impacts Scaphoid injuries from falls
Skiing	Skier's thumb (acute ulnar collateral ligament injury at first MCP joint) Proximal intersection syndrome
Rock climbing	Flexor pulley injuries (A2 and A3, middle and ring fingers) Collateral ligament injuries Lumbrical tears common in crimping positions TFCC injuries from dynamic movements
Rowing	De Quervain's tenosynovitis Extensor carpi ulnaris tendinopathy Proximal intersection syndrome Tendon overuse injuries
Cycling	Carpal tunnel syndrome (vibrations and repetitive direct force) Ulnar neuropathy (repetitive ulnar sided wrist compression) Handlebar palsy (compression of deep branch of ulnar nerve)
Weight training	De Quervain's tenosynovitis Extensor carpi ulnaris subsheath injury Proximal intersection syndrome
Break dancing	Triquetrum stress injuries
Handball	Keinbock's disease (osteonecrosis of lunate)
Horse riding	Proximal intersection syndrome
Gaming/esports	Carpal tunnel syndrome Tendinopathies from repetitive movements De Quervain's tenosynovitis in competitive gamers

Table 2 Injury mechanisms across multiple sports

Injury mechanism	Common injuries
Fall on outstretched hand	Scaphoid fractures Distal radius fractures Lunotriquetral ligament injuries TFCC injuries
Repetitive wrist movements	Proximal intersection syndrome Stress fractures Tendinopathies
Direct Impact/ collision	Metacarpal and phalangeal fractures Joint dislocations
Ball impact on fingertip	Mallet finger Coach finger

References

Abrahamsson SO, Sollerman C, Lundborg G (1990) Diagnosis of displaced ulnar collateral ligament of the metacarpophalangeal joint of the thumb. J Hand Surg [Am] 15(3):457–460

Albanese SA, Palmer AK, Kerr DR (1989) Wrist pain and distal growth plate closure of the radius in gymnasts. J Pediatr Orthop 9(1):23–28

Alter TH, Romeo PV, Bielicka DL, Monica JT (2023) Distal intersection syndrome between second and third dorsal compartments of the wrist. Cureus. [online] https://doi.org/10.7759/cureus.36919.

Aronowitz ER, Leddy JP (1998) Closed tendon injuries of the hand and wrist in athletes. Clin Sports Med 17(3):449–467

Batta NS, Abhinetri K, Batra V, Mittal M, Jain V (2023) Non-dominant leading wrist injuries in Indian professional cricketers. Indian J Musculoskelet Radiol 5:97–105

Bhairo NH, Nijsten MW, van Dalen KC, ten Duis HJ (1992) Hand injuries in volleyball. Int J Sports Med 13(4):351–354

Burkhart S, Wood M, Linscheid RL (1982) Post-traumatic recurrent subluxation of the extensor carpi ulnaris tendon. J Hand Surg 7(1):1–3

Capitani D, Beer S (2002) Handlebar palsy—a compression syndrome of the deep terminal (motor) branch of the ulnar nerve in biking. J Neurol 249(10):1441–1445

Carpo JT, Hasting H (1998) Metacarpal and phalangeal fractures in athletes. Clin Sports Med 17(3):491–511

Cerezal L, del Pinal F, Abascal F, Garcia-Valtuille R, Pereda T, Canga A (2002) Imaging findings in ulnar-sided wrist impaction syndromes. Radiographics 22(1):105–121

Chen NC, Jupiter JB, Jebson PJ (2009) Sports-related wrist injuries in adults. Sports Health 1(6):469–477

Cockenpot E, Lefebvre G, Demondion X, Chantelot C, Cotten A (2016) Imaging of sports-related hand and wrist injuries: sports imaging series. Radiology 279(3):674–692

Connell D, Page P, Wright W, Hoy G (2001) Magnetic resonance imaging of the wrist ligaments. Australas Radiol 45(4):411–422

Costa CR, Morrison WB, Carrino JA (2003) MRI features of intersection syndrome of the forearm. Am J Roentgenol 181(5):1245–1249

Deckey DG, Scott KL, Hinckley NB, Makovicka JL, Hassebrock JD, Tummala SV, Pena A, Asprey W, Chhabra A (2020) Hand and wrist injuries in men's and women's National Collegiate Athletic Association basketball. Orthop J Sports Med 8(9):2325967120946614

Elliott RA (1970) Injuries to the extensor mechanism of the hand. Orthop Clin N Am 1:335

Gabel GT (1998) Gymnastic wrist injuries. Clin Sports Med 17(3):611–621

Gil JA, Kakar S (2019) Hand and wrist injuries in tennis players. Curr Rev Musculoskelet Med 12(2):87–97

Holtzhausen LM, Noakes TD (1996) Elbow, forearm, wrist, and hand injuries among sport rock climbers. Clin J Sport Med 6(3):196–203

Howse C (1994) Wrist injuries in sport. Sports Med 17(3):163–175

Isani A, Melone CP (1986) Ligamentous injuries of the hand in athletes. Clin Sports Med 5(4):757–772

Lin JD, Strauch RJ (2014) Closed soft tissue extensor mechanism injuries (mallet, boutonniere, and sagittal band). J Hand Surg [Am] 39(5):1005–1011

Lin E, Tummala SV, Morikawa L, Vij N, Petty SB, McQuivey KS, Chhabra A (2023) Strains/sprains and fractures are the most common hand and wrist injuries in National Basketball Association athletes who return to preinjury player efficiency and equal or greater true shooting percentage within two years of injury. Arthrosc Sports Med Rehabil 5(6):e100829

Lisle DA, Shepherd GJ, Cowderoy GA, O'Connell PT (2009) MR imaging of traumatic and overuse injuries of the wrist and hand in athletes. Magn Reson Imaging Clin N Am 17(4):639–654

Lohman M, Kivisaari L, Partio EK (2003) Stress reaction in the carpal bones caused by breakdancing. Emerg Radiol 10:102–104

Loosemore M, Lightfoot J, Gatt I, Hayton M, Beardsley C (2017) Hand and wrist injuries in elite boxing: a longitudinal prospective study (2005–2012) of the Great Britain Olympic Boxing Squad. Hand 12(2):181–187

McCue FC, Andrews JR, Hakala M, Gieck JH (1974) The coach's finger. J Sports Med 2(5):270–275

Melone CP, Polatsch DB, Beldner S (2009) Disabling hand injuries in boxing: boxer's knuckle and traumatic carpal boss. Clin Sports Med 28(4):609–621

Murray PM, Cooney WP (1996) Golf-induced injuries of the wrist. Clin Sports Med 15(1):85–109

Oneson SR, Scales LM, Timins ME, Erickson SJ, Chamoy L (1996) MR imaging interpretation of the Palmer classification of triangular fibrocartilage complex lesions. Radiographics 16(1):97–106

Reinstein L (1983) de Quervain's stenosing tenosynovitis in a video games player. Arch Phys Med Rehabil 64(9):434–435

Rettig AC (2004) Athletic injuries of the wrist and hand: part II: overuse injuries of the wrist and traumatic injuries to the hand. Am J Sports Med 32(1): 262–273

Rossoni A, Vecchiato M, Brugin E, Tranchita E, Adami PE, Bartesaghi M, Cavarretta E, Palermi S (2023) The eSports medicine: pre-participation screening and injuries management-an update. Sports 11(2):34

Schöffl V, von Schroeder H, Lisse J, El-Sheikh Y, Küpper T, Klinder A, Lutter C (2023) Wrist injuries in climbers. Am J Sports Med 51(13):3416–3425

Shih C, Chang CY, Penn IW, Tiu CM, Chang T, Wu JJ (1995) Chronically stressed wrists in adolescent gymnasts: MR imaging appearance. Radiology 195(3):855–859

Tedesco LJ, Swindell HW, Anderson FL, Jang E, Wong TT, Kazam JK, Kadiyala RK, Popkin CA (2020) Evaluation and management of hand, wrist and elbow injuries in ice hockey. Open Access J Sports Med 11:93–103

Trumble TE, Katolik LI (2006) Treatment of Kienböck disease in athletes. Atlas Hand Clin 11(1):45–65

Waninger KN, Lombardo JA (1995) Stress fracture of index metacarpal in an adolescent tennis player. Clin J Sport Med 5(1):63–66

Werner SL, Plancher KD (1998) Biomechanics of wrist injuries in sports. Clin Sports Med 17(3):407–420

Yamabe E, Nakamura T, Pham P, Yoshioka H (2012) The athlete's wrist: ulnar-sided pain. Semin Musculoskelet Radiol 16(4):331–337

Tumours and Tumour-Like Lesions of Bone

Hasaam Uldin, Nikhil A. Kotnis, Mark A. Davies, Steven L. J. James, and Rajesh Botchu

Contents

H. Uldin (✉) · M. A. Davies · S. L. J. James · R. Botchu
Department of Radiology, Royal Orthopaedic Hospital, Birmingham, UK
e-mail: hasaam.uldin1@nhs.net

N. A. Kotnis
Department of Radiology, Sheffield Teaching Hospitals NHS Foundation Trust, Sheffield, UK

Abstract

Bone tumours affecting the hand and wrist are rare, making up for less than 5% of all bone tumours. Primary bone tumours are especially uncommon when compared with tumours arising in the soft tissues of the hand; Haber described 2321 tumours of the hand with only 38 cases involving bone.

1 Introduction

Bone tumours affecting the hand and wrist are uncommon, accounting for less than 5% of all skeletal tumours (Erdoğan and Gürkan 2020). The majority of bone tumours are benign, with most of these being enchondromas (Melamud et al. 2014; Payne and Merrell 2010). Despite this relative rarity, many clinicians will encounter such tumours, usually as incidental findings found in unrelated trauma although pathological fractures can also trigger presentation.

Radiographs are the mainstay first-line investigation to facilitate diagnosis. Further assessment with computed tomography (CT) allows characterization of tumour matrix and presence of bone destruction, while magnetic resonance imaging (MRI) provides information regarding the extent of marrow involvement and soft tissue invasion (Plate et al. 2003.

The majority (over 80% in several series) of bone tumours that affect the hand are benign, par-

Med Radiol Diagn Imaging (2025)
https://doi.org/10.1007/174_2025_576,
Published Online: 17 April 2025

ticularly when seen in younger patients (Campbell et al. 1995; Thomas et al. 2011). However, being able to distinguish benign entities from malignancy on initial presentation is crucial in directing the subsequent investigation and management (Hsu et al. 2007). The most frequent benign lesion is enchondroma, but there are a wide range of other benign tumours and tumour-like lesions to also consider, covered in more detail in this chapter (Albanese et al. 2024). Similarly, chondrosarcoma is the most common malignant tumour but metastases and a range of other primary tumours can also present.

This chapter reviews the most common benign and malignant bone neoplasms of the hand and wrist. The incidence, demographics, clinical presentation, and distribution as well as imaging characteristics of these tumours specific to this location are discussed.

2 Benign Bone Tumours of the Hand and Wrist

2.1 Benign Cartilaginous Tumours

2.1.1 Enchondroma

Enchondromas are the most common primary bone tumours found in the hand and wrist, arising more frequently here than in any other part of the body (Boriani et al. 2021). Histologically, these develop from hyaline cartilage within the medullary cavity which can subsequently expand (Nazarova et al. 2020; Nielsen 2021). Although radiologically most commonly seen in the hand, they are arguably more common in the proximal humerus and around the knee but radiologically less conspicuous in these areas (Davies et al. 2020). Overall, occurrence is typically in long bones (including phalanges) with sesamoid bones (e.g. the carpals) relatively rarely affected (Shimizu et al. 1997; Sollaci and Araújo 2019; Cavalcante et al. 2021).

Typically, the tumour is discovered incidentally on radiographs obtained for other reasons (Fig. 1). When not found incidentally, patients usually present with a pathological fracture following minor trauma with presentation with a slowly enlarging mass less common (Riester et al. 2016).

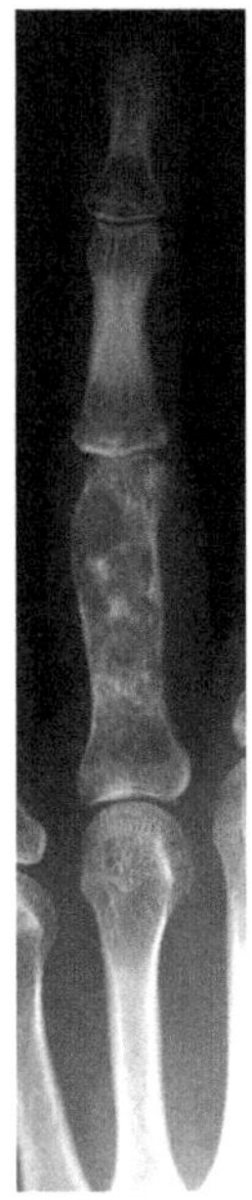

Fig. 1 Enchondroma. There is a lytic, mildly expansile tumour in the proximal phalanx containing punctate cartilage calcification

Multiple hand enchondromas may be encountered in association with several syndromes, most commonly either Ollier disease or Maffucci syndrome (Sharif et al. 2022). Ollier disease is characterized by multiple enchondromas alone (Fig. 2), whereas the additional presence of soft tissue haemangiomas is termed Maffucci syndrome (Fig. 3) (Kumar et al. 2015; Jurik 2020). The distribution of lesions tends to be in either a monomelic or hemimelic fashion and a skeletal deformity is often clinically apparent (Nazarova et al. 2021).

Enchondromas can undergo malignant transformation into chondrosarcoma (Çapkin et al. 2020; Nielsen 2021). Although this is rare in solitary enchondromas, several authors have reported that enchondromas arising from the aforementioned syndromes are more likely to develop into secondary chondrosarcoma (Fig. 4) with approx-

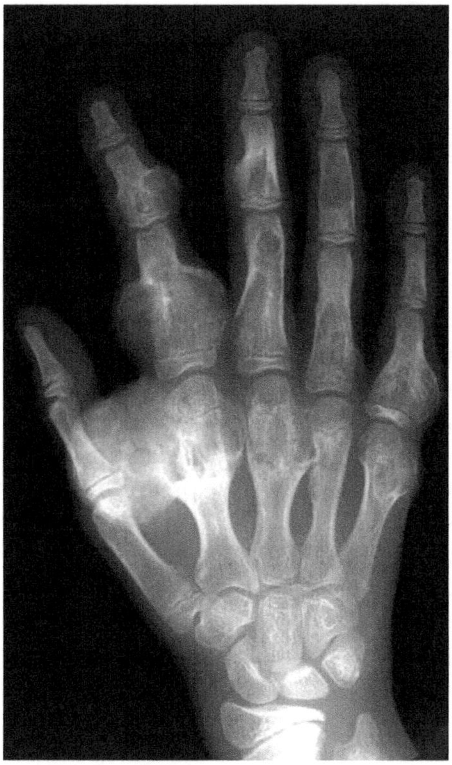

Fig. 2 Ollier disease. Multiple enchondromas arising in the metacarpals and phalanges

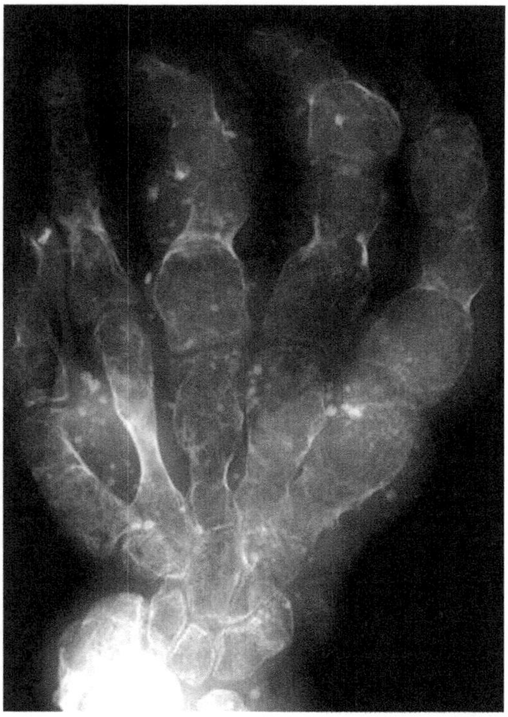

Fig. 3 Maffucci syndrome. Multiple enchondromas in association with soft tissue angiomas. Multiple calcified phleboliths are present

imately 40% of patients with Ollier disease being affected (Sharif et al. 2022; Jurik 2020; Çapkin et al. 2020). As discussed below, the difficulty in differentiating a benign enchondroma from a low-grade chondrosarcoma on radiology and histopathology can make epidemiology challenging.

On imaging, enchondromas are typically eccentrically located in the metaphyseal or diaphyseal regions of long bones, more in the former (Nayak et al. 2021). In the hand, a well-defined radiolucent intramedullary lesion containing thin internal trabeculations is typically seen (Fig. 1) (Boriani et al. 2021). Endosteal scalloping, cortical thinning and expansion of the bone are commonly identified (Douis et al. 2018). Associated chondroid calcifications are less common in enchondromas of the hand than at other skeletal locations. Cross-sectional imaging is rarely required to make the diagnosis but CT can clarify the presence of chondroid matrix and is superior to MRI at delineating endosteal scalloping. Enchondroma has a distinctive appearance on MR imaging, with hyaline cartilage content manifesting as multiple lobules of high signal intensity on T2W, fat suppressed and STIR sequences (Lubahn and Bachoura 2016). Low signal septae are often seen separating the lobules, corresponding to calcified chondroid matrix.

Radiographic features concerning for malignant transformation include cortical destruction and an associated soft tissue mass. Of note, the development of lucency in a previously mineralized cartilage lesion can rarely occur with benign resolution but is far more suspicious for malignant transformation (Sensarma et al. 2015). Imaging with MRI is useful in evaluating the extent of soft tissue extension in cases where malignant transformation is suspected.

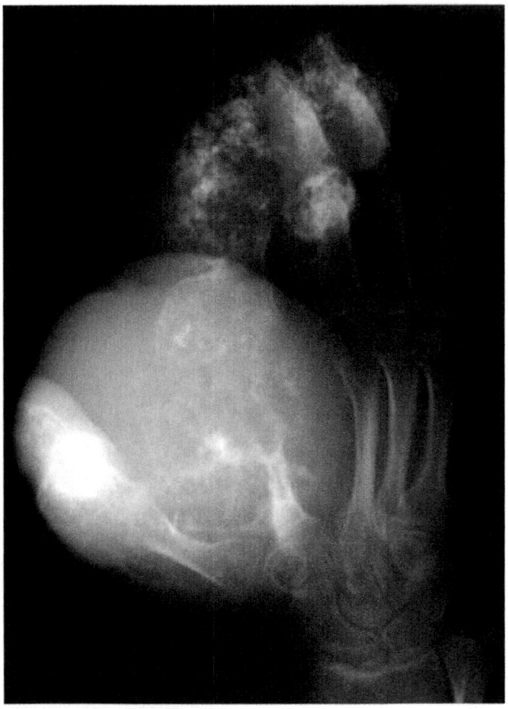

Fig. 4 Malignant transformation in Ollier disease. Multiple enchondromas with a large chondrosarcoma arising in the second metacarpal

Enchondroma can pose a diagnostic challenge both on imaging and pathology as it can be difficult to distinguish from a low-grade chondrosarcoma (Afonso et al. 2019). Thankfully, the treatment between both is the same (i.e. curettage) because the latter condition has a low metastatic potential (Lubahn and Bachoura 2016). However, higher grade chondrosarcomas are a different proposition as different diagnostic features and management mean identifying these lesions on radiology and histopathology is of utmost importance (Miwa et al. 2021).

2.1.2 Periosteal Chondroma

Periosteal chondroma (also termed juxtacortical chondroma) is a solitary, benign cartilaginous lesion arising in the periosteum and growing into adjacent soft tissue (Choi and Ro 2021; Pandey and Verma 2020). It is a rare tumour that was first described in 1959 and represents less than 2% of bone neoplasms (Lichtenstein and Hall 1952). Chondromas are most common in males usually presenting in the second decade of life but the age range is broad (Pandey and Verma 2020). The lesion most commonly affects the metaphyses or metadiaphyses of the long bones with the phalanges of the hands and feet often involved (Kurt et al. 2021).

Scalloping of the cortex is a typical radiographic feature and can range from minimal change to displacement of cortex into the medullary cavity (Fig. 5) (Pandey and Verma 2020). Sclerosis is typically present at the base of the lesion. Overhanging edges/buttressing seen at the margin may completely or partially encircle the lesion. A visible soft tissue mass with associated chondroid matrix is seen in about 50% of cases and is more commonly associated with small lesions of the hands and feet (Rabarin et al. 2014). CT and MRI are useful in demonstrating the presence of an outer periosteal shell, soft tissue mass and calcified matrix. MRI demonstrates a juxtacortical mass of low-to-intermediate T1 and high T2 signal reflecting the hyaline cartilage content of the lesion (Fig. 5c, d).

There are numerous differential diagnoses including other benign tumours, but differentiation from periosteal chondrosarcoma is most crucial (Pandey and Verma 2020; Kresse et al. 2023). Larger size (>3 cm) favours chondrosarcoma as does a large soft tissue component (Robinson et al. 2001; Bertoni et al. 1982). However, there is significant radiological and histopathological overlap, and features such as intramedullary extension and intramedullary oedema on MRI are less specific (Nakagawa et al. 2022).

2.1.3 Osteochondroma

Osteochondromas are benign bony projections capped by cartilaginous tissue, typically arising in long tubular bones. A characteristic medullary cavity within the lesion will be continuous with the medullary cavity of the bone from which it arises. Pathophysiologically, osteochondromas are similar to enchondromas as they develop from aberrant cartilaginous rests in the bone marrow but these grow beyond the periosteum whereas an enchondroma remains intramedullary (Chilvers et al. 2021; Bailescu et al. 2022).

Although osteochondromas are the most common benign bone tumour, occurrence in the upper

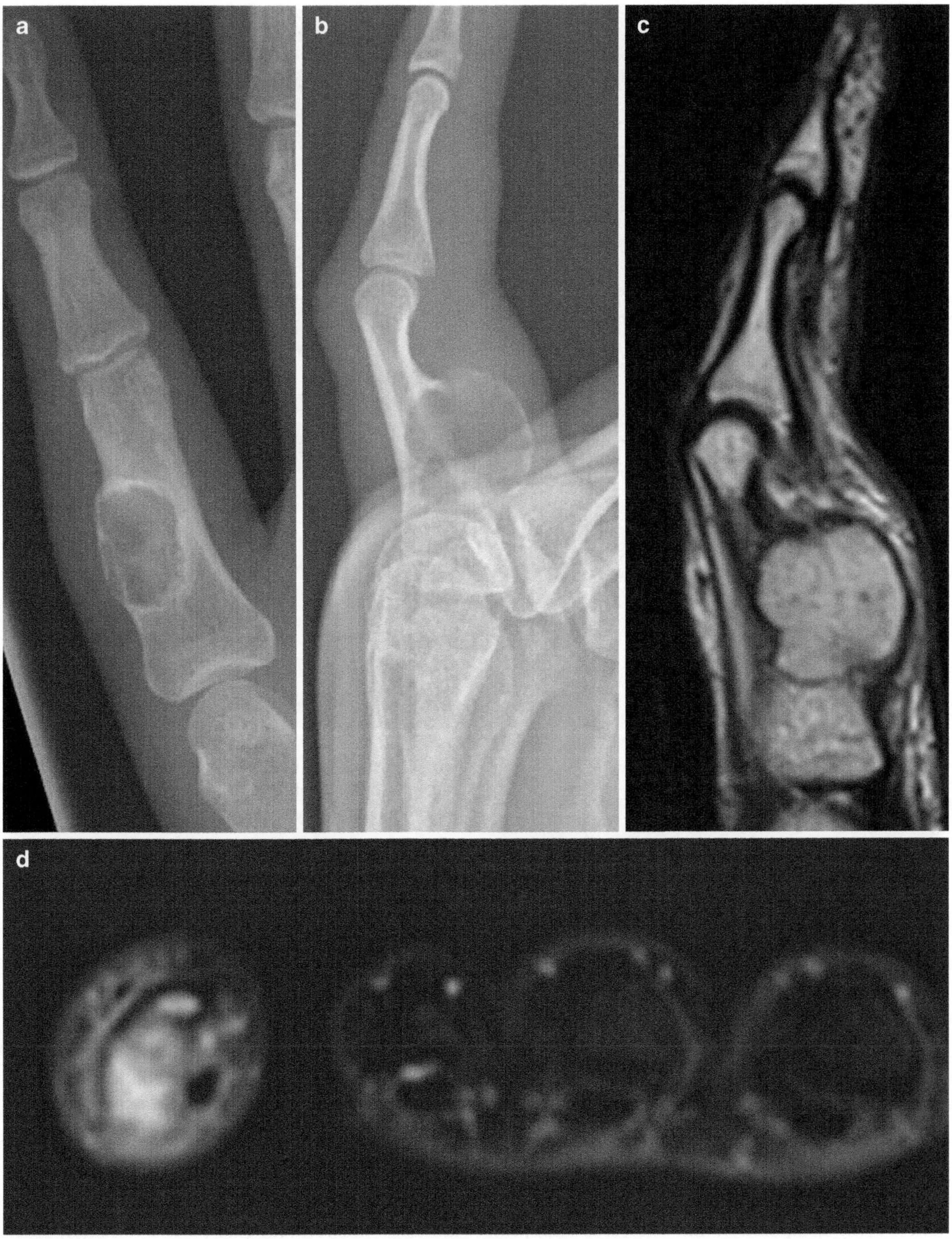

Fig. 5 Periosteal chondroma. (**a**, **b**) Eccentric lytic lesion arising in the shaft of the little finger proximal phalanx. On MRI, there is high signal on PD (**c**) and STIR (**d**) weighted sequences

limb and more specifically the hands is uncommon (Tepelenis et al. 2021; Gnoli et al. 2024). When osteochondroma does develop in the hand, the proximal phalanges are most commonly involved with metacarpal involvement rare and carpal lesions rarer still (Fig. 6) (Motomiya et al. 2020; Teodoreanu et al. 2022; Woodside et al. 2015). Since solitary osteochondroma of the

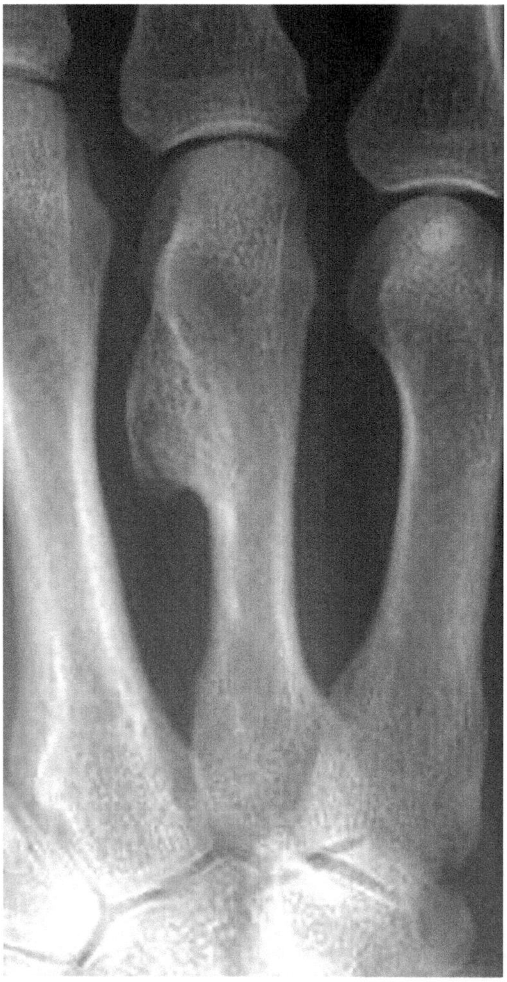

Fig. 6 Osteochondroma. It is arising from the surface of the distal 4th metacarpal. Note that there is continuity of trabeculae within the lesion and the underlying medullary bone

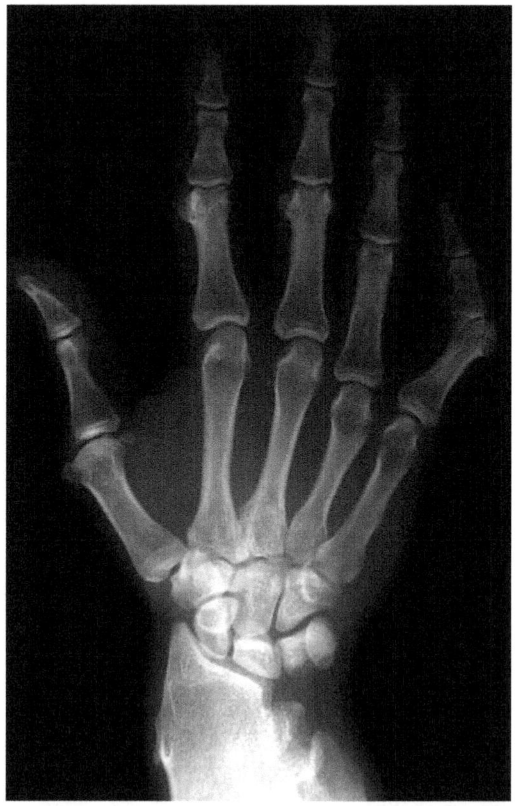

Fig. 7 Hereditary multiple exostoses (diaphyseal aclasis). Multiple small osteochondromas and a pseudo-Madelung deformity of the wrist

hand is unusual, patients should be assessed for hereditary multiple exostoses (HME) when a hand lesion is seen (Ohkuma et al. 2011).

Osteochondromas of the hand are usually asymptomatic and do not warrant treatment unless lying in a position that interferes with joint function or developing into a palpable mass (El-Sobky et al. 2018; Niemeler et al. 2022; Woodside et al. 2015). In children, trigger finger due to impingement of the flexor tendons may be the only presentation with small osteochondromas (de Oliveira et al. 2017). Disruption of the normal epiphyseal growth plate in HME leads to angular deformity at the ends of long bones and ulnar shortening at the wrist, leading to secondary bowing deformity of the distal radius giving rise to a pseudo-Madelung deformity (Fig. 7) (Hannan et al. 2019).

Most hand osteochondromas are seen with HME, an autosomal-dominant skeletal disorder characterized by formation of numerous cartilage-capped exostoses. Osteochondromas associated with this are more likely to undergo malignant transformation into chondrosarcoma, although this remains rare (2–5% in HME, otherwise 1%) (Teodoreanu et al. 2022; Neder Filho et al. 2024). The hand is commonly involved in HME and usually with multiple lesions, most typically around the metacarpophalangeal joints (Ohkuma et al. 2011).

A key risk of osteochondroma is malignant transformation of the cartilage cap into a secondary peripheral chondrosarcoma (Gnoli et al. 2024). In solitary osteochondroma, this risk ranges from approximately 1–8% (Righi et al. 2022; Ahmed et al. 2003; Tsuda et al. 2019). However, the risk is substantially higher (around 10%) with HME which is associated with EXT1/EXT2 gene mutations (Tepelenis et al. 2021; Gnoli et al. 2024; Sebastian et al. 2023). Because most of these studies originate from tertiary orthopaedic oncology referral centres, the true risk is probably lower than the published literature and is certainly lower for those lesions in the appendicular skeleton (Sonne-Holm et al. 2014). In the hand, there are only a few case reports of chondrosarcoma developing from osteochondroma (Fig. 8), of which all except one (described by Cash and Habermann) occurred with HME (Saunders et al. 1997; Cash and Habermann 1988; Stomeo et al. 2014; Ostlere et al. 1991). Although most osteochondromas occur in children, malignant transformation typically occurs in the third decade (Tepelenis et al. 2021; Avramidis et al. 2023).

On imaging, osteochondromas are typically sessile or pedunculated lesions which show continuity with the underlying medullary cavity of the bone of origin (Fig. 6) (Alghamdi et al. 2023; Tepelenis et al. 2021). Most are metaphyseal and characteristically point away from the physis (de Macedo Pontes et al. 2023). Radiographs are helpful in demonstrating complications of osteochondromas such as fracture, growth disturbance, osseous deformity and malignant change. Any increase in size of a lesion after skeletal maturity is concerning for sarcomatous change and necessitates further evaluation. Other concerning features are loss of a previously well-defined margin, lucency within a previously

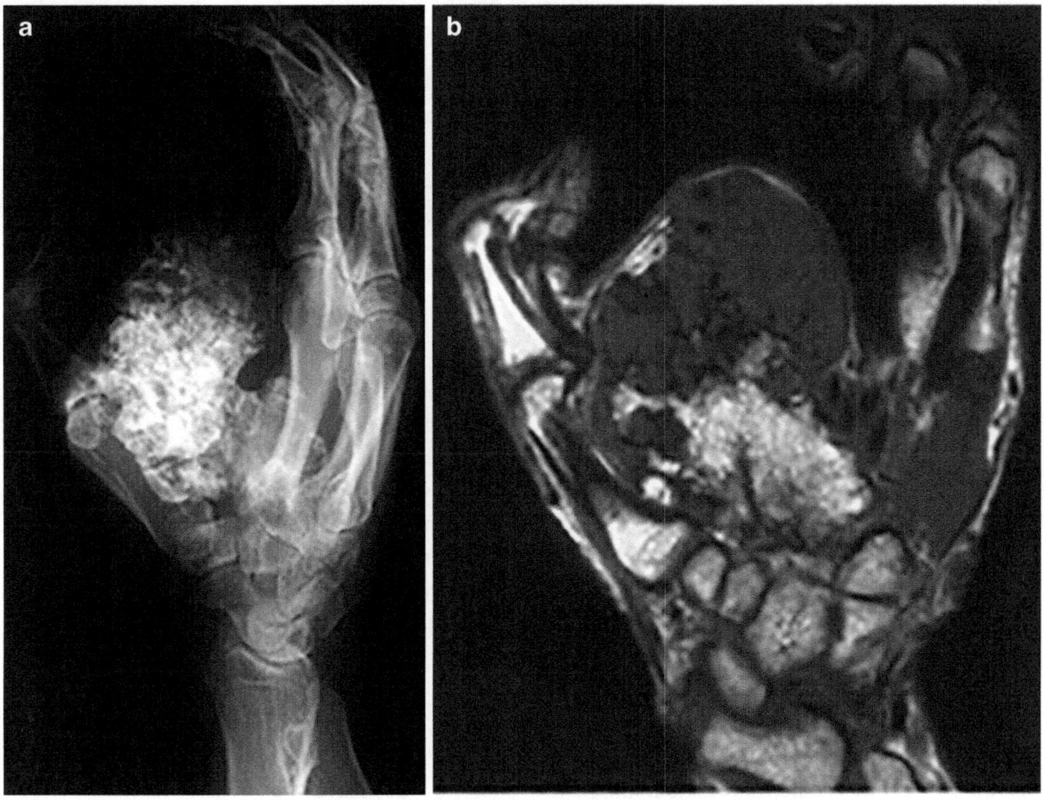

Fig. 8 Malignant transformation in hereditary multiple exostoses. (**a**) PA oblique radiograph and (**b**) coronal T1-weighted MR image showing a large peripheral low-grade chondrosarcoma arising from the second metacarpal. Note the thick cartilaginous cap in the MR image (>2 cm)

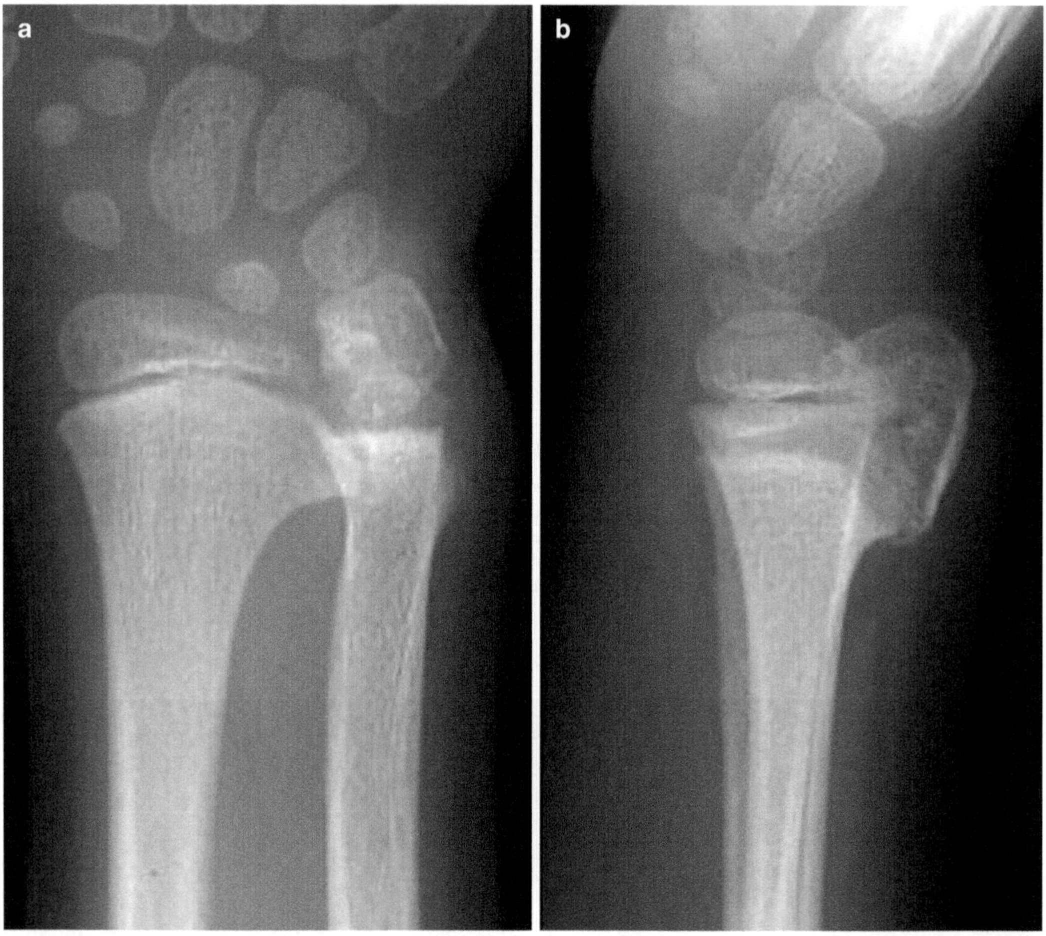

Fig. 9 Dysplasia epiphysealis hemimelica (Trevor disease). There is a modelling deformity with an osteochondroma-like mass arising from the distal ulnar epiphysis

mineralized area in the cartilage cap and a cap thickness larger than 2 cm (Fig. 8b) (Bailescu et al. 2022; Tepelenis et al. 2021). To complement radiography and CT evaluation, MRI provides precisely assessed thickness of the cartilage cap that has high signal intensity on T2 spin echo sequences as well as provides information regarding other complications such as reactive bursa formation, neural impingement and vascular compromise.

A key differential for osteochondroma is dysplasia epiphysealis hemimelica (Trevor disease), and the two entities share radiological and histological features (Degnan and Ho-Fung 2018). Cases have been reported at the proximal interphalangeal joint and distal radioulnar joint (Degnan and Ho-Fung 2018; Kopriva et al. 2020). The main differentiating feature is that rather than affecting the metaphysis, asymmetric excessive overgrowth of the epiphysis causes resultant bony protrusion (De Smet 2004). Radiographs demonstrate an osteochondroma-like protruberance arising from an epiphysis (Fig. 9).

2.2 Giant Cell Tumour of Bone and Giant Cell Reparative Granuloma

Giant cell tumour of bone (GCTB) is a locally aggressive primary tumour of bone. Although

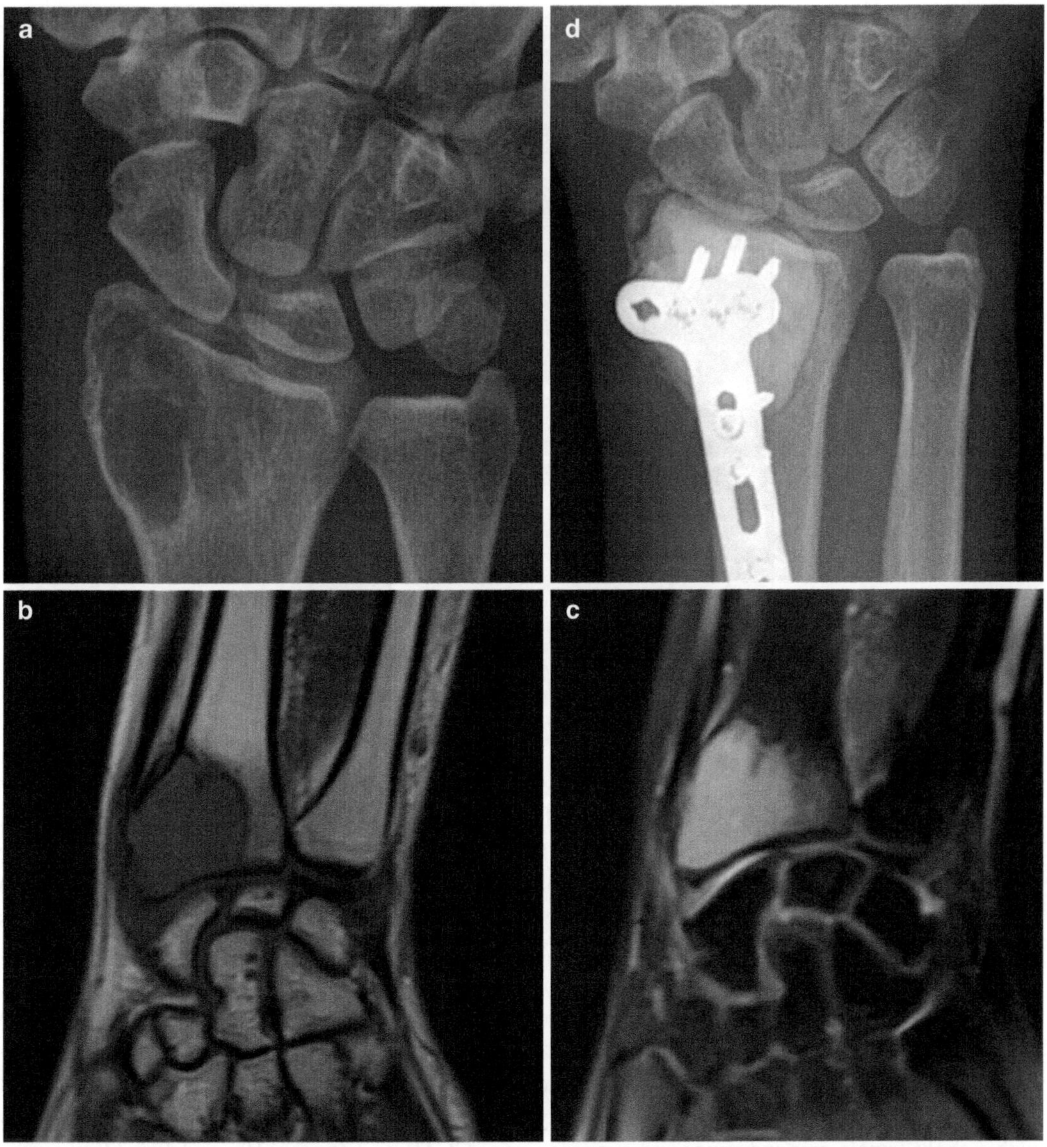

Fig. 10 Giant cell tumour. (**a**) PA radiograph showing a subarticular, expansile, lytic lesion in the distal radius with a trabeculated contour. (**b**) Coronal T1-weighted and (**c**) fluid-sensitive MR images showing the extent of the lesion and low signal areas due to the presence of haemosiderin. (**d**) PA radiograph showing internal fixation and cement augmentation following Denosumab treatment

the vast majority are benign, up to 4% of cases are either primary malignancy or have the risk of malignant transformation (Sobti et al. 2016; Palmerini et al. 2019). Histologically, the tumour is characterized by the diffuse presence of osteoclastic multinucleated giant cells in a background of mononuclear stromal cells (Sobti et al. 2016).

Approximately 5–6% of primary bone tumours and 20% of benign tumours are GCTB with a slight female predilection (Palmerini et al. 2019; Mavrogenis et al. 2017a). Most tumours affect the distal femur, proximal tibia and distal radius of skeletally mature individuals (Fig. 10) (Puri et al. 2021). Approximately 5% occur in the small bones of the hand and feet with 2% in the metacarpals

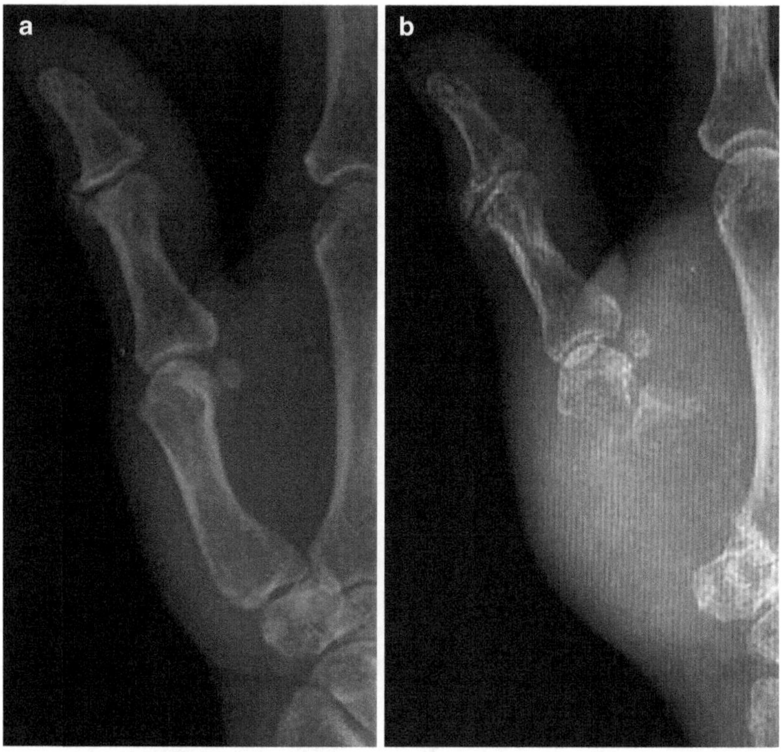

Fig. 11 Giant cell tumour. (**a**) PA radiograph at presentation showing a small area of permeative bone destruction in the proximal 1st metacarpal. (**b**) 4 months later without treatment, the tumour has enlarged dramatically and is destroying much of the metacarpal

(Fig. 11) and 1% in the phalanges (Puri et al. 2021; Averill et al. 1980; James and Davies 2005). However, the majority of lesions at the wrist involve the distal radius and ulna. Involvement of the carpal bones is very rare, involving only 15% of GCTB of the hand occurring in the carpus of which the hamate is most commonly involved (Shigematsu et al. 2006; Mier et al. 2024).

In terms of epidemiology, GCTB of the hand and wrist is similar to GCTB elsewhere in the body with a slight female preponderance and occurring most commonly in the third decade though the age range is wide (Berger et al. 2024). However, GCTB can rarely develop in skeletally immature patients (up to 6% of lesions) often as a mimic for aneurysmal bone cysts from which it must be distinguished, given the differences in management (Haseeb et al. 2020; Ambrosi et al. 2021). Symptoms are nonspecific and patients usually present with pain, local swelling, and reduced adjacent joint motion from the tumour itself but may also present with a pathological fracture (Meena et al. 2016).

Most GCTB cases are monostotic, but multicentric cases have been described including in the hands (Mavrogenis et al. 2017a; Puri et al. 2021). Multicentric lesions are more likely to involve atypical locations than monostotic lesions with about 60% of all described multicentric GCTs being in the hands and feet (Meena et al. 2016; James and Davies 2005; Oliveira et al. 2013).

Although generally considered a benign lesion, GCTB does have potential for local recurrence and metastasis particularly with risk of spread to the lung. The overall risk of metastasis in GCTB is between 1% and 9% (Tsukamoto et al. 2021; Xu and Choong 2022). The rate of local recurrence and metastases is higher than the 20% reported elsewhere. The literature suggests that the relatively fragile bones of the hand and distal radius are anatomically difficult to aggressively curettage and post-curettage local recurrence rates of up to 50% have been described (Tsukamoto et al. 2021; Oliveira et al. 2013). As with lesions elsewhere, the rate of recurrence is lowest for hand and wrist GCTB treated with resection followed by curettage with adjuvants, and the highest recurrence is from curettage alone (Teixeira et al. 2014).

Malignant GCTB can occur as a primary malignancy (in 1.6% of all cases), but more commonly (2.6% of all cases) it occurs as a secondary tumour with sarcomatous transformation following radiotherapy, a key trigger (Tsukamoto et al. 2021). Malignant GCTB has not, to the best of our knowledge, been reported in the small bones of the hand and wrist.

On radiography, GCTB in the long bones of the wrist and hand shares features with lesions elsewhere with an eccentric, expansile, lytic appearance, located in a subarticular position involving the epiphysis and metaphysis (Parmeggiani et al. 2021; Cecava et al. 2020) (Fig. 10a). However, GCTB of the long bones of the hand is more likely to involve metaphyses and diaphyses as well as central part of the bone (Meena et al. 2016). The few described cases of distal radial tumours in skeletally immature patients show the tumour is typically metaphyseal, though extension across the growth plate into the epiphysis is rarely observed (James and Davies 2005).

A narrow zone of transition is seen at the metaphyseal margin of the lesion, and there is typically no matrix mineralization. Thinning of the cortex and extension into the soft tissues are well recognized. Internal trabeculation is common but the pattern may vary from fine striations to coarse trabeculation (Fig. 10a). Periosteal reaction is suggestive of a locally aggressive lesion or a complicating fracture (Davies et al. 2020; Cecava et al. 2020). In current practice, preoperative Denosumab (a human monoclonal antibody used to inhibit osteolysis) is often employed for structural integrity which radiographically manifests as cortical sclerosis and matrix osteosclerosis (van Langevelde and McCarthy 2020).

The radiographic grading system described by Campanacci in 1987 remains in use in modern practice to describe imaging features that correlate with local aggressiveness of a GCTB (Campanacci et al. 1987). Stage I lesions do not distort or perforate the cortex, stage II lesions expand or distort the cortex but do not extend into soft tissues, and stage III lesions exhibit cortical destruction and soft tissue extension. Stage III tumours are associated with a higher rate of recurrence (Teixeira et al. 2014).

Technetium 99-m bone scintigraphy may demonstrate a classic "doughnut" configuration with avid uptake at and around the periphery of the tumour and a relatively photopenic centre (Levine et al. 1984; Patel et al. 1987; Utomo et al. 2019). Uptake can also be seen on FDG-PET (O'Connor et al. 2014). However, although scintigraphy can identify lesions, anatomical characterization is limited.

Lesions in the hand and wrist show similar MR imaging characteristics to GCTB elsewhere in the body (Fig. 10b). The main benefit of both CT and MRI is to define the intra- and extra-osseous extent of the tumour (Garcia and Bianchi 2001). Low signal intensity on all sequences can be seen which is indicative of chronic haemosiderin deposition in GCTB (Fig. 10c). Fluid–fluid levels may be demonstrated within the tumour mass indicating the presence of secondary aneurysmal bone cyst (ABC) formation.

Giant-cell reparative granuloma (GCRG) (also termed Central Giant Cell Granuloma) is a reactive pseudotumour that most commonly involves the mandible, maxilla and small bones of the hands and feet (Ventura-Parellada et al. 2021; Nackos et al. 2006). It shares imaging and histological characteristics with GCTB but does not share the latter's propensity to recurrence, metastasis, and malignant transformation (Gouin et al. 2003; Nackos et al. 2006). Histologically, GCRG is characterized by non-neoplastic vascular tissues, fibroblasts and clusters of multinucleated giant cells surrounded by foci of haemorrhage which may also contain areas of osteoid matrix and aneurysmal bone cyst formation (Macdonald et al. 2003; Arvind et al. 2023; Li et al. 2021).

In general, GCRG affects a younger age group than GCTB, with presentation often seen in skeletally immature patients (Arvind et al. 2023). As with GCTB, clinical presentation may be non-specific with swelling and pain. In the hand, GCRG most commonly affects the phalanges, followed by the metacarpals and carpal bones (Fig. 12) (Li et al. 2021). The tumours are metaphyseal in location, and unlike in GCTB, involvement of the epiphysis is rare (Chilla et al.

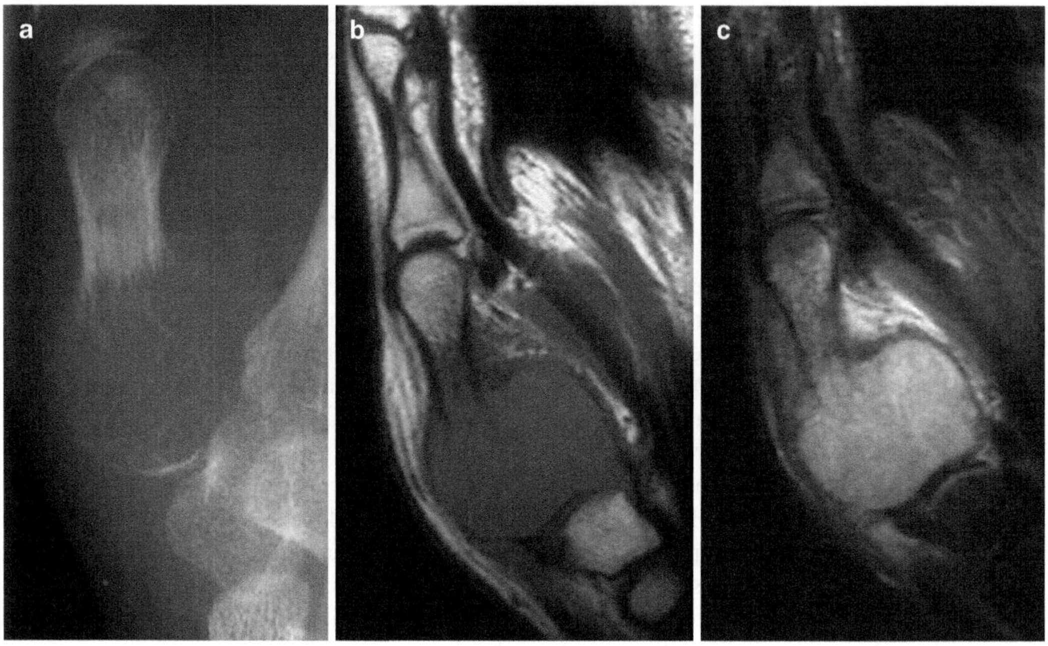

Fig. 12 Giant cell reparative granuloma. (**a**) PA radiograph, (**b**) coronal T1-weighted and (**c**) coronal STIR MR images showing a lytic, expansile lesion destroying the proximal third of the first metacarpal

2005). To our knowledge, extension of GCRG across an unfused physis has not been reported. The tumours may have an expansile, lytic radiographic appearance and may demonstrate cortical destruction (Fig. 11) (Li et al. 2021). Periosteal reaction is rarely seen but pathological fracture can rarely occur (Li et al. 2021).

2.3 Bone Cysts

Aneurysmal bone cyst (ABC) accounts for around 1% of all bone tumours (Restrepo et al. 2022) and between 5% and 6% of benign bone tumours (Athanasian 2004). The lesions are composed of blood-filled cavities with three microscopic components—osteoclast-like multinucleated giant cells, collagenous extracellular matrix and organic bone matrix deposited by osteoblasts (Choi and Ro 2021). The most common locations of ABC are the long bone metaphyses followed by the spine (Martinez and Sissons, 1988). Occurrence in the hand is rare with only approximately 6% of cases in the recently published literature present here (Pena-Burgos et al. 2023).

ABC most commonly presents in the second decade of life and has a slight female predilection (Restrepo et al. 2022). In the hand, ABC most commonly involves the metacarpals (52%) followed by the phalanges (36%) and carpal bones 4% (Platt and Klugman 1995). An unusual case of ABC arising in a sesamoid bone of the hand has been reported (Havulinna et al. 2005). Trauma is implicated in association with almost half of the published cases of hand ABC but may simply draw attention to a pre-existing lesion (Crowe et al. 2015). Typically, the patient presents with a slowly enlarging mass that may or may not be painful (Restrepo et al. 2022). On examination, there may be extensive swelling and warmth (Athanasian 2004; Crowe et al. 2015). Patients may present with a pathological fracture or with this as an incidental lesion.

Radiographs of the hand demonstrate a central, expansile, lytic lesion that causes cortical thinning (Restrepo et al. 2022). ABCs are normally epiphyseal or metaphyseal in location (Fig. 13). Subperiosteal ABCs are eccentrically located and tend to involve the metaphysis or

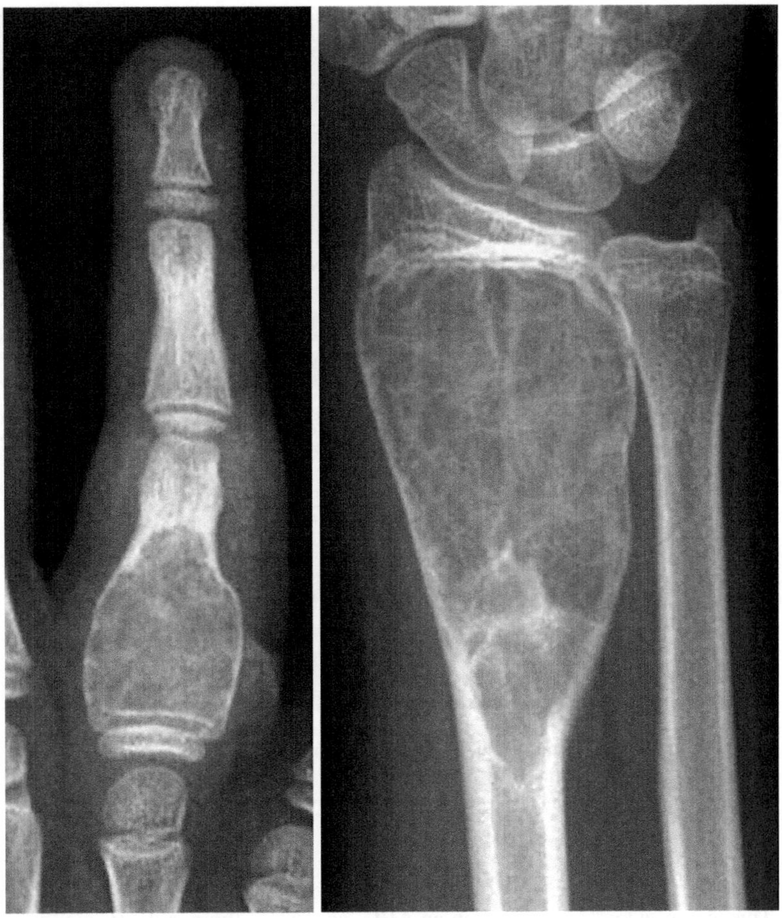

Fig. 13 Aneurysmal bone cyst. Two different cases both in children. Lytic, expansile, juxta-epiphyseal lesions arising in the proximal phalanx and distal radius

metadiaphysis. These lesions grow outside the confine of normal bone but are limited externally by periosteum and internally by endosteum (James and Davies 2005). Only a handful of cases of subperiosteal ABC have been reported in the hand involving metacarpals and a phalanx (Fig. 14a) (Nanda et al. 2018; Shimal et al. 2009; Maiya et al. 2002). A sclerotic margin may be seen (Gajewski et al. 2023). Matrix trabeculations are sometimes observed and may be mixed or lytic (Pai et al. 2021). Periosteal reaction is usually absent and its presence suggests a pathological cortical fracture (Noordin et al. 2019). When the lesion presents in the distal phalanx, significant bone destruction may occur (Leeson et al. 1988). The natural history of ABC is that of progressive enlargement and bone destruction, though some authors have described spontaneous healing or healing following minor disturbance such as fracture or biopsy (Mendenhall et al. 2006; Reddy et al. 2014).

On MR and CT imaging, fluid–fluid levels are suggestive but not diagnostic of ABC (Fig. 14b, c). The possibility of secondary ABC formation in a pre-existing lesion should always be considered. Both radiologically and histologically the lesion may be confused with telangiectatic osteosarcoma, although the latter entity is rarer than ABC in the hand (Zishan et al. 2020). Although ABC can be locally aggressive, it is not known to have metastatic potential. Local recurrence after curettage has been widely reported due to the difficulty of operating in the hand (Gajewski et al. 2023).

Simple bone cyst (also termed unicameral bone cyst) is a tumour-like lesion of unknown cause. Distinction from ABC is crucial given the differences in their management (Mascard et al. 2015).

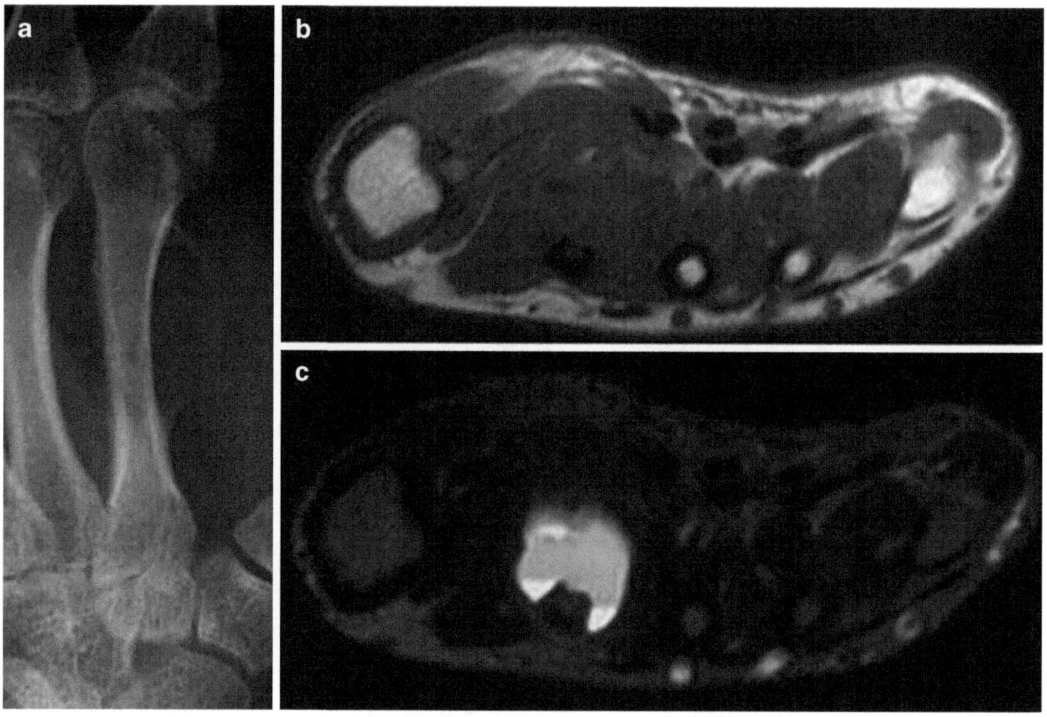

Fig. 14 Subperiosteal aneurysmal bone cyst. (**a**) Oblique radiograph showing a thin shell of periosteal new bone arising from the second metacarpal. (**b**) Axial T1- and (**c**) axial T2-weighted fat-suppressed MR images showing an eccentric lesion with fluid–fluid levels

This lesion is less complex than an ABC, consisting of a bony cavity, lined by a thin membrane and filled with serous fluid (Chebib et al. 2020). It most commonly arises in the proximal humerus and proximal femur with 85% occurring prior to completion of skeletal fusion. Involvement of the hand and wrist is rare (Kozlowski et al. 1988; Inozu et al. 2016). Radiographic features, irrespective of site, are those of a benign looking, lytic lesion arising in the metaphysis of a long bone. Frequently, cases present with a pathological fracture following only minor trauma which can introduce complexity to the structure and somewhat mimic an ABC (Fig. 15a) (Chebib et al. 2020; Wang et al. 2022). In time, the cyst will grow away from physis with the laying down of normal intervening trabecular bone, but resolution is usually incomplete, even by the time of skeletal maturity (Fig. 15b) (Donaldson and Wright 2015).

Intraosseous ganglia are benign non-neoplastic bone lesions that are histologically similar to their soft tissue counterpart (Sakamoto et al. 2013). The terms intraosseous ganglion, subchondral cyst and geode are often applied interchangeably, although the latter are more frequently used to describe juxta-articular lesions associated with degenerative or inflammatory joint disease (Williams et al. 2004). On imaging, these all appear as well-defined subarticular lytic lesions. When not associated with degenerative joint disease, they can mimic other juxta-articular lesions such as giant cell tumour (Fig. 16). Cases arising in the carpal bones are not uncommon—particularly in the proximal row—and can be multiple and bilateral (Osagie et al. 2015).

2.4 Osteoid Osteoma

Osteoid osteoma is a benign osteoblastic tumour that was first described in 1935 as a tumour consisting of an area of variably calcified osteoid tis-

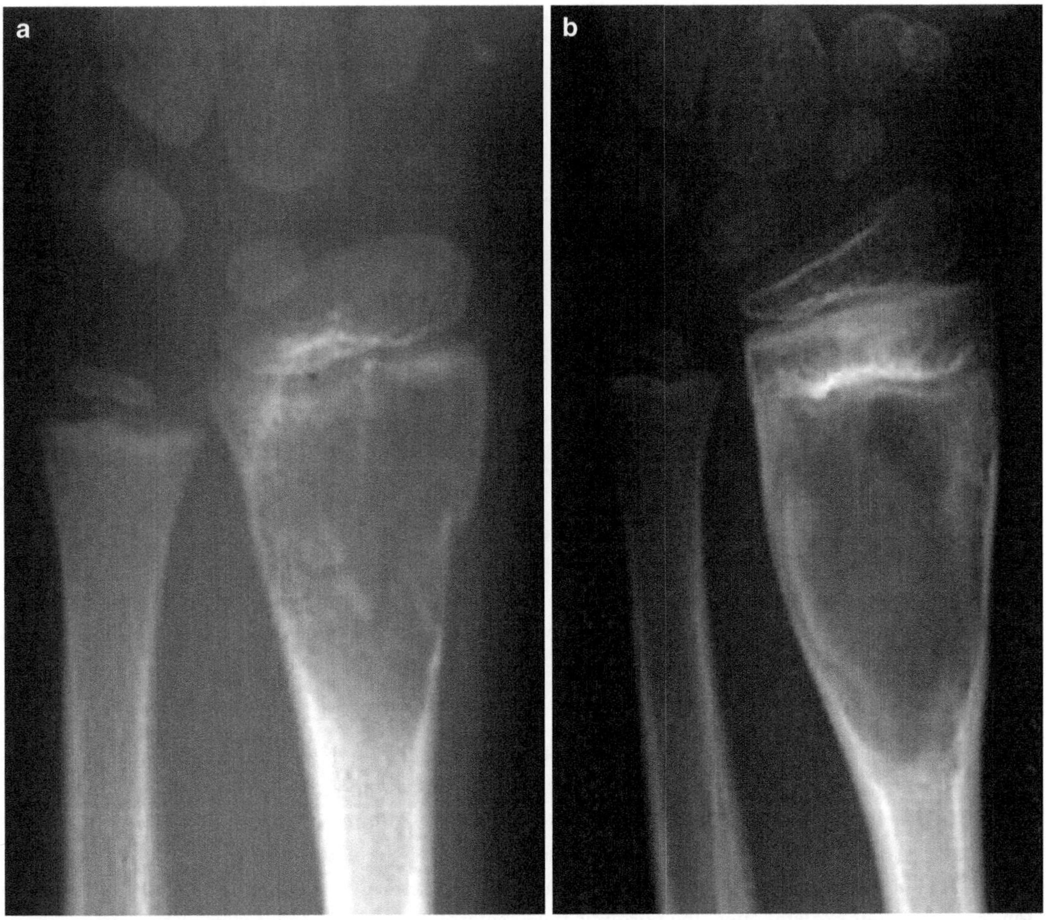

Fig. 15 Simple bone cyst. (**a**) PA radiograph showing a pathological fracture through a lytic lesion in the distal radial metaphysis. (**b**) 2 years later the fracture has healed. The lesion is mildly expansile and has started to grow away from the distal radial growth plate

sue within a stroma of relatively loose vascular connective tissue (Jaffe 1935). A rim of sclerotic reactive bone, less than 2 cm in diameter, surrounds the lesion and there may be a periosteal reaction. Approximately 10% of cases involve the hand and wrist with just over half of these in the phalanges and the remaining split between the metacarpal and carpal bones (Jafari et al. 2013). The middle phalanges are the least commonly affected bones in the hand (Marcuzzi et al. 2002; Meyer et al. 2023b).

In general, osteoid osteoma most commonly presents in the second decade of life and is generally reported to have a female predeliction (Jafari et al. 2013; Ambrosia et al. 1987). Typical clinical symptoms are of gradually increasing pain and swelling but juxta-articular lesions can lead to restriction of movement and muscle atrophy (Ambrosia et al. 1987; Marcuzzi et al. 2002). Physical signs often vary depending on the site of clinical symptoms. Proximal and middle phalanx involvement may be associated with a grossly enlarged phalanx with hypertrophy of the soft tissues, while distal phalanx involvement may lead to single finger clubbing and hypertrophy of the nail (Meyer et al. 2023a; Horiuchi et al. 2017). The average duration of symptoms for osteoid osteoma of the hand and wrist before diagnosis is between 13 and 15 months—painless osteoid osteoma appears to occur in the digits more fre-

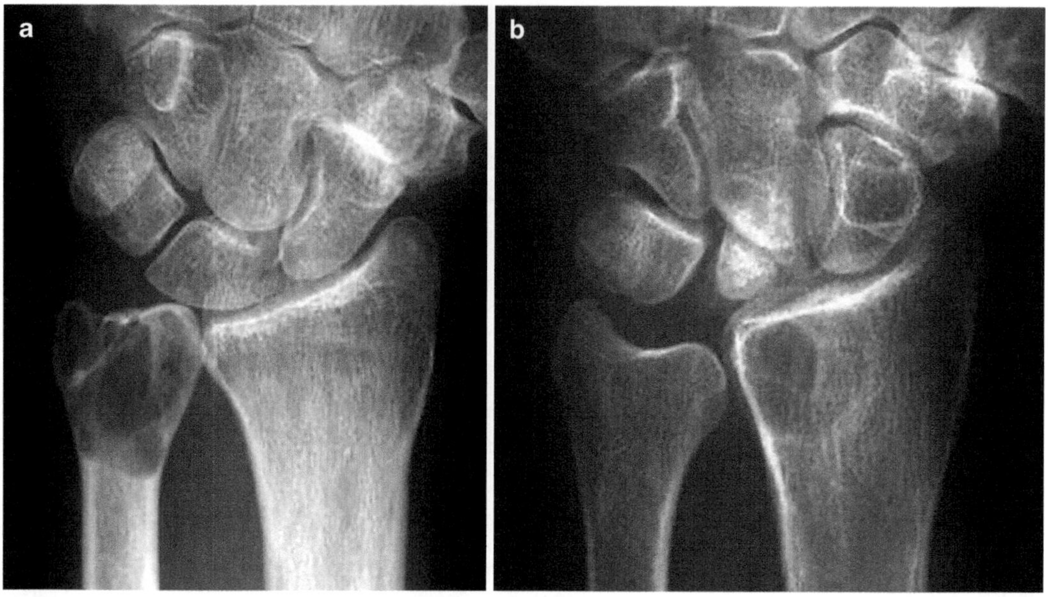

Fig. 16 Intraosseous ganglion. Two different cases showing subarticular lytic lesions involving (**a**) the distal ulna and (**b**) the distal radius. This second case also shows scapho-lunate disassociation

quently than in any other skeletal location (Marcuzzi et al. 2002; De Smet 2001; Claeys et al. 2016).

Osteoid osteomas may arise centrally in the medulla, in the cortex or in a subperiosteal location. As with other skeletal sites, the cortex is the most common location for osteoid osteomas of the hand and wrist. Subperiosteal lesions are extremely rare in the hand, with only a few reported cases (Meyer et al. 2023a, b).

The typical radiographic appearance is that of a small, radiolucent lesion or nidus surrounded by an area of bone sclerosis (Fig. 17). Lesions in the subperiosteum have atypical radiographic findings and may only be diagnosed as osteoid osteoma on histopathology (Fig. 18) (Shubinets et al. 2019). Radiographs can initially appear normal with bony abnormality taking up to 25 months to manifest (Marcuzzi et al. 2002).

As with other skeletal locations, bone scintigraphy of osteoid osteoma of the hand and wrist shows a well-defined focal area of increased activity during all three phases of a technetium-99 MDP scan (Streek et al. 1998). However, findings can also be non-specific with diffuse uptake of radionuclide in the area of the lesion, thus rendering this a supplementary modality (Meyer et al. 2023b). Computed tomography is the most specific and characteristically shows a lytic lesion with a central granular opacity surrounded by a sclerotic margin (Meyer et al. 2023a, b).

On MRI, the typical pattern is that of a lesion composed of a hypointense, sclerotic centre with a high T2 signal rim surrounded by marrow oedema (Meyer et al. 2023b). While MRI is the most sensitive imaging modality at identifying the florid oedema that accompanies osteoid osteomas; this can mask the nidus thus causing misdiagnosis in the absence of radiographs, CT, or radionuclide imaging (Meyer et al. 2023b; Carneiro et al. 2021). This limitation of specificity can be significant in differentiating osseous neoplasms like osteoid osteoma from low-grade infection and florid reactive periostitis.

Thermoablation is the first-line treatment option for osteoid osteoma, with radiofrequency ablation being the preferred technique at the authors tertiary centre (Motamedi et al. 2009; Uldin et al. 2024).

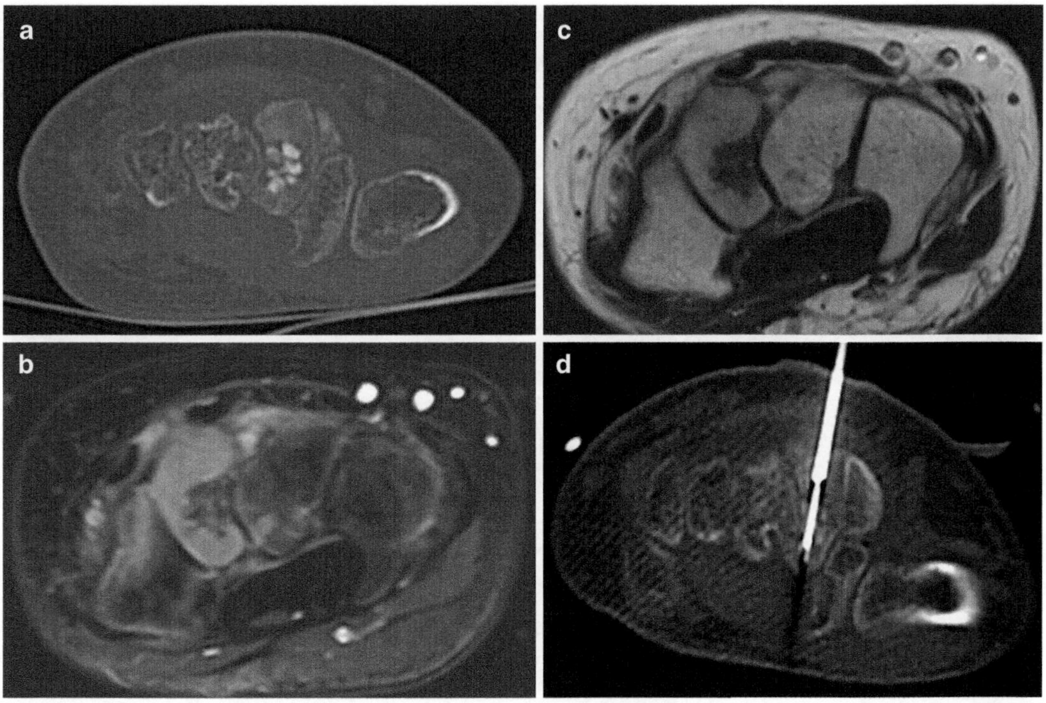

Fig. 17 Osteoid osteoma. (**a**) Focal calcification of the trapezoid bone with faint lucencies representing the nidus of the lesion. Axial (**b**) STIR and (**c**) PD sequences show extensive associated marrow oedema-like signal of the trapezoid as well as adjacent bony and soft tissue oedema. Radiofrequency ablation under CT guidance (**d**) is a key treatment option

2.5 Focal Proliferative Periosteal Processes

There are several focal benign proliferative periosteal processes of the hand (particularly the phalanges) which are important to understand but are often confusingly described (Tang et al. 2023). Florid reactive periostitis (FRP) was first reported in 1933 by Mallory, although this was not the term used to describe it (cited by Jambhekar et al. in 2004 amongst other authors). Subsequently, bizarre parosteal osteochondromatous proliferation (BPOP) of the phalanges was described as a new radiopathological entity by Nora et al. in 1983 (Nora et al. 1983). Initially, these two conditions were considered to represent two distinct processes. In 1992, Yuen et al. proposed a hypothesis that the two entities, along with turret exostosis, are part of a continuous spectrum of the same process and subsequent literature has supported this assessment (Yuen et al. 1992; Abramovici and Steiner 2002; Ribeiro et al. 2019). The work of these authors suggests that initial subperiosteal haemorrhage causes a localized fusiform periostitis consistent with FRP. Later, this periostitis becomes incorporated into cortex, and remodelling leads to a broad-based cancellous protuberance that is characteristic for BPOP.

2.5.1 Florid Reactive Periostitis

The term 'florid reactive periostitis' was first used by Spjut and Dorfman in their series of 12 cases to describe a painful osteoblastic proliferation arising from the periosteum of the small long bones of the hands and feet (Spjut and Dorfman 1981). The exact pathophysiology is not entirely clear (Tomori et al. 2016). Because of its histological resemblance to nodular fasciitis, other names used to describe the entity have included fasciitis ossificans and parosteal fasciitis (Marui

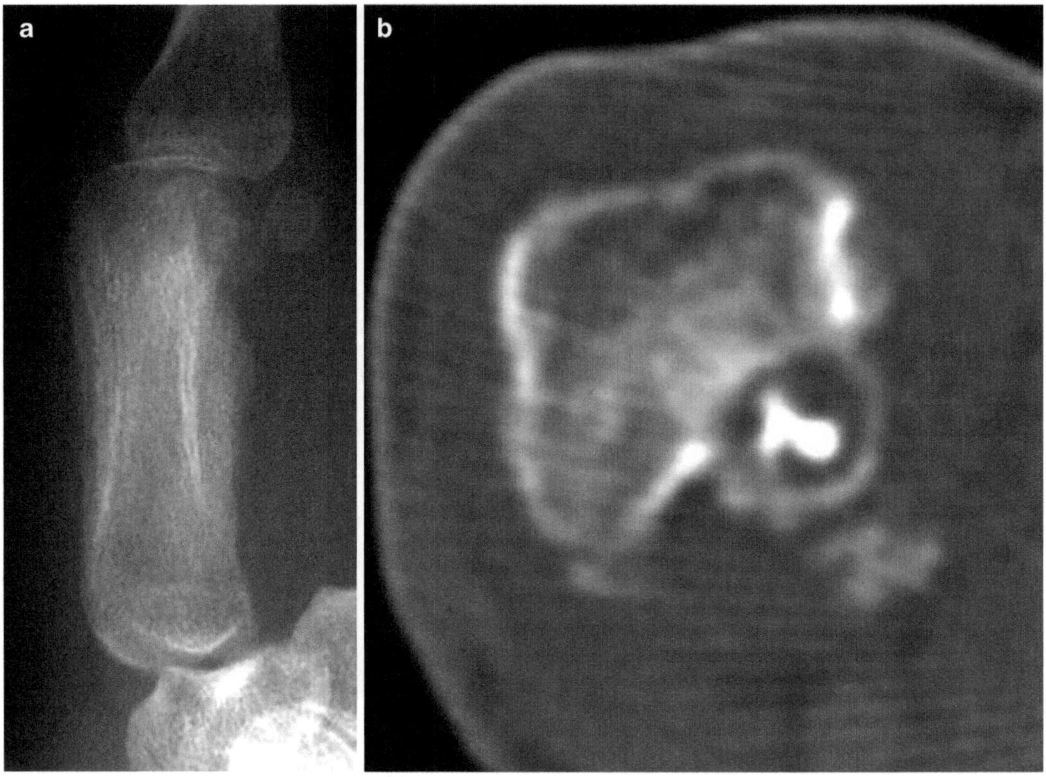

Fig. 18 Subperiosteal osteoid osteoma. (**a**) Radiograph showing periosteal new bone formation along the first metacarpal with a faint eccentric nidus located distally. (**b**) Axial CT reveals the nidus formed by the subperiosteal cavity and containing a small focus of calcification

et al. 2003; Dhillon et al. 2023). Dupree and Enzinger, in a series of 21 cases, used the term 'fibro-osseous pseudotumour of the digits' as they disputed its periosteal origin and suggested that it arises from soft tissues and surrounding fibrous structures (Dupree and Enzinger 1986).

FRP is typically seen in the second and third decades of life with a slight female preponderance (Solana et al. 2003). An antecedent history of trauma—including repetitive low-level trauma—is present in between 10% and 50% of cases of FRP (Tomori et al. 2016; Michelsen et al. 2004).

Unlike many of the lesions described until this point of this chapter, FRP is most frequent in the hands and feet (Mathew et al. 2011). The majority of cases involve the proximal phalanx, followed by the middle phalanx, metacarpal and distal phalanx in decreasing order of frequency (Tomori et al. 2016). Typically, only one bone is involved, although cases involving two contiguous phalanges have been described (Tomori et al. 2016).

Radiographs typically demonstrate soft tissue swelling with a variable degree of diffuse calcification (Olvi et al. 2020; Memon et al. 2022). Periosteal reaction is present in approximately 50% of cases and can either be lamellated or mature (Fig. 19a) (Jamshidi et al. 2017). Cortical erosions associated with FRP have been described in several series (Jamshidi). Both conservative treatment with rest and anti-inflammatory treatment as well as marginal resection have been described as effective treatments (Tomori et al. 2016; Jamshidi et al. 2017; Tang et al. 2023).

The main radiological differential diagnoses include osteomyelitis and parosteal osteosarcoma (Tomori et al. 2016). Concern regarding a delay in treatment for potential malignancy often leads to hastily performed surgical procedures (Jambhekar et al. 2004). Sundaram et al. advocate more prospective radiological diagnosis of FRP with close clinical and radiographic follow-up to allow more appropriate and timely intervention (Sundaram et al. 2001).

2.5.2 Bizarre Parosteal Osteochondromatous Proliferation (BPOP)

Since its initial description by Nora (and subsequent eponymization), several case series and case reports of BPOP have been published. This is a benign mineralized mass-like surface-based bone lesion proposed to be a sequela of FRP and develop through cartilaginous metaplasia (Gitto et al. 2023; Kastanis et al. 2024; Martínez Álvarez et al. 2021). Like FRP, this typically involves the tubular bones of the hand and feet (Washington et al. 2021). Though the age at which presentation occurs is wide and includes children, peak incidence tends to be in the third and fourth decades (Gitto et al. 2023; Edoardo et al. 2022; Dharmshaktu et al. 2022; Martínez Álvarez et al. 2021). There is no definite sex predilection in the existing literature.

An antecedent history of trauma is uncommon but is reported by some authors, and the post-traumatic reactive neoformative change has been considered a potential mechanism (Michelsen et al. 2004; Edoardo et al. 2022). Typically, presentation is insidious and characterized by a slow-growing mass causing functional restriction of motion and possibly pain (Kastanis et al. 2024).

Radiographs demonstrate a well-marginated mineralized mass arising from the cortical surface of the affected bone—cortex itself is classically unaffected and the absence of corticomedullary continuity is a key feature (Fig. 19b) (Nora et al. 1983; Kastanis et al. 2024). The lesion can measure up to 4 cm (Nora et al. 1983; Dhondt et al. 2006). The hand and foot are involved in 75% with far more in the former and approximately 50% of cases affecting the proximal phalanges, with the remainder evenly distributed between the middle phalanges and metacarpals (Torreggiani et al. 2001; Olvi et al. 2020; Simon et al. 2014). The distal phalanx tends not to be involved. The characteristic radiological findings that differentiate BPOP from osteochondroma are the lack of cortical flaring at the margin of the protruberance and the absence of continuity of the lesion with medulla of underlying bone (Kastanis et al. 2024; Olvi et al. 2020). However, Rybak et al. have reported cases of histologically proven BPOP cases where medullary communication was demonstrated leading them to hypothesize that a continuum also exists between BPOP and osteochondroma (Rybak et al. 2007). However, none of the cases in that series were in the hand.

Computed tomography is valuable in demonstrating the relationship between the lesion and underlying cortex and establishing that there is not continuity with the medullary cavity. There are many reports of the characteristic MRI appearances of BPOP (Gitto et al. 2023; Kastanis et al. 2024; Torreggiani et al. 2001; Orui et al. 2002). The lesion is of low signal intensity on T1-weighted images and high signal intensity on T2- and STIR-weighted images. The medulla and surrounding soft tissues are usually normal in appearance though there is a reported case with oedema in both the adjacent medulla and surrounding soft tissues (Orui et al. 2002).

Definitive treatment is surgical excision. The recurrence rate is however high with recurrence in 18 of the 35 cases in Nora's original series. Malignant transformation is exceedingly rare with no such reported cases in the hand, but isolated cases of transformation to fibrosarcoma and a recent case of high-grade metastatic pleomorphic sarcoma have been described in the literature (Choi et al. 2001; Ulrich et al. 2024).

2.5.3 Turret Exostosis

Turret exostosis is a rare complication of trivial trauma to the fingers. It is thought to result from traumatic breach of the periosteum with formation and subsequent ossification of subperiosteal haemorrhage (Casstevens et al. 2021; Wissinger et al. 1966). The index and little finger digits are most frequently involved (Kang et al. 2012). The phalanges are the typical location for the lesion, but cases involving metacarpals have been reported

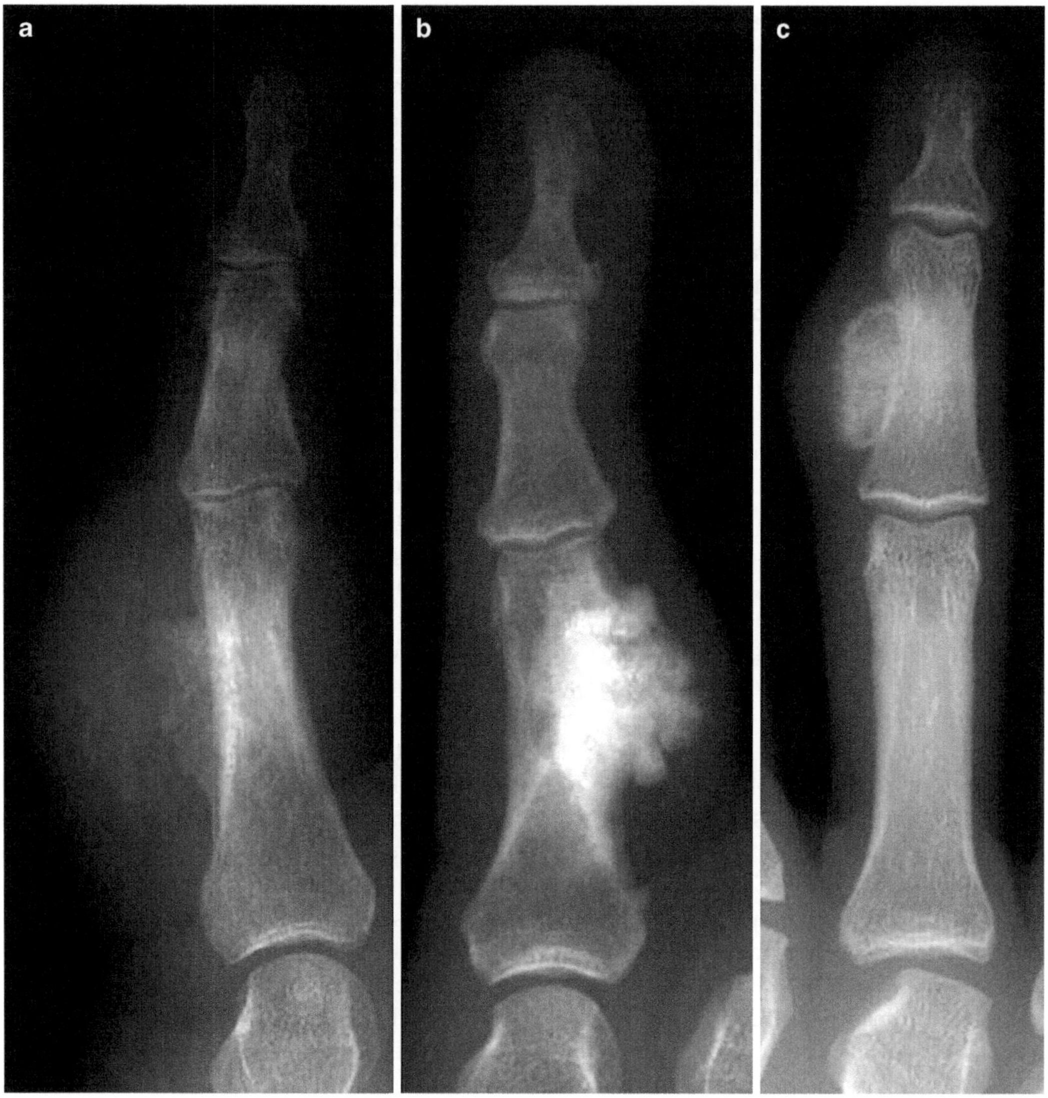

Fig. 19 Focal proliferative periosteal processes. (**a**) Florid reactive periostitis, (**b**) bizarre parosteal osteochondromatous proliferation and (**c**) turret exostosis

(Kang et al. 2012; Rubin and Steinberg 1996). The lesion usually occurs on the dorsal surface of the affected phalanx with only one case reported to date arising on the volar aspect (Rubin and Steinberg 1996; Mohanna et al. 2000).

A firm mass is usually palpable on clinical presentation, and there may be loss of function of the digit distal to the exostosis due to excursion of the extensor tendons (Mohanna et al. 2000). If large enough, flexor tendon function may also be impaired. There is almost always an antecedent history of trauma usually in the form of a laceration. Radiographically, the earliest finding is soft tissue swelling. A poorly defined, fragmented collection of subperiosteal new bone may be seen up to about 4 months from the initial injury (James and Davies 2005). The mature lesion demonstrates a narrow body with a smooth dome and usually lies deep to the extensor apparatus (Fig. 19c). Most authors recommend a 6-month period between the episode of trauma and local excision of the lesion, because excision of the lesion before it has fully matured may result in recurrence (Rubin and Steinberg 1996; Mohanna et al. 2000; Kontogeorgakos et al. 2007). Serial radiographs and bone scan can be used to assess maturity of the lesion which is indicated by well-defined cortical margins on radiographs and decreasing activity on bone scintigraphy (Rubin and Steinberg 1996; Kang et al. 2012).

2.5.4 Subungual Exostosis

Subungual exostosis is an uncommon benign condition arising in a distal phalanx beneath or adjacent to the nail bed. The lesion most commonly occurs in the great toe with only 10–20% of cases involving the fingers (Davis and Cohen 1996; Chiheb et al. 2021). There is no preponderance for a particular digit in the hand. More recent literature suggests that subungual exostosis has a similar incidence in females and males but larger older studies imply a female predisposition (Davis and Cohen 1996; Chiheb et al. 2021; Dąbrowski et al. 2023; Li et al. 2022). Patients usually present in the second and third decades of life, although it is also seen in children. Clinical presentation typically involves pain, swelling or surrounding ulceration of the nail bed which can result in secondary soft tissue infection (Pratap et al. 2019; Dave et al. 2004). The aetiology remains unclear but trauma and chronic irritation are probable precipitating factors (Russell et al. 2016; Turan et al. 2012).

The tumour is histologically characterized by mature trabecular bone and an overlying fibrocartilaginous cap which serves as the focus of growth (Yousefian 2021; Turan et al. 2012). This feature distinguishes the tumour from osteochondroma which has a hyaline cartilage. Radiographs demonstrate a mature trabecular bony excrescence arising from the dorsal aspect of the distal phalanx (Fig. 20). The fibrocartilage cap is radiolucent. The lesion may have a narrow or broad attachment, but there is no continuity with the underlying medulla, a distinguishing feature from osteochondroma. There should be no bony destruction (Pratap et al. 2019). Occasionally, the lesion may be strictly more paraungual than subungual in location (Fig. 20). No cases of malignant change have been reported in the literature, although the chronic irritation of skin associated with an exostosis has been proposed as an aetiological factor for skin squamous cell carcinoma development (Valero et al. 2014).

2.5.5 Periostitis Ossificans

Myositis ossificans occurring in the hand is an extremely rare entity. When it occurs in a juxtacortical location, it is termed periostitis ossificans and may mimic BPOP or FRP (Fig. 21) (James and Davies 2005; Saad et al. 2023). It is usually seen in young adults with a male predeliction (Saad et al. 2023). Patients may present with a rapid onset of pain, a palpable mass, oedema, joint contractures and decreased range of motion (Levy et al. 2021; Sundaram et al. 2001).

Initial radiographs may be normal or demonstrate a non-calcified soft tissue mass. The mass undergoes peripheral mineralization at 7–14 days. Unlike myositis ossificans, this focus of heterotopic ossification will be connected to the adjacent bone, and periosteal reaction may also be observed (Fig. 21). By 6–8 weeks, a densely calcified periphery develops and a lucent centre is observed on radiographs. As the lesion matures, it undergoes ossification from the margins inwards. This 'zoning' phenomenon is the hallmark of myositis ossificans and helps differentiate it from parosteal osteosarcoma both radiologically and histologically (Fig. 21c).

2.6 Miscellaneous Benign Tumours

Chondroblastoma (CB) is generally rare, accounting for less than 1% of all bone tumours (Choi et al. 2022; Davila et al. 2004). It is common in the tibia, femur and humerus but rare in the hand and wrist which account for approximately 10% of all CB (Wu et al. 2013; Ebeid et al. 2019). It typically occurs in an older age group to CB at other locations, most commonly presenting in the third decade of life (Davila et al. 2004). Cases of CB occurring in the phalanges, metacarpals and carpal bones have been documented (Wu et al. 2013). The clinical presentation, as at other locations, almost always

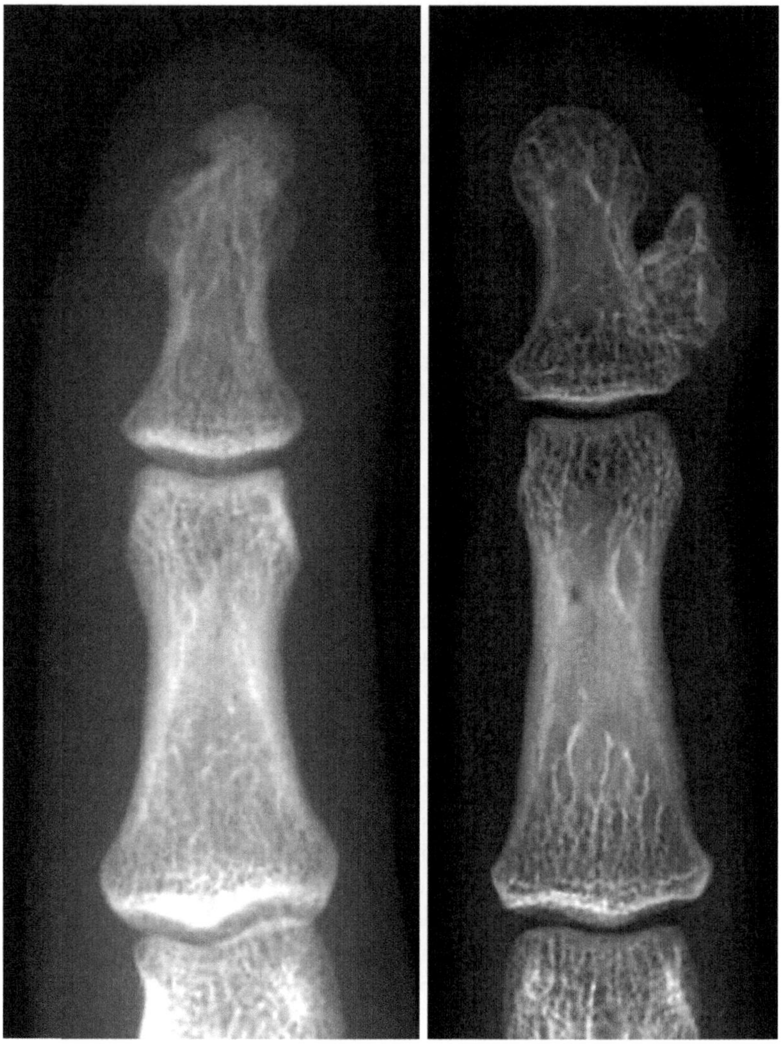

Fig. 20 Subungual and paraungual exostoses

involves pain (Wu et al. 2013; Xu et al. 2015). The typical radiographic appearance is of a lytic lesion with sclerotic margins, bony expansion, matrix mineralization and occasional septation (Wu et al. 2013; Davila et al. 2004). At MRI, a secondary aneurysmal bone cyst component is frequently present (more common than at other sites), and marrow oedema surrounding the lesion may be identified (Davila et al. 2004; Rhee et al. 2012; Chen and DiFrancesco 2017).

Osteoblastoma of the hand and wrist is also very rare and accounts for between 5% and 6% of all osteoblastomas (Adler 2000). On radiographs, osteoblastoma is typically eccentrically located and demonstrates a large focus of central osteolysis, between 4 and 10 cm in diameter, with a small area or peripheral sclerosis. In the short tubular bones, the lesions are much smaller, centrally located and expansile. They are well circumscribed and predominantly radiolucent (Afshar 2016). Osteoblastoma has been reported in carpal, metacarpal and phalangeal bones (Afshar 2016; Simon et al. 2014). It is usually a solitary tumour; however, cases of multifocal osteoblastoma involving the small bones of the hand and wrist have been reported (Muren et al. 1991; Adler 2000; Kyriakos et al. 2007).

Fibrous dysplasia of the hand and wrist is very uncommon (Attard et al. 2002; Kokkalis et al. 2010; Kinnunen et al. 2020). A large review of 1958 cases (almost exclusively monostotic) found that only 2.5% of cases affected the hands (Olson et al.

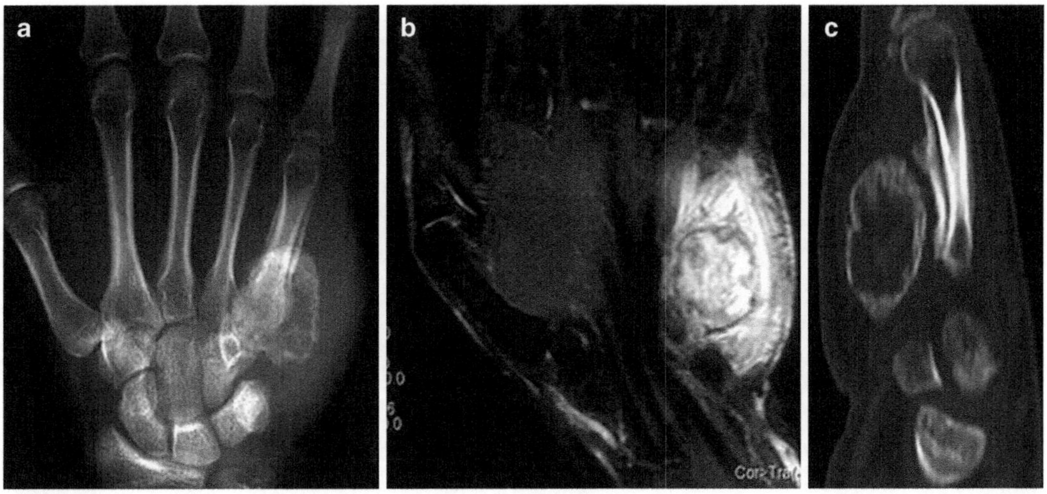

Fig. 21 Periostitis ossificans. (**a**) PA radiograph showing peripheral mineralization (zoning phenomenon) and reactive periosteal new bone. (**b**) Coronal STIR MR image showing the thin low signal intensity rim corresponding to the mineralization and a florid surrounding inflammatory response. (**c**) Sagittal CT reconstruction confirming the peripheral mineralization and periosteal reaction along the adjacent metacarpal

2021). There is a roughly equal distribution in the metacarpal bones and phalanges, although isolated cases involving phalanges are less common (Hatanaka 2007; Olson et al. 2021). Usually, an expansile, lytic lesion involving the shaft with a lobulated sclerotic border is described on radiographs, similar to other locations (Fig. 22) (Hatanaka 2007). Periosteal reaction and soft tissue extension as delineated on MRI have been reported but are uncommon (Chapurlat and Orcel 2008). Pathological fracture may be a presenting feature (Ozsen et al. 2018).

Intraosseous epidermal cysts, or epidermal inclusion cysts, are squamous epithelial-lined benign cysts within bone. These are rare and incidence is highest within the 25–50 age group with a male to female ratio of 3:1, the latter speculated to be secondary to increased risk of trauma in this group precipitating epidermal element implantation (Kim and Lee 2023). The distal phalanx is most affected (Kim and Noh 2023; Dumitru et al. 2020). On radiographs, they usually appear as a solitary well-defined, unilocular, osteolytic lesion with a sclerotic margin (Fig. 23) and may exhibit spotty calcifications (Dumitru et al. 2020; Patel et al. 2006). Enchondroma is the major differential diagnosis, but unlike intraosseous epidermal cysts, it is rarely symptomatic in the absence of a fracture and tends to be located more proximal in the bone (Ruchelsman et al. 2010).

Glomus tumours are benign hamartomas. They arise from the normal glomus apparatus within subcutaneous tissue. The tumours mainly occur in women and are most commonly located in the distal phalanx, usually in a subungual location (Fig. 24) (Dahlin et al. 2005). Intraosseous glomus tumours of the hand are extremely rare although related bony change such as scalloping as a result of the tumour growth is reasonably common (Kransdorf et al. 2024; Le Corroller et al. 2012). MRI has proved to be a valuable method of imaging glomus tumours although it can be limited in smaller lesions (Al-Qattan et al. 2005; Trehan et al. 2015). Most glomus tumours demonstrate high signal on spin echo T2-weighted sequences and avid enhancement post-gadolinium injection (Theumann et al. 2002). Cases have been reported where a tumour was present despite a negative MRI. On this basis, it has been suggested that in the correct clinical context, surgical exploration should be considered even if MRI findings do not support the diagnosis (Dahlin et al. 2005).

Bone islands (enostoses) are relatively frequently encountered on routine imaging of the hand and wrist for other indications. They represent a focus of mature compact bone and are best considered a benign tumour-like lesion (Dharmshaktu and Singh 2018; Greenspan 1995). Radiographs demonstrate a sclerotic focus that often has a round or oval appearance which blends with the adjacent

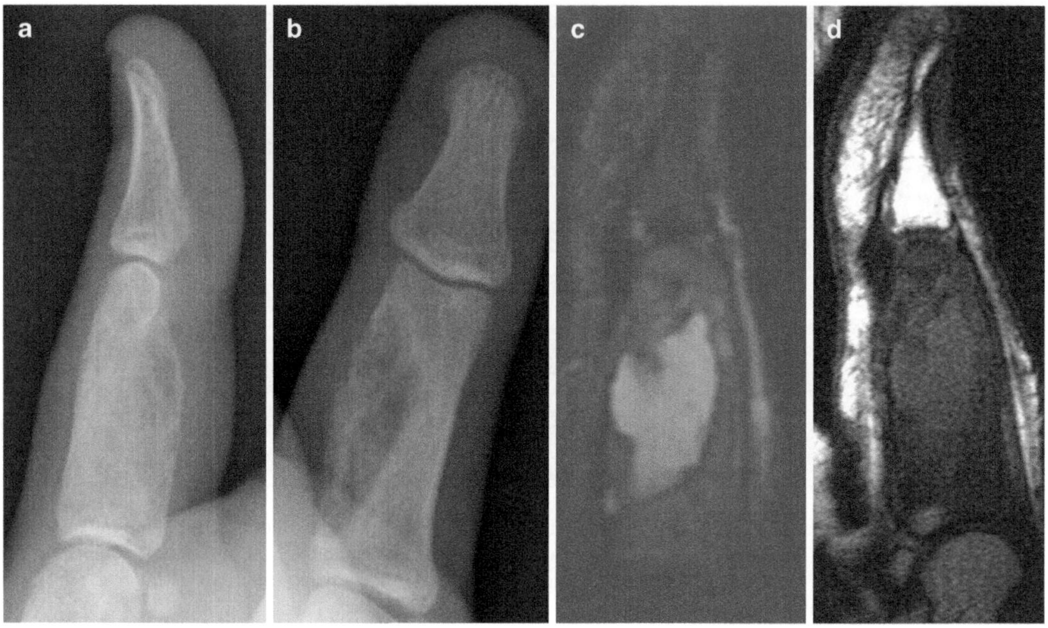

Fig. 22 Fibrous dysplasia. Lesion involving the proximal phalanx of the thumb with (**a**, **b**) radiography showing typical mild bony expansion with a ground glass matrix. MRI (**c**), STIR, and (**d**) T1 sagittal imaging show a lesion returning fluid-like signal appearances

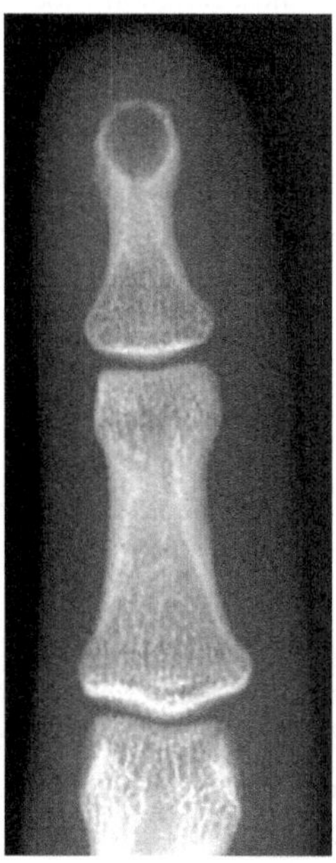

Fig. 23 Intraosseous epidermal cyst. Well-defined, rounded, lytic lesion in the tip of the terminal phalanx

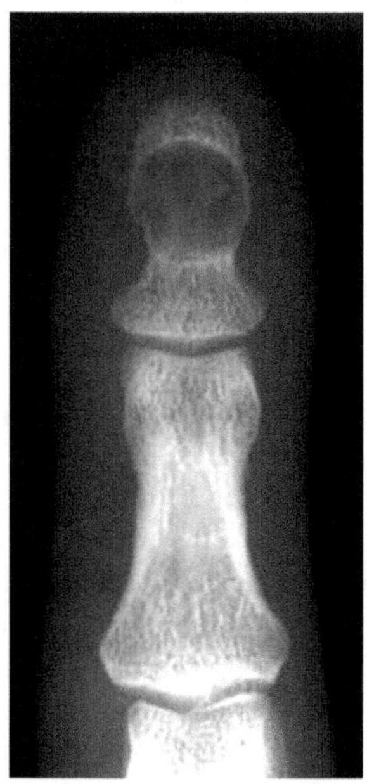

Fig. 24 Glomus tumour. Pathological fracture through well-defined lytic lesion in the terminal phalanx

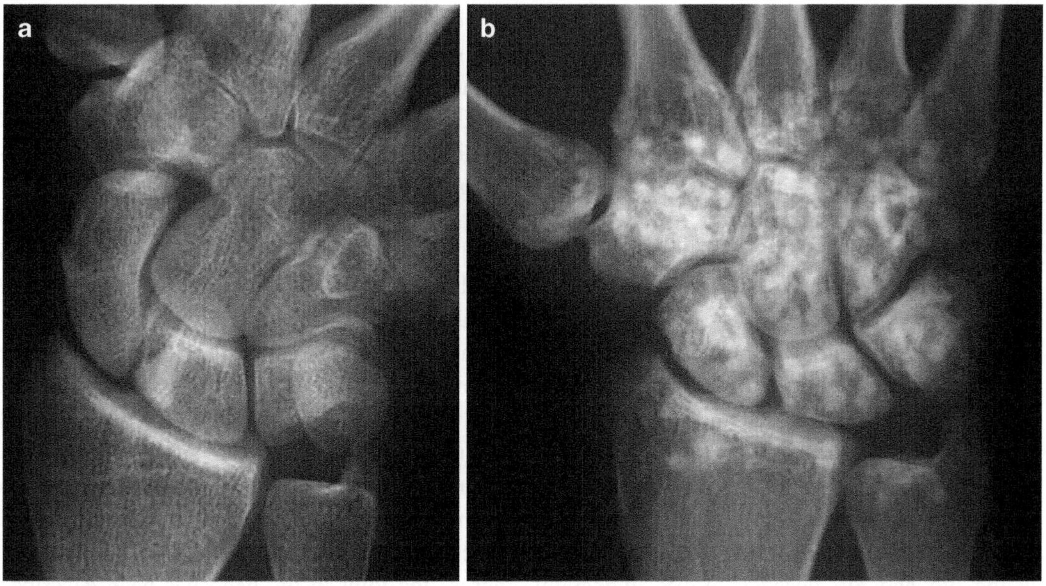

Fig. 25 Bone island. (**a**) Solitary sclerotic focus in the lunate, (**b**) Multiple small bone islands clustered around the bone ends (osteopoikilosis)

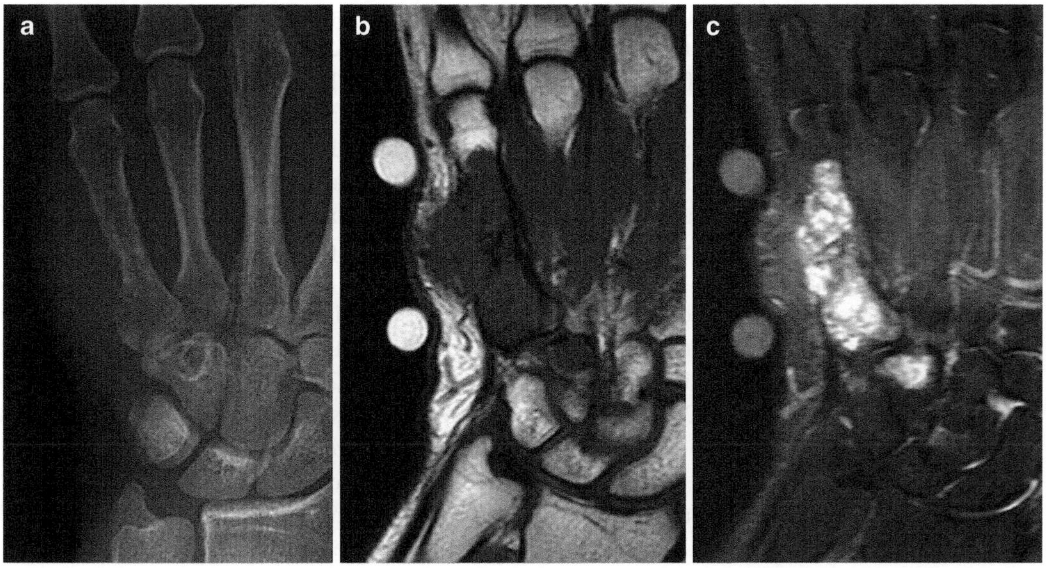

Fig. 26 Multifocal haemangioendothelioma. (**a**) PA radiograph, (**b**) coronal T1-weighted, and (**c**) STIR MR images showing extensive infiltration of the 5th metacarpal with a further focus of tumour in the hamate

cancellous bone (Fig. 25a). CT shows a localized spiculate margin to the lesion, and MRI will demonstrate the lesion to be low signal on all sequences. In the multiple form, osteopoikilosis, the bone islands are clustered around the bone ends (Fig. 25b).

There is a spectrum of vascular tumours that may arise in bone from benign haemangioma to malignant angiosarcoma. All are uncommon in the hand and wrist. Of particular note is that these lesions, including low-grade haemangioendothelioma, can be multicentric and so should be considered in the differential diagnosis when imaging reveals multiple lytic bony lesions (Fig. 26).

3 Malignant Bone Tumours of the Hand and Wrist

3.1 Chondrosarcoma

Chondrosarcoma of the hand accounts for fewer than 3% of all chondrosaromas (Stomeo et al. 2014; Atalay et al. 2018; Sridhar et al. 2014). However, they remain the most common malignant bone neoplasm of the hand and are considered to most commonly occur from malignant degeneration of a pre-existing lesion rather than as primary chondrosarcoma (Stomeo et al. 2014; O'Connor and Bancroft 2004).

Chondrosarcoma of the hand and wrist occurs in an older age group than chondrosarcoma at other locations with presentation most commonly in the 6th and 7th decades of life and slight female predeliction (Mavrogenis et al. 2017b; Saunders et al. 1997; Kask et al. 2021; Atalay et al. 2018). Typical clinical features are of pain and swelling though not always in combination and with variable duration of symptoms (Kask et al. 2021; O'Connor and Bancroft 2004; Atalay et al. 2018).

As already discussed in this chapter, chondrosarcomas arising from pre-existing solitary enchondromas or osteochondromas or in conditions of enchondromatosis or HME are well documented in the literature (Figs. 4 and 8). These "secondary" chondrosarcomas account for around a quarter of chondrosarcomas reported in the hand compared to approximately 15% in all locations (Brien et al. 1997; Sridhar et al. 2014; Saunders et al. 1997).

Chondrosarcoma of the hand is located at similar locations to enchondroma, originating near the site of the epiphyseal growth plate of the bone: proximally in the phalanx and distally in the metacarpal (Fig. 27) (Bovée et al. 1999; Mavrogenis et al. 2017b; Sridhar et al. 2014; Demíreli et al. 2006). The tumour most commonly occurs at the proximal phalanx and most commonly involves the 5th digit with the 4th least commonly involved (Mavrogenis et al. 2017b; Vasilakaki et al. 2012). Interestingly, the majority of distal phalangeal chondrosarcomas affect the thumb. Chondrosarcomas have been rarely described arising in the carpal bones (Ogose et al. 1997; Demíreli et al. 2006; Chaudhary et al. 2010).

Chondrosarcoma of the hand can be difficult to differentiate radiographically from benign cartilaginous tumours particularly in the absence of clear extension through the cortex and an associated soft tissue mass (Murphey et al. 2003). In a study of 160 cases of chondrosarcomas of the small bones of the hands and feet, endosteal erosion, cortical destruction, and expansion were observed in 90% of the 111 cases where imaging was available (Ogose et al. 1997). Other features included an associated soft tissue mass (80%), poor margination (79%), mineralization (74%), a permeative lytic pattern (50%), and a periosteal reaction (14%) (Fig. 27). Extension of tumour across the joint in the hand has been described (Patil et al. 2003; Bansal 2020). Pathological fractures and matrix calcification are observed in both enchondroma and chondrosarcoma. MRI better defines the extent of soft tissue involvement. Tumours classically demonstrate high signal on T2-weighted images and low signal on T1-weighted images, reflecting the hyaline cartilage content of the tumour (Fig. 27b, c).

The periosteal or juxtacortical type makes up an extremely rare subset of chondrosarcoma of the hand. Of 23 patients with chondrosarcoma of the small bones of the hand, Patil et al. identified one periosteal tumour but further cases have been described in later literature (Patil et al. 2003; Tilden et al. 2022). Multiple cases in the literature of chondrosarcoma with periosteal reaction in the hand have been described (Cecava et al. 2020). The degree of cortical destruction and soft tissue tumour has been shown to be less marked in periosteal chondrosarcoma than in conventional chondrosarcoma (Tilden et al. 2022). It is probably for this reason that the distinction between periosteal chondroma and low-grade juxtacortical chondrosarcoma is sometimes difficult to make.

Most published series suggests that chondrosarcoma of the hand is distinct from lesions elsewhere by a lower tendency to metastasis (Patil et al. 2003; Kask et al. 2021). However, one study by Ogose et al. of patients with chondrosarcoma

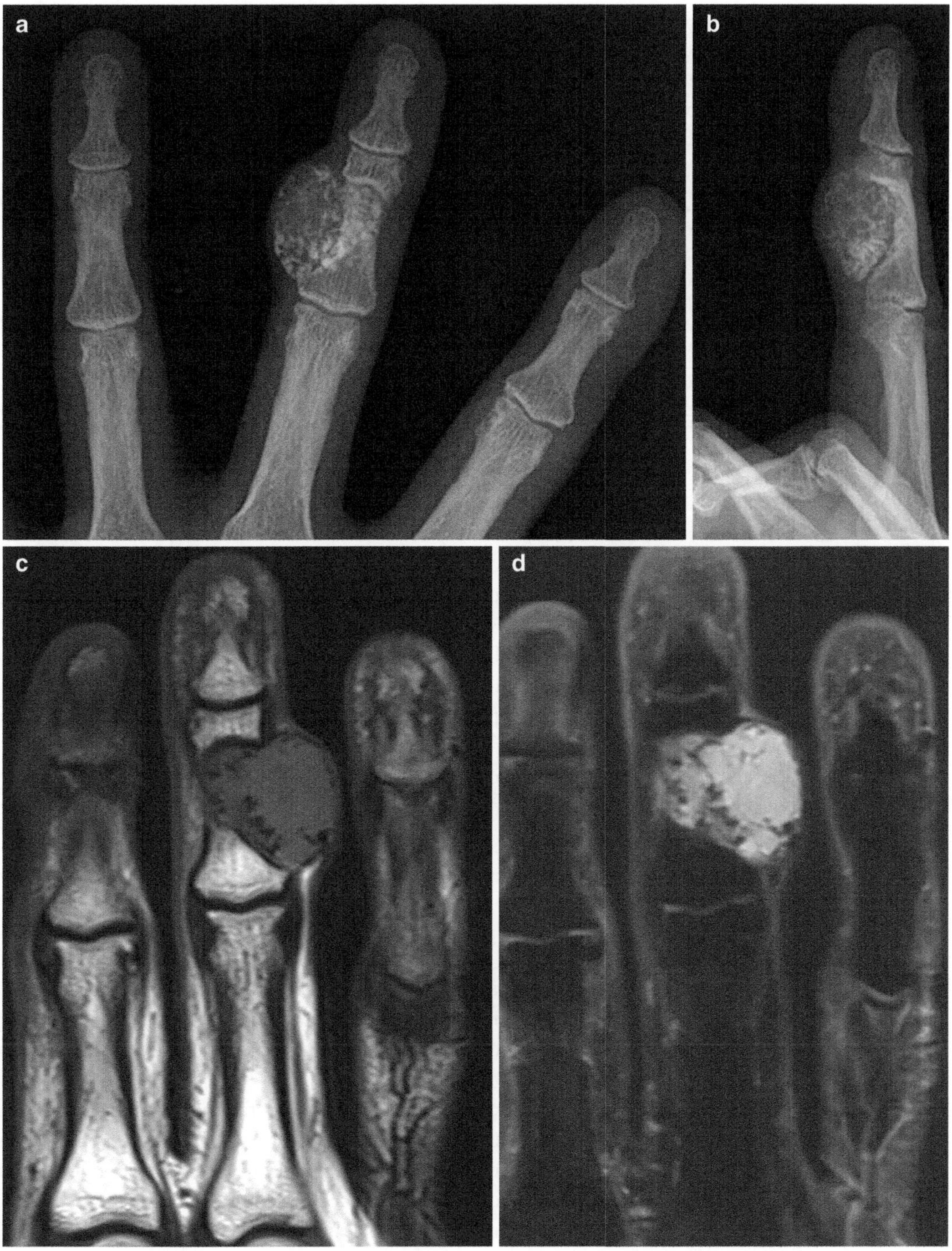

Fig. 27 Malignant chondrosarcoma. (**a**) AP and (**b**) lateral radiographs showing a lesion with a chondroid matrix from the middle finger middle phalanx. (**c**) Coronal T1-weighted and (**d**) coronal T2-weighted fat-saturated images show the extent of intraosseous and extraosseous spread

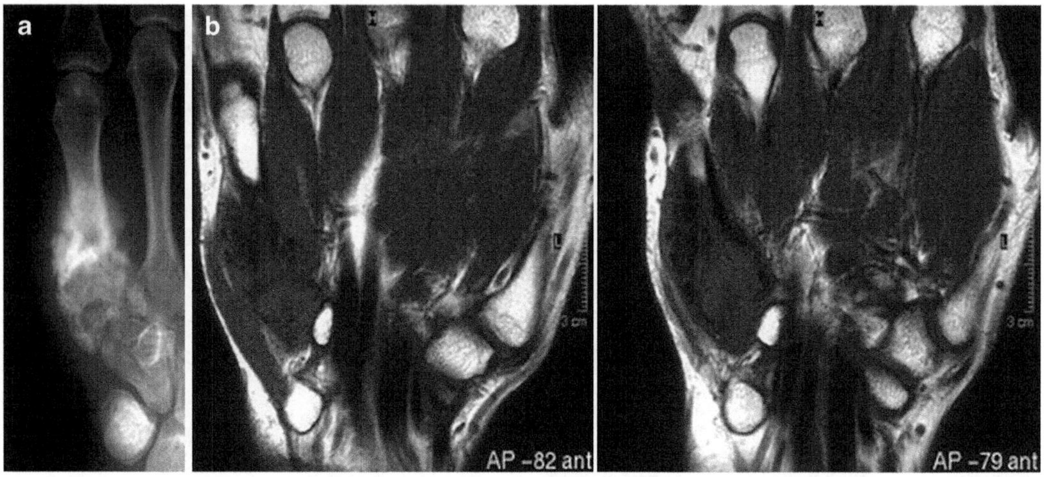

Fig. 28 Osteosarcoma. (**a**) Radiograph showing a mixed lytic and sclerotic lesion arising in the proximal half of the 5th metacarpal. (**b**) Coronal T1-weighted MR images showing the tumour infiltration and low signal intensity areas due to the malignant mineralization

of the small bones of the hands and feet reported 12 distant metastatic lesions from the 70 patients where follow-up was available (Ogose et al. 1997). The risks of local recurrence and metastases after surgery mean both long-term follow-up of these tumours and aggressive surgical treatment of high-grade lesions have been proposed as management options (O'Connor and Bancroft 2004; Kask et al. 2021).

3.2 Osteosarcoma

Osteosarcoma of the small bones of the hand is rare with multiple studies showing that less than 1% of skeletal osteosarcomas involves the hand (Rossetti et al. 2022; de la Guardia et al. 2023; Fowble et al. 2005; Mahdal et al. 2025; Ferrando et al. 2021). Osteosarcoma of the hand appears to affect an older age group than conventional osteosarcoma, the mean age being 42 years and almost 10 years older than osteosarcoma in long bones elsewhere in the body (Mahdal et al. 2025; de la Guardia et al. 2023). Risk factors identified in published cases include Paget's disease, previous radiation treatment, trauma, and metastasis from primary osteosarcoma located elsewhere in the skeleton (Mavrogenis et al. 2017b; Fowble et al. 2005). Clinical presentation is typically with pain and swelling (Mahdal et al. 2025; Mavrogenis et al. 2017b). The long duration of symptoms, long interval before local recurrence, and excellent response to treatment suggest that lesions in this location are less aggressive than conventional osteosarcomas.

Osteosarcoma of the hand shows a preferential distribution around the MCP joints, often sited within the metacarpal heads and bases of the proximal phalanges, with a slight predilection for the second and third digits (Mavrogenis et al. 2017b; Fowble et al. 2005). These sites represent the fastest growing growth plates and the longest bones of the hand. Only a handful of cases in the carpus have been reported, specifically in the trapezium and scaphoid (Ferrando et al. 2021; de la Guardia et al. 2023).

The radiographic findings are similar to the appearance of osteosarcoma at other sites with matrix mineralization, bone destruction, and florid periosteal reaction (Fig. 28) (Mathov et al. 2008). The tumour is generally intramedullary in location with extension into the soft tissues (Fig. 28b). The presence of intramedullary involvement is helpful in distinguishing the lesion from benign entities such as BPOP and FRP that can otherwise appear similar on radiographs (Jones et al. 2006). The absence of zonal organization in osteosarcomas as characterized by

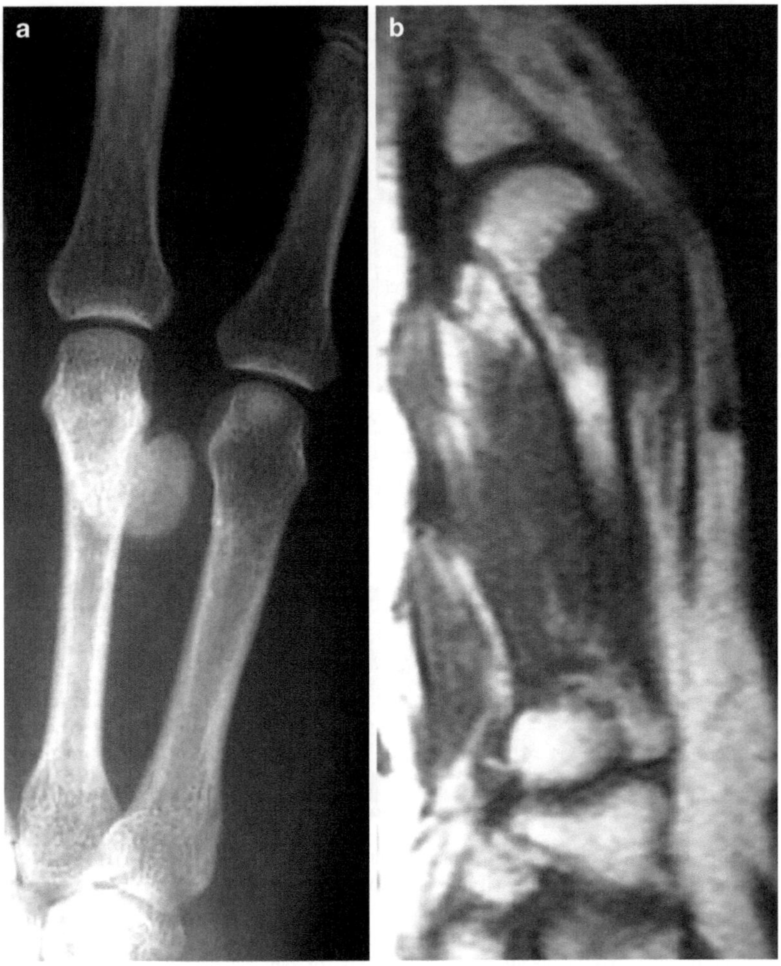

Fig. 29 Parosteal osteosarcoma. (**a**) The radiograph shows an ossified surface lesion arising from the 4th metacarpal. (**b**) Sagittal T1-weighted MR image showing the lesion invading the underlying medulla

peripheral density and central lucency can also help differentiate it from benign entities (Jones et al. 2006). MRI better assesses the soft tissue involvement and degree of intramedullary extension (Fig. 28b). The lesion is typically isointense on T1-weighted imaging and of high-signal intensity on T2-weighted imaging (Honoki et al. 2001).

There appears to be a greater propensity for lesions to arise from the surface of the bone when compared to osteosarcoma at other sites. The majority of these surface tumours are parosteal with only two reported periosteal osteosarcomas of the hand (James and Davies 2005; Jones et al. 2006; Muir et al. 2008; Rossetti et al. 2022). Surface osteosarcomas often appear as a densely calcified mass adjacent to a metacarpal or phalanx on radiographs (Fig. 29) (Cecava et al. 2020; Revell et al. 2000). They can be connected to bone by a stalk that may only be demonstrated on CT. These lesions may be difficult and sometimes impossible to differentiate from benign disorders on imaging although lucencies within the tumor and wrapping of the tumor around adjacent bone are suggestive of malignancy (Cecava et al. 2020). A rare variant of parosteal osteosarcoma is the osteochondroma-like parosteal osteosarcoma that has been reported in the hand and wrist (Fig. 30) (Sanghavi et al. 2017). On imaging, these lesions appear as a 'pasted on' ossified mass with an intact underlying cortex and no medullary involvement (Sanghavi et al. 2017). These features can lead to misdiagnosis as benign entities on both radiological and histological assessment.

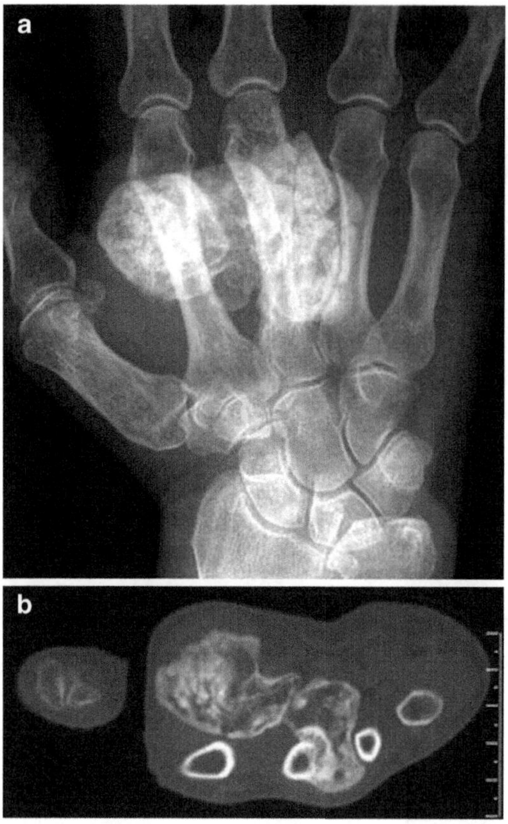

Fig. 30 Osteochondroma-like parosteal osteosarcoma. (**a**) The radiograph shows an ossifying mass overlying the metacarpals. (**b**) The CT shows it to be arising from the surface of the 3rd metacarpal, but there is no trabecular continuity that would exclude the diagnosis of an osteochondroma

3.3 Ewing Sarcoma

Ewing sarcoma (ES) of the hand has an incidence of between 0.3% and 1% of all ES of bone (Mavrogenis et al. 2017b; Baumhoer and Jundt 2010; Parida et al. 2012). Multiple series have shown that the hands are approximately three times less likely to be involved than the feet (Baraga et al. 2001; Damron et al. 2007). The demographics are similar to ES of bone at other sites with peak incidence in the second decade and males twice as commonly affected as females (Mavrogenis et al. 2017b; Baraga et al. 2001). Cases of ES in the hand are particularly rare (Skinner et al. 2019). Typical clinical features are nonspecific and consist of pain, swelling, systemic symptoms of fever and malaise (Mavrogenis et al. 2017b; Zarghooni et al. 2023; Parida et al. 2012). Presentation may be acute or insidious. An antecedent history of trauma is uncommon.

Ewing's sarcoma of the hand is most likely to occur in the metacarpal bones and phalanges (McBee et al. 2023; Parida et al. 2012). Most reported cases of phalangeal involvement describe involvement of the proximal phalanx (Babu et al. 2022; Baccari et al. 2012). To the best of our knowledge, ES has never been reported in a carpal bone though it is known to occur in the tarsal bones of the feet. The tumour typically occurs in the meta-diaphyseal region of the short tubular bones of the hands and feet but may occupy the whole length of the bone (Baraga et al. 2001; Skinner et al. 2019).

The classic radiographic findings of a permeative lytic lesion, with associated areas of sclerosis and a soft tissue mass, is commonly seen in ES of the small bones of the hands as well as at other locations (Fig. 31) (Mavrogenis et al. 2017b; Baraga et al. 2001). In the hand, it is less commonly a purely lytic lesion and more often demonstrates blastic or mixed change than at other sites (Baccari et al. 2012; Baraga et al. 2001; Mahan et al. 2016). Bone expansion is more commonly seen than elsewhere in the skeleton likely due to a smaller volume of bone (Baraga et al. 2001). Periosteal reaction is seen as at other locations but is not necessarily always present (Mahan et al. 2016; Baraga et al. 2001; Baccari et al. 2012). MRI can be used to accurately quantify the extent of the soft tissue mass both prior to and after chemotherapy (Baccari et al. 2012). The main differential diagnosis for ES in the small bones of the hands is osteomyelitis, and misdiagnosis can lead to significant delay in treatment (Mahan et al. 2016).

It has been proposed that ES arising at the hand has a better prognosis than at other sites but remains much worse than for osteosarcoma (Wang et al. 2018; Daecke et al. 2005). This is thought to be due to less soft tissue in the extremities allowing for comparatively early presentation, diagnosis and excision with a wide margin. Smaller tumour volume and a lower incidence of metastasis at presentation are also thought to be important factors. However, Akanwenze et al., in

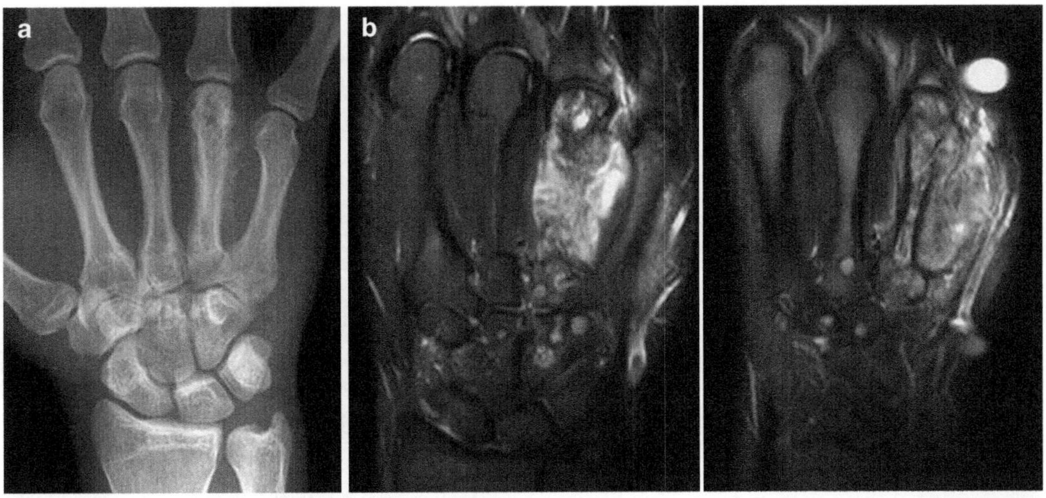

Fig. 31 Ewing sarcoma. (**a**) Radiograph showing typical features of an onion skin and spiculated periosteal reaction along the 4th metacarpal. (**b**) Two contiguous coronal STIR MR images showing extensive tumour infiltration of the metacarpal with soft tissue extension and multiple small skip metastases in the carpal bones and adjacent metacarpal

their series of 5 cases reported a similar survival rate to ES at other sites (Anakwenze et al. 2009).

3.4 Metastasis

Metastasis to the hand is rare and accounts for approximately 0.1% of all metastatic bone lesions (Mavrogenis et al. 2014; Umana et al. 2021; Muñoz-Mahamud et al. 2017). Metastasis to the hand may rarely be the initial presentation of occult malignancy (Muñoz-Mahamud et al. 2017). It is in this context in particular that acrometastasis can be misdiagnosed as other skeletal pathologies such as infection or inflammatory arthritis both clinically and radiologically and thus be associated with a poor prognosis.

Any bone in the hand and wrist can be involved, though the most commonly reported site is the terminal phalanx (Muñoz-Mahamud et al. 2017; Umana et al. 2021). This is proposed to be because arterial flow is greatest in this area of the hand (Flynn et al. 2008; Umana et al. 2021). The most commonly affected digit is conflictingly described as the thumb and middle finger in the existing literature (Flynn et al. 2008; Spiteri et al. 2008). The carpus is less commonly affected, involving less than 15% of bone metastases to the hand and wrist (El Abiad et al. 2019; Umana et al. 2021). The majority of patients are in their fifth decade or older (El Abiad et al. 2019; Umana et al. 2021).

Of skeletal wrist and hand metastases, 40–50% are from primary bronchial carcinoma (Fig. 32) (Muñoz-Mahamud et al. 2017; Umana et al. 2021). This is thought to be due to the fact that primary tumours in the lung can shed cells directly into the systemic arterial circulation, whereas potential secondaries from other sites pass through the capillary bed of the lung or liver first (Umana et al. 2021). Breast and renal cell carcinomas are also reasonably common, each accounting for around 10% of bone metastases to the hand and wrist and both placing as the second most common tumour in different studies (Dow et al. 2024; Muñoz-Mahamud et al. 2017; Sahoo et al. 2016). Subdiaphragmatic tumours are generally more likely to metastasize to the feet, although metastatic hand lesions from the prostate, stomach, cervix, and uterus have all been described (Muñoz-Mahamud et al. 2017; Linabury and Henley 2022; Dow et al. 2024). Sarcomatous metastases to the hand are much less frequent than metastases from carcinoma but have been described with both soft tissue and bone sarcomas (Morris et al. 2017; El Abiad et al. 2019).

Clinically, the patient may present with pain, swelling, and loss of function (Muñoz-Mahamud

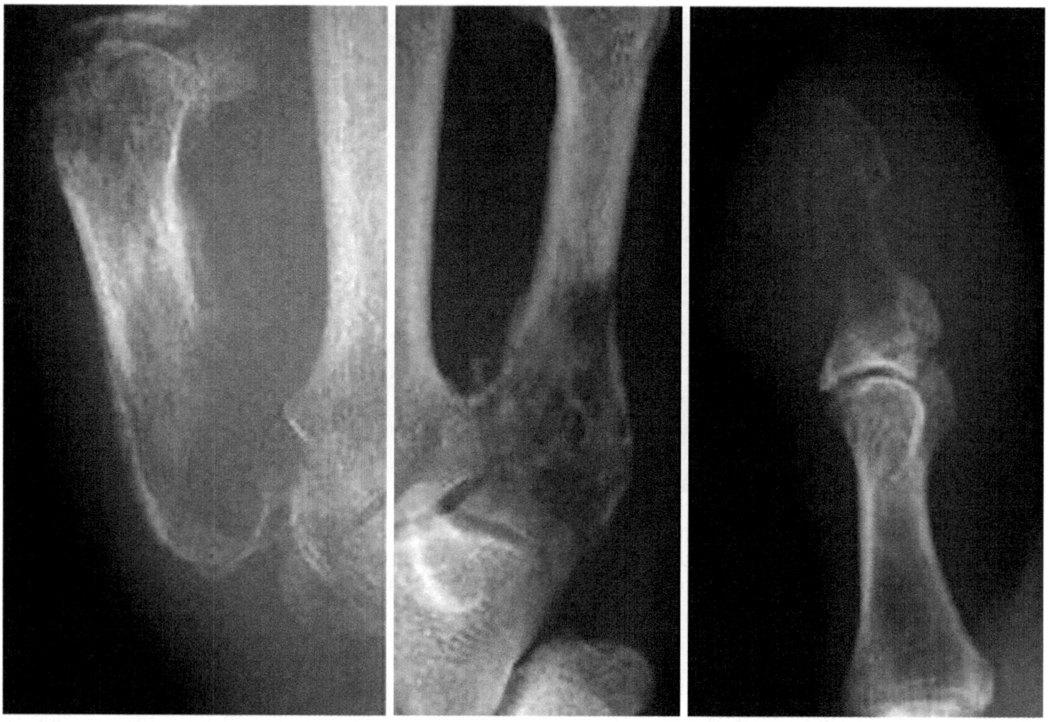

Fig. 32 Lytic metastases. Radiographs showing examples of bronchial metastases to the fingers in three different patients

et al. 2017; Umana et al. 2021; Sahoo et al. 2016). In the presence of widespread metastases at other locations, the diagnosis may be straightforward. However, in cases of occult malignancy, the lesion may clinically resemble osteomyelitis, septic arthritis, or acute monoarticular rheumatoid arthritis (Umana et al. 2021; Sahoo et al. 2016).

Metastases of the hand appear most frequently as nonspecific lytic, aggressive lesions (Fig. 32). The pattern of bone destruction varies but usually a thin rim of cortication is present around the lesion. The neoplasm may expand the cortical shell as it enlarges. Sclerotic forms have been described and are typical of metastatic osteosarcoma, but have also been seen with prostate and breast metastases (Fig. 33) (Umana et al. 2021). Periosteal reaction is uncommon (Sahoo et al. 2016). A soft tissue component is frequent (Puşcaşu et al. 2023). In juxta-articular lesions, subchondral bone is usually spared, and joint involvement is rare but involvement of both has been described (Flynn et al. 2008; Muñoz-Mahamud et al. 2017).

The prognosis for patients with metastases to the hand and wrist is extremely poor. To illustrate this, a 2021 study by Cattelan et al. of 482 patients gave a mean survival time of 7.2 months for a range of acrometastases to the hand (Cattelan and Dumontier 2021).

3.5 Lymphoma

Lymphoma involving bone usually occurs in the setting of widespread systemic disease. Non-Hodgkin lymphoma is the predominant type arising in bone, making up >95% of cases (Bhakta et al. 2023). However, primary bone lymphoma remains uncommon accounting for 3–7% of all extranodal lymphomas (Pinheiro et al. 2009; Bindal et al. 2020). In a review of 82 cases of primary lymphoma of bone, Beal et al. found the femur to be the most common site of presentation, followed by the pelvis and tibia with the hand rarely involved (Beal et al. 2006). Fewer than ten case reports of primary lymphoma of

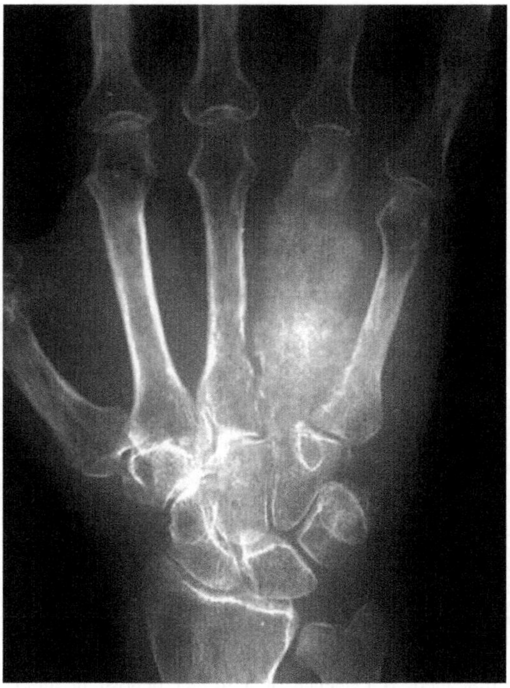

Fig. 33 Sclerotic metastasis. Radiograph showing a rare case in the 4th metacarpal from a primary mucinous adenocarcinoma of the colon

bone occurring in the small bones of the hand have been published reflecting it's rarity (Archer et al. 2009; Chua et al. 2009; Pinheiro et al. 2009; Barbon et al. 2024; Galati et al. 2018; Yeom et al. 2018; Gordon et al. 2014). All of these bar one were cases of unifocal disease, with only one of these reports showing polyostotic disease (Barbon et al. 2024).

Primary lymphoma mostly affects patients over 30 years old, generally in their fifth or sixth decades with males more frequently affected than females (Yeom et al. 2018). Clinical presentation in the hand typically involves pain and swelling, often at an affected joint, and may mimic a rhematological disorder (Archer et al. 2009; Barbon et al. 2024; Galati et al. 2018). Constitutional 'B' symptoms are rare in primary bone lymphoma (Symeonidis et al. 2019; Verma et al. 2020). Radiographs demonstrate a destructive lytic deposit with an associated soft tissue mass (Fig. 34). Despite the extensive destruction, pathological fractures are uncommon (Verma et al. 2020). Magnetic resonance imaging and CT may both demonstrate more extensive local disease than suggested on radiographs. A bone scan is required in all patients presenting with primary lymphoma of bone to assess for the presence of multifocal disease. Patients usually present with early stage disease, and with modern curative modalities, the prognosis is excellent (Beal et al. 2006).

3.6 Multiple Myeloma

Multiple myeloma is the malignant proliferation of plasma cells involving more than 10% of bone marrow. Involvement of the extremities is rare and seen in less than 1% of all solitary bone plasmacytomas (Celik et al. 1996). Osteolytic lesions involving the small bones of the hand, either isolated or associated with multiple lytic lesions at other sites, have rarely been reported in multiple myeloma and plasma cell leukaemia (Fig. 35) (Jafari et al. 2009; Daneshbod et al. 2014; Celik et al. 1996; Wandroo et al. 2005; Capalbo and Mascolo 2007). Lesions arising in the phalanges are most commonly described, but Capalbo and Moscolo have reported a case of multiple lesions involving the metacarpals and phalanges of both hands (Fig. 36).

Typical radiographic features are that of an expansile lytic lesion with cortical erosion. Patients may present with a pathological fracture through a lytic lesion which could be initially mistaken for an enchondroma (Heaton et al. 2015). Diagnosis is usually made by means of biopsy and routine haematological tests. A skeletal survey is mandatory once the diagnosis has been made to assess for synchronous lesions. Solitary bone plasmacytomas account for around 5% of all bone plasmacytomas and are more common in the axial skeleton (Jafari et al. 2009). Involvement of the hand is particularly rare with isolated plasmacytoma, but cases involving the digits are reasonably have been described (Jafari et al. 2009; Daneshbod et al. 2014).

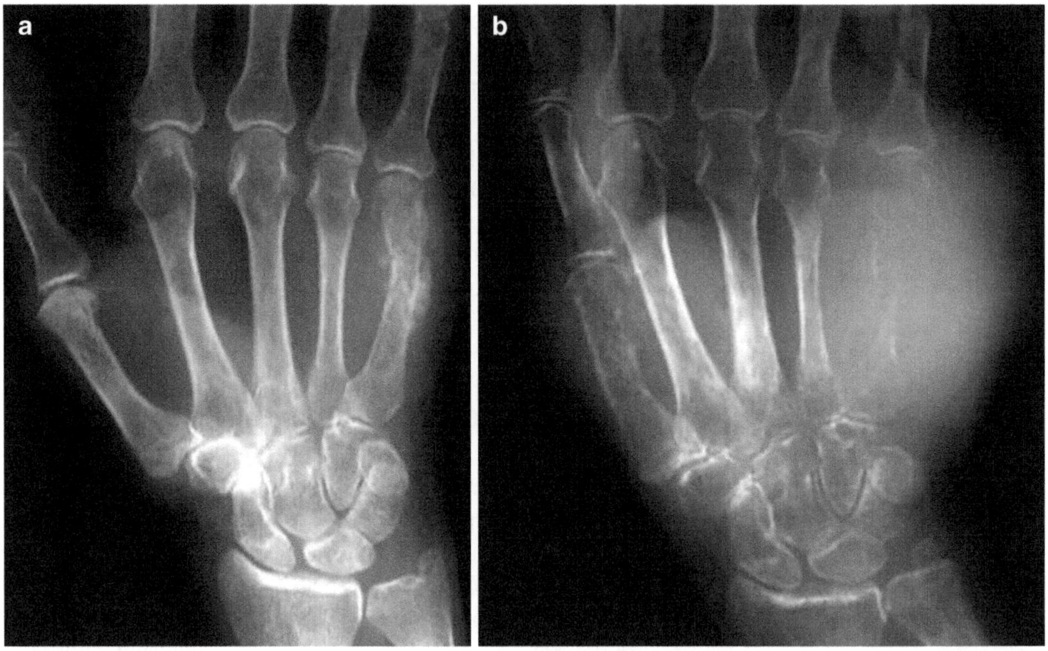

Fig. 34 Lymphoma. (**a**) Radiographs at presentation and (**b**) 4 months later. There is rapid progression of the permeative lytic lesion in the 5th metacarpal, and on the latter film, there is evidence of a further deposit in the 1st metacarpal

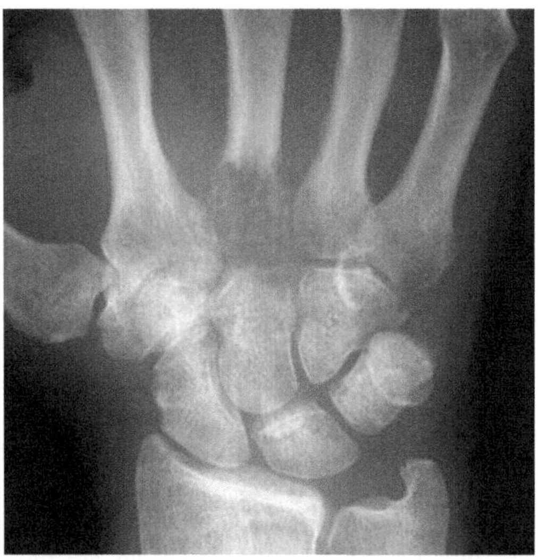

Fig. 35 Myeloma. There is a lytic lesion arising in the base of the 3rd metacarpal. The appearances are similar to both a metastasis and giant cell tumour

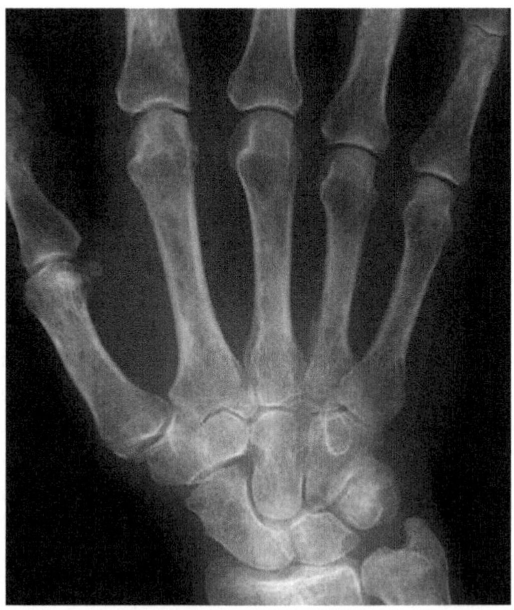

Fig. 36 Multiple myeloma. Multiple small cortical lucencies involving all the metacarpals

4 Conclusion

Bone tumours of the hand and wrist are infrequently encountered in general clinical practice. The clinical history, physical findings, and radiographic features are sufficient to make the diagnosis in the majority of cases. A wide variety of tumour and tumour-like lesions however can present in the hand and wrist. Due to their rare occurrence at this site, they present diagnostic challenges for both the radiologist and the clinician. Knowledge of the imaging characteristics specific to each lesion can facilitate more appropriate and timely management. The imaging findings should always be considered in conjunction with the demographics, clinical presentation, and distribution for each individual case.

The superficial location leads to earlier presentation, allowing expeditious diagnosis and treatment of malignant neoplasms. This often results in a better clinical outcome when compared to the same tumours at other skeletal sites. Though rare, it is important to remember the possibility of a malignant neoplasm when encountering an aggressive bone lesion in the hand or wrist. It is also important to consider benign lesions that radiographically appear aggressive and may be misdiagnosed as malignant tumours. Thorough evaluation of the clinical history, imaging findings, and any available histopathology should be made before arriving at a diagnosis in these cases.

5 Keypoints

- Though uncommon, a variety of tumour and tumour-like lesions may present in the bones of the hand and wrist.
- The majority are benign.
- Enchondroma is the commonest benign tumour.
- Chondrosarcoma is the commonest malignant primary tumour.
- A spectrum of benign proliferative disorders of the phalanges exists which may require close clinical and radiographic follow-up to avoid confusion with a malignant process.
- Malignant tumours of the hand frequently have a better prognosis than at other skeletal sites due to earlier presentation.
- The distribution of a lesion and demographic features of the patient should be considered in conjunction with the imaging findings when assessing bone lesions of the hand and wrist.

References

Abramovici L, Steiner GC (2002) Bizarre parosteal osteochondromatous proliferation (Nora's lesion): a retrospective study of 12 cases, 2 arising in long bones. Hum Pathol 33(12):1205–1210. Available at: https://doi.org/10.1053/hupa.2002.130103

Adler CP (2000) Multifocal osteoblastoma of the hand. Skeletal Radiol 29(10):601–604. Available at: https://doi.org/10.1007/s002560000257

Afonso PD, Isaac A, Villagrán JM (2019) Chondroid tumors as incidental findings and differential diagnosis between enchondromas and low-grade chondrosarcomas. Semin Musculoskelet Radiol 23(1):3–18. Available at: https://doi.org/10.1055/s-0038-1675550

Afshar A (2016) Osteoblastoma of the capitate bone. J Hand Microsurg 04:34–38. Available at: https://doi.org/10.1007/s12593-011-0050-y

Ahmed AR et al (2003) Secondary chondrosarcoma in osteochondroma: report of 107 patients. Clin Orthop Relat Res 411:193. Available at: https://doi.org/10.1097/01.blo.0000069888.31220.2b

Albanese KM et al (2024) Benign bone tumors of the hand: beyond enchondromas. JAAOS – J Am Acad Orthop Surg. Available at: https://journals.lww.com/jaaos/abstract/9900/benign_bone_tumors_of_the_hand__beyond.1137.aspx. Accessed 7 Dec 2024

Alghamdi FA et al (2023) Solitary osteochondroma at unusual sites: a case report and literature review. Cureus 15(11):e49582. Available at: https://doi.org/10.7759/cureus.49582

Al-Qattan MM et al (2005) Magnetic resonance imaging in the diagnosis of glomus tumours of the hand. J Hand Surg 30(5):535–540. Available at: https://doi.org/10.1016/j.jhsb.2005.06.009

Ambrosi F et al (2021) Giant cell tumor of bone in patients under 16 years old: A single-institution case series. Cancers 13(11):2585. Available at: https://doi.org/10.3390/cancers13112585

Ambrosia JM, Wold LE, Amadio PC (1987) Osteoid osteoma of the hand and wrist. J Hand Surg Am 12(5):794–800. Available at: https://doi.org/10.1016/S0363-5023(87)80072-2

Anakwenze OA et al (2009) Ewing's sarcoma of the hand. J Hand Surg (Eur Vol) 34(1):35–39. Available at: https://doi.org/10.1177/1753193408094922

Archer L, Wilson D, McCoubrie P (2009) Re: imaging features of primary extranodal lymphomas. Clin Radiol 64(9):948–950. Available at: https://doi.org/10.1016/j.crad.2009.05.003

Arvind V, Konigsberg MW, Strauch RJ (2023) Giant cell reparative granuloma in the thumb distal phalanx: a case report. Cureus 15(8):e43564. Available at: https://doi.org/10.7759/cureus.43564

Atalay İB et al (2018) Chondrosarcomas of the phalanges of the hand. Eklem Hastaliklari Ve Cerrahisi = Joint Dis Relat Surg 29(1):34–39. Available at: https://doi.org/10.5606/ehc.2018.58876

Athanasian EA (2004) Aneurysmal bone cyst and giant cell tumor of bone of the hand and distal radius. Hand Clin 20(3):269–281. Available at: https://doi.org/10.1016/j.hcl.2004.03.016

Attard G, Zammit J, Sciberras C (2002) Case of monostotic fibrous dysplasia in the hand. Available at: https://www.um.edu.mt/library/oar/handle/123456789/412. Accessed 31 Dec 2024

Averill RM, Smith RJ, Campbell CJ (1980) Giant-cell tumors of the bones of the hand. J Hand Surg Am 5(1):39–50. Available at: https://doi.org/10.1016/s0363-5023(80)80042-6

Avramidis K et al (2023) A solitary, large calcaneal osteochondroma growing extensively after skeletal maturity: a case report and review of the literature. Cureus 15(7):e42570. Available at: https://doi.org/10.7759/cureus.42570

Babu S et al (2022) Ewing sarcoma of phalanx—a common tumor with an uncommon presentation. Indian J Med Paediatr Oncol 43:189–192. Available at: https://doi.org/10.1055/s-0042-1742443

Baccari S et al (2012) Ewing's sarcoma of the finger: report of two cases and literature review. Orthop Traumatol Surg Res 98(2):233–237. Available at: https://doi.org/10.1016/j.otsr.2011.06.012

Bailescu I et al (2022) Diagnosis and evolution of the benign tumor osteochondroma. Exp Ther Med 23(1):1–6. Available at: https://doi.org/10.3892/etm.2021.11026

Bansal M (2020) Retrospective study to find the prevalence of neoplasia in swellings of hand and foot bones. Int J Orthop Traumatol Surg Sci 6(1):39–45. Available at: https://doi.org/10.47618/IJOTSS/v6i1.9

Baraga JJ et al (2001) Radiographic features of Ewing's sarcoma of the bones of the hands and feet. Skeletal Radiol 30(3):121–126. Available at: https://doi.org/10.1007/s002560100349

Barbon DA et al (2024) Primary lymphoma of bone of the little finger: a case report and review of the literature. Skeletal Radiol 53(8):1645–1650. Available at: https://doi.org/10.1007/s00256-024-04576-9

Baumhoer D, Jundt G (2010) Tumours of the hand: a review on histology of bone malignancies. J Hand Surg Eur Vol 35(5):354–361. Available at: https://doi.org/10.1177/1753193409358382

Beal K, Allen L, Yahalom J (2006) Primary bone lymphoma: treatment results and prognostic factors with long-term follow-up of 82 patients. Cancer 106(12):2652–2656. Available at: https://doi.org/10.1002/cncr.21930

Berger O et al (2024) Recurrence and risk factors of giant cell Tumors in hand bones: a systematic review. Plast Reconstr Surg Glob Open 12(10):e6253. Available at: https://doi.org/10.1097/GOX.0000000000006253

Bertoni F et al (1982) Periosteal chondrosarcoma and periosteal osteosarcoma. Two distinct entities. J Bone Joint Surg Br Vol 64(3):370–376. Available at: https://doi.org/10.1302/0301-620X.64B3.7096408

Bhakta P et al (2023) Pathological fracture due to primary bone lymphoma in a patient with a history of prostate cancer: a case report and review of literature. Front Oncol 13:1100559. Available at: https://doi.org/10.3389/fonc.2023.1100559

Bindal P et al (2020) Primary bone lymphoma: A case series and review of literature. Case Rep Hematol 2020(1):4254803. Available at: https://doi.org/10.1155/2020/4254803

Boriani F, Raposio E, Errani C (2021) Imaging Features of Primary Tumors of the Hand. Current Medical Imaging. 17(2):179–96.

Bovée JVMG et al (1999) Chondrosarcoma of the phalanx. Cancer 86(9):1724–1732. Available at: https://doi.org/10.1002/(SICI)1097-0142(19991101)86:9<1724::AID-CNCR14>3.0.CO;2-I

Brien EW, Mirra JM, Kerr R (1997) Benign and malignant cartilage tumors of bone and joint: their anatomic and theoretical basis with an emphasis on radiology, pathology and clinical biology. Skeletal Radiol 26(6):325–353. Available at: https://doi.org/10.1007/s002560050246

Campanacci M et al (1987) Giant-cell tumor of bone. JBJS 69(1):106

Campbell DA, Millner PA, Dreghorn CR (1995) Primary bone tumours of the hand and wrist. J Hand Surg 20(1):5–7. Available at: https://doi.org/10.1016/S0266-7681(05)80004-X

Capalbo S, Mascolo V (2007) Phalangeal lytic lesions in multiple myeloma. Clin Lymphoma Myeloma 7(9):597. Available at: https://doi.org/10.1016/s1557-9190(11)70113-5

Çapkin S et al (2020) Surgical treatment of solitary enchondromas of the hand. Cureus 12(4):e7497. Available at: https://doi.org/10.7759/cureus.7497

Carneiro BC et al (2021) Osteoid osteoma: the great mimicker. Insights Imaging 12(1):32. Available at: https://doi.org/10.1186/s13244-021-00978-8

Cash S, Habermann E (1988) Chondrosarcoma of the small bones of the hand: case report and review of the literature. Orthop Rev [Preprint]. Available at: https://www.semanticscholar.org/paper/Chondrosarcoma-of-the-small-bones-of-the-hand%3A-case-Cash-Habermann/99f5ea45e7228dd9b1fbe57ebe8bc2f4de94c657. Accessed 20 Dec 2024

Casstevens C, Hubbard J, Abrams R (2021) Impinging exostoses of the proximal radius: a report of two cases with distinct clinical features. JSES Rev Rep Tech

1(2):141–144. Available at: https://doi.org/10.1016/j.xrrt.2021.01.001

Cattelan M, Dumontier C (2021) Metastatic tumour of the hand – three new cases and a literature review. J Plast Reconstr Aesthet Surg 74(9):2163–2168. Available at: https://doi.org/10.1016/j.bjps.2021.03.084

Cavalcante MM et al (2021) Tumors and pseudotumors of foot and ankle: bone lesions. Foot 49:101845. Available at: https://doi.org/10.1016/j.foot.2021.101845

Cecava ND, Kephart DA, Bui-Mansfield LT (2020) Bone lesions of the hand and wrist: systematic approach to imaging evaluation. Contemp Diagn Radiol 43(5):1–7. Available at: https://doi.org/10.1097/01.CDR.0000655428.84944.40

Celik I et al (1996) Solitary phalanx plasmacytoma relapse with disseminated extramedullary plasmacytomas and myeloma after short duration of remission. Anticancer Res 16(2):959–962

Chapurlat RD, Orcel P (2008) Fibrous dysplasia of bone and McCune–Albright syndrome. Best Pract Res Clin Rheumatol 22(1):55–69. Available at: https://doi.org/10.1016/j.berh.2007.11.004

Chaudhary S, Singh D, Sen R (2010) Chondrosarcoma of distal radius- a case report and brief review of literature. Available at: https://www.researchgate.net/publication/48408371_Chondrosarcoma_Of_Distal_Radius-_A_Case_Report_And_Brief_Review_Of_Literature. Accessed 31 Dec 2024

Chebib I et al (2020) Histopathology of fibro-osseous and cystic tumors of bone. Diagn Histopathol 26(10):461–473. Available at: https://doi.org/10.1016/j.mpdhp.2020.07.003

Chen W, DiFrancesco LM (2017) Chondroblastoma: an update. Arch Pathol Lab Med 141(6):867–871. Available at: https://doi.org/10.5858/arpa.2016-0281-RS

Chiheb S et al (2021) Subungual exostosis: a case series of 48 patients. Skin Appendage Disord 7(6):475–479. Available at: https://doi.org/10.1159/000516660

Chilla BK et al (2005) Giant cell reparative granuloma of the distal phalanx: a review of osteolytic lesions of the phalanges and their radiologic differential diagnosis. J Am Soc Surg Hand 5(2):109–114. Available at: https://doi.org/10.1016/j.jassh.2005.02.001

Chilvers R et al (2021) An unusual example of hereditary multiple exostoses: a case report and review of the literature. BMC Musculoskelet Disord 22(1):96. Available at: https://doi.org/10.1186/s12891-021-03967-6

Choi JH, Ro JY (2021) The 2020 WHO Classification of Tumors of Bone: An Updated Review. Adv Anat Pathol. 28(3):119–38.

Choi JH et al (2001) Fibrosarcoma in bizarre parosteal osteochondromatous proliferation. Skeletal Radiol 30(1):44–47. Available at: https://doi.org/10.1007/s002560000265

Choi J et al (2022) Unusual chondroblastoma of the hand with large extraosseous soft tissue component. Radiol Case Rep 17(9):3214–3218. Available at: https://doi.org/10.1016/j.radcr.2022.06.024

Chua SC, Rozalli FI, O'Connor SR (2009) Imaging features of primary extranodal lymphomas. Clin Radiol 64(6):574–588. Available at: https://doi.org/10.1016/j.crad.2008.11.001

Claeys R et al (2016) Osteoid osteoma of the pisiform bone: a rare cause of wrist pain. Hand Surg Rehabil 35(4):296–298. Available at: https://doi.org/10.1016/j.hansur.2016.04.002

Crowe MM et al (2015) Aneurysmal bone cysts of the hand, wrist, and forearm. J Hand Surg Am 40(10):2052–2057. Available at: https://doi.org/10.1016/j.jhsa.2015.06.108

Dąbrowski M et al (2023) The influence of clinical factors on treatment outcome and a recurrence of surgically removed protruded subungual osteochondroma and subungual exostosis. J Clin Med 12(19):6413. Available at: https://doi.org/10.3390/jcm12196413

Daecke W et al (2005) Ewing's sarcoma and primitive neuroectodermal tumor of hand and forearm. Experience of the Cooperative Ewing's Sarcoma Study Group. J Cancer Res Clin Oncol 131(4):219–225. Available at: https://doi.org/10.1007/s00432-004-0637-9

Dahlin LB, Besjakov J, Veress B (2005) A glomus tumour: classic signs without magnetic resonance imaging findings. Scand J Plast Reconstr Surg Hand Surg [Preprint]. Available at: https://doi.org/10.1080/02844310410002993

Damron TA, Ward WG, Stewart A (2007) Osteosarcoma, chondrosarcoma, and Ewing's sarcoma: National Cancer Data Base Report. Clin Orthop Relat Res 459:40–47. Available at: https://doi.org/10.1097/BLO.0b013e318059b8c9

Daneshbod Y et al (2014) Solitary plasmacytoma of the index finger. J Clin Pathol [Preprint]. Available at: https://doi.org/10.1136/jclinpath-2014-202413

Dave S et al (2004) Subungual exostosis of the thumb. Dermatol Online J 10(1). Available at: https://doi.org/10.5070/D39959094x

Davies AM et al (2020) Are the tubular bones of the hand really the commonest site for an enchondroma? Clin Radiol 75(7):533–537. Available at: https://doi.org/10.1016/j.crad.2020.02.004

Davila JA et al (2004) Chondroblastoma of the hands and feet. Skeletal Radiol 33(10):582–587. Available at: https://doi.org/10.1007/s00256-004-0762-1

Davis D, Cohen P (1996) Subungual exostosis: case report and review of the literature. Pediatr Dermatol 13(3). Available at: https://doi.org/10.1111/j.1525-1470.1996.tb01205.x

de la Guardia V et al (2023) Osteogenic sarcomas of the hands: a case series with emphasis in its peculiarities and literature review. Pathol Res Pract 242:154326. Available at: https://doi.org/10.1016/j.prp.2023.154326

de Macedo Pontes ÍC et al (2023) Imaging of solitary and multiple osteochondromas: from head to toe — a review. Clin Imaging 103:109989. Available at: https://doi.org/10.1016/j.clinimag.2023.109989

de Oliveira RK, Delgado PJ, Geist JGB (2017) Pediatric trigger finger due to osteochondroma: a report of two cases. Hand 12(1):99–105. Available at: https://doi.org/10.1177/1558944715627634

De Smet L (2001) Osteoid osteoma of the wrist and hand. J Am Soc Surg Hand 1(4):267–274. Available at: https://doi.org/10.1053/jssh.2001.28804

De Smet L (2004) Dysplasia epiphysealis hemimelica of the hand: two cases at the proximal interphalangeal joint. J Pediatr Orthop B 13(5):323–325. Available at: https://doi.org/10.1097/01202412-200409000-00007

Degnan AJ, Ho-Fung VM (2018) More than epiphyseal osteochondromas: updated understanding of imaging findings in dysplasia epiphysealis hemimelica (Trevor disease). Am J Roentgenol 211(4):910–919. Available at: https://doi.org/10.2214/AJR.18.19712

Demíreli P et al (2006) Secondary chondrosarcoma arising from a solitary enchondroma at the index finger of the right hand: a case report. Turk J Pathol 22(1):053–056

Dharmshaktu GS, Singh B (2018) Bone island and hand involvement – a short review. Hand Microsurg 7(2):93–93. Available at: https://doi.org/10.5455/handmicrosurg.258665

Dharmshaktu GS et al (2022) Bizarre parosteal osteochondromatous proliferation or Nora's lesion affecting the extremities: A concise update. J Musculoskelet Surg Res 6(3):200–206. Available at: https://doi.org/10.25259/JMSR_66_2022

Dhillon P et al (2023) Fasciitis ossificans: imaging features, histology, and differential diagnosis. Clin Radiol 78(9). Available at: https://doi.org/10.1016/j.crad.2023.05.008

Dhondt E et al (2006) Nora's lesion, a distinct radiological entity? Skeletal Radiol 35(7):497–502. Available at: https://doi.org/10.1007/s00256-005-0041-9

Donaldson S, Wright JG (2015) Simple bone cysts: better with age? J Pediatr Orthop 35(1):108. Available at: https://doi.org/10.1097/BPO.0000000000000336

Douis H et al (2018) What are the differentiating clinical and MRI-features of enchondromas from low-grade chondrosarcomas? Eur Radiol 28(1):398–409. Available at: https://doi.org/10.1007/s00330-017-4947-0

Dow T et al (2024) Cancer metastases to the hand: a systematic review and meta-analysis. Hand 19(6):865–874. Available at: https://doi.org/10.1177/15589447231153175

Dumitru A et al (2020) Posttraumatic intraosseous epidermoid inclusion cyst. A case report and short literature review. Rom J Orthop Surg Traumatol 3(1):3–8. Available at: https://doi.org/10.2478/rojost-2020-0002

Dupree WB, Enzinger FM (1986) Fibro-osseous pseudotumor of the digits. Cancer. 58(9):2103–9

Ebeid WA et al (2019) Functional and oncological outcome after treatment of chondroblastoma with intralesional curettage. J Pediatr Orthop 39(4):e312. Available at: https://doi.org/10.1097/BPO.0000000000001293

Edoardo I et al (2022) bizarre parosteal osteochondromatous proliferation (Nora lesion): a narrative review. Acta Med Litu 29(2):176–193. Available at: https://doi.org/10.15388/Amed.2022.29.2.4

El Abiad JM et al (2019) Osseous metastatic disease to the hands and feet. Orthopedics 42(2):e197–e201. Available at: https://doi.org/10.3928/01477447-20181227-04

El-Sobky TA et al (2018) Current paediatric orthopaedic practice in hereditary multiple osteochondromas of the forearm: a systematic review. SICOT-J 4:10. Available at: https://doi.org/10.1051/sicotj/2018002

Erdoğan Ö, Gürkan V (2020) Benign bone tumors of hand and wrist: evaluation of diagnosis and treatment. Joint Dis Relat Surg 31(1):81–87. Available at: https://doi.org/10.5606/ehc.2020.72162

Ferrando E et al (2021) Osteosarcoma of the trapezium. J Hand Surg Am 46(8):717.e1–717.e5. Available at: https://doi.org/10.1016/j.jhsa.2020.10.011

Flynn CJ et al (2008) Two cases of acrometastasis to the hands and review of the literature. Curr Oncol 15(5):51–58

Fowble VA et al (2005) Case reports: osteosarcoma of the hand: one case and a literature review. Clin Orthop Relat Res 440:255–261. Available at: https://doi.org/10.1097/01.blo.0000180604.46228.6b

Gajewski CR et al (2023) Approach to the treatment of expansile metacarpal aneurysmal bone cysts: a report of two cases. J Hand Surg Glob Online 5(5):689–694. Available at: https://doi.org/10.1016/j.jhsg.2023.05.004

Galati V et al (2018) A rare manifestation of primary bone lymphoma: solitary diffuse large B-cell lymphoma of the little finger. J Hand Surg Am 43(8):779.e1–779.e4. Available at: https://doi.org/10.1016/j.jhsa.2017.12.007

Garcia J, Bianchi S (2001) Diagnostic imaging of tumors of the hand and wrist. Eur Radiol 11(8):1470–1482. Available at: https://doi.org/10.1007/s003300000751

Gitto S, Serpi F, Messina C, Albano D, Di Bernardo A, Armiraglio E, et al (2023) Bizarre parosteal osteochondromatous proliferation: an educational review. Insights Imaging. 14(1):109

Gnoli M et al (2024) Secondary peripheral chondrosarcoma in multiple osteochondromas: a retrospective single-institution case series. Orphanet J Rare Dis 19(1):63. Available at: https://doi.org/10.1186/s13023-023-03006-8

Gordon MJ, Peterson BA, Skubitz KM (2014) Lymphoma of the hands in a patient with rheumatoid arthritis: case report. J Hand Surg Am 39(4):728–731. Available at: https://doi.org/10.1016/j.jhsa.2014.01.034

Gouin F et al (2003) Metatarsal giant cell tumors and giant cell reparative granuloma are similar entities. Clin Orthop Relat Res 416:278–284. Available at: https://doi.org/10.1097/01.blo.0000093016.90435.f6

Greenspan A (1995) Bone island (enostosis): current concept — a review. Skeletal Radiol 24(2):111–115. Available at: https://doi.org/10.1007/BF00198072

Hannan M et al (2019) A young boy with multiple bony overgrowths. J Enam Med Coll 9(1):60–63. Available at: https://doi.org/10.3329/jemc.v9i1.39908

Haseeb A, Singh VA, Jayalakshmi P (2020) Can giant cell tumor of the bone occur in the skeletally immature?

J Am Podiatr Med Assoc. Available at: https://doi.org/10.7547/19-030

Hatanaka H (2007) Monostotic fibrous dysplasia of the middle phalanx. Hand Surg 12(02):91–95. Available at: https://doi.org/10.1142/S0218810407003432

Havulinna J, Parkkinen J, Laitinen M (2005) Aneurysmal bone cyst of the index sesamoid. J Hand Surg Am 30(5):1091–1093. Available at: https://doi.org/10.1016/j.jhsa.2005.06.009

Heaton D, Alexander H, Trumble TE (2015) Missed pathologic fracture from multiple myeloma. J Hand Surg Am 40(7):1501–1503. Available at: https://doi.org/10.1016/j.jhsa.2014.07.037

Honoki K et al (2001) Primary osteogenic sarcoma of a finger proximal phalanx: a case report and literature review. J Hand Surg Am 26(6):1151–1156. Available at: https://doi.org/10.1053/jhsu.2001.28945

Horiuchi K, Horiuchi Y, Ochi K (2017) Osteoid osteoma of the distal phalanx of the ring finger with clubbed finger deformity: a case report. J Hand Surg (Asian-Pac Vol) 22(02):248–250. Available at: https://doi.org/10.1142/S0218810417720170

Hsu CS, Hentz VR, Yao J (2007) Tumours of the hand. Lancet Oncol 8(2):157–166. Available at: https://doi.org/10.1016/S1470-2045(07)70035-9

Inozu E, Horoz U, Seven E, Ozakpinar HR, Tellioglu AT (2016) Fracture of phalanx from simple bone cyst: A rare bone lesion in the hand. Hand Microsurg 5(2):100–103. https://doi.org/10.5455/handmicrosurg.203499

Jafari D et al (2009) Solitary plasmacytoma of the thumb: arare case report. Med J Islam Repub Iran (MJIRI) 23(3):173–176

Jafari D et al (2013) Osteoid osteoma of the hand and wrist: a report of 25 cases. Med J Islam Repub Iran 27(2):62–66

Jaffe HL (1935) "Osteoid-osteoma": a benign osteoblastic tumor composed of osteoid and atypical bone. Arch Surg 31(5):709–728. Available at: https://doi.org/10.1001/archsurg.1935.01180170034003

Jambhekar NA et al (2004) Florid reactive periostitis of the hands. Skeletal Radiol 33(11):663–665. Available at: https://doi.org/10.1007/s00256-004-0760-3

James SLJ, Davies AM (2005) Giant-cell tumours of bone of the hand and wrist: a review of imaging findings and differential diagnoses. Eur Radiol 15(9):1855–1866. Available at: https://doi.org/10.1007/s00330-005-2762-5

Jamshidi K, Givehchian B, Mirzaei A (2017) Florid reactive periostitis of the long bone: a case series of seven patients. J Orthop Sci 22(3):560–565. Available at: https://doi.org/10.1016/j.jos.2016.12.015

Jones KB, Buckwalter JA, McCarthy EF (2006) Parosteal osteosarcoma of the thumb metacarpal: a case report. Iowa Orthop J 26:134–137

Jurik AG (2020) Multiple hereditary exostoses and enchondromatosis. Best Pract Res Clin Rheumatol 34(3):101505. Available at: https://doi.org/10.1016/j.berh.2020.101505

Kang ST, Kim TH, Kim HW (2012) Huge turret exostosis of metacarpus: a case report. J Korean Bone Joint Tumor Soc 18(2):109–112

Kask G et al (2021) Chondrosarcoma of the hands and feet: when to worry? Bone Joint J 103-B(3):562–568. Available at: https://doi.org/10.1302/0301-620X.103B3.BJJ-2020-1337.R1

Kastanis G et al (2024) Bizarre parosteal osteochondromatous proliferation of the hand: a report of an atypical case and current concepts. Cureus 16(3):e56392. Available at: https://doi.org/10.7759/cureus.56392

Kim J-H, Lee SK (2023) Classification of chondrosarcoma: from characteristic to challenging imaging findings. Cancers 15(6):1703. Available at: https://doi.org/10.3390/cancers15061703

Kim DH, Noh JH (2023) Intraosseous epidermoid cyst of distal phalanx—report of two cases. Clin Case Reports 11(8):e7738. Available at: https://doi.org/10.1002/ccr3.7738

Kinnunen A-R, Sironen R, Sipola P (2020) Magnetic resonance imaging characteristics in patients with histopathologically proven fibrous dysplasia—a systematic review. Skeletal Radiol 49(6):837–845. Available at: https://doi.org/10.1007/s00256-020-03388-x

Kokkalis ZT, Jain S, Sotereanos DG (2010) Fibrous dysplasia around the elbow. J Shoulder Elb Surg 19(1):e6–e11. Available at: https://doi.org/10.1016/j.jse.2009.06.006

Kontogeorgakos VA et al (2007) Turret exostosis of the hallux. J Foot Ankle Surg 46(2):130–132. Available at: https://doi.org/10.1053/j.jfas.2006.11.006

Kopriva JM et al (2020) Trevor's disease of the distal radioulnar joint in two children with achondroplasia. Am J Med Genet A 182(5):1249–1254. Available at: https://doi.org/10.1002/ajmg.a.61529

Kozlowski K et al (1988) Primary bone tumours of the hand. Pediatr Radiol 18(2):140–148. Available at: https://doi.org/10.1007/BF02387558

Kransdorf MJ et al (2024) Musculoskeletal glomus tumor: a review of 218 lesions in 176 patients. Skeletal Radiol [Preprint]. Available at: https://doi.org/10.1007/s00256-024-04743-y

Kresse ME et al (2023) Periosteal chondrosarcoma: an unusual juxtacortical sarcoma. Skeletal Radiol 52(3):623–631. Available at: https://doi.org/10.1007/s00256-022-04216-0

Kumar A et al (2015) Ollier disease: pathogenesis, diagnosis, and management. Orthopedics 38(6):e497–e506. Available at: https://doi.org/10.3928/01477447-20150603-58

Kurt CB et al (2021) Periosteal chondroma of rib at adulthood. Curr Thorac Surg 6(3). Available at: https://doi.org/10.26663/cts.2021.0025

Kyriakos M et al (2007) Osteoblastomatosis of bone. A benign, multifocal osteoblastic lesion, distinct from osteoid osteoma and osteoblastoma, radiologically simulating a vascular tumor. Skeletal Radiol 36(3):237–247. Available at: https://doi.org/10.1007/s00256-006-0113-5

Le Corroller T et al (2012) Primary intraosseous glomus tumor in a middle phalanx. Skeletal Radiol 41(2):227–230. Available at: https://doi.org/10.1007/s00256-011-1217-0

Leeson MC, Lowry L, McCue RW (1988) Aneurysmal bone cyst of the distal thumb phalanx: a case report and review of the literature. Orthopedics 11(4):601–604. Available at: https://doi.org/10.3928/0147-7447-19880401-11

Levine E et al (1984) Scintigraphic evaluation of giant cell tumor of bone. Am J Roentgenol 143(2):343–348. Available at: https://doi.org/10.2214/ajr.143.2.343

Levy JL et al (2021) Focal reactive periostitis ossificans in a long bone: radiologic and pathologic findings. Radiol Case Rep 16(12):3638–3642. Available at: https://doi.org/10.1016/j.radcr.2021.09.009

Li J, Zhang W, Wu G, Zhang zhan (2021) Resection and Reconstruction is the Procedure of Choice for Giant Cell Lesions of Small Bones: A Case Report and Literature Review [Internet]. Research Square [cited 2024 Dec 26]. Available from: https://doi.org/10.21203/rs.3.rs-633635/v1

Li H et al (2022) Clinical diagnosis and treatment of subungual exostosis in children. Front Pediatr 10. Available at: https://doi.org/10.3389/fped.2022.1075089

Lichtenstein L, Hall JE (1952) Periosteal chondroma; a distinctive benign cartilage tumor. J Bone Joint Surg Am Vol 24A(3):691–697

Linabury JF, Henley ND (2022) A woman with a rapidly expanding subungual mass: subungual endometrial carcinoma metastasis. Am J Dermatopathol 44(9):e103. Available at: https://doi.org/10.1097/DAD.0000000000002233

López-Pousa A et al (2015) Giant cell tumour of bone: new treatments in development. Clin Transl Oncol 17(6):419–430. Available at: https://doi.org/10.1007/s12094-014-1268-5

Lubahn JD, Bachoura A (2016) Enchondroma of the hand: evaluation and management. JAAOS – J Am Acad Orthop Surg 24(9):625. Available at: https://doi.org/10.5435/JAAOS-D-15-00452

Macdonald DF et al (2003) Giant cell reparative granuloma of the hand: case report and review of giant cell lesions of hands and feet. Can J Surg 46(6):471–473

Mahan MC et al (2016) Ewing sarcoma in the fifth metacarpal of an adult woman: a case report. JBJS Case Connect 6(4):e95. Available at: https://doi.org/10.2106/JBJS.CC.16.00051

Mahdal M et al (2025) Osteosarcomas of the hand and foot: a sarcoma-center case series experience. Oncol Lett 29(1):1–11. Available at: https://doi.org/10.3892/ol.2024.14800

Maiya S, Davies A, Evans N, Grimer R et al (2002) Surface aneurysmal bone cysts: a pictorial review. Eur Radiol 12(1). Available at: https://doi.org/10.1007/s003300101009

Marcuzzi A, Acciaro AL, Landi A (2002) Osteoid osteoma of the hand and wrist. J Bone Joint Surg Br Vol 27(5):440–443. Available at: https://doi.org/10.1054/jhsb.2002.0811

Martínez Álvarez S, Azorín Cuadrillero DL, Little KJ (2021) Bizarre parosteal osteochondromatous proliferation (Nora lesion) in pediatric phalanges. J Hand Surg Am 46(4):344.e1–344.e9. Available at: https://doi.org/10.1016/j.jhsa.2020.05.002

Martinez V, Sissons HA (1988) Aneurysmal bone cyst. A review of 123 cases including primary lesions and those secondary to other bone pathology. Cancer 61(11):2291–2304. Available at: https://doi.org/10.1002/1097-0142(19880601)61:11<2291::aid-cncr2820611125>3.0.co;2-v

Marui T et al (2003) Parosteal fasciitis of the scapula. J Shoulder Elb Surg 12(4):408–410. Available at: https://doi.org/10.1016/S1058-2746(02)00046-0

Mascard E, Gomez-Brouchet A, Lambot K (2015) Bone cysts: Unicameral and aneurysmal bone cyst. Orthopaedics & Traumatology: Surgery & Research. 101(1, Supplement):S119–27

Mathew SE et al (2011) Florid reactive periostitis of the forearm bones in a child. J Bone Joint Surg Br Vol 93-B(3):418–420. Available at: https://doi.org/10.1302/0301-620X.93B3.24955

Mathov SH, Bougie JD, Awad S (2008) Osteosarcoma of the hand: a rare case for radiographic appearance, location, and age. J Manip Physiol Ther 31(2):164–167. Available at: https://doi.org/10.1016/j.jmpt.2007.12.008

Mavrogenis AF et al (2014) Acrometastases. Eur J Orthop Surg Traumatol: Orthop Traumatol 24(3):279–283. Available at: https://doi.org/10.1007/s00590-013-1311-1

Mavrogenis AF, Igoumenou VG et al (2017a) Giant cell tumor of bone revisited. SICOT-J 3:54. Available at: https://doi.org/10.1051/sicotj/2017041

Mavrogenis AF, Panagopoulos GN et al (2017b) Tumors of the hand. Eur J Orthop Surg Traumatol 27(6):747–762. Available at: https://doi.org/10.1007/s00590-017-1984-y

McBee DB, Bentley HA, Toledanes G (2023) Ewing's sarcoma of the hand: an unusual presentation in a young Hispanic male. Cureus 15(11):e49140. Available at: https://doi.org/10.7759/cureus.49140

Meena UK, Sharma YK, Saini N, Meena DS, Gahlot N (2016) Giant Cell Tumours of Hand Bones: a Report of Two Cases. Journal of Hand and Microsurgery. 07:177–81.

Melamud K et al (2014) Diagnostic imaging of benign and malignant osseous tumors of the fingers. Radiographics 34(7):1954–1967. Available at: https://doi.org/10.1148/rg.347130031

Memon RA, Wei S, Siegal GP (2022) Some Reactive Lesions of Bone Are Probably Neoplasms: A Review. Archives of Pathology & Laboratory Medicine. 146(1):60–9

Mendenhall WM et al (2006) Aneurysmal bone cyst. Am J Clin Oncol 29(3):311–315. Available at: https://doi.org/10.1097/01.coc.0000204403.13451.52

Meyer J, Rolvien T et al (2023a) Osteoid osteoma in the bones of the hand: a systematic literature review. Arch

Orthop Trauma Surg 143(8):5437–5444. Available at: https://doi.org/10.1007/s00402-023-04839-5
Meyer J, Priemel M et al (2023b) The diagnostic challenge of osteoid osteoma in the bones of the hand—a case series. Diagnostics 13(7):1279. Available at: https://doi.org/10.3390/diagnostics13071279
Michelsen H et al (2004) Bizarre parosteal osteochondromatous proliferation (Nora's lesion) in the hand. J Hand Surg Am 29(3):520–525. Available at: https://doi.org/10.1016/j.jhsa.2004.02.002
Mier LCG et al (2024) Multifocal giant cell tumor of the carpus: unusual presentation. Case report and review of the literature. Int J Surg Case Rep 114:109127. Available at: https://doi.org/10.1016/j.ijscr.2023.109127
Miwa S et al (2021) A radiological scoring system for differentiation between enchondroma and chondrosarcoma. Cancers 13(14):3558. Available at: https://doi.org/10.3390/cancers13143558
Mohanna P-N, Moiemen NS, Frame JD (2000) Turret exostosis of the thumb. Br J Plast Surg 53(7):629–631. Available at: https://doi.org/10.1054/bjps.2000.3401
Morris G et al (2017) Bone metastases of the hand. Ann R Coll Surg Engl 99(7):563–567. Available at: https://doi.org/10.1308/rcsann.2017.0096
Motamedi D, Learch TJ, Ishimitsu DN, Motamedi K, Katz MD, Brien EW, Menendez L (2009) Thermal ablation of osteoid osteoma: overview and step-by-step guide. RadioGraphics 29(7):2127–2141
Motomiya M, Sakazaki T, Iwasaki N (2020) Atypical osteochondroma of the hamate that presented clinically as carpal tunnel syndrome: report of an extremely rare case and literature review. BMC Musculoskelet Disord 21(1):231. Available at: https://doi.org/10.1186/s12891-020-03272-8
Muir TM, Lehman TP, Meyer WH (2008) Periosteal osteosarcoma in the hand of a pediatric patient: a case report. J Hand Surg Am. 33(2):266–8.
Muñoz-Mahamud E, Combalia A, Carreño A, Arandes JM (2017) Five cases of acrometastasis to the hand from a carcinoma and review of the literature. Hand Surg Rehabil 36(1):12–16. Available at: https://doi.org/10.1016/j.hansur.2016.10.211
Muren C et al (1991) Osteoid osteomas of the hand. Report of three cases and review of the literature. Acta Radiol (Stockh, Swed: 1987) 32(1):62–66
Murphey MD et al (2003) From the archives of the AFIP: imaging of primary chondrosarcoma: radiologic-pathologic correlation. Radiographics 23(5):1245–1278. Available at: https://doi.org/10.1148/rg.235035134
Nackos JS, Wiggins RH, Harnsberger HR (2006) CT and MR imaging of giant cell granuloma of the craniofacial bones. Am J Neuroradiol 27(8):1651–1653
Nakagawa M et al (2022) Clinical, radiological, and histopathological characteristics of periosteal chondrosarcoma with a focus on the frequency of medullary invasion. J Clin Med 11(7):2062. Available at: https://doi.org/10.3390/jcm11072062
Nanda SN et al (2018) Aneurysmal bone cyst of 3rd metacarpal, management and follow-up: a case report. J Orthop Case Rep 8(2):9–12. Available at: https://doi.org/10.13107/jocr.2250-0685.1024
Nayak KR et al (2021) Enchondroma in the diaphysis of tibia – a case report and review of its characteristics and differentials in the diaphysis. J Orthop Case Rep 11(7):6–11. Available at: https://doi.org/10.13107/jocr.2021.v11.i07.2292
Nazarova NZ et al (2020) The distribution of chondromas: why the hand? Med Hypotheses 143:110132. Available at: https://doi.org/10.1016/j.mehy.2020.110132
Nazarova NZ et al (2021) The surgical management of the cavity and bone defects in enchondroma cases: a prospective randomized trial. Surg Oncol 37:101565. Available at: https://doi.org/10.1016/j.suronc.2021.101565
Neder Filho AT et al (2024) Hand tumors. Rev Assoc Med Bras 70:e2024S108. Available at: https://doi.org/10.1590/1806-9282.2024S108
Nielsen GP (2021) Bone tumor pathology, an issue of surgical pathology clinics. Elsevier Health Sciences
Niemeler JK, Melissa G, Nader P (2022) Rapidly growing solitary osteochondroma in the adult finger: a case report. Available at: https://www.proquest.com/openview/722c45ec6a6770c154801ef82e40e52c/1?pq-origsite=gscholar&cbl=1646346. Accessed 20 Dec 2024
Noordin S et al (2019) Aneurysmal bone cyst of the pelvis and extremities: contemporary management. IJS Oncol 4:e711. Available at: https://doi.org/10.1097/IJ9.0000000000000071
Nora FE, Dahlin DC, Beabout JW (1983) Bizarre parosteal osteochondromatous proliferations of the hands and feet. Am J Surg Pathol 7(3):245–250. Available at: https://doi.org/10.1097/00000478-198304000-00003
O'Connor MI, Bancroft LW (2004) Benign and malignant cartilage tumors of the hand. Hand Clin. 20(3):317–23:vi
O'Connor W et al (2014) The hypermetabolic giant: 18F-FDG avid giant cell tumor identified on PET-CT. J Radiol Case Rep 8(6):27–38. Available at: https://doi.org/10.3941/jrcr.v8i6.1328
Ogose A et al (1997) Chondrosarcoma of small bones of the hands and feet. Cancer 80(1):50–59
Ohkuma R, McCarthy EF, Deune EG (2011) Hereditary multiple exostoses in the hands and fingers: early presentation and early surgical treatment in family members. Case reports. Hand (New York, N.Y.) 6(2):209–216. Available at: https://doi.org/10.1007/s11552-010-9307-3
Oliveira VC et al (2013) Giant cell tumours of the small bones of the hands and feet: long-term results of 30 patients and a systematic literature review. Bone Joint J 95-B(6):838–845. Available at: https://doi.org/10.1302/0301-620X.95B6.30876
Olson NJ et al (2021) Fibrous dysplasia at unusual anatomic sites: a series of 86 cases with emphasis on histologic patterns. Int J Surg Pathol 29(7):704–709. Available at: https://doi.org/10.1177/1066896921997141

Olvi LG, Gonzalez ML, da Cunha IW, Santini-Araujo E, Kalil RK (2020) Bizarre Parosteal Osteochondromatous Proliferation. In: Santini-Araujo E, Kalil RK, Bertoni F, Park YK. Tumors and Tumor-Like Lesions of Bone [Internet]. Springer International Publishing; p. 811–9.

Orui H et al (2002) Magnetic resonance imaging characteristics of bizarre parosteal osteochondromatous proliferation of the hand: a case report. J Hand Surg Am 27(6):1104–1108. Available at: https://doi.org/10.1053/jhsu.2002.36526

Osagie L et al (2015) Intraosseous ganglion cysts of the carpus: current practice. Hand 10(4):598–601. Available at: https://doi.org/10.1007/s11552-015-9750-2

Ostlere SJ et al (1991) Case report 658: chondrosarcoma of the proximal phalanx of right fourth finger secondary to multiple hereditary exostoses (MHE). Skeletal Radiol 20(2):145–148. Available at: https://doi.org/10.1007/BF00193831

Ozsen M et al (2018) Fibrous dysplasia: clinicopathologic presentation of 36 cases. Turk J Pathol [Preprint]. Available at: https://doi.org/10.5146/tjpath.2018.01428

Pai SN, Rajappa S, Pavithra V (2021) Primary aneurysmal bone cyst of the phalanx. J Hand Microsurg 15:242–244. Available at: https://doi.org/10.1055/s-0041-1736005

Palmerini E et al (2019) Malignancy in giant cell tumor of bone: a review of the literature. Technol Cancer Res Treat 18:1533033819840000. Available at: https://doi.org/10.1177/1533033819840000

Pandey PK, Verma RR (2020) Periosteal chondroma of the radial diaphysis—rare presentation and review of literature. Indian J Surg Oncol 11(2):232–236. Available at: https://doi.org/10.1007/s13193-020-01186-4

Parida L et al (2012) Clinical management of Ewing sarcoma of the bones of the hands and feet: a retrospective single-institution review. J Pediatr Surg 47(10):1806–1810. Available at: https://doi.org/10.1016/j.jpedsurg.2012.05.022

Parmeggiani A et al (2021) State of the art and new concepts in giant cell tumor of bone: imaging features and tumor characteristics. Cancers 13(24):6298. Available at: https://doi.org/10.3390/cancers13246298

Patil S et al (2003) Chondrosarcoma of small bones of the hand. J Hand Surg Br Eur Vol 28(6):602–608. Available at: https://doi.org/10.1016/S0266-7681(03)00149-9

Patel MR, Desai SS, Gordon SL, Nimberg GA, Sclafani SJ, Vigorita VJ, et al. (1987) Management of skeletal giant cell tumors of the phalanges of the hand. The Journal of Hand Surgery 12(1):70–7.

Patel K, Bhuiya T, Chen S, Kenan S, Kahn L (2006) Epidermal inclusion cyst of phalanx: a case report and review of the literature. Skeletal Radiol 35(11):861–3.

Payne WT, Merrell G (2010) Benign bony and soft tissue tumors of the hand. J Hand Surg Am 35(11):1901–1910. Available at: https://doi.org/10.1016/j.jhsa.2010.08.015

Pena-Burgos EM et al (2023) Primary aneurysmal bone cyst of hands and feet: a series of 14 cases. Ann Diagn Pathol 66:152169. Available at: https://doi.org/10.1016/j.anndiagpath.2023.152169

Pinheiro RF et al (2009) Primary non-Hodgkin lymphoma of bone: an unusual presentation. J Cancer Res Ther 5(1):52–53. Available at: https://doi.org/10.4103/0973-1482.48772

Plate A-M, Steiner G, Posner MA (2006) Malignant tumors of the hand and wrist. JAAOS – J Am Acad Orthop Surg. Available at: https://journals.lww.com/jaaos/abstract/2006/11000/malignant_tumors_of_the_hand_and_wrist.13.aspx. Accessed 7 Dec 2024

Platt AJ, Klugman DJ (1995) Aneurysmal bone cyst of the capitate. J Hand Surg 20(1):8–11. Available at: https://doi.org/10.1016/S0266-7681(05)80005-1

Pratap D, Hasaan S, Kumar P (2019) Subungual exostosis – clinical, radiological, and histological findings – PMC. Available at: https://pmc.ncbi.nlm.nih.gov/articles/PMC6434752/. Accessed 7 Jan 2025

Puri A, Rajalbandi R, Gulia A (2021) Giant cell tumour of hand bones: outcomes of treatment. J Hand Surg (Eur Vol) 46(7):774–780. Available at: https://doi.org/10.1177/17531934211007820

Puşcaşu A-I et al (2023) Solitary acrometastasis of the phalanx as initial presentation of an oligometastatic Kirsten rat sarcoma viral oncogene homolog-mutated lung adenocarcinoma: a case report. J Med Case Rep 17(1):395. Available at: https://doi.org/10.1186/s13256-023-04127-1

Rabarin F et al (2014) Focal periosteal chondroma of the hand: a review of 24 cases. Orthop Traumatol Surg Res 100(6):617–620. Available at: https://doi.org/10.1016/j.otsr.2014.05.014

Reddy KIA et al (2014) Aneurysmal bone cysts: do simple treatments work? Clin Orthop Relat Res 472(6):1901–1910. Available at: https://doi.org/10.1007/s11999-014-3513-1

Restrepo R et al (2022) Update on aneurysmal bone cyst: pathophysiology, histology, imaging and treatment. Pediatr Radiol 52(9):1601–1614. Available at: https://doi.org/10.1007/s00247-022-05396-6

Revell MP, Mulligan PJ, Grimer RJ (2000) Parosteal osteosarcoma of the ring finger metacarpal in a semi-professional pianist. J Hand Surg (Edinb, Scotl) 25(3):314–316. Available at: https://doi.org/10.1054/jhsb.2000.0386

Rhee PC et al (2012) Chondroblastoma with secondary aneurysmal bone cyst of the hamate: case report. J Hand Surg Am 37(3):538–542. Available at: https://doi.org/10.1016/j.jhsa.2011.11.014

Ribeiro JNA et al (2019) Periostite reativa florida da falange proximal – relato de caso e revisão de literatura. Rev Bras Ortop 54(03):335–338. Available at: https://doi.org/10.1055/s-0039-1692430

Riester S et al (2016) Predicting fracture risk for enchondroma of the hand. Hand 11(2):206–210. Available at: https://doi.org/10.1177/1558944715626931

Righi A et al (2022) Secondary peripheral chondrosarcoma arising in solitary osteochondroma: variables influencing prognosis and survival. Orphanet J Rare Dis 17(1):74. Available at: https://doi.org/10.1186/s13023-022-02210-2

Robinson P et al (2001) Periosteal chondroid tumors: radiologic evaluation with pathologic correlation. AJR Am J Roentgenol 177(5):1183–1188. Available at: https://doi.org/10.2214/ajr.177.5.1771183

Rossetti A et al (2022) Parosteal osteosarcoma of the thumb: a case report and literature review. Hand Surg Rehabil 41(2):273–277. Available at: https://doi.org/10.1016/j.hansur.2022.01.005

Rubin JA, Steinberg DR (1996) Turret exostosis of the metacarpal: a case report. J Hand Surg Am 21(2):296–298. Available at: https://doi.org/10.1016/S0363-5023(96)80124-9

Ruchelsman DE et al (2010) Digital intraosseous epidermoid inclusion cyst of the distal phalanx. J Hand Microsurg 2(1):24–27. Available at: https://doi.org/10.1007/s12593-010-0001-z

Russell JD et al (2016) Subungual exostosis. Cutis 98(2):128–129

Rybak LD et al (2007) Cortico-medullary continuity in bizarre parosteal osteochondromatous proliferation mimicking osteochondroma on imaging. Skeletal Radiol 36(9):829–834. Available at: https://doi.org/10.1007/s00256-007-0300-z

Saad A et al (2023) Periostitis ossificans: largest case series with review of literature. Indian J Radiol Imaging 34:32–36. Available at: https://doi.org/10.1055/s-0043-1770723

Sahoo TK et al (2016) Digital acrometastasis as initial presentation in carcinoma of lung a case report and review of literature. J Clin Diagn Res: JCDR 10(6):XD01–XD02. Available at: https://doi.org/10.7860/JCDR/2016/16063.7951

Sakamoto A, Oda Y, Iwamoto Y (2013) Intraosseous ganglia: a series of 17 treated cases. Biomed Res Int 2013(1):462730. Available at: https://doi.org/10.1155/2013/462730

Sanghavi S et al (2017) Parosteal osteosarcoma of the distal radius mimicking an osteochondroma—a diagnostic misadventure. J Hand Surg Am 42(12):1038.e1–1038.e10. Available at: https://doi.org/10.1016/j.jhsa.2017.07.010

Saunders C, Szabo RM, Mora S (1997) Chondrosarcoma of the hand arising in a young patient with multiple hereditary exostoses. J Hand Surg Asian Pac Vol 22(2):237–242. Available at: https://doi.org/10.1016/S0266-7681(97)80072-1

Sebastian A et al (2023) Malignant transformation of a solitary osteochondroma of proximal humerus: a rare case report. J Curr Oncol 6(2):85–89. Available at: https://doi.org/10.1177/25898892241253375

Sensarma A et al (2015) Regression of an enchondroma: a case report and proposed etiology. Skeletal Radiol 44(5):739–742. Available at: https://doi.org/10.1007/s00256-014-2032-1

Sharif B, Lindsay D, Saifuddin A (2022) Update on the imaging features of the enchondromatosis syndromes. Skeletal Radiol 51(4):747–762. Available at: https://doi.org/10.1007/s00256-021-03870-0

Shigematsu K et al (2006) Giant-cell tumors of the carpus. J Hand Surg Am 31(7):1214–1219. Available at: https://doi.org/10.1016/j.jhsa.2006.04.012

Shimal A et al (2009) Subperiosteal aneurysmal bone cyst of the metacarpal. Eur J Radiol Extra 71(3):e117–e119. Available at: https://doi.org/10.1016/j.ejrex.2009.03.015

Shimizu K et al (1997) Enchondroma of the distal phalanx of the hand. JBJS 79(6):898

Shubinets V, Ben-Amotz O, Steinberg DR (2019) A subperiosteal proximal phalanx osteoid osteoma: a challenging diagnosis. J Hand Surg Asian Pac Vol 24(2):233–237. Available at: https://doi.org/10.1142/S2424835519720111

Simon MJ et al (2014) Incidence, histopathologic analysis and distribution of tumours of the hand. BMC Musculoskelet Disord 15(1):182. Available at: https://doi.org/10.1186/1471-2474-15-182

Skinner S, Conant S, Lansinger Y (2019) Ewing sarcoma in an infant metacarpal. J Hand Surg Am 44(8):701.e1–701.e5. Available at: https://doi.org/10.1016/j.jhsa.2018.09.001

Sobti A et al (2016) Giant cell tumor of bone – an overview. Arch Bone Joint Surg 4(1):2–9

Solana J, Bosch M, Español I (2003) Florid reactive periostitis of the thumb: a case report and review of the literature. Chir Main 22(2):99–103. Available at: https://doi.org/10.1016/S1297-3203(03)00019-2

Sollaci C, de Araújo GCS (2019) Enchondromas of the hand: a 20-year experience. Rev Bras Ortop 54:714–720. Available at: https://doi.org/10.1055/s-0039-1697970

Sonne-Holm E, Wong C, Sonne-Holm S (2014) Multiple cartilaginous exostoses and development of chondrosarcomas--a systematic review. Dan Med J 61(9):A4895

Spiteri V et al (2008) Managing acrometastases treatment strategy with a case illustration. Ann R Coll Surg Engl 90(7):W8–W11. Available at: https://doi.org/10.1308/147870808X303137

Spjut HJ, Dorfman HD (1981) Florid reactive periostitis of the tubular bones of the hands and feet. A benign lesion which may simulate osteosarcoma. Am J Surg Pathol. (5):423–33.

Sridhar H et al (2014) Chondrosarcoma arising in an enchondroma of the metacarpal bone – a case report. J Clin Diagn Res: JCDR 8(3):142–143. Available at: https://doi.org/10.7860/JCDR/2014/8142.4139

Stomeo D et al (2014) Chondrosarcoma of the hand: a literature review. J Cancer Ther 5(4):403–409. Available at: https://doi.org/10.4236/jct.2014.54046

Streek PV et al (1998) Upper extremity radionuclide bone imaging: the wrist and hand. Semin Nucl Med 28(1):14–24. Available at: https://doi.org/10.1016/S0001-2998(98)80016-0

Sundaram M et al (2001) Florid reactive periostitis and bizarre parosteal osteochondromatous proliferation: pre-biopsy imaging evolution, treatment and outcome.

Skeletal Radiol 30(4):192–198. Available at: https://doi.org/10.1007/s002560100343

Symeonidis A et al (2019) Primary bone non-Hodgkin's lymphoma: a specific clinical entity with aggressive clinical course and high cure rate – retrospective analysis of 102 patients from Greece. Blood 134(Supplement_1):5340. Available at: https://doi.org/10.1182/blood-2019-130219

Tang J et al (2023) Florid reactive periostitis of the clavicle: A case report and literature review. Medicine 102(50):e36674. Available at: https://doi.org/10.1097/MD.0000000000036674

Teixeira LEM et al (2014) Giant cell tumors of bone: nonsurgical factors associated with local recurrence. Acta Orthop Traumatol Turc 48(2):136–140. Available at: https://doi.org/10.3944/AOTT.2014.2714

Teodoreanu RN et al (2022) Benign cartilaginous tumors of the hand, a five-year retrospective study. Romanian J Morphol Embryol 63(4):625–632. Available at: https://doi.org/10.47162/RJME.63.4.04

Tepelenis K et al (2021) Osteochondromas: an updated review of epidemiology, pathogenesis, clinical presentation, radiological features and treatment options. In Vivo 35(2):681–691. Available at: https://doi.org/10.21873/invivo.12308

Theumann NH et al (2002) Recurrent glomus tumors of fingertips: MR imaging evaluation. Radiology 223(1):143–151. Available at: https://doi.org/10.1148/radiol.2231010977

Thomas BP et al (2011) Malignant tumours of the hand and wrist. Indian J Plast Surg 44(2):337–347. Available at: https://doi.org/10.4103/0970-0358.85355

Tilden W et al (2022) Peripheral and periosteal chondrosarcoma: MRI-pathological correlation in 58 cases. Skeletal Radiol 51(6):1189–1199. Available at: https://doi.org/10.1007/s00256-021-03947-w

Tomori Y et al (2016) Florid reactive periostitis in the fifth phalange of a professional boxer. Medicine 95(51):e5697. Available at: https://doi.org/10.1097/MD.0000000000005697

Torreggiani WC et al (2001) MR imaging features of bizarre parosteal osteochondromatous proliferation of bone (Nora's lesion). Eur J Radiol 40(3):224–231. Available at: https://doi.org/10.1016/s0720-048x(01)00362-x

Trehan SK et al (2015) Characteristics of glomus tumors in the hand not diagnosed on magnetic resonance imaging. J Hand Surg Am 40(3):542–545. Available at: https://doi.org/10.1016/j.jhsa.2014.12.002

Tsuda Y et al (2019) Secondary chondrosarcoma arising from osteochondroma: outcomes and prognostic factors. Bone Joint J 101-B(10):1313–1320. Available at: https://doi.org/10.1302/0301-620X.101B9.BJJ-2019-0190.R1

Tsukamoto S, Mavrogenis AF, Kido A, Errani C (2021) Current Concepts in the Treatment of Giant Cell Tumors of Bone. Cancers. 13(15):3647

Turan H, Uslu M, Erdem H (2012) A case of subungual exostosis. Indian J Dermatol Venereol Leprol 78(2):186. Available at: https://doi.org/10.4103/0378-6323.93638

Uldin H, Kanbour I, Patel A, Botchu R (2024) Image-guided musculoskeletal interventional radiology in the personalised management of musculoskeletal tumours. J Pers Med 14(12):1167. Available at: https://doi.org/10.3390/jpm14121167

Ulrich G, Wood R, Pearson J, Jiganti M, Tedesco N (2024) Bizarre Parosteal Osteochondromatous Proliferation With Malignant Transformation and Metastases. Orthopedics. 47(6):e322–6

Umana GE et al (2021) Acrometastases to the hand: a systematic review. Medicina 57(9):950. Available at: https://doi.org/10.3390/medicina57090950

Utomo P, Idulhaq M, Mudigdo A, Sentana OM (2019) Giant Cell Tumor of the Phalanx of Finger: Case Reports. Indonesian Journal of Medicine 4(1):65–74

Valero J et al (2014) Subungual squamous cell carcinoma and exostosis in third toe – case report and literature review. J Eur Acad Dermatol Venereol 28(10):1292–1297. Available at: https://doi.org/10.1111/jdv.12271

van Langevelde K, McCarthy CL (2020) Radiological findings of denosumab treatment for giant cell tumours of bone. Skeletal Radiol 49:1345–1358. https://doi.org/10.1007/s00256-020-03449-1

Vasilakaki T et al (2012) Chondrosarcoma of the proximal phalanx of the fourth digit: a rare location. Case Rep Oncol 5(3):566–569. Available at: https://doi.org/10.1159/000343915

Ventura-Parellada C, Martínez-Ruiz A, Subirà-i-Álvarez T (2021) Giant cell reparative granuloma of the phalanx in a violinist. Occup Med 71(4–5):231–233. Available at: https://doi.org/10.1093/occmed/kqab069

Verma S et al (2020) Primary lymphoma of long bones causing pathological fracture: a rare entity. J Case Rep 10(4):214–219. Available at: https://doi.org/10.17659/01.2020.0056

Wandroo FA et al (2005) Plasma cell leukaemia presenting with polyarthralgia and phalangeal lytic lesions. Clin Lab Haematol 27(3):203–205. Available at: https://doi.org/10.1111/j.1365-2257.2005.00669.x

Wang Z et al (2018) Prognostic factors for survival among patients with primary bone sarcomas of small bones. Cancer Manag Res 10(null):1191–1199. Available at: https://doi.org/10.2147/CMAR.S163229

Wang Y et al (2022) Risk factors for pathological fractures of simple bone cysts of the humerus in children: a retrospective cohort study. Transl Pediatr 11(7):1261–1266. Available at: https://doi.org/10.21037/tp-22-290

Washington E et al (2021) Bizarre parosteal osteochondromatous proliferation: rare case affecting distal ulna and review of literature. Clin Imaging 69:233–237. Available at: https://doi.org/10.1016/j.clinimag.2020.08.019

Williams HJ et al (2004) Imaging features of intraosseous ganglia: a report of 45 cases. Eur Radiol 14(10):1761–1769. Available at: https://doi.org/10.1007/s00330-004-2371-8

Wissinger HA, Mcclain EJ, Boyes JH (1966) Turret exostosis: ossifying hematoma of the phalanges. JBJS 48(1):105

Woodside JC, Ganey T, Gaston RG (2015) Multiple osteochondroma of the hand: initial and long-term follow-up study. Hand 10(4):616–620. Available at: https://doi.org/10.1007/s11552-015-9775-6

Wu C et al (2013) Chondroblastoma of the triquetrum – PubMed. Pediatr Neonatol 54(4):278–280

Xu R, Choong PFM (2022) Metastatic giant cell tumour of bone: a narrative review of management options and approaches. ANZ J Surg 92(4):691–696. Available at: https://doi.org/10.1111/ans.17520

Xu H et al (2015) Chondroblastoma of bone in the extremities: a multicenter retrospective study. J Bone Joint Surg 97(11):925–931. Available at: https://doi.org/10.2106/JBJS.N.00992

Yeom JA et al (2018) A rare manifestation of solitary primary bone lymphoma of the finger: a case report. Invest Magn Reson Imaging 22(4):240–244. Available at: https://doi.org/10.13104/imri.2018.22.4.240

Yousefian F (2021) Pediatric subungual exostosis. Cutis 108(5). Available at: https://doi.org/10.12788/cutis.0380

Yuen M et al (1992) Proliferative periosteal processes of phalanges: a unitary hypothesis. Skeletal Radiol 21(5):301–303. Available at: https://doi.org/10.1007/BF00241768

Zarghooni K et al (2023) The diagnosis and treatment of osteosarcoma and Ewing's sarcoma in children and adolescents. Dtsch Arztebl Int 120(24):405–412. Available at: https://doi.org/10.3238/arztebl.m2023.0079

Zishan US et al (2020) The differentiation between aneurysmal bone cyst and telangiectatic osteosarcoma: a clinical, radiographic and MRI study. Skeletal Radiol 49(9):1375–1386. Available at: https://doi.org/10.1007/s00256-020-03432-w

Tumor and Tumor-Like Lesions of Soft Tissue

Shashank Chapala, Hasaam Uldin, Filip M. Vanhoenacker, Robert U. Ashford, and Rajesh Botchu

Contents

S. Chapala (✉)
Department of Radiology, AIG Hospitals, Hyderabad, India

H. Uldin · R. Botchu
Department of Musculoskeletal Radiology, Royal Orthopedic Hospital, Birmingham, UK

F. M. Vanhoenacker
Department of Radiology, University Hospital Antwerp, Edegem, Belgium

Faculty of Medicine and Health Sciences, Universities of Antwerp and Ghent, Antwerp, Belgium

General Hospital Sint-Maarten Mechelen, Mechelen, Belgium

R. U. Ashford
Department of Orthopedics, University Hospitals of Leicester, Leicester, UK

Med Radiol Diagn Imaging (2025)
https://doi.org/10.1007/174_2025_586,
Published Online: 26 July 2025

Abstract

Masses of the hand and wrist are a common clinical problem. Soft-tissue tumors of the hand and wrist are far more frequent than bone tumors. If clinical examination is equivocal, imaging is often requested. Majority of the soft tissue tumors are benign and it is important to understand typical and atypical imaging features. This chapter aims to present an overview of the imaging characteristics of the most frequent tumors (both benign and malignant), tumor-like soft-tissue lesions, and infections of the hand and wrist.

1 Introduction

Mesodermal mesenchyme differentiates into tendon, muscle, nerves, skin, blood vessels, and synovial sheath. Tumors of hand can comprise of any of these soft tissues. Despite accounting for only a small percentage of the body's surface area and weight, the hands are prone to a relatively high number of soft tissue tumors, with 15% of all soft tissue tumors occurring in this area (Garcia and Bianchi 2001). Fortunately, the majority of hand tumors are benign, with 95% of those without skin involvement (Nepal et al. 2019). Due to their superficial location, tumors of hand and wrist are often detected early, contributing to a generally good prognosis. Malignant soft tissue tumors of the hand are rare, making up only 2% of all hand lesions (Nepal et al. 2019).

2 Benign Soft-Tissue Tumors

2.1 Synovial Cyst, Ganglion Cyst, and Tendon Sheath Cyst

2.1.1 Definition and Nosological Classification

Cystic lesions are the most common mass lesions arising in the hand and wrist, accounting for 50–70% of all soft-tissue tumors of the hand and wrist (De Beuckeleer et al. 2001; Angeledes 1999). The terminology of cystic lesions can be very confusing and depends on a combination of parameters such as topography, the presence or absence of joint communication, and the histologic composition.

The term *synovial cyst* describes a continuation or herniation of the synovial membrane through the joint capsule. In the French literature, the term "arthrosynovial" cyst is preferred, which refers to its intimate relationship with the adjacent joint. Indeed, there is always a communication with the adjacent joint and the histologic composition is identical to those of the joint cavity. It consists of a collection of intra-articular fluid lined by a continuous layer of "true" synovial cells. Usually associated joint diseases are present, like osteoarthrosis, inflammatory, and post-traumatic joint diseases. Thirty percent of the lesions are associated with underlying interosseous ligament injury (Lowden et al. 2005). The elevated intra-articular pressure due to an accumulation of joint fluid in these diseases causes herniation of joint fluid and synovium through a "locus minoris resistentiae" within the joint capsule.

Ganglion cysts are the most common type of soft-tissue tumor found in the hand, accounting for approximately 65% of all masses in the wrist and hand. They are more commonly found in females with a female-to-male ratio of almost 3:1. The most common locations for ganglion cysts are the dorsal wrist (70%), volar wrist (20%), and volar retinacular cysts (10%) (AbuMoussa et al. 2023).

Ganglia also contain mucinous fluid, but their wall consists of a (discontinuous) layer of flattened pseudosynovial cells surrounded by connective tissue (pseudocapsule).

A communication with the adjacent joint is not always present.

There remains much controversy in the literature concerning the pathogenesis of ganglion cysts. Several theories have been proposed including displacement of synovial tissue during embryogenesis, proliferation of pluripotential mesenchymal cells, degeneration of connective tissues after trauma, and migration of synovial fluid into the cyst (synovial herniation theory). The exact cause of ganglion cysts is not fully understood, but it is thought that repetitive stretching of the joint capsule and ligaments may stimulate the production of hyaluronic acid, leading to the formation of the cyst (Minotti and Taras 2002).

Based upon the similar appearances of synovial cysts and ganglion cysts on imaging and macroscopically at surgery, we believe that the synovial herniation hypothesis is the most satisfactory. According to this theory, synovial cysts or ganglion cysts are formed by a herniation of synovium through a breach in the adjacent articulation.

Whereas a synovial cyst has a continuous synovial lining of true synovial cells, the wall composition of a ganglion cyst consists of a discontinuous layer of pseudosynovial cells, cuboidal epithelium.

A ganglion cyst may represent an advanced stage of a degenerated synovial cyst, in which the continuous synovial lining and the communication with the joint may be lost during the process of degeneration (Vanhoenacker et al. 2006b). These are pseudocysts with jelly like fluid as content lined by fattened cells and arise from joint or tendon sheath following synovial fluid extension to adjacent soft tissues (Wigley et al. 2019).

A tendon sheath cyst consists of a special subtype of a ganglion cyst located on the course of a tendon sheath. Intratendinous ganglion cysts (ITGC) are very rare, as reported by (Saad et al. 2023), and can extend into muscle belly.

2.1.2 Clinical Findings

Cystic lesions of the hand and wrist occur most frequently between 20 and 40 years of age but may arise in the pediatric population and the elderly (Nahra and Bucchieri 2004; Wang and Hutchinson 2001). There is a female predominance (Nahra and Bucchieri 2004). Half of the patients are asymptomatic (Lowden et al. 2005), whereas the remainder suffer from chronic wrist pain, tenderness, or functional impairment (Peh et al. 1995).

The lesion may fluctuate in size, particularly during flexion of the wrist.

The majority of ganglion cysts are located at the dorsal aspect of the wrist adjacent to the scapholunate ligament (60–70%), whereas volar wrist cysts account for approximately 18–20%. Approximately two-thirds of volar ganglions arise from the radiocarpal joint and one-third arise from the scaphotrapezial joint (Greendyke et al. 1992). Volar cysts may cause median and ulnar nerve palsies (Kobayashi et al. 2001; Christiaanse et al. 2010). Some cysts may adhere directly to the tendon sheath (Nahra and Bucchieri 2004). Rarely, cysts arise from the dorsal aspect of the interphalangeal joints, often secondary to Heberden osteoarthritis in elderly patients (Nahra and Bucchieri 2004).

2.1.3 Imaging Findings

The role of imaging is to define the cystic nature of those lesions and to demonstrate a possible communication with the joint. This is important for the surgeon, because the resection of the communicating stalk with the joint is essential to avoid postsurgical recurrence of the cyst.

2.1.4 Conventional Radiography

Standard radiography is nonspecific and may reveal an ill-defined or rounded, noncalcified soft-tissue mass. Rarely, gas or calcified loose bodies may be seen within a communicating cyst.

2.1.5 Ultrasound

On US, synovial cysts and ganglion cysts appear as anechoic masses (Fig. 1) and may have a visible communication with a joint (Figs. 1 and 2) or tendon sheath (Figs. 2a and 3). The lesion may be multiseptated and may contain some fine internal septations. Ultrasound is an accurate technique to define the cystic nature in superficial cysts around the wrist and the hand, but it has limited ability to visualize deeper lying structures and their relationship with the adjacent joint. Furthermore, cysts containing debris or hyperplastic synovium may simulate solid mass lesions on ultrasound examinations (Vanhoenacker et al. 2006b).

2.1.6 CT

Due to its low soft-tissue contrast, CT is of limited value in assessing soft-tissue lesions. Para-articular cysts are typically of lower attenuation than muscle and of higher attenuation than fat. Rim enhancement is seen after intravenous contrast administration (Steiner et al. 1996). A possible communication with the joint can be difficult to define on axial images.

2.1.7 MRI

MR imaging demonstrates the exact location and extent of the cystic lesion and its relationship to the joint and surrounding structures (Fig. 2). The diagnosis of a cystic mass is usually straightforward by analysis of the signal intensities of the lesion. They are typically hypo- or iso-intense to muscle on T1-weighted images and homogeneously hyperintense on T2-weighted images. However, there are some pitfalls. For example, atypical cyst content due to debris or hemorrhage may alter the imaging appearance of the cysts. Chronic inflammation may cause marked thickening of the synovial membrane and, therefore, mimic a solid soft-tissue mass. Cystic lesions are well-circumscribed but may be lobulated or multicystic with internal septae. A communicating neck with the adjacent joint may be visible. Ruptured cysts, due to an elevated pressure, are irregularly delineated and must be differentiated from other soft-tissue tumors and hemorrhagic or inflammatory lesions.

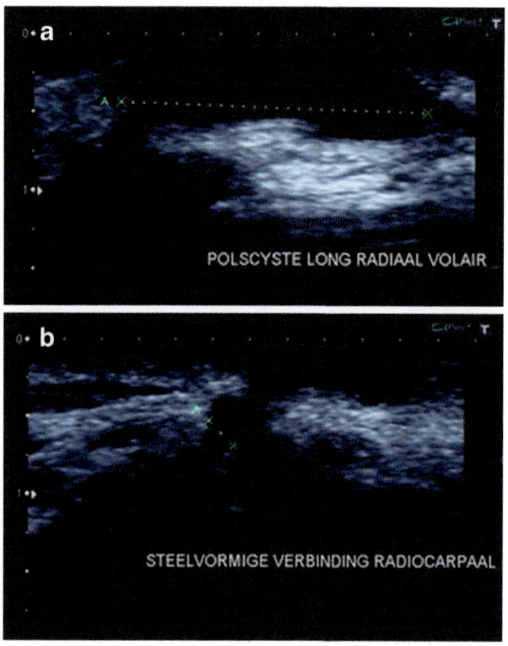

Fig. 1 Ganglion cyst. Longitudinal ultrasound (**a**) shows a well-defined anechoic structure at the palmar aspect of the carpus; (**b**) shows a stalk-like connection with the adjacent radiocarpal joint

After gadolinium contrast administration, subtle rim enhancement of the peripheral fibrovascular tissue in the cyst wall is seen, but there is never central enhancement unlike in other well-delineated soft-tissue lesions with high signal intensity on T2-weighted images such as myxoma, myxoid liposarcoma, hemangioma, synovial sarcoma, and mucinosis.

Although not true ganglion cysts, it is worth noting that mucoid cysts of the distal interphalangeal (DIP) joints are common and are associated with osteoarthritis and marginal osteophytes (Heberden's nodes) (Fig. 4). While not truly ganglion cysts, they share similar characteristics and are often treated similarly.

Small rents in a joint capsule allow accumulation of synovial fluid in the ganglion. Ganglion cysts of dorsal wrist arise from scapholunate joint, whereas volar ganglion cysts arise from radio-scapholunate interval and scaphotrapezial joint. Retinacular cysts along the flexor tendon sheaths originate from the A1 and A2 pulley (Jebson and Spencer 2007).

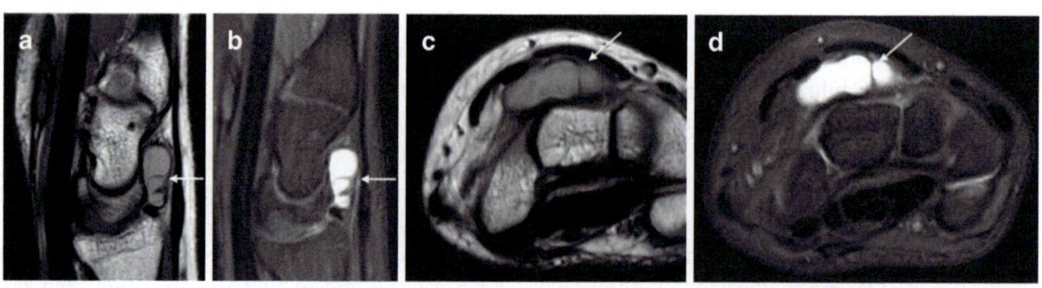

Fig. 2 Sagittal PD (**a**), PDFS (**b**), axial PD (**c**), and PDFS (**d**) showing dorsal wrist ganglion (arrows)

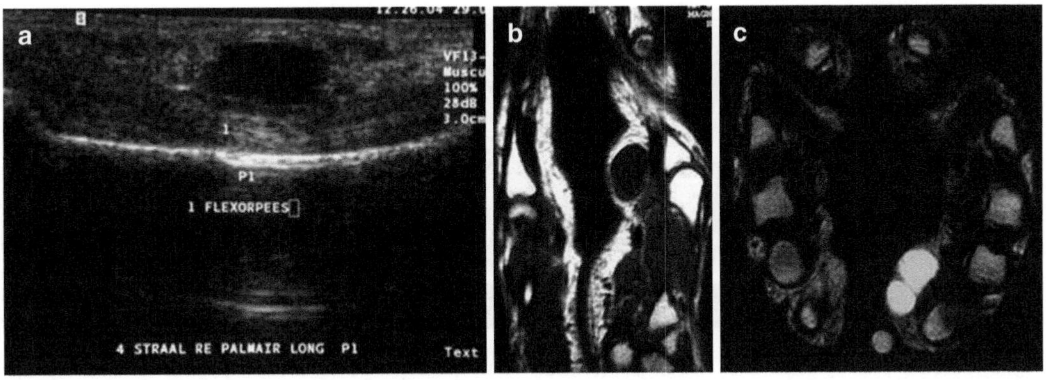

Fig. 3 Cyst of the tendon sheath. (**a**) Longitudinal ultrasound showing a well-delineated sonolucent structure on the course of the flexor tendon of right fourth finger. (**b**) Sagittal SE T1-weighted image. (**c**) Axial TSE T2-weighted image in another patient with a tendon sheath cyst of the flexor tendon. The lesion is isointense to muscle on T1-weighted images (**b**) and hyperintense on T2-weighted images (**c**)

Fig. 4 Sagittal T1 (**a**), STIR (**b**), axial T1 (**c**), and STIR (**d**) showing mucinous cyst (arrow) in relation to the dorsal aspect of the DIPJ

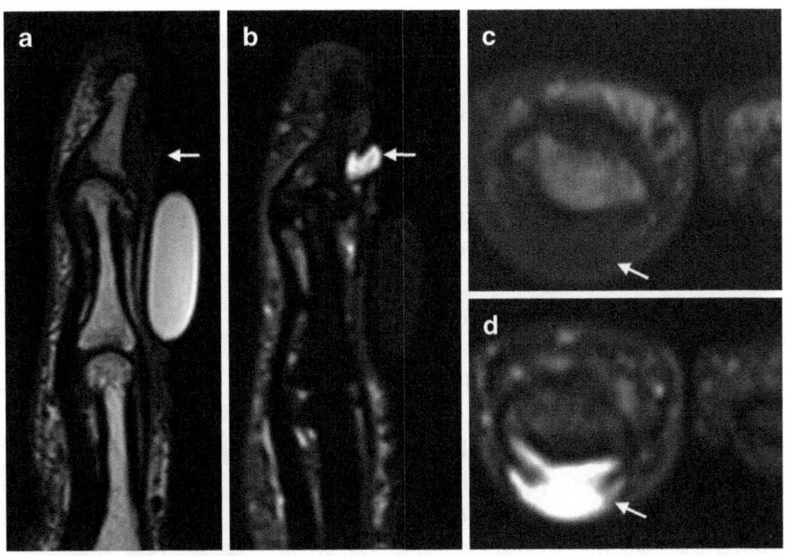

2.2 Epidermoid Cyst

2.2.1 Definition and Histopathology

An epidermoid cyst, also known as epidermal inclusion cyst or infundibular cyst, results from the proliferation of surface epidermal cells within the dermis. The lesion is typically located within the subcutaneous tissue and is often secondary to trauma where epithelial tissue can implant itself into soft tissue or bone (Rajakulasingam et al. 2019a). It is more frequently seen in men than in women (Nahra and Bucchieri 2004).

Macroscopically, the lesion is filled with keratin (Ergun et al. 2010). The walls of the cyst resemble follicular epithelium (Murphy and Elder 1991). The cyst wall may rupture with secondary foreign body-type reaction, granulomatous reaction, granulation tissue, or abscess formation (Murphy and Elder 1991; Jin et al. 2008).

2.2.2 Imaging

On plain radiographs, epidermal cysts may be located in the subcutaneous tissue or within the bone (most frequently at the terminal phalanges

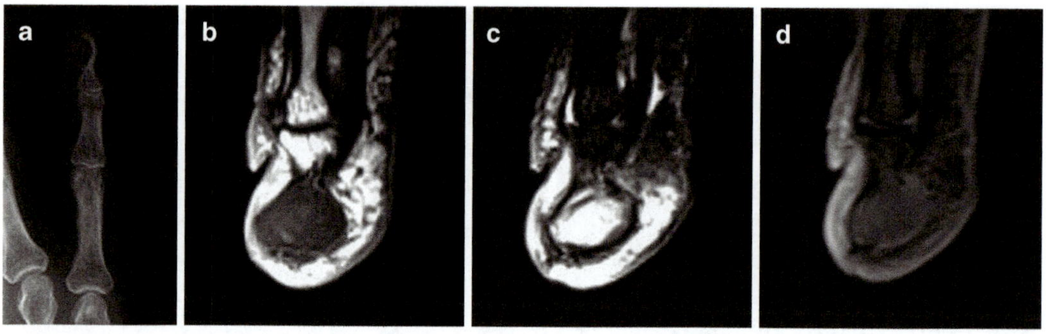

Fig. 5 Subcutaneous epidermoid cyst with involvement of the adjacent bone of the terminal phalanx of the right fifth finger. (**a**) Plain radiograph showing a well-defined osteolytic defect at the radial side of the distal phalanx. Note cortical destruction of the radial cortex. (**b**) Coronal SE T1-weighted image. The lesion is of intermediate signal intensity with some internal areas of relatively high signal. (**c**) Coronal TSE T2-weighted image. High signal intensity of the lesion. (**d**) Coronal SE T1-weighted image after intravenous injection of gadolinium contrast. There is only subtle peripheral enhancement of the lesion. (Case courtesy of C. Kenis, Antwerp)

of the fingers). Lesions located within the dermis may cause well-defined remodeling of the adjacent bone (Fig. 5a).

Ultrasound is more sensitive than clinical examination for the diagnosis of an epidermoid cyst (after palpation, 93.5%; after ultrasonography, 99.3%) (Kuwano et al. 2009). The lesion is usually well defined. Echogenicity varies with the content of the cyst. The lesions are usually hypoechoic, with posterior acoustic enhancement. Large lesions may show intralesional hyperechoic debris or keratin clusters (Fig. 6) (Gielen et al. 2006). Rupture of the cysts may result in changes in shapes (either lobulations, protrusions, or abscess pocket formations), pericystic changes, and increased vascularity on power Doppler ultrasound (Jin et al. 2008).

In the case of epidermoid inclusion cysts occurring in the fingertips, there may be bony involvement in which the cyst erodes into the bone causing a lytic lesion within the distal phalanx. Cortical destruction and osteolysis may mimic a malignant or infectious process (Nahra and Bucchieri 2004).

On CT and MRI, the lesion is well defined. MRI features depend on the chemical composition of cholesterol and keratin content. Lesions with a high lipid content are hyperintense on both pulse sequences, whereas a crystalline form of cholesterol and the presence of keratin and microcalcifications may result in a low signal on T2-weighted images. After administration of intravenous gadolinium contrast, there is no enhancement in noncomplicated epidermoid cysts (Fig. 5b–d) (Ergun et al. 2010).

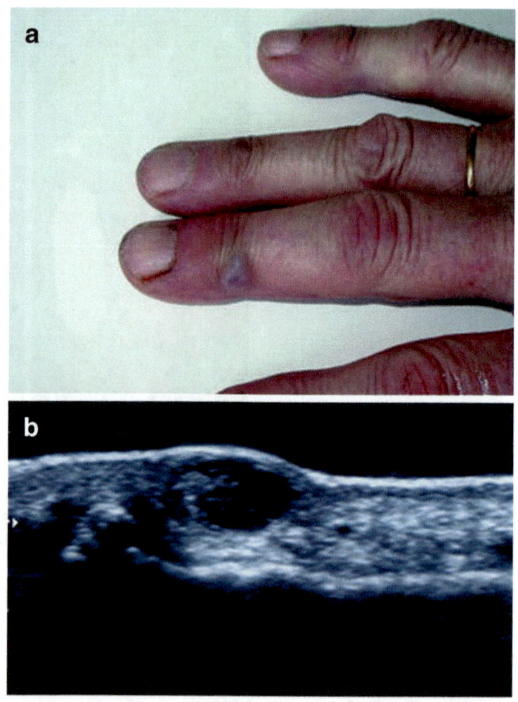

Fig. 6 Subcutaneous epidermoid cyst. (**a**) Clinical picture showing a small soft-tissue lesion with bluish skin discoloration at the third finger. (**b**) Longitudinal ultrasound showing a well-defined subcutaneous lesion with variable echogenicity (anechoic components and some internal hyperechoic debris)

Pilomatrixoma is a benign tumor that originates from the cortex of a hair follicle. It is most common in children under 2 years old but can occur at any age, typically in the head and neck region or extremities. On ultrasound, it appears as a well-defined, oval, hypoechoic mass with internal matrix calcification, often in a scattered dot pattern (Choo et al. 2010), and with a hypoechoic peripheral rim representing a connective tissue capsule. It may exhibit posterior acoustic shadowing and intermediate internal vascularity in 50% of cases. In contrast, an epidermoid cyst (a potential differential diagnosis) typically shows internal anechoic cysts, linear hyperechoic strands, posterior acoustic enhancement, a laminated concentric ring "target" pattern, and a pseudotestis appearance (Huang et al. 2011) but lacks internal vascularity.

2.3 Lipoma

2.3.1 Definition

Lipomas are well-encapsulated masses composed of mature adipose cells. They are the most frequently encountered benign lipomatous lesions of the hand (Peh et al. 1995; Ergun et al. 2010).

2.3.2 Clinical Findings

Lipomas are most frequently located under the skin (superficial lipoma) but can also be seen in muscles (often within thenar or hypothenar muscles), bones, and tendons (deep seated lipoma) (Peh et al. 1995; Ergun et al. 2010), rarely intra-articularly (Mettu et al. 2024) and intrasynovial lipoma of flexors of fingers (Vidoni et al. 2020). The lesions are usually asymptomatic but may occasionally compress adjacent nerves, vessels, or tendons (Peh et al. 1995). Most frequently, lipoma affects patients in the fifth to sixth decade of life (De Beuckeleer et al. 2001).

2.3.3 Imaging

Radiographs are usually normal, but a low to intermediate density may be seen in larger lesions (Murphey et al. 2004).

On ultrasound, superficial lipomas have an elongated shape and are usually parallel to the skin. Intramuscular lesions are often more difficult to distinguish from the surrounding muscle fibers. The reflectivity is highly variable ranging from hypo- to hyper-reflective compared to subcutaneous fat.

CT shows a homogeneous mass with low density (−60 to −130 HU). Intramuscular lesions may contain thin fibromuscular septa. There is no significant contrast enhancement.

On MRI, the lesion has similar signal characteristics to subcutaneous fat on all pulse sequences. Fat-suppression techniques show homogeneous suppression. Minor (<2 mm) internal septa and a low signal intensity capsule may be seen. After administration of intravenous gadolinium contrast, there is no contrast enhancement, except for the peripheral fibrous capsule or the subtle internal septa (Fig. 7) (Ergun et al. 2010).

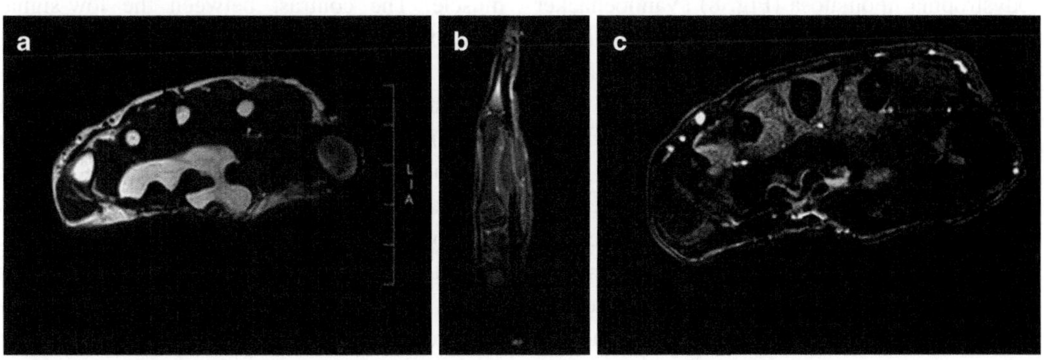

Fig. 7 Deep-seated lipoma of the hand in a 43-year-old women. (**a**) Axial SE T1-weighted image. Note the presence of a dumbbell shaped mass at the flexor compartment of the hand. The lesion is well defined and isointense to subcutaneous fat. (**b**) Sagittal fatsuppressed TSE T2-weighted image. There is homogeneous fat suppression of the lesion. (**c**) Axial fatsuppressed SE T1-weighted image after intravenous injection of gadolinium contrast. There is absence of enhancement of the lesion

2.4 Lipomatosis of Nerve

2.4.1 Definition

Lipomatosis of nerve has also been termed previously as fibrolipomatous hamartoma, fibrofatty overgrowth, lipomatous hamartoma, lipofibroma, neurolipoma, intraneural lipoma, fatty infiltration of the nerve, and neural fibrolipoma. In 2002, the WHO adopted the designation of "lipomatosis of nerve" (Christopher et al. 2002). It is a very rare tumor, characterized by a proliferation of fatty and fibrous components that surround the thickened nerve bundles and infiltrates both the epineurium and the perineurium. The cause is unknown, but some consider this condition as a congenital lesion since it is occasionally present at birth, whereas others believe there is a causative relationship with prior trauma.

2.4.2 Clinical Findings

This tumor affects predominantly children or young adults. Males are affected more frequently than females

Lipomatosis of nerve occurs chiefly in the volar aspects of the hands, wrist, and forearm and usually involves the median nerve. A soft-tissue mass is frequently present for several years before onset of symptoms. Lipomatosis of nerve usually gives rise to pain, paresthesia, or decreased sensation or muscle strength in the area innervated by the affected nerves. It may be associated with bone overgrowth and macrodactyly of the fingers, a condition described as macrodystrophia lipomatosa (Fig. 8) (Vanhoenacker et al. 2005, 2006a, b). Intraneural lipoma can cause radiculopathy-like pain posing a diagnostic dilemma (Jeyaraman et al. 2023)

2.4.3 Imaging

On plain radiographs, lipomatosis of nerve may manifest as a soft-tissue mass or only be suspected by indirect signs such as the presence of macrodactyly, usually affecting the second and third digits of the hand. There is soft-tissue and osseous hypertrophy including long, broad, and splayed phalanges (Fig. 9).

CT and MRI can identify the nervous origin of the tumor due to the presence of tortuous tubular structures, corresponding to enlarged nerve bundles within a predominantly fatty mass (Fig. 7). These structures, clearly depicted on MRI, show low signal intensity on both T1- and T2-weighted images according to their fibrous content. The tumor tends to spread along the branches of the nerve with a significant variation in the distribution of fat along the nerves and their innervated muscle. The contrast between the low-signal nerve fascicles and surrounding high-signal fat results in a "co-axial cable-like" appearance of the tumor when visualized on axial planes on T1-weighted MR images (Fig. 10) and a "spaghetti-like" appearance on coronal planes (Shirodkar et al. 2025). The MR imaging findings of lipomatosis of nerve are very characteristic, obviating the need for biopsy (Marom and Helms 1999). Lipomatosis of nerve must be differentiated from a nerve sheath lipoma associated with altered sensibility along the course of some nerves. MRI allows differentiation between these two entities since lipoma manifests as a focal mass separated from the nerve bundles.

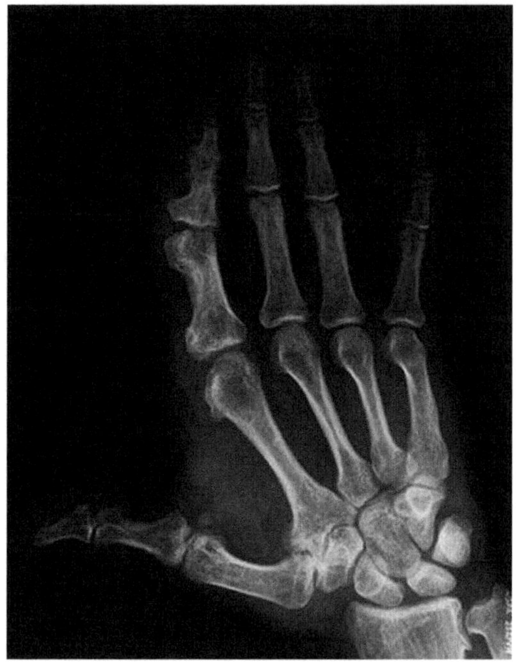

Fig. 8 Macrodystophia lipomatosa. Posterioanterior radiograph of the right hand. Note osseous and soft-tissue enlargement affecting the second finger

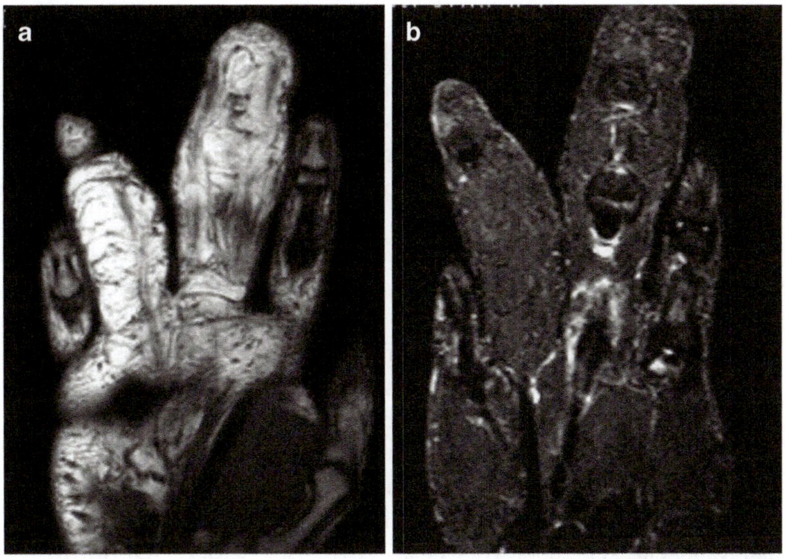

Fig. 9 T1 (**a**) and STIR (**b**) coronal showing classic lipomatous macrodystrophy

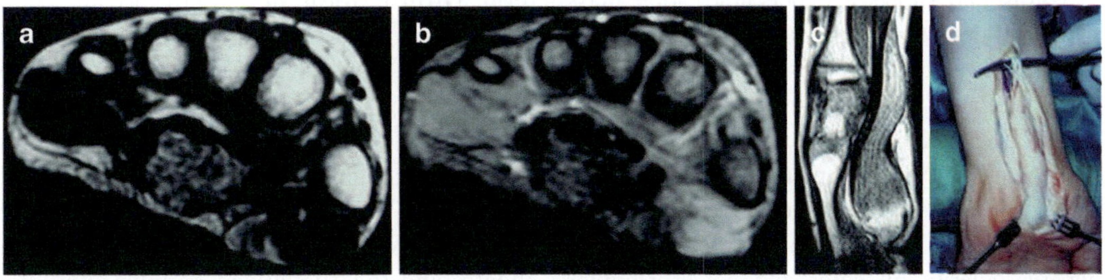

Fig. 10 Lipomatosis of nerve of the median nerve at the level of the carpal tunnel in a 40-year-old man. (**a**) Axial SE T1-weighted MR image. (**b**) Axial gradient echo T2*-weighted MR image. (**c**) Sagittal SE T1-weighted MR image and corresponding preoperative view (**d**) of the median nerve. A heterogeneous mass is seen within the carpal tunnel. There is a mixed signal intensity of fatty components, fibrous components, and neural fascicles (**a–c**). The signal intensity and localization are highly characteristic of lipomatosis of the median nerve. Note fusiform thickening of the median nerve with a cable-like appearance (**d**)

2.5 Giant Cell Tumor of Tendon Sheath (GCTTS)

2.5.1 Definition

Tenosynovial giant cell tumors (GCT)/tenosynovial tumors of tendon sheath are fibrohistiocytic tumors typically benign tumors that originate from the synovium of joints, bursae, or tendon sheaths (Sbaraglia et al. 2020). Despite having the similar histological characteristics, there are two distinct subtypes: (1) localized form and (2) diffused form of GCT that differ in their clinical presentation and require different treatment approaches (Bansal et al. 2021; Jeong et al. 2023). GCTTS are benign proliferative lesions of synovial origin. In the hand and the wrist, this is the second most common soft-tissue lesion after a ganglion cyst. The pathogenesis remains unclear but is probably due to a reactive inflammatory process. GCTTS may arise from the tendon sheath, joint capsule, bursae, fascia, or ligaments (Nguyon et al. 2004; Peh et al. 1995). Histologically, they are composed of histiocytes, macrophages, multinucleated giant cells, and hemosiderin due to repeated hemorrhage (Nguyon et al. 2004; Peh et al. 1995; Wan et al. 2010).

2.5.2 Clinical Findings

The lesions are more common in the fingers than in the wrist and palm. The most affected site is the volar aspect of the first three digits (Ushijima et al. 1986). They are usually well-circumscribed firm masses that grow slowly and are typically painless. If located near a joint, they may cause decreased joint motion (Capelastegui et al. 1999).

2.5.3 Imaging

Standard radiography may be normal or display a well-circumscribed soft-tissue mass in about half of the patients. Pressure erosions at the underlying bone are present in about 20% of patients, while periosteal reaction, calcifications, and cystic changes are extremely unusual (De Beuckeleer and Vanhoenacker 2006; Wan et al. 2010; De Schepper et al. 2007).

Ultrasound shows a hypoechoic, solid mass with well-defined margins usually located near tendons (Fig. 11). Bone erosions due to pressure of the tumor on the cortex may be demonstrated as well. The tendon usually exhibits normal shape and echogenicity. Contrary to ganglia, the giant cell tumor lacks posterior acoustic enhancement, presents always with internal echoes, and shows hypervascularity on color and power Doppler imaging (Wan et al. 2010).

MR images typically show a well-defined mass adjacent to or enveloping a tendon, with a signal intensity similar to or less than that of skeletal muscle on T1-weighted images. On T2-weighted images, the signal intensity is predominantly low, with a variable degree of heterogeneity. Blooming artifact is seen on gradient-echo sequences due to the presence of hemosiderin (Wan et al. 2010). GCTTS usually enhance after gadolinium contrast administration (Fig. 12).

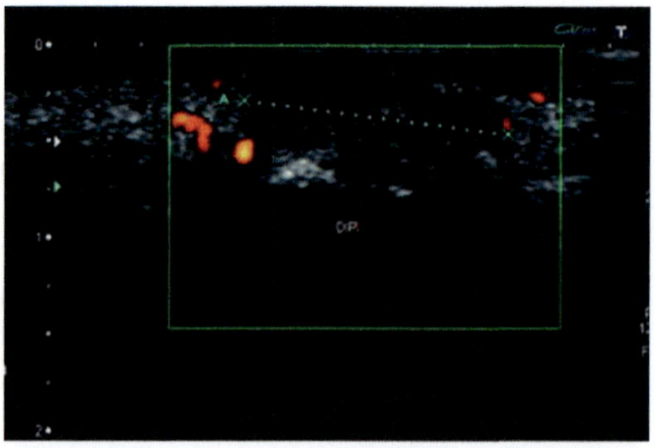

Fig. 11 Giant cell tumor of the tendon sheath. Longitudinal ultrasound showing a well-defined hypoechoic mass adjacent to the flexor tendon. There is increased Doppler signal at the periphery of the lesion

Fibroma of the tendon sheath may have a similar presentation as GCTTS on MR imaging (Sect. 2.10), but it lacks giant cells (Nguyon et al. 2004).

2.6 Pigmented Villonodular Synovitis

2.6.1 Definition

The 2020 WHO classification uses the term Diffuse form of "Tenosynovial giant cell tumor" to describe this condition, with "Giant cell tumor of tendon sheath" also being acceptable (Sbaraglia et al. 2020). Previously, it was known by other names such as pigmented villonodular tumor of the tendon sheath PVNTS, extra-articular pigmented villonodular tumor of the tendon sheath, and focal/localized nodular synovitis (Nepal et al. 2019), but term PVNS is no longer recommended (Nepal et al. 2019).

PVNS is a benign, rare monoarticular arthropathy that usually occurs between the ages of 20 and 50 with a peak incidence between the third and the fourth decades of life. There is no sex predilection. Occasionally it is polyarticular.

It usually involves the knee (80%) or the hip, while the ankle, elbow, shoulder, and wrist are less frequent locations.

2.6.2 Clinical Findings

The clinical picture is characterized by the insidious onset of monoarticular swelling in young adults, stiffness, and progressive pain. Symptoms tend to be continuous, but exacerbations occur from time to time. Aspirated synovial fluid is typically xanthochromic or serosanguineous.

Tenosynovial giant cell tumor, formerly known as PVNS, can be focal or diffuse and can be intra-articular or extra-articular

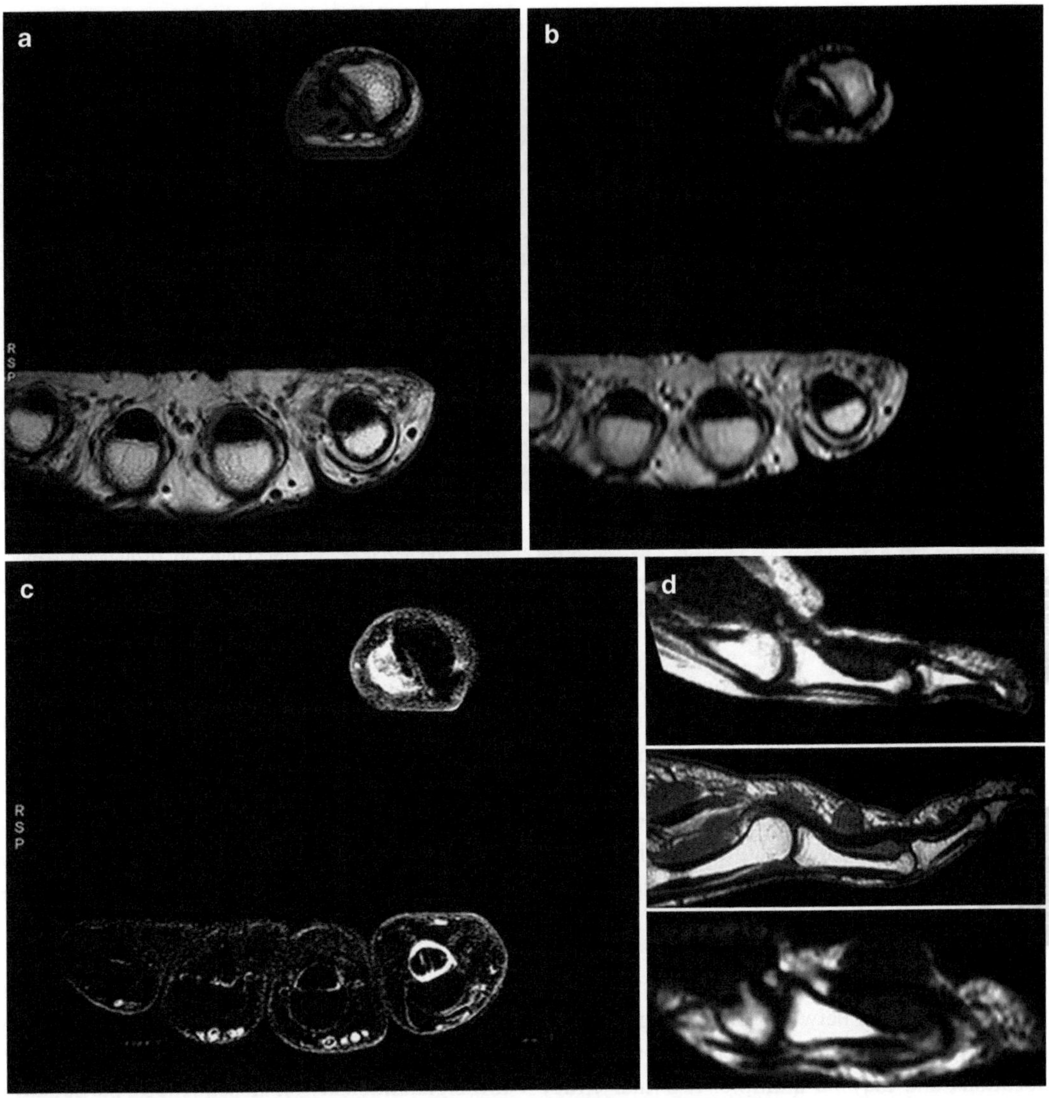

Fig. 12 Giant cell tumor of the tendon sheath. (**a**) Axial SE T1-weighted image. A hypointense structure surrounds the flexor tendons of the thumb. (**b**) Axial TSE T2-weighted image. The lesion is of low signal intensity. (**c**) Axial SE T1-weighted image after intravenous injection of gadolinium contrast (subtraction image). There is marked inhomogeneous enhancement of the lesion. (**d**) Sagittal SE T1-weighted image in another patient with a giant cell tumor of tendon sheath. A hypointense structure is surrounding the flexor tendon, which is a typical location for a GCTTS

(Rajakulasingam et al. 2019b) Microscopically, the lesions are composed of solid or finger-like masses of hyperplastic synovium with multinucleated giant cells, xanthoma cells, and intra-and extracellular hemosiderin, all lying in a fibrous stroma. Long-standing lesions show fibrosis and hyalinization.

When the villi become matted together, clefts lined by synovial cells are seen and may give an appearance alarmingly similar to synovial sarcoma.

2.6.3 Imaging Findings

Conventional radiographs may be normal or show a nonspecific periarticular soft-tissue mass and associated joint effusion. Visible calcifications are extremely unusual. The presence of calcifications should suggest an alternative diagnosis

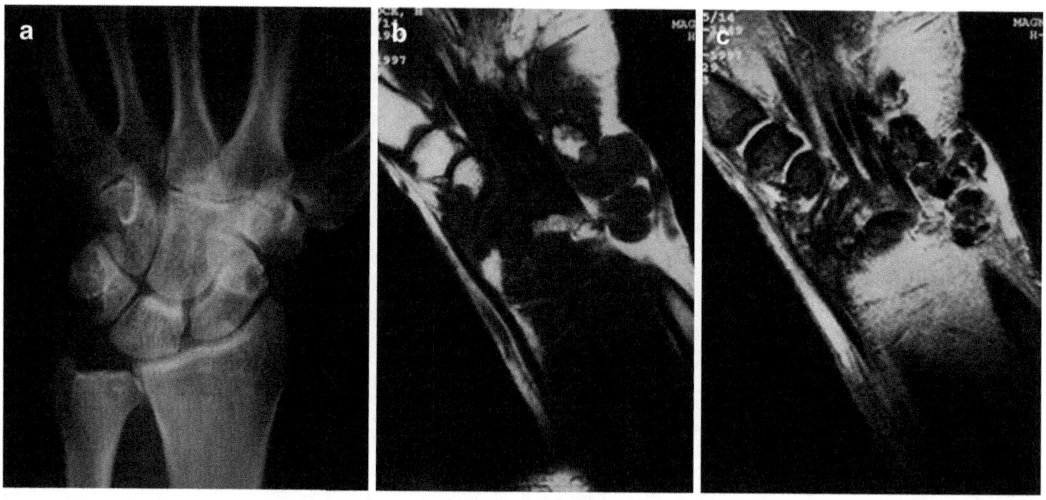

Fig. 13 Pigmented villonodular synovitis. (**a**) Plain radiograph of the left wrist. There are multiple erosions at the distal aspect of the scaphoid bone and at the proximal aspect of the triquetral bone. (**b**) Coronal SE T1-weighted image. The lesion is located intra-articularly within the wrist joint and is of low signal intensity (isointense to muscle). Note also erosions at the carpal bones. (**c**) Coronal gradient T2* image showing blooming artifact of the lesion

such as synovial osteochondromatosis. Despite the absence of calcification in this, high iron content may be present within the synovium, producing a higher radiodensity than adjacent joint effusion or soft tissue. Associated bone erosions (Fig. 13a) with sclerotic margins may be present on both sides of the affected joints, particularly in joints with a tight capsule, such as the wrist. These erosive changes are probably due to a pressure phenomenon resulting from entrapment of soft-tissue masses between articulating surfaces. These lesions are usually present in nonmarginal locations and may be multiple. If solitary, they may mimic primary osteolytic bone neoplasms. The preservation of the articular space until late in the disease and the absence of peri-articular osteopenia are helpful in the differential diagnosis from an inflammatory synovitis. Retained or neglected foreign bodies surrounding joints may mimic PVNS (Kumar et al. 2024).

Ultrasonography shows a heterogeneous mass lesion. Sometimes, related enlarged synovial cysts or bursae with internal septa are noted.

CT is able to sharply define lytic bone lesions associated with PVNS. Associated intraosseous soft-tissue masses extending with a narrow pedicle to the synovium are easily visualized. Joint effusion is atypical and the tumoral mass itself is also not as characteristic as on MR imaging. Sometimes a high attenuation tissue is identified within the joint due to the presence of hemosiderin. The differential diagnosis includes calcification and iron deposition in the joint due to hemophilia or chronic bleeding and calcification. Enhancement after intravenous contrast administration appears to be the rule.

The MR appearance of PVNS is quite characteristic due to the presence of hemosiderin within the synovial masses. A heterogeneous, hyperplastic synovial process with significant areas of low signal intensity on all sequences, particularly T2-weighted images, is typical. The presence of hemosiderin causes local changes in susceptibility and therefore loss of MR signal. This is especially true for gradient-echo sequences and at high field strengths. This decreased signal intensity is most prominent in the periphery of the lesions (the so-called "blooming" artifact) (Fig. 13b, c). Figures 13 and 14 show tenosynovial giant cell tumor (formerly PVNS) of the flexor tendons). Occasionally, intralesional areas of high signal intensity on both pulse sequences may be present due to fat, edema, or inflammation. Joint effusion appears as hyperintense areas entrapped between the low signal intensity areas on T2-weighted images.

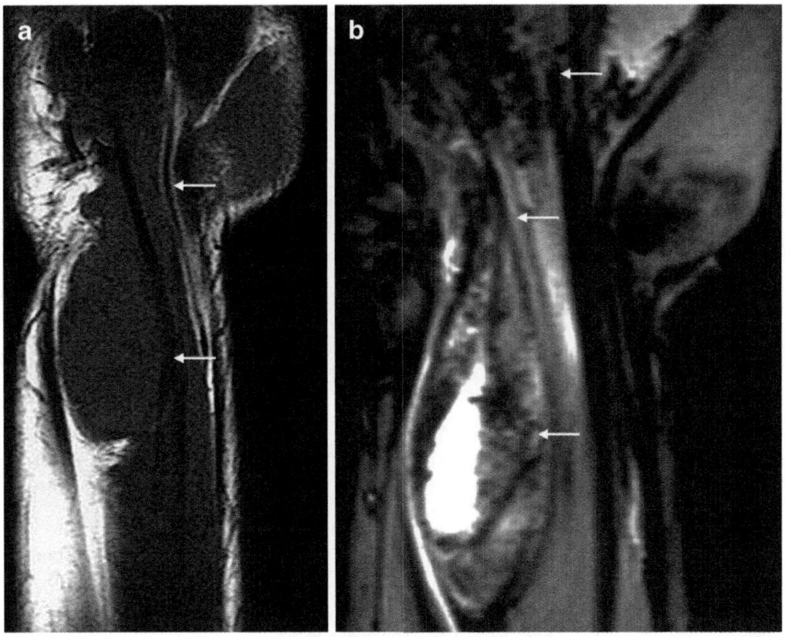

Fig. 14 Coronal T1 (**a**) and T2 (**b**) showing extensive PVNS of the flexor tendons (arrow)

After gadolinium contrast administration, homogeneous or septal enhancement may be observed. The differential diagnosis on MR imaging includes other causes of chronic hemarthrosis such as chronic trauma, hemophilia, synovial hemangioma and "burnt out" rheumatoid pannus, and amyloid arthropathy. These disorders can be separated on the basis of clinical history, laboratory findings, and enhancement pattern. In hemophilia, there are usually diffuse changes in cartilage and bone including cartilaginous and subchondral erosions as well as joint space narrowing. Synovial chondromatosis can simulate PVNS on MR, and in general this is true for all low signal intensity masses with calcified or ossified components. This should not pose an issue since these areas are well recognized on plain films and CT. Synovial chondromatosis and Tophaceous gout may also mimic PVNS if there is a high concentration of calcium within the tophus, with exception in the initial stages on Radiography wherein calcification is not pronounced (Eurorad.org n.d.). Finally, desmoid tumors, benign fibrous histiocytoma, and sclerosing hemangioma could be mistaken for PVNS due to their low signal on MR imaging given their dense fibrous content. The lack of intra-articular changes should alert one to consider another diagnosis besides pigmented villonodular synovitis.

MR is the imaging technique of choice to evaluate the possible extra-articular extension and areas of the joint which are difficult to see arthroscopically.

2.7 Vascular Tumors and Lymphatic Tumors

2.7.1 Definition

Vascular tumors and malformations in the hand can be categorized into two main types: low-flow and high-flow lesions. Low-flow malformations include venous malformations (VMs), capillary malformations (CMs), and lymphatic or veno-lymphatic malformations (LMs or VLMs) (Cox et al. 2014). These lesions are typically characterized by a soft-tissue mass that may be painful, especially with activity or cold weather, and may have a bluish tint (AbuMoussa et al. 2023). VMs often increase in size when the arm is in a dependent position and decrease in size when the arm is elevated. High-flow lesions, such as arteriovenous malformations (AVMs), are often warm,

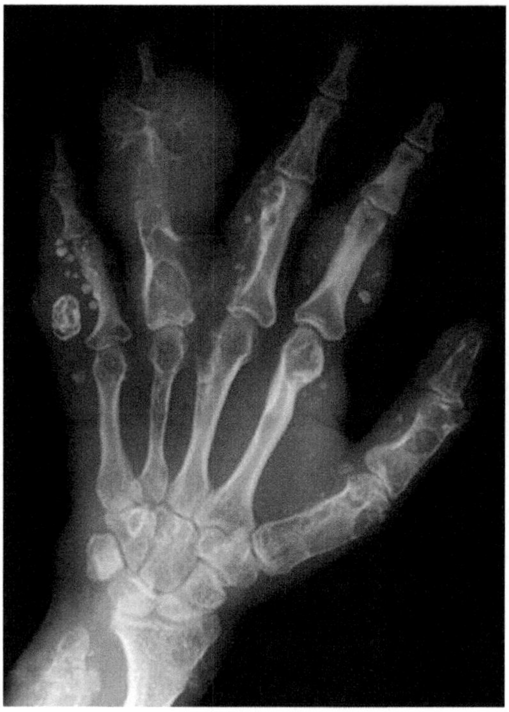

Fig. 15 Maffucci syndrome. Plain radiograph of the left hand. Note multiple enchondromas and soft-tissue hemangiomas with intralesional phleboliths

pulsatile masses with associated bruits and thrills due to arterialized blood flow through engorged veins.

In radiology literature and clinical practice historically, the term "hemangioma" has been used to describe venous malformations. Benign vascular tumors are common benign soft-tissue masses, which include localized hemangioma and diffuse angiomatosis. Klippel-Trénaunay syndrome is a separate entity in which hemangiomas are accompanied by unilateral hypertrophy of the extremity. Maffucci's syndrome consists of the combination of hemangiomas and enchondromatosis (Fig. 15). Semimalignant vascular tumors include hemangioendotheliomas (Nguyon et al. 2004; Peh et al. 1995; Ergun et al. 2010). Hemangiomas represent a broad spectrum of vascular tumors which may be classified by vessel size into capillary, cavernous, venous, or arteriovenous malformations (Ergun et al. 2010). Apart from vessels, the lesions contain variable amounts of nonvascular elements including thrombus, fat, fibrous tissue, bone, and muscular tissue (Nguyon et al. 2004; Schmitt 2008; Ergun et al. 2010). Lymphangiomas of hand are rare.

2.7.2 Clinical Findings

Vascular malformations may cause compression of nearby nerves, leading to paresthesia, pain, or weakness. Lymphatic malformations, on the other hand, have a classic rubbery texture and may have overlying skin dimpling. Capillary malformations present as red or pink cutaneous discolorations, commonly referred to as port-wine stains (AbuMoussa et al. 2023).

Most hemangiomas are asymptomatic, but they may present at an early age secondary to cosmetic deformity or pain. Women are more affected than men with incidence peaking in early adulthood. A familial disposition may occur (Schmitt 2008). The hand is frequently affected. The cutaneous and subcutaneous compartments are often involved and there is frequently an overlying skin discoloration (Fig. 16a). Less often, the lesion is found in tendon sheaths (Fig. 16), muscles, or the median nerve (Nguyon et al. 2004; Schmitt 2008). Figure 17 shows vascular malformation of dorsal aspect of wrist.

Capillary hemangiomas are most frequent and are usually located in the skin and subcutaneous tissue. Clinically, they are characterized as port-wine spot lesions. Because of the superficial location, the diagnosis is often made clinically and imaging is rarely required.

Conversely, venous hemangiomas typically involve the deep structures (Ergun et al. 2010).

2.7.3 Imaging

Radiographs often provide little information. Phleboliths are sometimes seen (Fig. 17). Linear or arciform calcifications are less common (Nguyon et al. 2004; Schmitt 2008). Adjacent osseous remodeling can occur (Fig. 18a) including erosion, overgrowth, periosteal reaction, and osteoporosis (Nguyon et al. 2004).

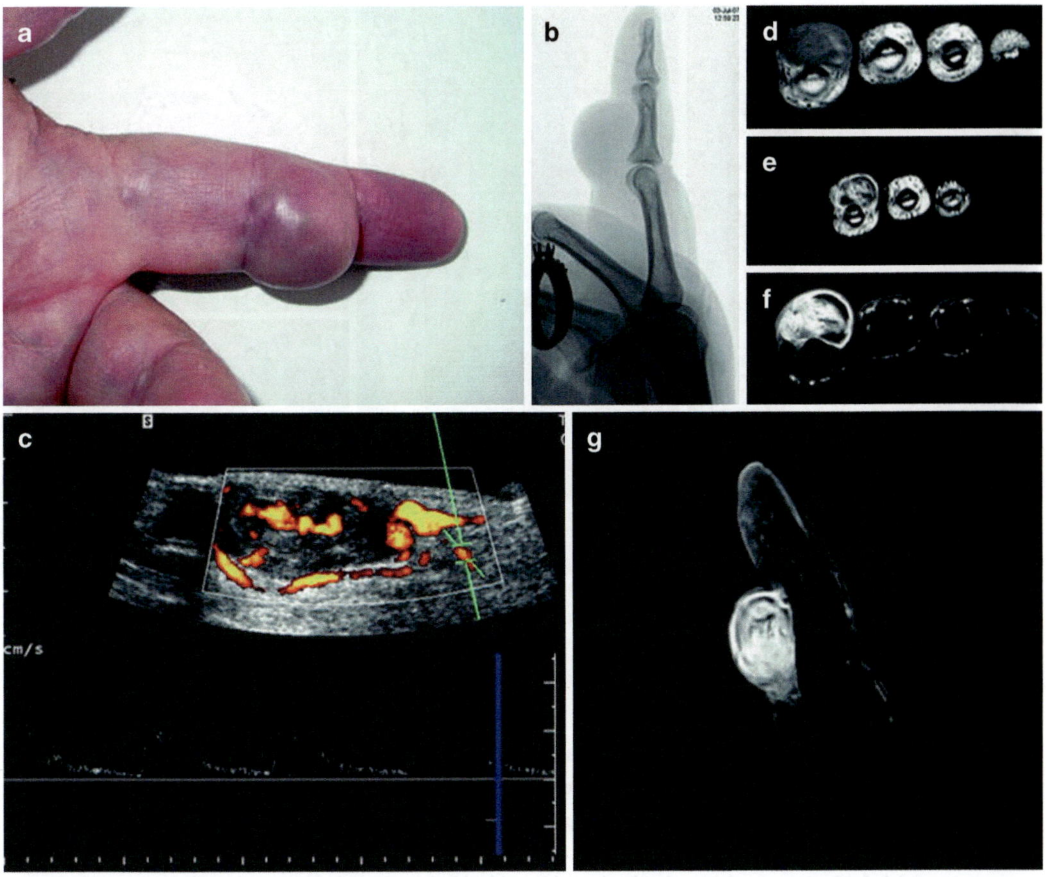

Fig. 16 Partially thrombosed arteriovenous malformation adjacent to the flexor tendon. (**a**) Clinical image showing a soft-tissue mass at the palmar aspect of the index. There is bluish discoloration of the overlying skin. (**b**) Plain radiograph (lateral view) demonstrates a nonspecific soft-tissue mass at the palmar aspect of the index. (**c**) Longitudinal ultrasound showing an oval shaped hypoechoic structure with increased intralesional power Doppler signal and an arterial feeder at the proximal side of the lesion. (**d**) Axial T1-weighted images shows that the lesion is of heterogeneous signal intensity. Areas of high signal intensity may correspond to thrombosis. (**e**) Axial TSE T2-weighted image. The lesion is heterogeneous with areas of high and low signal intensity. (**f, g**) Axial and sagittal fat-suppressed T1-weighted images after intravenous injection of gadolinium contrast. There is heterogeneous enhancement of the lesion. Areas of nonenhancement may correspond to thrombosis of vascular structures

On ultrasound, hemangiomas have a variable appearance, presenting as circumscribed or diffuse, homogeneous, or inhomogeneous lesions. Doppler reveals blood flow within the lesion (Fig. 18c) (Nguyon et al. 2004).

On MRI, arteriovenous malformation often appears as an enlarged vascular channel without a discrete soft-tissue mass (Ergun et al. 2010).

Cavernous hemangiomas are well-circumscribed lobulated masses which are usually isointense to muscle on T1-weighted images, with variable areas of interspersed hyperintense fat (Fig. 18b). On T2-weighted sequences, the lesion is heterogeneously hyperintense (Fig. 18c), as a result of the mixed amounts of fat and pooled blood in larger vessels. Thrombotic vessel segments have different signal intensities depending on the age of thrombosis. Fast blood flow generally causes a flow void with a dark lumen, whereas a slow or stagnant flow in dilated or tor-

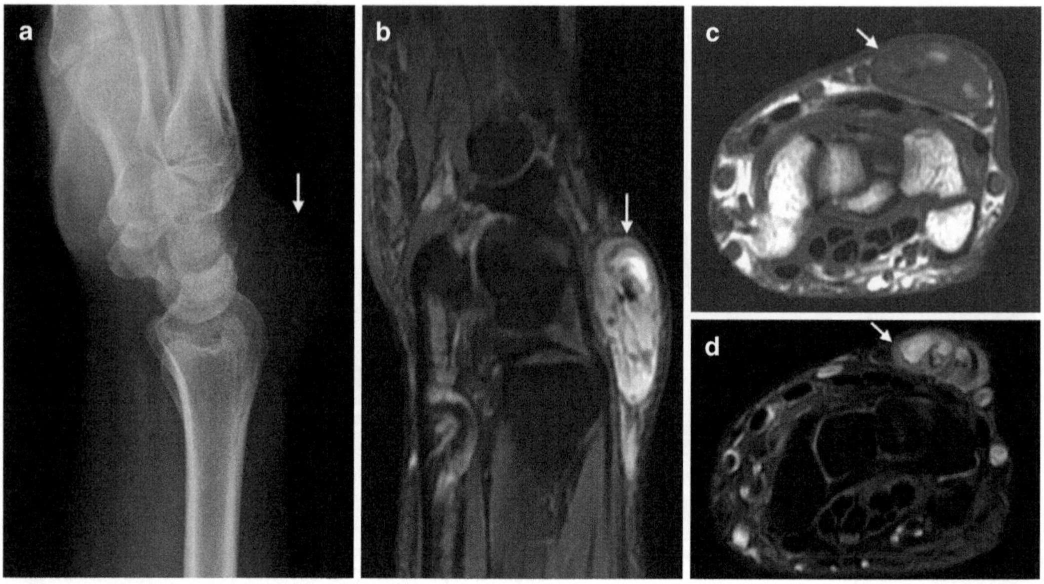

Fig. 17 Lateral radiograph (**a**), sagittal T2 fat suppressed (**b**), axial T1 (**c**), STIR (**d**) showing vascular malformation in relation to the dorsal aspect of wrist (arrow)

tuous vessels can cause increased signal ("paradoxical enhancement"). Linear or serpiginous flow voids with round filing defects may be demonstrated on both pulse sequences, indicating the presence of high-flow vessels and phleboliths (Fig. 19). Smaller cavernous hemangiomas are more likely to have an atypical appearance (Nguyon et al. 2004).

After intravenous injection of gadolinium contrast, occasionally the arterial feeders and draining veins may be seen both on CT- (Fig. 20) and MR Angiography. Delayed imaging after a few minutes allows evaluation of the precise extent of the tumor (Schmitt 2008) (Fig. 13d, e).

On CT, lymphangiomas usually have a negative attenuation due to high lipid content of the lymphatic fluid.

On T1-weighted MR images, the lesion is of intermediate signal intensity and typically hyperintense on T2-weighted images.

2.8 Benign Neurogenic Tumors

2.8.1 Definition

The most frequent subtypes of neurogenic tumors in the hand and wrist are neurinomas (schwannomas) and neurofibromas.

Schwannomas originate from the Schwann cells surrounding the peripheral nerves. The lesions are eccentric to the nerve of origin and are surrounded by a capsule of connective tissue. A schwannoma originates usually from the deeper and broader nerves of the hand and wrist and is primarily located at the palmar side (Schmitt 2008; Ergun et al. 2010).

Neurofibromas cause diffuse thickening of the nerve sheath. The nerve fascicles run through the concentric tumor. The lesion involves the smaller cutaneous nerves and has no capsule. Neurofibromas occur as solitary lesions or in conjunction with von Recklinghausen disease (neurofibromatosis type I). Multiple schwan-

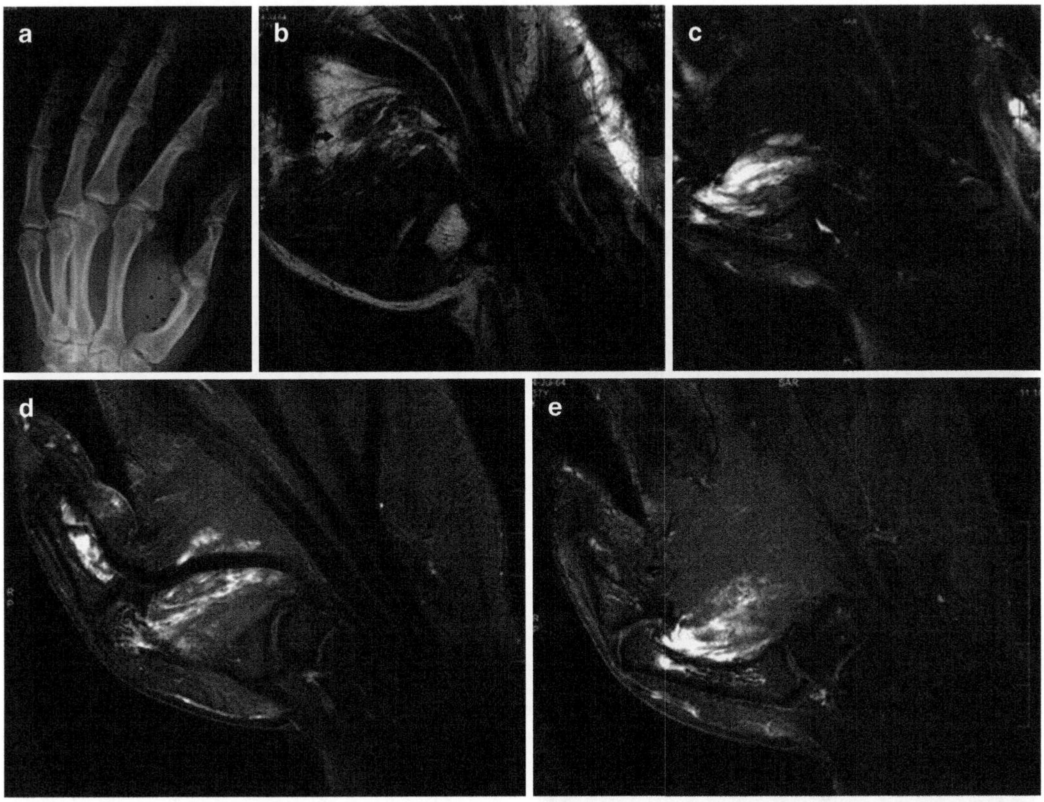

Fig. 18 Hemangioma of the thenar muscle. (**a**) Plain radiograph of the left hand. There is a nonspecific soft-tissue mass (asterisks), containing some streaks of fat and causing pressure erosion of the ulnar side of the first metacarpal and proximal phalanx of the thumb (*arrows*). (**b**) Coronal SE T1-weighted image shows a well-defined lobulated mass in the thenar muscle (*arrows*) with areas of interspersed fat. (**c**) Coronal fatsuppressed TSE T2-weighted image. The lesion is located within the thenar muscles and has a heterogeneous high signal intensity. There is also osseous remodeling of the ulnar side of the cortex of metacarpal 1. Note some streaks of high signal within the medullary bone of metacarpal 1, due to intra-osseous extension in the metacarpal bone. (**d**, **e**) Coronal SE fatsuppressed T1-weighted images after intravenous injection of gadolinium contrast. There is marked serpiginous enhancement of the intramuscular and intraosseous components of the lesion (metacarpal 1 and proximal phalanx of the thumb)

nomas as part of schwannomatosis is much more rare.

Traumatic neuroma is a non-neoplastic growth that occurs when a nerve is injured or transected, either partially or completely. It is characterized by the abnormal proliferation of nerve tissue at the site of injury in proximal segment of nerve in 1–12 months after the initial trauma. There are two types of traumatic neuromas: (1) spindle neuromas, which form around an intact nerve that has been chronically irritated, and (2) stump neuromas, which form at the end of a partially or completely severed nerve (Nepal et al. 2019).

2.8.2 Clinical Findings

Patients present with a palpable mass (Fig. 21a) and rarely complain of pain. Pain may be elicited by percussion of the mass (Hoffmann-Tinel sign).

2.8.3 Imaging Findings

Plain radiographs are usually normal, but paraosseous neurogenic tumors can cause scalloping of the adjacent bone.

On ultrasound, schwannomas are located eccentric to the surrounding nerve, whereas neurofibromas are concentric in relation to the affected nerve. The Hoffman-Tinel sign can be provoked by sonographic palpation of the affected nerve.

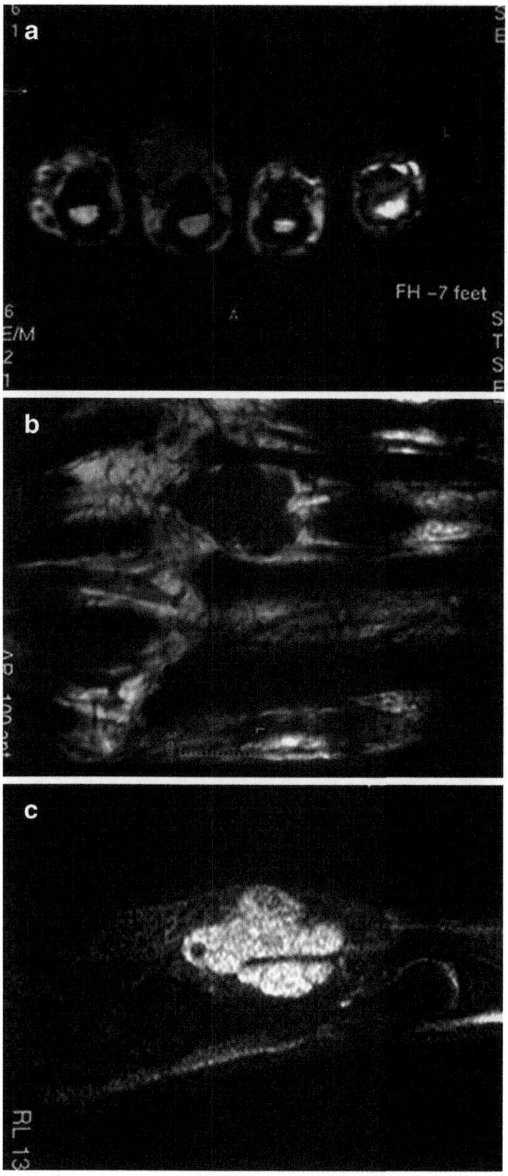

Fig. 19 Hemangioma of the finger. (**a**) Axial SE T1-weighted image and (**b**) coronal SE T1-weighted image shows a well-defined lobulated at the flexor side of the third finger. (**c**) Coronal fatsuppressed TSE T2-weighted image. The lesion is predominantly of high signal intensity. Note also some intralesional round areas of low signal intensity (phleboliths)

On MRI, benign nerve sheath tumors are well-demarcated masses. The lesions are isointense or slightly hyperintense to muscle on T1-weighted images and heterogeneously hyperintense on T2-weighted images. A target sign consisting of a central low signal and a hyperintense periphery is highly suggestive for a neurogenic tumor (Fig. 21). Other morphological signs of neurogenic tumors are the split fat sign (displaced fat around the mass on the neurovascular bundle), the fascicular sign (nerve fascicles on the course of the tumor), and the presence of a fusiform mass on the course of the involved nerve (Schmitt 2008; Ergun et al. 2010).

Traumatic neuroma can appear as a hypoechoic nodule or a T2 hyperintense mass that resembles a baseball shaped mass giving a balloon on a string or a green onion appearance. The presence of surrounding scarring and the lack of a split fat sign or target sign can help distinguish a traumatic neuroma from a neurogenic tumor. However, traumatic neuromas can occasionally enhance on imaging, making them appear nonspecific.

2.9 Glomus Tumor

2.9.1 Definition

Glomus tumors are a type of perivascular neoplasm arising from the glomus body, a neuroarterial structure located in the distal phalanx and subungual region of the finger. These structures are responsible for thermoregulation and are typically found underneath the nails or in the pulp of the finger. Most glomus tumors are benign, but some can be malignant and exhibit aggressive behavior. Glomus tumors account for approximately 1–5% of hand tumors and typically present in individuals between the ages of 40 and 60 years old (Carroll and Berman 1972). They are slightly more common in females than males and their etiology is often idiopathic. The lesion shows both muscle fibers and epithelial-appearing glomus cells (Enzinger and Weiss 1995).

2.9.2 Clinical Findings

The most common location is the subungual tissue at the tip of the finger. At this location, there is a striking female predominance. Glomus tumors are also seen at the palm, wrist, forearm, and foot. Multiple lesions may be present, espe-

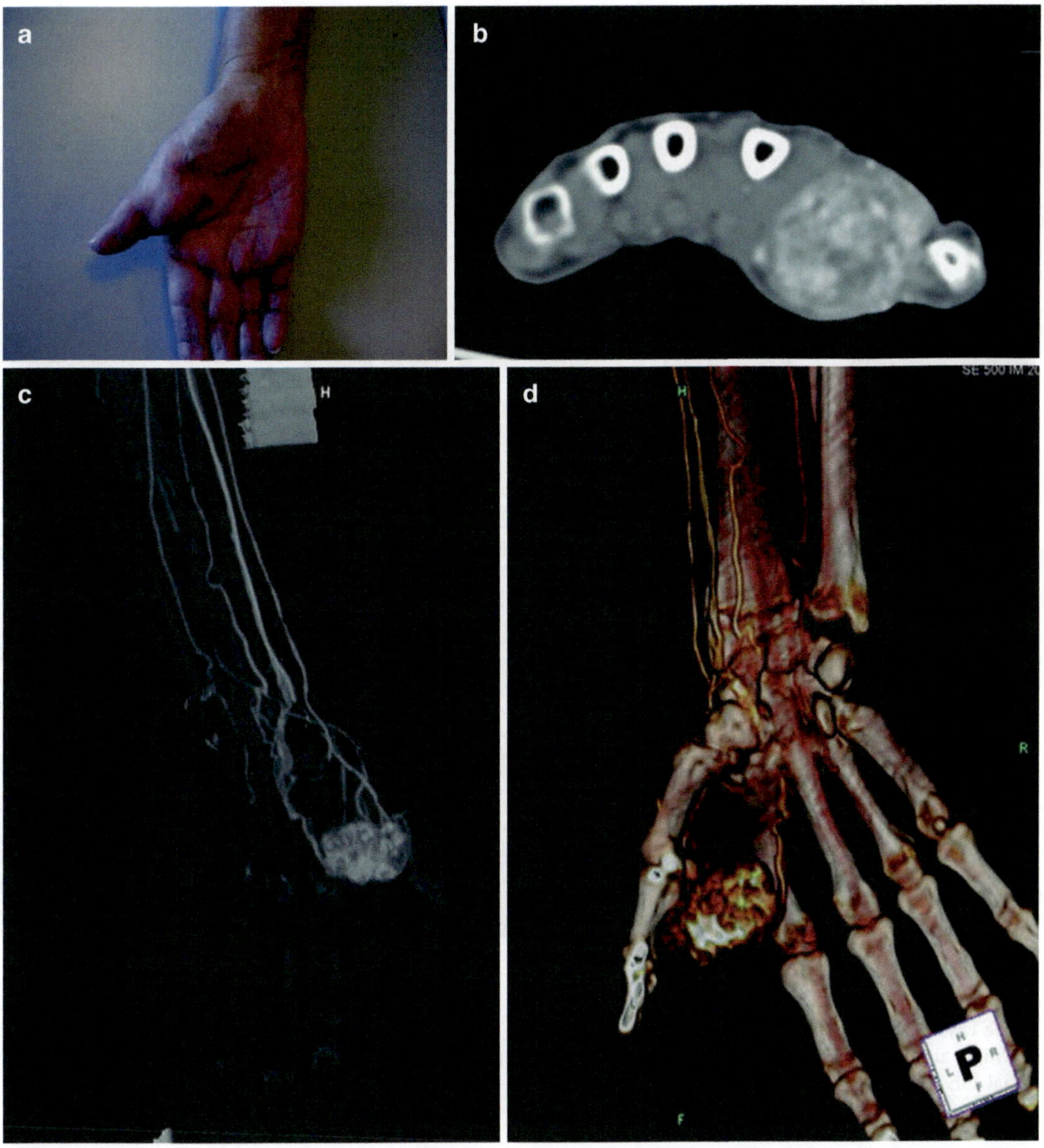

Fig. 20 Arteriovenous malformation of the thumb. (**a**) Clinical image showing a soft-tissue mass at the palmar aspect of the thumb. (**b**) Axial contrast-enhanced CT showing an intramuscular thenar mass with heterogeneous contrast enhancement. (**c**, **d**) CT-angiography (MIP and VRT image) showing the feeding arteries and draining veins

cially during childhood. Glomus tumors cause a radiating pain which is elicited by a change in temperature. Clinical examination usually reveals a characteristic blue-red nodule. Therapy aims at complete excision, still leaving a recurrence rate of 10% (Enzinger and Weiss 1995). Subungual and phalangeal glomus tumors are usually small, measuring less than 1 cm in size, and present with a classic triad of symptoms: local sensitivity, pain on exposure to cold, and severe pain following minor trauma (Macharia and Nthumba 2015). Subungual involvement can also lead to discoloration or deformation of the nail plate (AbuMoussa et al. 2023).

2.9.3 Imaging

Plain films may show a small mass at the dorsal aspect of the finger, associated with a small ero-

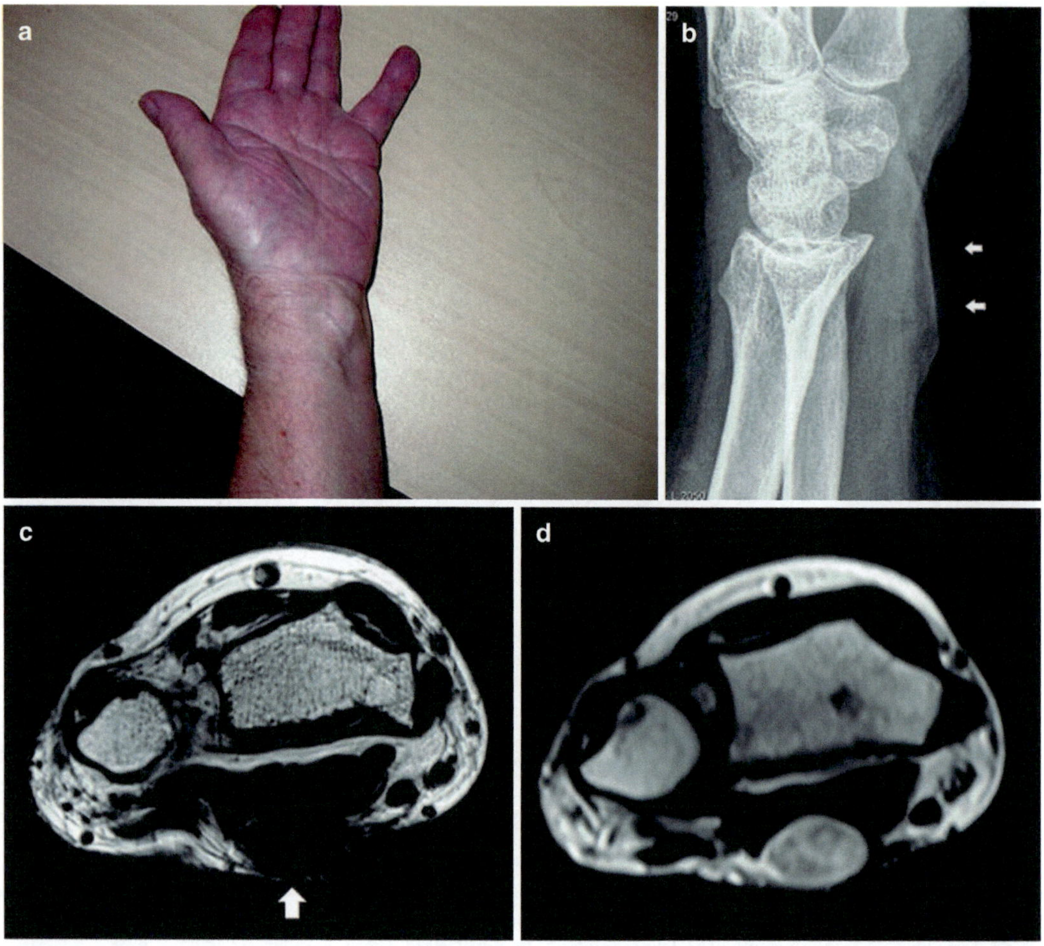

Fig. 21 Schwannoma of the median nerve. (**a**) Clinical image showing a soft-tissue mass at the palmar aspect of the wrist. (**b**) Plain radiograph. Nonspecific soft-tissue mass at the palmar aspect of the wrist (*arrows*). (**c**) Axial SE T1-weighted image. Well-defined hypointense mass on the course of the median nerve (*arrow*). (**d**) Axial fat-suppressed TSE T2-weighted image. Target-like appearance consisting of a hyperintense periphery and central areas of relatively hypointense signal

sion of the adjacent bone. However, this sign is nonspecific and is only found in 12–60% of glomus tumors (Drape et al. 2009). Ultrasound may detect lesions as small as 2 mm (Drape et al. 2009; Matsunga et al. 2007). Ultrasound is more sensitive than plain films to detect cortical erosions at the dorsal aspect of the distal phalanx in up to 78% of cases (Drape et al. 2009). Ultrasound is able to detect 92% of glomus tumors (Drape et al. 2009; Marchadier et al. 2006). The lesion is usually rounded and the echogenicity may be variable (usually hypoechoic to the subungual region). Most glomus tumors are hypervascular on power Doppler (Fig. 22a, b), but 21% of the lesions may be hypovascular (Drape et al. 2009).

On MRI, glomus tumors are of low to intermediate signal intensity on T1-weighted images and of high signal intensity on T2-weighted images. After intravenous administration of gadolinium contrast, moderate-to-strong enhancement is seen (Fig. 22c–f) (Fig. 23 glomus tumor of distal phalanx). MR angiography is a very useful technique to demonstrate the hypervascular nature of the lesion and an entangled arteriovenous anastomosis. Delayed imaging is sometimes

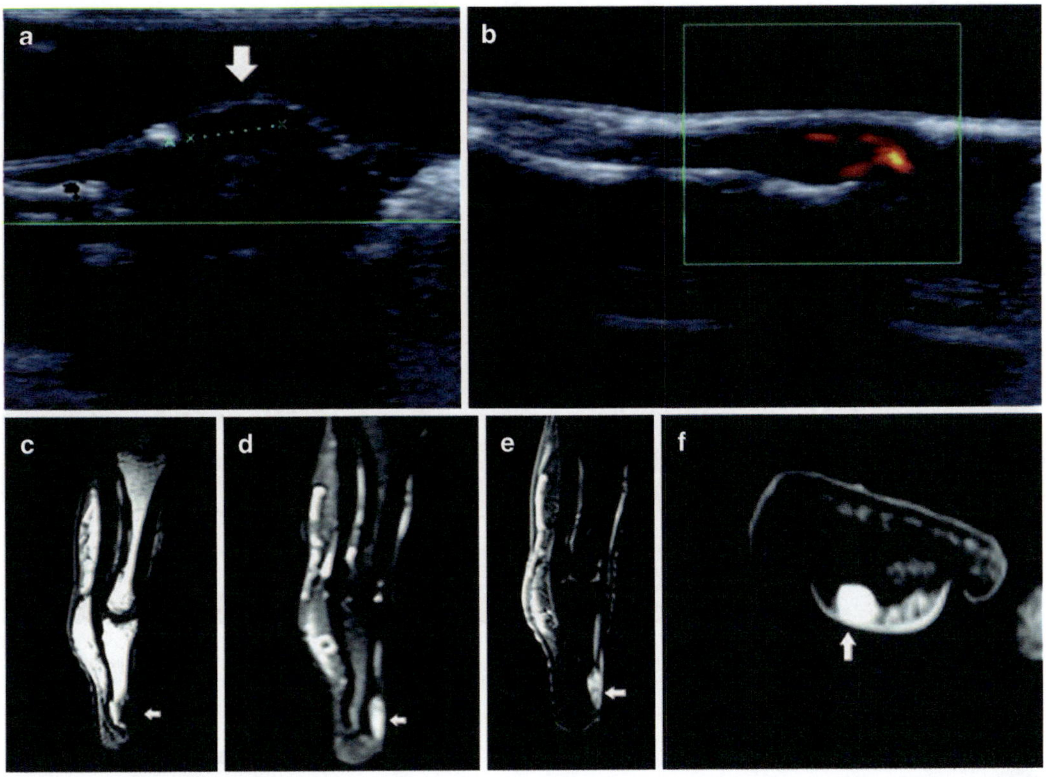

Fig. 22 Subungual glomus tumor. (**a**) Transverse ultrasound. Small hypoechoic subungual lesion causing cortical erosion of the dorsal aspect of the distal phalanx (*arrow*). (**b**) Longitudinal ultrasound showing increased intralesional power Doppler signal. (**c**) Sagittal SE T1-weighted image. There is a well-defined subungual hypointense lesion (*arrow*), causing cortical erosion of the distal phalanx. (**d**) Sagittal fat-suppressed TSE T2-weighted image. Hyperintense signal of the lesion (*arrow*). (**e, f**) Sagittal and axial SE fat-suppressed T1-weighted images after intravenous injection of gadolinium contrast. Marked enhancement of the tumor (*arrow*)

required to demonstrate the hypervascular nature of some lesions (late interstitial diffusion of a minority of lesions) (Drape et al. 2009).

2.10 Fibroma of the Tendon Sheath

2.10.1 Definition

Fibroma of the tendon sheath (FTS) is a benign soft tissue tumor that occurs adjacent to the tendon sheath, typically in adults between the second and fifth decades of life (Nepal et al. 2019). It is characterized by reactive fibrosis, which leads to the formation of a slow-growing mildly painful mass. The mass is usually located on the flexor surface of the hand or wrist, often in relation to an annular pulley. Approximately 82% of FTS occur in the hand and wrist region (Nepal et al. 2019). Fibroma is rarely larger than 2 cm in diameter, attached to the tendon sheath of the digits. The thumb is the most commonly involved digit (Nguyon et al. 2004; Plate et al. 2003). Histologically, the lesion is composed of scattered benign fibroblasts with dense collagen but lacks giants cells and xanthoma cells, in contradistinction to GCTTS (Nguyon et al. 2004; Peh et al. 1995; Wan et al. 2010).

2.10.2 Clinical Findings

They are less common than GCTTS and they often present as slow-growing, firm, and non-tender masses. The mean age of presentation is 42 years (Nguyon et al. 2004). Lesions are typically located on the flexor surfaces, occurring most often in men (75%) (Fox et al. 2003).

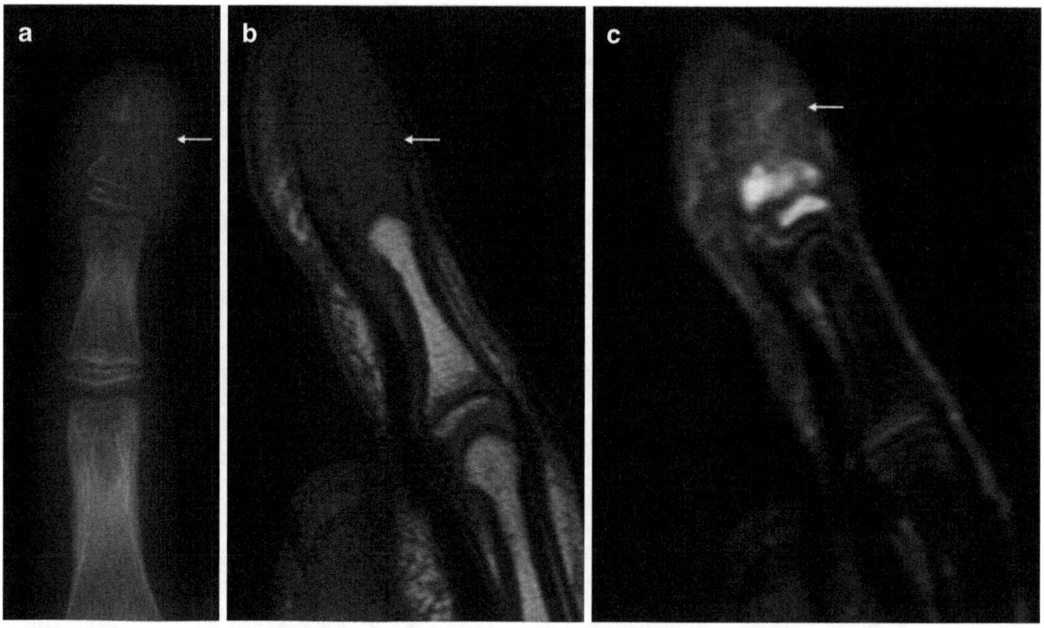

Fig. 23 Lateral radiograph (**a**), sagittal T1 (**b**), and STIR (**c**) showing glomus tumor of distal phalanx (arrow)

2.10.3 Imaging Findings

Pressure erosion of the underlying bone on plain films is very rare. Ultrasound shows a nonspecific hypoechoic mass adjacent to the tendon sheath (Fig. 24a). The lesion is usually hypointense on MR sequences, and no or minimal enhancement is seen.

Increased capillary vascularity near the lesion surface may cause minor peripheral enhancement (Figs. 24 and 25). The MRI findings vary when areas of increased cellularity or myxoid change occur within the lesion; myxoid changes within the lesion may cause an intermediate-to-high signal intensity on T2-weighted images, whereas areas of increased cellularity may enhance (Ergun et al. 2010; Fox et al. 2003). In these instances, differentiation of FTS from other tumors such as giant cell tumor of the tendon sheath is problematic (Fig. 24d). TSGCT typically shows susceptibility artifacts on gradient echo (GRE) images and adjacent cortical erosion on plain radiographs, which are absent in FTS. Nodular fasciitis is usually subcutaneous and not associated with the tendon sheath, helping to distinguish it from FTS.

2.11 Palmar Fibromatosis (Dupuytren Disease)

2.11.1 Definition

Palmar fibromatosis was originally described in 1831 by the French physician Dupuytren and is often referred to as Dupuytren disease or contracture. It is the most common of the superficial fibromatoses, affecting 1–2% of the general population. The disease is seen almost exclusively in Caucasians and is rare in populations of African or Asian descent.

The etiology of palmar fibromatosis is not completely understood, but it is thought to be multifactorial, including associations with trauma, microvascular injury, immunologic processes, and genetic factors (Murphey et al. 2009).

2.11.2 Clinical Features

The disease most commonly occurs in patients over 65 years of age with a frequency of 20% in this age group. Men are three to four times more likely to be affected by the disease than women, and lesions are bilateral in 40–60% of patients. Patients present clinically with painless, subcuta-

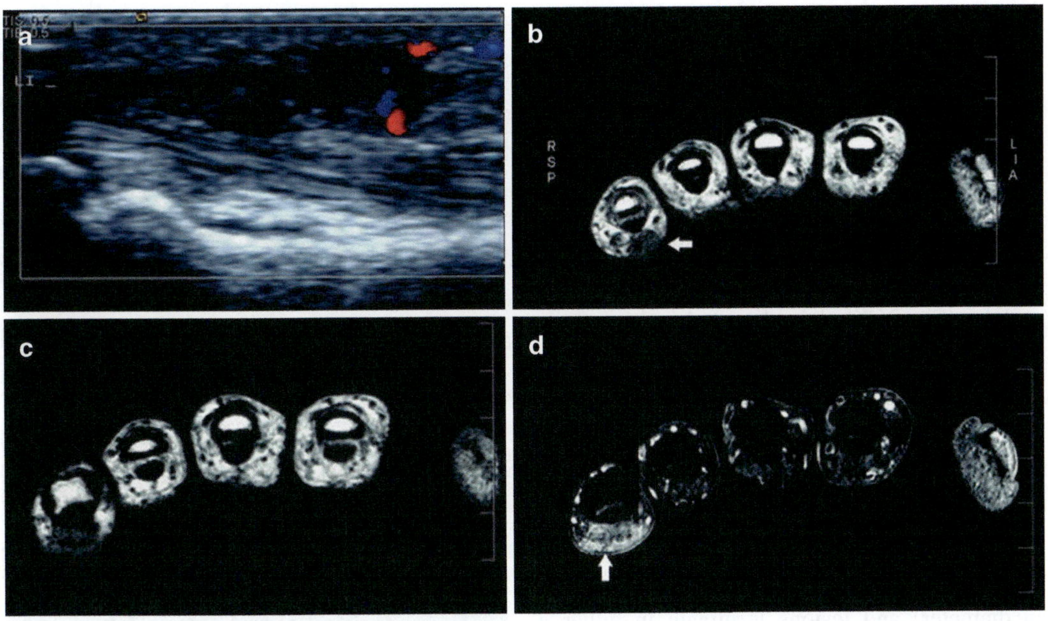

Fig. 24 Fibroma of the tendon sheath of the left fifth finger. (**a**) Longitudinal ultrasound. Polylobular hypoechoic lesion adjacent to the flexor tendons. Note some increased power Doppler signal at the proximal part of the lesion. (**b**) Axial SE T1-weighted image. The lesion is isointense to muscle (*arrow*). (**c**) Axial TSE T2-weighted image. The lesion remains of low signal intensity. (**d**) Axial SE fat-suppressed T1-weighted images after intravenous injection of gadolinium contrast. There is moderate enhancement of the lesion (*arrow*). In cases with contrast enhancement, differentiation of a tendon sheath fibroma from a GCTTS may be difficult

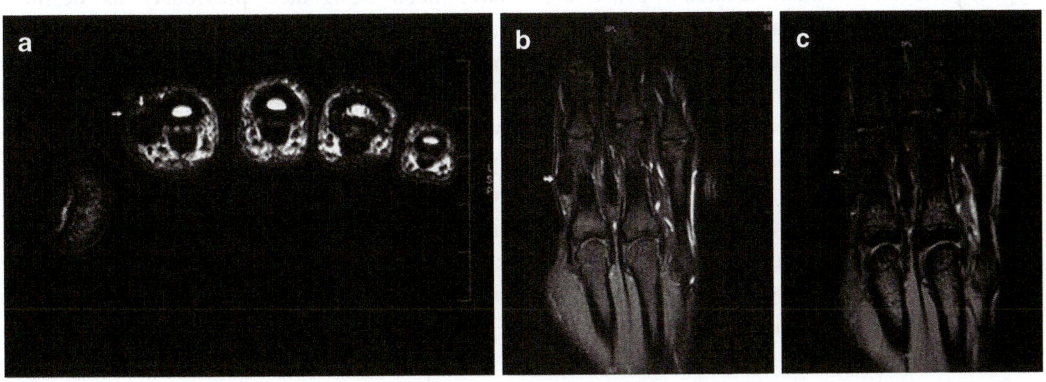

Fig. 25 Typical MR characteristics of a fibroma of the index. (**a**) Axial SE T1-weighted image. The lesion is hypointense to muscle (*arrows*). (**b**) Coronal fatsuppressed TSE T2-weighted image. The lesion remains of low signal intensity (*arrow*). (**c**) Coronal gradient echo T2*-weighted image. There is absence of blooming artifact (*arrow*)

neous nodules (Murphey et al. 2009). These nodules may progress slowly to fibrous cords or bands that attach to and cause traction on the underlying flexor tendons, resulting in flexion contractures of the digits. The fourth and fifth digits are most commonly involved. Patients commonly have related diseases such as plantar fibromatosis (5–20%), Peyronie disease, and knuckle pad fibromatosis. Other associated diseases include diabetes mellitus (20% of patients), epilepsy (50% of male patients and 25% of female patients), alcoholism (particularly liver disease related to alcoholism), and keloid (Murphey et al. 2009).

2.11.3 Imaging Findings

Plain radiographs are typically normal, other than the flexion contractures.

Ultrasound reveals hypervascular, hypoechoic nodules (Fig. 26) in the palmar subcutaneous tissues, superficial to the flexor tendons.

CT shows nonspecific, nodular soft-tissue thickening.

On MRI, there are multiple nodular or cord-like, superficial soft-tissue masses that arise from the proximal palmar aponeurosis and extend superficially in parallel with the flexor tendons. Lesion length varies from 10 to 55 mm (2–10 mm in diameter) and lesions terminate in either a branching or nodular configuration at the level of the distal metacarpal.

The signal intensity of palmar fibromatosis is variable along with the cellularity and the collagen content of the lesion. Lesions of low signal intensity on all pulse sequences are relatively hypocellular and contain abundant dense collagen (Fig. 27). In contradistinction, the lesions of intermediate signal intensity on both T1- and T2-weighted images are more cellular or mixed, with less abundant collagen (Murphey et al. 2009; Yacoe et al. 1993). Lesions with a higher cellular component have been shown to have a higher local recurrence rate following local excision. This information is important because preoperative MR imaging may assist the surgeon in determining the appropriate timing for excision (Yacoe et al. 1993; Robbin et al. 2001). After intravenous administration of gadolinium contrast, hypercellular lesions are enhancing more avidly than hypocellular lesions (Murphey et al. 2009).

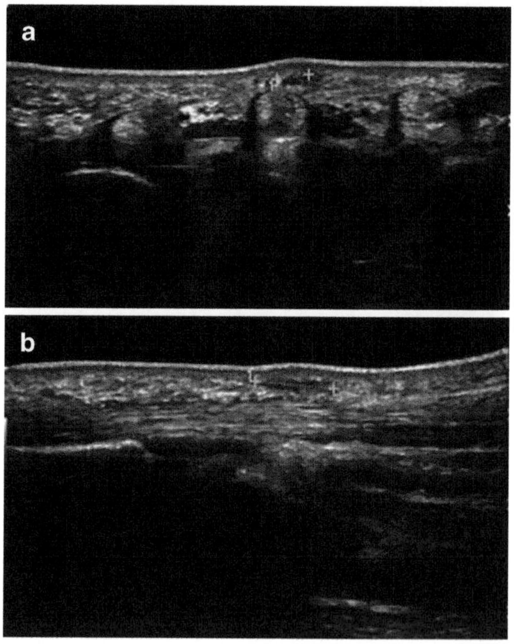

Fig. 26 Palmar fibromatosis. (**a**) Transverse ultrasound. (**b**) Longitudinal ultrasound. Hypoechoic nodule adjacent to the third flexor tendon of the palm of the hand

2.12 Desmoid Tumors (Desmoid Type Fibromatosis)

2.12.1 Definition

Extra-abdominal desmoids are rare benign soft-tissue tumors arising from connective tissue of muscle, overlying fascia, or aponeurosis. They have been designated previously as desmoid tumor, aggressive fibromatosis, or musculoaponeurotic fibromatosis. The term “desmoid” means band-like or tendon-like lesion (De Schepper and Vandevenne 2006). Currently, the term desmoid-type fibromatosis is used. The lesions can be regarded as deep seated fibromatosis in contradistinction to palmar fibromatosis which is a superficially located. Desmoid fibromas are infiltrative tumors, known for their frequent recurrences. Complete surgical excision is often difficult.

2.12.2 Clinical Features

The most commonly encountered locations are the upper arm (28%), chest wall and paraspinal area (17%), thigh (12%), neck (8%), knee (7%), pelvis or buttock (6%), lower leg (5%). The hand and forearm is rarely affected in up to 5% (Murphey et al. 2009; Berthe et al. 2003). Desmoids occur most frequently in patients in the second to fourth decades of life, with a peak incidence between the ages of 25 and 35 years (Murphey et al. 2009). The lesion is typically

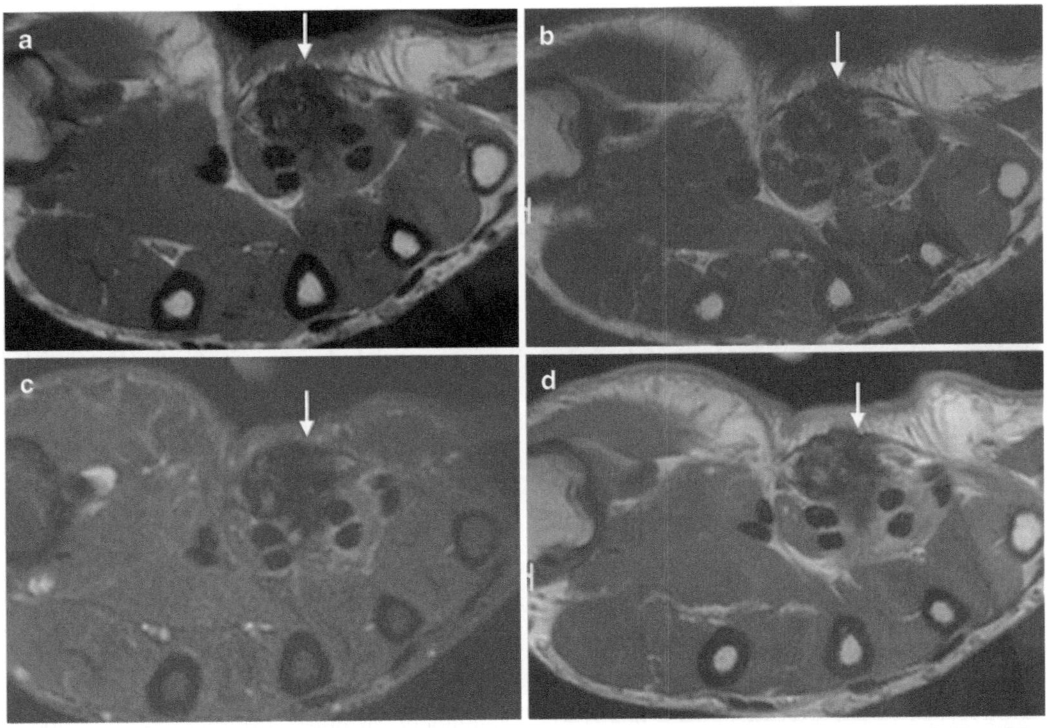

Fig. 27 Axial T1 (**a**), T2 (**b**), STIR (**c**), and T1 postcontrast (**d**) showing fibromatosis (arrow)

deeply seated and poorly circumscribed. Slow insidious growth is the rule, and most lesions are painless (Murphey et al. 2009).

2.12.3 Imaging Findings

Plain radiographs are often normal. A nonspecific soft-tissue mass may be apparent in patients with larger lesions. Calcification is uncommon, although underlying pressure erosion or cortical scalloping may be seen.

The US appearance of desmoid-type fibromatosis has not been extensively described. Ultrasound may demonstrate a nonspecific poorly defined, hypoechoic soft-tissue mass. Large lesions may demonstrate posterior acoustic shadowing. Increased vascularity is seen on Doppler-ultrasound (Murphey et al. 2009).

On CT, the lesion has a variable attenuation and enhancement (up to 110 HU). The attenuation is usually similar to that of skeletal muscle, but lesions with more prominent collagen content may reveal mildly higher attenuation. Low attenuation is rare and is associated with myxoid components. The margins are often indistinct (Murphey et al. 2009).

On MRI, the lesion may be well-demarcated or ill-defined. The signal intensity of desmoid-type fibromatosis is variable, dependent on the extent of collagen and degree of cellularity of the lesion. Low signal intensity areas on T2-weighted images correspond histologically to hypocellular and collagen-rich portions of the tumor, whereas more cellular areas with a large extracellular space are of high signal on T2-weighted images. In addition, high T2 signal may be seen in myxoid portions.

Postcontrast MR images typically reveal heterogeneous and often moderate to marked enhancement of these lesions. Hypocellular, collagenized bands do not enhance and therefore are often accentuated at postcontrast MR imaging (Fig. 28) (Murphey et al. 2009).

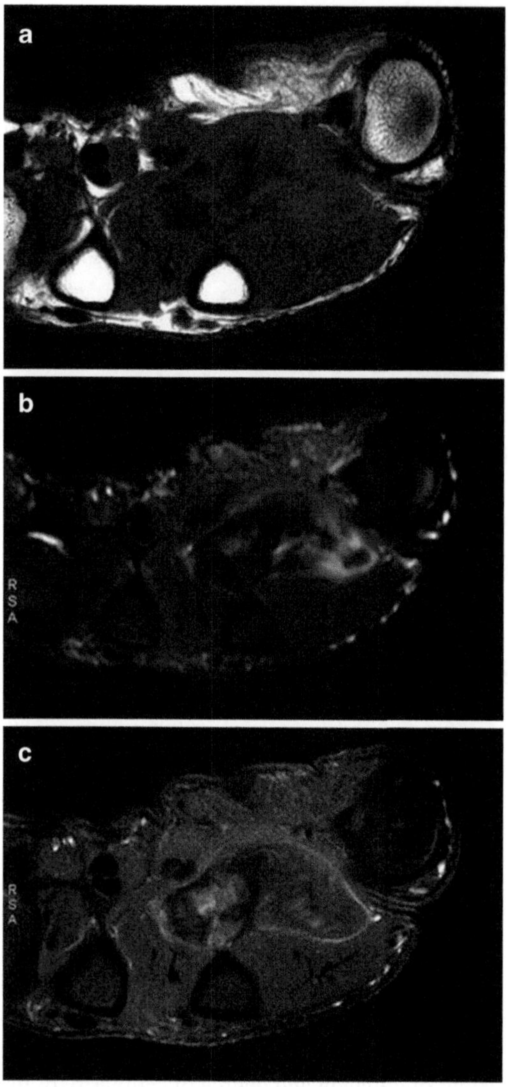

Fig. 28 Desmoid tumor. (**a**) Axial SE T1-weighted image. Ill-defined intramuscular lesion in the thenar compartment. The mass is of heterogeneous signal with isointense and hypointense areas compared to muscle. (**b**) Axial fat-suppressed TSE T2-weighted image. Heterogeneous signal intensity with areas of low and intermediate signal. The areas of low signal intensity on both pulse sequences correspond to areas of hypocellularity and collagenized areas. (**c**) Axial SE fat-suppressed T1-weighted images after intravenous injection of gadolinium contrast. Hypocellular, collagenized areas do not enhance

2.13 Synovial Chondromatosis

2.13.1 Definition

Primary synovial chondromatosis represents an uncommon benign neoplastic process with hyaline cartilage nodules in the subsynovial tissue of a joint, tendon sheath (Fig. 29), or bursa. The nodules may enlarge and detach from the synovium (Murphey et al. 2007). Synovial chondromatosis may be divided into primary and secondary forms. Secondary chondromatosis represents a nontumoral condition associated with underlying degenerative, destructive, or post-traumatic joint disease that causes intra-articular chondral bodies. On the contrary, primary synovial chondromatosis can be regarded as a true benign neoplastic disorder (Murphey et al. 2007; Buddingh et al. 2003).

2.13.2 Clinical Findings

Male adults are the most commonly affected patient population.

Primary chondromatosis usually involves large joints such as the knee and hip. The metacarpophalangeal, interphalangeal, and distal radioulnar joints of the hand and wrist are less commonly involved (Murphey et al. 2007). Primary synovial chondromatosis can also involve extra-articular sites (Murphey et al. 2007). This subtype arises probably in synovium about the tendons or bursa and is frequently referred to as tenosynovial (Fig. 29) or bursal chondromatosis, respectively (Murphey et al. 2007). Figures 30 and 31 show synovial chondromatosis of wrist and interphalangeal joint of thumb.

2.13.3 Imaging

Radiologic findings are frequently pathognomonic. Radiographs reveal multiple intra-articular calcifications (70–95% of cases) of similar size and shape, distributed throughout the joint, with typical chondroid "ring-and-arc" pattern of mineralization. Extrinsic erosion of bone is seen in 20–50% of cases. The joint space is typically maintained, unless the disease is complicated by secondary osteoarthritis.

Ultrasound shows a heterogeneous mass containing foci of hyperechogenicity, representing either chondral fragments or fronds of synovium with underlying cartilage nodule formation. The nodules are usually multiple and have a lobular contour. If the lesion contains sufficient mineralization or enchondral ossification, posterior

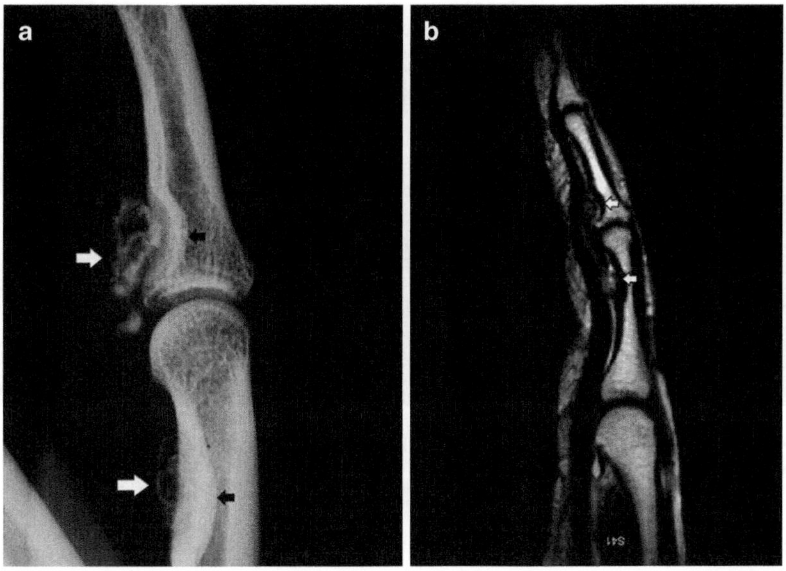

Fig. 29 Tenosynovial chondromatosis of the finger. (**a**) Plain radiograph. Chondroid-like calcifications adjacent to the flexor side of the proximal and middle phalanx (*white arrows*). There is scalloping of the adjacent cortical bone (*black arrows*). (**b**) Sagittal TSE T2-weighted image. The lesions are of variable signal intensity corresponding to calcified and noncalcified chondroid areas. Note the intimate relationship with the flexor tendons and the presence of cortical erosions (*arrows*)

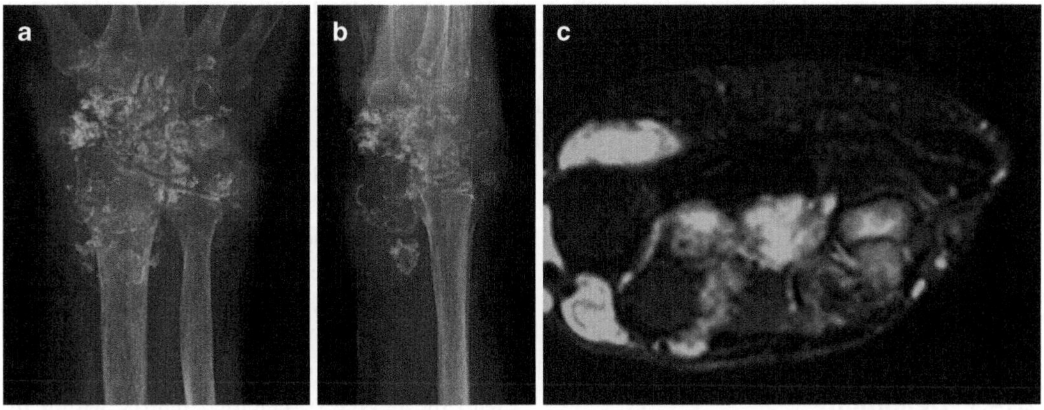

Fig. 30 Anteroposterior (**a**) and lateral (**b**) radiographs of the wrist and axial STIR (**c**) showing extensive synovial chondromatosis of the wrist

acoustic shadowing may be present (Murphey et al. 2007). Synovial chondromatosis is avascular on power Doppler (Roberts et al. 2004).

Computed tomography (CT) may depict calcified intra-articular fragments and more subtle extrinsic bone erosion.

Findings on MRI are more variable, depending on the degree of mineralization, although the most common pattern (77% of cases) (Murphey et al. 2007) reveals low-to-intermediate signal intensity with T1-weighting and very high signal intensity with T2-weighting with hypointense calcifications. These signal intensity characteristics on MR images and low attenuation of the nonmineralized regions on CT scans reflect the high water content of the cartilaginous lesions. CT and MRI depict the extent of the synovial disease (particularly surrounding soft-tissue involvement) and lobular

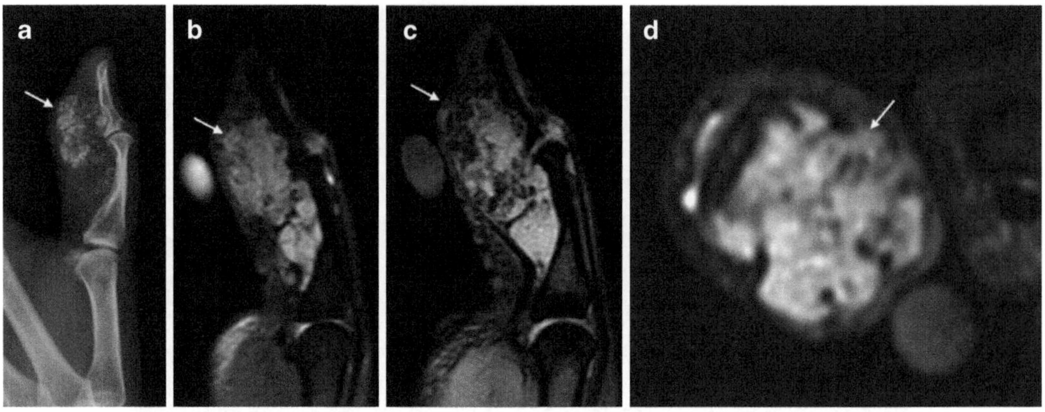

Fig. 31 Lateral radiograph (**a**), Sagittal STIR (**b**), and T2 (**c**) and axial STIR (**d**) showing synovial chondromatosis (arrows) of the interphalangeal joint of the thumb

growth. Following intravenous administration of contrast, peripheral or arc-like enhancement may be observed (Wittkop et al. 2002). With delayed imaging after intravenous contrast administration, an indirect MR arthrographic effect may be obtained, showing multiple intra-articular nodules within the joint cavity (Brassens and Cotten 2010).

Secondary synovial chondromatosis can be distinguished from primary disease both radiologically (underlying articular disease and fewer chondral bodies of variable size and shape) and pathologically (concentric rings of growth) (Murphey et al. 2007).

2.14 Soft-Tissue Chondroma (Tenosynovial Chondromatosis)

2.14.1 Definition

Soft-tissue chondroma, also known as extraskeletal chondroma or chondroma of soft-tissue parts, is a rare soft-tissue tumor accounting for only 1.5% of benign soft-tissue tumors (Hondar Wu et al. 2006). The origin is not known but is assumed to be synovial since the lesion is typically attached to the synovial capsule or tendon sheath (Ergun et al. 2010).

2.14.2 Clinical Features

Soft-tissue chondroma occurs at almost any age, but most commonly in 30- to 60-year-old patients. The tumor occurs most commonly in the hands and feet (Hondar Wu et al. 2006). Men are affected more often than women in the third decades of life. When the disease is diagnosed in older patients (after the fifth decade), there is a female predominance (Murphey et al. 2007). The patient most frequently presents with a painless mass or only mild tenderness upon palpation of the lesion. Duration of the symptoms ranges between 5 and 18 years with a median of 2 years (Fetsch et al. 2003).

2.14.3 Imaging Features

Plain films demonstrate calcifications in 33–80% of soft-tissue chondromas. The pattern of calcifications is variable, including curvilinear, punctate, mixed, and dystrophic or focal dense pattern (Fig. 29) (Hondar Wu et al. 2006).

On MRI, the signal intensity varies along with the degree of calcified matrix within the lesion (Fig. 29). Highly calcified lesions are of low signal intensity on both pulse sequences, whereas noncalcified lesions are of intermediate signal intensity on T1-weighted images and of high signal on T2-weighted images. The high signal is due to a high water content of the mucopolysaccharide/myxoid component (Hondar Wu et al. 2006). Following intravenous administration of contrast, septal or peripheral enhancement may be observed, corresponding to fibrovascular tissue surrounding the avascular nodules (Ergun et al. 2010).

2.15 Leiomyoma of Hand

2.15.1 Definition

Leiomyoma is a benign tumor that arises from smooth muscle cells and is typically slow-growing. It is most commonly found in uterus, esophagus, pleura, gastrointestinal system, and lower extremities. Leiomyomas are more common in women than in men and usually occur in 30 and 40 years of age (Boutayeb et al. 2008). Three types of leiomyomas described by Enzinger and Weiss (Enzinger and Weiss's Soft Tissue Tumors – ClinicalKey n.d.) are vascular, cutaneous, and deep soft tissue (Sayit et al. 2014). Vascular leiomyomas originate from the tunica media layer of walls of veins, and cutaneous leiomyomas are intradermal and originate from erector pili muscle and deep soft tissue leiomyomas from the unstriated muscles and vessels of the lower extremities (Kulkarni et al. 2009). The lower leg is the most common location for leiomyomas, accounting for 50–70% of cases, while the hand is a less common location, making up less than 10% of cases (Hwang et al. 1998).

2.15.2 Imaging

Radiography shows a soft tissue mass with mild swelling but no bone involvement or calcification. On MRI, the mass appears similar in intensity to muscle on T1-weighted images and slightly hyperintense to muscle and nonhomogenous on T2-weighted image. The lesion is devoid of fat tissue within.

3 Malignant Soft-Tissue Tumors

Soft-tissue malignancies in the hand are relatively rare, accounting for only about 20% of all soft-tissue sarcomas (Sayit et al. 2014). Malignant soft-tissue tumors are much more rare than benign tumors and tumor-like conditions in the hand and wrist (de La Kethulle de Ryhove et al. 2000; Capelastegui et al. 1999). These tumors arise from mesenchymal tissues and can be classified into different types including fibrosarcomas, rhabdomyosarcomas, epithelioid sarcomas, and synovial sarcomas. In adults, the most common types of malignant soft-tissue sarcomas in the hand are epithelioid sarcomas, synovial sarcomas, and undifferentiated pleomorphic sarcomas (Duran-Moreno et al. 2019). In the pediatric age group, fibrosarcoma and rhabdomyosarcoma are most common (AbuMoussa et al. 2023).

Soft-tissue sarcomas of the hand may be found in young adults and clinical symptoms are usually nonspecific as most patients present with a painless mass without functional deficit.

Plain radiographs and CT are usually nondiagnostic. Amorphous (synovial sarcoma, extraskeletal osteosarcoma) or arc-like (extraskeletal chondrosarcoma) calcifications may be seen in certain malignant tumors. Destruction of the adjacent bone is very rare.

Most malignant soft-tissue tumors are hypoechoic on ultrasound and may show intralesional necrosis. The tumor extent cannot be reliably determined on ultrasound.

Soft-tissue sarcomas typically present as a painless growing mass and patients may attribute incidental local trauma. MRI is the imaging modality of choice for grading (differentiation between benign and malignant tumors and assessment of malignancy grade) and local staging of malignant soft-tissue tumors of the hand and wrist. MRI is essential in evaluating the extent of the tumor and its involvement with surrounding structures such as neurovasculature, tendons, and bone. The imaging characteristics of soft-tissue sarcomas include low signal on T1-weighted images and heterogeneous high signal on T2 sequences. In higher-grade tumors, a nonenhancing necrotic center with a peripheral enhancing zone of viable tumor may be observed, which can be mischaracterized as an abscess.

Important grading parameters, which may suggest malignancy based on MR imaging (Figs. 32 and 33), are summarized in Table 1. There are some exceptions to these rules of thumb as some malignant tumors may have relatively well-defined margins and may demonstrate homogeneous enhancement (e.g., clear cell sarcoma). Given the relatively low predictive value of each individual parameter, correct differentiation requires a combination of multiple parameters (Gielen et al. 2004; Van Rijswijk

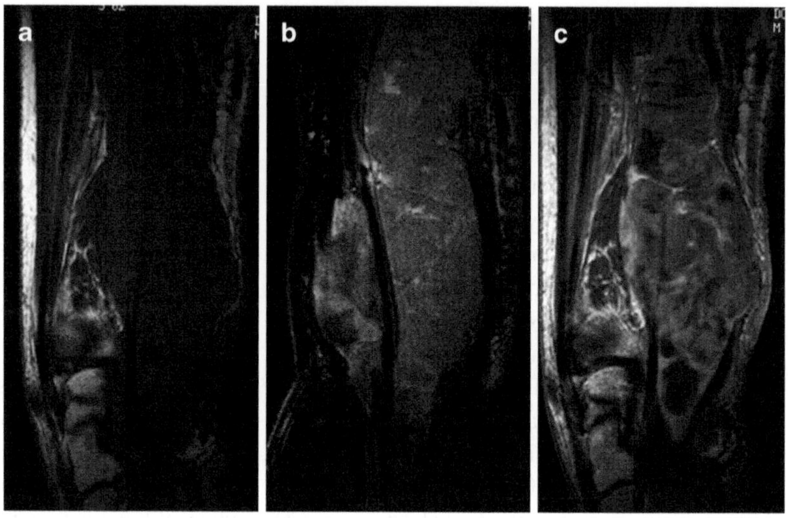

Fig. 32 Typical example of a malignant soft-tissue tumor of the wrist (highly malignant sarcoma NOS). (**a**) Sagittal SE T1-weighted image. (**b**) Sagittal fatsuppressed TSE T2-weighted image. (**c**) Sagittal fat-suppressed SE T1-weighted images after intravenous injection of gadolinium contrast. The lesion is large, inhomogeneous on T2-weighted images and shows marked and inhomogeneous enhancement

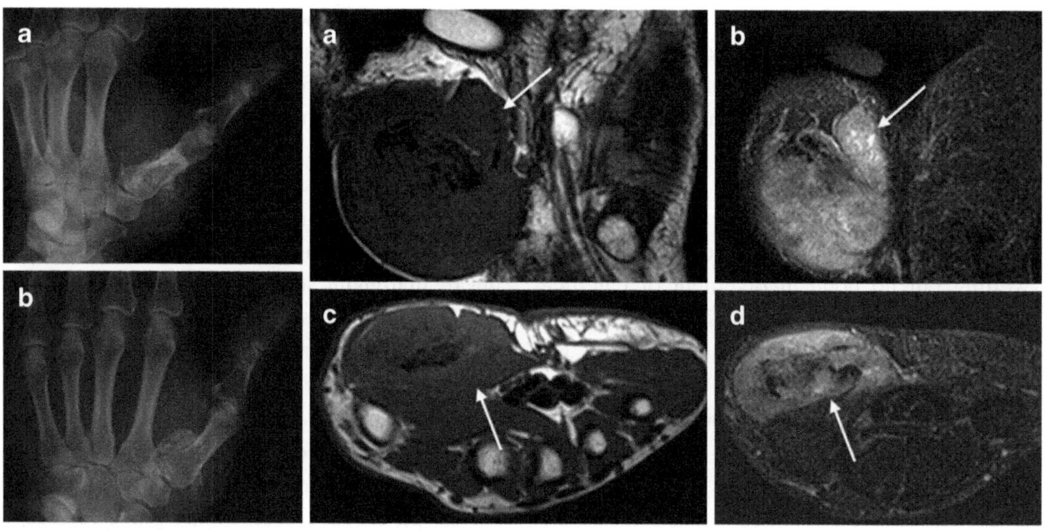

Fig. 33 Synovial sarcoma. Coronal T1 (**a**), STIR (**b**), axial T1 (**c**), and STIR (**d**) showing synovial sarcoma involving the thenar musclesOblique (**a**) and anteroposterior radiograph (**b**) of the hand showing soft tissue tumor with calcification in the thenar eminence

et al. 2004). Although a correct histologic diagnosis (tissue specific diagnosis) of malignant soft-tissue tumors cannot be reached based on imaging studies alone, the radiologist can help identify any soft tissue that may be potentially malignant. These lesions should be further evaluated with biopsy without jeopardizing definitive treatment options (Terek and Brien 1995).

Table 1 MR Imaging features that may suggest malignancy

Large volume (any lesion exceeding 3 cm in Hand and wrist
Ill defined margins
Inhomogeneity on all pulse sequences
Intralesional hemorrhage
Intralesional necrosis
Extensive and peripheral enhancement pattern (with papillary projections) on static contrast examination
Rapid enhancement with steep slope on dynamic contrast examination
Extracompartmental extension
Invasion of adjacent bones and neurovascular bundles.

Modified from De Schepper and Bloem (2007)

As the imaging features of these histologic subtypes are often nonspecific, further discussion is beyond the scope of this chapter. The goal of treatment is to achieve wide negative tumor margins which may necessitate radical resection and reconstruction of tendon, bone, nerve, and skin. In some cases, ray amputation may be required for limb salvage.

4 Pseudotumoral Lesions

4.1 Myositis Ossificans

Myositis ossificans (MO) is a benign condition of heterotopic bone formation which can mimic soft-tissue malignancies. It is rarely seen in the hand region (Chadha and Agarwal 2007; Van Zwieten et al. 2007). The ossification on plain films is centripetal (in contrast to the central ossification in extraskeletal osteosarcoma).

Zonal pattern is the typical imaging characteristic (Fig. 34) (Ergun et al. 2010). Detailed discussion of the imaging features of MO is beyond the scope of this chapter.

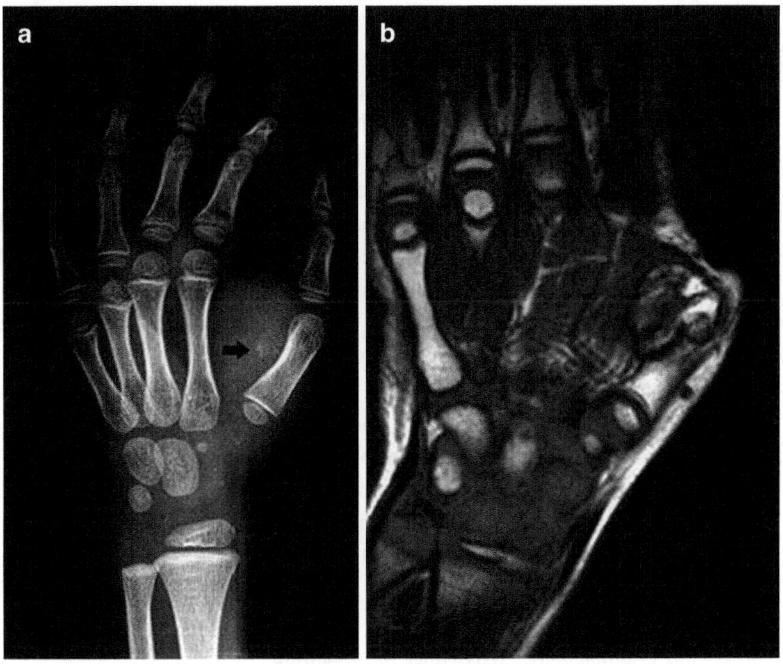

Fig. 34 Thenar myositis ossificans in a 7-year-old boy, presenting with pain and swelling at the thumb. (**a**) Plain radiograph. Note calcifications in the thenar (*arrow*). (**b**) Coronal SE T1-weighted image 9 month later shows an intramuscular ossified mass with central high signal intensity (fatty bone marrow) with peripheral and central areas of low signal. (Courtesy of J. Vandevenne, Genk)

4.2 Foreign-Body Granuloma

4.2.1 Definition
Foreign body granuloma is usually observed due to previous penetrating trauma in which the foreign body is not properly retrieved.

4.2.2 Clinical Findings
Most patients will present with a palpable mass, pain, and discomfort.

4.2.3 Imaging Findings
Plain radiographs are only capable of demonstrating radio-opaque foreign bodies, where ultrasound is the imaging technique of choice to demonstrate non-radio-opaque foreign bodies and the surrounding inflammatory reaction (Fig. 35).

In the early course of the lesion, MRI depicts high T2-signal and contrast enhancement surrounding the foreign body, while the granulation tissue may be of low T2-signal without contrast uptake in the chronic stage of the disease (Ergun et al. 2010).

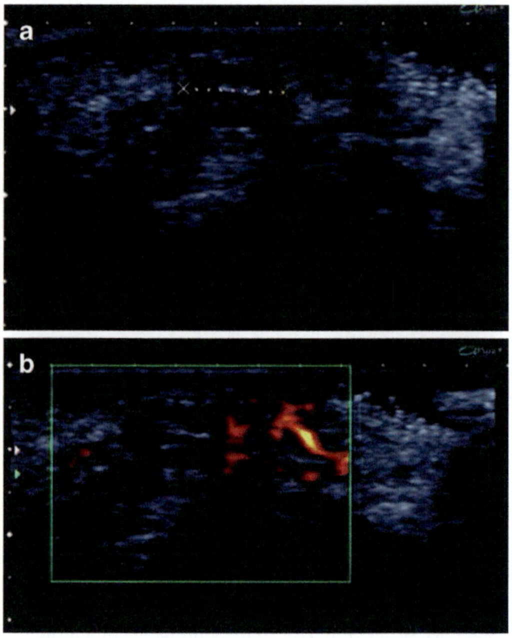

Fig. 35 Foreign body (wood). (**a**) Ultrasound shows a central hyperechoic wood fragment surrounded by a hypoechoic inflammatory reaction. (**b**) On power Doppler examination, there is increased signal at the periphery of the lesion

4.3 Rheumatoid Nodule

4.3.1 Definition
Rheumatoid nodules may be rarely observed in cases of long-standing RA or other rheumatic disease such as lupus, spondyloarthropathy, agammaglobulinemia, and rheumatic fever. Rarely, it may precede the articular manifestations of rheumatic disease. Histologically, the lesion consists of chronic inflammation, with or without central necrosis.

4.3.2 Clinical Findings
The lesions are usually located at the dorsal aspect of the hand within the subcutaneous tissue (particularly at sites of pressure or repetitive trauma), but bursae, joints, tendons and ligaments may be involved as well (Ergun et al. 2010).

4.3.3 Imaging Findings
Ultrasound is nonspecific. MRI may demonstrate iso- to hypo-intense lesions compared to muscle on T1-weighted images. Solid lesions are hypointense on T2-weighted images, whereas cystic lesions are hyperintense. The enhancement pattern is variable ranging from marked in solid lesions to peripheral ring-like in cystic lesions (Ergun et al. 2010).

4.4 Gout, Tophaceous Pseudogout, and Other Metabolic Disease

Crystal disease such as gout and pseudogout (hydroxyapatite and calcium pyrophosphate dehydrate deposition disease) and amyloid deposition may occasionally present as peri-articular soft-tissue masses (Fig. 36). Imaging findings are discussed in another chapter of this book.

4.5 Tenosynovitis and Soft-Tissue Abscess

Tenosynovitis consists of inflammation of the tendon sheath. The etiology may include acute

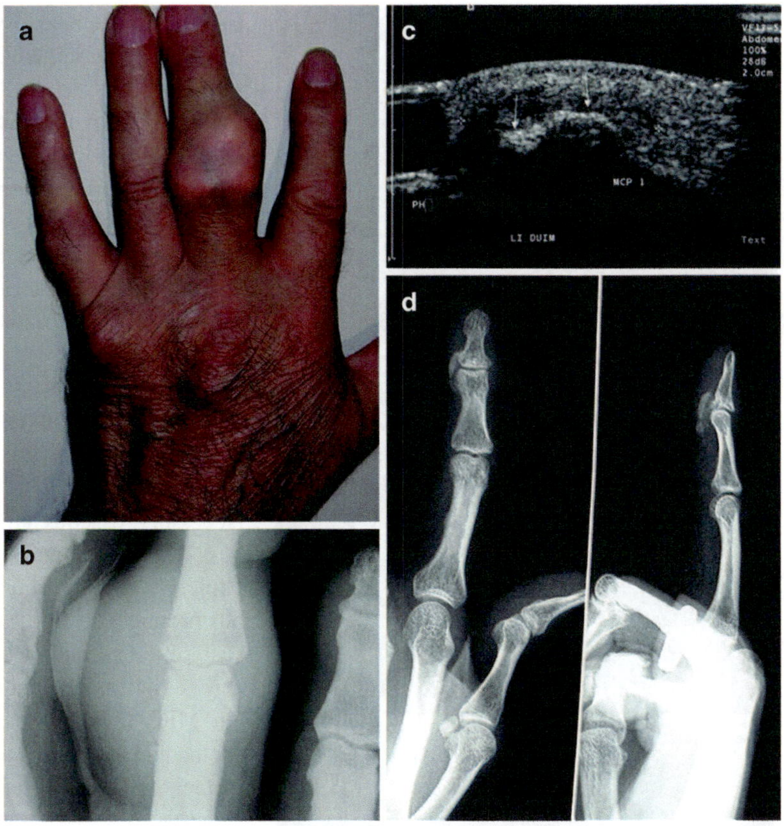

Fig. 36 Examples of pseudomasses due to metabolic diseases. (**a**) Clinical picture of tophaceous gout. Peri-articular soft-tissue swelling best seen at the proximal interphalangeal joint of the third finger. (**b**) Corresponding plain radiograph showing the soft-tissue swelling and adjacent periosteal new bone formation. (**c**) On ultrasound, there is a hypoechoic mass with intralesional reflections with retro-acoustic shadowing due to urate deposition. (**d**) Pseudogout (hydroxyapatite deposition disease) in another patient. Plain radiograph showing linear and amorphous calcifications at the joint capsule of the distal interphalangeal joint of the index

and chronic trauma, infection, or inflammatory or metabolic disease (Figs. 37 and 38).

Infection of the hand and wrist can rapidly spread along the numerous tendon sheaths, fascial planes, and lymphatics of the hand. Infectious tenosynovitis is an orthopedic emergency in which inflammation occurs in tendon sheath (Spinnato et al. 2022). The flexor tendon sheaths are the most common location for this condition, often resulting from increased compartmental pressures (in closed compartments) either due to trauma or infection (Altmayer et al. 2020). If left untreated, infectious tenosynovitis can cause significant morbidity and disability due to contracture of the affected musculature.

The most common microorganisms responsible for infectious tenosynovitis include *Staphylococcus aureus*, *Pasteurella multocida*, *Neisseria gonorrhoeae*, *Eikenella corrodens*, and *Mycobacteria tuberculosis* (Spann et al. 2004). MRI is the most sensitive and specific diagnostic imaging modality for infectious tenosynovitis (Spinnato et al. 2022) due to its high contrast resolution. It can detect fluid accumulation within the tendon sheaths, synovial hyperplasia, and other signs of inflammation. In cases of tenosynovitis caused by *Mycobacteria tuberculosis* “rice-bodies” may be seen on MRI (Fig. 39). Contrast-enhanced MRI with gadolinium can demonstrate paratendinous contrast enhancement indicating diffuse inflammation. Additionally, CT scans with contrast can show tendon thickening, edema, and abscesses.

4.6 Anomalous and Accessory Muscles

4.6.1 Definition

Accessory muscles are congenital anatomic variants that may clinically simulate mass lesions. The most encountered accessory muscles of the

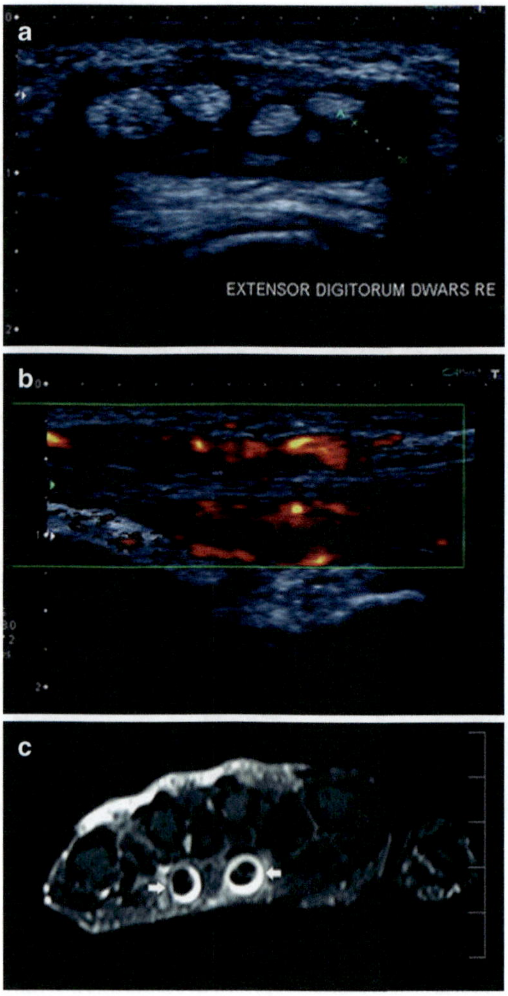

Fig. 37 Tenosynovitis. (**a**) Transverse ultrasound of the extensor tendons of the wrist showing fluid surrounding the extensor tendons of compartment 4. (**b**) Longitudinal power Doppler examination shows increased signal within the tendon sheath and tendons. (**c**) Axial fat-suppressed TSE T2-weighted image showing increased fluid around the flexor tendons of the third and fourth finger (*arrows*) in another patient with known rheumatoid arthritis

hand and wrist are the accessory palmaris longus muscle, extensor digitorum brevis muscle, accessory abductor pollicis minimi muscle, and the anomalies of the flexor digitorum muscles.

4.6.2 Clinical Findings

The lesion may present as a wrist mass. Palmaris longus and accessory flexor digitorum superficialis muscle may be associated with median or ulnar nerve entrapment.

4.6.3 Imaging Findings

Ultrasound shows a hypoechoic structure with a typical striated appearance of muscle. Dynamic ultrasound will show changes in the shape of the mass with active muscle contraction. Signal characteristics of accessory muscles are identical to muscles on all MR pulse sequences.

4.7 Anomalous Osseous Structures

Accessory osseous structures such as a carpal boss may sometimes simulate soft-tissue masses clinically. A carpal boss consists of a firm osseous prominence on the dorsum of the hand at the base of the second or third metacarpal and adjacent to the capitate and trapezoid bone (Fig. 40). On MRI, there may be reactive bone marrow edema and associated joint effusion at the carpometacarpal joint (Nguyon et al. 2004).

4.8 Bizarre Parosteal Osteochondromatous Proliferation (BPOP)

This reactive lesion and other surface lesions of bone are discussed in "Tumours and Tumour-Like Lesions of Bone."

4.9 Knuckle Pads

Knuckle pads are caused by focal fibrous thickening dorsally at the proximal interphalangeal (PIP) or metacarpophalangeal (MCP) joint and may precede the development of palmar fibromatosis. They are usually asymptomatic. Imaging features are nonspecific. On MRI, a nodular thickening is seen at the dorsal aspect of the PIP or MCP joint, with intermediate signal intensity compared to muscle on both pulse sequences and moderate enhancement (Murphey et al. 2009).

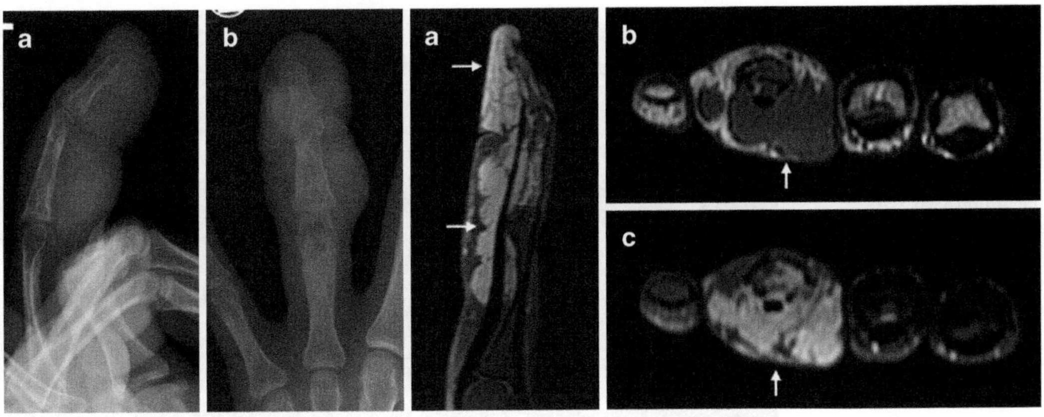

Fig. 38 Tubercular tenosynovitis: Lateral (**a**) and anteroposterior (**b**) radiographs shows marked soft tissue swelling of the finger; Sagittal STIR (**a**), axial T1 (**b**), and STIR (**c**) showing large amount of fluid in the within the ring finger flexor tendon sheath (arrow)

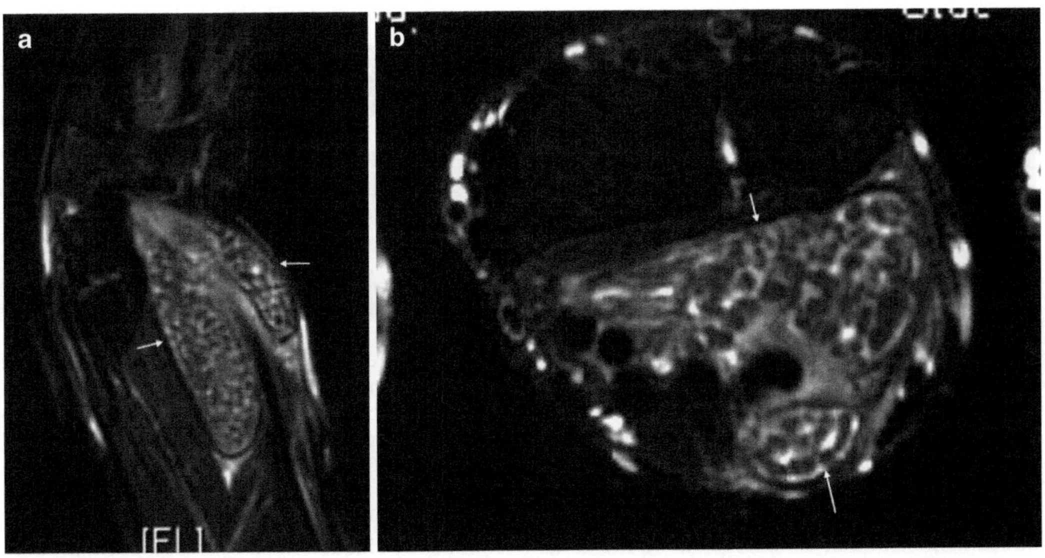

Fig. 39 Tubercular tenosynovitis: STIR sagittal (**a**) and axial (**b**) showing multiple loose bodies in the flexor tendon sheaths of the hand and wrist

4.10 Subcutaneous Granuloma Annulare

Subcutaneous granuloma annulare is a rare inflammatory dermatosis that may be encountered in children, usually located in the pretibial area or the scalp. The lesion presents as an ill-demarcated fast-growing painless subcutaneous lesion with variable signal intensity and contrast enhancement.

4.11 Hypothenar Hammer Syndrome

A post-traumatic partially thrombosed palmar aneurysm resulting from repeated trauma to the wrist (hypothenar hammer syndrome) may mimic a soft-tissue tumor (Van Zwieten et al. 2007).

The typical location of the lesion is at the ulnar artery distal to the hamulus of the hamate. The history of repeated trauma, the signal inten-

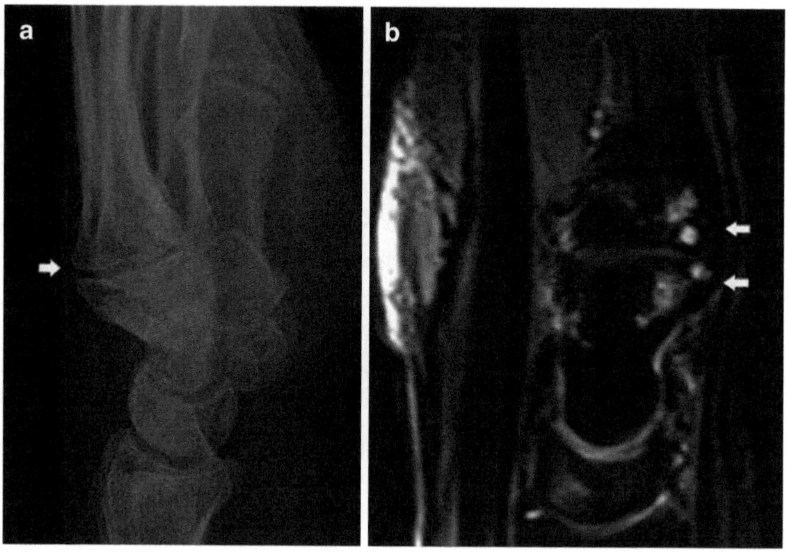

Fig. 40 Carpal boss. (**a**) Plain radiograph (*lateral view*) showing a bony prominence at the dorsal aspect of the carpometacarpal joint (*arrow*). (**b**) Sagittal fat-suppressed TSE T2-weighted image. Note bone marrow edema and subchondral cyst formation at the carpo-metacarpal joint (*arrows*)

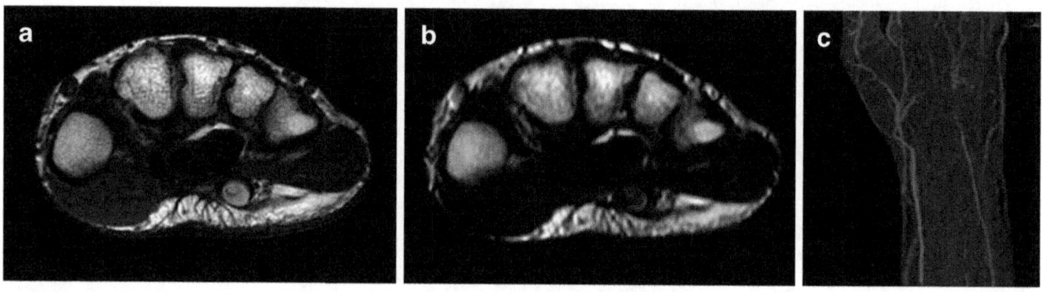

Fig. 41 Hypothenar hammer syndrome. (**a**) Axial SE T1-weighted image shows a well-defined oval mass superficial to the flexor tendons and immediately distal to the hamulus of the hamate. The lesion is of high signal with central area of lower signal intensity. (**b**) Axial TSE T2-weighted image shows comparable signal intensities, consistent with thrombosis. (**c**) CT-angiography shows occlusion of the ulnar artery

sity of the lesion (indicative of thrombosis), and direct demonstration of occlusion of the ulnar artery on different imaging modalities (Doppler-ultrasound, MR and CT-angiography) facilitate a correct diagnosis (Fig. 41).

5 Conclusion

Most benign soft-tissue tumors or tumor-like conditions of the hand have a predilection for certain locations in the hand or wrist and may present with characteristic imaging features. This applies particularly for ganglion cysts, epidermoid inclusion cysts, lipoma, hemangiomas, glomus tumors, and nerve sheath tumors. These lesions can be confidently characterized by imaging. On the contrary, malignant tumors and certain locally aggressive tumors such as desmoid tumor present with nonspecific imaging features. Further histologic confirmation is mandatory in order to allow proper management of these lesions.

Appendix A. Key Points

- Soft-tissue tumors of the hand and wrist (H&W) are more frequent than bone tumors.
- Benign tumors outnumber their malignant counterparts.

- Some tumors preferentially involve the hand and wrist, including ganglion cysts, GCTTS, lipomatosis of nerve etc.
- Benign tumors mostly have distinctive features on MRI as seen in cysts, GCTTS, hemangiomas, lipomas, neurogenic tumors, etc.
- Ultrasound is the initial technique for evaluation of superficial cystic lesions and may have role in the evaluation of small glomus tumors.
- MRI is the preferred technique in detection, staging, grading, and characterization of soft-tissue tumors. There is only a limited role for plain radiography or CT scan.
- The main uses of MRI are to characterize benign tumors and to advocate direct biopsy in MRI-nonspecific lesions.

References

AbuMoussa S, Roshan MP, Souza FF, Daley D, Rosenberg A, Pretell J, Fullerton N, Subhawong T (2023) Soft tissue masses of the hand: a review of clinical presentation and imaging features. Curr Oncol 30:2032–2048. https://doi.org/10.3390/curroncol30020158

Altmayer S, Verma N, Dicks EA, Oliveira A (2020) Imaging musculoskeletal soft tissue infections. Semin Ultrasound CT MR 41:85–98. https://doi.org/10.1053/j.sult.2019.09.005

Angeledes AC (1999) Ganglions of the hand and wrist. In: Green DP, Hotchkiss RN, Pederson WC (eds) Operative hand surgery. Churchill Livingstone, New York, pp 2171–2183

Bansal A, Goyal S, Goyal A, Jana M (2021) WHO classification of soft tissue tumours 2020: an update and simplified approach for radiologists. Eur J Radiol 143. https://doi.org/10.1016/j.ejrad.2021.109937

Berthe JV, Loréa P, De Prez C, De Mey A (2003) A case report of desmoid tumor of the finger. Chir Main 22(6):312–314

Boutayeb F, El Ibrahimi A, Chraibi F, Znati K (2008) Leiomyoma in an index finger: report of case and review of literature. Hand (N Y) 3:210–211. https://doi.org/10.1007/s11552-008-9084-4

Brassens H, Cotten A (2010) Chondromatose synoviale. In: Cotten A, Malghem J (eds) 10èmes mises au point en imagerie ostéo-articulaire. Bruxelles Lille, pp 111–125

Buddingh EP, Krallman P, Neff JR, Nelson M, Liu J, Bridge JA (2003) Chromosome 6 abnormalities are recurrent in synovial chondromatosis. Cancer Genet Cytogenet 1:18–22

Capelastegui A, Astigarraga E, Fernandez-Canton G et al (1999) Masses and pseudomasses of the hand and wrist: MR findings in 134 cases. Skeletal Radiol 28:498–507

Carroll RE, Berman AT (1972) Glomus tumors of the hand: review of the literature and report on twenty-eight cases. J Bone Joint Surg Am 54:691–703

Chadha M, Agarwal A (2007) Myositis ossificans traumatica of the hand. Can J Surg 50(6):E21–E22

Choo HJ, Lee SJ, Lee YH, Lee JH, Oh M, Kim MH, Lee EJ, Song JW, Kim SJ, Kim DW (2010) Pilomatricomas: the diagnostic value of ultrasound. Skeletal Radiol 39:243–250. https://doi.org/10.1007/s00256-009-0678-x

Christiaanse ECY, Jager T, Vanhoenacker FM, Van Hedent E, Van Damme R (2010) Piso-Hamate hiatus syndrome. JBR-BTR 93:34

Christopher D, Unni K, Mertens F (2002) Adipocytic tumors. WHO Classification of tumors. Pathology and genetics: tumors of soft tissue and bone. IARC, Lyon, pp 19–46

Cox JA, Bartlett E, Lee EI (2014) Vascular malformations: a review. Semin Plast Surg 28:58–63. https://doi.org/10.1055/s-0034-1376263

De Beuckeleer LHL, Vanhoenacker FM (2006) Lipomatous tumors. In: De Schepper AM, Vanhoenacker F, Parizel PM, Gielen J (eds) Imaging of soft tissue tumors. Springer, Berlin, Heidelberg, New York, pp 203–226

De Beuckeleer LH, De Schepper AM, de La Kethulle de Ryhove D, Nishimura H (2001) Imaging of soft tissue tumors of the hand and wrist. In: Guglielmi G, Van Kuijk C, Genant HK (eds) Fundamentals of hand and wrist imaging. Springer, Berlin, Heidelberg, New York, pp 331–363

de La Kethulle de Ryhove D, De Beuckeleer L, De Schepper A (2000) Magnetic resonance imaging of soft tissue tumors of the hand and wrist. J Radiol 81(5):493–507

De Schepper AM, Bloem JL (2007) Soft tissue tumors: grading, staging, and tissue-specific diagnosis. Top Magn Reson Imaging 18(6):431–444

De Schepper AM, Vandevenne JE (2006) Tumors of connective tissue. In: De Schepper AM, Vanhoenacker F, Parizel PM, Gielen J (eds) Imaging of soft tissue tumors. Springer, Berlin, Heidelberg, New York, pp 167–202

De Schepper AM, Hogendoorn PC, Bloem JL (2007) Giant cell tumors of the tendon sheath may present radiologically as intrinsic osseous lesions. Eur Radiol 17(2):499–502

Drape JL, Rousseau J, Guerini H, Feydy A, Chevrot A (2009) Tumeurs glomiques sous-ungéales: confrontations echo-IRM. In: Drape JL et al (eds) Poignet et main. SIMS, Sauramps Medical, Montpellier, pp 327–332

Duran-Moreno J, Kontogeorgakos V, Koumarianou A (2019) Soft tissue sarcomas of the upper extremities: maximizing treatment opportunities and outcomes. Oncol Lett 18:2179–2191. https://doi.org/10.3892/ol.2019.10575

Enzinger and Weiss's Soft Tissue Tumors – ClinicalKey [WWW Document] (n.d.). URL https://www.clinicalkey.com/#!/browse/book/3-s2.0-C20170011588. Accessed 3 Oct 2025

Enzinger FM, Weis SW (1995) Perivascular tumors. In: Enzinger FM, Weis SW (eds) Soft tissue tumors, 3rd edn. Mosby, St Louis, pp 701–755

Ergun TE, Lakadamyali H, Derincek A, Tarhan NC, Ozturk A (2010) Magnetic resonance imaging in the visualization of benign tumors and tumor-like lesions of hand and wrist. Curr Probl Diagn Radiol 39:1–16

Eurorad.org [WWW Document] (n.d.) Eurorad – brought you ESR. URL https://www.eurorad.org/case/17774. Accessed 3 Oct 2025

Fetsch JF, Vinh TN, Remotti F, Walker EA, Murphey MD, Sweet DE (2003) Tenosynovial (extraarticular) chondromatosis: an analysis of 37 cases of an underrecognized clinicopathologic entity with a strong predilection for the hands and feet and a high local recurrence rate. Am J Surg Pathol 27:1260–1268

Fox MG, Kransdorf MJ, Bancroft LW, Peterson JJ, Flemming DJ (2003) MR imaging of fibroma of the tendon sheath. AJR Am J Roentgenol 180:1449–1453

Garcia J, Bianchi S (2001) Diagnostic imaging of tumors of the hand and wrist. Eur Radiol 11:1470–1482. https://doi.org/10.1007/s003300000751

Gielen JL, De Schepper AM, Vanhoenacker F, Parizel PM, Wang XL, Sciot R, Weyler J (2004) Accuracy of MRI in characterization of soft tissue tumors and tumor-like lesions. A prospective study in 548 patients. Eur Radiol 14(12):2320–2330

Gielen J, Ceulemans R, van Holsbeeck M (2006) Ultrasound of soft tissue tumors. In: De Schepper AM, Vanhoenacker F, Parizel PM, Gielen J (eds) Imaging of soft tissue tumors. Springer, Berlin, Heidelberg, New York, pp 3–18

Greendyke SD, Wilson M, Shepier TR (1992) Anterior wrist ganglia from the from the scaphotrapezial joint. J Hand Surg Am 17(3):487–490

Hondar Wu HT, Chen W, Lee O, Chang CY (2006) Imaging and pathological correlation of soft-tissue chondroma: a serial five-case study and literature review. Clin Imaging 30(1):32–36

Huang C-C, Ko S-F, Huang H-Y, Ng S-H, Lee T-Y, Lee Y-W, Chen M-C (2011) Epidermal cysts in the superficial soft tissue: sonographic features with an emphasis on the pseudotestis pattern. J Ultrasound Med 30:11–17. https://doi.org/10.7863/jum.2011.30.1.11

Hwang JW, Ahn JM, Kang HS, Suh JS, Kim SM, Seo JW (1998) Vascular leiomyoma of an extremity: MR imaging-pathology correlation. AJR Am J Roentgenol 171:981–985. https://doi.org/10.2214/ajr.171.4.9762979

Jebson PJL, Spencer EE (2007) Flexor tendon sheath ganglions: results of surgical excision. Hand (N Y) 2:94–100. https://doi.org/10.1007/s11552-007-9028-4

Jeong HS, Lee SK, Kim J-Y, Yoo C, Joo MW, Kim J-H (2023) Tenosynovial giant cell tumors of digits: MRI differentiation between localized types and diffuse types with pathology correlation. Skeletal Radiol 52:593–603. https://doi.org/10.1007/s00256-022-04170-x

Jeyaraman M, Iyengar KP, Beale D, Botchu R (2023) Ischiofemoral impingement caused by an intrapelvic lipoma of the sciatic nerve – a rare case presentation. J Orthop Rep 2:100165. https://doi.org/10.1016/j.jorep.2023.100165

Jin W, Ryu KN, Kim GY, Kim HC, Lee JH, Park JS (2008) Sonographic findings of ruptured epidermal inclusion cysts in superficial soft tissue: emphasis on shapes, pericystic changes, and pericystic vascularity. J Ultrasound Med 27(2):171–176; quiz 177–178

Kobayashi N, Koshino T, Nakazawa A, Saito T (2001) Neuropathy of motor branch of median or ulnar nerve induced by midpalm ganglion. J Hand Surg [Am] 26:474

Kulkarni AR, Haase SC, Chung KC (2009) Leiomyoma of the hand. Hand (N Y) 4:145–149. https://doi.org/10.1007/s11552-008-9143-x

Kumar N, Singh DK, Hassan M, Rustagi A, Batta NS, Botchu R (2024) Thorn-induced injury of the knee mimicking pigmented villonodular synovitis (PVNS): a case report. Apollo Med 21:S55–S58. https://doi.org/10.1177/09760016241270099

Kuwano Y, Ishizaki K, Watanabe R, Nanko H (2009) Efficacy of diagnostic ultrasonography of lipomas, epidermal cysts, and ganglions. Arch Dermatol 145(7):761–764

Lowden CM, Attiah M, Gravin G, Macdermid JC, Osman S, Farber KJ (2005) The prevalence of wrist ganglia in a asymptomatic population: magnetic resonance evaluation. J Hand Surg (Br) 30B(3):302–306

Macharia C, Nthumba PM (2015) Glomus tumor presenting as complex regional pain syndrome of the left upper limb: a case report. J Med Case Rep 9:293. https://doi.org/10.1186/s13256-015-0793-3

Marchadier A, Cohen M, Legre R (2006) Subungual glomus tumors of the fingers: ultrasound diagnosis. Chir Main 25:16–21

Marom EM, Helms CA (1999) Fibrolipomatous hamartoma: pathognomonic on MR imaging. Skeletal Radiol 28:260–264

Matsunga A, Ochiai T, Abe I et al (2007) Subungual glomus tumour: evaluation of ultrasound imaging in preoperative assessment. Eur J Dermatol 17:67–69

Mettu S, Gavvala SN, Shirodkar K, Iyengar KP, Papineni VRK, Botchu R (2024) Intra-articular lipoma of the pisotriquetral joint: a rare case report. Indian J Radiol Imaging 34:558–561. https://doi.org/10.1055/s-0044-1779521

Minotti P, Taras JS (2002) Ganglion cysts of the wrist. J Am Soc Surg Hand 2:102–107. https://doi.org/10.1053/jssh.2002.33318

Murphey MD, Carroll JF, Flemming DJ, Pope TL, Gannon FH, Kransdorf MJ (2004) From the archives of the AFIP. Benign musculoskeletal lipomatous lesions. Radiographics 24:1433–1466

Murphey MD, Vidal JA, Fanburg-Smith JC, Gajewski DA (2007) Imaging of synovial chondromatosis with

radiologic-pathologic correlation. Radiographics 27:1465–1488. https://doi.org/10.1148/rg.275075116
Murphey MD, Ruble CM, Tyszko SM, Zbojniewicz AM, Potter BK, Miettinen M (2009) From the archives of the AFIP: musculoskeletal fibromatoses: radiologic-pathologic correlation. Radiographics 29(7):2143–2173
Murphy GE, Elder DE (1991) Atlas of tumor pathology: non-melanotic tumors of the skin. Armed Forces Institute of Pathology, Washington
Nahra ME, Bucchieri JS (2004) Ganglion cysts and other tumor related conditions of the hand and wrist. Hand Clin 20:249–260
Nepal P, Songmen S, Alam SI, Gandhi D, Ghimire N, Ojili V (2019) Common soft tissue tumors involving the hand with histopathological correlation. J Clin Imaging Sci 9:15. https://doi.org/10.25259/JCIS-6-2019
Nguyon V, Choi J, Davis KW (2004) Imaging of Wrist masses. Curr Probl Diagn Radiol 33:147–160
Peh WCG, Truong NP, Totty WG, Gilula LA (1995) Pictorial review: magnetic resonance imaging of benign soft tissue masses of the hand and wrist. Clin Radiol 50:519–525
Plate AM, Lee SJ, Steiner G, Posner M (2003) Tumorlike lesions and benign tumors of the hand and wrist. J Am Acad Orthop Surg 11:129–141
Rajakulasingam R, Azzopardi C, Murphy J, Davies M, Toms A, James S, Botchu R (2019a) Lesions of the distal phalanx: imaging overview. Indian J Musculoskelet Radiol 1:47–56. https://doi.org/10.25259/IJMSR_13_2019
Rajakulasingam R, Murphy J, Badreddine I, James S, Botchu R (2019b) Pigmented villonodular synovitis masquerading as a metastasis: imaging features and coaxial needle biopsy technique. Iowa Orthop J 39:73–75
Robbin MR, Murphey MD, Temple HT, Kransdorf MJ, Choi JJ (2001) Imaging of musculoskeletal fibromatosis. Radiographics 21(3):585–600
Roberts D, Miller TT, Erlanger SM (2004) Sonographic appearance of primary synovial chondromatosis of the knee. J Ultrasound Med 23:707–709
Saad A, Iyengar KP, Botchu R (2023) A rare case of an intratendinous ganglion cyst extending into the muscle belly of flexor carpi radialis: a case report and review of the literature. J Ultrasound 26:919–922. https://doi.org/10.1007/s40477-023-00784-6
Sayit E, Sayit AT, Zan E, Bakirtas M, Akpinar H, Gunbey HP (2014) Vascular leiomyoma of an extremity: report of two cases with MRI and histopathologic correlation. J Clin Orthop Trauma 5:110–114. https://doi.org/10.1016/j.jcot.2014.04.001
Sbaraglia M, Bellan E, Dei Tos AP (2020) The 2020 WHO classification of soft tissue tumours: news and perspectives. Pathologica 113:70–84. https://doi.org/10.32074/1591-951X-213
Schmitt R (2008) Soft-tissue tumors. In: Schmitt R, Lanz U (eds) Diagnostic imaging of the hand. Georg Thieme Verlag, Stuttgart, pp 502–521
Shirodkar K, Hussein M, Reddy PS, Shah AB, Raniga S, Pal D, Iyengar KP, Botchu R (2025) Imaging of peripheral intraneural tumors: a comprehensive review for radiologists. Cancers 17:246. https://doi.org/10.3390/cancers17020246
Spann M, Talmor M, Nolan WB (2004) Hand infections: basic principles and management. Surg Infect 5:210–220. https://doi.org/10.1089/sur.2004.5.210
Spinnato P, Patel DB, Di Carlo M, Bartoloni A, Cevolani L, Matcuk GR, Crombé A (2022) Imaging of musculoskeletal soft-tissue infections in clinical practice: a comprehensive updated review. Microorganisms 10:2329. https://doi.org/10.3390/microorganisms10122329
Steiner E, Steinbach LS, Schnarkowski P, Tirman PF, Genant HK (1996) Ganglia and cysts around joints. Radiol Clin North Am 34:395–425
Terek RM, Brien EW (1995) Soft-tissue sarcomas of the hand and wrist. Hand Clin 11(2):287–305
Ushijima M, Hashimoto H, Tsuneyoshi M et al (1986) Giant cell tumor of the tendon sheath (nodular tenosynovitis). A study of 207 cases to compare the large joint group with the common digit group. Cancer 15:875–884
van Rijswijk CS, Geirnaerdt MJ, Hogendoorn PC, Taminiau AH, van Coevorden F, Zwinderman AH, Pope TL, Bloem JL (2004) Soft-tissue tumors: value of static and dynamic gadopentetate dimeglumine-enhanced MR imaging in prediction of malignancy. Radiology 233(2):493–502
Van Zwieten KJ, Brys P, Van Rietvelde F et al (2007) Imaging of the hand, techniques and pathology: a pictorial essay. JBR-BTR 90(5):395–455
Vanhoenacker FM, De Schepper AM, Gielen JL, Parizel PM (2005) MR imaging in the diagnosis and management of inheritable musculoskeletal disorders. Clin Radiol 60:160–170
Vanhoenacker FM, Marques MC, Garcia H (2006a) Lipomatous tumors. In: De Schepper AM, Vanhoenacker F, Parizel PM, Gielen J (eds) Imaging of soft tissue tumors. Springer, Berlin, Heidelberg, New York, pp 227–261
Vanhoenacker FM, Van Goethem JWM, Vandevenne JE, Shahabpour M (2006b) Synovial tumors. In: De Schepper AM, Vanhoenacker F, Parizel PM, Gielen J (eds) Imaging of soft tissue tumors. Springer, Berlin, Heidelberg, New York, pp 311–324
Vidoni A, Shrivastava M, Botchu R (2020) Intrasynovial spindle cell lipoma of the deep flexor of the middle finger causing intermittent carpal tunnel syndrome–case report and review of the literature. J Ultrasound 23:419–423. https://doi.org/10.1007/s40477-018-0281-x
Wan JM, Magarelli N, Peh WC, Guglielmi G, Shek TW (2010) Imaging of giant cell tumour of the tendon sheath. Radiol Med 115:141–151
Wang AA, Hutchinson DT (2001) Longitudinal observation of pediatric hand and wrist ganglia. J Hand Surg [Am] 26:599–602

Wigley C, Morris G, Evans S, Botchu R (2019) A case of an extraosseous pretibial ganglion cyst. Indian J Musculoskelet Radiol 1:114–116. https://doi.org/10.25259/IJMSR_12_2019

Wittkop AM, Davies AM, Mangham DC (2002) Primary synovial chondromatosis and synovial chondrosarcoma. Eur Radiol 12:2112–2219

Yacoe ME, Bergman AG, Ladd AL, Hellman BH (1993) Dupuytren's contracture: MR imaging findings and correlation between MR signal intensity and cellularity of lesions. AJR Am J Roentgenol 160(4):813–817

Miscellaneous Conditions with Manifestations in the Hand and Wrist

Shashank Chapala, A. Mark Davies, Ramy Mansour, Steven L. James, and Rajesh Botchu

Contents

S. Chapala (✉)
Department of Radiology, AIG Hospitals,
Hyderabad, India

A. M. Davies · S. L. James · R. Botchu
Department of Musculoskeletal Radiology,
Royal Orthopaedic Hospital, Birmingham, UK

R. Mansour
Department of Radiology, University of Ottawa,
Ottawa, ON, Canada

Med Radiol Diagn Imaging (2025)
https://doi.org/10.1007/174_2025_613,
Published Online: 17 September 2025

Abstract

In any textbook dealing with conditions affecting a particular anatomical site, there will be some which do not fit conveniently under the standard chapter headings. The purpose of this chapter is to review these miscellaneous localised and systemic disorders that may affect the hand and wrist.

1 Introduction

In any textbook dealing with conditions affecting a particular anatomical site, there will be some which do not fit conveniently under the standard chapter headings. The purpose of this chapter is to review these miscellaneous localised and systemic disorders that may affect the hand and wrist.

2 Paget's Disease

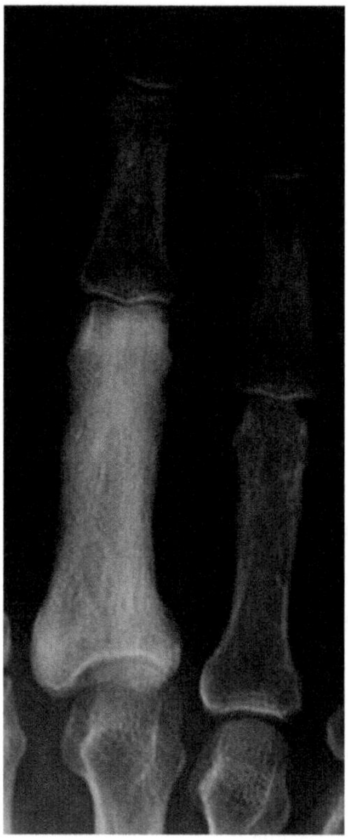

Fig. 1 Paget's disease. There is bony sclerosis and expansion of the proximal phalanx of the middle finger

Paget's disease of bone is a benign disorder affecting 3%–4% of the population over 40 years of age predominantly in Caucasian races (Smith et al. 2002). There is recent evidence of decreasing prevalence (Cundy 2006). The abnormality in Paget's disease is osteoclastic bone resorption and compensatory excess osteoblastic activation (Cortis et al. 2011). Three pathologic phases have been described: the lytic phase, the mixed phase and the blastic phase. Initially there is osteolysis, followed by trabecular and cortical thickening and enlargement in the mixed phase of the disease, followed by sclerosis in the blastic phase. Paget's disease is usually polyostotic and asymmetric. Polyostotic disease (65%–90%) is more frequent than monostotic disease.

Involvement in the hand and wrist has been reported infrequently, although bone scintigraphy studies reveal hand localisation varying from 6.4% to 11.6% (Friedman et al. 1982). Clinically, Paget's disease in the hands is usually asymptomatic; however, several cases with pain in the hands have been reported (Friedman et al. 1982). When Paget's disease occurs in the hand, there is usually a polyostotic involvement (Haverbush et al. 1972). Monostotic localisation in the hand is less frequent (Rodriguez-Peralto et al. 1994; Calif et al. 2007). It typically affects the phalanges and metacarpals, with carpal involvement rare and distal phalangeal involvement almost unknown. The most common radiographic pattern of disease in the hand is sclerosis (Fig. 1; Haverbush et al. 1972) and is seen in 45% of cases (Friedman et al. 1982). However, all patterns as found elsewhere in the body (cortical destruction, bone expansion, coarsened trabeculae and bone sclerosis) may be seen in the hand (Friedman et al. 1982). Sarcomatous transformation is the most sinister complication of Paget's disease and is rarely seen in the hand. A review by Lopez et al. (2003) looked at 340 cases of Paget's sarcoma in the literature and identified no cases in the hand and wrist. Isolated cases of

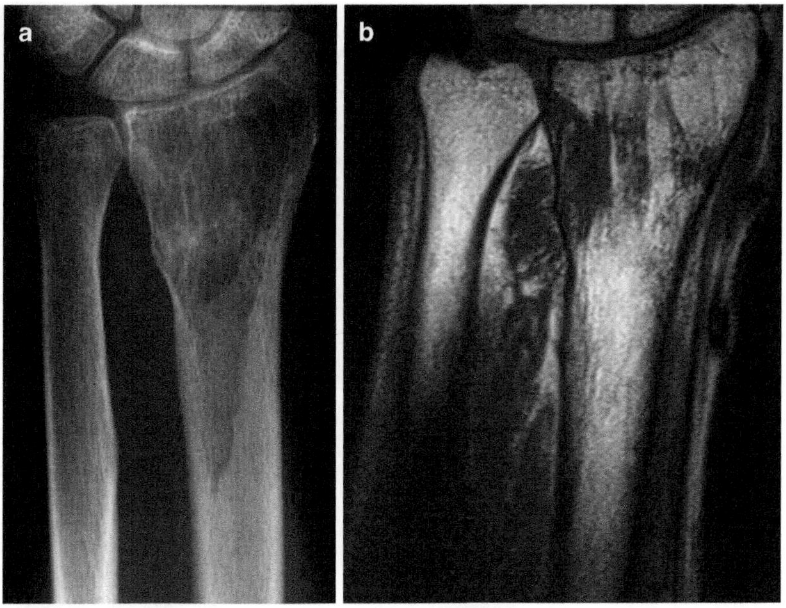

Fig. 2 (**a**) Radiograph and (**b**) coronal T1-weighted MR imaging of Paget's disease of the distal radius. The radiograph was initially misinterpreted as showing a giant cell tumour but the preservation of the hyperintense marrow signal in **b** is highly suggestive of Paget's disease

malignant transformation have, however, been recorded (Friedman et al. 1982). The MR imaging appearances of Pagetic marrow can be variable (Smith et al. 2002) but a useful diagnostic sign is the preservation of the hyperintense marrow signal on T1-weighted images (Fig. 2; Boutin et al. 1998; Kaufmann et al. 1991; Sundaram et al. 2001; Vande Berg et al. 2001).

3 Sarcoid

Sarcoidosis is a granulomatous disorder of unknown cause that affects multiple organ systems (Rajakulasingam et al. 2019). It is characterised by the presence of multiple non-caseating granulomas, most commonly seen in the lungs, lymph nodes, skin and eyes. The diagnosis is made by a combination of clinical, radiological and histological features.

Skeletal involvement has been reported in 1%–13% of patients with the disease. Radiographic evaluation is often limited to the hands or feet, which demonstrate predominantly osteolytic lesions. The hand is the commonest site of skeletal sarcoidosis. The lesions may be unilateral or bilateral, but symmetrical involvement is unusual. Lesions in the hand are most commonly seen in the middle and distal phalanges, and less often in the proximal phalanges and metacarpals (Van Linthoudt and Ott 1986). There are several types of lesion that are seen. The characteristic lesion is the alteration of the trabecular lattice resulting in a honeycomb lytic appearance (Fig. 3). Cystic lesions may also occur leading to a punched-out appearance that may be located centrally or eccentrically (Fig. 3). Osseous destruction may appear rapidly if these lesions are associated with cortical erosion, which can lead to pathological fracture (Neville et al. 1976, 1977). Periosteal new bone formation is uncommon.

Acro-osteolysis (terminal phalangeal resorption) has been reported in sarcoid involvement of the hands (Fig. 4). The finding is non-specific. In both the hand and the wrist, tenosynovitis is a recognised complication of sarcoidosis (Katzman et al. 1997; Moore 2003). Other soft tissue changes can be seen on MR imaging. These include focal and diffuse muscle lesions, soft tissue infiltration and masses (Moore 2003). MR imaging may also be useful in the differential diagnosis, for example in the evaluation of soft tissue nodules distinguishing gout from sarcoid-

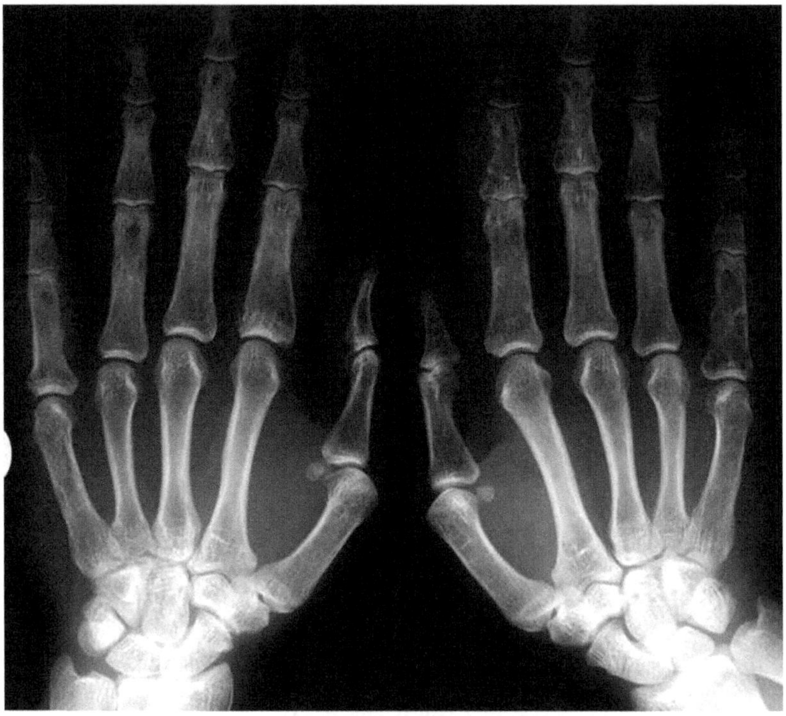

Fig. 3 Sarcoidosis. There is involvement of the proximal and middle phalanges of both hands. The appearances are more punched-out on the *left* with honeycomb osteolysis on the *right*

osis. Intermediate-weighted MR images typically show tophi as hypointense, whereas sarcoid nodules will usually be hyperintense.

Lofgren syndrome is a well-recognised manifestation of sarcoidosis, with patients exhibiting arthralgias, erythema nodosum and bilateral hilar lymphadenopathy. Polyarthritis involving the interphalangeal joints, wrists, elbows, knees or ankles is common. Monoarthritis and effusion are uncommon. Ten to thirty-five percentage of sarcoidosis patients will also experience joint symptoms due to granulomatous arthritis with a chronic transient or relapsing arthropathy. Sausage-like dactylitis of the fingers can also occur (Fig. 4). Pain is usually not severe. The uptake of FDG in PET scanning from sarcoid tissue is non-specific. However, Brudin et al. (1994) have described how the degree of FDG uptake correlates with disease activity, and although FDG PET is not useful for initial diagnosis, it could be used for evaluating the extent of active disease and monitoring response to therapy (Love et al. 2005).

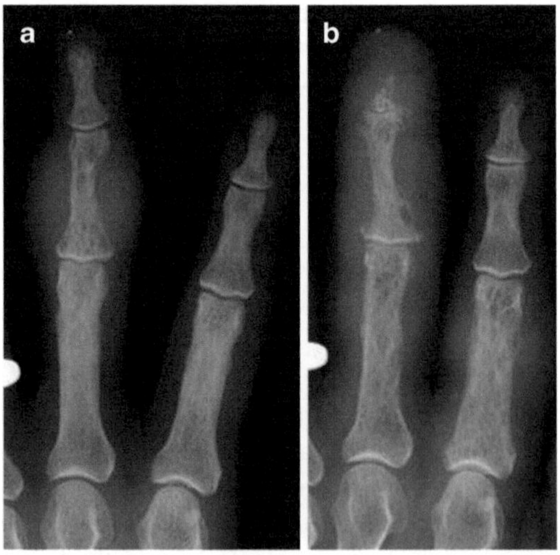

Fig. 4 Sarcoidosis. At presentation, (**a**) showing eccentric soft tissue swelling and lacy osteolysis of the middle phalanx of the middle finger; 14 years later, (**b**) showing soft tissue swelling of both index and middle fingers and progression of disease with terminal phalangeal resorption and further destruction of the middle phalanx of the middle finger. There is now also involvement of the proximal phalanges of both fingers

4 Reflex Sympathetic Dystrophy

Reflex sympathetic dystrophy (RSD) is a distinct condition that occurs in a variety of clinical situations. There are several terms that are used to describe the same condition including: causalgia, algodystrophy, Sudeck's atrophy, post-traumatic osteoporosis and complex regional pain syndrome (Agha and Jawad 2011). Although the cause is often idiopathic, many visceral, musculoskeletal, neurological and vascular conditions can cause RSD with trauma the most common. The most frequent site for RSD is in the hand. Clinical symptoms include stiffness, pain, tenderness and weakness. Radiographic changes range from soft tissue swelling with juxta-articular osteopenia (Fig. 5) to a more generalised osteopenia (Fig. 6). The former can mimic the presentation of an acute inflammatory arthropathy but in RSD there is no joint space narrowing or erosions. Both three-phase bone scintigraphy and MR imaging can be used to assess the "activity" of this disorder over time (Park et al. 2009).

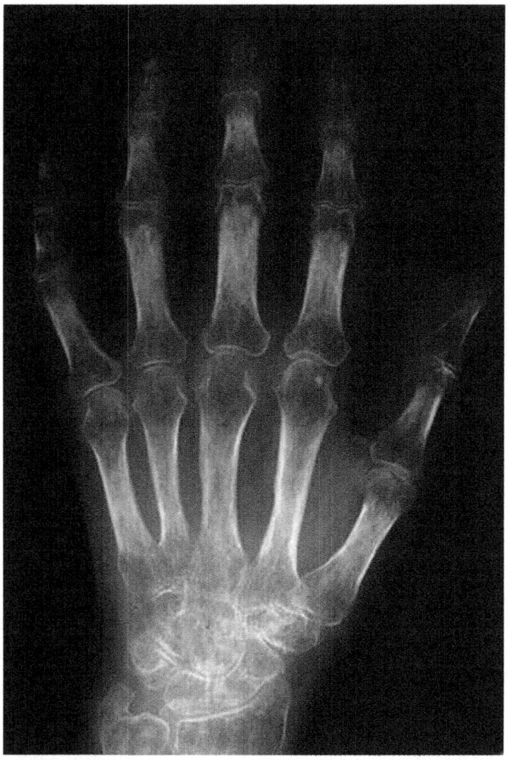

Fig. 5 Reflex sympathetic dystrophy. There is intense juxta-articular osteopenia mimicking an acute inflammatory arthropathy

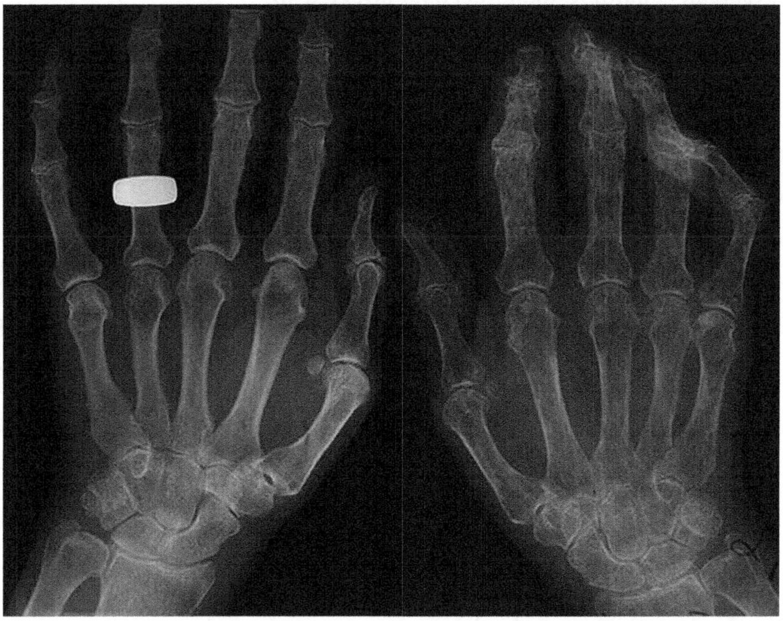

Fig. 6 Reflex sympathetic dystrophy. In this chronic case affecting the right hand, there is intense generalised osteopenia with multiple intracortical lucencies. Note the normal bone density of the unaffected left hand

5 Haematological and Marrow Disorders

This section covers the imaging manifestations in the hand and wrist of haematological and marrow disorders including haemophilia, sickle cell anaemia and thalassaemia.

5.1 Haemophilia

Haemophilia and related bleeding disorders are a group of conditions that are characterised by abnormality in blood coagulation caused by deficiency in certain plasma clotting factors. The two most common types associated with intraosseous and intraarticular bleeding are haemophilia A (deficiency in clotting factor VIII) and haemophilia B (deficiency in clotting factor IX). Haemarthrosis occurs in 75%–90% of people with haemophilia and in time leads to a haemophilic arthropathy. This begins between the ages of 2–3 years and increases in frequency till the ages of 8–13 years. The joints most commonly affected include the knee, elbow, ankle, hip and shoulder. Usually, a single joint is involved in each episode, though eventually multiple joints become affected in this disease. Intraarticular bleeding is rare in the hand and wrist. A well-recognised but rare complication occurring in approximately 2% of patients with severe haemophilia is the so-called haemophilic pseudotumour. These result from chronic recurrent haemorrhage that may be intraosseous (Cross et al. 2013), subperiosteal or arise in the soft tissues. The bones most frequently involved, in order of decreasing frequency, are the femur, pelvis, tibia and the small bones of the hand (Park and Ryu 2004). Cases have also been reported affecting the distal forearm bones (Ahlberg 1975; Shaheen and Alasha 2005). Cases involving the hand and wrist are usually of intraosseous origin, whereas pseudotumours arising in the lower limbs and pelvis tend to be extraosseous with secondary pressure erosion of adjacent bones. In the long bones of the hand, intraosseous haemophilic pseudotumour shows an expansile benign-appearing lytic lesion mimicking amongst other pathologies an aneurysmal bone cyst (Fig. 7; Shaw and Wilson 1993).

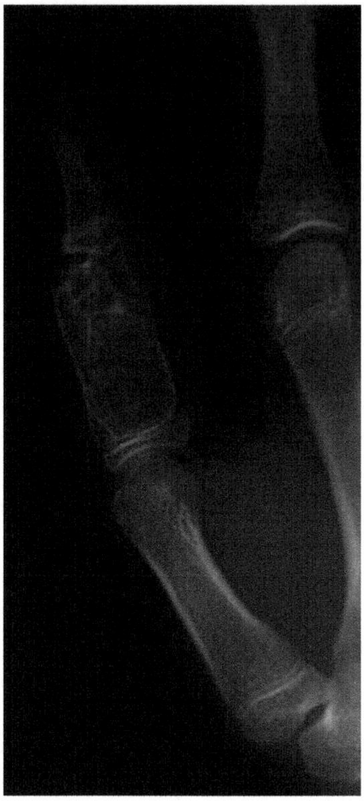

Fig. 7 Haemophilic pseudotumour proximal phalanx of the thumb. The age of the patient and the radiographic appearances mimic an aneurysmal bone cyst

5.2 Sickle Cell Disease

Sickle cell disease is one of the hereditary haemoglobinopathies characterised by an abnormal haemoglobin chain (HbS). Clinical manifestations of the disease include painful crises affecting the bones and joints of the extremities (Solomon et al. 2022). In children with sickle cell anaemia, 30% will present with hand–foot syndrome between the ages of 6–24 months with pain and swelling of the hands due to marrow infarction (Watson et al. 1963). The radiographic changes are those of a dactylitis with osteolysis and periosteal new bone formation (Fig. 8; Bohrer 1970). Hand–foot syndrome is rare after

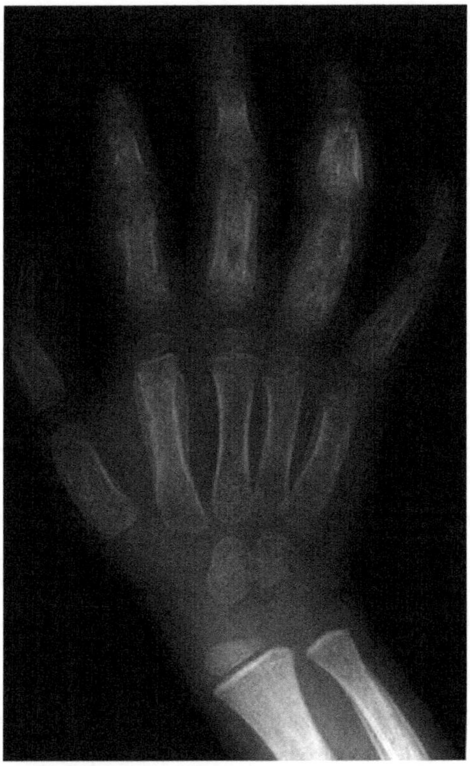

Fig. 8 Sickle cell disease. A young child with severe hand–foot syndrome showing medullary lucencies and periosteal new bone formation involving all the long bones of the hand and the distal ulna. The visible mineralised carpal bones are not involved

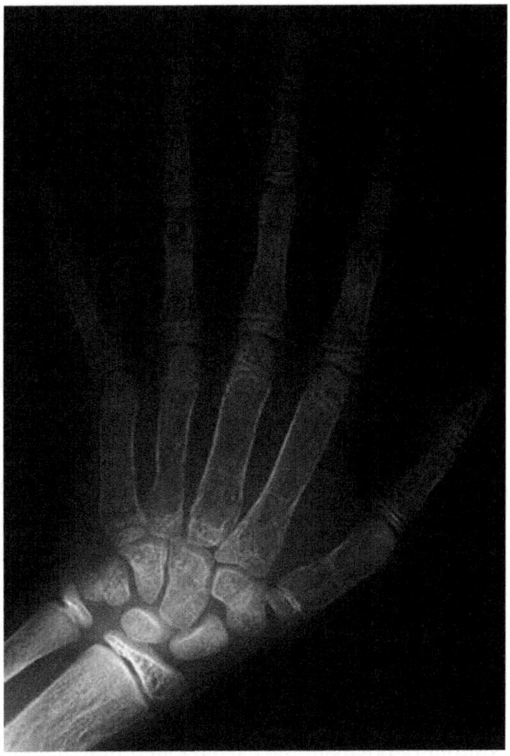

Fig. 9 Thalassaemia. The marrow hyperplasia is causing severe generalised osteopenia, trabeculation and minor expansion of the long bones

6 years of age because the red marrow recedes from the distal tubular bones of the hand and is replaced by yellow marrow with reduced oxygen requirements. Severe dactylitis may cause premature growth plate fusion thereby causing relative shortening of one or more long bones of the hand (Cockshott 1963). Ischaemic changes in the carpal bones are uncommon (Lanzer et al. 1984).

5.3 Thalassaemia

Thalassaemia is a hereditary haemoglobinopathy with an abnormality in the globin chain production of the red blood cell. This can involve a deficiency in alpha-globin chain synthesis or beta-globin chain synthesis. In severe untreated cases, there is generalised osteopenia and the tubular bones of the hand are expanded secondary to marrow hyperplasia (Fig. 9; Caffey 1957; Middlemiss and Raper 1966). There is also cortical thinning with a coarse, trabeculated appearance. When MR imaging is used in the assessment of the tubular bones of the hand, the findings may include an indistinct physeal–metaphyseal junction, altered signal intensity in the metaphysis, physeal widening and metadiaphyseal and epiphyseal lesions. Severe radiographic changes are not often seen in the developed world these days as most cases are treated from early infancy with repeated blood transfusions thereby reducing the marrow hyperplasia.

5.4 Other Marrow Disorders

The radiographic appearances in the hands of other marrow and deposition disorders such as Gaucher's disease and Niemann-Pick disease are relatively minor when compared with changes elsewhere in the skeleton. The authors have reported a single case of Erdheim–Chester disease presenting with a lytic lesion in a metacarpal mimicking a giant cell tumour or metastasis (Davies et al. 2010). Marrow malignancies are covered in the chapter "Tumours and Tumour-like Lesions of Bone".

6 Amyloidosis

Amyloidosis is the deposition of abnormal insoluble proteins in soft tissues and bone. It is not a single disease entity with to-date over 20 variants identified. The World Health Organization has proposed a classification based on the precursor fibril protein (Westermark et al. 2002). This includes primary systemic, secondary systemic, familial, dialysis-related, etc. Soft tissue amyloid deposition produces nodules that are often prominent over the joints of the hand and wrist. Similar deposits in the carpal canal may lead to carpal tunnel syndrome. Ten to thirty percentage of patients with primary amyloidosis have carpal tunnel syndrome. Typically, a bilateral distribution is seen, and signs and symptoms related to carpal tunnel syndrome often precede other manifestations of the disease. Amyloid deposition has also been documented in the wrists of patients on dialysis for chronic renal failure with carpal tunnel syndrome. The radiographic findings of amyloidosis in the hand and wrist include asymmetric soft tissue masses, peri-articular osteoporosis, widening of the articular spaces and subchondral cysts and erosions (Connor and Hole 2025). The appearance differs from rheumatoid disease of the hands and wrist as there is preservation of the joint space with soft tissue nodular masses. Extensive joint destruction is occasionally encountered in amyloidosis resulting from neuropathic arthropathy or osteonecrosis of the epiphyseal surfaces. On MR imaging, the amyloid deposits tend to be iso- or slightly hypointense with respect to muscle (Cobby et al. 1991; Kiss et al. 2005).

7 Haemochromatosis

Haemochromatosis results from excessive iron storage in the soft tissues. It may be primary, inherited as an autosomal recessive disorder, or secondary to chronic anaemias with multiple transfusions and dietary iron overload. In the hand and wrist, calcium pyrophosphate dihydrate (CPPD) crystal deposition causes chondrocalcinosis of the triangular fibrocartilage in up to 60% of cases. In chronic cases, particularly the primary form, a structural arthropathy develops with a predilection for the second and third metacarpophalangeal joints with joint space narrowing and hook-like exostoses on the radial aspect of the metacarpal heads (Heilmeier et al. 2023).

8 Phakomatoses

The phakomatoses are a group of neurocutaneous syndromes typified by the development of benign tumours and malformations, especially in organs of ectodermal origin. The two such conditions that may manifest in the hands are neurofibromatosis and tuberous sclerosis. In neurofibromatosis, this includes soft tissue masses, bone erosion from adjacent neurofibromas and localised gigantism (macrodactyly; Fig. 10) (Patel and Stacy 2012). In tuberous sclerosis, there may be multiple cyst-like radiolucencies, periosteal thickening and localised gigantism (Fig. 11; Bernauer et al. 2001).

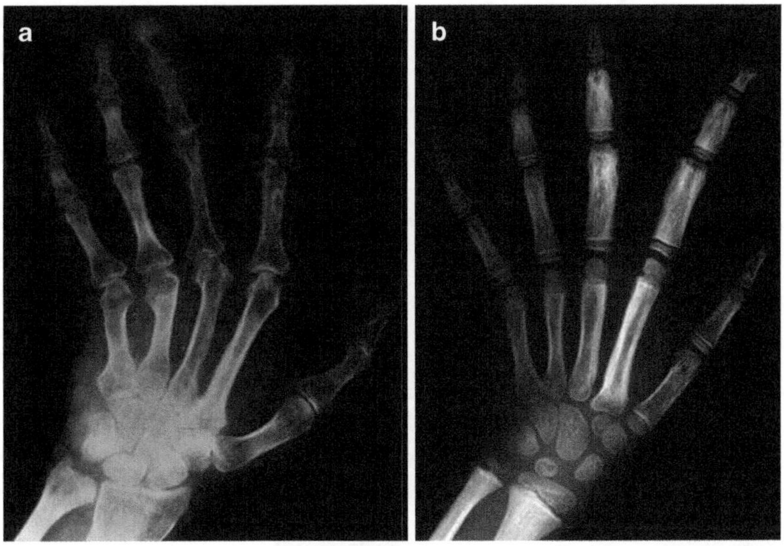

Fig. 10 Two different cases of neurofibromatosis. (**a**) Multiple soft tissue lumps due to subcutaneous neurofibromas and bone erosions in the index and middle fingers. (**b**) There is focal gigantism and sclerosis of the index and middle metacarpals and fingers

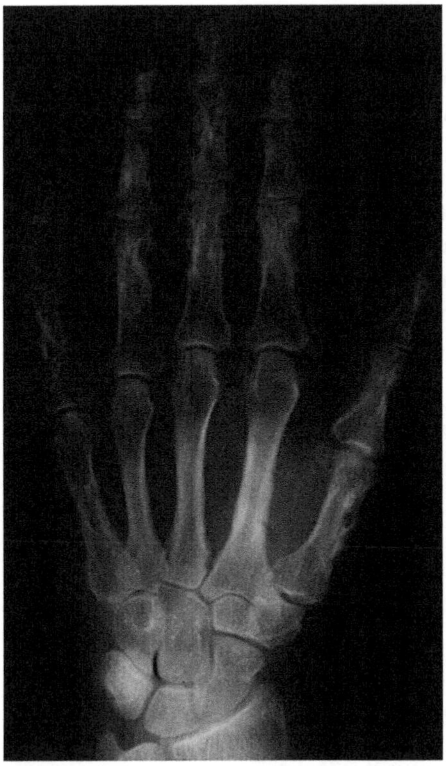

Fig. 11 Tuberous sclerosis. Multiple cyst-like radiolucencies involving the first and fifth metacarpals and all the fingers

9 Macrodystrophia Lipomatosa

This is a rare congenital form of localised gigantism due to overgrowth of the mesenchymal tissues particularly hypertrophy of adipose tissue (Mehra et al. 2017). This results in enlargement of one or more adjacent digits (Fig. 12; Hildebrandt et al. 1993). Most of the reported lesions are present at birth and are associated with a high incidence of local anomalies including syndactyly, polydactyly and clinodactyly. In the adult, the bony hypertrophy can be associated with periarticular exostoses (Fig. 13). The condition may also be associated with carpal tunnel syndrome (Ranawat et al. 1968).

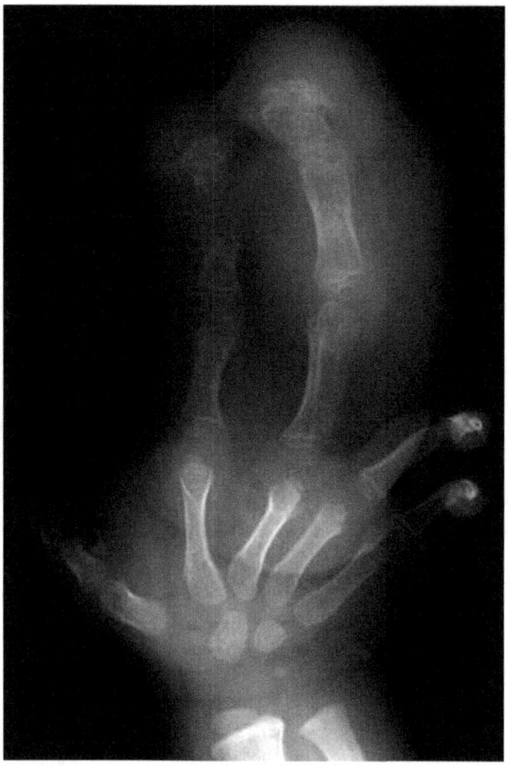

Fig. 12 Macrodystrophia lipomatosa in a child. Focal gigantism of the index and middle fingers with bony overgrowth and soft tissue syndactyly

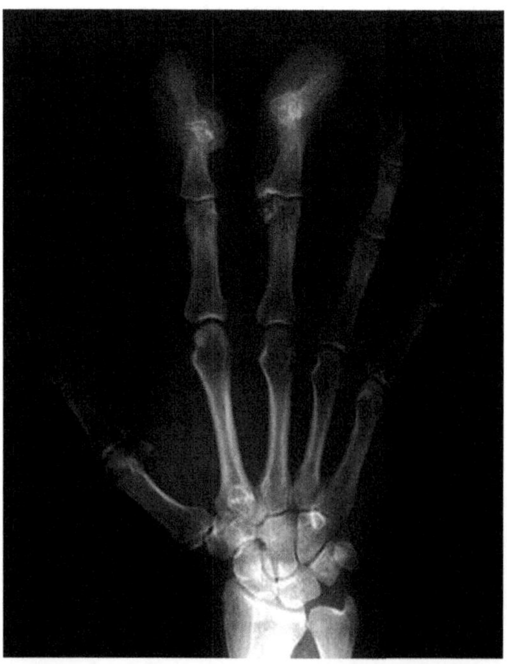

Fig. 13 Macrodystrophia lipomatosa in an adult: focal gigantism of the index and middle fingers with periarticular exostoses

10 Hypertrophic Osteoarthropathy

Originally called hypertrophic pulmonary osteoarthropathy, this condition was first described in the French literature at the end of the nineteenth century (Marie 1890). Clinical presentation is with pain and tenderness of the extremities with digital clubbing. Although most commonly associated with lung diseases, classically bronchogenic carcinoma, the term pulmonary has been dropped in recognition of the non-pulmonary associations (Table 1). The typical radiographic appearance is symmetrical periosteal new bone formation along the tubular bones. This occurs in the diaphyses of the radius and ulna, and less frequently in the metacarpals and phalanges (Yap et al. 2017). The severity can vary from simple elevation of the periosteum (Fig. 14), to a lamellated "onion-skin" appearance, to irregular periosteal "cloaking" with an undulating contour (Fig. 15; Ali et al. 1980; Pineda et al. 1987). The differential diagnosis for hypertrophic pulmonary osteoarthropathy includes pachydermoperiostitis sometimes referred to as primary hypertrophic osteoarthropathy. This is a rare, often familial, lesion predominantly of

Table 1 Diseases associated with hypertrophic osteoarthropathy

Pulmonary
Bronchogenic carcinoma
Metastases
Mesothelioma
Pulmonary abscess
Tuberculosis
Bronchiectasis
Cystic fibrosis
Cardiac
Cyanotic heart disease
Bacterial endocarditis
Gastrointestinal
Inflammatory bowel disease
Biliary atresia
Cirrhosis
Miscellaneous
Nasopharyngeal carcinoma
Hodgkin's lymphoma
AIDS

Modified from Gibson et al. (2008)

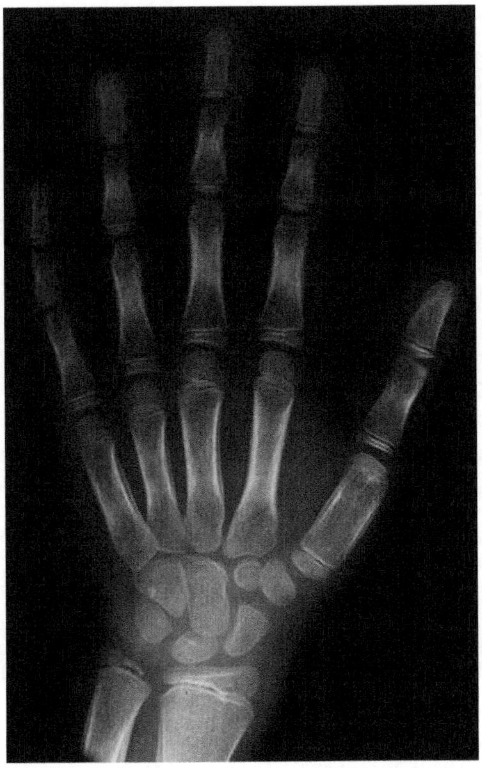

Fig. 14 Hypertrophic osteoarthropathy. Child with long-standing, untreated cyanotic heart disease. There is a single-layer lamellar periosteal reaction along the distal radius and ulna, the metacarpals and to a lesser extent the phalanges. There is also evidence of digital clubbing

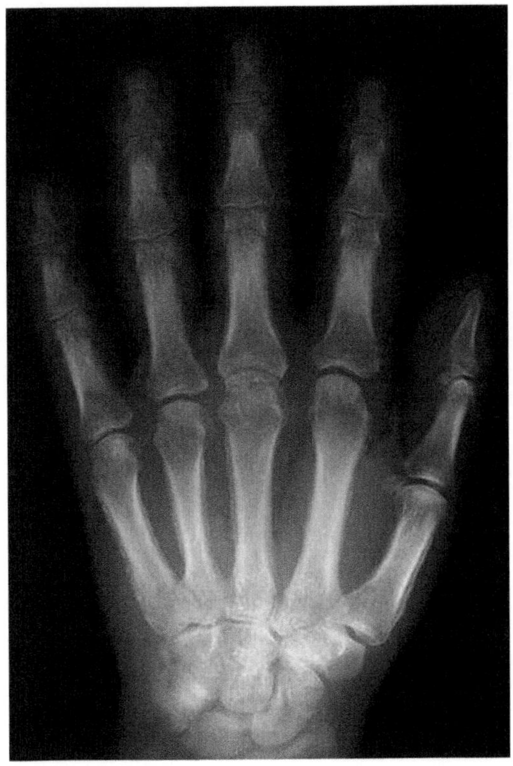

Fig. 15 Hypertrophic osteoarthropathy. Adult with known bronchogenic carcinoma. There is symmetrical coarse periosteal new bone formation along all the metacarpals and to a lesser extent the phalanges

males with a predisposition for Afro-Caribbean populations. Clinically, there is clubbing of the fingers, thickening of the skin and hyperhydrosis. Compared with hypertrophic pulmonary osteoarthropathy, it is relatively pain free. The bones most commonly affected are the radius and ulna, followed by the tubular bones of the hands. The periosteal reaction is similar to hypertrophic pulmonary osteoarthropathy but is more solid and spiculated and also involves the epiphyses to produce outgrowths around joints (Fig. 16).

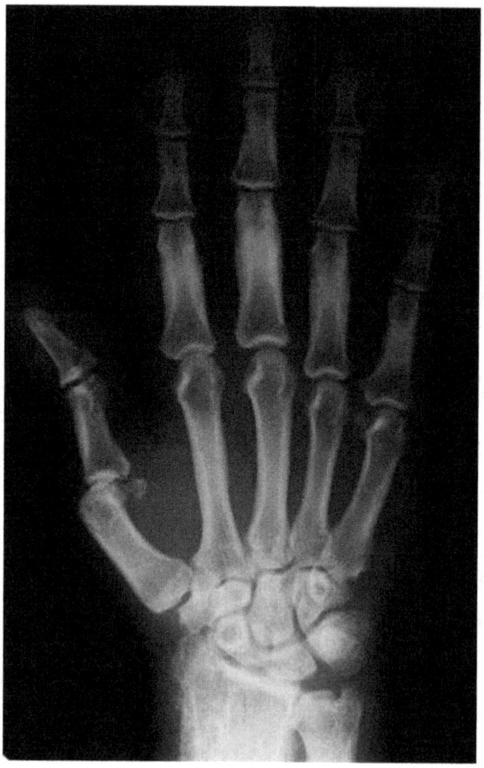

Fig. 16 Pachydermoperiostosis in an adult of Afro-Caribbean ethnic origin. Digital clubbing with coarse periosteal new bone formation along the distal radius and proximal phalanges

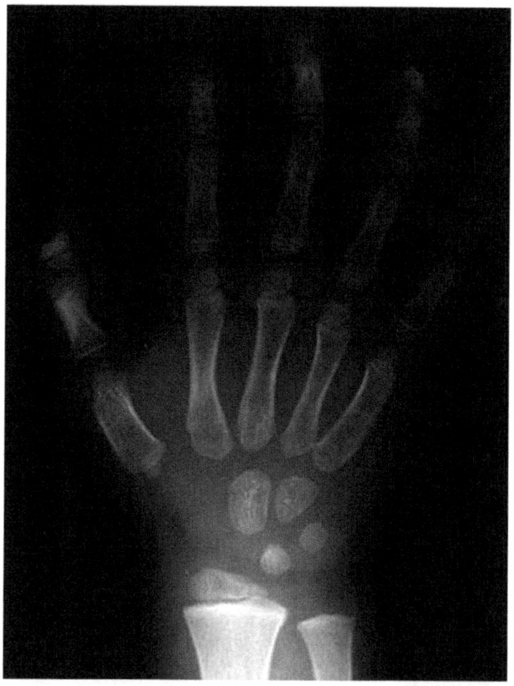

Fig. 17 Congenital insensitivity to pain. There is extensive terminal phalangeal resorption (acro-osteolysis) secondary to the underlying neuropathy. The appearances are non-specific and may be seen in other causes of neuropathy such as leprosy or following "trauma" such as frostbite

11 Congenital Insensitivity to Pain

Congenital insensitivity to pain, first described in 1932 (Dearbon 1932), is a rare hereditary sensory and autonomic neuropathy characterised by the congenital inability to register pain or temperature changes (Rahalkar et al. 2008; Reilly 2009). The principal orthopaedic manifestations are recurrent fractures, neuropathic joints and osteomyelitis (Silverman and Gilden 1959; Siegelman et al. 1966; Karmani et al. 2001). The changes in the hand include acro-osteolysis, amputations and secondary osteomyelitis (Fig. 17; Gwathmey and House 1984). Most of skeletal manifestations are secondary to neuropathic arthropathy rather than fractures (Mifsud et al. 2019). In children, epiphyseal separation and growth plate fragmentation may occur at the wrist.

12 Toxic Agents and Pharmacological Agents

Toxic effects manifested in the hand may be localised or systemic. An example of a localised toxic effect is soft tissue necrosis and contractures secondary to snake bite venom (Huang et al. 1978). Snake and scorpion venom have also both been reported as causing acro-osteolysis (Qteishat et al. 1985). Osteolysis resulting from secondary infections due to animal bites is well recognised. The animals include domestic pets, rodents, exotic animals such as camels (Al-Boukai et al. 1989) and of course humans (Resnick et al. 1985).

Systemic toxic effects include lead poisoning seen in the past in children who had ingested lead-based paints. Radiographs show a radiodense line paralleling the growth plates in the metaphyses of the distal radius and small tubular bones of the hand (Fig. 18; Leone Jr 1968; Sachs 1981). Multiple lead lines may be seen if the exposure to the lead has been repeated. The differential diagnosis of radiodense lines in the distal radial metaphysis includes other forms of heavy metal poisoning (e.g. bismuth and phosphorus) and the healing phase of rickets and scurvy and treated leukaemia. A toxic cause of more generalised bony sclerosis is fluorosis that is endemic in certain areas of India. In children, this may be associated with rickets-like changes (Christie 1980). An unusual form of occupational acro-osteolysis has been described in polyvinylchloride (PVC) poisoning (Gama and Meira 1978). The typical radiographic feature is a band of osteolysis through the terminal phalanges (Fig. 19a). With removal of exposure to the PVC manufacturing process, there is healing of the defects with shortening and widening of the terminal phalanges (Fig. 19b). A similar appearance may be seen with familial acro-osteolysis (Hajdu–Cheney syndrome) and has also been reported in a guitarist (Destouet and Murphy 1981).

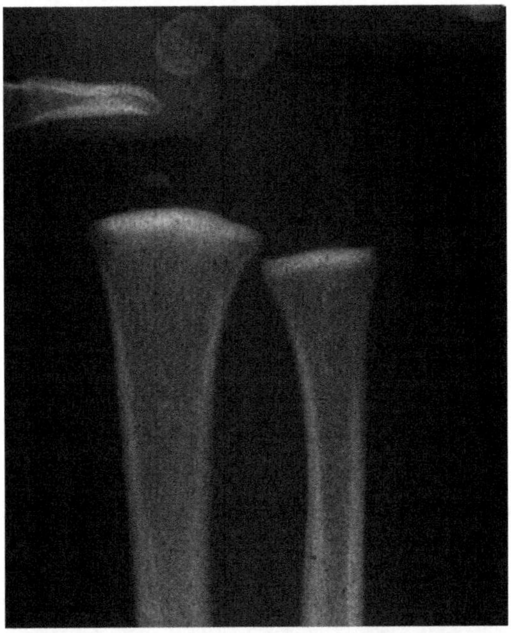

Fig. 18 Lead poisoning. An infant with a radiodense "lead line" in the distal radial and ulnar metaphyses

Prolonged and excessive exposure to numerous pharmacological agents may cause skeletal abnormalities identifiable on radiographs of the hand. These range from the devastating teratogenic effects of thalidomide (Fig. 20) to the rickets-like or osteomalacia pattern associated with phenytoin,

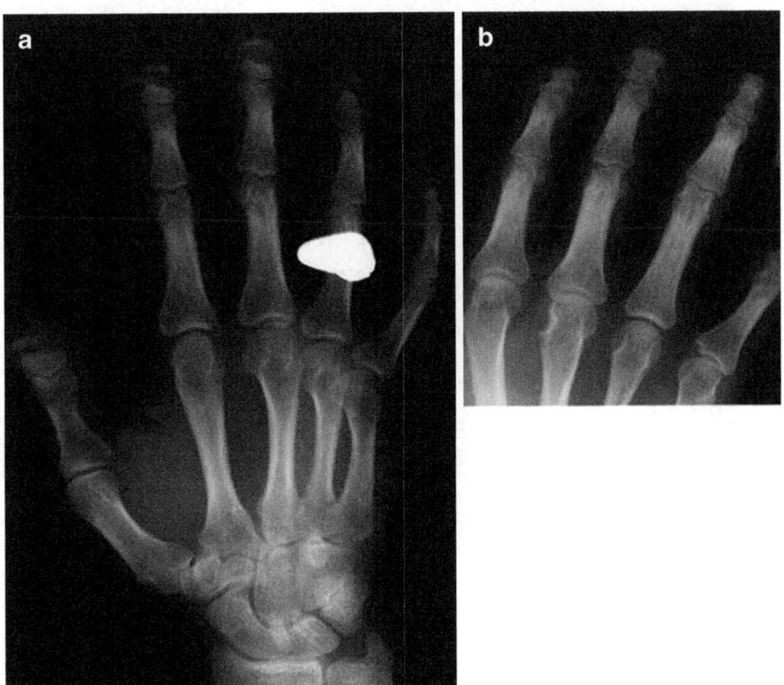

Fig. 19 Polyvinylchloride (PVC) poisoning. (**a**) Typical band-like acro-osteolysis across the terminal phalanges. (**b**) On removal from exposure to the PVC manufacturing process, there has been healing of the defects with shortening and widening of the terminal phalanges

phenobarbital, deferoxamine, diphosphonates and dialysis-related aluminium toxicity (Fig. 21). Hypervitaminosis A can cause generalised periosteal reactions (Caffey 1951) and hypervitaminosis D sclerotic metaphyseal bands (De Wind 1961).

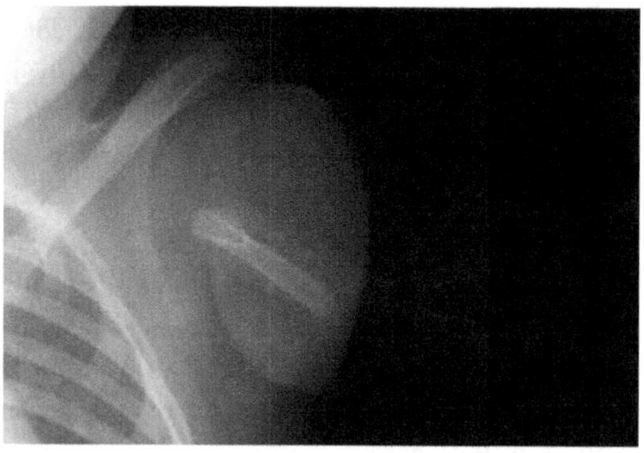

Fig. 20 Teratogenic effects of thalidomide therapy during pregnancy. The child has been born with proximal phocomelia and severe skeletal abnormalities of the hand

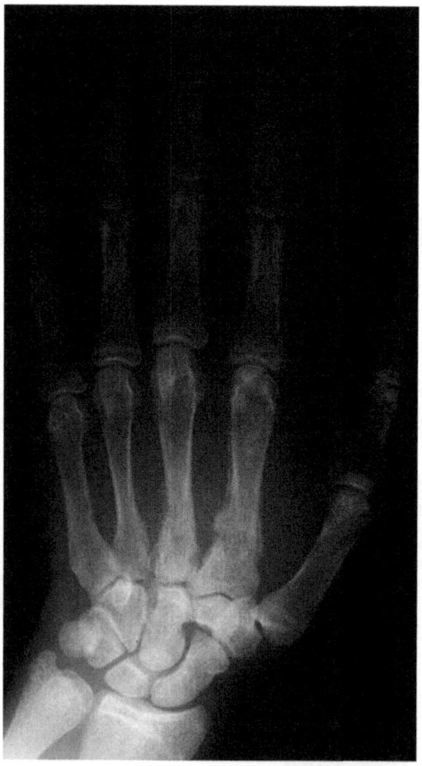

Fig. 21 Dialysis-related aluminium bone disease. Osteomalacic pattern with Looser's zone in the 2nd and 3rd metacarpals

13 Radiation Changes

It was not long after the discovery of X-rays in 1895 by Wilhelm Roentgen that the deleterious effects were being reported. An eminent British Radiologist, John Hall-Edwards, working at the General Hospital in Birmingham was one of the first to give a comprehensive description of the adverse effects of X-rays on the bones of the hand—using his own hands for case material (Hall-Edwards 1908). Complications include radiation-induced dermatitis with an increased risk of malignant transformation, growth plate damage in children and radionecrosis of the bones (Fig. 22; Steen et al. 2020). Radiation-induced damage to the hands from diagnostic X-rays is mercifully rare in this day and age but modern radiologists do need to be aware of the

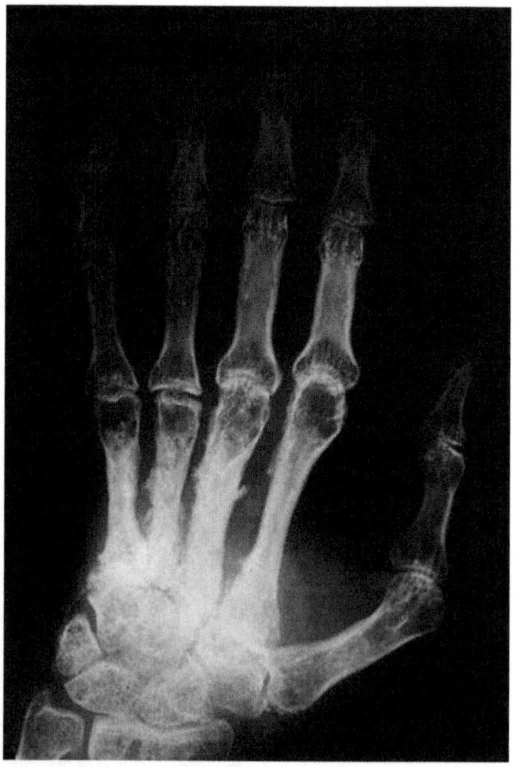

Fig. 22 Radionecrosis. Historical case of a seamstress who underwent protracted fluoroscopy for the removal of a sewing needle embedded in the soft tissues. This caused skin ulceration and contractures and radionecrosis of the metacarpals. (From the collection of Dr Philip Jacobs—deceased)

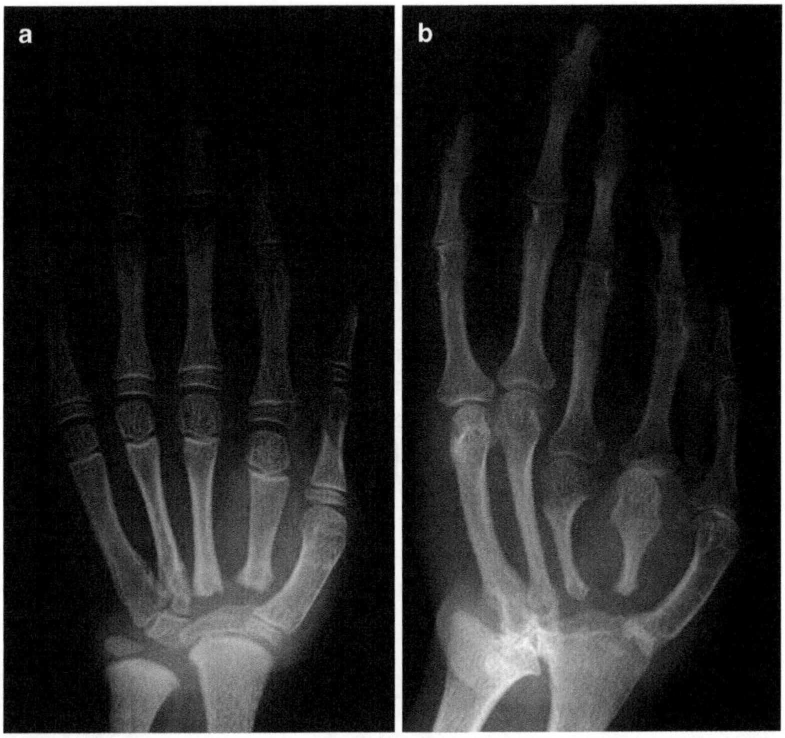

Fig. 23 Idiopathic multicentric osteolysis (Carpal-Tarsal Osteolysis). (**a**) Child showing marked resorption of the carpal bones with involvement of the bases of the 2nd and 3rd metacarpals. (**b**) Same case as an adult showing disease progression with further involvement of the metacarpals

potential increase in radiation dose to the hands when undertaking interventional procedures under either fluoroscopic or CT control. Radiation-induced tumours of the hand following radiotherapy are rare (Libshitz and Cohen 1982). It is possible that the incidence of radiation-induced osteochondromas in the hands may rise due to the increasing use of whole-body irradiation in children as part of the preparative regimen for haematopoietic stem cell (bone marrow) transplantation.

14 Massive Osteolysis

Bone destruction is a non-specific feature of numerous different bone conditions. There is a rare group of idiopathic disorders causing significant bone destruction that can be categorised under the title of primary osteolysis syndromes (Resnick 2002). The commonest is known as Gorham's disease or Massive Osteolysis characterised by uncontrolled, destructive proliferation of vascular or lymphatic vessels within bone and the surrounding soft tissues (Gorham and Stout 1955). Radiographs show dramatic, progressive resorption of bone that can cross joints and involve adjacent bones (Ozbayrak et al. 2013). The shoulder and the pelvis are the most common sites of involvement but cases have been reported in the hand (Patel 2005). Another rarer form of primary osteolysis is Idiopathic Multicentric Osteolysis also known as Carpal-Tarsal Osteolysis. Radiographs show progressive carpal bone resorption with in time involvement of the metacarpals (Fig. 23). Cases may be associated with a nephropathy (Warady et al. 1991).

15 Hydroxyapatite Deposition Disease (HADD)/Calcium Pyrophosphate Dihydrate Deposition Disease (CPPD)

Hydroxyapatite deposition disease (HADD) is a cell-mediated inflammation characterised by the accumulation of hydroxyapatite crystals in or around tendons (Hayes and Conway 1990).

The exact cause is unclear, but repetitive microtrauma and local ischemia are thought to contribute to its development other associations include end-stage renal disease, collagenosis and tumour calcinosis (Hongsmatip et al. 2019). HADD can affect the wrist, particularly in the flexor carpi ulnaris tendon proximal to pisiform and PIP, MCP joints (Ruban and Albert 2015). The condition progresses through four stages: precalcific, calcific, resorptive, and postcalcific (Benvenuto and Locas 2020). During the calcific stage, dense calcifications form, which can lead to an acute painful phase during the resorptive stage as the calcifications break down and cause inflammation. In post calcific phase, calcifications disappear. Most cases resolve spontaneously, but some may experience persistent pain and functional impairment due to ongoing inflammation or impingement (Doumas et al. 2007; Reddy et al. 2015) Soft tissue inflammation in acute phase of HADD might be misdiagnosed, as cellulitis, infectious arthritis or gout (Doumas et al. 2007). Unlike with calcium pyrophosphate dihydrate deposition disease (CPPD), a HA (hydroxyapatite) deposit usually presents as solitary amorphous calcification in the course of tendons. HA deposits are thus in contrast to the linear, granular/crumbly CPPD deposits (Schmitt et al. 2005) (Figs. 24, 25, and 26). Oral NSAIDs are usually the first-line drugs to alleviate pain and shorten acute inflammatory phase. Other options include oral corticosteroids or ultrasound-guided calcific lavage, in cases of calcifications over 1 cm (Reddy et al. 2015), image-guided local injection of corticosteroids.

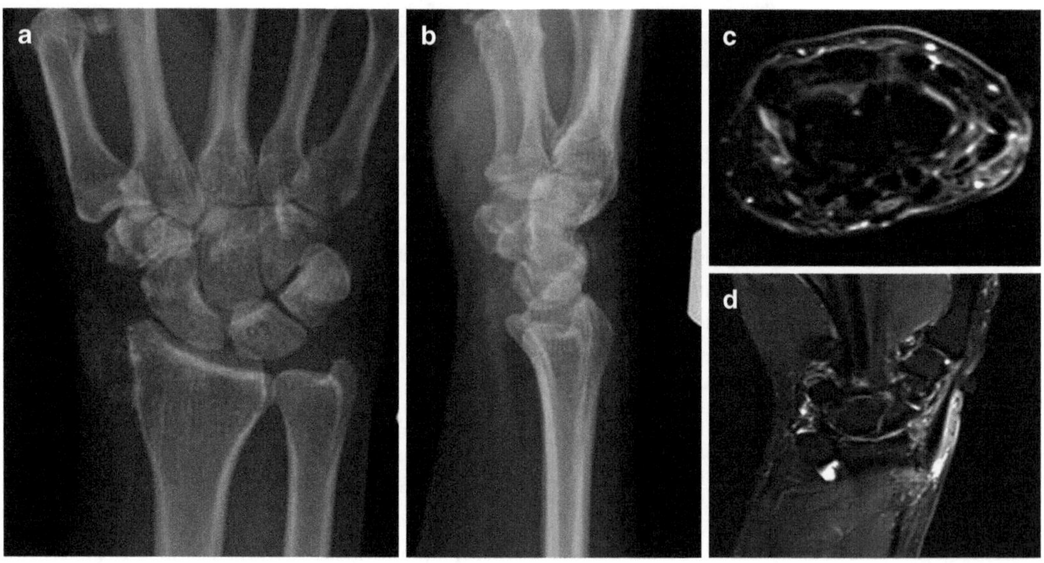

Fig. 24 AP (**a**) and lateral (**b**) radiographs of the right wrist show HADD (arrow). STIR axial (**c**) and coronal (**d**) show ill-defined oedema at the site of HADD

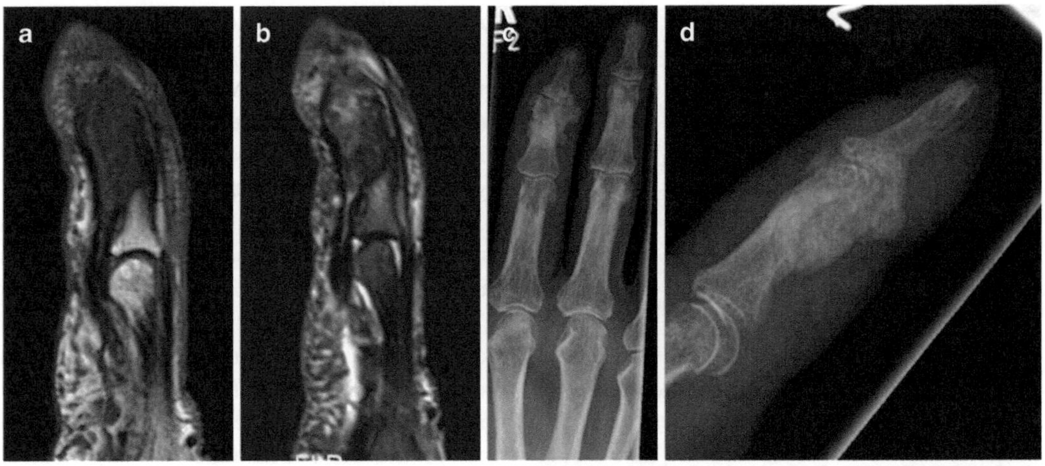

Fig. 25 Sagittal T1 (**a**) and STIR (**b**) show destruction with oedema involving the distal interphalangeal joint of index finger. AP (**c**) and lateral (**d**) radiographs demonstrated CPPD involving the distal interphalangeal joint of index finger

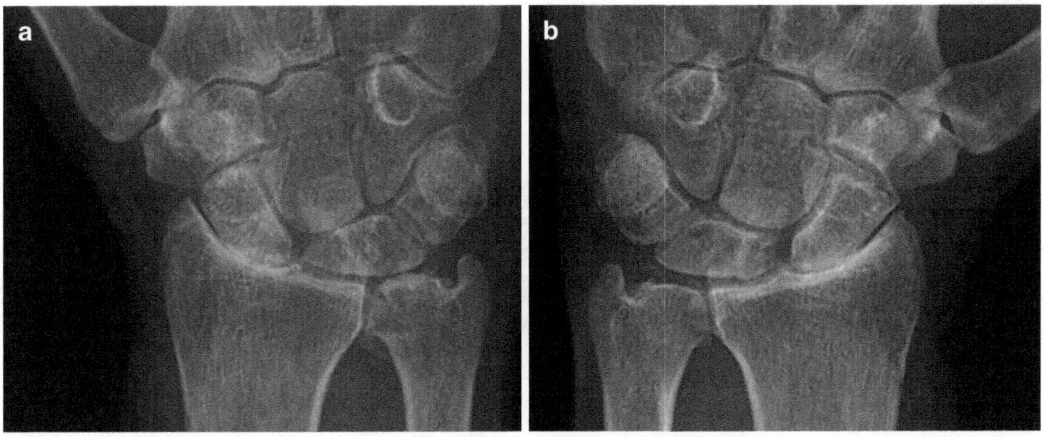

Fig. 26 (**a**, **b**) AP Radiograph of both wrists showing CPPD with severe radiocarpal degenerative changes

16 Ivory Phalanx

Ivory phalanx refers to a radiographic finding where a phalanx becomes denser due to endosteal and periosteal bone formation. This sign is specific to psoriatic arthritis, particularly useful when other bone or joint abnormalities of psoriatic arthritis are absent (Ory et al. 2005), and is often linked to nail disease in the same digit (Fig. 27).

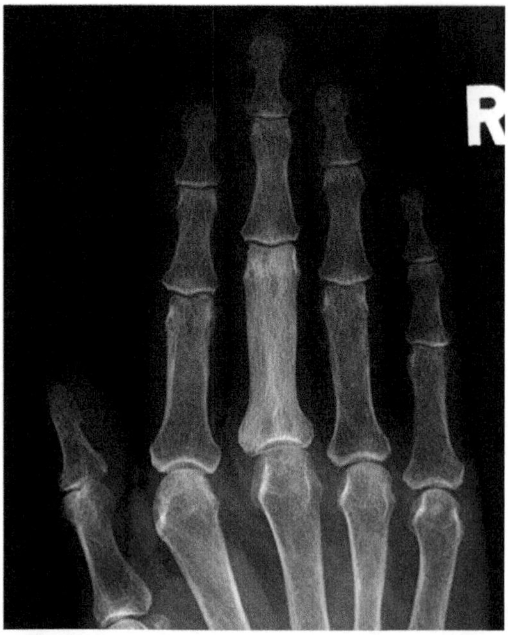

Fig. 27 AP radiograph of the right hand shows ivory phalanx involving the proximal phalanx of the middle finger

17 Finger Clubbing

Finger clubbing is a clinical sign where the distal phalanges of the fingers become enlarged, resembling drumsticks, often associated with underlying heart or lung disease (Fig. 28).

18 Acromegaly

Acromegaly causes characteristic changes in the fingers, including soft tissue thickening and bone enlargement, particularly in the terminal tufts of the distal phalanges from periosteal bone formation resulting in a spade-like appearance (Chang et al. 2016; Resnick et al. 2024) (Fig. 29). This can also lead to the formation of a pseudoforamen. However, similar changes can occur as normal variants, especially in manual labourers and the elderly (Resnick et al. 2024). Simultaneous formation

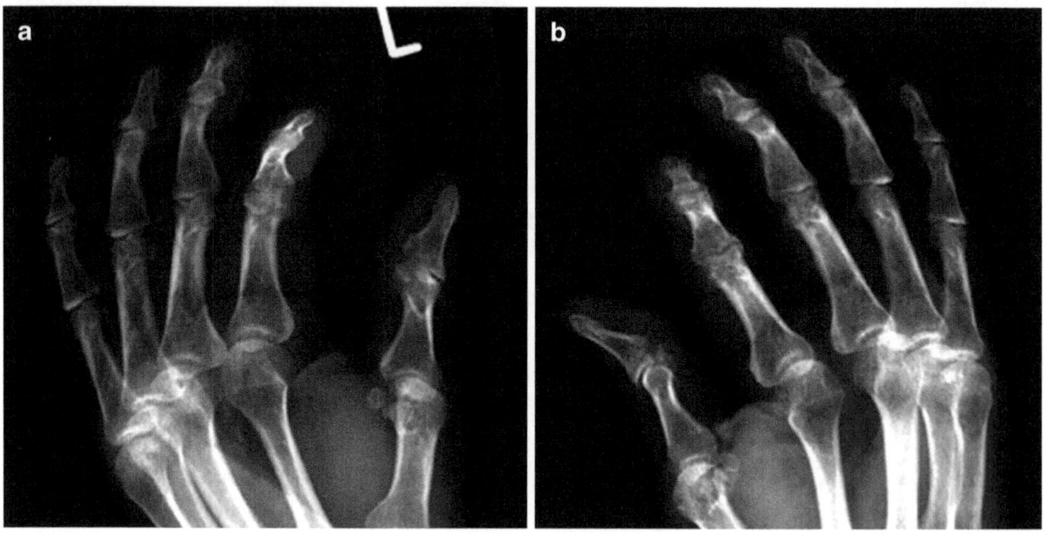

Fig. 28 (**a**, **b**) Obliqur radiograph showing soft tissue swelling of distal phalanges (distal part) of fingers

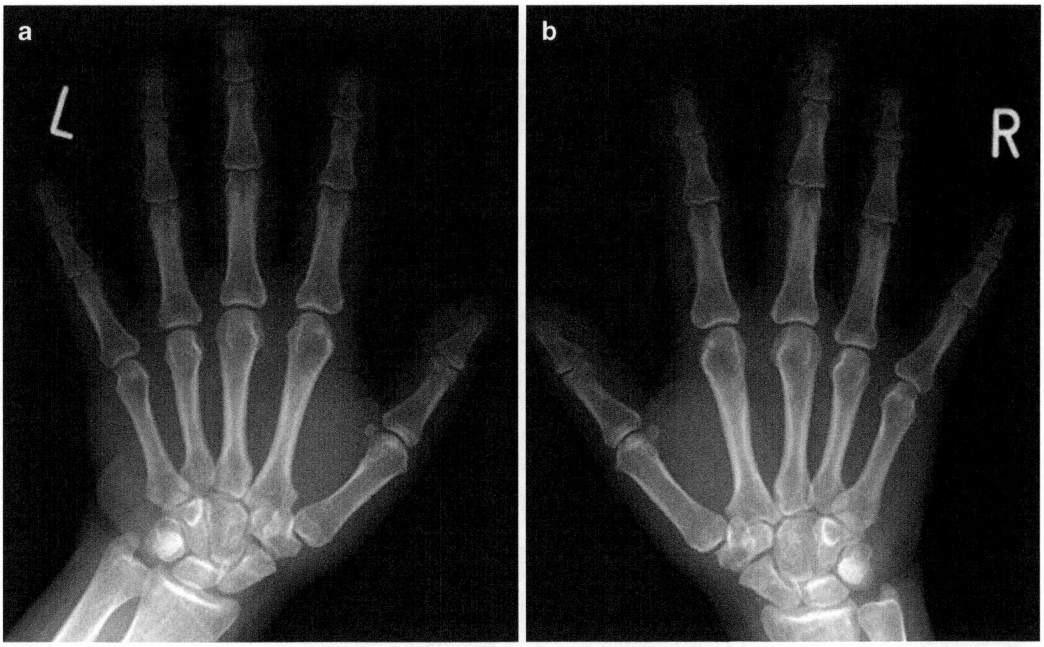

Fig. 29 (**a**, **b**) AP radiograph of both hands showing tifting of distal phalanx and soft tissue swelling of fingers

and resorption of bone causes hyper constriction of phalangeal diaphysis.

19 Achondroplasia

Achondroplasia is a genetic disorder (FGFR3 gene mutation) (Pauli 2019; Webster and Donoghue 1996) and most common cause of rhizomelic dwarfism characterised by distinctive radiographic features. It affects bones formed by endochondral ossification, leading to skeletal abnormalities, while bones formed by membranous ossification, like the skull vault, develop normally. Features in hand and wrist include short metacarpal, phalangeal bones, trident hand and pseudo epiphyses or accessory epiphyses (Gök et al. 2022) (Fig. 30). Individuals with achondroplasia typically have normal intelligence and motor function, may present with delayed motor milestones.

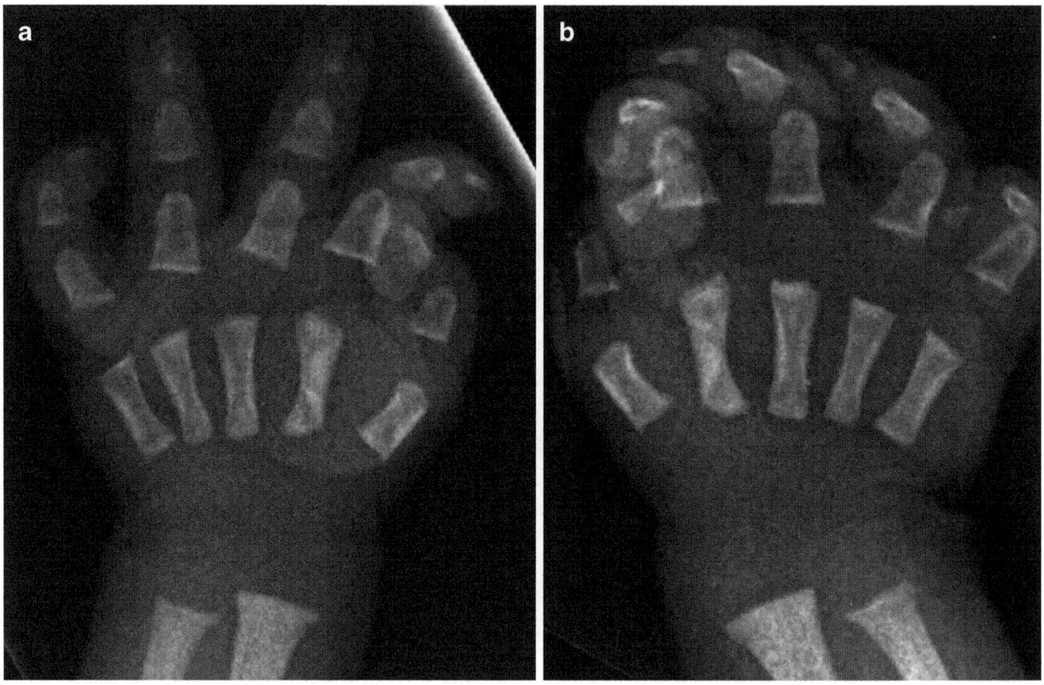

Fig. 30 (**a**, **b**) X-ray images of a child's hand, showing bone structure. Panel (**a**) displays an open hand with visible phalanges and metacarpals. Panel (**b**) shows a closed fist, highlighting the same bones from a different angle. The images are labeled with letters a and b in the top left corners

Fig. 31 AP radiographs of both hands show subtle increase density of bones and decrease in medullary cavity in particular of the metacarpals

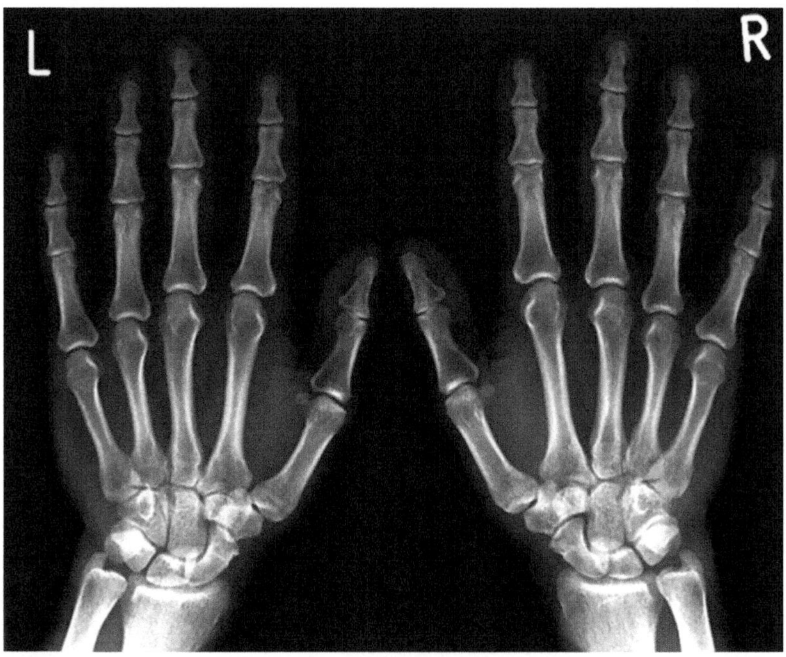

20 Osteopetrosis

Osteopetrosis, or marble bone disease, is a rare genetic disorder caused by defective osteoclasts, leading to dense but brittle bones prone to fractures (Fig. 31). There are two subtypes: infantile autosomal recessive and benign adult autosomal dominant. The condition results in weakened bones, bone marrow dysfunction, anaemia, and hepatosplenomegaly due to extramedullary haematopoiesis.

Appendix A. Key Points

- The hand is the commonest site of bone involvement with sarcoid.
- The hand is the commonest site for reflex sympathetic dystrophy (complex regional pain syndrome).
- Dactylitis may be seen in numerous diseases including sarcoidosis and sickle cell anaemia.
- Hypertrophic osteoarthropathy may be associated with both pulmonary and non-pulmonary disorders.

References

Agha M, Jawad A (2011) Complex regional pain syndrome of the right wrist – type I (CRPS-I). Egypt J Radiol Nucl Med 42:367–371. https://doi.org/10.1016/j.ejrnm.2011.10.002

Ahlberg AK (1975) On the natural history of hemophilic pseudotumor. J Bone Joint Surg Am 57A:1133–1136

Al-Boukai AA, Hawass NE, Patel PJ, Kolawole TM (1989) Camel bites: report of severe osteolysis as late bone complications. Postgrad Med J 65:900–904

Ali A, Tetalman MR, Fordham EW et al (1980) Distribution of hypertrophic pulmonary osteoarthropathy. AJR Am J Roentgenol 134:771–780

Benvenuto P, Locas S (2020) Hydroxyapatite deposition disease: a common disease in an uncommon location. Intern Emerg Med 15:333–334. https://doi.org/10.1007/s11739-019-02235-9

Bernauer TA, Mirowski GW, Caldemeyer KS (2001) Tuberous sclerosis: II. Musculoskeletal and visceral findings. J Am Acad Dermatol 45:450–452

Bohrer SP (1970) Acute long bone diaphyseal infarcts in sickle cell disease. Br J Radiol 43:685–697

Boutin RD, Spitz DJ, Newman JS, Lenchik L, Steinbach LS (1998) Complications in Paget disease at MR imaging. Radiology 209:641–651

Brudin L, Valind S, Rhodes C et al (1994) Fluorine-18 deoxyglucose uptake in sarcoidosis measured with positron emission tomography. Eur J Nucl Med 21:297–305

Caffey J (1951) Chronic poisoning due to excess vitamin A. AJR Am J Roentgenol 65:12–26

Caffey J (1957) Cooley's anemia: a review of the roentgenographic findings in the skeleton. Hickey Lecture. AJR Am J Roentgenol 78:381–391

Calif E, Vlodavsky E, Stahl S (2007) Ivory fingers: monostotic Paget's disease of the phalanges. J Clin Endocrinol Metab 92:1590–1591

Chang CY, Rosenthal DI, Mitchell DM, Handa A, Kattapuram SV, Huang AJ (2016) Imaging findings of metabolic bone disease. Radiogr Rev Publ Radiol Soc N Am Inc 36:1871–1887. https://doi.org/10.1148/rg.2016160004

Christie DP (1980) The spectrum of radiographic bone changes in children with fluorosis. Radiology 136:85–90

Cobby MJ, Adler RS, Swartz R, Martel W (1991) Dialysis-related amyloid arthropathy: MR findings in four patients. AJR Am J Roentgenol 157:1023–1027

Cockshott WP (1963) Dactylitis and growth disorders. Br J Radiol 36:19–26

Connor T, Hole S (2025) Musculoskeletal amyloidosis imaging. In: StatPearls. StatPearls Publishing, Treasure Island (FL)

Cortis K, Micallef K, Mizzi A (2011) Imaging Paget's disease of bone—from head to toe. Clin Radiol 66:662–672. https://doi.org/10.1016/j.crad.2010.12.016

Cross S, Vaidya S, Fotiadis N (2013) Hemophilic arthropathy: a review of imaging and staging. Semin Ultrasound CT MRI, Radiological Imaging in Hematological Disorders 34:516–524. https://doi.org/10.1053/j.sult.2013.05.007

Cundy T (2006) Is Paget's disease of bone disappearing. Skeletal Radiol 35:350–351

Davies AM, Colley SP, James SLJ, Sumathi VP, Grimer RJ (2010) Erdheim–Chester disease presenting with destruction of a metacarpal. Clin Radiol 65:250–253

De Wind LT (1961) Hypervitaminosis D with osteosclerosis. Arch Dis Child 36:373–380

Dearbon GV (1932) A case of congenital general pure analgesia. J Nerv Ment Dis 75:612

Destouet JM, Murphy WA (1981) Guitar player acro-osteolysis. Skeletal Radiol 6:275–277

Doumas C, Vazirani RM, Clifford PD, Owens P (2007) Acute calcific periarthritis of the hand and wrist: a series and review of the literature. Emerg Radiol 14:199–203

Friedman A, Orcutt J, Madewell J (1982) Paget disease of the hand: radiographic spectrum. Am J Roentgenol 138(4):691–693

Gama C, Meira JB (1978) Occupational acro-osteolysis. J Bone Joint Surg Am 60A:86–90

Gibson MS, Jennings BT, Murphey MD (2008) Hypertrophic osteoarthropathy. In: Pope TL Jr, Bloem HL, Beltran J, Morrison WB, Wilson DJ (eds) Imaging of the musculoskeletal system, vol 2. Saunders Elsevier, Philadelphia, p 1612

Gök M, Güneş S, Anık A (2022) Frequency and characteristics of metacarpal pseudoepiphyses in healthy children aged 5–15 years. Turk Arch Pediatr 57:651–655

Gorham LW, Stout AP (1955) Massive osteolysis (acute spontaneous absorption of bone, phantom bone, disappearing bone): its relation to haemangiomatosis. J Bone Joint Surg Am 37A:985–1004

Gwathmey FW, House JH (1984) Clinical manifestations of congenital insensitivity of the hand and classification of syndromes. J Hand Surg [Am] 9A:863–869

Hall-Edwards J (1908) The effects upon bone due to prolonged exposure to X-rays. Arch Roentgen Ray 13:44

Haverbush T, Wilde A, Phalen G (1972) The hand in Paget's disease of bone: report of two cases. J Bone Joint Surg Am 54A:173–175

Hayes CW, Conway WF (1990) Calcium hydroxyapatite deposition disease. Radiographics 10:1031–1048. https://doi.org/10.1148/radiographics.10.6.2175444

Heilmeier U, Burghardt AJ, Tse JJ, Kapoor P, Stok KS, Manske S, Voll RE, Schett G, Finzel S (2023) Analysis of hand joint space morphology in women and men with hereditary hemochromatosis. Calcif Tissue Int 112:440–451. https://doi.org/10.1007/s00223-022-01050-3

Hildebrandt JW, Olson P, Paratainen H, Griffiths H (1993) Macrodystrophia lipomatosa. Orthopedics 16:1075–1077

Hongsmatip P, Cheng KY, Kim C, Lawrence DA, Rivera R, Smitaman E (2019) Calcium hydroxyapatite deposition disease: imaging features and presentations mimicking other pathologies. Eur J Radiol 120:108653. https://doi.org/10.1016/j.ejrad.2019.108653

Huang TT, Blackwell SJ, Lewis SR (1978) Hand deformities in patients with snake bite. Plast Reconstr Surg 62:32–36

Karmani S, Shedden R, De Sousa C (2001) Orthopaedic manifestations of congenital insensitivity to pain. J R Soc Med 94:139–140

Katzman BM, Caligiuri DA, Klein DM, Perrier G, Dauterman PA (1997) Sarcoid flexor tenosynovitis of the wrist: a case report. J Hand Surg Am 22:336–337

Kaufmann GA, Sundaram M, McDonald DJ (1991) MR imaging in symptomatic Paget's disease. Skeletal Radiol 20:413–418

Kiss E, Keusch G, Zanetti M, Jung T, Schwarz A, Schocke M, Jaschke W, Czermak BV (2005) Dialysis-related amyloidosis revisited. AJR Am J Roentgenol 185:1460–1470

Lanzer W, Szabo R, Gelberman R (1984) Avascular necrosis of the lunate and sickle cell anemia: a case report. Clin Orthop Relat Res 187:168–171

Leone AJ Jr (1968) On lead lines. AJR Am J Roentgenol 103:165–167

Libshitz HI, Cohen MA (1982) Radiation-induced osteochondromas. Radiology 142:643–647

Lopez C, Thomas DV, Davies AM (2003) Neoplastic transformation and tumour-like lesions in Paget's disease of bone: a pictorial review. Eur Radiol 13:L151–L163

Love C, Tomas M, Tronco G et al (2005) FDG PET of infection and inflammation. Radiographics 25:1357–1368

Marie P (1890) De l'osteoarthropathie hypertrophiante pneumonique. Rev Med (Paris) 10:1–36

Mehra R, Bhartiya R, Agrawal P, Kumari N (2017) Macrodystrophia lipomatosa: clinico-patho-radiological correlation. Indian J Med Paediatr Oncol 38:559–562. https://doi.org/10.4103/ijmpo.ijmpo_65_16

Middlemiss JH, Raper AB (1966) Skeletal changes in the haemoglobinopathies. J Bone Joint Surg Br 48B:693–701

Mifsud M, Spiteri M, Camilleri K, Bonello M, Azzopardi T, Abela M (2019) The orthopedic manifestations of congenital insensitivity to pain: a population-based study. Indian J Orthop 53:665–673. https://doi.org/10.4103/ortho.IJOrtho_378_18

Moore S (2003) Musculoskeletal sarcoidosis: spectrum of appearances at MR imaging. Radiographics 23:1389–1399

Neville E, Carstairs LS, James DG (1976) Bone sarcoidosis. Ann N Y Acad Sci 278:475–487

Neville EW, Carstairs LS, James DG (1977) Sarcoidosis of bone. Q J Med 46:215–217

Ory PA, Gladman DD, Mease PJ (2005) Psoriatic arthritis and imaging. Ann Rheum Dis 64:ii55–ii57. https://doi.org/10.1136/ard.2004.033928

Ozbayrak M, Yilmaz MH, Kantarci F, Ozer H, Harmanci K, Babacan M, Dervisoglu S (2013) A case of an idiopathic massive osteolysis with skip lesions. Korean J Radiol 14(6):946–950

Park JS, Ryu KN (2004) Hemophilic pseudotumor involving the musculoskeletal system: spectrum of radiologic findings. AJR Am J Roentgenol 183:55–61

Park SA, Yang CY, Shin YI, Oh GJ, Lee M (2009) Patterns of three-phase bone scintigraphy according to the time course of complex regional pain syndrome type 1 after a stroke or traumatic brain injury. Clin Nucl Med 34:773–776

Patel DV (2005) Gorham's disease or massive osteolysis. Clin Med Res 3:65–74

Patel NB, Stacy GS (2012) Musculoskeletal manifestations of neurofibromatosis type 1. Am J Roentgenol 199:W99–W106. https://doi.org/10.2214/AJR.11.7811

Pauli RM (2019) Achondroplasia: a comprehensive clinical review. Orphanet J Rare Dis 14:1. https://doi.org/10.1186/s13023-018-0972-6

Pineda CJ, Martinez-Lavin M, Goodbar JE et al (1987) Periostitis in hypertrophic osteoarthropathy: relationship to disease duration. AJR Am J Roentgenol 148:773–778

Qteishat WA, Whitehouse GH, Hawass N (1985) Acro-osteolysis following snake and scorpion envenomisation. Br J Radiol 58:1035–1039

Rahalkar MD, Rahalkar AM, Joshi SK (2008) Case series: congenital insensitivity to pain and anhidrosis. Indian J Radiol Imaging 18:132–134

Rajakulasingam R, Azzopardi C, Murphy J, Davies M, Toms A, James S, Botchu R (2019) Lesions of the distal phalanx: imaging overview. Indian J Musculoskelet Radiol 1:47–56. https://doi.org/10.25259/IJMSR_13_2019

Ranawat CS, Arora MM, Singh RG (1968) Macrodystrophia lipomatosa with carpal tunnel syndrome: a case report. J Bone Joint Surg Am 50A:1242–1244

Reddy G, Hodgson N, Peach C, Phillips NJ (2015) Plain radiographic evidence of stages of calcifying tendinitis of supraspinatus tendon of shoulder. Emerg Med J 32:582–583. https://doi.org/10.1136/emermed-2013-203387

Reilly MM (2009) Classification and diagnosis of inherited neuropathies. Ann Indian Acad Neurol 12:80–88

Resnick D (2002) Osteolysis and chondrolysis. In: Resnick D (ed) Diagnosis of bone and joint disorders, 4th edn. WB Saunders Co., Philadelphia, pp 4920–4944

Resnick D, Pineda CJ, Weisman HM, Kerr R (1985) Osteomyelitis and septic arthritis of the hand following human bites. Skeletal Radiol 14:263–266

Resnick D et al (2024) Resnick's bone and joint imaging, 4th edn. Elsevier, St. Louis

Rodriguez-Peralto J, Ro J, McCabe K et al (1994) Case report 806: monostotic Paget's disease of the hand. Skeletal Radiol 23:55–57

Ruban TN, Albert L (2015) Wrist involvement of calcium hydroxyapatite deposition disease. J Rheumatol 42:1724–1725. https://doi.org/10.3899/jrheum.150178

Sachs H (1981) The evolution of the radiologic lead line. Radiology 139:81–85

Schmitt R, Christopoulos G, Kalb K, Coblenz G, Fröhner S, Brunner H, Krimmer H, Lanz U (2005) Differential diagnosis of the signal-compromised lunate in MRI. Rofo 177:358–366. https://doi.org/10.1055/s-2004-813931

Shaheen S, Alasha E (2005) Hemophilic pseudotumor of the distal parts of the radius and ulna: a case report. J Bone Joint Surg Am 87A:2546–2549

Shaw JA, Wilson SC (1993) Multiple hemophilic bone cysts in the hand. J Hand Surg Am 18:262–264

Siegelman SS, Heimann WG, Manin MC (1966) Congenital indifference to pain. AJR Am J Roentgenol 97:242–247

Silverman FN, Gilden JJ (1959) Congenital insensitivity to pain: a neurologic syndrome with bizarre skeletal lesions. Radiology 72:176–190

Smith S, Murphey M, Motamedi K et al (2002) Radiologic spectrum of Paget's disease of bone and its complications with pathologic correlation. Radiographics 22:1191–1216

Solomon N, Segaran N, Badawy M, Elsayes KM, Pellerito JS, Katz DS, Moshiri M, Revzin MV (2022) Manifestations of sickle cell disorder at abdominal and pelvic imaging. Radiographics 42:1103–1122. https://doi.org/10.1148/rg.210154

Steen K, Hayward V, Novak C, Anastakis D, McCabe S (2020) Secondary effects of radiation therapy to the hand for benign conditions. Hand (N Y) 15:341–347. https://doi.org/10.1177/1558944718810891

Sundaram M, Khanna G, El-Khoury GY (2001) T1-weighteds MR imaging for distinguishing large osteolysis of Paget's disease from sarcomatous degeneration. Skeletal Radiol 30:378–383

Van Linthoudt D, Ott H (1986) An unusual case of sarcoid dactylitis. Br J Rheumatol 25:222–224

Vande Berg B, Malghem J, Lecouvet F et al (2001) Magnetic resonance appearance of uncomplicated Paget's disease of bone. Semin Musculoskelet Radiol 1:69–77

Warady BA, Haug SJ, Lindsley CB (1991) Multicentric osteolysis: an infrequently recognized renal-rheumatologic syndrome. J Rheumatol 18:142–145

Watson RJ, Burko H, Megas H, Robinson M (1963) The hand–foot syndrome in sickle cell disease in young children. Pediatrics 31:975–982

Webster MK, Donoghue DJ (1996) Constitutive activation of fibroblast growth factor receptor 3 by the transmembrane domain point mutation found in achondroplasia. EMBO J 15:520–527

Westermark P, Benson MD, Buxbaum JN et al (2002) Amyloid fibril protein nomenclature. Amyloid J Protein Folding Disord 9:197–200

Yap FY, Skalski MR, Patel DB, Schein AJ, White EA, Tomasian A, Masih S, Matcuk GR (2017) Hypertrophic osteoarthropathy: clinical and imaging features. Radiographics 37:157–195. https://doi.org/10.1148/rg.2017160052

Post-operative Imaging of the Hand: Techniques and Applications

David Temperley and Raj Murali

Contents

D. Temperley · R. Murali (✉)
Wrightington Hospital, Appley Bridge, Wigan, UK
e-mail: David.Temperley@wwl.nhs.uk; raj.murali@wwl.nhs.uk

Abstract

Musculoskeletal (MSK) radiology plays a crucial role in the post-operative imaging of hand and wrist conditions. Apart from plain radiography, evolving and emerging radiology modalities such as computed tomography (CT), magnetic resonance imaging (MRI) and ultrasound (US) imaging provide the ability to assess fracture healing, detect post-operative complications, implant or hardware failures and monitor orthopaedic procedures. These abilities are fundamental to support clinical decision-making process and effective patient management.

In this chapter, focussing particularly on post-operative imaging of hand and wrist conditions, we provide an overview of a spectrum of pathologies MSK radiology is able to aid hand surgeons in Clinical Practice.

1 Introduction

This chapter focusses on the post-operative imaging of the hand. Needless to state that the radiological findings have to be interpreted only after a thorough clinical history and examination has been carried out as this will be of paramount importance to ensure that the radiological changes match the clinical findings.

Med Radiol Diagn Imaging (2025)
https://doi.org/10.1007/174_2025_614,
Published Online: 01 November 2025

2 Imaging Techniques in Post-operative Evaluation of Hand

2.1 Plain Radiography (X-ray)

The most important initial imaging examination in post-operative bone or joint surgical procedures is the hand X-ray. It is normal to obtain two projections of any bony structure, usually PA, and either lateral or oblique views. These show the metacarpals and phalanges and can assess bony alignment and assess for displacement of orthopaedic metal work or implants as well as loosening of joint prosthesis. A lateral X-ray will show overlapping metacarpals and phalanges but is useful to assess post-operative metacarpal bony alignment. Lateral X-rays of the individual fingers are performed by fanning the fingers so that each individual finger can be seen or by flexing the non-operated fingers out of the X-ray field (Whitley et al. 2005).

2.2 Computed Tomography (CT)

CT is useful in the post-operative hand to assess bony alignment and particularly fracture or osteotomy healing where X-ray does not give sufficient detail. Accurate demonstration of the position of fixation screws or wires, or joint prostheses can be obtained particularly where displaced. Thin section axial slices on modern CT scanners can be reconstructed into coronal and sagittal, or any required oblique plane without loss of image quality. 3D reconstructions performed by the scanner, or using a picture archiving and communication system (PACS) software, show a road map of the overall position of bones and orthopaedic implants. Metal implants lead to degradation of image quality through artefact because the metal absorbs photons so much more efficiently than bone or soft tissue, leading to streak artefacts. This can be compensated by increasing the tube KV, using a dual-energy CT X-ray technique and by other processing methods. The radiographer needs to be aware of the metal hardware to apply these procedures in obtaining the scan (Katsura et al. 2018).

2.3 Magnetic Resonance Imaging (MRI)

MRI is invaluable in assessing the soft tissue structures in the post-operative hand (Fig. 1). Unlike plain X-ray and CT, MRI shows excellent contrast resolution contrast resolution between different soft tissues. Tendon integrity and tendon sheath fluid can be readily demonstrated along with muscle abnormalities and fluid collections. MRI is very sensitive for soft tissue and bone marrow oedema, which is non-specific, but alerts the reporting radiologist to the presence of trauma, inflammation or infection. Hand MRI scans are performed with the patient prone in the 'superman' position within the scanner, or with the arm by the patient side if this is not possible. Dedicated hand and wrist coils should be used to obtain a small anatomical field of view and thus obtain high-resolution images. A combination of T1 and T2 weighted along with frequency selective fat suppression sequences are used to optimise demonstration of anatomy and pathological processes. Metal artefact is also a problem in MRI and is reduced by performing short tau inversion recovery (STIR) sequences (instead of frequency selective fat suppression), Dixon sequences, or using standard spin echo sequences with increased bandwidth and other metal artefact reduction techniques (Gupta et al. 2015).

2.4 Ultrasound (US)

Ultrasound is also useful in assessment of the soft tissues of the post-operative hand. Like MRI it can distinguish tendons, muscles and joints. Ultrasound is also used to assess masses and is particularly useful in distinguishing cystic from soft tissue lesions. In contrast to MRI, it can be used for dynamic assessment, which can be carried out along with clinical evaluation. It can sometimes be difficult to assess the integrity of a tendon on MRI, particularly in the post-operative situation. Using dynamic scanning movement of the finger or wrist while scanning will assess whether the tendon is moving and therefore whether it is intact. Tendons may be seen to

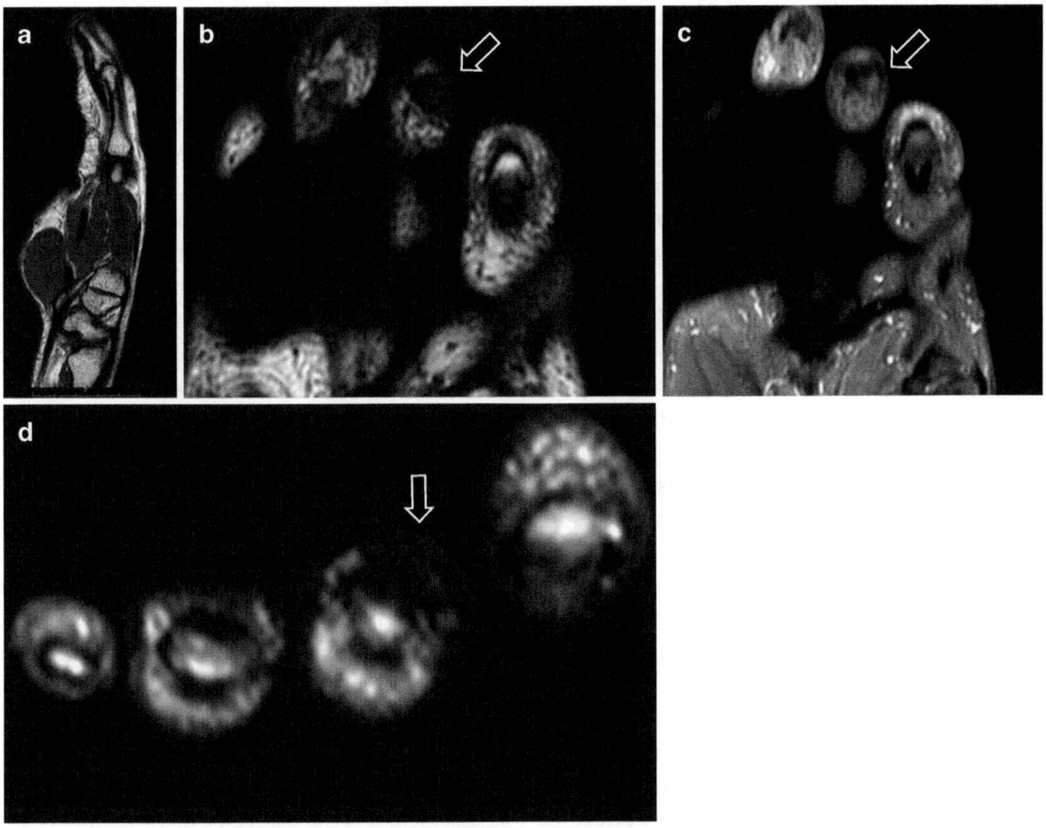

Fig. 1 (**a**–**d**) Neuroma after amputation of distal phalanx of a finger: Sagittal T1 MRI through the middle finger (**a**) shows evidence of amputation performed 12 years earlier. The patient presented with intense pain at the amputation tip. T1 coronal (**b**), PD fat suppressed coronal (**c**) and T2 TSE axial sequences show neuroma close to the tip of the amputation. (Arrows)

'catch' or move in an irregular manner. Ultrasound gives a clear representation of the internal fibrillar structure of a tendon, unlike MRI which just shows homogeneous low signal. Fluid in the tendon sheath is readily visualised. Ultrasound is particularly useful in the context of post-operative infection, and in particular to visualise collections that might need aspiration or drainage. Power and colour Doppler assess the vascularity of a lesion or tissue, which can be useful to assess for inflammation. Careful assessment of the hand bones will show fracture discontinuity, but it will be preferred in most cases to use X-ray to assess fracture or fracture nonunion. Ultrasound is commonly used to guide injections and aspiration in the hand.

3 Radiological Evaluation of Hand Fractures After Surgery

Fractures of the phalanges and metacarpals are common and represent 40% of all upper extremity fractures (Chung et al. 2019). Nonunion and particularly malunion are common. Tendon complications, either from the initial injury or as a complication of surgery, may occur, leading to adhesions limiting tendon and finger movement, and also tendon rupture. Infection is, as ever, a dreaded complication, fortunately uncommon when the fracture is closed, even if treated surgically, but deep infection rate can be up to 11% in open fractures (McLain et al. 1991).

Radiology plays an essential role in assessing these complications.

Operative treatment may be with 'K' (Kirschner) wire, plate and screws, screws alone, or non-surgical. Plain X-rays are the mainstay of post-operative assessment, and metal work should be carefully assessed for position and integrity, particularly where there are clinical complications.

The commonest complication of metacarpal or phalangeal fractures is malunion. An adequate X-ray series is excellent for assessing angular malalignment or shortening. The patient may be able to compensate for residual angular deformity, but rotational deformity transmits to the entire digit distal to the injury and will make, for example, making fist or fine finger movements impossible. On X-ray, it is important to assess the alignment of the distal part of the bone with the proximal, but even so it may be impossible to pick up small but important degrees of rotational deformity. CT may be required for this, and other complex post-operative fracture deformities. It is essential to assess whether the malunion involves the articular surface, because this may affect the nature of the corrective surgery, as the articular surface will need to be made congruent.

Nonunion and delayed union of the tubular bones, when they occur, will be associated with significant functional problems. Nonunion can also occur after attempted arthrodesis, particularly of the first carpo-metacarpal (CMC) joint (Fig. 2). Management of nonunion will depend on the site of the fracture and associated disability. Depending on this treatment can be with reoperation to achieve bony union, arthrodesis, arthroplasty or amputation. On occasion, operation may be deemed unnecessary (Jupiter et al. 1985). The value of radiology is to diagnose the nonunion or assess the degree of bony union. This can be achieved with plain X-ray, or if the presence or degree of union is not obvious on the X-ray, CT should be performed. It is important to note the presence of any metal work when referring for CT, as an extended Hounsfield range can be used when performing the CT scan, to reduce metal artefact. The presence of nonunion or the degree of union can be accurately assessed on CT, despite the presence of metal work. Partial bony union can be assessed in approximate percentage terms. A CT reconstruction plane perpendicular to the fracture is assessed, and the degree of bony continuity for each slice is estimated as a percent of the total, and then an average taken (Singh et al. 2005).

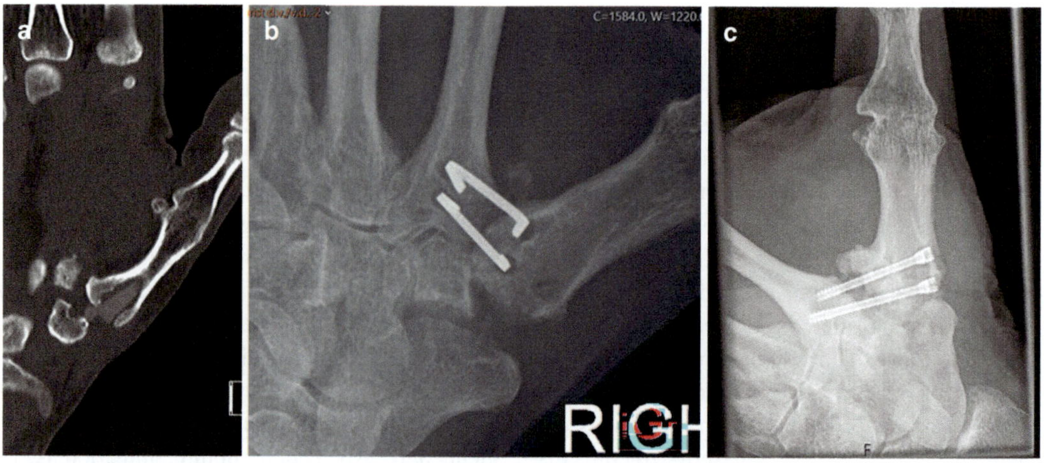

Fig. 2 (**a–c**) Nonunion following fusion: (**a**) CT, sagittally orientated with respect to the thumb, shows displaced, loose silastic 1st CMC joint replacement. (**b**, **c**) X-rays of the base of the thumb show successive attempts to fuse the base of the first and second metatarsal bones

Stiffness is a common complication after hand fractures and is more likely after more serious or open fractures. Periosteal stripping and neurovascular injuries associated with the trauma contribute to a complex pattern of injury which is often associated with stiffness. Plate and screw fusion may be associated with tendon adhesions, attrition or ruptures. Early mobilisation is important in the prevention of post-operative stiffness, along with adequate pain relief to allow this (Balaram and Bednar 2010). The main role of imaging in this context is to assess tendon integrity and movement. This is best achieved with ultrasound, which can assess dynamically for tendon mobility, tendon rupture and tenosynovitis.

Infection is a serious complication of hand fractures, or any hand injury. It is most uncommon in closed fractures, or those with minor soft tissue injuries, even if treated surgically. However, in open fractures with significant soft tissue injury the incidence is much higher.

Radiological investigations are essential in order to help early diagnosis in order to allow treatment before widespread infection takes hold, which may require amputation. Initial radiological investigation is with X-ray, looking for signs of bony erosion or resorption particularly around surgical metal work. Displacement of metal work may give a clue to underlying infection. MRI is invaluable to assess the extent of soft tissue and bony inflammation and infection. The hallmark of acute infection on MRI is prominent soft tissue or bone marrow oedema. MRI will distinguish fluid collections in the soft tissues or tendon sheaths, which may indicate the need for surgical debridement.

4 Post-operative Infection in Hand Surgery: Evaluation and Assessment

Post-operative infection in hand surgery is a serious complication. Fortunately, it is uncommon, occurring in 1.2% in a series of over 10,000 cases (Lipira et al. 2015). Risk factors for infection in hand surgery include older patients, diabetes, cardio-respiratory disease and increasing American Society of Anaesthesiologists (ASA) class. Patients with contaminated wounds, emergency surgery and longer operating time are more likely to suffer post-operative infections, while elective and outpatient surgery is associated with a significantly lower risk, Infection is more likely in cases where external fixation is used (Chung and Spilson 2001). In these cases, infection is most likely to occur along the pin or screw track.

In assessing soft tissue infection in the hand, a knowledge of the communicating anatomical spaces is useful. On the palmar side the flexor tendon sheaths to the thumb and little finger tendon sheaths communicate with the radial and ulnar wrist bursae respectively. The ulnar wrist bursa encloses the flexor tendons to the index, middle and ring fingers at the level of the wrist and carpus but is separate from the finger tendon sheaths further distally (Patel et al. 2014). Anatomical variants are common, and in particular the radial and ulnar wrist bursae may communicate (Fussey et al. 2009).

Deep to the flexor tendon sheets there are three palmar spaces, the thenar space, the mid palmar space and the hypothenar space which are separated by septa.

On the dorsal surface of the wrist there are separate synovial sheaths for each of the six extensor compartments which extend from distal radius and ulnar level to the proximal metacarpals. Separate potential spaces exist superficial to the extensor tendons (the subcutaneous layer), and also between the extensor tendons and the periosteum.

At the level of the distal phalanx of the fingers infection can spread from the nail bed to the pulp space, and vice versa (Patel et al. 2014).

Radiological investigation of potential post-operative hand infection should commence with plain X-ray. This will show bony and articular surface erosion in cases of osteomyelitis or septic arthritis. In cases where wire or screw tracks have become infected the X-ray will show

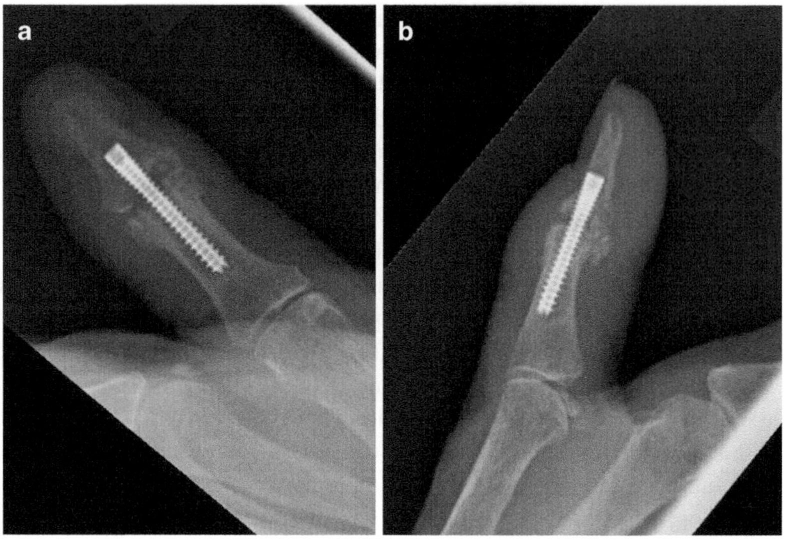

Fig. 3 (**a**, **b**) Infection nonunion. This X-ray is 8 weeks following routine arthrodesis of the interphalangeal joint and could suggest both infection and nonunion. This highlights the need for thorough clinical assessment supported by blood tests

lucency and bony destruction around the metal work (Fig. 3). It should be noted that the X-ray may be normal in cases of osteomyelitis for 2 weeks. Investigation of suspected post-operative hand infection should proceed to MRI. This will show evidence of bony or soft tissue infection at the earliest stage. Particularly useful is the presence of bone marrow and soft tissue oedema which are sensitive for the presence of infection, and specific with appropriate clinical findings (Fig. 4). MRI will show the extent and anatomical spaces involved with infection. There can be difficulty in distinguishing between infective cellulitis and reactive or non-infective causes of oedema. MRI with intravenous contrast may be necessary to distinguish fluid collections, as these do not enhance with contrast, while inflammatory changes show marked contrast enhancement. Ultrasound is particularly useful to distinguish fluid collections, including abscesses, tendon sheath fluid and joint effusions (Fig. 5). Doppler ultrasound can show increased vascularity which, like oedema on the MRI scan, is a marker for inflammation.

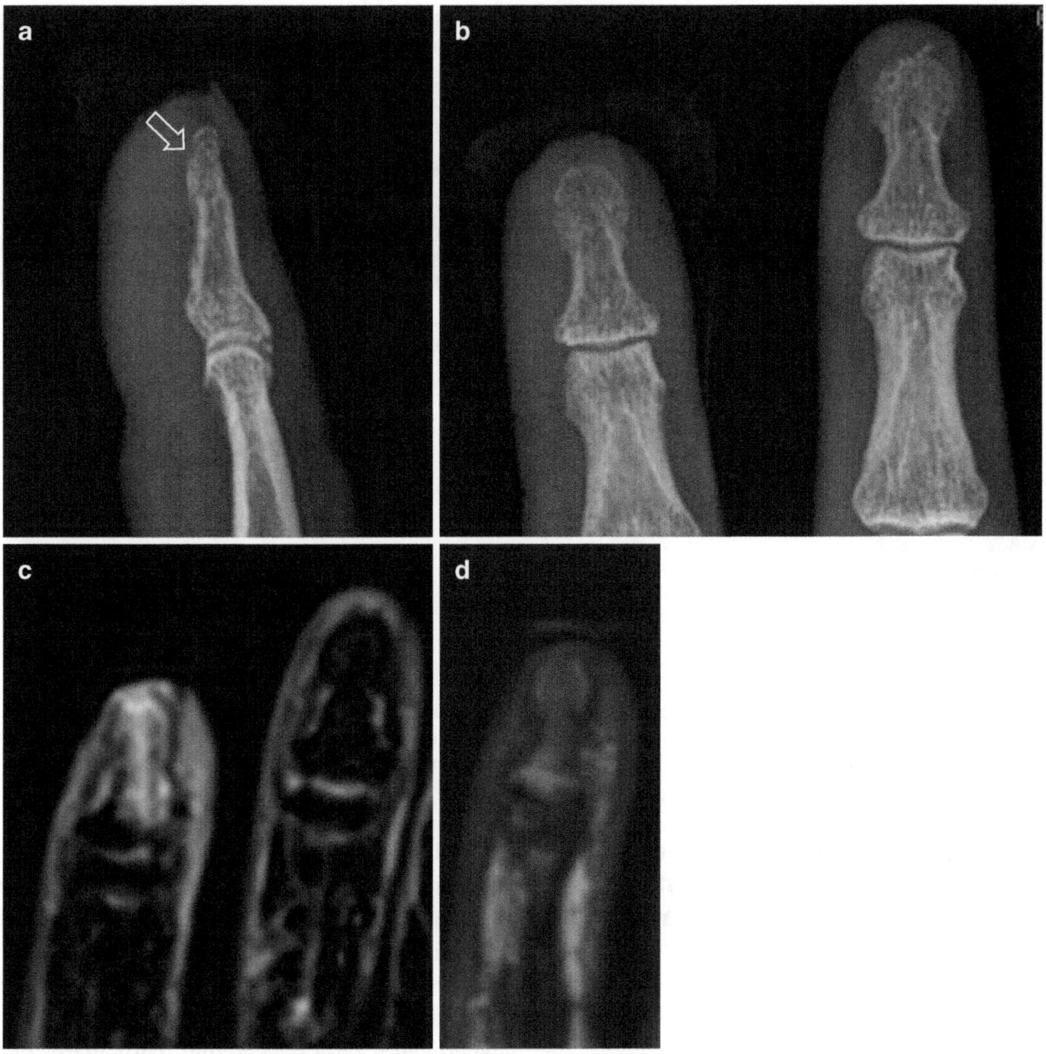

Fig. 4 (**a–d**) Osteomyelitis of the distal phalanx of the index finger in a patient with mixed connective tissue disease: (**a**). Lateral X-ray shows subtle erosion at the tip of the distal phalanx (arrow). (**b**). DP X-ray shows loss of bone density in the distal phalanx of the index finger compared with the middle finger. Coronal STIR and T1 MRI of the distal phalanx shows bone marrow oedema, confirming osteomyelitis (**c**, **d**)

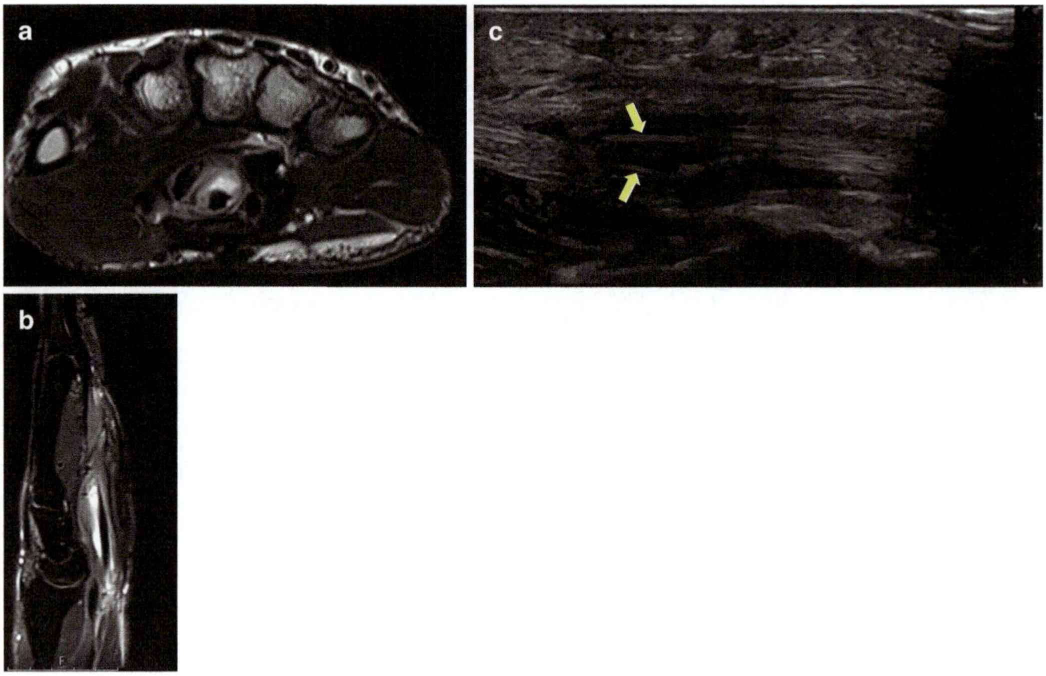

Fig. 5 (**a**–**c**) Post-operative infection following repair of the median nerve and flexor digitorum profundus tendon of index finger: (**a**) Axial T2 TSE and (**b**) Sagittal PDFS MRI images show fluid in the index FDP tendon sheath. The tendon is intact. (**c**) sagittal ultrasound image shows fluid in the tendon sheath, along with suture material

5 Radiological Assessment of Common Hand Tumours. Post-operative Evaluation

5.1 Recurrence of Glomus Tumours

The glomus body is a highly specialised arteriovenous anastomosis, which has a role in thermal regulation. Glomus bodies are present in the dermis throughout the body, but are more common in the fingers, the palms and the soles of the feet. Tumours of the glomus bodies represent about 2% of hand tumours, and around 2% of them are multiple (Theumann et al. 2002). They present clinically with severe and sometimes pulsating pain, and with tenderness and cold sensitivity. They may be raised with a pinkish or blueish colour. Clinical diagnosis is aided by Love's pin test (exquisite tenderness on pressing the nail with a pinhead) and Hildreth's test (pain relief by applying a tourniquet to the arm) (Morey et al. 2016).

Although clinical assessment may be suggestive, imaging is often required to help confirm the diagnosis. MRI is the most helpful radiological modality. The tumours show low signal intensity or are isointense on T1-weighted images. Because of their strong vascularity they are typically hyperintense on T2 weighting, particularly fat-suppressed T2-weighted images. Again, because of vascularity, they almost always strongly enhance (Koç et al. 2007). 75% are found in a subungual location and can also occur in the nail bed and in the pulp of the finger.

Ultrasound can be helpful and was the only cross-sectional imaging modality available prior to the development of high-resolution peripheral MRI scanning. Lesions as small as 3 mm can be seen, but ultrasound is operator-dependent and artefact from the nail can obscure visualisation of the lesion. Generally, ultrasound is considered less accurate than MRI.

The only curative treatment for glomus tumours of the hand is surgical excision.

The incidence of recurrence of glomus tumours after surgical excision has varied from 5% to 50% in literature studies. In general, early recurrence, within 1 year, is associated with incomplete resection of the tumour, or occasionally a second tumour that was not diagnosed pre or intraoperatively. Late recurrence, occurring after several years, is most commonly associated with a new tumour. MRI shows post-operative scar tissue in most cases which is of low signal on T1- and T2-weighted images. Scar tissue can enhance, but this is uncommon. Recurrent glomus tumours, on the other hand, almost always show features typical of the pre-operative lesion, with hypointense, isointense or occasionally hyperintense appearances on T1 weighting, and are hyperintense on T2-weighted sequences. Enhancement is usually, but not always, strong. Tumours are typically between 1.5 and 10 mm. On MRI imaging the recurrent tumours are more likely to be ill defined than the non-operated tumour (Theumann et al. 2002).

5.2 Giant Cell Tumour of the Tendon Sheath

Giant cell tumours of the tendon sheath are part of a series of benign proliferative tumours of synovial origin, sharing similar histology. *Tenosynovial giant cell tumours (TGCT)* are a group of non-malignant tumours involving the synovium, bursae or tendon sheaths. They do not metastasise but can be locally aggressive and can recur. Two main forms of this condition are defined: localised and diffuse. Diffuse TGCT encompass pigmented villonodular synovitis, generally occurring in large joints, most commonly the knee. Giant cell tumours of the tendon sheath are defined as localised TGCT. There is also a more localised form of TGCT in large joints, presenting with a solitary mass rather than diffuse disease (National Association for Rare Diseases 2023).

Giant cell tumour of the tendon sheath arises from the synovia of the tendon sheath of the hand, particularly on the volar aspects of the fingers. They are the second most common tumour of the hand after ganglion cysts. Typically found in the third to fifth decades presentation is with a slow-growing mass, usually painless. The tumour is benign; malignancy is considered an extreme rarity. A characteristic histological and radiological feature is the presence of haemosiderin as a result of haemorrhage into the tumour. This is extremely helpful in radiological diagnosis (Wan et al. 2010).

MRI is typically of low to intermediate signal on T1-weighted images and intermediate to high signal on T2-weighted images (Wang et al. 2017). Relatively low signal on T2-weighted images for a tumour are associated with collagen and hemosiderin. Hemosiderin is visualised as small, scattered foci of signal void on all sequences, i.e. black on MRI. This is accentuated on gradient echo sequences due to magnetic susceptibility leading to 'blooming' of the signal void areas. The tumour is vascular, and there is generally prominent contrast enhancement. Giant cell tumours of the tendon sheath typically show a lobulated outline, and in the fingers it often surrounds the flexor tendons which is helpful in differentiating from other soft tissue tumours. Ganglion cysts are easily distinguished as they show homogeneous high signal on T2-weighted sequences.

Ultrasound appearances are variable, and giant cell tumours of the tendon sheath have been described as hypoechoic, hyperechoic and either heterogeneous or homogeneous. Increased vascularity on Doppler is typical. X-ray and CT may show well-defined bony erosion, while CT and ultrasound are useful for guiding biopsy (Wan et al. 2010).

Recurrence rate of giant cell tumour of the tendon sheath has been reported between 9% and 44%. Complete tumour resection is the key to preventing recurrence, and it has been reported that interphalangeal joint disease, bony pressure erosions on X-ray and degenerative joint disease are associated with higher recurrence rates. Recurrence is more likely if the tumour is more diffuse or multicentric. Microscopic surgery has been advocated to prevent recurrence (Suresh and Zaki 2016). MRI is the mainstay of post-operative diagnosis of TGCT recurrence (Choi et al. 2024). Tumours will show similar characteristics to the pre-operative scan, with intermediate to low signal on T1-weighted images, and often low signal on T2. Areas of hemosiderin will show signal void particularly on gradient echo sequences. Ultrasound can be used to detect discrete lesions, assess for multiple lesions and to assess whether they are solid or cystic.

6 Post-operative Assessment of Metacarpophalangeal (MCP) Joint Replacement

MCP joint replacements are routinely performed in advanced hand arthritis to treat pain and improve function. Generally, silastic implants are used for inflammatory arthritis, particularly rheumatoid arthritis, whilst pyrocarbon implants are used in cases of osteoarthritis and post-traumatic arthritis.

The MCP joints are the most commonly affected joints in rheumatoid arthritis (RA) and can progress to significant deformity. In this systemic disease multiple MCP joints are often affected together, and on both sides—the symmetrical involvement that is the hallmark of rheumatoid arthritis. The joints become destroyed with ulnar deviation and subluxation and are painful. Joint replacement at this stage is associated with functional improvement and reduced pain (Parkkila et al. 2006).

The frequency of surgical intervention for rheumatoid arthritis of the hand has reduced by at least 50% over the last 20 years (Tominaga et al. 2023). This is because of improved treatment protocols, the early use of disease-modifying anti-rheumatic drugs (DMARDs), particularly methotrexate, and the more recent use of monoclonal antibody 'biologic' treatments and targeted synthetic DMARDs. These treatments prevent the progression of disease to joint destruction and deformity, with a consequent reduction in the requirement for surgery.

Nevertheless, arthroplasty still has a central and vital role in the treatment of advanced rheumatoid arthritis of the hand.

Silastic joint replacements have been found to give the best results in MCP arthroplasty in rheumatoid arthritis and are most commonly used in these patients. Silastic is a silicon polymer. On x-ray, silicon joint replacements are relatively radiolucent. They are visible as they are slightly denser than soft tissues on x-rays. They can be used with grommets, titanium 'caps' placed over the metacarpal and phalangeal stems. These are radio-opaque on X-ray. They aim to improve the durability of the implant by preventing bone edges from tearing the silastic. Long-term outcome of silastic metacarpal joint replacements is good, with nearly 2/3 implant survival at 17 years (Trail et al. 2004), although complications are common.

By far the most common complication is an implant fracture. In long-term follow up most silastic implants fracture. They are subjected to considerable stress over long periods of time on MCP joint flexion, particularly with excessive flexion (Ikari et al. 2020). They are most likely to fracture at the hinge stem junction, and this can progress to complete fragmentation. The rate of implant fracture is much greater than that of revision surgery. This is because radiographic evidence of fracture does not always cause recurrence of pain and loss of function, and therefore revision is commonly not required (Koenuma et al. 2024).

Other complications of silastic joint replacements include progression of implant fracture and failure to joint deformity, usually ulnar deviation, and subluxation, stiffness, silicon synovitis, loosening and rarely infection (Trail et al. 2004). Silicon synovitis has been reported with varying frequency after silastic finger joint replacements but generally considered uncommon although well reported. Sloughing of microparticles can set off an intense inflammatory reaction leading to synovitis which can invade the bone adjacent to the prosthesis. This leads to bone destruction with osteolysis and bony cavities forming around the silicon prosthesis (Randall 1992).

In cases of osteoarthritis, including post-traumatic osteoarthritis and calcium pyrophosphate arthritis of the metacarpal phalangeal joints, pyrocarbon implants are used. Pyrocarbon is a synthetic material manufactured by covering a graphite base with a thin layer of heated pyrolytic carbon. This leads to a substance that has a high compression strength, and elasticity similar to that of cortical bone. It is very hard wearing (Bellemère 2018). On X-ray pyrocarbon is radiodense, but less so than metal. In the total MCP joint replacement metacarpal and phalangeal components simulate the MCP ball and socket joint. Alternatively, a hemiarthroplasty can be performed, where a spherical pyrocarbon sphere is used to replace the metacarpal head (the HAPY prosthesis). Clinical outcome is good, with pain reduction, increased grip strength and increased mobility in most cases, and patient satisfaction of over 90%. Reoperation rate is around 10% at 5 years. Bone erosion, implant subsidence and radiolucent lines are common (Figs. 6, 7, and 8), but do not correlate with outcome. Intra-operative fracture can occur but is not common (Atkinson and Smith 1986).

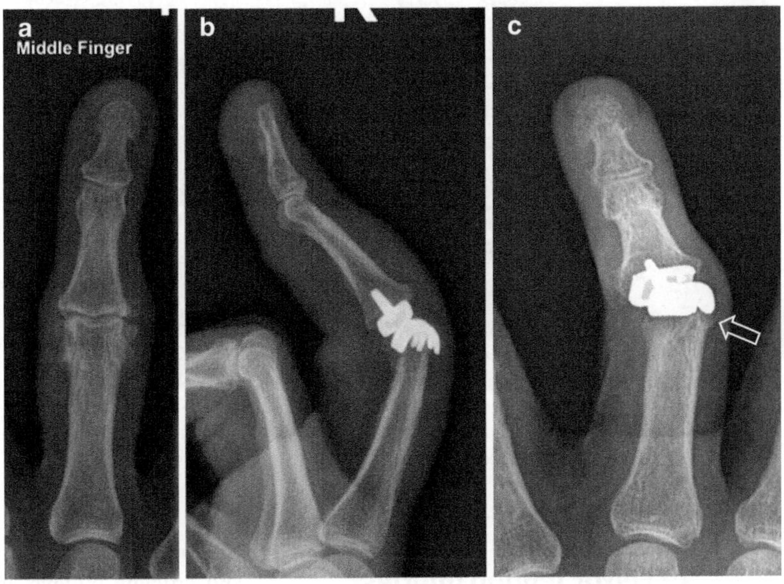

Fig. 6 (**a**–**c**) Failed PIP joint replacement: Pre-operative X-ray (**a**) shows osteoarthritis of the pip joint of the middle finger. Lateral and DP X-ray 15 months post-op (**b**, **c**) show flexion and ulnar deviation deformity with early bony lucency of the proximal phalanx component (arrow)

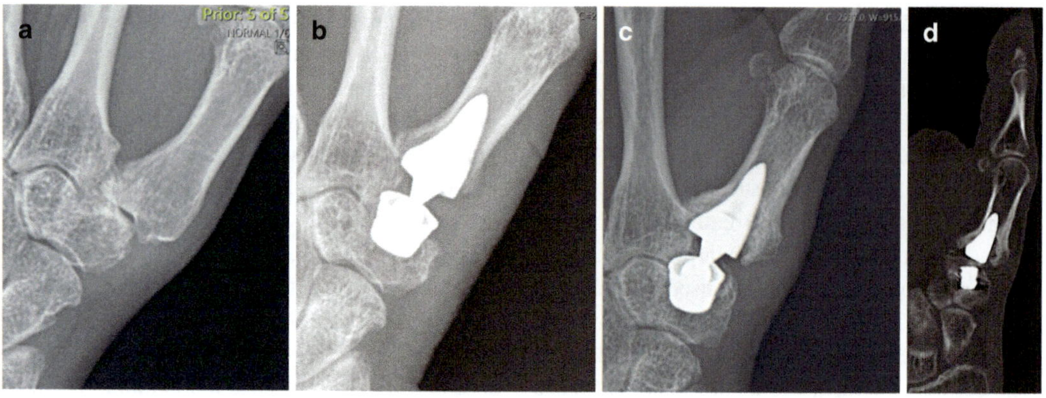

Fig. 7 (**a–d**) Progressive loosening of CMC joint implant: Pre-op X-ray (**a**) shows osteoarthritis of the first CMC joint. X-ray soon after operation (**b**) shows position of implant. X-ray 3 years later (**c**) shows loosening at the base of the metacarpal component, and subsidence of the trapezium component. CT (**d**) shows loosening in greater detail

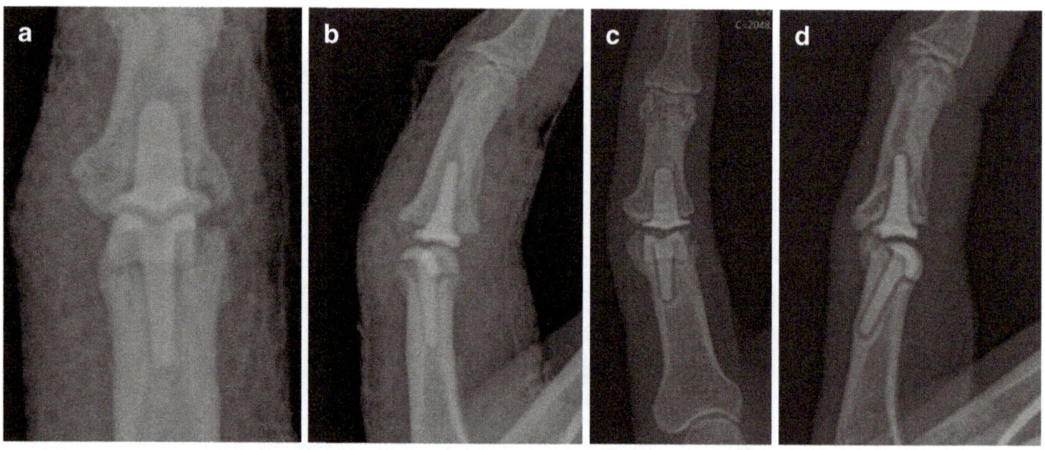

Fig. 8 **a** (AP and lateral), **b** (AP and lateral): Aseptic loosening of index finger PIP joint replacement: Immediate post-operative X-ray of index finger (**a**, **b**) followed by loosening within 42 months (**c**, **d**)

7 Post-operative Assessment of Flexor Tendon Injuries

There are two flexor tendons to each of the index, middle, ring and little fingers, one tendon each from the flexor digitorum superficialis (FDS) and the flexor digitorum profundus (FDP). The FDS tendon travels superficial to the FDP tendon until the level of the metacarpophalangeal (MCP) joint where the FDS tendon bifurcates, with one slip passing on the radial and one slip on the ulnar side of the FDP tendon to insert onto the base of the middle phalanx. The FDP tendon continues to the base of the distal phalanx. The tendons are supported superficially by a number of annular and cruciate pulleys, fibrous bands that support the tendons superficially, and prevent them from moving away from the bone.

Most flexor tendon injuries are acute, but can occur due to repetitive strain, particularly in patients with rheumatoid arthritis.

Flexor tendon injuries can occur at the level of the middle phalanx (zone 1), the proximal phalanx (zone 2) or further proximally. Zone 3 injuries occur distal to the carpal tunnel, zone 4 at the level of the carpal tunnel and zone 5 proximal to the carpal tunnel. Zone 1 tears may have an associated avulsion fracture of the distal phalanx.

Tears of the flexor tendons may be due to hyperextension injury of the distal interphalangeal joint, typically zone 1 injuries of the FDP tendon, or laceration, typically for injuries more proximally. The most important aim of pre-operative imaging is to diagnose the level of the tear and the degree of retraction of the proximal tendon. This can be assessed with MRI or ultrasound, with plain X-ray to review any bony injuries (Daniels et al. 2024).

Tendon repair is generally indicated for full-thickness tears, and high-grade partial-thickness tears, where more than 50% of the tendon is torn. Primary surgical tendon repair is preferred, if possible, with direct reattachment of the two tendon ends. If there is too much tendon damage to achieve a primary repair the tendon will need to be reconstructed. This may be by a two-stage procedure; in the first stage the damaged tendon is resected, and a silicon implant (Hunter rod) is inserted into the tendon bed. This allows for formation of a pseudo tendon sheath. At least 3 months later, the Hunter rod is removed and a tendon graft, often from the palmaris longus or plantaris tendons, is inserted into the torn tendon gap. The Hunter rod is sufficiently radio-dense to be visible on plain X-ray. Zone 2 tendon tears may involve the FDP tendon only, or both the FDP and FDS tendons. They are generally the most difficult tears to treat surgically, because the repair has to be fitted into a restricted space. Zone 3, 4 and 5 injuries are generally treated with direct repair, with good outcomes. They are less common as they are protected by overlying muscles or the flexor retinaculum, but may be associated with other injuries, including nerve injuries, when present (Daniels et al. 2024).

Post-operative imaging of tendon repairs is not usually performed routinely but is used to assess complications. The two major complications are recurrent tears and adhesions, which can be difficult to differentiate clinically. Recurrent tears occur in about 4% of primary tendon repairs and 14% of two-stage reconstructions. Adhesions also occur in about 4% of primary repairs (Dy et al. 2012). Zone 2 repairs are most susceptible to adhesions. Recurrent tears may require further surgery, while adhesions can be treated with physiotherapy initially, although may need tenolysis if restriction in movement persists.

Ultrasound is the primary modality used for post-operative assessment. While MRI may be better at viewing a tendon gap, there is often, on both modalities, hypoechoic or low signal post-surgical soft tissue thickening, or oedema which can obscure the visualisation of the tendon. Ultrasound has the advantage of allowing dynamic assessment on flexion of the finger. This will assess whether the tendon moves with passive or active flexion and is therefore intact. Individual joint movement can be assessed, for example passively flexing the DIP joint while fixing the PIP and MCP joints, although care should be taken not to overstress a recently repaired tendon. If the flexor tendons are intact, their movement can be assessed on finger flexion and extension to assess for adhesions. Adhesions are directly visualised as soft tissue thickening/scarring around the tendons, but direct diagnosis is difficult as there will be post-surgical soft tissue thickening anyway (Daniels et al. 2024).

Infection is uncommon, and is more likely with two-stage tendon reconstructions than one-stage operations. MRI is advised in suspected post-operative infection. This will assess the amount of oedema and fluid, the degree to which the infection has spread and any bony involvement. Bone involvement will be seen initially by marrow oedema followed by bony erosion in aggressive infections. Post-contrast scans may be required to assess for defined abscess collections that may require surgical debridement.

The thumb is different from the other fingers, in that there is only one flexor tendon, the flexor pollicis longus (FPL). FPL rupture is relatively uncommon but as with any flexor tendon tear in the hand can significantly disrupt hand function. Tears may be caused by direct laceration, acute wrist trauma or repetitive strain. Some cases are associated with volar plate fixation of distal radius fractures. The tendon can be repaired directly, or with a graft from the palmaris longus tendon. Like other flexor tendons, the main complications are formation of adhesions, nonunion of the tendon graft or re-rupture, and infection (Shih et al. 2023).

8 Post-operative Assessment of Extensor Tendon Injuries

The extensor tendons crossing the dorsum of the wrist are divided into six separate compartments:

1. Abductor pollicis longus and extensor pollicis brevis.
2. Extensor carpi radialis longus and extensor carpi radialis brevis.
3. Extensor pollicis longus.
4. Extensor digitorum communis and extensor indicis.
5. Extensor digiti minimi.
6. Extensor carpi ulnaris.

Thus there are two extensor tendons each to the thumb, index finger and little fingers and one extensor tendon to the middle and ring fingers.

Extensor tendon injuries can be open or closed. Open lacerations are typically lacerations associated with sharp objects, including glass. Closed tendon tears are more likely to be associated with attritional damage in patients with arthritis or crystal deposition disease, or from previous surgical metal work (Tos et al. 2016).

Traumatic extensor tendon injuries at the distal phalanx are associated with inability to extend the distal phalanx (mallet finger) and may be associated with a dorsal distal phalanx avulsion (bony injury). A tear of the central slip of the extensor tendon at the level of the proximal interphalangeal joint (PIPJ) is associated with a boutonniere deformity (flexion of the PIP joint and hyperextension at the distal interphalangeal joint (DIP) joint).

As with flexor tendon injuries, pre-operative assessment will be with X-ray to assess for fractures, and MRI or ultrasound to assess tendon discontinuity may be needed.

Post-operative radiology for an extensor tendon injury typically involves high-resolution ultrasound imaging to assess the integrity of the repaired tendon, looking for signs of healing, potential complications like re-rupture, or any peritendinous adhesions that might limit movement, often with dynamic ultrasound to evaluate tendon function during movement. In some cases, MRI may be used for more detailed evaluation of the surrounding soft tissues and bone structures.

As with the flexor tendons, the most common complications of extensor tendon repair are re-rupture, adhesions and infection. High-resolution ultrasound is advised for imaging assessment. This will show post-operative tendon thickening, and the normal tubular structure of the tendon may not be obvious. Ultrasound offers the opportunity of dynamic assessment. If the tendon is seen to move with active or passive finger movement, it is not ruptured. Occasionally adhesions may form but will be difficult to distinguish on ultrasound or MRI from normal post-operative soft tissue thickening but the normal gliding movement of the tendon on finger flexion can be sought on ultrasound. The presence of fluid around the tendon may indicate inflammation or infection. MRI will be useful to assess soft tissue spread of infection and also osseous involvement.

9 Conclusion

The various modalities of imaging play a key supportive role in the management of patients with suspected post-operative complications. The authors would stress again that the clinical context must always be considered when interpreting the findings noted in the imaging modalities to diagnose post-operative conditions in the hand.

References

Atkinson RE, Smith RJ (1986) Silicone synovitis following silicone implant arthroplasty. Hand Clin 2(2):291–299

Balaram AK, Bednar MS (2010) Complications after the fractures of metacarpal and phalanges. Hand Clin 26(2):169–177. https://doi.org/10.1016/j.hcl.2010.01.005

Bellemère P (2018) Pyrocarbon implants for the hand and wrist. Hand Surg Rehabil 37(3):129–154. https://doi.org/10.1016/j.hansur.2018.03.001

Choi WS, Lee SK, Kim J-Y, Kim Y (2024) Diffuse-type tenosynovial giant cell tumor: what are the important findings on the initial and follow-up MRI? Cancers (Basel) 16(2):402. https://doi.org/10.3390/cancers16020402

Chung KC, Spilson SV (2001) The frequency and epidemiology of hand and forearm fractures in the United

States. J Hand Surg 26(5):908–915. https://doi.org/10.1053/jhsu.2001.26322

Chung KC, Malay S, Shauver MJ, Kim HM (2019) Assessment of distal radius fracture complications among adults 60 years or older. JAMA Netw Open 2(1):e187053. https://doi.org/10.1001/jamanetworkopen.2018

Daniels SP, Kirby D, De Tolla J (2024) Diagnosis and treatment of flexor tendon injuries of the hand: what the radiologist needs to know. Skeletal Radiol 53:597–608. https://doi.org/10.1007/s00256-023-04460-y

Dy CJ, Hernandez-Soria A, Ma Y, Roberts TR, Daluiski A (2012) Complications after flexor tendon repair: a systematic review and meta-analysis. J Hand Surg 37(3):543–551.e1. https://doi.org/10.1016/j.jhsa.2011.11.006

Fussey JM, Chin KF, Gogi N, Gella S, Deshmukh SC (2009) An anatomic study of flexor tendon sheaths: a cadaveric study. J Hand Surg (Eur Vol) 34(6):762–765. https://doi.org/10.1177/1753193409344529

Gupta A, Subhas N, Primak AN, Nittka M, Liu K (2015) Metal artifact reduction. Radiol Clin North Am 53(3):531–547. https://doi.org/10.1016/j.rcl.2014.12.005

Ikari K, Iwamoto T, Ishii K, Suzuki T, Kimura H, Matsumura N, Sato K (2020) Risk factors contributing to early implant fracture in silicone metacarpophalangeal joint arthroplasty for patients with rheumatoid arthritis. J Hand Surg [Am]. https://doi.org/10.1016/j.jhsa.2020.09.002

Jupiter JB, Koniuch MP, Smith RJ (1985) The management of delayed union and nonunion of the metacarpals and phalanges. J Hand Surg 10(4):457–466. https://doi.org/10.1016/s0363-5023(85)80066-6

Katsura M, Sato J, Akahane M, Kunimatsu A, Abe O (2018) Current and novel techniques for metal artifact reduction at CT: practical guide for radiologists. Radiographics 38(2):450–461. https://doi.org/10.1148/rg.2018170102

Koç O, Kivrak A, Paksoy Y (2007) Subungual glomus tumour: magnetic resonance imaging findings. Australas Radiol 51:B107–B109. https://doi.org/10.1111/j.1440-1673.2007.01797.x

Koenuma N, Ikari K, Oh K, Iwakura N, Okazaki K (2024) Long-term implant fracture rates following silicone metacarpophalangeal joint arthroplasty in rheumatoid arthritis. J Hand Surg [Am]. https://doi.org/10.1016/j.jhsa.2024.01.009

Lipira AB, Sood RF, Tatman PD, Davis JI, Morrison SD, Ko JH (2015) Complications within 30 days of hand surgery: an analysis of 10,646 patients. J Hand Surg [Am] 40(9):1852–59.e3

McLain RF, Steyers C, Stoddard M (1991) Infections in open fractures of the hand. J Hand Surg 16(1):108–112. https://doi.org/10.1016/s0363-5023(10)80022-x

Morey VM, Garg B, Kotwal PP (2016) Glomus tumours of the hand: review of literature. J Clin Orthop Trauma 7(4):286–291. https://doi.org/10.1016/j.jcot.2016.04.00

National Association for Rare Diseases (2023) Tenosynovial giant cell tumor. https://rarediseases.org/clinical-trial/tenosynovial-giant-cell-tumor-tgct/

Parkkila DTJ, Belt EA, Hakala M, Kautiainen HJ, Leppilahti J (2006) Survival and complications are similar after Swanson and Sutter implant replacement of metacarpophalangeal joints in patients with rheumatoid arthritis. Scand J Plast Reconstr Surg Hand Surg 40(1):49–53. https://doi.org/10.1080/02844310500327753

Patel DB, Emmanuel NB, Stevanovic MV, Matcuk GR, Gottsegen CJ, Forrester DM, White EA (2014) Hand infections: anatomy, types and spread of infection, imaging findings, and treatment options. Radiographics 34(7):1968–1986. https://doi.org/10.1148/rg.347130101

Randall T (1992) Surgeons grapple with synovitis, fractures around silicone implants for hand and wrist. JAMA 268(1):13–18

Shih Y-S, Chang Y-J, Cheng Y-T, Chang C-S, Lin Y-H (2023) Flexor pollicis longus tendon rupture: a case series on palmaris longus tendon graft reconstruction after volar plate fixation. J Surg Case Rep 7:1–4. https://doi.org/10.1093/jscr/rjad399

Singh HP et al (2005) Partial union of acute scaphoid fractures. J Hand Surg (Eur Vol) 30(5). https://doi.org/10.1016/j.jhsb.2005.05.007

Suresh S, Zaki H (2016) Giant cell tumor of tendon sheath: case series and review of literature. J Hand Microsurg 2(2):67–71. https://doi.org/10.1007/s12593-010-0020-9

Theumann NH, Goettmann S, Le Viet D, Resnick D, Chung CB, Bittoun J, Drapé J-L (2002) Recurrent glomus tumours of fingertips: MR imaging evaluation. Radiology 223(1):143–151. https://doi.org/10.1148/radiol.223101097

Tominaga A, Ikari K, Yano K, Tanaka E, Inoue E, Harigai M, Okazaki K (2023) Surgical intervention for patients with rheumatoid arthritis is declining except for foot and ankle surgery: a single-centre, 20-year observational cohort study. Mod Rheumatol 33(3):509–516. https://doi.org/10.1093/mr/roac042

Tos P, Battiston B, Merolla G, Porcellini G, Artiaco S, Colzani G (2016) Traumatic extensor tendon injuries to the hand: clinical anatomy, biomechanics, and surgical procedure review. J Hand Microsurg 8(1):2–12. https://doi.org/10.1055/s-0036-1572534

Trail IA, Martin JA, Nuttall D, Stanley JK (2004) Seventeen-year survivorship analysis of silastic metacarpophalangeal joint replacement. J Bone Joint Surg Br 86-B:1002–1006. https://doi.org/10.1302/0301-620X.86B7

Wan JMC, Magarelli N, Peh WCG, Guglielmi G, Shek TWH (2010) Imaging of giant cell tumour of the tendon sheath. Radiol Med 115(1):141–151. https://doi.org/10.1007/s11547-010-0515-2

Wang C, Song R-R, Kuang P-D, Wang L-H, Zhang M-M (2017) Giant cell tumor of the tendon sheath: magnetic resonance imaging findings in 38 patients. Oncol Lett 13(6):4459–4462. https://doi.org/10.3892/ol.2017.6011

Whitley AS, Sloane C, Hoadley G et al (2005) Clark's positioning in radiography. Hodder Arnold Publication. ISBN: 0340763906

Post-operative Imaging: Wrist

Jasmeet Jhaj, Manish Gupta, Gemma Smith,
Feiran Wu, Rajive Jose, Karan Mangat,
and Rajesh Botchu

Contents

J. Jhaj (✉) · M. Gupta · G. Smith · F. Wu · R. Jose
The Birmingham Hand Centre, University Hospitals
Birmingham NHS Foundation Trust,
Birmingham, UK

K. Mangat
South Warwickshire NHS Foundation Trust,
South Warwickshire, UK

R. Botchu
The Royal Orthopaedic Hospital NHS Foundation
Trust, Birmingham, UK

Med Radiol Diagn Imaging (2025)
https://doi.org/10.1007/174_2025_616,
Published Online: 12 November 2025

Abstract

Post-operative imaging of the wrist is essential for assessing surgical outcomes, identifying complications, and guiding ongoing management. As surgical techniques and orthopaedic implants continue to evolve, radiologists must be able to recognise the wide range of post-operative appearances. The aim of this chapter is to provide the radiologist with an overview of common traumatic and degenerative surgical wrist interventions, the imaging modalities required for assessment, and common complications to recognise. Guidance is also offered on what to include in the structured radiology report to support clinical decision-making.

1 Introduction

The wrist is a complex joint made up of multiple bony articulations and stabilising ligaments, all of which contribute to its wide range of movement and functional stability. Traumatic and degenerative wrist conditions make up a considerable proportion of the hand surgeon's practice, with many conditions requiring surgical intervention. With advancing surgical techniques and the increasing diversity of orthopaedic implants, it is imperative that radiologists are familiar with the expected post-operative imaging appearances. Accurate and timely identification and reporting of radiographic complications such as nonunion, delayed union, infection and metalwork failure is critical in supporting clinical decision-making and improving patient outcomes.

2 Scaphoid Waist Fractures

The scaphoid is the most commonly fractured carpal bone, accounting for 15% of all acute wrist injuries (Leslie and Dickson 1981; Shenoy et al. 2007). Of these, 60% occur at the scaphoid waist, which is biomechanically the weakest part (Clementson et al. 2020). This is often due to a high-energy fall onto an outstretched hand. Minimally displaced scaphoid waist fractures (<2 mm) can often be managed nonoperatively with cast immobilisation (Dias et al. 2020). Post-operative imaging with a computed tomography (CT) scan is recommended with timely reporting on the presence of union, as nounion would warrant surgical fixation. Partial union, where there is at least 25% bridging trabecular bone across the fracture, has been shown to be predictive of full union with conservative management (Singh et al. 2005). For acute displaced waist fractures (>2 mm), fixation is recommended. This can be achieved with a headless compression screw (Fig. 1), Kirschner wires (k-wires) or plate fixation. A headless compression screw has differential pitch across the head and shaft to generate

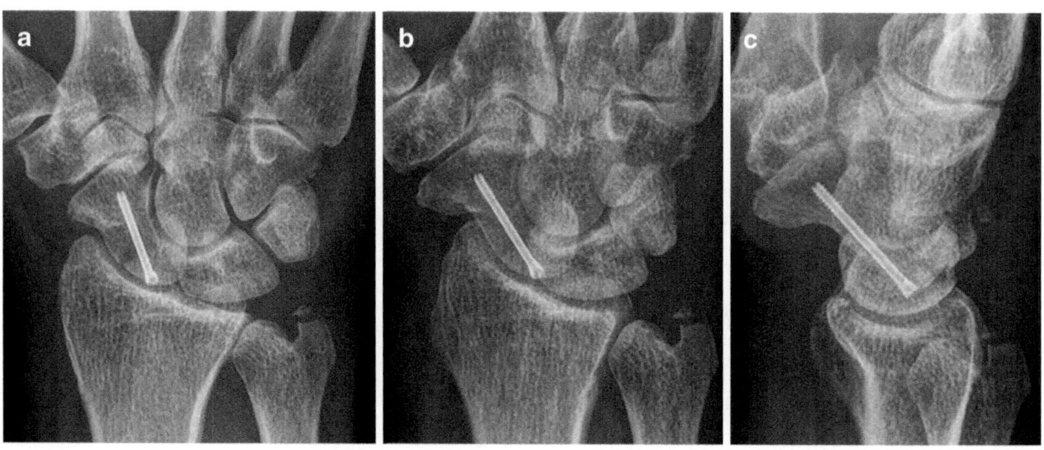

Fig. 1 (a–c) PA, oblique and lateral radiographs showing antegrade screw fixation of a scaphoid waist fracture

compression across the fracture and can be inserted either antegrade to retrograde to provide stability and allow union. The ideal position of the screw is central to the long axis of the scaphoid with no cortical breach.

Complications: screw/k-wire length too long, nonunion, malunion, infection.

What to include in the radiology report:

- Report on the metalwork (screw/k-wire length, joint penetration, lucency)
- Report on the screw placement (positioning the screw along the central longitudinal axis of the scaphoid is associated with improved biomechanical stability and higher union rates, Kupperman et al. 2018)
- Report on evidence of fracture healing, in particular the percentage of bridging trabeculae

3 Scaphoid Nonunion

Due to several biomechanical factors scaphoid waist and proximal pole fractures can go onto nonunion. 14% of scaphoid waist fractures treated with plaster cast immobilisation went onto nonunion and 34% for proximal pole fractures (Clay et al. 1991). Even after surgical treatment the nonunion rate for waist fractures is 1.5% (Eastley et al. 2013), and up to 90% for proximal pole fractures (Majeed 2014). Timely fixation is essential to prevent the predictable degenerative changes of scaphoid nonunion advanced collapse (SNAC) (Pinder et al. 2015). In Fig. 2b the hand surgeon used autologous bone graft from the distal radius followed by fixation with a retrograde screw. K-wire fixation can also be used instead of screw fixation, with no reported differences in union rates (Brogan et al. 2015). Bone graft can either be vascularised or non-vascularised. At 6–8 weeks post-operatively a CT scan is usually requested to check for bony union (Fig. 2c).

Complications: nonunion, delayed union, malunion, graft extrusion, infection (seen by subtle lucency around the metalwork).

What to include in the radiology report:

- Report on whether the graft is in place (compare with intraoperative fluoroscopy if available)

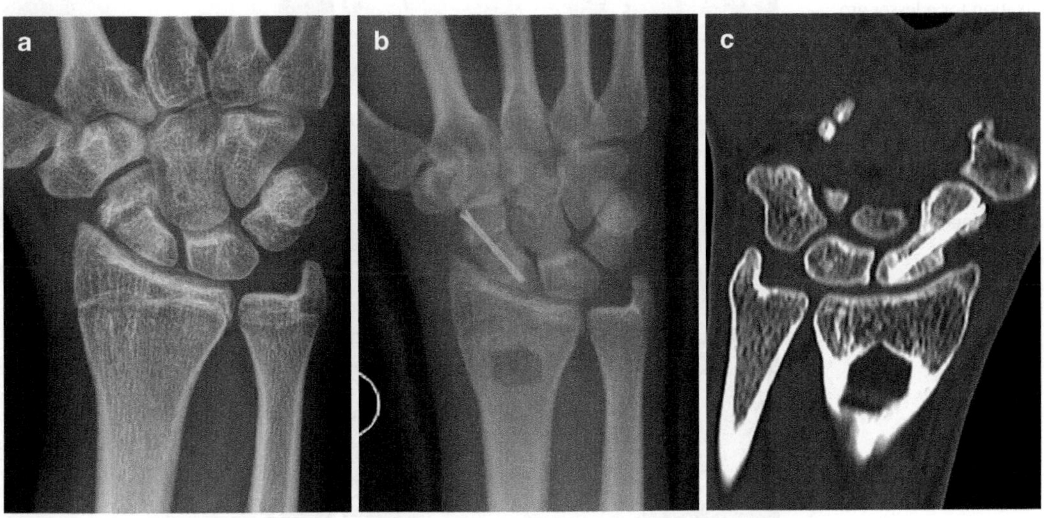

Fig. 2 (**a**) Pre-operative images of a scaphoid waist nonunion. Here the fracture line is clearly visible with sclerotic changes. There are no degenerative changes to suggest a SNAC wrist. (**b**) The scaphoid nonunion was treated with cancellous bone graft from the distal radius and retrograde screw fixation (**c**) a CT scan obtained 10 weeks post-operatively shows 100% union, evidenced by 100% bridging trabeculae. The bony void in the distal radius fills in over time and does not require further follow-up

- Report on evidence of fracture healing, in particular the percentage of bridging trabeculae
- Report on any metalwork complications (screw/k-wire length, joint penetration, lucency)
- Report on the graft donor site location (a complication could be if the graft is taken too close to the articular surface)
- Report on any evidence of SNAC wrist changes—arthritis affecting the radial styloid, scaphocapitate and lunocapitate joints
- Report on the carpal alignment, in particular a dorsal intercalated segmental instability (DISI)

4 Peri-Lunate Injuries

Peri-lunate injuries account for approximately 7% of acute carpal injuries and typically result from high-energy trauma (Najarian et al. 2011). These injuries involve disruption of the intercarpal ligaments, most notably the scapholunate ligament, and can be associated with fractures of the carpal bones. They are classified into two types: lesser arc injuries (Fig. 3), which affect only the interosseous ligaments and greater arc injuries (Fig. 4), which involve both ligamentous disruption and carpal fractures.

Surgical management has been shown to yield superior outcomes compared to closed reduction and immobilisation by reducing the risk of carpal instability and the development of post-traumatic arthritis (Apergis et al. 1997). The goal of surgery is to restore normal carpal alignment and promote ligamentous healing (Herzberg 2000). Post-operative imaging typically includes posteroanterior (PA) and lateral radiographs of the wrist at 6–8 weeks to assess carpal alignment and monitor fracture healing. When fixation of carpal bones is performed a CT scan is often indicated at follow-up to evaluate bony union, particularly when radiographs are inconclusive (Fig. 5).

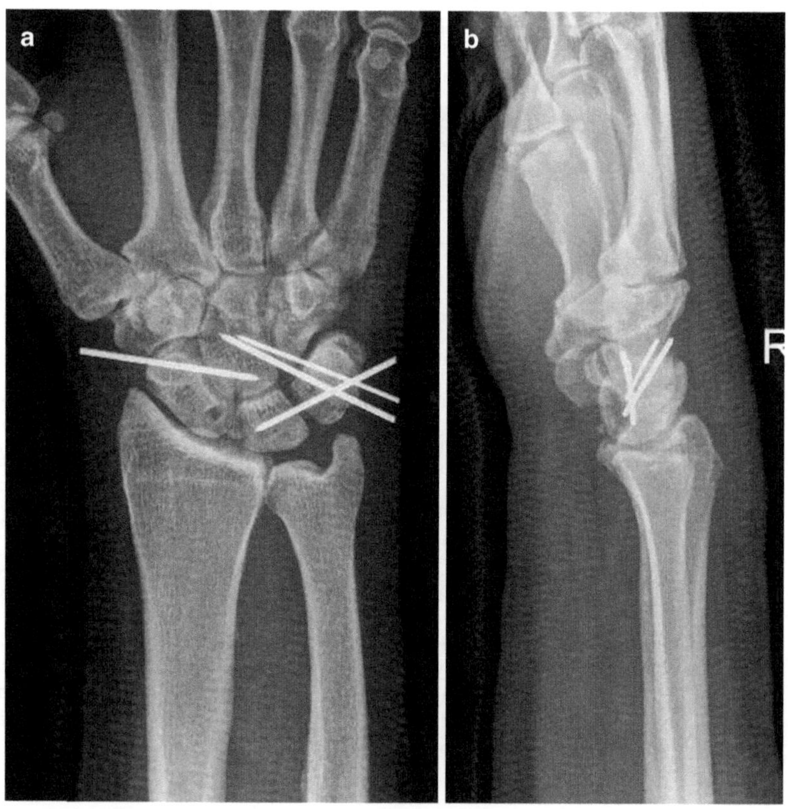

Fig. 3 Case 1 (**a**, **b**) Post-operative PA and lateral radiographs after fixation for a lesser arc injury. The purpose of the k-wires is to stabilise the carpus to prevent movement and allow interosseous ligament healing. The wires are removed at approximately 8 weeks post-surgery

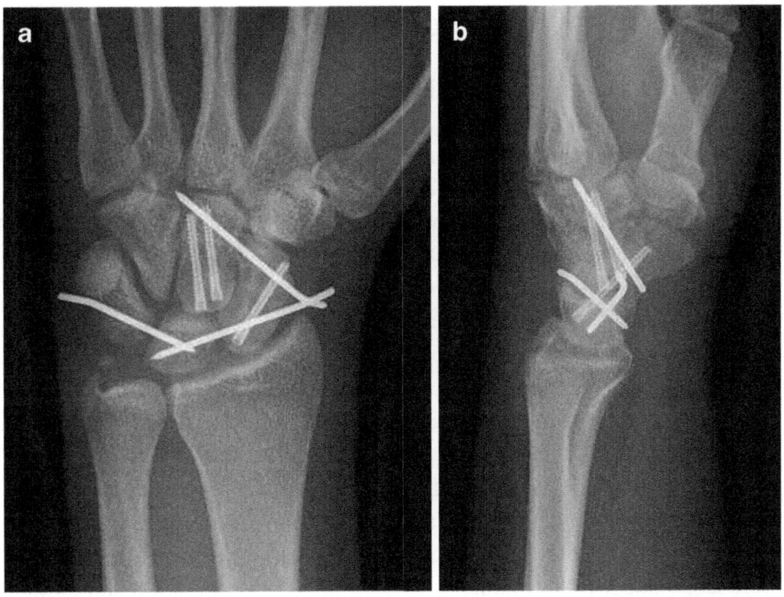

Fig. 4 Case 1 (**a**, **b**) PA and lateral radiographs of the wrist showing antegrade screw fixation of the capitate and scaphoid and k-wire stabilisation of the carpus. These radiographs demonstrate fixation after a greater arc injury

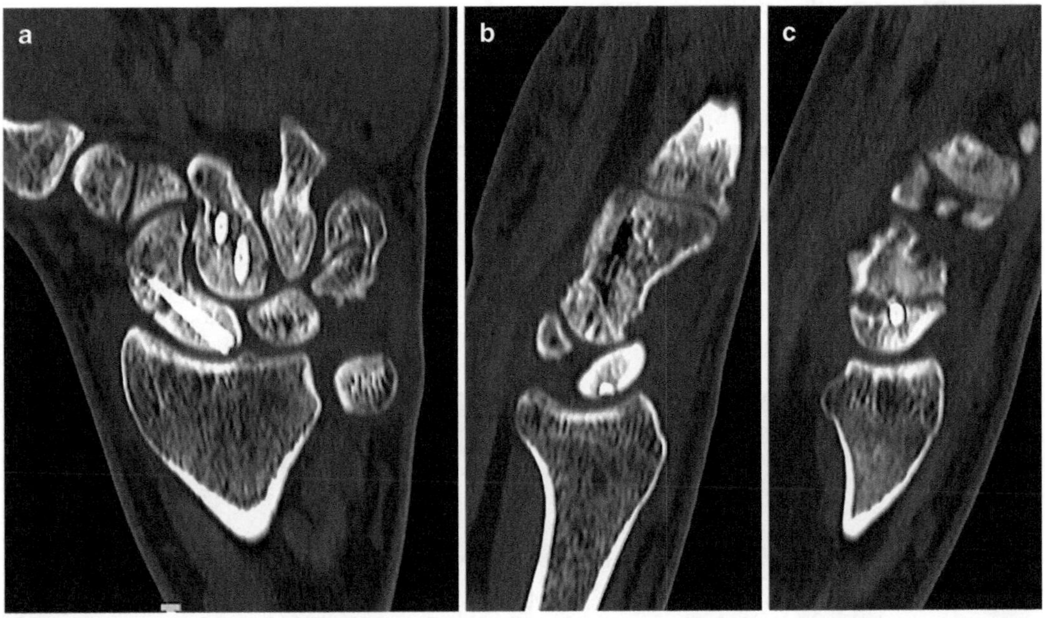

Fig. 5 Case 1 (**a**–**c**) CT slices at 3 months post-op. The capitate has gone onto 100% union evidenced by complete bridging trabecular across the fracture site but the scaphoid has yet to show signs of union, with no bridging trabeculae seen

What to include in the radiology report:

- Report on the general carpal alignment, is there a DISI deformity?
- Report on the scapholunate gap on PA radiographs (normal <2 mm) (Said et al. 2018)
- Report on the scapholunate angle on lateral radiographs (normal 36°–66°) (Larsen et al. 1991)
- Report on the capito-lunate angles (normal <15°) (Larsen et al. 1991)
- Report on evidence of fracture healing, in particular the percentage of bridging trabeculae
- Report on any metalwork complications (screw/k-wire length and migration close to neurovascular structures, joint penetration, lucency)—compare with intraoperative fluoroscopy images if available.

5 Distal Radius Fractures (DRF)

An estimated 70,000 adult men and women sustain a DRF each year in the UK, which is one of the most common orthopaedic injuries (O'Neill et al. 2001). DRFs account for 18% of all fractures in adults over 65 years (Baron et al. 1996), making this a common injury seen by the orthopaedic surgeon and reporting radiologist. A range of stabilisation techniques may be used depending on the fracture configuration and patient-specific factors. These include manipulation under anaesthesia (MUA) with cast immobilisation (Fig. 6), k-wire fixation (Fig. 7), open reduction and internal fixation (ORIF) using volar (Figs. 8 and 9) or dorsal plating (Fig. 10) and in more complex cases, with extensive bony comminution, dorsal bridge plating across the wrist joint to restore distal radius length and alignment (Fig. 11).

Dorsally displaced fractures, termed Colles fractures, and volar displaced fractures, termed Smith's fractures represent two of the most common DRF patterns. Colles fracture was first described by Abraham Colles in 1814, this is an extra-articular dorsally angulated fracture typically resulting from a fall onto an outstretched hand. They are commonly seen in the elderly population and come under the umbrella of fragility fractures (Haentjens et al. 2004). Higher energy trauma is associated with the younger population. Treatment options are dependent on fracture and patient-specific factors, which include manipulation under anaesthesia (MUA) with plaster immobilisation, to open reduction internal fixation (ORIF), or k-wire stabilisation (Kapandji 1976). In contrast, Smith fractures are volar-angulated. These are intra-articular fractures typically sustained by falling onto a flexed wrist. They are less common than Colles fractures but are inherently more unstable, often

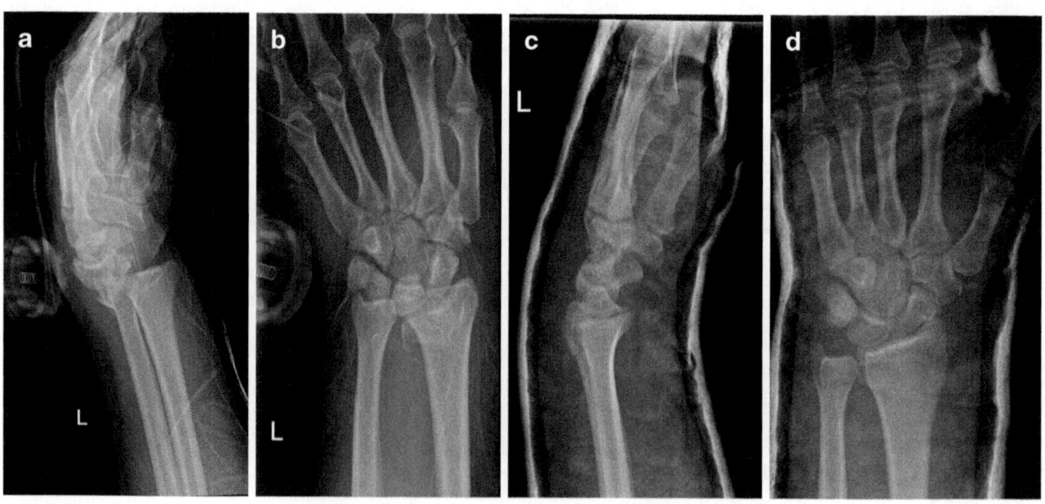

Fig. 6 (**a**, **b**) Pre-manipulation radiographs. (**c**, **d**) post-manipulation radiographs

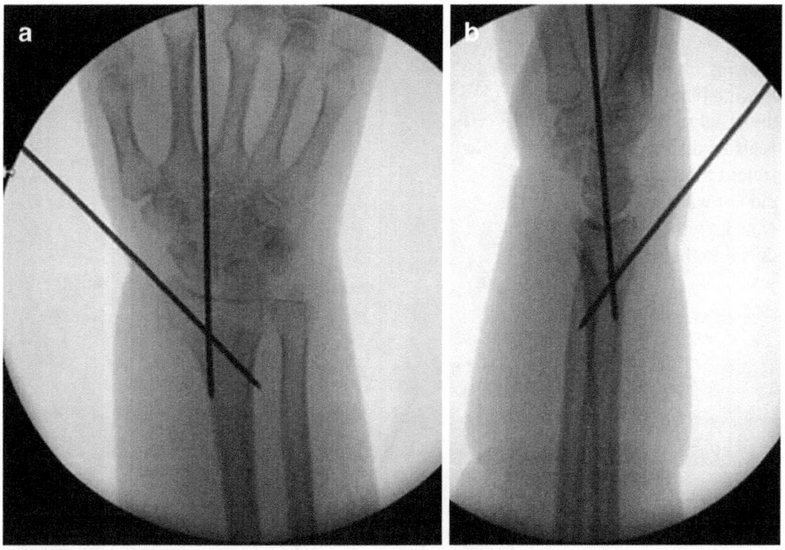

Fig. 7 (**a**, **b**) PA and lateral fluoroscopy images showing K-wire fixation for a dorsally displaced distal radius fracture

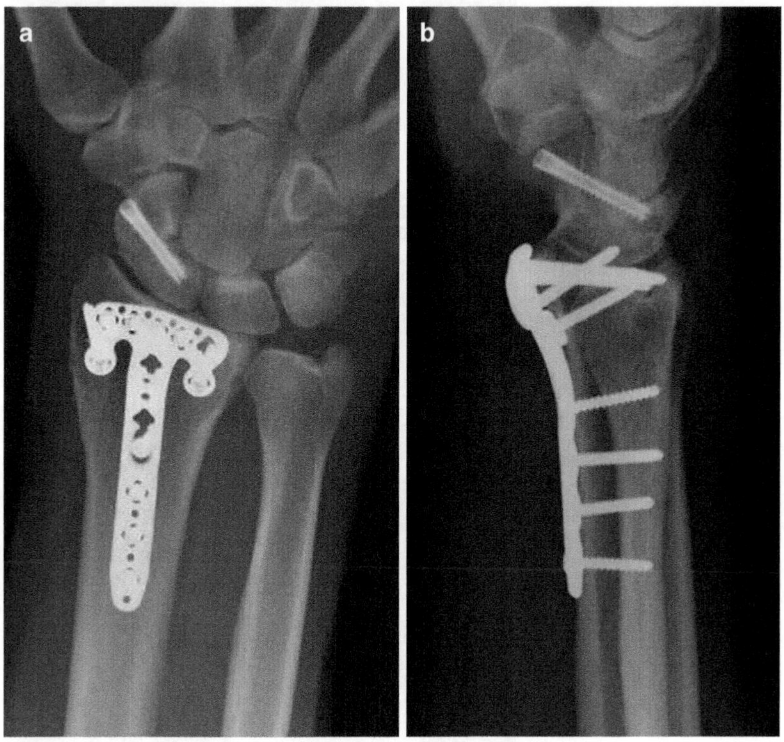

Fig. 8 (**a**, **b**) PA and lateral radiographs showing volar locking rim plate fixation for a DRF and a scaphoid waist fracture treated with a retrograde screw. Volar rim plates are often used to treat very distal fractures involving the distal radius. They are placed volar to the watershed line allowing locking screw position closer to the perpendicular angle of the plate. However, there is a higher incidence of FPL tendon injury associated with a more volar plate position

necessitating surgical fixation using volar locking plates. Post-operative follow-up includes PA and lateral radiographs. Complications of both fracture types include hardware issues, tendon injury, nonunion, malunion, loss of reduction or infection. Specific complications include extensor tendon rupture, specifically extensor pollicis longus (EPL) due to prominent screws (Perry et al. 2011) and flexor pollicis longus (FPL) tendon rupture, both related to volar plating. FPL ruptures are particularly seen in cases where the plate is positioned volar to the watershed line, classified as Soong grade 2 (Soong et al. 2011).

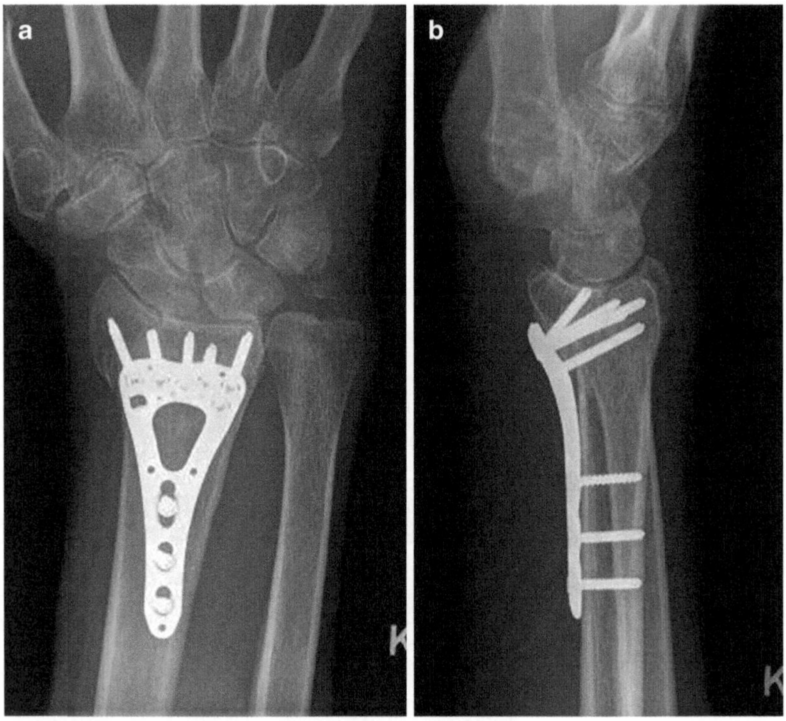

Fig. 9 (**a**, **b**) PA and lateral radiographs showing a standard volar locking plate fixation of the distal radius. There is also a displaced ulna styloid fracture which did not warrant fixation. Note how the plate sits dorsal to the watershed line

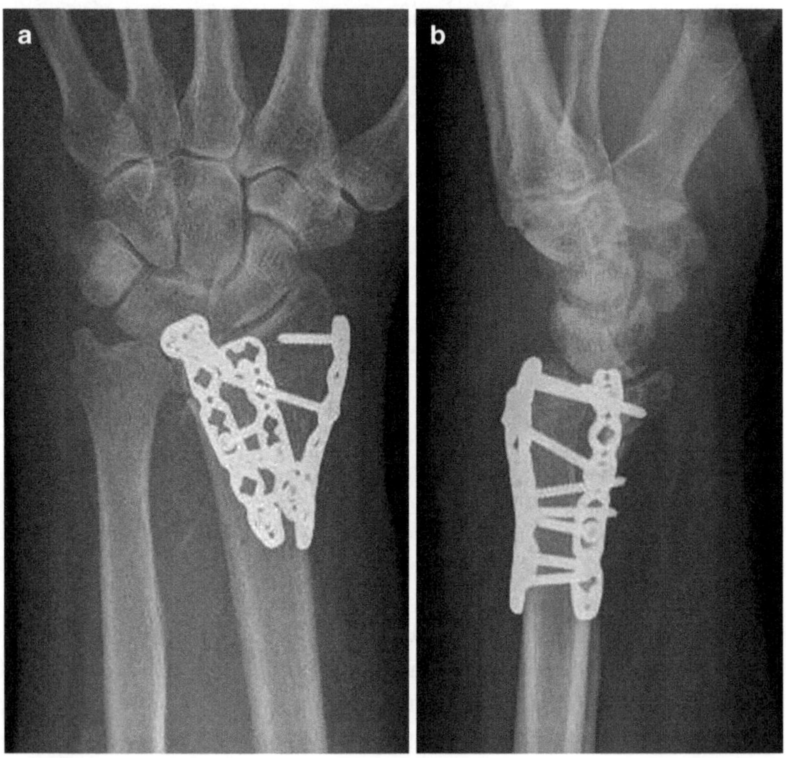

Fig. 10 (**a**, **b**) PA and lateral radiographs showing dorsal plate and radial styloid fixation of the distal radius

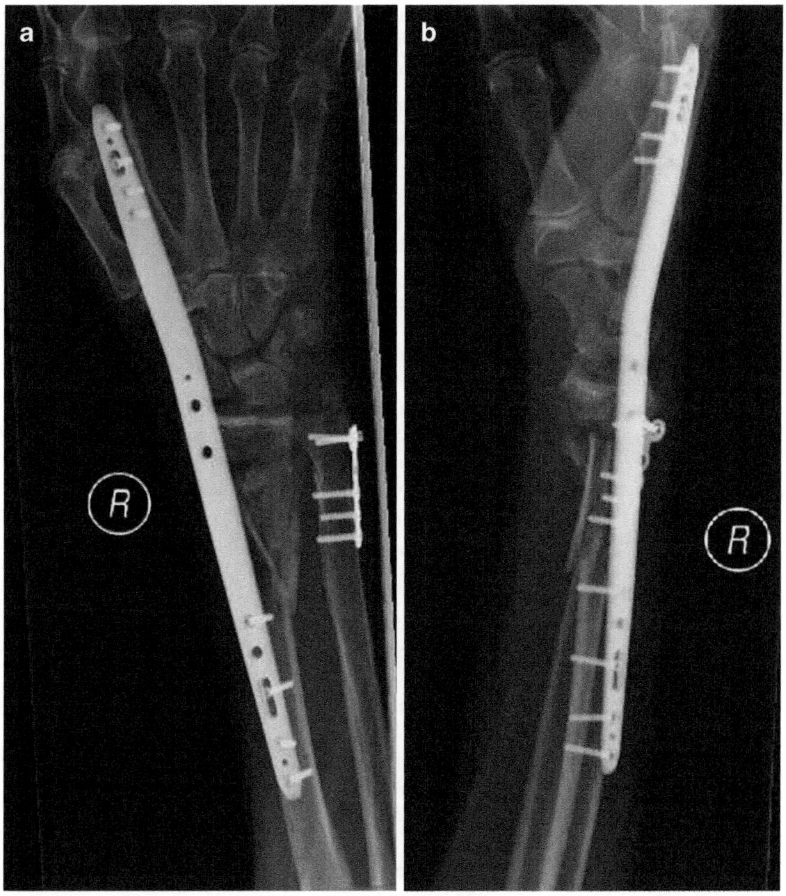

Fig. 11 (**a**, **b**) PA and lateral radiographs showing a dorsal bridge plate (DBP) fixation with a distal ulna fracture fixation. DBPs are served for highly comminuted fractures not amenable to fragment-specific plate fixation. As the name suggests, it bridges the fracture across the wrist joint to allow healing by secondary intention. The aim of the surgery is to restore length and alignment. The distal radius bridge plate is typically removed once the fracture unites

Nonoperative management with MUA and POP (plaster of Paris) remains appropriate for minimally displaced or stable fractures, especially in older patients, with some evidence supporting this as the gold standard for those over 65 years (Arora et al. 2011). Weekly radiographs are crucial in the first 2 weeks to monitor for displacement. K-wire stabilisation of dorsally displaced fractures is a cost-effective alternative to ORIF as supported by the multicentre DRAFFT trial (Costa et al. 2014), which showed equivalent long-term outcomes. However, it carries risks such as pin-site infection, wire migration, and loss of reduction, requiring close radiographic monitoring at 1–2 weeks and again at 4 weeks prior to wire removal. For more complex fracture patterns with dorsal comminution, dorsal distal radius plating (DDRP) may be preferred to buttress unstable dorsal fragments. Though less commonly used than volar plates, DDRP is essential in select cases, with lateral radiographs critical post-operatively to assess for hardware prominence, which may cause extensor tendon irritation and rupture.

Regardless of the fixation methods used, the same reporting radiographic parameters are required. Radial height, radial inclination, volar tilt, ulna variance, carpal alignment and intra-articular steps need to be reported.

What to include in the radiology report:

- Report on the parameters mentioned in Table 1
- Report on the position of the plates (volar plates placed volar to the watershed line are known to have a higher incidence of flexor pollicis longus tendon rupture) (Vasara et al. 2023)

Table 1 All distal radius fractures should have the following parameters included in the radiology report

Parameter	Normal range/ Mean ± SD	Description
Volar tilt (°)	Mean: 15.4° ± 4.3°	The angle between the distal radial articular surface and a line perpendicular to the radial shaft on a lateral radiograph
Radial inclination (°)	Mean: 26.7° ± 3.3°	The angle between a line from the radial styloid to the ulnar corner of the distal radius and a line perpendicular to the radial shaft on a PA radiograph
Radial height (mm)	Mean: 13.6 ± 2.1 mm	The distance from the tip of the radial styloid to the ulna corner of the distal radius on a PA radiograph
Ulna variance (mm)	Mean: 0.8 ± 1.9 mm	The vertical distance between the distal articular surfaces of the radius and ulna; positive values indicate a longer ulna
Radiocarpal angle (°)	Mean: 11.6° ± 3.1°	The angle between the longitudinal axis of the radius and a line connecting the radial and ulna styloid tips on a PA radiograph

- Report on screw or K-wire positioning, in particular if they are too long or close to neurovascular structures
- Report on the degree of fracture healing, including malunion

Volar Tilt (°)—on the lateral radiograph two lines are drawn. The first line is drawn tangentially between the dorsal and volar articular margins. The second line is drawn perpendicular to the long axis of the radius. The angle between these two lines will give you the volar tilt. The average normal value is 11° (Fig. 12).

Radial Inclination (°)—on the PA view two lines are drawn. The first line is drawn from the tip of the radial styloid to the medial edge of the distal radius. The second line is drawn perpendicularly to the longitudinal axis of the distal radius. The angle between the two lines is measured as the radial inclination. The average normal value is 22° (Fig. 13).

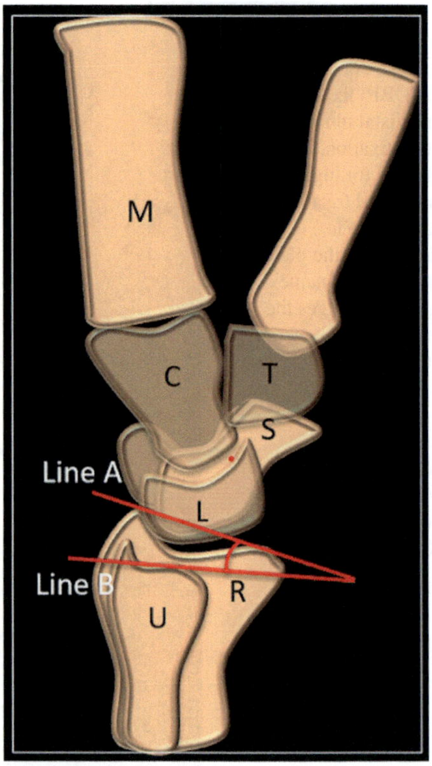

Fig. 12 Schematic showing measurement of volar tilt—angle between line A and line B

Ulna Variance (mm)—on the PA view two lines are drawn. The first line is drawn perpendicular to the longitudinal axis of the distal radius at the level of the distal articular surface of the lunate fossa. The second line is drawn perpendicular to the longitudinal axis of the ulna at the level of the distal cortical margin. The distance between the two lines is measured as an ulna variance. A positive ulna variance occurs when the ulna is longer than the distal radius and a negative ulna variance when the ulna is shorter than the distal radius (Fig. 14).

Radial Height (mm)—on the PA view two lines are drawn. The first line is drawn perpendicular to the longitudinal axis of the distal radius

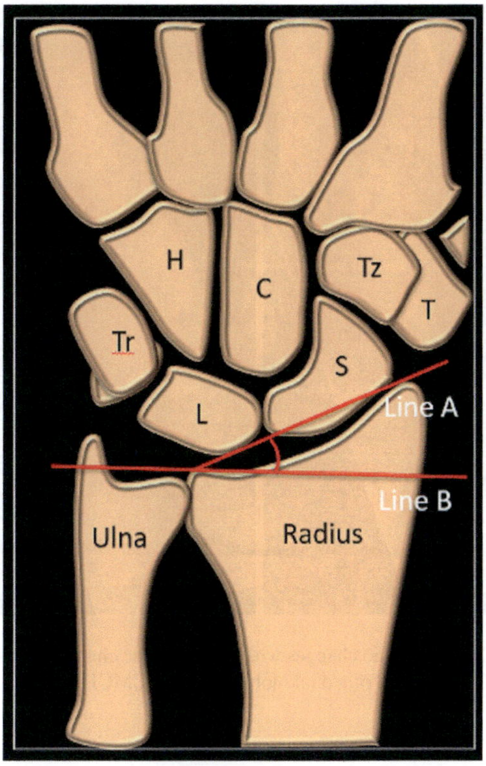

Fig. 13 Schematic showing measurement of radial inclination—angle between line A and line B

at the level of the tip of the styloid process. The second line is drawn perpendicular to the long axis of the radius at the level of the lunate fossa. The distance between the two lines is measured as the radial height. The normal average value is 12 mm.

6 Thumb Carpometacarpal Joint (CMCJ) Replacement

Thumb carpometacarpal joint (CMCJ) arthritis is a painful and debilitating condition with a preponderance for women and clinically affecting around 1.4% of the population (Moriatis Wolf et al. 2014). Surgical treatment options include trapeziectomy, interposition arthroplasty, arthrodesis, or total joint replacement. Thumb CMCJ replacement comprises of a ball and socket joint, similar to that of a total hip replacement. The most common indication is thumb CMCJ osteoarthritis (Moriatis Wolf et al. 2014). Thumb CMCJ replacement was first described as a single mobility implant in 1979 by de la Caffinière and Aucouturier and then went onto

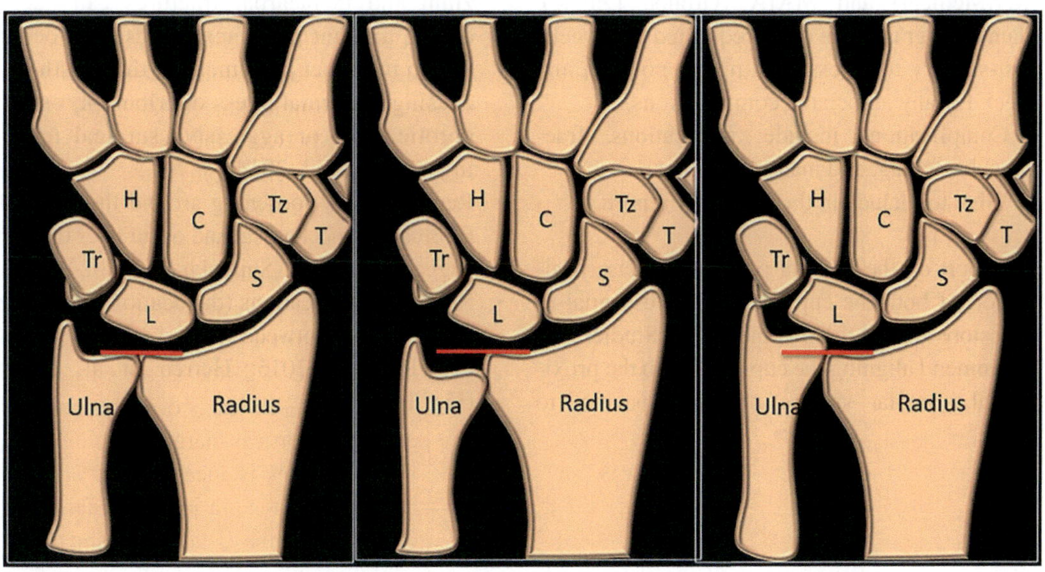

Fig. 14 Schematic showing measurement of ulna variance. The first image shows a neutral ulna variance, the second image a negative ulna variance, and the third image a positive ulna variance

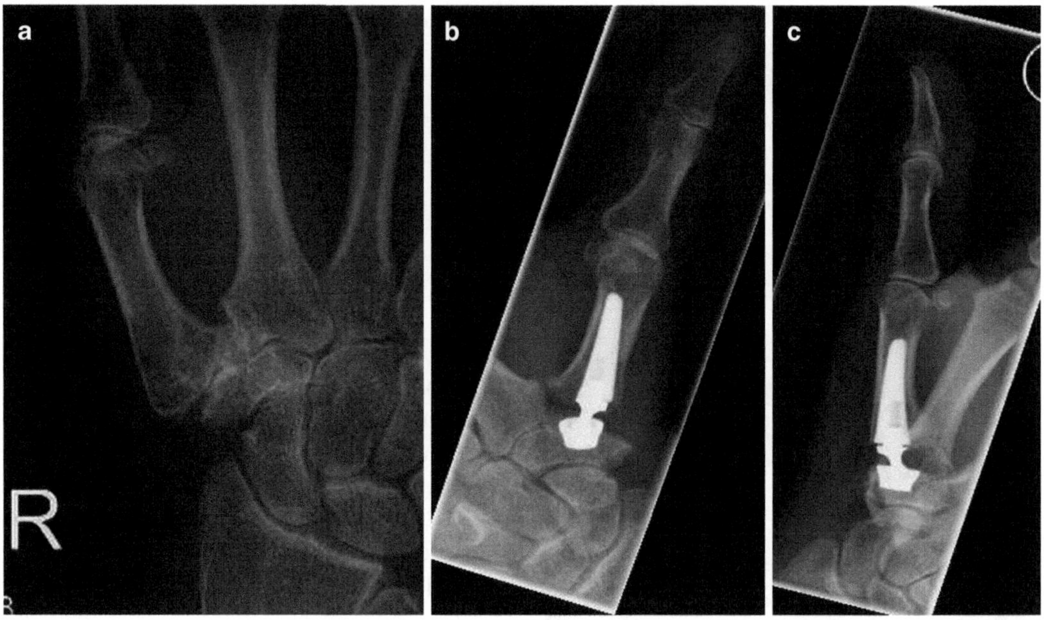

Fig. 15 Case 1 (**a**) PA radiograph showing advanced thumb CMCJ arthritic changes with mild arthritic changes within the scaphotrapezio-trapezoid joint (STT) (**b**, **c**) PA and lateral radiographs of a dual mobility thumb CMCJ implant

the third-generation dual-mobility implants we use today (Fig. 15). In the UK the two most commonly used implants today are the TOUCH (KeriMedical) and MAIA (Groupe Lépine). Plain radiographs are often requested at 6 weeks post-surgery to assess the implant position and check for any associated complications.

Complications include: dislocations, fractures, loosening, and mal-positioning.

What to include in the radiology report:

- Report on the implant position (precise position of both the cup and stem is essential to restore normal thumb kinematics. Studies recommend aligning the cup parallel to the proximal articular surface of the trapezium to prevent mechanical impingement and ensure joint stability) (Murai et al. 2022)
- Report on any associated fractures (trapezium and metacarpal fractures can occur during implant placement. These can occur due to incorrect placement of the prosthesis causing abnormal stress distribution, osteoporotic bone or aggressive surgical reaming) (Chug et al. 2014)
- Report on any loosening around the implant (this can be mechanical and occur over time or suggest infection) (Shintaku et al. 2024)
- Report on dislocations (dislocation rates have been reported between 1% and 4.5%) (Bricout and Rezzouk 2016; Herren et al. 2023) (Fig. 16).

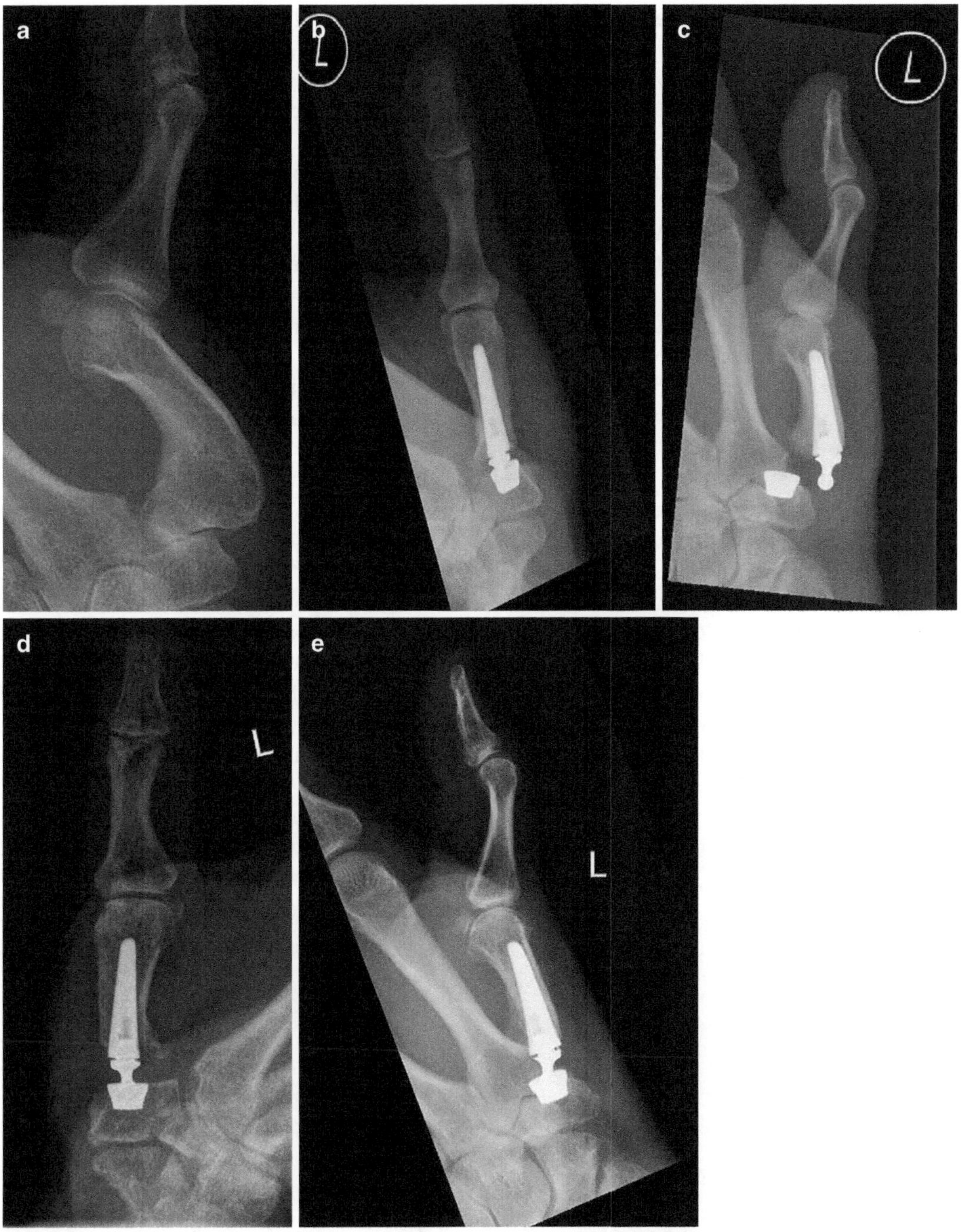

Fig. 16 Case 2—This patient fell onto an outstretched hand 2 weeks after their thumb CMCJ replacement, sustaining a dislocation. (**a**) Pre-operative images show arthritic changes with the thumb CMCJ on a background of a previous thumb metacarpal fracture malunion. (**b**) A thumb CMCJ arthroplasty was performed. (**c**) Radiographs showing a dislocation of the prosthesis. (**d**, **e**) PA and lateral radiographs post revision surgery

7 Distal Radius Osteotomy

Fractures of the distal radius are common injuries, comprising of up to 17% of all injuries (Nana et al. 2005). Malunion of distal radius fractures is the most common complication with a 24% incidence with those treated in plaster cast immobilisation (McGrory and Amadio 1998). Up to 83% of malunions can result in some form of functional disability, pain and arthritis (Cooney 3rd et al. 1980). A distal radius osteotomy is an elective procedure carried out to correct the distal radius alignment to improve wrist biomechanics, function and pain. Standard wrist radiographs (PA and true lateral) with the forearm held in neutral rotation should be obtained preoperatively. A true lateral view can provide better visualisation of the articular surface and lunate facet (Katt et al. 2020). The distal radius osteotomy can involve an opening or closing wedge and may use bone grafts. Both volar (Fig. 17) and dorsal plates can be used depending on the malunion configuration and surgeon choice. For dorsally displaced fractures a volar plate will require a closing wedge osteotomy and a dorsal plate for an opening wedge osteotomy. Post-operative radiographs include a PA and lateral views centred on the wrist which are requested at the follow-up appointments.

Complications: nonunion, metalwork failure, graft resorption, persistent malunion.

What to include in the radiology report:

- Report on the distal radius alignment parameters (see Table 1). Pre-operative images can be used for comparison.
- Report on the osteotomy site healing including bone graft incorporation if used.
- Report on the implant position (see distal radius section)
- Report on any metalwork complications

8 Ulna Shortening Osteotomy

Ulna impaction syndrome (UIS) is a common cause of ulna-sided wrist pain. UIS is a painful degenerative wrist condition caused by ulna head impaction with the ulna side of the carpus. Abnormal loads are placed through the ulna side

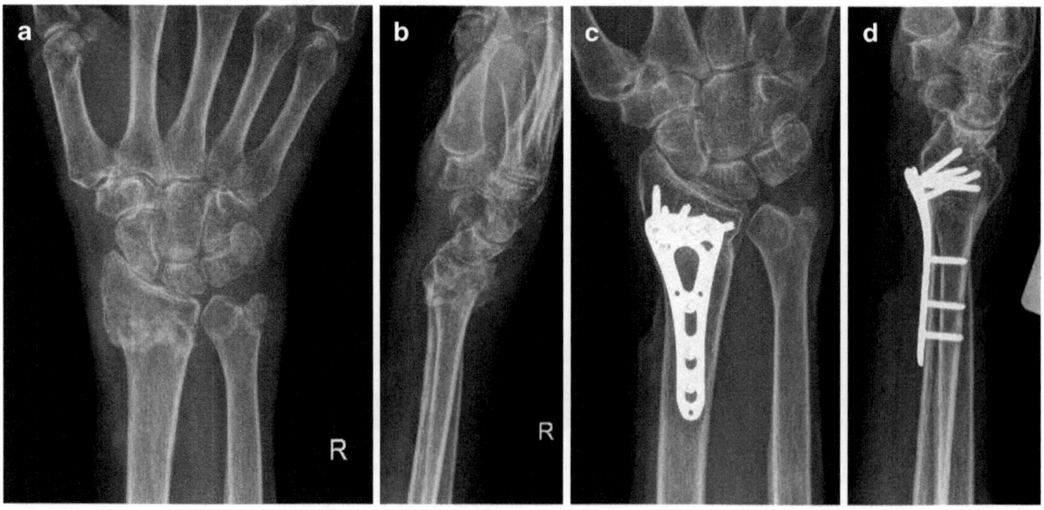

Fig. 17 (**a**, **b**) PA and lateral radiographs of the wrist showing a malunited dorsally displaced distal radius fracture. (**c**, **d**) PA and lateral radiographs of the malunion correction with a closing wedge osteotomy and volar locking plate. The distal radius alignment has been corrected, and the fracture has gone onto full union. (Note both lateral images are not true lateral)

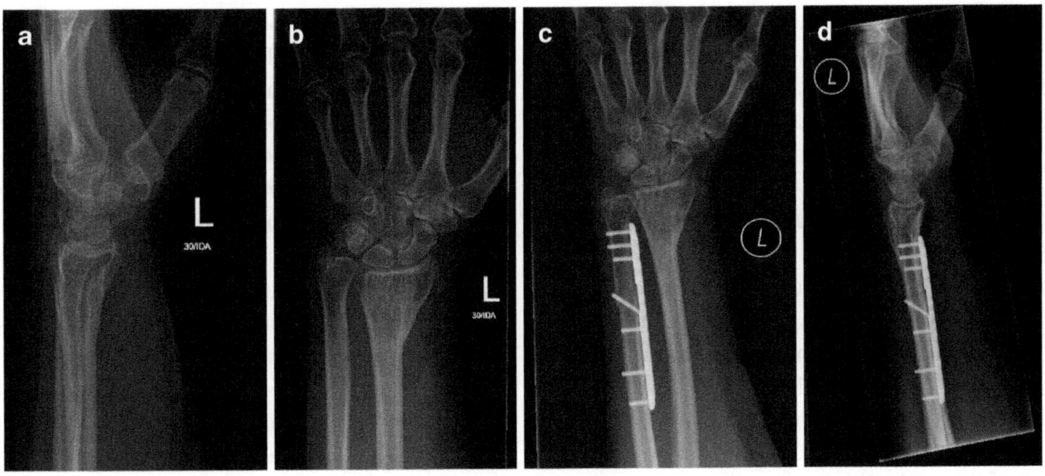

Fig. 18 (**a**, **b**) Pre-operative lateral and PA radiographs showing a malunited distal radius fracture with a positive ulna variance. (**c**, **d**) PA and lateral radiographs showing compression plate fixation of the ulna with correction of the positive ulna variance. The DRUJ is also aligned on the lateral view

of the wrist resulting in triangular fibrocartilage complex (TFCC) degeneration, lunate and ulna head chondromalacia, and lunotriquetral ligament disruption (Yu et al. 2022). Causes of UIS include distal radius malunion, radial head resection, premature radial physeal closure or congenital wrist abnormalities. An ulna-shortening osteotomy (Fig. 18) is one of the most common procedures performed for UIS (Terzis et al. 2020). This is an elective procedure with the aim of offloading the ulnocarpal joint and restoring distal radial ulna joint (DRUJ) congruence. The procedure involves creating an osteotomy site in the diaphyseal part of the ulna and fixation with a straight compression plate to shorten the length of the ulna.

Complications: delayed union, nonunion, metalwork failure, overcorrection leading to a negative ulna variance and DRUJ incongruity.

What to include in the radiology report:

- Report on the ulna variance when comparing to pre-operative radiographs (ulna variance is a critical reporting parameter. It is measured on PA radiographs with the forearm in neutral rotation. The method involves drawing lines perpendicular to the longitudinal axes of the radius and ulna at their distal ends and measuring the distance between these lines) (Kox et al. 2020) (Fig. 14)
- Report on the osteotomy site healing (nonunion rates range from 4% to 10%) (Owens et al. 2019)
- Report on metalwork complications (Zhang et al. in 2025 reported a hardware removal rate up to 30%)

9 3D Planning with CT

Traditionally plain radiographs have been used to plan the distal radius osteotomy, however the limitation of this is that complex multiplanar corrections can be difficult to address (Vroemen et al. 2013). Von Campe et al. in 2006 reported that 60% of osteotomies carried out using plain radiographs do not obtain the desired correction. 3-D CT-assisted planning with custom-made guides has been shown to improve the accuracy of the correction (Miyake et al. 2011). The 3D planning involves three steps (de Muinck Keizer et al. 2017): Step 1: a CT scan is obtained of the malunited distal radius and contralateral healthy forearm. Step 2: Virtual models are created of both radii using 3D planning software, both images are superimposed (the malunited radius on a mirrored version of the healthy contralateral side). Step 3: Virtual corrections or more advanced 3D custom-made cutting jigs are designed to allow for accurate on table corrections (Materialise).

10 Four Corner Fusions (4CF)

A 4CF is an elective salvage procedure to treat advanced degenerative arthritis. Common indications include scapho-lunate advanced collapse (SLAC) or scaphoid nonunion advanced collapse (SNAC) with the aim of preserving partial wrist motion. 4CF was first described by Watson and Ballet in 1984 (Watson and Ballet 1984) and since its introduction a variety of fixation methods have been described; K-wires, staples (Fig. 19), plates (Fig. 20) and headless compression screws (Andronic et al. 2022). The surgery often involves excision of the scaphoid and fusion of the lunate, triquetrum, hamate, and capitate. Cancellous bone graft is often taken from the distal radius to facilitate bony union. Post-operative imaging with PA and lateral radiographs is required to assess union, check for metalwork complications such as impingement, and evaluate for progressive arthritis. (Mulford et al. 2009). Radiographs can often be difficult to interpret to assess union and metalwork complications due to the overlapping structures, so it is not uncommon for hand surgeons to also request a CT scan in the post-operative follow-up period. A study by Ekelund et al. in 2007 showed a 64-slice CT to provide effective evaluation of healing after 4CFs despite the presence of metallic artifacts from fixation devices.

Complications: nonunion, metalwork malpositioning leading to dorsal impingement, metalwork failure, loosening, and secondary arthritis in the radiocarpal joint.

What to include in the radiology report:

- Report on the position of the implant
- Report on the alignment of the carpus
- Report on degenerative changes within the radio-lunate joint (the load of the wrist is transferred primarily through the radio-lunate joint which can lead to degenerative changes over time. A 10-year follow-up study by Traverso et al. in 2017 reported up to 73% of patients having radiographic changes with the radio-lunate joint but very few were clinically symptomatic with high patient satisfaction scores).
- Report on the presence of bony union (generally union rates are high after a 4CF with stud-

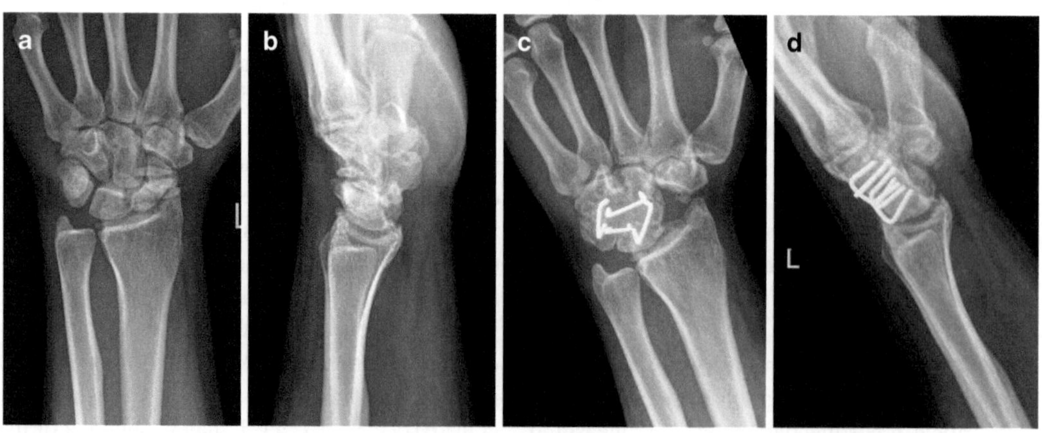

Fig. 19 (**a**, **b**) PA and lateral radiographs showing a scaphoid nonunion with radiocarpal degenerative changes (SNAC wrist). (**c**, **d**) Post-operative PA and lateral radiographs showing excision of the scaphoid and staple fixation of the lunate, triquetrum, hamate, and capitate. 100% bony union has been achieved with normal alignment of the carpus

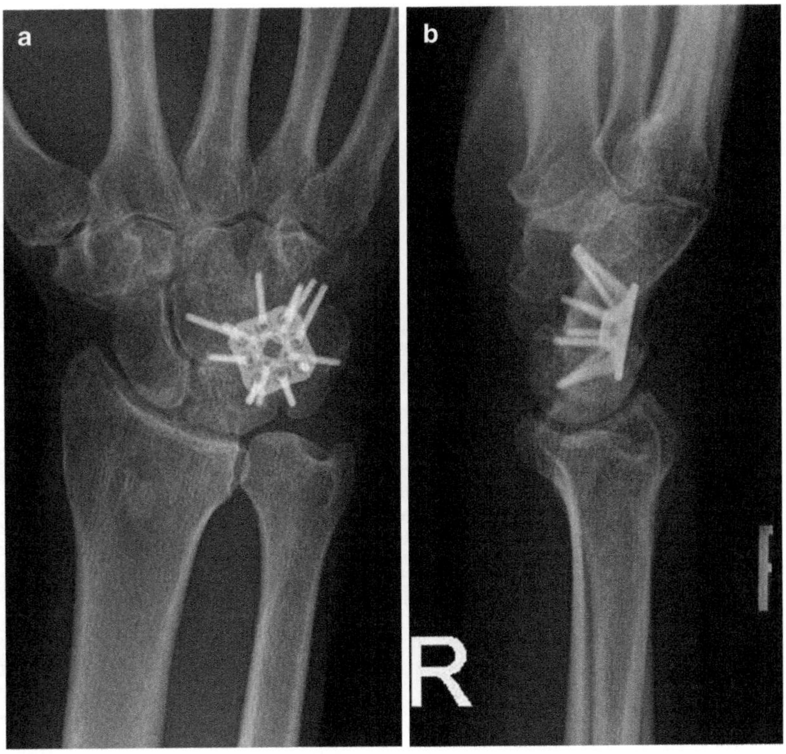

Fig. 20 (**a**, **b**) PA and lateral radiographs of a four-corner fusion with a "spider plate" fixation. In this case the scaphoid was not excised. Note the plate is flush with the bone reducing the incidence of dorsal impingement

ies reporting rates of 87%–100%) (Hayes et al. 2022)

- Report on metalwork complications (studies have reported incidences of dorsal plate impingement - 25% and broken screws - 13%) (Shindle et al. 2007)

11 Proximal Row Carpectomy (PRC)

A PRC is a motion-preserving procedure where the whole proximal carpal row is removed. The scaphoid, lunate, and triquetrum are removed allowing the capitate to rest in the lunate fossa (Fig. 21), therefore it is important that there is no evidence of mid-carpal arthritis before proceeding with this operation. Common indications for PRC include SLAC, SNAC, Kienbocks disease, and chronic peri-lunate dislocations. PRC can also be performed in conjunction with a wrist arthrodesis for end-stage arthritis or severe flexion contractures, placing the hand in a more functional position (Wall and Stern 2013). PA and lateral radiographs are often gained in the follow-up period to ensure carpal alignment is maintained and to monitor for mid-carpal degenerative changes in symptomatic patients that return to clinic.

Complications: capitate migration, radiocapitate arthritis.

What to include in the radiology report:

- Report on which bones have been removed
- Report on the position of the capitate, it should sit within the lunate fossa
- Report on signs of degenerative changes in the radiocapitate joint, particularly important for symptomatic patients that return to clinic.

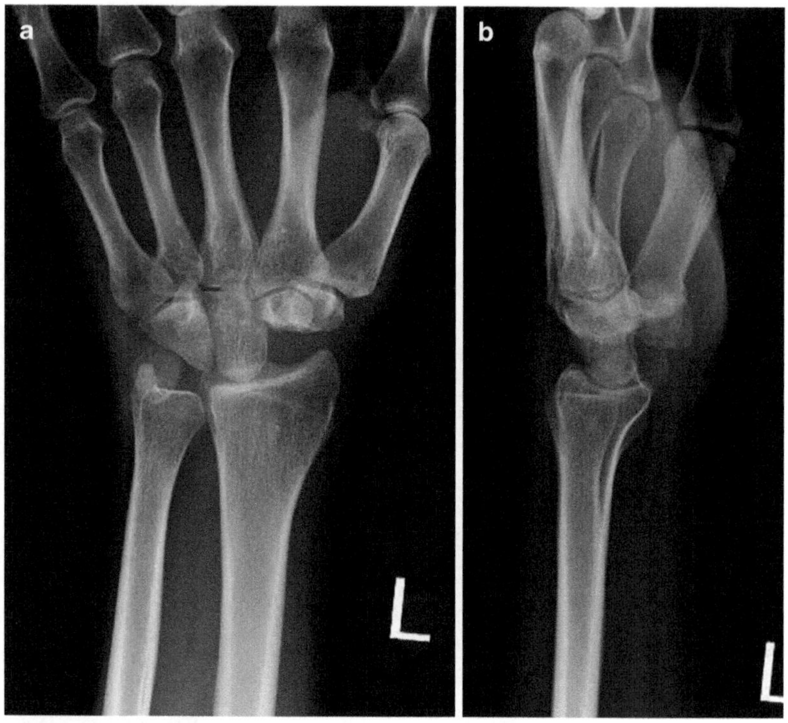

Fig. 21 (**a**, **b**) PA and lateral radiographs showing a proximal row carpectomy. The proximal capitate now rests in its new position within the lunate fossa. This is why any pre-operative degenerative changes within the mid-carpal joint are a contraindication for this procedure

12 Scaphotrapeziotrapezoid (STT) Fusion

STT fusion is a partial fusion procedure. Indications include isolated STT osteoarthritis, scaphoid instability, or Kienbocks disease (Deans et al. 2017). A variety of implants can be used to carry out the fusion, e.g. specific plates (Fig. 22), screws, staples, or headless compression screws. PA and lateral radiographs are requested at approximately 6 weeks clinic follow-up.

Complications: nonunion, delayed union, metalwork complications (breakage, loosening, misplacement)

What to include in the radiology report:

- Report on the positioning of the metalwork
- Report on the presence of bony union
- Report on evidence of degenerative changes in adjacent carpal joints

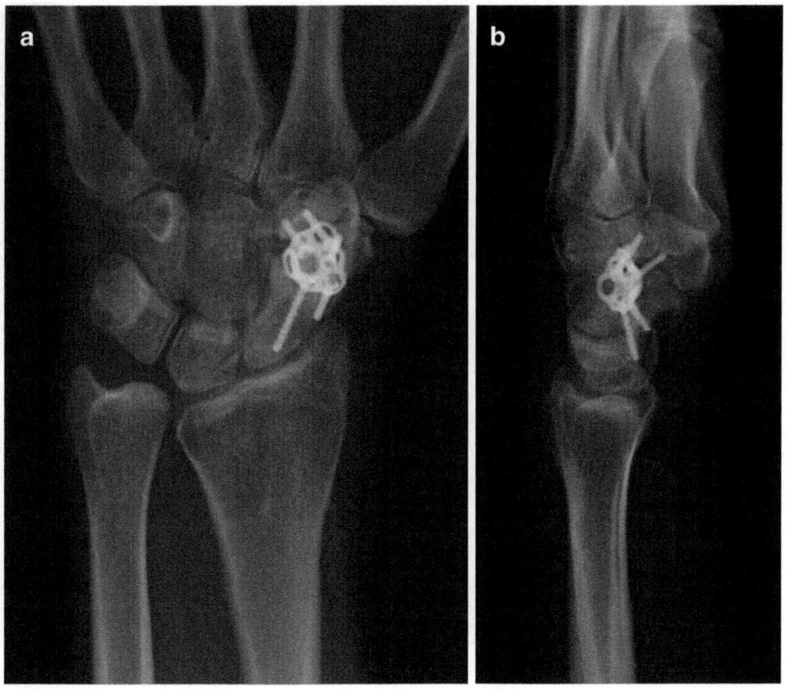

Fig. 22 (**a**, **b**) PA and lateral radiographs showing plate fixation for STT arthritis

13 Open Reduction Internal Fixation (ORIF) of Other Carpal Bones (e.g. Hamate/Capitate)

ORIF of carpal bones such as the capitate and hamate are often associated with high-energy trauma. They can be associated with carpal fracture dislocations. They often require fixation to help restore normal wrist biomechanics. Fixation techniques can include plates (Fig. 23), headless compression screws (Fig. 24), or K-wires depending on the fracture configuration. PA and lateral radiographs of the wrist are requested in the follow-up period to assess alignment and fracture healing.

Complications: nonunion, metalwork failure, avascular necrosis, post-traumatic arthritis, ulna nerve injury after hamate fixation (Bansal et al. 2017), flexor tendon rupture—flexor digitorum profundus (FDP) to the small finger.

What to include in the radiology report:

- Report on the type of implant used
- Report on the general carpal alignment
- Report on the fracture healing status
- Report on any metalwork complications

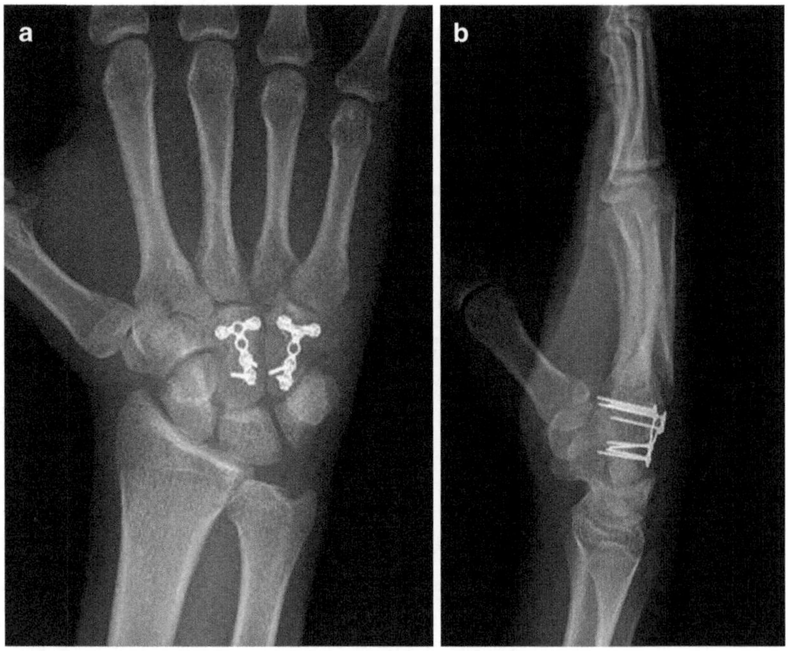

Fig. 23 (**a**, **b**) PA and lateral radiographs demonstrating plate fixation of the hamate and capitate

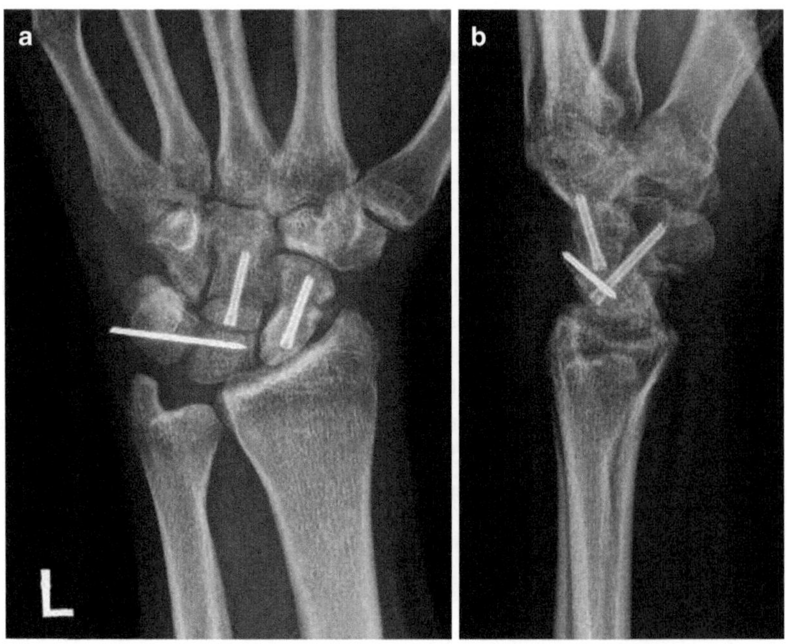

Fig. 24 (**a**, **b**) PA and lateral radiographs showing antegrade screw fixation of the capitate and hamate and K-wire stabilisation of the lunotriquetral joint, to allow interosseous ligament healing

14 Total Wrist Fusion (TWF)

TWF is an elective salvage procedure where the entire radiocarpal joint is fused. The main indications include end-stage degenerative or inflammatory arthritis (Berber et al. 2018). Other indications include failed total wrist arthroplasty or advanced carpal instability (Adams et al. 2016). A spanning dorsal plate (Fig. 25) is often used to fuse the wrist in a functional position, typically in a neutral or slightly extended position with 5–10° of ulna deviation (Hinds et al. 2016). This position allows for optimum grip strength and comfort in everyday resting and working postures. Post-operative imaging includes PA and lateral radiographs centred on the wrist with a CT scan often required to assess bony union with accuracy.

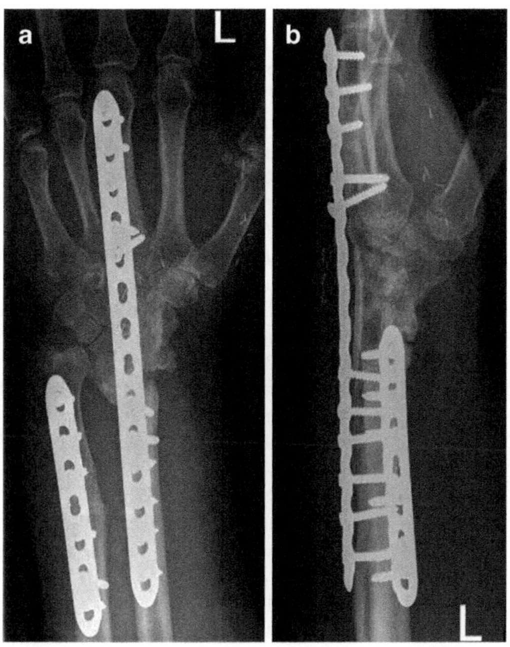

Fig. 25 (**a**, **b**) PA and lateral radiographs showing a total wrist fusion using a dorsal spanning plate. For this case the patient also underwent an ulna shortening osteotomy and a vascularised bone graft from the medial femoral condyle (MFC). Full bony union has taken place as evidenced on the lateral radiographs. The metallic clips seen in the images were used to as part of the free vascularised MFC bone graft which was anastomosed to the first dorsal metacarpal artery

Complications: nonunion, delayed union, metalwork failure or prominence, infection

What to include in the radiology report:

- Report on the plate positioning, typically the dorsal plate spans across to the third metacarpal
- Report on any lucency seen around the screws or evidence of screws backing out
- Report on the degree of bony union. A CT scan is often required to assess this with accuracy. Union rates have been reported as high as 98% (Hastings 2nd et al. 1996)
- Report on the general alignment of the carpus

15 Total Wrist Replacement (TWR)

TWR is a motion-preserving elective procedure and an alternative to a total wrist fusion. Indications for TWR include end-stage degenerative, inflammatory, or traumatic arthritis or failed partial midcarpal fusions. TWR was first introduced by Swanson in 1973 with a silicone prosthesis, but these had high failure rates, secondary mechanical failure, and silicone disintegration (Smith et al. 1985). We have now moved onto the current fourth generation of implants like the MOTEC (Swemac) prosthesis (Fig. 26). These have shown promising results with up to 86% survival at 10 years (Zijlker et al. 2021). The prosthesis compromises of a modular, uncemented system with radial and carpal components fixed with intramedullary stems. TWR is typically reserved for low functional demand patients as the weight restrictions to repetitive loading are typically up to 5 kg (Weiss and Akelman 2012). This is to help prevent implant loosening or dislocation, improving implant longevity. A proximal row carpectomy is also typically carried out in the same procedure, this has been shown to reduce the incidence of radial impaction syndrome and overall complications (Froschauer et al. 2021). Post-operative PA and lateral radiographs centred on the wrist are required at patient follow-up.

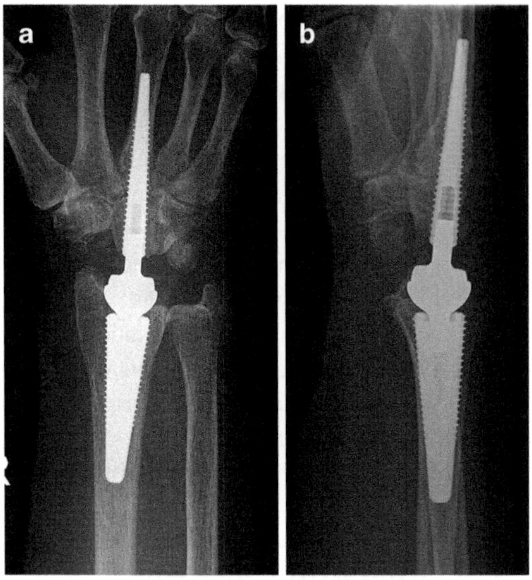

Fig. 26 (**a**, **b**) PA and lateral radiographs showing a Motec (Swemac) total wrist replacement. A proximal row carpectomy has also been performed

Complications: component loosening/osteolysis, subsidence, dislocation, periprosthetic fracture, infection.

What to include in the radiology report:

- Report on the presence of carpal or metacarpal osteolysis or lucency. Rates up to 9.5% have been reported (Krukhaug et al. 2011)
- Report on the implant position, the stems should sit down the central axis of the metacarpal and radius
- Report on any periprosthetic fractures. A 2% incidence for intra-operative and post-operative periprosthetic fractures has been reported (Wagner et al. 2017).
- To identify early failure report on evidence of osteolysis or changes in component alignment in comparison to previous radiographs

References

Adams BD, Kleinhenz BP, Guan JJ (2016) Wrist arthrodesis for failed total wrist arthroplasty. J Hand Surg [Am] 41(6):673–679. https://doi.org/10.1016/j.jhsa.2016.02.012

Andronic O, Nagy L, Burkhard MD et al (2022) Long-term outcomes of the four-corner fusion of the wrist: a systematic review. World J Orthop 13(1):112–121. https://doi.org/10.5312/wjo.v13.i1.112

Apergis E, Maris J, Theodoratos G, Pavlakis D, Antoniou N (1997) Perilunate dislocations and fracture-dislocations: closed and early open reduction compared in 28 cases. Acta Orthop Scand 275(Suppl):55–59

Arora R, Lutz M, Deml C, Krappinger D, Haug L, Gabl M (2011) A prospective randomized trial comparing nonoperative treatment with volar locking plate fixation for displaced and unstable distal radial fractures in patients sixty-five years of age and older. J Bone Joint Surg Am Vol 93(23):2146–2153. https://doi.org/10.2106/JBJS.J.01597

Bansal A, Carlan D, Moley J, Goodson H, Goldfarb CA (2017) Return to play and complications after hook of the hamate fracture surgery. J Hand Surg [Am] 42(10):803–809. https://doi.org/10.1016/j.jhsa.2017.06.108

Baron JA, Karagas M, Barrett J et al (1996) Basic epidemiology of fractures of the upper and lower limb among Americans over 65 years of age. Epidemiology 7(6):612–618. https://doi.org/10.1097/00001648-199611000-00008

Berber O, Garagnani L, Gidwani S (2018) Systematic review of total wrist arthroplasty and arthrodesis in wrist arthritis. J Wrist Surg 7(5):424–440. https://doi.org/10.1055/s-0038-1646956

Bricout M, Rezzouk J (2016) Complications and failures of the trapeziometacarpal Maia® prosthesis: a series of 156 cases. Hand Surg Rehabil 35(3):190–198. https://doi.org/10.1016/j.hansur.2016.02.005

Brogan DM, Moran SL, Shin AY (2015) Outcomes of open reduction and internal fixation of acute proximal pole scaphoid fractures. Hand (New York) 10(2):227–232. https://doi.org/10.1007/s11552-014-9689-8

Chug M, Williams N, Benn D, Brindley S (2014) Outcome of uncemented trapeziometacarpal prosthesis for treatment of thumb carpometacarpal joint arthritis. Indian J Orthop 48(4):394–398. https://doi.org/10.4103/0019-5413.136270

Clay NR, Dias JJ, Costigan PS, Gregg PJ, Barton NJ (1991) Need the thumb be immobilised in scaphoid fractures? A randomised prospective trial. J Bone Joint Surg Br Vol 73(5):828–832. https://doi.org/10.1302/0301-620X.73B5.1894676

Clementson M, Björkman A, Thomsen NOB (2020) Acute scaphoid fractures: guidelines for diagnosis and treatment. EFORT Open Rev 5(2):96–103. https://doi.org/10.1302/2058-5241.5.190025

Cooney WP 3rd, Dobyns JH, Linscheid RL (1980) Complications of Colles' fractures. J Bone Joint Surg (Am Vol) 62(4):613–619

Costa ML, Achten J, Parsons NR et al (2014) Percutaneous fixation with Kirschner wires versus volar locking plate fixation in adults with dorsally displaced fracture of distal radius: randomised controlled trial. BMJ 349:g4807. https://doi.org/10.1136/bmj.g4807

de la Caffinière JY, Aucouturier P (1979) Trapezio-metacarpal arthroplasty by total prosthesis.

Hand 11(1):41–46. https://doi.org/10.1016/S0072-968X(79)80007-8
de Muinck Keizer RJO, Lechner KM, Mulders MAM, Schep NWL, Eygendaal D, Goslings JC (2017) Three-dimensional virtual planning of corrective osteotomies of distal radius malunions: a systematic review and meta-analysis. Strategies Trauma Limb Reconstr 12(2):77–89. https://doi.org/10.1007/s11751-017-0284
Deans VM, Naqui Z, Muir LT (2017) Scaphotrapeziotrapezoidal joint osteoarthritis: a systematic review of surgical treatment. J Hand Surg Asian Pac Vol 22(1):1–9. https://doi.org/10.1142/S0218810417300017
Dias JJ, Brealey SD, Fairhurst C et al (2020) Surgery versus cast immobilisation for adults with a bicortical fracture of the scaphoid waist (SWIFFT): a pragmatic, multicentre, open-label, randomised superiority trial. Lancet 396(10248):390–401. https://doi.org/10.1016/S0140-6736(20)30931-4
Eastley N, Singh H, Dias JJ, Taub N (2013) Union rates after proximal scaphoid fractures: meta-analyses and review of available evidence. J Hand Surg Eur Vol 38(8):888–897. https://doi.org/10.1177/1753193412451424
Ekelund L, Hagberg L, Hörberg L, Jörgsholm P, Gunnarsson M (2007) Imaging of four-corner fusion (SLAC arthrodesis) of the wrist with 64-slice computed tomography. Acta Radiol 48(1):76–79. https://doi.org/10.1080/02841850601026450
Froschauer SM, Holzbauer M, Hager D, Kwasny O, Duscher D (2021) Proximal row carpectomy with total scaphoidectomy vs. conventional carpal resection for ReMotion total wrist arthroplasty. J Clin Med 10(9):1865. https://doi.org/10.3390/jcm10091865
Haentjens P, Johnell O, Kanis JA et al (2004) Evidence from data searches and life-table analyses for gender-related differences in absolute risk of hip fracture after Colles' or spine fracture: Colles' fracture as an early and sensitive marker of skeletal fragility in white men. J Bone Miner Res 19(12):1933–1944. https://doi.org/10.1359/JBMR.040917
Hastings H 2nd, Weiss AP, Quenzer D, Wiedeman GP, Hanington KR, Strickland JW (1996) Arthrodesis of the wrist for post-traumatic disorders. J Bone Joint Surg (Am Vol) 78(6):897–902. https://doi.org/10.2106/00004623-199606000-00013
Hayes E, Cheng Y, Sauder D, Sims L (2022) Four-corner arthrodesis with differing methods of osteosynthesis: a systematic review. J Hand Surg [Am] 47(5):477.e1–477.e9. https://doi.org/10.1016/j.jhsa.2021.06.002
Herren DB, Marks M, Neumeister S, Schindele S (2023) Low complication rate and high implant survival at 2 years after Touch® trapeziometacarpal joint arthroplasty. J Hand Surg (Eur Vol) 48(9):877–883. https://doi.org/10.1177/17531934231179581
Herzberg G (2000) Acute dorsal trans-scaphoid perilunate dislocations: open reduction and internal fixation. Tech Hand Upper Extrem Surg 4:2–13
Hinds RM, Melamed E, O'Connell A, Cherry F, Seu M, Capo JT (2016) Assessment of wrist function after simulated total wrist arthrodesis: a comparison of 6 wrist positions. Hand (N Y) 11(4):464–468. https://doi.org/10.1177/1558944715626930
Kapandji A (1976) L'ostéosynthèse par double embrochage intra-focal. Traitement fonctionnel des fractures non articulaires de l'extrémité inférieure du radius [Internal fixation by double intrafocal pinning. Functional treatment of non-articular fractures of the lower end of the radius (author's transl)]. Ann Chir 30(11–12):903–908
Katt B, Seigerman D, Lutsky K, Beredjiklian P (2020) Distal radius malunion. J Hand Surg [Am] 45(5):433–442. https://doi.org/10.1016/j.jhsa.2020.02.008
Kox LS, Jens S, Lauf K, Smithuis FF, van Rijn RR, Maas M (2020) Well-founded practice or personal preference: a comparison of established techniques for measuring ulnar variance in healthy children and adolescents. Eur Radiol 30(1):151–162. https://doi.org/10.1007/s00330-019-06354
Krukhaug Y, Lie SA, Havelin LI, Furnes O, Hove LM (2011) Results of 189 wrist replacements: a report from the Norwegian Arthroplasty Register. Acta Orthop 82(4):405–409. https://doi.org/10.3109/17453674.2011.588858
Kupperman A, Breighner R, Saltzman E, Sneag D, Wolfe S, Lee S (2018) Ideal starting point and trajectory of a screw for the dorsal approach to scaphoid fractures. J Hand Surg [Am] 43(11):993–999. https://doi.org/10.1016/j.jhsa.2018.03.044
Larsen CF, Mathiesen FK, Lindequist S (1991) Measurements of carpal bone angles on lateral wrist radiographs. J Hand Surg [Am] 16(5):888–893. https://doi.org/10.1016/s0363-5023(10)80156
Leslie IJ, Dickson RA (1981) The fractured carpal scaphoid: natural history and factors influencing outcome. J Bone Joint Surg Br Vol 63-B(2):225–230. https://doi.org/10.1302/0301-620X.63B2.7217146
Majeed H (2014) Non-operative treatment versus percutaneous fixation for minimally displaced scaphoid waist fractures in high demand young manual workers. J Orthop Traumatol 15(4):239–244. https://doi.org/10.1007/s10195-014-0293
McGrory BJ, Amadio PC (1998) Malunion of the distal radius. In: Cooney WP, Linscheid RL, Dobyns JH (eds) The wrist: diagnosis and operative treatment. Mosby, St. Louis, pp 356–384
Miyake J, Murase T, Moritomo H, Sugamoto K, Yoshikawa H (2011) Distal radius osteotomy with volar locking plates based on computer simulation. Clin Orthop Relat Res 469(6):1766–1773. https://doi.org/10.1007/s11999-010-1748
Moriatis Wolf J, Turkiewicz A, Atroshi I, Englund M (2014) Prevalence of doctor-diagnosed thumb carpometacarpal joint osteoarthritis: an analysis of Swedish health care. Arthritis Care Res 66(6):961–965. https://doi.org/10.1002/acr.22250

Mulford JS, Ceulemans LJ, Nam D, Axelrod TS (2009) Proximal row carpectomy vs four corner fusion for scapholunate (SLAC) or scaphoid nonunion advanced collapse (SNAC) wrists: a systematic review of outcomes. J Hand Surg (Eur Vol) 34(2):256–263. https://doi.org/10.1177/1753193408100954

Murai A, Kurosawa A, Tada K, Yamamoto T, Yamada K, Iijima H, Watanabe T (2022) Optimal center of rotation for ball-and-socket thumb carpometacarpal arthroplasty identified using three-dimensional kinematic analysis: a pilot study. Front Bioeng Biotechnol 10:868150. https://doi.org/10.3389/fbioe.2022.868150

Najarian R, Nourbakhsh A, Capo J, Tan V (2011) Perilunate injuries. Hand (New York) 6:1–7. https://doi.org/10.1007/S11552-010-9293-5

Nana AD, Joshi A, Lichtman DM (2005) Plating of the distal radius. J Am Acad Orthop Surg 13(3):159–171

O'Neill TW, Cooper C, Finn JD et al (2001) Incidence of distal forearm fracture in British men and women. Osteoporos Int 12(7):555–558. https://doi.org/10.1007/s001980170076

Owens J, Compton J, Day M, Glass N, Lawler E (2019) Nonunion rates among ulnar-shortening osteotomy for ulnar impaction syndrome: a systematic review. J Hand Surg [Am] 44(7):612.e1–612.e12. https://doi.org/10.1016/j.jhsa.2018.08.018

Perry DC, Machin DM, Casaletto JA, Brown DJ (2011) Minimising the risk of extensor pollicis longus rupture following volar plate fixation of distal radius fractures: a cadaveric study. Ann R Coll Surg Engl 93(1):57–60. https://doi.org/10.1308/003588411X12851639107151

Pinder RM, Brkljac M, Rix L, Muir L, Brewster M (2015) Treatment of scaphoid nonunion: a systematic review of the existing evidence. J Hand Surg [Am] 40(9):1797–1805.e3. https://doi.org/10.1016/j.jhsa.2015.05.003

Said J, Baker K, Fernandez L, Komatsu DE, Gould E, Hurst LC (2018) The optimal location to measure scapholunate diastasis on screening radiographs. Hand (New York) 13(6):671–677. https://doi.org/10.1177/1558944717729219

Shenoy R, Pillai A, Hadidi M (2007) Scaphoid fractures: variation in radiographic views – a survey of current practice in the West of Scotland region. Eur J Emerg Med 14(1):2–5. https://doi.org/10.1097/01.mej.0000228445.63523.b7

Shindle MK, Burton KJ, Weiland AJ, Domb BG, Wolfe SW (2007) Complications of circular plate fixation for four-corner arthrodesis. J Hand Surg (Eur Vol) 32(1):50–53. https://doi.org/10.1016/j.jhsb.2006.08.016

Shintaku T, Nakayama M, Ishii H, Yagi M, Ikegami H (2024) Long-term outcome over 15 years of prosthesis for thumb carpometacarpal joint arthritis: a case series. Cureus 16(11):e73480. https://doi.org/10.7759/cureus.73480

Singh HP, Forward D, Davis TR, Dawson JS, Oni JA, Downing ND (2005) Partial union of acute scaphoid fractures. J Hand Surg (Br Eur Vol) 30(5):440–445. https://doi.org/10.1016/j.jhsb.2005.05.007

Smith RJ, Atkinson RE, Jupiter JB (1985) Silicone synovitis of the wrist. J Hand Surg [Am] 10(1):47–60. https://doi.org/10.1016/s0363-5023(85)80247

Soong M, Earp BE, Bishop G, Leung A, Blazar P (2011) Volar locking plate implant prominence and flexor tendon rupture. J Bone Joint Surg (Am Vol) 93(4):328–335. https://doi.org/10.2106/JBJS.J.00193

Terzis A, Koehler S, Sebald J, Sauerbier M (2020) Ulnar shortening osteotomy as a treatment of symptomatic ulnar impaction syndrome after malunited distal radius fractures. Arch Orthop Trauma Surg 140(5):681–695. https://doi.org/10.1007/s00402-020-03374

Traverso P, Wong A, Wollstein R, Carlson L, Ashmead D, Watson HK (2017) Ten-year minimum follow-up of 4-corner fusion for SLAC and SNAC wrist. Hand (New York) 12(6):568–572. https://doi.org/10.1177/1558944716681949

Vasara H, Tarkiainen P, Stenroos A, Kosola J, Anttila T, Aavikko A, Nordback PH, Aspinen S (2023) Higher Soong grade predicts flexor tendon issues after volar plating of distal radius fractures: a retrospective cohort study. BMC Musculoskelet Disord 24(1):271. https://doi.org/10.1186/s12891-023-06313-0

Von Campe A, Nagy L, Arbab D, Dumont CE (2006) Corrective osteotomies in malunions of the distal radius: do we get what we planned? Clin Orthop Relat Res 450:179–185. https://doi.org/10.1097/01.blo.0000223994.79894.17

Vroemen JC, Dobbe JG, Sierevelt IN, Strackee SD, Streekstra GJ (2013) Accuracy of distal radius positioning using an anatomical plate. Orthopedics 36(4):e457–e462. https://doi.org/10.3928/01477447-20130327-22

Wagner ER, Srnec JJ, Mehrotra K, Rizzo M (2017) What are the risk factors and complications associated with intraoperative and post-operative fractures in total wrist arthroplasty? Clin Orthop Relat Res 475(11):2694–2700. https://doi.org/10.1007/s11999-017-5442

Wall LB, Stern PJ (2013) Proximal row carpectomy. Hand Clin 29(1):69–78. https://doi.org/10.1016/j.hcl.2012.08.022

Watson HK, Ballet FL (1984) The SLAC wrist: scapholunate advanced collapse pattern of degenerative arthritis. J Hand Surg [Am] 9(3):358–365. https://doi.org/10.1016/s0363-5023(84)80223

Weiss AP, Akelman E (2012) Total wrist replacement. Med Health R I 95(4):117–119

Yu H, Wang T, Wang Y, Zhu Y (2022) Ulnar shortening osteotomy vs. wafer resection for ulnar impaction syndrome: a systematic review and meta-analysis. Int J Surg 104:106725. https://doi.org/10.1016/j.ijsu.2022.106725

Zhang Y, Grewal R, Vergouwen M, Lu S, White N, WECan (2025) Risk factors for complications in ulnar shortening osteotomies: a multicenter retrospective review. J Hand Surg [Am] 50(1):104.e1–104.e7. https://doi.org/10.1016/j.jhsa.2023.06.001

Zijlker HJA, Ritt MJPF, Beumer A (2021) Fourth-generation total wrist arthroplasty: a systematic review of clinical outcomes. J Wrist Surg 11(5):456–464. https://doi.org/10.1055/s-0041-1735840

Artificial Intelligence in Hand and Wrist Imaging: Enhancing Diagnostics and Workflow

Pranav Ajmera, Girish Gandikota, and Amit Kharat

Contents

P. Ajmera (✉) · G. Gandikota
Division of Musculoskeletal Radiology, The University of North Carolina at Chapel Hill, Chapel Hill, NC, USA

A. Kharat
DeepTek Inc., Pune, India

Abstract

Artificial intelligence (AI) is rapidly reshaping hand and wrist radiology by augmenting the diagnostic process and streamlining clinical workflows. Advanced deep learning models are being gradually deployed to detect and classify fractures, evaluate arthritic changes, and analyze soft tissue abnormalities with remarkable precision. In practical terms, AI works like a diligent assistant—it carefully highlights the areas of potential concern on radiographic images, ensuring that no subtle detail goes unnoticed. In its preliminary role, AI reviews imaging studies and flags likely abnormalities, which frees up radiologists to focus on the tougher, more ambiguous cases. In busy or emergency settings, it serves as a prioritizer by quickly identifying urgent cases so that critical findings receive prompt attention.

Beyond these day-to-day functions, AI supports more advanced imaging techniques by enabling precise 3D reconstructions and detailed quantitative analyses. These capabilities enhance treatment planning and surgical decision-making. Although these developments hold tremendous potential for increasing diagnostic efficiency and accuracy, challenges with data diversity, bias reduction, and streamlined integration with current systems still exist. The necessity of continuous cooperation between radiologists, AI develop-

Med Radiol Diagn Imaging (2025)
https://doi.org/10.1007/174_2025_581,
Published Online: 10 May 2025

ers, and legislators is highlighted by ethical and legal considerations, especially with regard to patient privacy and accountability. In the end, AI has the potential to usher in a new era of personalized, data-driven radiology by augmenting human expertise. This will modify both routine diagnostics and intricate clinical decision-making in musculoskeletal imaging.

1 Introduction

Hand and wrist imaging plays a critical role in diagnosing a wide range of conditions, encompassing traumatic injuries, degenerative disorders, and soft tissue abnormalities. The complex anatomy of the hand and wrist, with its intricate network of bones, joints, tendons, ligaments, and neurovascular structures, presents unique challenges for radiological interpretation (Pinto et al. 2016; Sahu et al. 2014). Subtle pathological changes, such as hairline fractures or early signs of arthritis, often require a high degree of expertise and meticulous attention to detail. Even with advances in imaging modalities, the potential for misdiagnosis or missed findings remains a concern, particularly in high-volume clinical settings where radiologists face time constraints (Sharma 2023; Lee et al. 2023; Ajmera et al. 2021). Artificial intelligence (AI) has emerged as a transformative tool in medical imaging, offering the potential to enhance diagnostic accuracy, streamline workflows, and improve patient outcomes (Sharma 2023). This chapter attempts to give a thorough summary of the state of artificial intelligence (AI) in hand and wrist radiography, including its uses, constraints, and potential future developments. We aim to clarify how AI is influencing the direction of musculoskeletal imaging and its potential to transform patient care in this specialized field by examining the most recent studies and use cases.

2 Fundamentals of AI in Medical Imaging

A combination of cutting-edge computational techniques and clinical expertise, artificial intelligence (AI) in medical imaging aims to improve the precision and effectiveness of diagnostic procedures. AI is fundamentally the application of algorithms to mimic human intellect, and the two primary subfields driving medical imaging are machine learning (ML) and deep learning (DL) (Pesapane et al. 2018; Ajmera et al. 2021). DL is a subset of ML, which itself is a subset of AI. In recent times, there has been development of generative learning, which is a further advancement of DL techniques. A relationship between these differing yet overlapping technologies is shown in Fig. 1.

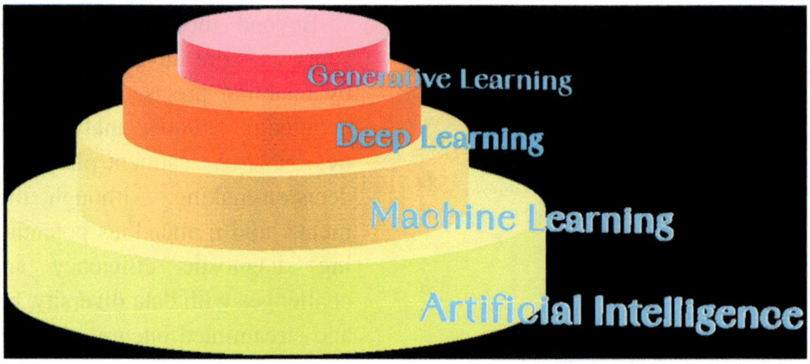

Fig. 1 An illustration depicting the progression and interconnected nature of artificial intelligence technologies. Each subsequent technology builds upon advancements from previous innovations or approaches problems in a distinct, iterative manner, while still remaining a subset of earlier frameworks

Machine learning is a subset of AI that allows systems to learn patterns from data and make predictions or decisions without being explicitly programmed. Traditional ML techniques rely on handcrafted features—specific image attributes identified by experts—to develop predictive models. For example, in the context of musculoskeletal radiology, an ML algorithm might analyze texture, shape, or intensity features to identify abnormalities in bone structure. While effective in some cases and offering the advantage of processing complex non-linear relationships, these methods often require extensive domain knowledge and are limited by their dependence on predefined features (Bulstra and Machine Learning 2022).

By doing away with the necessity for manual feature extraction, deep learning—a more sophisticated subset of machine learning—has completely transformed AI applications in radiology. Convolutional neural networks (CNNs), a type of deep learning model, are specifically engineered to automatically recognize and learn hierarchical features straight from unprocessed image data. Since CNNs can interpret both visual and spatial information, they are particularly well-suited for medical imaging tasks. For instance, a CNN analyzing an X-ray of the hand can learn to detect fractures by recognizing patterns such as discontinuities in cortical bone or abnormal alignment of joints (Alzubaidi et al. 2024; Raisuddin et al. 2021). During the training phase of creating these models, the algorithm is exposed to enormous collections of medical picture annotations. The model achieves high levels of accuracy by iteratively adjusting its internal parameters to minimize prediction mistakes. The dataset used to train and validate models is a crucial part of AI in medical imaging. Superior, annotated datasets are necessary to create reliable algorithms. Diverse and representative datasets are essential to ensure that AI models function consistently across various patient demographics and imaging devices.

Beyond CNNs, other deep learning architectures, such as recurrent neural networks (RNNs) and transformers, are also being explored for their potential applications in medical imaging. RNNs, which excel at processing sequential data, may have utility in analyzing temporal changes in imaging studies, such as monitoring disease progression on serial radiographs (Hosny et al. 2018). Transformers, known for their success in natural language processing, are being adapted for image analysis tasks, offering new avenues for innovation. Moreover, iterations such as data efficient image transformers (DeiT), have an additional benefit of reducing the risk of hidden stratification often seen in CNN models, due to which there is often a discrepancy in performance of the CNN models in different datasets, thus impacting their generalizability and widespread adoption. In a comparative performance analysis between the two, Murphy et al. (2022) demonstrated that while the DeiT had slightly lower performance for upper extremity radiographs, the actual clinical impact was negligible, but these were more resilient to hidden stratification.

These advancements have profound implications for musculoskeletal imaging, where early and accurate diagnosis is paramount for effective patient management. The application of AI in hand and wrist radiology is a relatively nascent but rapidly growing area of research and clinical interest. Moreover, AI applications extend beyond diagnostic assistance to include workflow optimization and decision support. By automating routine tasks, such as image segmentation and preliminary reporting, AI can alleviate the burden on radiologists and allow them to focus on more complex cases. Hospitals and imaging centers worldwide are beginning to integrate AI into their Picture Archiving and Communication Systems (PACS) to streamline operations and improve diagnostic efficiency. For example, the implementation of AI-driven triage systems has been shown to reduce turnaround times for critical findings, such as fractures or infections, thereby expediting patient care. A table summarizing majority of the artificial intelligence models being utilized in the hand and wrist domain (Table 1).

Table 1 Summary of AI models developed to tackle imaging challenges relating to imaging of hand and wrist

Publications	Purpose
Fractures	
Lindsey et al. (2018)	Identifying fractures on wrist radiographs
Kim and MacKinnon (2018)	Classify each image as "fracture" or "no fracture" on wrist radiographs
Yahalomi et al. (2019)	Accuracy for wrist fracture detection
Thian et al. (2019)	Radius and ulna fractures
Gan et al. (2019)	Presence or absence of a distal radius fracture
Langerhuizen et al. (2020)	Occult scaphoid fracture
Yoon et al. (2021)	Occult scaphoid fractures on radiographs
Raisuddin et al. (2021)	Wrist fracture detection
Ozkaya et al. (2022)	Scaphoid fracture
Lee et al. (2023)	Distal radius, ulnar styloid, and scaphoid fractures
Min et al. (2023)	Intra- versus extra-articular distal radius fractures
Arthritis	
Overgaard et al. (2024)	Segmentation and semiquantitative scoring of osteophytes on ultrasound images
Gitto et al. (2024)	Identifying and grading abnormal findings of osteoarthritis, as well as predicting the onset or progression of the disease
Soft Tissue Analysis	
Khatun et al. (2024)	To delineate tendon and ligament structures on MRI or ultrasound images
Droppelmann et al. (2024)	Evaluate tendon integrity in situations like tendinopathy or following surgical repair
Tumor and Mass Identification	
Sabeghi et al. (2024)	Differentiate between benign and malignant soft tissue tumors in MRI scans
Xu et al. (2024)	Differentiate between benign and malignant soft tissue tumors in MRI scans

3 Applications in Hand and Wrist Radiology

3.1 Fracture Detection and Classification

One of the most well-known uses of artificial intelligence (AI) in hand and wrist radiology is fracture identification. Perhaps the most prevalent cause of imaging investigations in this anatomical area is trauma, which includes fractures of the distal radius, scaphoid, and metacarpals. Even while fractures occur often, they can be difficult to find, particularly if they are subtle or situated in anatomically complicated places. Advanced diagnostic technologies are essential because misdiagnosis or missing fractures can result in poor patient outcomes and delayed treatment. There are multiple ways AI can be utilized to optimize workflow—it can serve as "an aid," an assistant, assisting the scan reader by demarcating suspected site(s) of involvement, saving them time and effort on each scan. It can serve as "a pre-reader," essentially identifying the pathology and keeping the reports dictated, freeing up significant time for each radiologist, time which can be better spent on particularly borderline or complicated cases. Another important role that can be played by AI, particularly in emergency setting, is that of a "Flagger," flagging all high-priority studies for faster reporting and slotting them ahead of the potentially normal ones. This approach allows the scan reader to direct their attention towards the "high values studies," studies which are pathological, but without which the system would have needed to wait in queue. Thus, this allows for a potentially faster turn-around-time (TAT) for pathological scans over the standard TAT for studies, which are not emergent (Fig. 2).

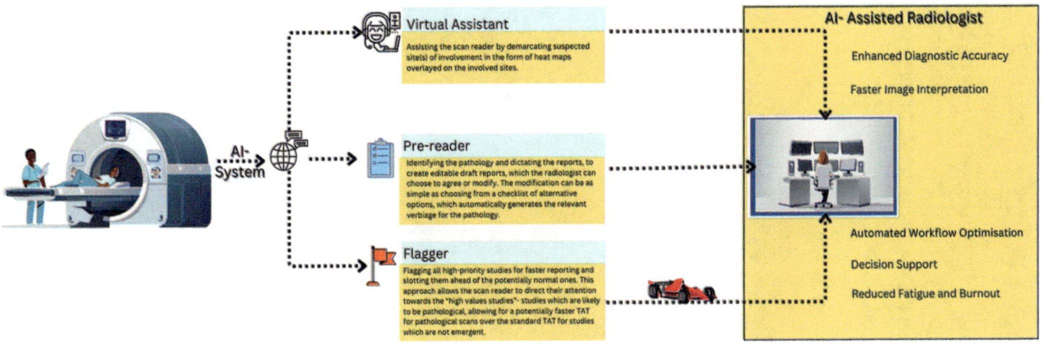

Fig. 2 An illustration showcasing the diverse roles an AI model can play in real-world radiology reporting

Before we get in depth of the various studies done so far and their specific regions of interest, we have for our readers a few examples of a commercially available model identifying fractures in upper extremity radiographs (Figs. 3, 4, and 5).

AI algorithms, particularly convolutional neural networks (CNNs), have demonstrated exceptional accuracy in fracture detection. For instance, Lindsey et al. (2018) developed a deep CNN model capable of identifying fractures on wrist radiographs, and the study concluded that the AI-assisted clinicians had a nearly 47% cut in misinterpretation rate with comparatively higher sensitivity and specificity. Yahalomi et al. (2019) on a faster R-CNN model determined their models accuracy for wrist fracture detection as 96%, much better than that of clinicians in their study. Thian et al. demonstrated the feasibility of fracture detection and localization on wrist radiographs utilizing an Inception Res-Net faster R-CNN (Thian et al. 2019), which revealed that the model correctly localized radius and ulna fractures in 91.2% and 96.3% cases. Langerhuizen et al. (2020) developed a DL model, which performed exceptionally well in detecting occult scaphoid fracture, but a subpar performance for detecting obvious scaphoid radiographs. Ozkaya et al. (2022) validated a CNN model for scaphoid fracture determination and found mixed results, with the model performance in between that of a less experience and more experienced clinician. In a later validation study of another deep CNN model by Yoon et al. (2021), to detect occult scaphoid fractures on radiographs, they found that their model could identify 90% of the occult fractures on wrist radiographs. Raisuddin et al. (2021) built a DL model for wrist fracture detection, but they also went a step further in comparing the model performance on a mixed difficulty dataset with that on a predominantly challenging dataset and documented an area-under the curve (AOC) of 0.99 versus 0.84, respectively. Lee et al. (2023) utilized their DL model for the detection of the three most common wrist fractures—distal radius, ulnar styloid, and scaphoid—and found an AUC of 0.9, 0.92, and 0.8, respectively. A comparison of "unaided" versus "aided" radiologists revealed a definitive jump in AUC for the detection of scaphoid fractures.

Kim and MacKinnon (2018) deployed a CNN model in a potential role as "flagger," to classify each image as "fracture" or "no fracture" on wrist radiographs with an AUC of 0.954. In another study by Gan et al. (2019) utilizing a fast object detection CNN algorithm, to classify the presence or absence of a distal radius fracture, the model had an AUC of 0.96, slightly superior to that of the radiologists in the study.

In addition to detection, AI has been employed for fracture classification, which involves categorizing fractures based on their type, location, and severity. Accurate classification is critical for guiding treatment decisions, such as conservative management versus surgical intervention. Min et al. (2023) developed a two-step Ensemble DL model for categorization of intra- versus extra-articular distal radius fractures, and they achieved an AUC and accuracy of 0.82 and 0.81, respectively, demonstrating a potentially scalable use case.

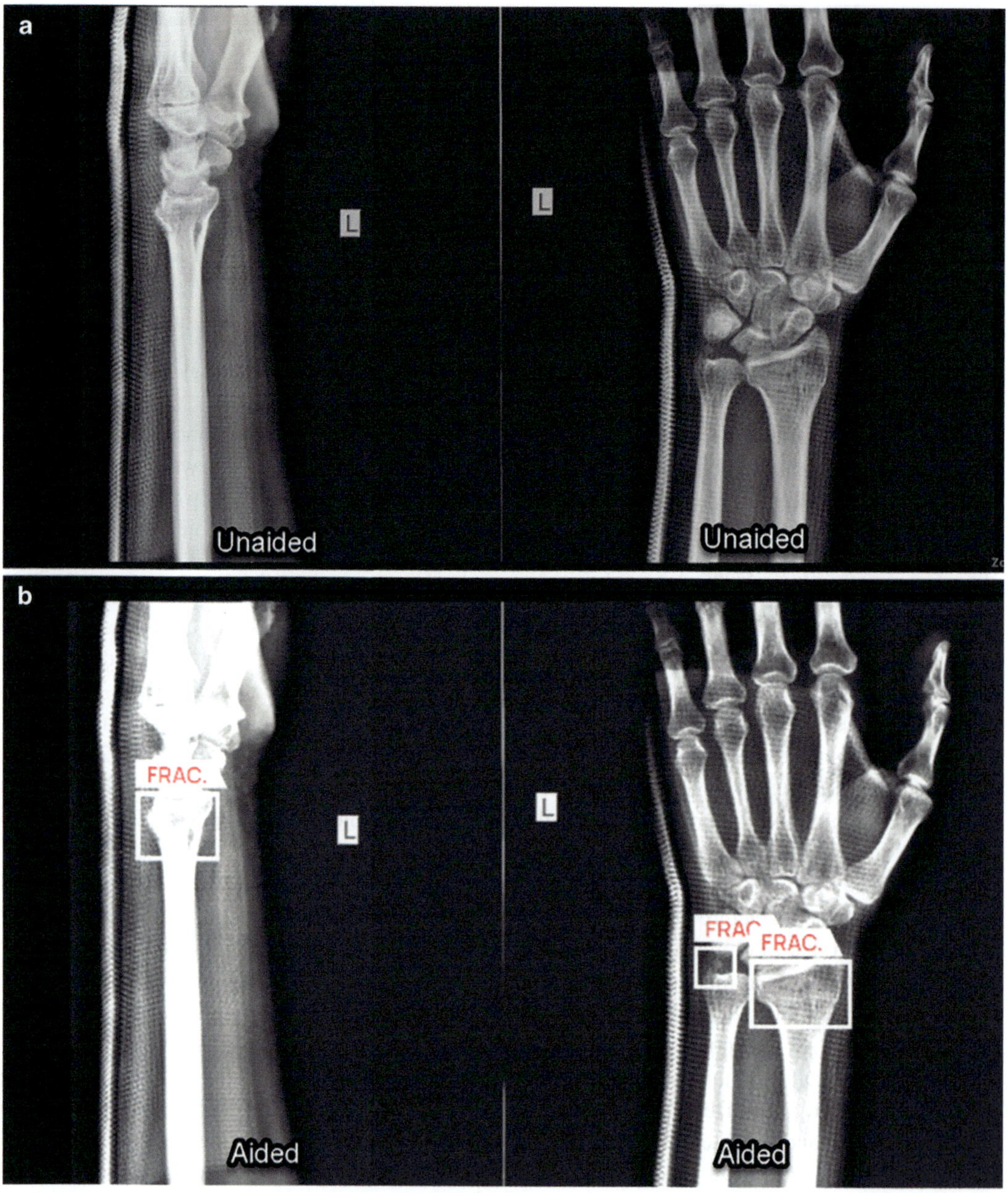

Fig. 3 A real-world example of an AI model being utilized to detect wrist fractures. (Image courtesy of AZ Med). (**a**) Radiographs without any aid of the AI model, that would be interpreted by the radiologist, as such. (**b**) Radiographs with the AI model, aiding the radiologist by identifying the suspected sites of fractures

Advanced AI models have also been integrated with three-dimensional (3D) imaging modalities, such as computed tomography (CT), to provide more detailed fracture characterization.

3.2 Arthritis Evaluation

AI applications in assessing rheumatoid arthritis and osteoarthritis are emerging, with algorithms

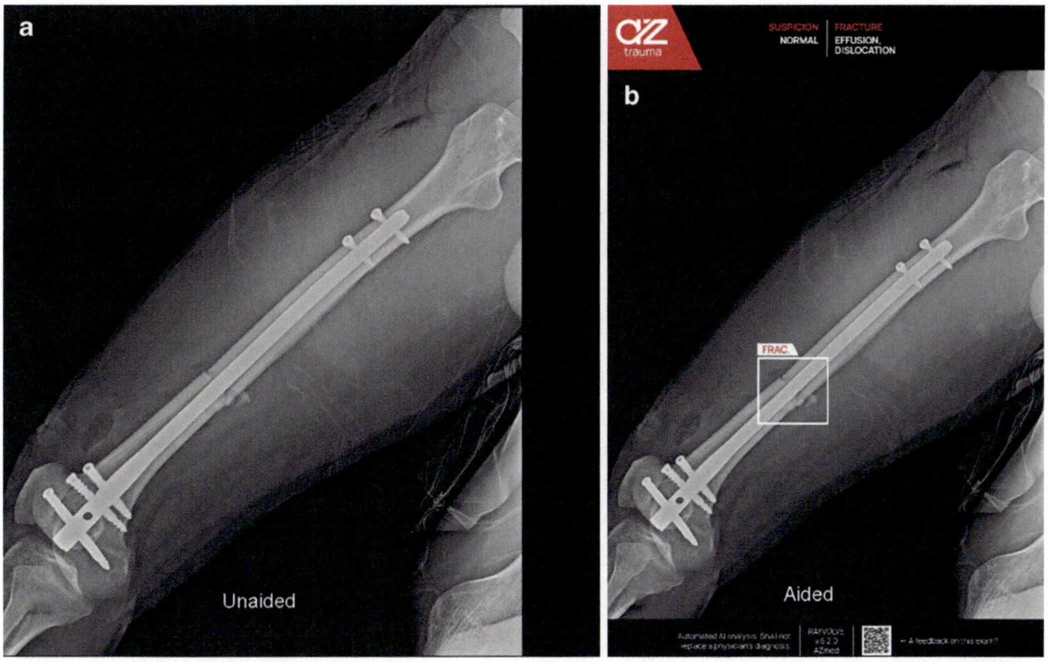

Fig. 4 A real-world example of an AI model being utilized to detect peri-prosthetic fracture of the humerus. (Image courtesy of AZ Med). (**a**) Radiographs without any aid of the AI model, that would be interpreted by the radiologist, as such. (**b**) Radiographs with the AI model, aiding the radiologist by identifying the suspected sites of fractures

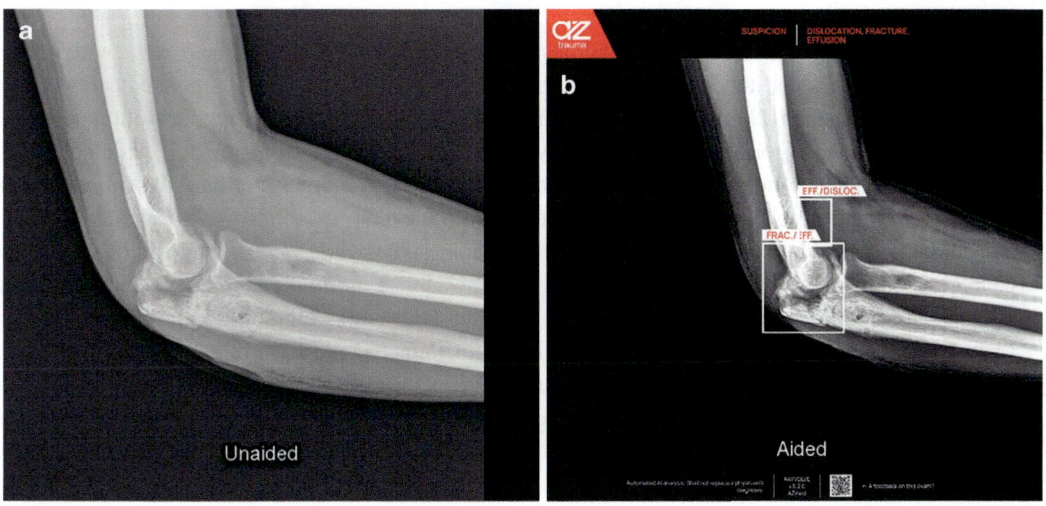

Fig. 5 A real-world example of an AI model being utilized to detect elbow fractures. (Image courtesy of AZ Med). (**a**) Radiographs without any aid of the AI model, that would be interpreted by the radiologist, as such. (**b**) Radiographs with the AI model, aiding the radiologist by identifying the suspected sites of fractures

being developed to evaluate joint space narrowing, erosions, and other arthritic changes. These tools aim to provide quantitative assessments that can aid in monitoring disease progression and treatment response. AI may potentially aid radiologists in identifying and grading abnormal findings of osteoarthritis, as well as predicting the onset or progression of the disease (Gitto et al. 2024). For example, A U-Net++ based CNN model for segmentation and semiquantitative scoring of osteophytes on ultrasound images was developed by Overgaard et al. (2024), and they reported that the model had a percentage exact agreement (PEA) of 50%, 76%, 70%, and 59% for CMC, MCP, PIP, and DIP joints, respectively. However, overall, the ability to automate scoring on radiographs still remains challenging because of multiple barriers, the foremost of which happens to be a lack of multi-center, multi-scanner pathological radiographs from geographically distinct sites, allowing for training of AI algorithms which are much more redundant, less biased, and more generalizable (Overgaard et al. 2024; Bird et al. 2022). Development of such models apart from the effort saving benefits also had the added benefit of standardization. As of now, there usually is poor interobserver agreement between readers adjudicating pathological radiographs, often heavily reliant on experience in the field (Bird et al. 2022).

3.3 Soft Tissue Analysis

AI's role in detecting soft tissue abnormalities, such as ligament tears and tendon injuries, is an area of ongoing research. By analyzing MRI or ultrasound images, AI algorithms can potentially identify subtle changes indicative of soft tissue pathology, assisting radiologists in making more accurate diagnoses. AI has applications in musculoskeletal radiology, including improving sensitivity in identifying ligament tears and fractures.

Among the most common indications for MRI of wrist and hands is injury to the triangular fibrocartilage (TFCC), intrinsic ligaments of the wrist, tendon, and ligament injuries, such as those involving the flexor tendons, extensor tendons, and scapholunate ligament (Vassa et al. 2020). AI algorithms have shown potential in augmenting diagnostic accuracy by identifying subtle abnormalities that may be overlooked on imaging. For instance, deep learning models trained on MRI datasets have been developed to recognize tendon tears and inflammation with high sensitivity. These models utilize advanced CNNs to detect patterns in imaging data that correlate with pathology, such as signal intensity changes or abnormal contouring of tendons and ligaments.

Moreover, automated segmentation algorithms have been employed to delineate tendon and ligament structures on MRI or ultrasound images (Khatun et al. 2024). By creating precise maps of these structures, AI can assist clinicians in identifying partial or complete ruptures and monitoring post-repair healing. The application of AI to measure structural alterations over time is gaining traction as an approach to dynamically evaluate tendon integrity in situations like tendinopathy or following surgical repair (Droppelmann et al. 2024).

3.4 Bone Age Assessment

Attempts to utilize some form of computer assisted detection (CAD) for the detection of bone age have been ongoing since 1990s, but more recently newer systems have been developed of this task. BoneXpert is utilized widely across Europe. Other solutions such as VUNO Med-BoneAge and HH-boneage.io are semiautomatic and fully automated systems, respectively. All the models deployed so far have variable success rate, as their performance varies across ethnicities and is limited in cases with bone abnormalities or previously operated cases (Gitto et al. 2024). Continued refinement of models will allow development of algorithms which are reliable across ethnicities, perhaps algorithms which also consider associated clinical and demographic data while interpreting the bone age, to allow for a normalized output, one which is redundant across ethnicities. In such cases, the algorithms need to be highly reliable because bone age assessments are often linked to a medico-legal issue, and an incorrect adjudication can have serious consequences for the patient under review, increasing the risk of being sued for incorrect results. Radiologists can benefit significantly from such an algorithm because most graduating radiologists often have very limited experience in bone age assessment.

3.5 Tumor and Mass Identification

AI-assisted hand and wrist mass and bone tumor identification is a new area of study. Based on imaging features, algorithms are being taught to distinguish between benign and malignant tumors. Diagnosing soft tissue masses, such as tumors, lipomas, and ganglion cysts, can be difficult, especially when separating benign from malignant lesions. A technique to improve the characterization of these lesions is AI-based radiomics, which utilizes quantitative features from medical images. Features such as texture, shape, and heterogeneity can be analyzed using machine learning models to provide non-invasive insights into tumor behavior (Zhou et al. 2022; Ong et al. 2023).

This application holds promise for early detection and appropriate management of bone tumors. AI tools have the capability to assist radiologists in tasks ranging from image segmentation to lesion detection in bone and soft tissue tumors (Ong et al. 2023; Von Schacky et al. 2021).

For example, researchers have trained AI models to differentiate between benign and malignant soft tissue tumors in MRI scans, achieving a high AUC value (Xu et al. 2024). These tools not only assist in early detection but also aid in surgical planning by providing detailed maps of tumor margins and their relationship to adjacent anatomical structures (Sabeghi et al. 2024; Xu et al. 2024).

4 Role of AI in Advanced Imaging Modalities

4.1 MRI-Based Applications

AI has been applied to accelerate MRI acquisition and improve image quality (Koch et al. 2021; Herrmann et al. 2023; Kim et al. 2022). While these have been evaluated for joints such as the shoulder, hip, knee, ankle, for some time, the development of an AI-assisted MRI sequence in hand and wrist is only recent. Herrmann et al. (2023) undertook a comparative study of routine TSE sequence with DL-assisted TSE sequence and found that the DL-assisted TSE reduce the examination time by nearly 60%. These advancements can lead to more accurate diagnoses and improved patient outcomes. Thus, deep learning-based reconstruction techniques have been evaluated for turbo spin echo sequences of the hand and wrist, showing potential in enhancing image quality and visualization of anatomical structures

4.2 CT-Based Applications

In computed tomography (CT), AI algorithms assist in 3D reconstruction and volumetric analysis, aiding in the assessment of complex fractures and preoperative planning. DL-based tools can help lower patient dose of radiation by limiting exposure time or intensity (Rozema et al. 2021) and relying instead on algorithms to acquire high-quality images (Koetzier et al. 2023). They provide detailed insights into bone architecture, facilitating better surgical outcomes. AI can also help in detecting metastatic bone lesions and monitoring their progression on serial scans.

5 Performance and Validation of AI Models

The performance of AI models in hand and wrist radiology is typically evaluated using metrics such as sensitivity, specificity, and area under the receiver operating characteristic curve (AUC-ROC). Studies have demonstrated that AI can achieve high diagnostic accuracy, with some models performing at the level of experienced radiologists. For example, an AI algorithm for scaphoid fracture detection achieved performance comparable to musculoskeletal radiologists. However, it is crucial to note that AI performance can vary depending on the complexity of cases. A study evaluating deep neural networks for wrist fracture detection found that while the model performed well on general test sets, its performance declined on challenging cases requiring CT confirmation, highlighting the need for meticulous analysis before clinical deployment.

6 Clinical Implementation and Challenges

6.1 Workflow Integration

Artificial intelligence (AI) has the ability to fundamentally alter patient care, diagnostic accuracy, and efficiency when included into clinical processes for hand and wrist imaging. However, a comprehensive approach that tackles both operational and technological issues is necessary for a smooth deployment.

The capture and processing of images is a crucial area where AI can have a profound impact. AI-powered solutions can streamline MRI or CT scan parameters such as contrast levels, exposure times, and slice thickness, thereby optimizing imaging methods. In addition to enhancing image quality, this also reduces down on radiation exposure and scan durations. For instance, sophisticated algorithms are able to identify motion artifacts in real time and flag or alter for them, ensuring that consistently diagnostically meaningful pictures are acquired. Additionally, AI-driven reconstruction algorithms have demonstrated potential in generating high-quality images from low-dose data, which is especially advantageous in scenarios involving repeat imaging or pediatric patients.

By automating initial processes like image segmentation and annotation, AI systems can optimize radiologists' operations when imaging is completed. Delineating the flexor tendons, scapholunate ligament, or carpal bones on MRI, for example, is a laborious procedure that may now be automated with remarkable precision. Radiologists can increase productivity by concentrating on interpretation instead of tedious manual procedures thanks to these pre-segmented pictures. Additionally, automated triage systems are being utilized, giving priority to cases with significant findings such tendon ruptures or fractures. According to studies, AI-driven triage ensures prompt response for patients with acute injuries by cutting down on turnaround times for critical situations.

Successful workflow integration demands robust interoperability between AI tools and existing Picture Archiving and Communication Systems (PACS). This requires seamless software integration and adherence to standards such as DICOM and HL7.

6.2 Ethical and Medicolegal Issues

The adoption of artificial intelligence (AI) in hand and wrist radiology introduces several ethical and legal challenges that demand careful attention to ensure responsible and fair use. As AI tools become increasingly integrated into clinical workflows, addressing these issues is essential for building trust and promoting equitable outcomes.

One major ethical concern is safeguarding patient privacy. AI systems require access to substantial datasets for training and validation, which often include sensitive patient information, such as medical imaging and associated health details. To protect confidentiality, it is crucial to implement de-identification processes while maintaining the clinical utility of the data. Additionally, stringent data security measures, including encryption and secure transfer protocols, must be in place to prevent data breaches or unauthorized access. Adherence to regulations like the Health Insurance Portability and Accountability Act (HIPAA), the General Data Protection Regulation (GDPR), and acts such as the European Unions' AI act is also imperative for ensuring patient data is handled appropriately.

Another significant ethical issue is the transparency of AI systems. Many AI algorithms, particularly those using deep learning, operate as "black boxes," offering limited insight into their decision-making processes. This lack of interpretability can create challenges for radiologists, who remain responsible for the final diagnosis. Developing explainable AI (XAI) frameworks that clarify how algorithms reach their conclusions is essential to foster trust among clinicians and patients. Such transparency ensures that AI recommendations can be understood, validated, and integrated into clinical decision-making.

The use of AI in radiology raises ethical and medicolegal considerations, including issues of accountability, patient consent, and data privacy. Determining liability in cases of AI diagnostic errors and ensuring patient data confidentiality are critical challenges that need to be addressed (Ajmera et al. 2021). From a legal perspective, questions around liability and accountability remain unresolved. When an AI system makes an incorrect prediction or fails to detect a critical finding, determining responsibility becomes complex. Is the liability borne by the software developer, the radiologist using the tool, or the healthcare institution implementing it? Establishing clear guidelines and legal frameworks is essential to address these scenarios and protect all stakeholders, including patients.

6.3 Biases in AI Models

Biases in artificial intelligence (AI) models represent a critical issue in hand and wrist radiology, as they can compromise diagnostic accuracy, perpetuate healthcare disparities, and impact patient outcomes. These biases often originate from the training data and the methodologies employed in developing AI algorithms.

A major contributor to bias is the lack of diversity in training datasets. Many radiology AI models are built using data that disproportionately represents specific populations, such as those from certain geographic locations, ethnic groups, or healthcare systems. For instance, a model trained primarily on adult imaging data may underperform when applied to pediatric patients, whose anatomy and pathology differ significantly. Similarly, algorithms trained on high-resolution images from advanced facilities may not generalize well to lower-quality images from resource-limited environments, widening gaps in care delivery.

Bias can be worsened by imbalances in how conditions are represented in training datasets. For instance, the model can have trouble identifying unusual or minor fractures in clinical practice if they are underrepresented. This significantly limits the algorithm's clinical value in hand and wrist radiography by causing it to overlook or incorrectly categorize less prevalent injuries.

Additionally, biases in the data may be unintentionally reinforced by algorithmic design. CNNs, for instance, could make inaccurate predictions due to their emphasis on non-clinical image factors. This could manifest in musculoskeletal radiology as an over dependence on demographic correlations or imaging artifacts that are not consistent with disease. To mitigate these biases, a multipronged strategy is essential. Foremost, among these are developing datasets that are diverse, inclusive, and representative of different patient populations and clinical scenarios. Collaborative efforts across institutions can help ensure models are trained on a wide range of imaging modalities and demographic data. Moreover, techniques like data augmentation and transfer learning can enhance model performance across varied scenarios. Explainable AI (XAI) tools are also important, as they can provide transparency into algorithmic decision-making, helping clinicians identify and address any biases (Borys et al. 2023).

Regular monitoring and validation of AI systems in real-world settings are equally important. Post-deployment analysis can reveal biases that may not have been apparent during the training and testing phases. Moreover, establishing regulatory standards and guidelines for fairness, transparency, and accountability in AI is crucial to ensure ethical implementation.

Addressing biases in AI models is fundamental to achieving accurate and equitable outcomes in hand and wrist radiology. By focusing on inclusivity, transparency, and continuous improvement, we can ensure these technologies deliver reliable benefits across diverse patient populations and maintain their reliability and fairness (Ricci Lara et al. 2022).

7 Future Directions

7.1 Personalized Medicine in Musculoskeletal Imaging

The innovation of artificial intelligence creates a multitude of opportunities in personalizing medicine through individualized imaging evaluations and specific treatment strategies for the patients. In hand and wrist radiology, AI could review and systematically integrate the patient's known genetic factors, medical history, and advanced imaging studies to more accurately predict disease risk and outcomes. Personalized AI-driven models could also help in determination of best treatment approaches for different types of musculoskeletal disorders for better patient outcomes and satisfaction.

7.2 Predicting Treatment Outcomes

Many AI algorithms are currently being designed to predict treatment efforts, especially for cases with an operative approach. For instance, with scaphoid fractures or wrist arthritis, AI would do analyze preoperative imaging and then offer prediction regarding successful surgical management and possible complications. Likewise, AI could evaluate post-treatment imaging to assess the effectiveness of therapy and determine if data-driven changes would need to be made to the treatment plan. Such developments would improve the quality of care provided to patients.

7.3 Emerging Technologies

The use of AI in hand and wrist radiology is about to undergo yet another revolution due to emerging technologies like explainable AI (XAI) and federated learning. Federated learning solves issues with data sharing and confidentiality by enabling AI models to learn from data spread across several institutions while protecting patient privacy (Rehman et al. 2023). In order to help radiologists and clinicians comprehend the reasoning behind AI-driven diagnoses and recommendations, explainable AI aims to increase the transparency of AI models' decision-making process (Borys et al. 2023).

The combination of AI algorithms and natural language processing (NLP) for radiology reporting is another exciting field. Radiologists and referring physicians can communicate more effectively and with less variability when NLP techniques are used to create structured, standardized reports based on imaging findings.

7.4 Real-Time Decision Support

AI's ability to provide real-time decision support could be a game-changer in clinical practice. For instance, during complex surgical procedures involving the hand and wrist, AI-driven tools could provide real-time feedback based on intraoperative imaging, helping surgeons achieve optimal outcomes. Similarly, point-of-care ultrasound devices integrated with AI could assist clinicians in quickly diagnosing conditions such as tenosynovitis or masses in outpatient settings.

8 Conclusion

Artificial intelligence (AI) technology functions as a transformational element in the practice of hand and wrist radiology by changing how medical professionals perform and evaluate musculoskeletal imaging for clinical applications. AI delivers transformative capabilities through better detection of fractures and characterization of soft tissue injuries alongside workflow management improvements and advanced image analysis methods. The system demonstrates vast potential to boost diagnostic precision while decreasing radiologists' workload ultimately leading to better patient outcomes because of its fast and exact handling of imaging data analysis. The application of AI in hand and wrist radiology exists currently in its initial development phase even though significant progress has been made. The persistence of algorithmic biases alongside requirements for diverse datasets and understandable AI systems drives ongoing research and development. The successful deployment of AI systems requires resolving ethical and legal concerns including data privacy issues alongside accountability standards and fair access benefits.

Future advancements in AI applications for hand and wrist radiology depend on integrated work between medical professionals including radiologists and data scientists together with healthcare policy makers. The development of trustworthy AI models which explain their decisions will be essential as radiologists' expertise needs complementary support in the future. The successful realization of AI potential in healthcare delivery will depend on ongoing efforts to integrate AI into clinical environments and provide radiologists with training to utilize these tools effectively.

Ultimately, while challenges remain, the future of AI in hand and wrist radiology is promising. As the field continues to innovate, AI has the potential to revolutionize musculoskeletal imaging, driving improvements in diagnostic precision, operational efficiency, and patient care in the years to come (Fig. 6).

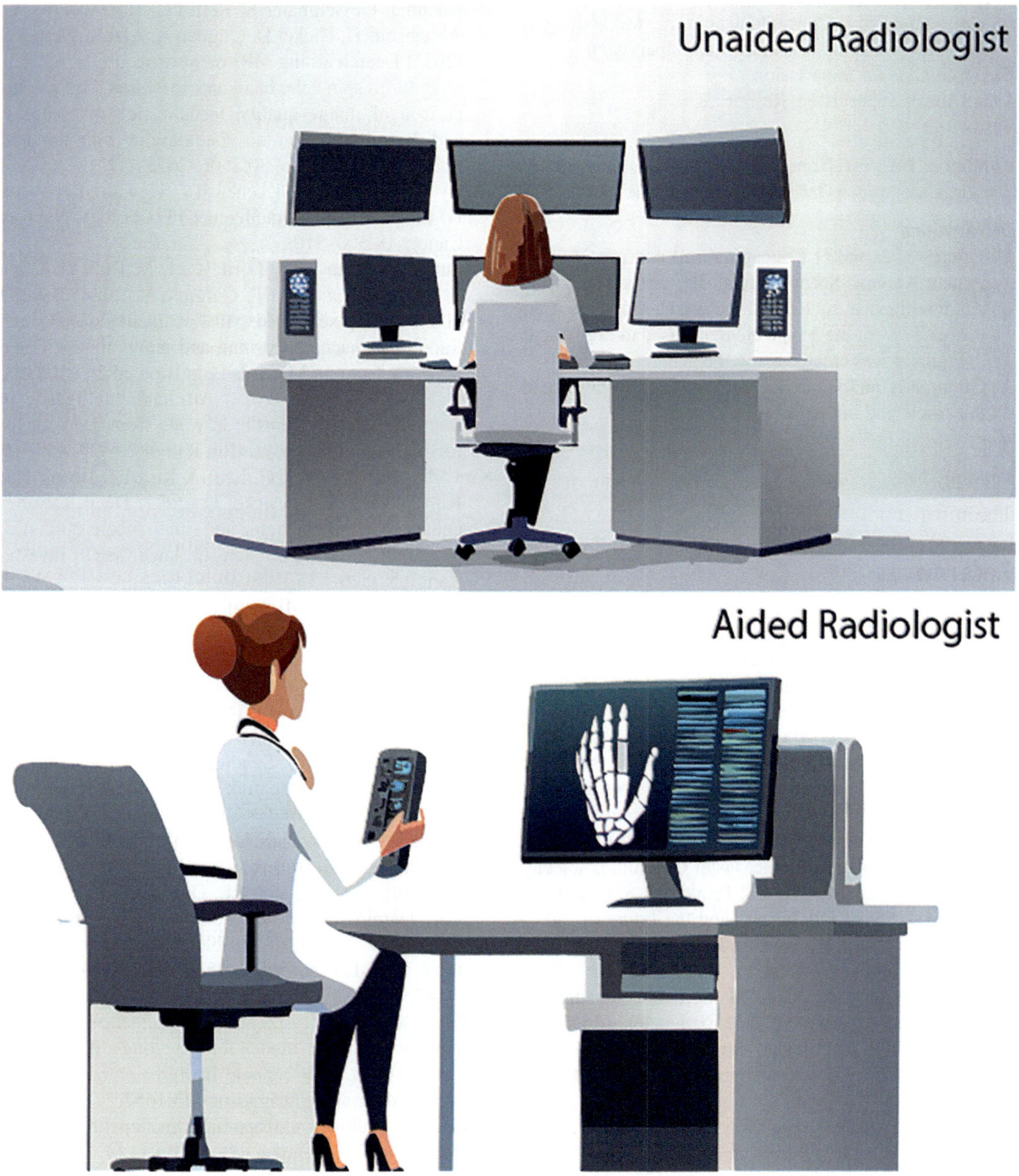

Fig. 6 A rendition of how an aided radiologist would potentially have a more systematic workflow where his attention will need to be directed at filtered information provided by the AI aid. This will effectively declutter a radiologists' environment

Acknowledgements We appreciate the role of Mr Shivam, Sales head at AZ Med, for providing Figs. 3, 4, and 5—the set of sample images, both with and without AI Output generated by AZ Med Trauma software and provided to us for use in this chapter.

Credit Authorship Contribution
Pranav Ajmera: Conceptualization, Methodology, Resources, Writing, Visualization, Supervision
Girish Gandikota: Supervision
Amit Kharat: Supervision, Resources

Conflict of Interest None relevant to this manuscript.

Declarations
1. Figures 1, 2, and 6: Conceptualized and prepared by Pranav Ajmera. Software featuring generative artificial intelligence, such as Adobe and Canva, were used to create few of the design elements used in Figs. 1 and 2. Figure 6 was created using the generative feature.
2. Grammarly and ChatGPT were utilized to proofread the article and improvise the syntax.

Funding None to declare

References

Ajmera P, Kharat A, Botchu R, Gupta H, Kulkarni V (2021) Real-world analysis of artificial intelligence in musculoskeletal trauma. J Clin Orthop Trauma 22:101573

Alzubaidi L, Khamael AD, Salhi A, Alammar Z, Fadhel MA, Albahri A, Alamoodi A, Albahri O, Hasan AF, Bai J (2024) Comprehensive review of deep learning in orthopaedics: applications, challenges, trustworthiness, and fusion. Artif Intell Med 155:102935

Bird A, Oakden-Rayner L, McMaster C, Smith LA, Zeng M, Wechalekar MD, Ray S, Proudman S, Palmer LJ (2022) Artificial intelligence and the future of radiographic scoring in rheumatoid arthritis: a viewpoint. Arthritis Res Ther 24:268

Borys K, Schmitt YA, Nauta M, Seifert C, Krämer N, Friedrich CM, Nensa F (2023) Explainable AI in medical imaging: an overview for clinical practitioners–beyond saliency-based XAI approaches. Eur J Radiol 162:110786

Bulstra AEJ, Machine Learning C (2022) A machine learning algorithm to estimate the probability of a true scaphoid fracture after wrist trauma. J Hand Surg Am 47:709–718

Droppelmann G, Rodríguez C, Smague D, Jorquera C, Feijoo F (2024) Deep learning models for tendinopathy detection: a systematic review and meta-analysis of diagnostic tests. EFORT Open Rev 9:941–952

Gan K, Xu D, Lin Y, Shen Y, Zhang T, Hu K, Zhou K, Bi M, Pan L, Wu W (2019) Artificial intelligence detection of distal radius fractures: a comparison between the convolutional neural network and professional assessments. Acta Orthop 90:394–400

Gitto S, Serpi F, Albano D, Risoleo G, Fusco S, Messina C, Sconfienza LM (2024) AI applications in musculoskeletal imaging: a narrative review. Eur Radiol Exp 8:22

Herrmann J, Gassenmaier S, Keller G, Koerzdoerfer G, Almansour H, Nickel D, Othman A, Afat S, Werner S (2023) Deep learning MRI reconstruction for accelerating turbo spin echo hand and wrist imaging: a comparison of image quality, visualization of anatomy, and detection of common pathologies with standard imaging. Acad Radiol 30:2606–2615

Hosny A, Parmar C, Quackenbush J, Schwartz LH, Aerts HJ (2018) Artificial intelligence in radiology. Nat Rev Cancer 18:500–510

Khatun Z, Jónsson H Jr, Tsirilaki M, Maffulli N, Oliva F, Daval P, Tortorella F, Gargiulo P (2024) Beyond pixel: superpixel-based MRI segmentation through traditional machine learning and graph convolutional network. Comput Methods Prog Biomed 256:108398

Kim D, Mackinnon T (2018) Artificial intelligence in fracture detection: transfer learning from deep convolutional neural networks. Clin Radiol 73:439–445

Kim M, Lee S-M, Park C, Lee D, Kim KS, Jeong HS, Kim S, Choi M-H, Nickel D (2022) Deep learning-enhanced parallel imaging and simultaneous multislice acceleration reconstruction in knee MRI. Investig Radiol 57:826–833

Koch KM, Sherafati M, Arpinar VE, Bhave S, Ausman R, Nencka AS, Lebel RM, McKinnon G, Kaushik SS, Vierck D (2021) Analysis and evaluation of a deep learning reconstruction approach with denoising for orthopedic MRI. Radiol Artif Intell 3:e200278

Koetzier LR, Mastrodicasa D, Szczykutowicz TP, Van Der Werf NR, Wang AS, Sandfort V, Van Der Molen AJ, Fleischmann D, Willemink MJ (2023) Deep learning image reconstruction for CT: technical principles and clinical prospects. Radiology 306:e221257

Langerhuizen DW, Bulstra AEJ, Janssen SJ, Ring D, Kerkhoffs GM, Jaarsma RL, Doornberg JN (2020) Is deep learning on par with human observers for detection of radiographically visible and occult fractures of the scaphoid? Clin Orthop Relat Res 478:2653–2659

Lee K-C, Choi IC, Kang CH, Ahn K-S, Yoon H, Lee J-J, Kim BH, Shim E (2023) Clinical validation of an artificial intelligence model for detecting distal radius, ulnar styloid, and scaphoid fractures on conventional wrist radiographs. Diagnostics 13:1657

Lindsey R, Daluiski A, Chopra S, Lachapelle A, Mozer M, Sicular S, Hanel D, Gardner M, Gupta A, Hotchkiss R (2018) Deep neural network improves fracture detection by clinicians. Proc Natl Acad Sci 115:11591–11596

Min H, Rabi Y, Wadhawan A, Bourgeat P, Dowling J, White J, Tchernegovski A, Formanek B, Schuetz M, Mitchell G (2023) Automatic classification of distal radius fracture using a two-stage ensemble deep learning framework. Phys Eng Sci Med 46:877–886

Murphy ZR, Venkatesh K, Sulam J, Yi PH (2022) Visual transformers and convolutional neural networks for disease classification on radiographs: a comparison of performance, sample efficiency, and hidden stratification. Radiol Artif Intell 4:e220012

Ong W, Zhu L, Tan YL, Teo EC, Tan JH, Kumar N, Vellayappan BA, Ooi BC, Quek ST, Makmur A (2023) Application of machine learning for differentiating bone malignancy on imaging: a systematic review. Cancers 15:1837

Overgaard BS, Christensen ABH, Terslev L, Savarimuthu TR, Just SA (2024) Artificial intelligence model for segmentation and severity scoring of osteophytes in hand osteoarthritis on ultrasound images. Front Med 11:1297088

Ozkaya E, Topal FE, Bulut T, Gursoy M, Ozuysal M, Karakaya Z (2022) Evaluation of an artificial intelligence system for diagnosing scaphoid fracture on direct radiography. Eur J Trauma Emerg Surg 48:585–592

Pesapane F, Codari M, Sardanelli F (2018) Artificial intelligence in medical imaging: threat or opportunity? Radiologists again at the forefront of innovation in medicine. Eur Radiol Exp 2:35

Pinto A, Reginelli A, Pinto F, Lo Re G, Midiri F, Muzj C, Romano L, Brunese L (2016) Errors in imaging patients in the emergency setting. Br J Radiol 89:20150914

Raisuddin AM, Vaattovaara E, Nevalainen M, Nikki M, Järvenpää E, Makkonen K, Pinola P, Palsio T, Niemensivu A, Tervonen O (2021) Critical evaluation of deep neural networks for wrist fracture detection. Sci Rep 11:6006

Rehman MHU, Hugo Lopez Pinaya W, Nachev P, Teo JT, Ourselin S, Cardoso MJ (2023) Federated learning for medical imaging radiology. Br J Radiol 96:20220890

Ricci Lara MA, Echeveste R, Ferrante E (2022) Addressing fairness in artificial intelligence for medical imaging. Nat Commun 13:4581

Rozema R, Kruitbosch HT, Van Minnen B, Dorgelo B, Kraeima J, Van Ooijen PM (2021) Iterative reconstruction and deep learning algorithms for enabling low-dose computed tomography in midfacial trauma. Oral Surg Oral Med Oral Pathol Oral Radiol 132:247–254

Sabeghi P, Kinkar KK, Castaneda GDR, Eibschutz LS, Fields BK, Varghese BA, Patel DB, Gholamrezanezhad A (2024) Artificial intelligence and machine learning applications for the imaging of bone and soft tissue tumors. Front Radiol 4:1332535

Sahu A, Pang C, Lynch J, Suresh P (2014) A review of radiological imaging in the hand and wrist. Orthop Trauma 28:172–186

Sharma S (2023) Artificial intelligence for fracture diagnosis in orthopedic X-rays: current developments and future potential. SICOT J 9:21

Thian YL, Li Y, Jagmohan P, Sia D, Chan VEY, Tan RT (2019) Convolutional neural networks for automated fracture detection and localization on wrist radiographs. Radiol Artif Intell 1:e180001

Vassa R, Garg A, Omar IM (2020) Magnetic resonance imaging of the wrist and hand. Pol J Radiol 85:e461

Von Schacky CE, Wilhelm NJ, Schäfer VS, Leonhardt Y, Gassert FG, Foreman SC, Gassert FT, Jung M, Jungmann PM, Russe MF (2021) Multitask deep learning for segmentation and classification of primary bone tumors on radiographs. Radiology 301:398–406

Xu L, Wang M-Y, Qi L, Zou Y-F, Fei-Yun W, Sun X-L (2024) Radiomics approach to distinguish between benign and malignant soft tissue tumors on magnetic resonance imaging. Eur J Radiol Open 12:100555

Yahalomi E, Chernofsky M, Werman M (2019) Detection of distal radius fractures trained by a small set of X-ray images and Faster R-CNN. In: Intelligent computing: proceedings of the 2019 computing conference, vol 1. Springer, pp 971–981

Yoon AP, Lee Y-L, Kane RL, Kuo C-F, Lin C, Chung KC (2021) Development and validation of a deep learning model using convolutional neural networks to identify scaphoid fractures in radiographs. JAMA Netw Open 4:e216096

Zhou X, Wang H, Feng C, Xu R, He Y, Li L, Tu C (2022) Emerging applications of deep learning in bone tumors: current advances and challenges. Front Oncol 12:908873

GPSR Compliance

The European Union's (EU) General Product Safety Regulation (GPSR) is a set of rules that requires consumer products to be safe and our obligations to ensure this.

If you have any concerns about our products, you can contact us on ProductSafety@springernature.com

In case Publisher is established outside the EU, the EU authorized representative is:

Springer Nature Customer Service Center GmbH
Europaplatz 3
69115 Heidelberg, Germany

Batch number: 10450419

Printed by Printforce, the Netherlands